Contemporary Bioethics

A Reader with Cases

Jessica Pierce

*University of
Colorado Health Sciences Center*

George Randels

University of the Pacific

New York   Oxford
OXFORD UNIVERSITY PRESS
2010

Oxford University Press, Inc., publishes works that further
Oxford University's objective of excellence
in research, scholarship, and education.

Oxford   New York
Auckland   Cape Town   Dar es Salaam   Hong Kong   Karachi
Kuala Lumpur   Madrid   Melbourne   Mexico City   Nairobi
New Delhi   Shanghai   Taipei   Toronto

With offices in
Argentina   Austria   Brazil   Chile   Czech Republic   France   Greece
Guatemala   Hungary   Italy   Japan   Poland   Portugal   Singapore
South Korea   Switzerland   Thailand   Turkey   Ukraine   Vietnam

Published by Oxford University Press, Inc.
198 Madison Avenue, New York, New York 10016
http://www.oup.com

Oxford is a registered trademark of Oxford University Press

Library of Congress Cataloging-in-Publication Data
Contemporary bioethics : a reader with cases / [edited by] Jessica Pierce, George Randels.
    p.   cm.
Includes bibliographical references and index.
ISBN 978-0-19-531382-6 (textbook) — ISBN 978-0-19-973637-9 (instructor's manual on CD)
I. Pierce, Jessica, 1965– II. Randels, George.
QH332.C658 2010
174'.957—dc22   2009032268

Printing number: 9 8 7 6 5 4 3 2 1

Printed in the United States of America
on acid-free paper

BRIEF CONTENTS

CONTENTS

Chapter 6. Biomedical Research 487

Chapter 7. Genetics, Biotechnology, and Posthuman Possibilities 581

Welcome to *Contemporary Bioethics*

Our subject is *bioethics*, which is a broadly interdisciplinary field of inquiry concerning the application of the biomedical sciences to health and life. Bioethics addresses a wide range of moral issues. Some of the questions under discussion recently include the following: When should life-sustaining medical care be discontinued? Should physicians be involved in capital punishment? Is it ethical for parents to genetically alter their child? Who should be the first to get vaccinated in the event of a pandemic—the young or the elderly? What, if anything, makes humans different from other animals, and what do those similarities and differences mean for medical research? How should health care practices be evaluated in relation to the environment? Should there be more emphasis on healthy environments than on health care?

We are biased, of course, but we consider bioethics to be one of the most dynamic and exciting fields of inquiry taking place today. The subject matter is both fascinating and immediately relevant to each of us. We are dealing with big questions of life and death, what makes us human, and what manipulations of the body and mind go too far or not far enough. Bioethics is not about abstract questions, but about real issues confronting patients, health professionals, and humanity. Bioethics rides the crest of the wave of technological innovation and medical advance, making it timely and exciting.

Not only does bioethics unite different disciplines (law, medicine, philosophy, theology, sociology, biology, genetics), but it dynamically brings together a vast array of different perspectives and worldviews—or what, in this book, we call "voices": global bioethics, feminist bioethics, Asian bioethics, developing world bioethics, African bioethics, environmental bioethics. Bioethics also incorporates the voices of nonscholars—of activists and patients and students. Just about everyone has opinions about the issues on the table, and all are invited to contribute.

Unlike many academic disciplines which remain, well, simply academic, bioethics engages the real world. Bioethics has a real impact on practices in health care and research (for example, work by bioethicists has helped increase patient autonomy in medical decision making and influenced in numerous ways government regulation of human subjects research). Engaging these issues will undoubtedly have an impact on you, as well. As you read this book, you may find yourself struggling with moral issues of deep personal concern, and you will find yourself able to start a bioethics conversation with nearly everyone you meet. (Try it!) Although many people are unfamiliar with the term "bioethics," and may look puzzled or concerned when you say that is what you are studying, nearly everyone has engaged in bioethics and will find the subject matter interesting.

Let us outline for you what you will find in *Contemporary Bioethics*. This book provides a snapshot of the current field of bioethics. The topics are current, the readings drawn primarily from the past few years. We have included a wide number of perspectives (secular, religious, Western, non-Western, feminist, environmental, etc.) on a variety of topics.

Here is what to expect in this book:

Chapter One: An Introduction to Bioethics is an introduction and invitation to the field of bioethics. Our goal in this chapter is to give you a sense of how the field developed and provide you with some background for understanding and analyzing the reading selections and case studies in the subsequent chapters.

Chapters 2–8 explore some of the core issues in the field of bioethics. We have arranged the chapters topically, beginning with the issue that is arguably the most historically basic to bioethics—the doctor-patient relationship—and ending, finally, with the recent challenge posed to medicine by global warming and other emerging environmental problems. As you will see, the topics have considerable overlap (for example, environmental issues challenge some conventional ideas about the moral relationship between doctor and patient), so the organization into topical groups should be understood as a matter of convenience, rather than suggesting rigid disciplinary distinctions.

Because bioethics is an enormous field, we have had to leave out many important topics. For example, whole chapters could be devoted to public health, developing world bioethics, feminist bioethics, and global bioethics.

Chapters 2–8 include three core elements: an introduction to the topical area being covered, a selection of readings by scholars, and a collection of case studies. Here is what these three sections try to accomplish:

CHAPTER INTRODUCTIONS

The chapter introduction gives you a brief overview of how bioethical reflection in the area developed, including some of the landmark legal decisions, medical or technological advances that have influenced debate, and mention of particularly significant bioethics writings in the area.

Although this is a book in contemporary bioethics, the historical development of ideas is crucial. Bioethics lives in the moment, but it does so within the context of history. For example, the Terri Schiavo case is just a few years old, but the history of bioethical reflection on end-of-life care goes back at least several decades, and is critical to understanding Schiavo. You will want to know, for example, about Quinlan, Cruzan, and Wendland, as well as about the development of the bioethics literature on withdrawal and withholding of life-sustaining treatment, and the issue of artificial nutrition and hydration. Even the most seemingly futuristic issues—such as the application of advances in neuroscience to alter memory—connect with deeply rooted discussions ("What does it mean to be a person?").

READING SELECTIONS

What bioethicists do, at a most basic level, is engage in moral reasoning or argumentation. They try to discern and explore moral problems in a particular sphere (medicine and medical research), and through careful reasoning and argumentation they try to enlarge the understanding of others, alter practices, and change perceptions. Each of the reading selections is an example of careful moral reasoning, aimed to convince the reader to adopt the author's position or to view an issue from a new perspective.

We have chosen readings that represent the most current issues and ideas in bioethics. This means that we have not included some of the historically influential writings in each area. We have mentioned these important contributions within chapter introductions, and have given you a list of readings at each chapter's end which include particularly significant publications. Most of these are easily available online or through the library.

Look for a diversity of viewpoints in the reading selections. The reading selections are not strictly "pro" and "con" (which would imply only two possible positions on an issue), but rather represent a broad span of moral and political viewpoints, from the more conservative to the more liberal to the moderate. Many of them outline alternative perspectives on the topic, providing an access point into the larger conversation. We have included a diverse range of "voices" from within bioethics, from mainstream theoretical convictions to different voices such as feminist, Asian, developing world, and so forth.

DISCUSSION QUESTIONS

Several discussion questions follow each reading. These questions offer a way for readers to test their understanding of each particular essay, and can serve as a launching point for class discussion.

CASE STUDIES

A *case* is a real-life ethical problem—literally, a set of circumstances requiring investigation or action. Cases contain, as any good story does, a moral conflict. A single case can have tremendous power. Terri Schiavo's case began as a quiet tragedy within one family, but rose to become a political lightning rod and the center of a national debate in the United States about end-of-life care. Cases can set precedents in medicine, and can become the basis for changes in the law. As with Schiavo, cases often take on a life of their own. Even though Terri is dead, the Schiavo case is still very much alive in the ongoing conversation about end-of-life care and decision making.

When cases are used in a teaching setting they are often called *case studies*. In this book we have given a central place to case studies because they are a wonderful learning tool. Each chapter contains a selection of cases. The reading selections provide you with examples of thoughtful moral reasoning; the case studies offer further examples of the kinds of moral problems emerging in this particular topical area, and they give you a chance to engage in moral reasoning yourself. You can practice forming careful arguments of your own, and assessing and responding to the arguments of others. The idea behind using cases is that you learn by doing. They are like exercises for the moral muscles. Through engaging in moral reasoning, your moral muscles gain flexibility and strength. Cases also give you an opportunity to test out and develop your own views and values. There is more at stake than in the discussion, say, of an abstract piece of philosophical reasoning—personal views are part of the territory; you do not have to pretend to be an "objective" outside agent. You can build your capacity for empathy, objectivity, and respect for other views.

All of the cases in this book are real, or based on real-life events. They are drawn from newspapers, medical journals, government policies, and the personal experiences of physicians. These cases are not designed as problems for you to solve so much as problems that will get you thinking, and stretch your powers of moral reasoning.

INSTRUCTOR'S MANUAL AND COMPANION WEBSITE

This text is supplemented by an Instructor's Manual, available on CD, and a Companion Website. The Instructor's Manual and Website help professors design effective courses using *Contemporary Bioethics*, by providing test questions in various formats (multiple choice, true/false, short answer, essay), a glossary of important terms (with definitions), additional cases with discussion questions, and useful adjunct teaching material such as ideas for literature and movies, and lists of useful websites. The Website provides students with chapter summaries, practice tests, vocabulary flash cards, and additional resources to assist with research projects and papers.

ACKNOWLEDGEMENTS

Before we close, we would like to take a moment to thank those who have helped in the production of this book. First, we would like to thank Robert Miller, our editor at Oxford University Press, for his patient support, and perceptive counsel. Thanks, also, to Kristin Maffei, Yelena Bromberg, and Miriam Sicilia at Oxford, who have been the organizing force behind this book. We are most grateful to the reviewers who read and commented on our initial book proposal and those who read through an early (and entirely too long) draft of this book. Their generous and detailed advice helped us greatly improve the manuscript. Thanks to:

Robert Daumiller, Xavier University
James J. Fletcher, George Mason University
Anna Gotlib, Binghamton University
Dien Ho, Massachusetts College of Pharmacy and Health Sciences
Daniel Holbrook, Washington State University
Aline Kalbian, Florida State University
Karen Lebacqz, Pacific School of Religion
Maureen Sander-Staudt, Arizona State University
Ellen Suckiel, University of California—Santa Cruz
Mark van Roojen, University of Nebraska—Lincoln

And we must, of course, acknowledge and thank our spouses and families for their indulgence on many fronts during this whole process.

Without further ado, we now invite you into the world of bioethics.

Bioethics: An Introduction to the Discipline

Terri Schiavo

In the dark early morning hours of February 25, 1990, a twenty-six-year-old woman named Terri Schiavo collapsed, unconscious, in the hallway of her St. Petersburg, Florida, apartment. Her husband Michael rushed to call 911, but by the time the paramedics arrived and resuscitated her, Terri's brain had been deprived of oxygen for over ten minutes—more than long enough to cause severe and irreversible brain injury. Terri had not died, yet she also had not regained consciousness. After several years of therapy and attempts at rehabilitation, her condition was still unchanged. Terri lived in what doctors call a persistent vegetative state (PVS). Her heart still beat, yet she apparently had no awareness of herself or her surroundings. She breathed on her own, but had no swallowing reflex. Because she was unable to eat or drink on her own, Terri was given a percutaneous endoscopic gastrostomy (PEG) tube—a small piece of plastic tubing inserted into the wall of her abdomen through which she would receive liquid food and water. It was this small piece of tubing that marked the line between life and death for Terri Schiavo, and that became the center of a bitter struggle.

After seven years of care, testing, and attempts at therapy, Terri's condition remained unchanged. Michael Schiavo asked a Florida court to declare that Terri's PEG should be removed. Once the tube was removed, Terri would then be allowed to die of dehydration and starvation, over the course of several days to weeks. (In 1990, the U.S. Supreme Court ruled in the *Cruzan* case that just as a competent person has the right to refuse lifesaving medical treatment, including nutrition and hydration, an incompetent person could also refuse through a surrogate decision maker.) Michael insisted that although Terri had no living will (a document indicating people's intentions and desires regarding medical treatment, should they become unable to speak for themselves), she would not want to live under such circumstances, based on what she had told him while she was alive and well.

Terri's parents, Robert and Mary Schindler, opposed removing the tube, claiming that Terri would want to be kept alive. They further argued that Terri's doctors were wrong—she was not actually in PVS, and could recover with the appropriate therapy. As early as 1993, they sought to have Michael disqualified as Terri's guardian, and continued to ask courts to declare them to be Terri's legal guardians. Terri's court-appointed guardian *ad litem* (a person appointed by the court to protect the interests of an incompetent adult) issued a report concluding that Terri was in PVS with no chance of improvement.

Finally, ten years after Terri's accident, Michael won a judgment allowing removal of the PEG. The judge, George Greer, concluded that Michael had provided clear and convincing evidence that Terri would not want to be kept alive in PVS. Although the Schindlers made several appeals to state and federal courts, Terri's PEG was removed in April 2001, only to be reinserted two days later, pending a new legal claim filed by the Schindlers.

In October 2003, after many court hearings and appeals, the tube was once again removed. Within a week, the Florida state legislature passed "Terri's Law," allowing Governor Jeb Bush to order the tube reinserted, which he did. Terri's Law was declared unconstitutional, and that judgment was upheld on appeal. In March 2004, Pope John Paul II issued a statement supporting life-sustaining treatments for PVS patients, and the Schindlers insisted that as a Catholic, Terri would follow the pope's statement and choose to receive artificial nutrition and hydration. After additional litigation, allegations that Michael had abused Terri, refusal of the U.S. Supreme Court to hear the case, and attempts in the Florida legislature and by the U.S. Congress to support the Schindlers, Terri's PEG was again removed on March 18, 2005. Terri finally died thirteen days later, on March 31, while hundreds of protesters held a vigil outside of the hospice.

WHAT IS BIOETHICS?

The case of Terri Schiavo riveted the nation and was carefully watched throughout the world. Indeed, it was the largest, loudest and most public battle yet over the ethics of end-of-life care. The central point of controversy, of course, was whether or not the discontinuation of a "life-sustaining therapy" like a PEG can ever be ethically justified. For some, the obvious answer is "of course." Quality of life matters more than mere quantity, and mechanically keeping a person alive in PVS, with no awareness of herself or those around her, is cruel and dehumanizing. A PEG should not be labeled "life-sustaining" or "therapeutic"; it is simply one among many possible medical interventions. For others, the constant and unconditional care of the severely ill and disabled is a mark of our humanity. We cannot know or judge the quality of life for the PVS patient; therefore we must err on the side of life. The PEG holds particular moral significance because providing food and water is the most basic form of human tending; it is not medical "treatment" but rather the fulfillment of a person's most elementary needs.

The Schiavo case made ripples well beyond the question of withdrawing life support from PVS patients. It raised more general questions about end-of-life care, guardianship, living wills, and allocation of medical resources. It brought into relief questions about the role of religion in shaping health law and policy. It reverberated into the bitter cultural battle over abortion, and provided grist for those in the pro-life movement who view protecting the sanctity of life (by prolonging life) for the severely ill and handicapped as continuous with protecting fetal life. It even spilled over into the debate about human embryonic stem cells in research. The field of *bioethics* explores the kinds of issues raised by the Schiavo case.

Defining Bioethics

The term "bioethics" was first used by biologist Van Rensselaer Potter in his 1971 book *Bioethics: Bridge to the Future*. Potter viewed bioethics as the integration of biology, and values into a "science for survival." He sought to make the values dimension of biological science explicit and to shape the values of science in service of human and environmental well-being. The normative vision guiding the field is this: biology, and especially medical science, can be used to promote and sustain health and well-being for all people, coupled with broad respect for human rights, animal welfare, and ecological viability. This field of inquiry is sometimes also referred to as *medical ethics* or *biomedical ethics*. All three terms will be used throughout this text, and are often used interchangeably, although bioethics is a more contemporary term, and is broader in scope than medical practice. Other related terms include *health care ethics*, which (though largely still interchangeable with medical ethics) connotes a somewhat broader inquiry into the allied health professions such as nursing and pharmacy, and *clinical ethics*, which connotes an institutional setting (a hospital or health clinic).

The Beginnings of Bioethics

The roots of ethical reflection and writing about medicine in the Western tradition—the tradition of central interest in this book—can be traced to Greek and Roman medicine. Western medicine is often called Hippocratic medicine because of the profound influence of the Hippocratic Collection—seventy treatises on illness, healing, and medical ethics, attributed to Hippocrates of the Asklepians and written around the fifth century BCE. The Hippocratic Oath is probably the most famous document in medical ethics,

Bioethics as a distinct academic field, and as a coordinated discussion of certain kinds of moral problems, emerged in the late 1960s and early 1970s. It arose in response to a series of highly visible and acute developments in biology and medicine, including dangerous experiments with human subjects, James Watson and Francis Crick's discovery of DNA, the expanding practice of organ transplantation, and the advent of oral contraceptives and *in vitro* fertilization.

These events thrust into public view the unique moral problems emerging from advances in medical knowledge and technology. Philosophers and theologians stepped in to address these challenges. Bringing with them the concepts and methods from their respective disciplines, they began working closely with scientists and physicians to explore the ethical implications of advances in knowledge and technology. In the 1970s, philosophers and theologians began to publish carefully articulated responses to these emerging moral challenges, framed in the language and concepts of their disciplines. Slowly, a body of literature began to accumulate. Academic departments devoted to the study of bioethics began popping up. Philosophers and theologians began taking jobs in medical schools; physicians began studying philosophy, and some even went back to school for formal training in moral philosophy. Conferences and professional bioethics organizations formed. Bioethics had come into its own.

Although philosophy and theology were the initial core disciplines, the field of bioethics is interdisciplinary like almost no other and continues to benefit from interactions with diverse fields. Scholars from many other disciplines—including medicine, nursing, law, sociology, anthropology, genetics, and biology—have made significant contributions.

The field has also been shaped in important ways by the work of activists. For example, the women's health movement has strongly influenced the development of bioethics, especially in the areas of reproduction and research. Through challenging the medical status quo—for instance, the exclusion of women from clinical trials—activists, alongside feminist scholars, have reshaped research practices and at the same time made crucial contributions to the bioethics literature. Disability activists have similarly helped to shape discourse about issues such as treatment of severely handicapped newborns, and have helped bioethics evolve a more nuanced dialogue about the meanings of health, illness, and disability.

Bioethics has achieved a high public profile. Bioethicists are routinely quoted in newspapers and magazines, are invited to speak to public audiences, and are even consulted by U.S. presidents and Congress. As early as 1968, Congress sought the advice of a national advisory commission on ethical issues arising from biomedical research and technologies. In 1974, the first public advisory commission, the National Commission for the Protection of Human Subjects of Biomedical and Behavioral Research, was officially mandated by Congress. The commission active as of our writing of this book was appointed by President George W. Bush in 2001, and is called the President's Council on Bioethics. This council's term expires in September of 2009. It is unclear at the time of our writing whether President Barack Obama will appoint a new bioethics commission. (Obama has appointed a chief science advisor, who advises on science policy.)

BIOETHICS: THEORY AND METHOD

Bioethics is the exploration of *ethics* in the realm of health, medicine, biology, and environment. But what does it mean to explore ethics or be an ethicist? For philosophers, it means trying to understand what exactly morality is, why values are important to us, why different people can hold divergent beliefs about what is right or good, why we should behave in certain ways and not others, and why for most people the question "How ought I to live?" is compelling. (Philosophers sometimes distinguish between morality and ethics, but for our purposes we will consider the two terms interchangeable.)

Most of the work done by bioethicists falls under the umbrella of *normative ethics*, the branch of moral philosophy that seeks to identify moral standards of right and wrong conduct. Normative ethics, in turn, can be divided into two general branches: *moral theory* and *practical ethics* (also called *applied ethics*). Most of the published literature in bioethics—and what you will be reading in this text—reflects interplay between theoretical and practical ethics, and the two are not neatly separated. But it is worth drawing the distinction, for now. Moral theory does not concern itself with the rightness or wrongness of particular acts, so much as it seeks to provide an overarching and systematic account of morality as a whole—to provide a *theory* of ethics. Practical ethics, on the other hand, concerns the concrete matters of life and attempts to justify both a particular way of living and resolutions to moral conflict. Crafting an argument regarding appropriate protocol for the doctor-patient relationship is practical ethics, and so is crafting an argument regarding whether the normal duty of patient confidentiality may be breached in a particular case.

How do they work together? Practical ethics works upon a background of theory, with theory providing a framework for helping discern what might make a particular course of action or a particular policy right. In turn, dialogue about particular ways of living or about moral problems often sheds light on theoretical debates and informs theory in important ways. Thus, moral theory and practical ethics work together in a constant back and forth dialogue, mutually informing one another.

The readings in this book are about particular moral problems, but you cannot really do practical ethics without some awareness of the theoretical backdrop. What we do in the next section is give you a brief introduction to moral theory, with attention to three of the most prominent theories within the Western philosophical tradition: utilitarian theory, deontological theory, and virtue theory. We explain each of these theories and talk about their strengths and weaknesses. We are especially interested, of course, in how each of these theories has influenced the field of bioethics. We also explore why bioethics both incorporates and has moved beyond these theoretical options, and how the landscape is evolving as we write.

Moral Theory in Bioethics

Because morality is such a crucial component of our social lives, and because morality is deeply puzzling (Why do most people feel compelled to do good, even if no one is watching? Where do standards of right and wrong come from?), it has been a subject of intense interest to philosophers. One of the long-standing projects of Western moral philosophy has been the attempt to construct a comprehensive theory of morality. Philosophers have believed that a moral theory should be able to provide a formal, systematic account of what morality is and how it works. It should provide a framework for analyzing moral issues, a logical basis for moral decision making, and grounds for justifying those decisions. Normative claims, which guide action, would come from within the theory's framework.

The three most prominent categories of moral theory are utilitarian, deontological, and virtue. As you read the essays in the chapters that follow, you will find many explicit and unspoken references to these theoretical accounts of morality and to the philosophers who made them famous. These three theories, individually and as a group, have faced serious objections, particularly over the past three decades. Challenges have come from philosophers who seek a framework attuned to the experiences of women, of minorities, and of non-Westerners, and from those who believe that bioethics is better off without theory. Many of the essays represent these alternative perspectives. As you read, try to stay attuned to each author's theoretical commitments.

Utilitarianism: A Theory of Consequences

Utilitarianism considers actions to be justified or unjustified on the basis of their consequences. (There are other consequentialist theories, but utilitarianism is the most prominent one.) This theory was first developed by Jeremy Bentham and was refined by his godson, John Stuart Mill. It evaluates actions using the single, absolute principle of utility, which focuses on promoting human happiness. The common shorthand expression is that actions are justified if they tend to produce the greatest good for the greatest number of people. The actor may not privilege his or her own well-being over that of anyone else when determining the morally best course of action.

Utilitarianism sounds very simple, but it immediately presents several difficulties, three of which we mention here. First, it requires that people anticipate the potential consequences of their actions, which is no small task. Not every possible result can be predicted, of course, but utilitarianism does demand that people make good-faith efforts to gain the knowledge that they need to produce the best outcome. Some contemporary versions of utilitarianism recognize that the difficulty in determining the good can be alleviated through the use of certain principles and rules. Because following these principles and rules generally brings about the greatest good for the greatest number of people, we can rely on them to guide our actions, and avoid the difficult task of trying to predict possible consequences in every case. Second, there is the question of whether good consequences must actually be produced in order for an action to be considered good, or if it is sufficient that the person intended to produce good consequences. For example, suppose you give a homeless man five dollars to eat at a fast-food restaurant, but before he can reach the entrance he is hit by a car speeding through the drive-up lane. Your actions could be considered morally good, because you intended to provide him with food, which would have been a good consequence. Or they could be considered morally wrong, because the man is now severely injured, and would not have been if you had not given him the money to go to the restaurant. Third, the principle of utility begs the question What counts as good? Here, Bentham and Mill disagree. Bentham thinks that the good consists of happiness understood as pleasure. He holds that pleasure could be measured and evaluated in various ways, such as intensity, duration, and certainty of its occurrence, but that there otherwise should be no discrimination regarding what causes pleasure. People have different tastes, and so receive pleasure from different things. Mill agrees with Bentham that happiness is determined by receiving pleasure and avoiding pain, but holds that some pleasures are objectively superior to others. For example, Mill thinks that intellectual pleasures are superior to physical pleasures. People who are capable of experiencing different types of pleasure are the only ones in a position to judge which are superior. Some contemporary utilitarians reject this focus on pleasure in favor of pluralism regarding the good: they think there are important values, such as health, that cannot be reduced to pleasure. Bringing about the greatest good means attending to this range of values.

Utilitarianism remains an important ethical theory in bioethics today, and can be seen in the work of Peter Singer. Perhaps best known for his rejection of animal experimentation and support for human euthanasia, Singer bases his arguments on a utilitarian view of ethics. (His article "Voluntary Euthanasia: A Utilitarian Perspective" appears in chapter 3.) We can also see utilitarian influence in particular areas of bioethics, even without a full-fledged commitment to the theory itself. For example, when making treatment decisions for noncompetent patients, the *best interests* standard requires that surrogate decision makers consider the benefits and burdens of each option to the patient (see "Standards for Surrogate Decision Making" by Beauchamp and Childress, in chapter 2). And in the allocation of scarce medical resources, utilitarian considerations frequently are used to determine how to do the most good with the available resources (see chapter 5).

John Stuart Mill, *Utilitarianism*

The creed which accepts as the foundation of morals, Utility, or the Greatest Happiness Principle, holds that actions are right in proportion as they tend to promote happiness, wrong as they tend to produce the reverse of happiness. By happiness is intended pleasure, and the absence of pain; by unhappiness, pain, and the privation of pleasure. To give a clear view of the moral standard set up by the theory, much more requires to be said; in particular, what things it includes in the ideas of pain and pleasure; and to what extent this is left an open question. But these supplementary explanations do not affect the theory of life on which this theory of morality is grounded—

namely, that pleasure, and freedom from pain, are the only things desirable as ends; and that all desirable things (which are as numerous in the utilitarian as in any other scheme) are desirable either for the pleasure inherent in themselves, or as means to the promotion of pleasure and the prevention of pain.…

The happiness which forms the utilitarian standard of what is right in conduct is not the agent's own happiness, but that of all concerned. As between his own happiness and that of others, utilitarianism requires him to be as strictly impartial as a disinterested and benevolent spectator. In the golden rule of Jesus of Nazareth, we read the complete spirit of the ethics of utility. To do as you would be done by, and to love your neighbor as yourself, constitute the ideal perfection of utilitarian morality. As the means of making the nearest approach to this ideal, utility would enjoin, first, that laws and social arrangements should place the happiness, or (as speaking practically it may be called) the interest, of every individual, as nearly as possible in harmony with the interest of the whole; and secondly, that education and opinion, which have so vast a power over human character, should so use that power as to establish in the mind of every individual an indissoluble association between his own happiness and the good of the whole; especially between his own happiness and the practice of such modes of conduct, negative and positive, as regard for the universal happiness prescribes; so that not only he may be unable to conceive the possibility of happiness to himself, consistently with conduct opposed to the general good, but also that a direct impulse to promote the general good may be in every individual one of the habitual motives of action, and the sentiments connected therewith may fill a large and prominent place in every human being's sentient existence.

Deontology: A Theory of Duty

Deontology (from the Greek word *deon*, meaning duty) is a theory that focuses on the nature of actions, holding that something about an action itself makes it right or wrong. Consequences are not necessarily irrelevant, but by themselves do not determine an action's worth. This theory has been strongly influenced by Immanuel Kant, and often is called Kantianism, although many supporters of deontology subscribe to more moderate formulations than did Kant himself.

Kant thinks that actions have moral value only if they proceed from a pure motive of moral duty. Nothing is good in itself except a good will, and a truly good will reflects that the person is motivated by the duty to follow the moral law. It is the intention that flows from this good will that is morally important, even if an action accomplishes nothing. "Its usefulness or fruitfulness can neither add nor take away anything from this value." For Kant, morality is based on reason, rather than on sentiment or intuition, and flows from a single, basic principle that he calls the *categorical imperative*. It is categorical in the sense that it is absolute, and imperative because it must be followed under all circumstances. Kant articulates this principle in several, arguably different, ways. The first version claims that the maxim or rule that justifies an action must be *universalizable*, meaning that everyone should follow the same rule. Would it be legitimate to borrow money and promise to repay the loan, knowing that you could not do so? Kant says no, because it would be irrational to accept a rule that permits breaking promises that you know you cannot keep. Such a practice would mean that promises would be meaningless, and no one would believe them. The second version of the categorical imperative entails equal respect for ourselves and other people as autonomous beings; we are always to "treat every person as an *ends*, and never merely as a *means*." That is not to say that we can never be a means to the purposes of others, or they to ours, but we should never be treated or treat others as mere objects.

It is clear that Kant views the categorical imperative and the rules that flow directly from it as absolute. They are binding in all circumstances. While certain people have also been absolutists about moral rules, and many people are absolutists about a few particular rules, most deontologists reject Kant as too extreme on this point. They hold that there are exceptions to most, if not all, moral rules; there are times when promise breaking, lying, and other seemingly immoral actions are legitimate. We could universalize breaking the rules against them in similar, exceptional circumstances, but maintain that they are forbidden most of the time. An important deontologist who thinks along these lines is W. D. Ross. Ross claims that moral rules are *prima facie* ("at first sight") binding, rather than absolutely so; they are binding unless a competing moral obligation makes a stronger claim. For example, the rule of promise keeping typically requires you to keep your promises, such as meeting a friend for lunch. Your actual duty, however, may be very different in some cases, and require you to break that promise. If another friend becomes ill and needs a ride to the health clinic, then your duty to help one friend would be stronger than your duty to keep your promise to another.

Deontology's influence can be seen in contemporary bioethics, with the language of ends and means that figures prominently in various discussions, and with the notion of *prima facie* moral principles and rules. In particular, deontology often frames discussions about patient autonomy in treatment decisions (see chapters 2 and 3) and about medical research (see chapter 6). Many contemporary adherents come from religious perspectives. For example, Gilbert Meilaender (Protestant Christianity) and David Novak (Judaism, although directly influenced by Kant as well) are both deontologists. Secular versions of deontology can be seen in the work of Norman Daniels and H. Tristram Engelhardt (see their articles in chapter 5).

Immanuel Kant, *Groundwork for the Metaphysics of Morals*

We can now end where we started at the beginning, namely, with the conception of a will unconditionally good. That will is absolutely good which cannot be evil—in other words, whose maxim, if made a universal law, could never contradict itself. This principle, then, is its supreme law: "Act always on such a maxim as thou canst at the same time will to be a universal law"; this is the sole condition under which a will can never contradict itself; and such an imperative is categorical. Since the validity of the will as a universal law for possible actions is analogous to the universal connection of the existence of things by general laws, which is the formal notion of nature in general, the categorical imperative can also be expressed thus: "Act on maxims which can at the same time have for their object themselves as universal laws of nature." Such then is the formula of an absolutely good will.

Rational nature is distinguished from the rest of nature by this, that it sets before itself an end. This end would be the matter of every good will. But since in the idea of a will that is absolutely good without being limited by any condition (of attaining this or that end) we must abstract wholly from every end to be effected (since this would make every will only relatively good), it follows that in this case the end must be conceived, not as an end to be effected, but as an independently existing end. Consequently it is conceived only negatively, i.e., as that which we must never act against and which, therefore, must never be regarded merely as means, but must in every volition be esteemed as an end likewise. Now this end can be nothing but the subject of all possible ends, since this is also the subject of a possible absolutely good will; for such a will cannot without contradiction be postponed to any other object. The principle: "So act in regard to every rational being (thyself and others), that he may always have place in thy maxim as an end in himself," is accordingly essentially identical with this other: "Act upon a maxim which, at the same time, involves its own universal validity for every rational being." For that in using means for every end I should limit my maxim by the condition of its holding good as a law for every subject, this comes to the same thing as that the fundamental principle of all maxims of action must be that the subject of all ends, i.e., the rational being himself, be never employed merely as means, but as the supreme condition restricting the use of all means, that is in every case as an end likewise.

A Theory of Virtue

Virtue ethics is a theory that focuses on personal character and the traits that lead people to act in particular ways. In the West, it originates in the classical Greek tradition, especially in the work of Plato and Aristotle. In the ancient East, Confucius was similarly influential in promoting the importance of character and virtue. Virtue is any kind of excellence, and moral virtues are praiseworthy character traits that lead people to act well. Examples of moral virtues include courage, generosity, honesty, and temperance. Character traits can also be negative, and moral vices are traits that lead people to act in morally deficient ways. Examples of moral vices include cowardice, foolhardiness, stinginess, and prodigality. Aristotle thought that virtue fell in the mean between two extremes. The virtue of courage thus has two opposites—cowardice and foolhardiness—rather than just one. It is possible to have too much fear and too little. Some dangers should be faced, while others should be avoided. People become morally virtuous similar to the way in which people acquire other excellences and skills, such as driving a car or playing golf, that is, through practice. Good drivers are not born, but instead develop the skills and instincts necessary to act intuitively while on the road. Moral virtues are dispositions that form passions and create moral habits. According to Aristotle, they are a kind of second nature that disposes us to do the right thing, and even to gain pleasure from it. An honest person tells the truth automatically; a generous person is inclined to share things with others.

Contemporary virtue theorists emphasize that virtues are developed through particular practices and within communities that have shared purposes. (The ethical perspective called *communitarianism* is an offshoot of virtue theory.) Practices require the development of skills and character traits, and community members direct this development.

In contemporary bioethics, Edmund Pellegrino and David Thomasma view medicine through the lens of virtue theory. They understand medicine as a practice that trains people in the development of skills and virtues; the people involved in the practice share the goals of medicine, and so compose a community. While they admit of a correspondence between virtues and various principles and rules, they view the virtues as primary. Many bioethicists disagree with this emphasis, but they do recognize the importance of the virtues in developing our ideals for good physicians, nurses, and other medical professionals. They also tend to agree that the virtues are important for encouraging moral behavior and attaining good consequences. (For examples of articles that emphasize virtue theory, see the article by Wynia et al. in chapter 2 and Björkman in chapter 5.)

Aristotle, *Nicomachean Ethics*

Virtue, then, being of two kinds, intellectual and moral, intellectual virtue in the main owes both its birth and its growth to teaching (for which reason it requires experience and time), while moral virtue comes about as a result of habit, whence also its name (*ethike*) is one that is formed by a slight variation from the word *ethos* (habit). From this it is also plain that none of the moral virtues arises in us by nature; for nothing that exists by nature can form a habit contrary to its nature. For instance the stone which by nature moves downwards cannot be habituated to move upwards, not even if one tries to train it by throwing it up ten thousand times; nor can fire be habituated to move downwards, nor can anything else that by nature behaves in one way be trained to behave in another. Neither by nature, then, nor contrary to nature do the virtues arise in us; rather we are adapted by nature to receive them, and are made perfect by habit.

Again, of all the things that come to us by nature we first acquire the potentiality and later exhibit the activity (this is plain in the case of the senses; for it was not by often seeing or often hearing that we got these senses, but on the contrary we had them before we used them, and did not come to have them by using them); but the virtues we get by first exercising them, as also happens in the case of the arts as well. For the things we have to learn before we can do them, we learn by doing them, e.g., men become builders by building and lyre-players by playing the lyre; so too we become just by doing just acts, temperate by doing temperate acts, brave by doing brave acts....

Again, it is from the same causes and by the same means that every virtue is both produced and destroyed, and similarly every art; for it is from playing the lyre that both good and bad lyre-players are produced. And the corresponding statement is true of builders and of all the rest; men will be good or bad builders as a result of building well or badly. For if this were not so, there would have been no need of a teacher, but all men would have been born good or bad at their craft. This, then, is the case with the virtues also; by doing the acts that we do in our transactions with other men we become just or unjust, and by doing the acts that we do in the presence of danger, and being habituated to feel fear or confidence, we become brave or cowardly. The same is true of appetites and feelings of anger; some men become temperate and good-tempered, others self-indulgent and irascible, by behaving in one way or the other in the appropriate circumstances. Thus, in one word, states of character arise out of like activities. This is why the activities we exhibit must be of a certain kind; it is because the states of character correspond to the differences between these. It makes no small difference, then, whether we form habits of one kind or of another from our very youth; it makes a very great difference, or rather all the difference....

Virtue, then, is a state of character concerned with choice, lying in a mean, i.e., the mean relative to us, this being determined by a rational principle, and by that principle by which the man of practical wisdom would determine it. Now it is a mean between two vices, that which depends on excess and that which depends on defect; and again it is a mean because the vices respectively fall short of or exceed what is right in both passions and actions, while virtue both finds and chooses that which is intermediate. Hence in respect of its substance and the definition which states its essence virtue is a mean, with regard to what is best and right an extreme.

Other Theoretical Possibilities

Utilitarianism, deontology, and virtue ethics have been extremely important in the development of bioethics, and of moral philosophy more generally. They have been important not only because many people have subscribed to them, but also because dissatisfaction with them has led to innovation and evolution in philosophical thought. For example, some of the most important innovations in moral philosophy have come from feminist philosophers who argued that mainstream moral theories were sexist in some of their basic assumptions. Dissatisfaction with traditional moral theory began to build momentum after the publication of Harvard psychologist Carol Gilligan's enormously influential 1982 book *In a Different Voice*. Gilligan observes that the field of developmental psychology had based its assumptions about human moral development solely on the experiences of men. This, she argues, is not only unjust, but represents bad science. Gilligan contends that women develop differently than men, and that their moral capacities are shaped through their experiences of relationship and through their attention to care. Rather than being morally underdeveloped (as her colleague Lawrence Kohlberg saw them), perhaps women were differently developed.

Building on Gilligan's work, many philosophers (feminist and nonfeminist alike) began to question some of the bedrock assumptions of ethics. For example, the traditional split between reason and emotion (with reason being the province of men, and emotion of women) was given serious reconsideration. These philosophers joined the handful of their contemporaries who were writing about emotion, drawing upon the work of earlier thinkers such as David Hume and Adam Smith. This shift opened up a whole new world of theoretical options. These included a much more nuanced picture of emotion and reason as two complementary and equally important modes of moral experience. Furthermore, the traditional emphasis on individualistic, rights-oriented, and contractual ethics (framed in the language of obligation) was balanced by attention to relationships, care, love, and trust. This approach to ethics is sometimes called an ethics of response, or relational ethics. When there is a particular focus on women, it is often called the *feminist ethic of care*, or, more broadly, *feminist ethics*. Prominent feminist voices in bioethics include Mary Mahowald, Susan Sherwin, Rosemarie Tong, and Susan Wolf. (A selection by Wolf appears in chapter 3, and one by Mahowald appears in chapter 4.)

In addition to gender, bioethics has become more attentive to issues of race, social class, religion, cultural identity, disability, and environment (though there is still much work to be done in all these areas). Bioethics is extremely diverse in its "voices," and this diversity is what makes the field so dynamic and relevant. We say more about this diversity in the last section of this chapter.

Three Methods for Guiding Conduct: Using Principles, Cases, and Stories

As we noted at the outset of this section, moral theory is a systematic attempt to describe how morality works and to provide grounds for moral justification. Theory, though, has its limits. One theory can provide only a partial description of ethics, leading to an analytical framework that is incomplete and decisions that are insufficiently considered and inadequately justified. Deontology, for example, may have an insufficient appreciation for consequences or personal character. Furthermore, theories exist on the level of abstraction, and so often are inadequate on their own to guide conduct in concrete situations.

Theories can provide useful ways of conceptualizing moral problems and their resolution, and can help highlight differences in the way people understand what morality is and how it works. But philosophers generally agree that each theory has limitations, and none provides a complete or perfect account of the moral life. Moreover, because they are abstract and incomplete, theories cannot solve moral problems.

Development of "Principlism" in Bioethics

Because bioethics has always been a practical discipline, there needed to be some way to move past philosophical disagreements about theory so that real work on the issues at hand could move forward. Early bioethicists found that although they often disagreed about which moral theory was correct, they nevertheless could agree on how to resolve particular cases because they shared a commitment to several core ethical principles. What's more, these principles could be recognized and understood not just by philosophers, but by everyone involved in the dialogue—by theologians, lawyers, doctors, nurses, and even patients.

Thus emerged the language of *principles* and the method of analysis called "principlism." The idea was that a system of ethics could be built around a set of principles that all people—not just philosophers—could recognize and understand. A principle, in this context, is a broad action-guide or rule of conduct, for example: treat people fairly, tell the truth, do not cause people unnecessary harm. Principles are general—"be kind" or "be honest"—and leave room for individual interpretation and judgment.

Four principles have been at the core of bioethics: *nonmaleficence* (do no harm), *beneficence* (seek to benefit others), *respect for autonomy* (treat other people as intrinsically valuable subjects in their own right rather than merely as objects who may or may not have instrumental value for you), and *justice* (distribute benefits and burdens fairly). These principles seem to provide a clear and generally agreed-upon framework for doing normative ethics in the context of medicine.

The Core Principles of Bioethics

The first clear development of principles in the bioethics context came with two landmark publications in 1979. One was *The Belmont Report*, the work of the first National Commission for bioethics, which was charged with identifying the ethical principles that should govern human subject research. *The Belmont Report* proposed three principles: respect for persons, beneficence, and justice. The second publication was Tom L. Beauchamp and James F. Childress's *Principles of Biomedical Ethics* (now in its sixth edition). This book more fully developed the principles, and articulated four rather than three by distinguishing beneficence from nonmaleficence. *Principles of Biomedical Ethics* remains the single most influential publication in bioethics today. It remains so not merely because of its historical importance, but because no other single approach has proved superior in a pluralistic society like the United States. Recent scholarship has also found the principles at work in traditions as diverse as Islam and Confucianism. (An excerpt from *The Belmont Report* appears in chapter 6, and excerpts from *Principles of Biomedical Ethics* are included in chapter 2.)

We would like to spend some time now examining each of the four principles. This will be important background for you, as you approach the readings and cases in this book. You will frequently come across a discussion of one or another principle as it relates to a particular topic.

The first principle is **respect for autonomy**. Autonomy basically means self-rule, and this principle has been very important for bioethics. It supports patients making their own decisions regarding their health care and their participation in biomedical research projects, rather than those decisions being made by physicians and other authorities. Respecting autonomy means recognizing a person's right to choose regarding health care, but does not require forcing a person to make choices directly. Citing a study about family-centered decision making, Beauchamp and Childress claim that while some patients may defer to others regarding their health care, doing so can be an autonomous choice rather than representing undue control by others. This emphasis on freedom from coercion should not, however, construe respect for autonomy as strictly a negative principle. It also entails positive obligations on the part of health care professionals; for example, they should provide the information necessary for autonomous choice (diagnosis, prognosis, and treatment options) and ensure adequate understanding of that information.

Sometimes, as in *The Belmont Report*, this principle is expressed as "respect for persons" rather than respect for autonomy, reflecting the idea that Beauchamp and Childress's terminology is too narrow, because there are other ways that we can respect people in addition to their capacity as self-directed choosers. But arguably the language of autonomy remains fitting. One way this fittingness can be shown is by the decision-making standards used for incompetent patients. For previously competent patients, surrogate decision makers use either the explicit instructions or general values of the patient, thus respecting that patient's autonomy. For never-competent patients, or for incapacitated patients whose wishes and values are either unclear or unknown, surrogate decision makers use the best interests standard (what actions are in the best interests of the patient). It is impossible to respect autonomy in such cases, and so appeals are made to other principles, such as nonmaleficence and beneficence. The existence of these other, distinct principles makes it unnecessary to expand this first principle further.

The second principle is **nonmaleficence**, which derives from both moral theory and the Hippocratic medical tradition. Nonmaleficence is an obligation against harming others, with harm generally understood as bodily injury, but also as "setbacks to significant interests." Besides actual harm, nonmaleficence also includes an obligation not to impose risks of harm on others.

The third principle is **beneficence**, which is an obligation to provide benefits to other people. This principle usually concerns actions that are morally required, although other beneficent acts would be morally praiseworthy. For example, there is no moral obligation to rescue someone if the attempt would pose a significant risk to the rescuer. People who voluntarily take on such risks to benefit others would be moral heroes, but those who refrain are not morally blameworthy. Some philosophers have proposed a distinction between general and specific beneficence. *Specific beneficence* pertains to obligations that arise out of special relationships, such as that of doctor and patient, while *general beneficence* concerns obligations a person has to anyone. Medical professionals arguably have role-related or specific duties of beneficence in the care of the sick and injured that laypeople do not have.

The fourth and probably most complex principle is *justice*. In the context of bioethics, the concept refers to distributive justice—the fair and equitable distribution of benefits and burdens—rather than to other types of justice, such as criminal (or retributive) justice. Justice can be understood as a "super principle" in that it includes several related principles. One such principle is "formal" in nature: treat like cases alike. It is formal in that it does not determine how specific cases should be treated, only that fairness requires consistency. There are several "material" principles of justice, which indicate how benefits and burdens ought to be distributed. These principles include distribution according to need, or effort, or merit. Various material principles can be ethically appropriate in different contexts, but they often conflict with one another. More than one may be viable in the health care context. The selection of a material principle may reflect a more comprehensive underlying theory of justice (e.g., libertarian or egalitarian).

Conflicts Among the Principles

While each of the four principles embodies a general moral obligation, the principles unfortunately do not always work harmoniously. Conflicts may arise. An obvious example in the health care setting is the potential conflict between beneficence and respect for autonomy. Doctors are obligated to provide beneficial medical treatment; they are also obligated to respect the autonomy of patients. But patients may reject treatments that doctors think will provide benefit. To resolve such conflicts, Beauchamp and Childress could have given the principles a rank ordering (for example, "beneficence always trumps autonomy"). Instead, they view the four principles as pluralistic. Their relative strength depends upon particular contexts, and cannot be determined in the abstract. Because of the potential for conflict, the principles obviously cannot be absolutely binding. Sometimes one principle will be overridden by another. Thus they are *prima facie* binding.

Applying the Principles: Specification and Balancing

These principles are general and abstract—so can they also be practical? Can they help guide ethical judgment in concrete cases? Beauchamp and Childress contend that the principles can help us make ethical decisions through a process of specification and balancing. *Specification* involves the discernment of more specific rules that would be relevant in a particular case. Specifications of the principle of respect for autonomy include telling the truth to patients and obtaining their consent for treatment. Specifications of nonmaleficence include not killing innocent people and not causing pain and suffering. The process of specification can help reduce moral uncertainty and conflict, but specifications of principles must be justified, which can be problematic in itself, and competing specifications may emerge. In the Schiavo case, competing specifications of beneficence might be "Food and drink should be available to everyone, using artificial means if necessary" and "Only provide artificial nutrition and hydration to patients whose medical care is not futile." Competing specifications of nonmaleficence might be "Retaining the PEG causes harm, so it should be removed" and "Removing the PEG causes harm, so it should be retained."

When specification alone fails to determine an ethical course of action, then balancing becomes necessary. *Balancing* is "deliberation and judgment about the relative weights or strengths of norms" in concrete cases. Balancing, too, must be justified. In the Schiavo case, Michael argues that respect for Terri's wishes (autonomy) trumps any obligation to provide life-sustaining treatment (beneficence), whereas the Schindlers claim that beneficence outweighs other considerations, in addition to disputing Michael's assessment of Terri's wishes. Both parties must provide supporting reasons for their claims.

Beauchamp and Childress rely on a "coherence theory" of justification, in which the primary principles, specification, and balancing must cohere with our "considered judgments," that is, "the moral convictions in which we have the highest confidence and believe to have the lowest level of bias." Unfortunately, the processes of specification and balancing will only reduce, not eliminate, moral conflict. People may disagree about such things as factual matters, relevant norms, and the relative weight of norms, all of which occurred in the Terri Schiavo case. Judgments can also change over time. For example, before the 1970s, it was standard medical practice to avoid informing patients about terminal diagnoses like cancer. It was justified on the basis of avoiding harm to patients who might become depressed by the news that they likely would die from the disease. Today, the standard practice is to inform patients, on the basis of respect for their autonomy. This change in practice indicates a shift in our "reflective equilibrium."

Case Analysis in Bioethics

The principles method of resolving moral conflict begins with a kind of "top-down" approach, articulating broad moral principles and deductively applying them within particular situations. The use of principles allows ethicists, clinicians, and other decision makers to move beyond the abstraction of moral theory, and acknowledges that the battle, say, between deontology and utilitarianism, does little to help with real issues like whether to remove Terri Schiavo's PEG. But even though the principles are supposed to provide a method for resolving dilemmas that arise in medicine and the biomedical sciences, many bioethicists contend that the principles are still too abstract to have any real bite. The work of bioethics does not really begin, they argue, until we are confronted with actual moral conflict. And rather than working top down, it makes more sense to work from the bottom up. Ethics should begin with the concrete (experiences, persons, relationships, communities, etc.) and develop contextual norms from these specific vantage points. A "norm" is a culturally specific rule about how people ought to behave in a given situation; norms are generally enforced through social sanctioning (peer pressure, ostracism). A norm is more detailed and specific than a principle, and is considered "true" only relative to its contextual setting.

A case-based method, sometimes called *casuistry*, has been championed by Albert Jonsen and Stephen Toulmin's influential book, *The Abuse of Casuistry: A History of Moral Reasoning*, as well as subsequent publications by Jonsen, Carson Strong, and others. As Jonsen and Toulmin note from their own experience on the committee that drafted *The Belmont Report*, people can more readily agree on resolving practical matters than they can on the basis for the resolution. Grand ethical theory is unnecessary—and even detrimental—for ethical practice. So rather than begin with moral theory or principles and apply them deductively to practical matters, the case approach follows a philosophical tradition similar to the common law: it begins with cases and reasons inductively from them to maxims that determine how to resolve the case. Certain cases come to serve as paradigm cases, and analogical reasoning is used to discern the relevant similarities and differences between current cases and these precedents. Maxims from the paradigm cases are then utilized, modified, or rejected, depending upon how the cases compare. Context is critical for casuistry, because judgments depend upon factual matters rather than theoretical constructs. Case analysis has a link to virtue theory in that it requires the virtue of practical wisdom, also known as prudence or *phronesis*, in order to make good judgments regarding cases.

Bioethicists have tried to provide a structured approach to case resolution, giving a reliable method for identifying, analyzing, and resolving moral dilemmas. Perhaps the most prominent is called the "four box method," which was developed by Albert Jonsen, Mark Siegler, and William Winslade, and designed for use by physicians working in clinical medicine. Jonsen, Siegler, and Winslade believe that certain features are present in every clinical encounter, and that systematic attention to these features will facilitate adequate resolution of moral problems. (For a sample case analysis, and for more information on the use of the four box method in clinical ethics, visit the Ethics in Medicine [at the University of Washington School of Medicine] website: http://depts.washington.edu/bioethx/tools/index.html)

The Four Box Method

Medical Indications	Patient Preferences
What is the medical condition and proposed treatments? Will treatment fulfill the goals of medicine? Will it work?	Do we know the patient's preferences? (Does the patient have decision-making capacity?) Is the patient giving informed consent?
Quality of Life	**Contextual Features**
What is the patient's quality of life (in the patient's own terms)? How do family and caregivers assess the patient's quality of life?	Are there social, legal, economic, or institutional features that might influence decisions?
	Drawn from Jonsen, Siegler, and Winslade, *Clinical Ethics* (2006).

Because it was designed for use in the clinical setting, the four box method does not apply as neatly to broader issues like health care reform or biomedical research. Many of the case studies in the book you are reading—for example, those that explore a particular new technology or a proposed piece of legislation or a large-scale research study—could not easily be assessed using this method.

The focus on practice is undoubtedly casuistry's greatest strength, because bioethics must be of practical use. Furthermore, it is obvious that cases are important in medical practice, and there is clear evidence that key paradigm cases have been authoritative in shaping biomedical ethics: the Karen Ann Quinlan case shaped the rules for surrogate decision-making regarding life-sustaining treatment, and the Tuskeegee and Willowbrook experiments have shaped the rules for conducting human subject research. But casuistry is also problematic as a method for doing ethics. At issue is, who reasons, and by what standards? How do people interpret and describe the facts of the case they encounter? Consider, again, the Shiavo case. Terri's husband and her parents both described her situation differently, and viewed the removal of her PEG very differently (honoring Terri's wishes versus starving her to death). They would answer the questions in each of the four boxes differently. They invoked rival maxims for resolving the case. Here we have an example of disagreement on the practical issues resulting from their different approaches to the case.

Casuistry as a method clearly needs some content to justify its results, and, as a practical matter, utilizes and develops principles and rules. Its convergence with principlism is apparent. Both invoke a bidirectional movement between principles and cases through the process of specification and balancing. Jonsen as well as Beauchamp and Childress recognize the overlap between their methods, and Jonsen has acknowledged the need for principles; they are embedded in cases, and linked to the resulting maxims of the casuistic method.

Stories in Bioethics

A second, prominent methodological alternative to principlism is **narrative ethics**. Narrative is any type of story, including novels, history, parables, and film. Narrative ethics overlaps to some extent with casuistry as a method, in that cases are stories, and analogical reasoning is used to compare narratives to current situations. Narrative is much richer than casuistry, however, in that it includes stories that are more complex than the typical medical ethics case, and, more importantly, stories often reach far beyond the medical context.

While cases are vitally important for all aspects of medical education, including ethics, Robert Coles and others have championed the use of literature in medical education, and also view medicine itself as a narrative practice. This should not be a surprising development, because people generally relate to others through stories, and learn readily through stories. Furthermore, our most basic moral lessons are typically conveyed that way. For example, children learn the importance of truth telling from a story such as "The Boy Who Cried Wolf." Stories extend our life experience vicariously, opening us up to new insights. They are arguably a more effective means of communicating ethical truths and norms, and of getting people to accept those truths and norms as their own. Yet narrative ethics goes beyond moral lessons or insights that could be taught in other ways. As Martha Nussbaum puts it, there is a link between form and content. Narrative can convey certain perspectives, ideas, and feelings more "fully and fittingly" than a text like the one you are reading ever could. Literature is "indispensable to a philosophical inquiry in the ethical sphere,...[providing] sources of insight without which the inquiry cannot be complete."

Furthermore, narratives can help develop moral imagination in two ways. They can enhance perception (that is, the ability to see a rich ethical landscape) and the ability to recognize moral issues and their significance. They can also boost creativity, improving one's ability to develop possible solutions to various situations. Narratives appeal not just to our capacity to reason, but also to emotion and intuition.

Perhaps the most important stories that shape our moral judgments are those that comprise our worldview. These stories shape how we view the world morally *and* factually. In relation to the conflict between Terri Schiavo's husband and parents, their perception of the facts of the case differed, in large part, because of differing worldviews. Religious traditions provide stories and overarching narrative frameworks that orient followers in particular ways, shaping their ethical vision and practice. There are also secular stories that provide vision about humanity as a whole (e.g., Thomas Hobbes's *Leviathan*) or some part of it (e.g., stories about the founding of the United States). Many stories, sacred and secular, can contribute to a person's worldview.

While it is appealing as a way to find context and meaning, narrative ethics also presents serious difficulties. One key issue is the problem of story selection. What counts as a good story? What makes a particular story appropriate in a given context? Whose narrative is it? Who makes the selection, and for what purposes? The President's Council on Bioethics began its work in 2002 by discussing Nathaniel Hawthorne's "The Birthmark" before proceeding to a general discussion of biomedical ethics and to the problem of human cloning. Council Chair Leon Kass set this agenda, and his selection of this story was not without criticism. Many people asked whether "The Birthmark" was an appropriate lens for viewing human cloning and other biomedical issues. The selection and construction of narratives, whether they are short stories, cases, or other forms, invoke the perspective of the teller and/or chooser. Stories also involve problems of interpretation. As Garak, a character on the television show *Star Trek: Deep Space Nine* suggests, the moral of "The Boy Who Cried Wolf" is not necessarily the conventional understanding "Never tell a lie, or no one will believe anything you say," but instead could be "Never tell the same lie twice." What counts as a viable interpretation of a narrative? Is there more than one viable interpretation? Is one superior? What insights does the narrative provide for medicine and other aspects of life?

Like casuistry, narrative ethics focuses on the particular and rejects the deductive application of ethical theory. It also rejects rationalism (a philosophical doctrine in which reason is the sole source of knowledge and justification) in favor of including the emotions when making ethical judgments, and supports the development of moral imagination. Also like casuistry, narrative ethics can work very well with principlism. The processes of specification and balancing could include the use of stories and would be enhanced by more highly developed moral perception and imagination.

RELIGION AND BIOETHICS

If you were to conduct a survey to determine where people derive their sense of ethics, you likely would discover that religion plays a prominent role for many people, although not necessarily an exclusive one. You might also discover that a significant number of people believe it impossible for morality to be divorced from religious belief; they view the two as necessarily linked. Other people might not go so far as this, but still think that some connection between religion and morality exists, at least historically, and perhaps in terms of personal motivation to engage in moral behavior. This perceived correlation makes it important to consider religion in relation to morality, and to explore the differences and similarities between religious ethics and secular ethics. Furthermore, many of the issues in bioethics have deep religious significance to believers, as the Terri Schiavo case illustrates, and so there cannot be an adequate conversation about these issues without including religious voices. Indeed, it is simply not possible to explore most of the pressing issues in bioethics without talking about religion.

Religious Ethics: How Does It Differ from Secular Ethics?

Like morality, religion regulates behavior (religion is from the Latin *religare*, to bind), but usually does so relative to some notion of ultimate reality, such as God or the cosmic structure of the universe, as opposed to a secular perspective that makes no other-worldly references. Some of that regulated conduct obviously pertains to religious practice (e.g., ritual behavior). More importantly for our purposes here, religion also mandates certain moral conduct, and may even require supererogatory acts that secular ethics would view as voluntary. (*Supererogation* is going beyond the call of duty, such as self-sacrifice to the point of martyrdom. It comes from Latin *supererogatio*, meaning payment beyond what is due or asked, deriving from *super*, beyond, and *erogare*, to pay out).

In many respects, religious ethics operates similarly to the secular, philosophical accounts outlined earlier, utilizing some of the same broad ethical categories, concepts, and methods as secular morality. Religious traditions have their own versions of the moral theories, such as a deontological emphasis on certain rules (e.g., Judaism and the Ten Commandments among 613 *mitzvoh*). They may also have a concern for virtue, as in Josef Pieper's influential articulation of the four cardinal virtues (prudence, justice, fortitude, and temperance) and three theological virtues (faith, hope, and love) from a Catholic perspective, or the Dalai Lama's grounding of the virtues in a spirituality that reaches beyond Buddhism. Regarding method, some commentators have argued that the four bioethical principles have analogues in religious traditions as diverse as Confucianism and Islam, and religions have additional principles that they might invoke. For example, the Roman Catholic tradition makes a distinction between *ordinary* and *extraordinary* medical care, with ordinary care always being required, and extraordinary care being optional. What counts as ordinary or extraordinary care depends upon the particular context, and part of the issue in the Schiavo case was whether the PEG constituted ordinary or extraordinary care for Terri.

Sources of Moral Authority in Religious Ethics

Behind the superficial agreements on theory and method lie significant differences between secular and religious accounts of ethics. One of the key differences arises in relation to the sources of moral authority. As we saw in earlier sections, philosophical ethics looks to moral theory as the source for moral authority (as that which publicly justifies particular moral norms or principles and as that which makes them binding on us), or else bypasses foundational questions (i.e., theory) and moves straight into the resolution of moral problems using general principles or case analysis. Religious ethics deals with moral authority differently. There are several sources at use in religious traditions, although not all of them are accepted by all religious traditions.

The most obvious authority in religion is *sacred text*. Most religions have some type of sacred text that is authoritative in matters of faith and morals. Christians have the New Testament, Muslims have the Qur'an, Hindus have the Vedas, and Buddhists have the Tripitaka. How exactly a sacred text is understood to impart moral guidance varies considerably from one religion to another. Texts do not always provide clear guidance, and are subject to various interpretations, including the nature of the ethical norms that are advocated. Norms might be exact laws that must always be followed, general principles that are less specific, or ideals that set goals rather than strict standards. These norms might be precisely listed, or they might be illustrated through metaphor or story. One view of how morality is derived from sacred text is *divine command*. God's commands are issued to an intermediary of some type (prophet, messenger, or lawgiver) and then communicated to others. For example, Muslims believe that Muhammad received God's message from the angel Gabriel.

Another important source of moral norms in religious ethics is *natural law*. (Natural law is not exclusive to religious ethics; it also is used in some secular accounts of ethics.) According to natural law theory, objective moral standards can be derived from our nature as human beings and from the structure of the universe. Our most essential moral standards are knowable to everyone; no special revelation, such as a sacred text, or cultural training is necessary. Everyone is morally accountable for following the moral standards associated with natural law, whatever their religious beliefs might be. Natural law thinking can be found in many religions, but one of the most famous accounts of natural law comes from St. Thomas Aquinas, whose work remains strongly influential in Roman Catholic Christianity. According to Aquinas, the natural law contains self-evident first principles, knowable to us because we possess the capacity to reason and because they are part of our natural human inclinations. The foundational moral precept of the natural law is to do good and avoid evil. Several more specific principles follow from this: (1) self-preservation, (2) procreation and the education of offspring, and (3) knowing the truth about God and living in society. Certain moral conclusions are then drawn from the natural law. For example, suicide is prohibited because it violates the natural inclination toward self-preservation. This conclusion is important in Catholic bioethics because it leads to a rejection of physician-assisted suicide and a rejection of a patient's right to refuse ordinary care that is life sustaining.

A third source in religious ethics is *tradition*, which is the ongoing wisdom and standards of a religious community, passed down over time. Sacred texts and the ethical guidance that they provide require interpretation, as does the natural law, other important texts, and the ongoing experience of the community. The Jewish Talmud provides a historical example and Catholic social thought a contemporary one, of this type of reflection and interpretation. Other types of authoritative documents or sayings that would fall into this category include noncanonical texts or stories, such as Muslim *hadith*, which are narrations of the life and teaching of Muhammad not found in the Qur'an. A religion's tradition sometimes can provide guidance regarding bioethics issues, because it involves historical reflection on moral precepts and on particular issues.

A fourth source in religious ethics is the teaching and example of *charismatic leaders*. These leaders possess a moral authority that goes beyond human reason—they are considered to be linked to the Divine or Ultimate. They often do not possess any formal position of authority, but nevertheless show and tell humans the right way to live. They often challenge the authority of contemporary leaders and the religion's tradition, although their teachings and lives can eventually become part of that same tradition. A historical example is Gandhi, the Hindu champion of nonviolent resistance.

Finally, religious ethics may appeal to sources outside of the religion itself as part of its own conversation about morality. For example, religious ethics often appeals to knowledge gained through the social and natural sciences, and utilizes concepts from secular philosophy. It might also appeal to the lived experience of members of the religious community. Religious ethics, then, is a confluence of several sources of authority.

Secular and Religious Ethics: Is Conversation Possible?

As a discipline, bioethics has been marked by its open embrace of diversity. Religious perspectives have, for the most part, been welcomed into the dialogue and religiously informed scholars wield considerable influence. Nevertheless, some bioethicists have argued that when it comes to *public* debate about moral issues in medicine, religious perspectives should be left behind, as a coat might be left by the door before entering a public banquet. Given that the sources of moral authority in religious ethics will carry force only for believers, and will differ from one religion to another, we need to look past these foundations and find a common language that everyone, religious or nonreligious, Catholic or Hindu, can speak. When coming to the roundtable of bioethics discourse, we should express our values using concepts and terms that are shared in common with others in the room, such as the moral principles of justice and nonmaleficence. (This should sound familiar—recall the move past theoretical disagreements in philosophy and the common idiom of four principles.)

One compelling reason to bracket religious beliefs when participating in public debates is effectiveness. If an argument is based on premises that most people—secular and from various religions alike—can understand and accept (like the four principles), there will be considerably more buy-in, and more persuasiveness. For example, in talking about abortion, the most mileage seems to come from conversations that focus on shared values such as the tragedy of unwanted pregnancy and the inestimable value of children.

Yet the call to leave religion at the door is also deeply problematic, and we believe it is both unrealistic and undesirable. Of course, we acknowledge that moral discourse between religious and nonreligious perspectives is challenging. The sources of moral authority and even the vocabulary used to talk about values are often so different that it is hard to find common ground. But we believe that it seems difficult to find common ground primarily because people often just do not look for it. They see obvious disagreement ("pro-life" versus "pro-choice"), and that is where the conversation ends.

But the reasons why religious perspectives must be included are many. First of all, religion is important to the vast majority of people. Polls consistently show that eighty to ninety percent of Americans believe in the existence of God, though there is enormous diversity in how people understand the nature of God and what belief in God means in relation to human action. Furthermore, whether or not a person professes belief in a god, everyone, consciously or not, operates out of a belief system; everyone has beliefs about the nature of reality. So in this broad sense, everyone lives from within a "religious" perspective.

Second, "secular" and "religious" are identifying terms that tend to simplify and reduce moral perspectives. The fact is that most people utilize some blend of secular and religious ethics, and most ideas (even the most seemingly secular) are composites, at least historically. Religions are unavoidably shaped by the larger social and cultural context within which they function, and at the same time are also shapers of those contexts. This mutual influence is evident in the United States, where Protestant Christianity has a very blurry boundary with secular American ideals like liberty and democracy.

Third, the influence of religion on the development of medicine cannot be understated. For centuries, medicine was a religious practice, and many of our contemporary practices were developed in context of religion. Western medicine is a synthesis of many different strands of thought, not all of them "orthodox" (folk remedies and magical beliefs have had considerable influence). This diverse background should remind us that the medical traditions that we know today are a pastiche of worldviews and beliefs. Within clinics and hospitals, religious voices have played a more vocal role than a strictly secular bioethics would permit. Health professionals are increasingly attentive to the religious and cultural beliefs of their patients, particularly where these beliefs may impinge on healing and treatment. In addition, health professionals are also realizing that their own spiritual and cultural traditions have relevance within health care, meaning that they should not be disembodied practitioners, but whole people.

Finally, one simply cannot talk about bioethics without reference to religion. As we explained in our brief history of the development of bioethics, many of the formative voices have been scholars situated within religious traditions, and the debates about key issues such as abortion, end-of-life care, and human enhancement have been shaped in crucial ways by religious voices. Religion plays a critical role in the Schiavo case, because Terri's parents based their desire to continue her treatment on their Catholic beliefs, and many of their supporters were also religiously motivated. Furthermore, many of the historical objections to innovations in medicine and biology have come from religious perspectives, and these objections cannot be understood or assessed without some reference to religion. Current controversies are similarly shaped by religious perspectives. Take, for example, President George W. Bush's speech announcing a moratorium on federal funding for embryonic stem cell research on new cell lines: "My position on these issues is shaped by deeply held beliefs.... [I] believe human life is a sacred gift from our Creator. I worry about a culture that devalues life, and believe as your President I have an important obligation to foster and encourage respect for life in America and throughout the world."

Religious sensibilities also frequently support advances in medicine, even regarding the same issues that spark religious objections. In contrast to President Bush, President Barack Obama issued an executive order in 2009 to promote embryonic stem cell research, saying: "As a person of faith, I believe we are called to care for each other and work to ease human suffering. I believe we have been given the capacity and will to pursue this research – and the humanity and conscience to do so responsibly."

Even if people cannot agree on the ultimate source of their moral beliefs, there are still many opportunities to find common ground. Secular and religious viewpoints can converge, for example, on the importance of justice as a moral norm. They may have very different understandings of why justice is important— for a Christian, justice may be an extension of Jesus's "preferential option for the poor," while for an atheist the principle may be grounded in a commitment to human rights based on a secular notion of human dignity. But taking the time to understand the shared concern for justice may not only lead to points of agreement ("we should help the poor"), but will also increase civility and mutual understanding.

Religious values and beliefs cannot always be adequately translated into a secular language. Neither can many "alternative" perspectives incorporated by bioethics. In embracing diversity, bioethics must relinquish strong distinctions between secular and religious and find creative ways to encourage dialogue among people from different backgrounds. Bioethics is a dynamic and influential field precisely because it brings together a mosaic of perspectives and voices. As the field develops, this diversity will undoubtedly continue to blossom.

BIOETHICS COMES OF AGE: AN EXPANDING MORAL FRAMEWORK AND VOCABULARY

We have in place the theoretical backdrop of bioethics, as well as the central moral vocabulary of the field. We have also explored the role of religious perspectives in the development of the field. But all this is merely a review of where bioethics has been. As the field moves further into the twenty-first century, the theories and methods of bioethics continue to evolve as new voices seek to be heard, and as new developments in technology and medical science raise new moral quandaries or put new twists on old issues. We want to conclude this introduction to the field of bioethics with a sketch of some of the emerging voices in the field.

Western industrialized medicine—and the bioethics framework that has evolved along with it—is only one small piece of a much larger global picture of health and illness. Bioethics is just now beginning to take stock of this global, environmental context within which Western industrialized health care sits. It is now clear that environmental degradation has profound implications for health, and that health care itself puts significant strain on the very ecosystems on which human health relies. It is also clear that there are staggering inequities in health status around the world, and that the privileged lives of the well-off (including our excellent health services) are not unconnected from squalor and suffering in many parts of the world. Poverty and injustice are health issues, too.

To keep pace with the technological and economic globalization, bioethics has also been going global. Although the early focus of bioethics was really at the bedside, the scope of moral concern has continued to expand. In addition to bringing a host of new practical moral problems under discussion—for example, the impact of trade agreements on the ability of nations to access affordable medicines—globalization has also raised theoretical questions. For example, some believe that the four core principles of bioethics are universally valid, and that American bioethics can essentially be exported for use elsewhere. Others consider this yet another example of cultural imperialism. Bioethical values need to emerge from within each culture in order to be compelling and useful therein. For example, a recent collection of essays under the rubric of Latin American bioethics argues that traditional interpretations of respect for autonomy and truth telling do not translate neatly into the cultural milieu of Latin American culture. Thus, there are fledgling subfields within bioethics: Asian bioethics, African bioethics, Latin American bioethics—each seeking to define a unique bioethical voice.

Global environmental change has also posed a challenge to bioethics. Scholars have argued that bioethics has been slow to acknowledge the profound importance of global climate change, loss of biodiversity, and other environmental threats to health and well-being because the dominant theoretical paradigm is both individualistic and anthropocentric (human-centered). Furthermore, the moral vocabulary of bioethics is too thin to adequately incorporate concern for the global environment. In addition to the four core principles, surely the field must also integrate the moral principles such as sustainability, interconnection, modesty, and restraint.

The impacts of environmental degradation and economic globalization are felt most acutely by those with the least capacity to respond and adapt. In addition to gaining sensitivity to the global scope of bioethical issues, bioethics has begun (reluctantly, some have argued) to open itself to the experiences of the world's least well-off. Debates in the United States about who most deserves a new liver—the alcoholic famous baseball player or an unknown retired librarian—seem oddly off-point in the context of global poverty, where millions of children die each year from lack of basic health necessities like clean water. The work of physician and activist Paul Farmer, who has spent his career working with Haiti's poor, has helped inspire a new theoretical challenge: bioethics from below. Bioethics from below seeks to give voice to the worlds' marginalized, and challenges us to think about social justice on a global scale. One example of how bioethics principles evolve is the push to frame health as a basic human right, and to include environmental and economic concerns as part of a comprehensive human rights framework.

Feminists continue to pose theoretical and practical challenges within bioethics, often in collaboration with those working in the areas of global bioethics, human rights, and environmental bioethics. Women are still pressing bioethics to pay more attention to contextual detail: to the social structures within which health care functions, and to the unequal representation of the needs of women, the poor, and other marginalized groups. Feminists complain that bioethicists have allied themselves with the powerful—becoming comfortably "institutionalized" within academic health centers and hospital ethics committees—and have thus lost their willingness to challenge the status quo and speak for the oppressed or ignored. Feminists argue, as one example, that more attention must be given to "housekeeping" issues in medicine (the work of caregivers, nurses, home health workers); these jobs pay almost nothing, and receive little attention from bioethicists.

In addition to these various challenges to bioethics, the past decade has seen more interest in and attention to diverse religious perspectives. Although Catholic, Protestant, and Jewish perspectives have been most prominent, Islam, Hinduism, Buddhism, and other religions are beginning to develop a coherent and rich literature. The next decade will undoubtedly see growth in perspectives that until recently have been underemphasized in bioethics.

REFERENCES AND FURTHER READING

What Is Bioethics?

Baker, Robert, and Lawrence McCullough, eds. *The Cambridge World History of Medical Ethics*. Cambridge: Cambridge University Press, 2008.

Callahan, Daniel. *Abortion: Law, Choice, and Morality*. New York: Macmillan, 1970.

Caplan, Arthur L., James J. McCartney, and Dominic A. Sisti. *The Case of Terri Schiavo: Ethics at the End of Life*. Amherst, New York: Prometheus Press, 2006.

Curran, Charles E. *Contemporary Problems in Moral Theology*. Notre Dame, IN: Fides Publishers, 1970.

Fletcher, Joseph. *Morals and Medicine*. Princeton, NJ: Princeton University Press, 1954.

Jecker, Nancy S., Albert R. Jonsen, and Robert A. Pearlman. *Bioethics: An Introduction to the History, Methods, and Practice*. 2nd ed. Sudbury, MA: Jones and Bartlett, 2007.

Jonas, Hans. "Philosophical Reflections on Experimenting with Human Subjects." *Daedalus* 98, no. 2 (1969): 219–47.

Jonsen, Albert R. *A Short History of Medical Ethics*. New York: Oxford University Press, 2000.

———. *The Birth of Bioethics*. New York: Oxford University Press, 2003.

May, William F. *The Physician's Covenant*. 2nd ed. Philadelphia: Westminster John Knox, 2000.

McCormick, Richard, S.J. *How Brave a New World?* Washington, DC: Georgetown University Press, 1981.

Porter, Roy. *The Greatest Benefit to Mankind: A Medical History of Humanity*. New York: W.W. Norton, 1997.

Ramsey, Paul. *The Patient as Person*. New Haven, CT: Yale University Press, 1970.

Thielicke, Helmut. *The Ethics of Sex*. New York: Harper & Row, 1964.

Bioethics: Theory and Method

Aristotle. *Nicomachean Ethics*. Translated by W.D.Ross. Adelaide, Australia: eBooks@ Adelaide 2006. http://etext.library.adelaide.edu.au/a/aristotle/nicomachean.

Beauchamp, Tom L. "Does Ethical Theory Have a Future in Bioethics?" *Journal of Law, Medicine, & Ethics* 32 (2004): 209–217.

_____ and James F. Childress. *Principles of Biomedical Ethics*. 6th ed. New York: Oxford University Press, 2009.

Bentham, Jeremy. *The Principles of Morals and Legislation*. New ed. Amherst, NY: Prometheus Books, 1988.

Charon, Rita. *Narrative Medicine: Honoring the Stories of Illness*. New York: Oxford University Press, 2006.

Coles, Robert. *The Call of Stories: Teaching and the Moral Imagination*. Boston: Houghton Mifflin, 1989.

Gert, Benard M., Charles M. Culver, and K. Danner Clouser. *Bioethics: A Systematic Approach*. 2nd ed. New York: Oxford University Press, 2006.

Gilligan, Carol. *In a Different Voice*. Cambridge, MA: Harvard University Press, 1982.

Goering, Sara. "'You Say You're Happy, but…': Contested Quality of Life Judgments in Bioethics and Disability Studies." *Bioethical Inquiry* 5 (2008): 125–35.

Held, Virginia. *Feminist Morality*. Chicago: University of Chicago Press, 1993.

Holmes, H.B., and Laura M. Purdy, eds. *Feminist Perspectives in Medical Ethics*. Bloomington: Indiana University Press, 1992.

Jonsen, Albert R., Mark Siegler, and William J. Winslade. *Clinical Ethics: A Practical Approach to Ethical Decisions in Clinical Medicine*. 6th ed. New York: McGraw-Hill, 2006.

Jonsen, Albert R., and Stephen Toulmin. *The Abuse of Casuistry: A History of Moral Reasoning*. Berkeley: University of California Press, 1988.

Kant, Immanuel. *Fundamental Principles of the Metaphysics of Morals*. Translated by Thomas Kingsmill Abbott. Adelaide, Australia: eBooks@Adelaide 2004. http://etext.library.adelaide.edu.au/k/kant/immanuel/k16prm.

Kuczewski, Mark. "Disability: An Agenda for Bioethics." *American Journal of Bioethics* 1, no. 3 (2001): 36–44.

Little, Margaret. "Why a Feminist Approach to Bioethics." *Kennedy Institute of Ethics Journal* 6, no. 1 (1996): 1–18.

MacKenzie, C., and N. Stoljar, eds. *Relational Autonomy: Feminist Perspectives on Autonomy, Agency, and the Social Self*. New York: Oxford University Press, 2000.

Mahowald, Mary B. *Bioethics and Women: Across the Life Span*. New York: Oxford University Press, 2006.

Meilaender, Gilbert. *Bioethics: A Primer for Christians*. 2nd ed. Grand Rapids, MI: Wm. B. Eerdmans, 2004.

Mill, John Stuart. *On Liberty*. New ed. New Haven, CT: Yale University Press, 2003.

_____. *Utilitarianism*. Adelaide, Australia: eBooks@Adelaide. 2004. http://etext.library.adelaide.edu.au/m/mill/john_stuart/m645u.

Miller, Richard B. *Casuistry and Modern Ethics: A Poetics of Practical Reasoning*. Chicago: University of Chicago Press, 1996.

Novak, David. *Jewish Social Ethics*. New York: Oxford University Press, 1992.

Nussbaum, Martha. 1990. *Love's Knowledge: Essays on Philosophy and Literature*. New York: Oxford University Press, 1990.

_____. *Upheavals of Thought: The Intelligence of the Emotions*. Cambridge: Cambridge University Press, 2001.

Oliver, Mary. *Understanding Disability: From Theory to Practice*. New York: St. Martin's Press, 1996.

Ross, W.D. *The Right and the Good*. New York: Oxford University Press, 1930.

Shakespeare, Tom. *Disability Rights and Wrongs*. New York: Routledge, 2006.

Smith, Adam. *The Theory of Moral Sentiments*. The Glasgow Edition of the Works and Correspondence of Adam Smith, edited by D.D. Raphael and A.L. Macfie. New York: Oxford University Press, 1976.

Solomon, Robert. *The Passions: Emotions and the Meaning of Life*. Garden City, NY: Anchor Press, 1976.

Strong, Carson. "Critiques of Casuistry and Why They Are Mistaken." *Theoretical Medicine and Bioethics* 20 (1999): 395–411.

Tong, Rosemary. *Feminist Approaches to Bioethics: Theoretical Reflections and Practical Applications*. Boulder, CO: Westview Press, 1997.

Wolf, Susan, ed. *Feminism and Bioethics: Beyond Reproduction*. New York: Oxford University Press, 1996.

Religion and Bioethics

Aksoy, Sahin, and Ali Tenik. "'Four Principles of Bioethics' as Found in Islamlic Tradition." *Medicine and Law Journal* 21 (2002): 211–224.

Aquinas, Thomas. *Summa Theologiae* I-II, 94. In *St. Thomas Aquinas on Politics and Ethics*. Norton Critical Editions, translated by Paul E. Sigmund. New York: W. W. Norton, 1987.

Crawford, S. Cromwell. *Hindu Bioethics for the Twenty-First Century*. Albany, NY: SUNY Press, 2003.

Curran, Charles. E., and Richard A. McCormick, eds. *The Use of Scripture in Moral Theology*. Readings in Moral Theology, no. 4. New York: Paulist Press, 1984.

Dalai Lama. *Ethics for the New Millenium*. New York: Riverhead Books, 1999.

Dorff, Elliot N. *Matters of Life and Death: A Jewish Approach to Modern Medical Ethics*. Philadelphia, PA: Jewish Publication Society of America, 2004.

Keown, Damien. *Buddhism and Bioethics*. New York, NY: Palgrave Macmillan, 2001.

Lammers, Stephen E. "The Marginalization of Religious Voices in Bioethics." In *Religion and Medical Ethics: Looking Forward, Looking Back*, edited by Allen Verhey. Grand Rapids, MI: Wm. B. Eerdmans, 1996.

Lindbeck, George. *The Nature of Doctrine: Religion and Theology in a Post-Liberal Age*. Louisville, KY: Westminster John Knox Press, 1984.

McCormick, Richard A. "Theology and Bioethics." *Hastings Center Report* 19, no. 3 (1989): 5–10.

Pieper, Josef. *The Four Cardinal Virtues*. Notre Dame, IN: University of Notre Dame Press, 1966.

Rae, Scott B., and Paul M. Cox. *Bioethics: A Christian Approach in a Pluralistic Age*. Grand Rapids, MI: William B. Eerdmans, 1999.

Smith, David W. "Religion and the Roots of the Bioethics Revival." In *Religion and Medical Ethics: Looking Forward, Looking Back*, edited by Allen Verhey. Grand Rapids, MI: Wm. B. Eerdmans, 1996.

Strandberg, Hugo. *The Possibility of Discussion: Relativism, Truth and Criticism of Religious Beliefs*. Burlington, VT: Ashgate, 2006.

Tsai, D. F-C. "The Bioethical Principles and Confucius' Moral Philosophy." *Journal of Medical Ethics* 31 (2005): 159–63.

Yoder, John Howard. *The Priestly Kingdom: Social Ethics as Gospel*. Notre Dame, IN: University of Notre Dame Press, 1984.

Bioethics Comes of Age

Alora, Angeles Tan, and Josephine M. Lumitao. *Beyond a Western Bioethics: Voices from the Developing World*. Washington, DC: Georgetown University Press, 2001.

Bertameu, Maria Julia, and Arleen L.F. Salles, eds. *Bioethics: Latin American Perspectives*. New York: Rodopi, 2002.

Fadiman, Anne. *The Spirit Catches You and You Fall Down*. New York: Farrar, Straus and Giroux, 1997.

Farmer, Paul. *Pathologies of Power: Health, Human Rights, and the New War on the Poor*. New ed. University of California Press, 2004.

Luna, Florencia, and Peter Herissone-Kelly, eds. *Bioethics and Vulnerability: A Latin American View*. New York: Rodopi, 2006.

Tong, Rosemarie, Anne Donchin, and Susan Dodds, eds. *Linking Visions: Feminist Bioethics, Human Rights, and the Developing World*. Lanham, MD: Rowman & Littlefield, 2004.

CHAPTER 2

Doctors and Patients

INTRODUCTION

This chapter explores the profession of medicine and the special relationship between physician and patient. The first section of readings focuses on being a medical professional: what it means to take the Hippocratic Oath, what general ethical principles guide the profession of medicine, and how the notion of professionalism shapes the daily work of doctors. The second and third sections explore the *doctor-patient relationship*—the special obligations physicians have toward their patients and the responsibilities patients bear in the medical encounter. The final section looks beyond the doctor-patient dyad to the proper role of the physician in society.

The Profession of Medicine

To profess, from the Latin *pro*, "forth", and *fateri*, "acknowledge, confess," is to make a public declaration. A *profession* is a highly specialized body of knowledge and skills that a person publicly claims or professes to practice for the good of others. These others are vulnerable in some capacity, and must be able to trust the professional to act on their behalf and not for other purposes. That medicine is a profession tells us that it is not a run-of-the-mill job. A person cannot simply wake up one morning and hang a shingle on the door saying "The doctor is in." To enter the profession of medicine, a person must go through an arduous training and must prove that he or she has mastered a huge and very specific body of knowledge. In addition, when one becomes a doctor, one professes a commitment to a certain set of ethical principles.

The most obvious public avowal of this professional ethic is the famous *Hippocratic Oath*. The short reading by **Howard Markel**, which includes a translation of the Hippocratic Oath, explores the oath's historical background and current status. The oath was probably not authored by Hippocrates himself, and may not even represent the mainstream ethical values and medical practices of Hippocrates' time. For example, the oath prohibits aiding a patient in suicide or performing an abortion. Yet both of these practices were acceptable in the Greek and Roman era. Markel argues that physicians should disregard the specific moral rules (regarding, for example, suicide and abortion) because they are historical artifacts, and should focus only on the oath's larger symbolic importance. Others insist that the specific moral rules should hold value today, precisely because of their deep historical roots in Western medical ethics.

The larger symbolic importance of the Hippocratic Oath seems to motivate most modern oath-taking by doctors. Almost all medical schools require students to take an oath, though very few use the original Hippocratic text. Many schools use a modernized version of the Hippocratic Oath written by **Louis Lasagna** in 1964, and some schools require each class of graduating medical students to write their own oath. Modern medical oaths typically avoid articulating specific obligations or prohibitions, and stick instead with fairly generic moral maxims. For example, very few modern oaths prohibit euthanasia or abortion, nor do they offer an explicit prohibition against doctors having sexual relations with patients. Some believe this "watering down" of the oath reflects a general corrosion of the professional ethic of medicine. Others, however, view the updates as crucial, because they reflect the modern context just as the original reflected ancient Greece. We no longer worship Apollo and other gods, and we view surgery as a legitimate form of medical practice.

Professional ethics are moral standards or codes of conduct developed by and for practitioners of a particular profession, such as medicine. Many professions have an internal ethic: engineering, law, ministry, and even athletics. There may be overlap among different professional codes (lawyers, doctors, and priests all share an obligation of confidentiality), as well as some norms that are peculiar to a profession. Doctors are not—at least not according to the code of the American Medical Society—allowed to participate in capital punishment, nor are they allowed to accept gifts from patients. Athletes are not allowed to take steroids or "dope" their blood prior to a competition.

The professional ethic of medicine is embodied not only in the oath taken by graduating medical students, but also in various documents and codes put forth by professional organizations. We have included the **American Medical Association's** (AMA) "Principles of Medical Ethics." The AMA's "Principles" represent the basic moral standards that define the practice of an honorable and virtuous physician. Rather than a personal oath ("I promise..."), the AMA's principles define the guiding principles of the medical profession ("The physician should...").

Codes of ethics are a way of establishing professional identity, and reflect society's expectations of physicians. For example, when we go to a doctor we assume that he or she will act in our best interests, and not recommend a treatment that will be profitable to him or her but unnecessary or harmful to us. We assume that the drugs the doctor prescribes are safe and effective. We assume that the personal information we disclose will be kept private, and that the doctor will not laugh about our problems over dinner with friends. We assume that our doctor works hard to stay current on new medical knowledge, so that we are receiving optimal care.

It may seem, with the prevalence of oaths and codes of ethics, that professionalism is alive and well in medicine. But bioethicists worry that the long-standing values of medicine are under strain. Medicine is increasingly commercialized, and clinics and hospitals are increasingly run like businesses. Consider, for example, the profound influence of pharmaceutical companies on the practice of medicine. Pharmaceutical companies shape medical education by offering grand rounds, including free pizza lunch, to "educate" about their products. They shape the daily practice of doctors by providing free samples of medications alongside pens and notepads adorned with brand-name drugs, not to mention the doughnuts and Starbucks coffee. Even patient behavior is shaped by advertising; consumers are told to "ask their doctor" about this drug or that, and research shows that they do. Doctors and patients alike are "branded" and are more likely, respectively, to prescribe or take drugs that have been introduced by advertising. Some doctors see the commercialization of medicine as a natural process. Medicine, for them, is a business just like any other.

Yet others are concerned about the fading of professional values within the medicine-as-business framework. Physicians may no longer see themselves in a fiduciary relationship with their patients (a relationship of trust), and *caveat emptor*—"let the buyer beware"—may become the reigning ethic. The essay by **Matthew Wynia** and colleagues argues that there is an essential role for professionalism in a health care system largely driven by market forces and government control. Wynia and colleagues define professionalism as "an activity that involves both the distribution of a commodity and the fair allocation of a social good but that is uniquely defined according to moral relationships." (This definition comes from part of the essay that is not reprinted in this text.) There are three core elements of professionalism: (1) a moral commitment to the ethic of medical service and its values, (2) public profession of this ethic (in oaths and codes of ethics), and (3) engagement in a political process of negotiation, where professionals advocate for health care values. Professionalism, they argue, is a morally protective force in society and will help maintain decency and stability not just in medicine but in society as a whole.

We return later to the role of medical professionals within a decent and stable society. But let us now focus attention on the specific moral values which physicians are thought to protect and promote in their treatment of individual patients.

The Obligations of Doctors to Their Patients

The moral relationship between a doctor and patient is complex and many-layered, with rights and responsibilities flowing in both directions. Most of the attention in medical ethics has been focused on the moral obligations of the physician to the patient—the essence of the Hippocratic Oath and the various codes and standards of ethics that guide the profession. Although the specifics of codes and oaths vary, certain moral values and concepts are common to them all and could be said to form the core ethical commitments of the physician: respect for patient autonomy and dignity, as well as the need for informed consent, confidentiality, veracity, and fairness. The first reading in this section will give you a sense of how these basic moral obligations are articulated by the **American Medical Association**.

Respect for Autonomy and Informed Consent

Two conceptions of medicine have, at different times, framed the physician-patient relationship. In one view, medicine is a value-free and objective science. The doctor is a technician. He or she gives the patient all the relevant information about treatment, and lets the patient decide what to do with it. The patient is a consumer, with his or her own freely chosen subjective preferences and desires. In the other view, the doctor is omniscient and omnipotent. The doctor alone can understand the medical intricacies of a given patient, and the doctor alone can make a wise choice about what course of treatment the patient should follow. The first view might be called "strong autonomy," while the second might be called "strong paternalism."

Autonomy, from the Greek *auto* (self) and *nomos* (law), refers to a person's capacity for self-rule. An autonomous person freely acts in accordance with a self-chosen plan. To act autonomously, a person needs liberty, or independence from controlling influences, and agency, or the capacity for intentional action. To respect an autonomous agent is to acknowledge that person's right to hold views, make choices, and take actions based on personal values and beliefs. We act autonomously when our choices and actions are self-made, rather than coerced. When someone holds a knife to our back and tells us to jump, we are not jumping autonomously. Respect for autonomy has been one of—if not *the*—guiding principle in medical ethics, and has even become a kind of trump card over other values.

Autonomy is often placed in contrast to or tension with what is called *paternalism*. Paternalism in medicine is defined as acting for the welfare of the patient, often interfering with or ignoring patient autonomy. Like a father guiding a child, a paternalistic doctor might restrict a patient's freedom of choice by withholding information or even going against the patient's stated desires, in order to benefit the patient. "I know you don't like this, but it's for your own good." Paternalistic physicians act as if they alone ought to determine what is in the best interests of the patient. (Note that the term *parentalism* is sometimes used, to remove some of the gender bias of the term paternalism.) The practice of medicine in the West was for a long time framed within a strongly paternalistic model, until the pendulum began to swing in the 1960s and 1970s toward a framework of strong autonomy.

There is also a middle path, which over time has emerged in the medical ethics literature. In this view, medicine is a humanistic enterprise, and the doctor much more than a technician. This rich understanding of physician responsibility goes beyond simply presenting information to the patient, to include also helping patients to understand their own values, cope with their fears, and learn to live with pain and suffering. At the same time, the concept of patient autonomy is nuanced and complex, recognizing that patients often have limited understanding and knowledge, may be psychologically (emotionally or cognitively) affected by their illnesses and injuries, and may have psychosocial barriers to understanding their problems or possibilities for treatment. Autonomous decision making, then, is much more than simply giving a diagnosis and a list of treatment options to a patient and waiting for an answer.

The excerpt "Respect for Autonomy" from **Tom Beauchamp and James Childress's** *Principles of Biomedical Ethics* explores the importance of the concept of autonomy in medicine, and shows how and why medical ethics has paved this middle path between the extremes of strong paternalism and strong autonomy. While firmly establishing respect for autonomy as a core principle of medical ethics, Beauchamp and Childress offer a nuanced and realistic account of how autonomy actually functions within the health care setting. As the concept of autonomy has been carefully specified within the philosophical tradition, it has become clear that there is no such thing as what we might call "perfect autonomy." Illness and pain can compromise autonomy, both physically and psychologically. But even if autonomy is not "pure," it is still meaningful.

One of the most important practical aspects of respect for patient autonomy is consent, to which Beauchamp and Childress give careful attention in the excerpt "The Meaning and Justification of Informed Consent." They explain the concept of informed consent in medicine, and explore the intricacies of and difficulties with obtaining consent. For example, there are countless situations in medicine where a patient's capacity for autonomous choice is impaired—a patient may appear irrational, may be heavily sedated, or may be in severe pain. In such instances, judgments must be made about the patient's competence to make medical decisions. Beauchamp and Childress define competence (and the related term "capacity") and explore the standards that are used to judge a patient's competence and how these balance against the need to respect autonomy. Beauchamp and Childress also discuss disclosure: how do we judge just how much and what kind of information a patient needs in order to give informed consent.

Sometimes a patient is unable to make autonomous choices—perhaps the patient is a young child, or perhaps the patient is unconscious. When we cannot obtain informed consent from a patient, some kind of surrogate decision making must occur, and how and by whom such decisions should be made has been an area of profound controversy in medical ethics. In the excerpt "A Framework of Standards for Surrogate Decision Making," Beauchamp and Childress explore competing paradigms—*best interests*, *pure autonomy*, and *substituted judgment*—for surrogate decision making. Questions about surrogate decision making will figure large in the next chapter, on end-of-life care.

Confidentiality and Privacy

One of the most famous lines in the Hippocratic Oath states: "What I may see or hear in the course of the treatment or even outside of the treatment in regard to the life of men, which on no account one must spread abroad, I will keep to myself holding such things shameful to be spoken about." This "keeping to oneself" the private information of patients is generally referred to as confidentiality. The duty to maintain confidentiality, which applies also to certain other professionals such as lawyers, clergy, psychologists, and other therapists is a legal requirement, a practical necessity, and a moral obligation. The concepts of informed consent and confidentiality both deal with the sharing of information between doctor and patient. While informed consent deals primarily with information that flows from doctor to patient, confidentiality concerns information that the doctor receives from the patient.

The moral obligation to protect confidentiality stems from valuing the patient's dignity and privacy. The public expectation that private information will remain confidential is strong enough to constitute an implicit promise by physicians to uphold this principle. Confidentiality is closely related to the value of privacy, though privacy is a much broader concept.

Why is confidentiality so important from a practical standpoint? In order to treat patients well, health professionals need to have information of a highly personal and private nature. If patients do not trust doctors to keep this information to themselves, patients will be unlikely to reveal sensitive information. Full disclosure thus is important to good care.

A number of laws establish and protect "privileged communications" between doctor and patient. A doctor cannot, for example, be compelled to testify against a patient. Nor can a doctor reveal patient information to others—friends, insurance companies, advertisers—without express permission from the patient. Although laws protect privileged information, they also establish exceptions to the rule. These exceptions are designed primarily to protect third parties—individuals or the public—from harm. For example, physicians are required to report to the state health departments the names of patients with serious communicable diseases such as tuberculosis and gonorrhea. Doctors are also required to report suspected child abuse. **The American Medical Association's** excerpt on patient confidentiality discusses the ethical and legal duty, and outlines some of the circumstances under which breaches of confidentiality are permitted.

Kenneth Kipnis in his essay "A Defense of Unqualified Medical Confidentiality" takes up the issue of breaching confidentiality, and argues that the conventional wisdom in medical ethics—that breaches are sometimes ethically acceptable or even obligatory—is probably wrong. Confidentiality in medicine is closer to an absolute obligation than has generally been argued. In making his argument, he relies on a distinction between professional obligation and personal morality. Although personal morality might seem to dictate breaches of confidentiality in certain circumstances, these situations should be guided by professional ethics. His discussion of professional obligation fits in nicely with the first section of readings on professionalism.

Although confidentiality is considered essential to effective and respectful care, the realities of modern health care put confidentiality under a constant state of siege. Health care, particularly in hospital settings, is carried out by large teams of people, and it is essential to good care that information flow freely and quickly among these health professionals. The move toward electronic medical records, which is sweeping through all aspects of health care from small clinics to large hospitals, is a double-edged sword as far as confidentiality is concerned. Electronic records offer a way to make medical information immediately and widely available to health care workers, but there are risks, too, since no system is completely protected from intrusion.

HIPAA

If you have had any contact with a medical professional—whether a visit to the clinic for a physical or a trip to the ER with a broken leg—you will have signed a HIPAA waiver. The Health Insurance Portability and Accountability Act was enacted in 1996. HIPAA required the Department of Health and Human Services to issue national standards for the protection of certain private health information. These standards—called The Privacy Rule—were issued in 2000, and aim to provide adequate protection of individual health information while at the same time allowing health information to flow freely enough to promote high quality care and protect public health. Various entities are covered by the rule, including health insurance companies, health care providers, health care clearinghouses (such as billing companies), and any business that handles individually identifiable health information. The rule covers all "individually identifiable health information," which includes any information related to a certain person's past, present, or future mental or physical health, what kind of treatment they have received, and whether and how they paid for this treatment. The Privacy Rule also includes a long and complicated list of permitted uses and disclosures of protected health information.

Truth Telling

Traditional codes of medical ethics, while speaking to the confidentiality of patient information, were often silent on the issue of truth telling, or veracity. But modern medical ethics gives truth telling a central place. Truth telling is connected to the principle of respect for autonomy and is derived from it; patients can only make autonomous and informed decisions if they have all the relevant information at hand. Truth telling is not only a kind of negative obligation: do not lie or otherwise deceive a patient. There are also positive obligations regarding the truth: telling patients enough (everything is probably too rigorous a standard) that they can make autonomous, informed decisions.

Still, although the obligation to tell the truth seems straightforward, it is not always. For example, how much should a doctor tell a patient in order to convey the truth (since withholding information can be a form of deception)? It is easy in theory to say that physicians must truthfully disclose all risks of a medical treatment or drug to a patient. But in reality both physicians and patients struggle to understand and communicate risks. And how exactly physicians communicate—what words they choose—can have enormous influence. Studies have shown, for example, that patients "read" the same risk differently depending on whether it is presented in terms of risk of death or potential for success.

We have used the issue of truth telling in medicine to offer some perspective on how the core obligations of physicians might be understood quite differently in other cultural contexts. The article by **Ruiping Fan and Benfu Li** suggests that medical ethics may be culture-bound in important ways, and that for patients from other cultures telling the truth might *not* be just what the doctor (or ethicist) ordered. Fan and Li offer a Confucian view of truth telling in medicine. Chinese medical ethics, they say, is committed to hiding the truth from patients as well as lying to patients when necessary to achieve what the family views as the patient's best interest. The basic moral commitments within the Chinese framework are familial, rather than individualistic, and these framing commitments generate a different ethic of truthfulness and deception. Fan and Li's article suggests the possibility that other core values in Western medical ethics are culture-bound as well.

Other Values

Although we have singled out several core obligations that doctors have toward patients, there are many other values that shape the doctor-patient relationship. For example, the notion of fidelity captures, in its kaleidoscope of meanings, various facets of the doctor's professional obligation: the idea that physicians owe to their patients a certain kind of loyalty, that they are loyal to their professional commitments, and that they will be true to their promises. Another concept of central importance is trust or trustworthiness. Patients are vulnerable: they are sick or hurt, and have often exposed to their doctor the most intimate details of their lives. They trust that their doctor acts for their benefit, is competent, and will maintain confidentiality. At the same time, the physician must trust the patient: has the patient revealed, truthfully and fully, the important details of his or her physical and emotional condition? Will the patient follow through on the doctor's careful recommendations?

(There is one core value that we have not discussed: fairness or justice. We will not attend to this core value here, but put off focused discussion until chapter 5, "Distributing and Procuring Health Care Resources.")

Other Health Professionals

We have focused attention on the physician-patient relationship, but it is important to remember that health care involves many other professions. Although the literature on ethics in these other health professions is not as large as that about medicine itself, it is nevertheless robust and interesting, and each profession has taken its moral responsibilities seriously. Nursing and the various "allied health" professions such as pharmacy, perfusion, and physical therapy would have their own set of ethical standards, their own special relationship with the patient, and their own unique ethical challenges.

Responsibilities of Patients

The doctor stared thoughtfully at Charles. He had just set a little test to probe his guest's mind. And it had revealed what he had expected. He turned and went to the bookshelves by his desk and then came back with the same volume he had shown Charles before: Darwin's great work. He sat before him across the fire; then with a smile and a look at Charles over his glasses, he laid his hand, as if swearing on a Bible, on *The Origin of Species*.

"Nothing that has been said in this room or that remains to be said shall go beyond its walls." Then he put the book aside.
"My dear Doctor, that was not necessary."
"Confidence in the practitioner is half of medicine."
Charles smiled wanly. "And the other half?"
"Confidence in the patient."

—John Fowles, *The French Lieutenant's Woman*

Physicians have a long list of role-related responsibilities toward their patients. But what about patients? Do they have any responsibilities toward their doctors? Are there any special responsibilities generated by their participation in the health care system? As the preceding dialogue from John Fowles's novel suggests, something is expected of the patient, too.

Truth telling, for example, cuts both ways. Patients are expected to tell their doctors the truth about their physical and even psychological symptoms. Given that all aspects of lifestyle—for example, the quality of relationships, types of leisure activity—can impact health, patients are expected to reveal a great deal of very personal information. But patients rarely tell all there is to tell, or they shade the truth in various ways. Patients not only fail to disclose, but often outright lie. Patients lie, for example, to obtain prescriptions: for example, a college student, after some careful Internet research, presents himself to the doctor with all the classic symptoms of attention-deficit/hyperactivity disorder. What the student wants is a prescription for Adderall, which will help him study long hours with little sleep. A woman with drug dependency on opioids fakes back pain in order to get a prescription for OxyContin.

Not only do patients deliberately deceive doctors, they also in various small ways undercut the good work of their physicians. They fail to take medication that their doctor prescribes, or refuse to cut back on the cheeseburgers or get more exercise, despite their high cholesterol. They fail to show up for appointments, often with no call of warning or apology. They expect their doctor to fix them up, blaming the doctor for their ills and sapping their doctor's time and energy with little regard.

If the physician-patient relationship carries such moral weight, surely this is not borne completely by the physician. What, then, are the responsibilities that patients themselves might bear? Do they, for example, have a responsibility to do what the doctor tells them? Have they any responsibility to carry through on treatment plans, finish their course of prescribed antibiotics, stop smoking, get more exercise? Must they tell the truth to their doctor? There are many facets to these questions.

The first reading in this section is the **American Medical Association's** report "Patient Responsibilities." The report explores the moral grounds for patient responsibilities (the principle of autonomy, as well as the therapeutic partnership between physician and patient), and outlines some of the key responsibilities of patients such as communicating openly with their physician and abiding by recommended treatment plans (sometimes called "compliance"). Compare this report with the AMA's "Fundamental Elements of the Physician-Patient Relationship" and notice how patient rights correlate with patient responsibilities. Also, ask yourself: what rights do physicians have in the doctor-patient relationship?

"The Patient's Work," by bioethicists **Leonard Groopman, Franklin Miller, and Joseph Fins**, explores the patient's role in the healing process. The healing process is collaborative—the patient is not a piece of clay, but an active participant. Medical treatment almost always requires some work by the patient, whether taking a prescribed medicine or deciding upon a treatment plan. And the patient can fail to work, or can work poorly. Noncompliance is the most well-known form of failure, but there are also failures of passivity, dependence, and indecisiveness. The authors explore three relational models of doctor-patient relationship, with different views of patient's work: paternalism, autonomy, and mutualism. All three give the doctor and the patient moral work to do.

Recent attempts to draw up lists of patient responsibilities reflect physicians' frustration with the burden of clinical and legal responsibility for patient health. Yet although the idea of patient responsibility has intuitive appeal, **Maureen Kelley** argues in her essay for a cautious approach. While patients do clearly have responsibilities in the medical encounter, Kelley argues that these are less strong than the physician's. There has been, and she believes should be, an asymmetry in the medical profession: there ought to be greater emphasis on professional responsibility than on patient responsibility. There is an inherent imbalance in the relationship between doctor and patient, because the doctor is an expert and the patient is a layperson. This imbalance makes the relationship susceptible to subtle (and gross) forms of paternalism. She thinks that being a "responsible patient" will be too easily confused with being a compliant patient. The value of protecting the right to refuse treatment and arguments against paternalism block a more expansive account of patient responsibility. She also says we should emphasize prospective rather than retrospective notions of responsibility in clinical practice.

It's a Hard Life

Although many people's stereotype of the doctor boils down to a golf course and a nice car, the realities for those in the profession of medicine are often quite different. Family practice doctors, in particular, often have to struggle to make ends meet for their own families, and find themselves working extraordinary hours for only a modest salary. Not only are the financial rewards often relatively small, the work itself is extremely difficult and stressful. For example, a doctor writing in the *Journal of the American Medical Association* described what he thought might be "HMO-related hypertension." During his work days, Dr. W.R. Phillips frequently had to interrupt patient care in order to request authorization of services from his HMO. He noted high levels of stress during these often contentious and frustrating phone calls. He measured his blood pressure throughout the day, and recorded spikes in his measurements after these phone calls, but not after other professional activities, including major surgery. He developed hypertension, requiring drug treatment, as a direct result, he believes, of dealing with HMOs.

Doctors have the highest rate of suicide of any profession. Every year, between three hundred and four hundred doctors take their own lives. Many more suffer from depression. What makes things even worse is that many doctors are reluctant to seek psychiatric treatment for themselves. The worry is that if they admit to having a mental health problem and seek treatment for it, they could lose the respect and confidence of colleagues and patients. Furthermore, doctors are intimately acquainted with the insurance industry and know that a diagnosis of mental illness is a permanent black mark that will lead to increased premiums and difficulty buying insurance policies for themselves and their families.

The documentary "Struggling in Silence" explores the problem of depression and suicide in doctors. The website doctorswithdepression.com also hopes to raise awareness of this issue.

Doctors and Society

Challenges to professional integrity are everywhere. The boundaries of medicine are porous, and the duties of health professionals difficult to define precisely. In this final section of readings, we focus on two particular kinds of challenge to professional integrity. We consider, with the first reading, questions about contested therapies and the proper scope of medical care. Some procedures and treatments—most notably cosmetic surgery—are contested, in the sense that some people believe they fall outside the scope of appropriate medical treatment. Physicians who perform these therapies may, according to some, be acting unprofessionally and unethically. The second reading raises questions about what might be called "dual loyalties"— situations in which physicians are asked to fulfill a social duty that seems to conflict with the basic moral commitments of medicine. We explore one particularly controversial role that physicians are asked to fill: as physician-soldiers in war.

Contested Therapies

A man who goes by the name of Stalking Cat has had countless surgical modifications to achieve oneness with his Native American totem, the tiger. He has had, among other things, his teeth removed and replaced with fangs, stainless steel mounts implanted into his forehead, and his lip split to resemble a cat. Although most of these modifications have been performed by an artist, not a practicing surgeon, they raise the question: would performing such procedures, at the request of a patient, go beyond the ken of appropriate medical treatment? And how different are these extreme modifications from the teenage girl who asks the doctor for breast implants, or the short-statured boy whose parents ask that he be given growth hormones to add an inch or two to his height?

Most medical care is obviously appropriate; it conforms with broadly accepted goals of medicine. But some kinds of treatments push the boundaries. These contested therapies are the focus of the essay by **Franklin Miller, Howard Brody, and Kevin Chung**, who argue that medicine is not a morally neutral technique; rather, it is a professional practice governed by a moral framework consisting of goals proper to medicine, role-specific duties, and clinical virtues. This framework is what they call the "internal morality of medicine." Their essay maps the moral domain of medicine, and provides a framework for distinguishing between legitimate medical practice and those procedures and practices that fall outside the moral domain and are thus unethical for a physician to perform.

Miller and colleagues raise some difficult questions: Is it morally appropriate for physicians to offer treatments that fall beyond the scope of preventing or treating disease or impairment? Who determines what "appropriate medical services" include—doctors or consumers? What are the proper goals of medicine? These issues will resurface in later chapters. For example, chapter 7 explores genetic and pharmaceutical enhancements, and the problematic distinction between enhancement and therapy. A recurring theme within each chapter is how properly to understand "disease" and "health"—for a great deal rests on how we define these concepts. All of the chapters, in one way or another, take up the question of medicine's moral domain—what practices are legitimate and ethical, and which are not (abortion? assisted suicide?).

Dual Loyalties

The medical professional is sometimes asked to serve some social purpose at odds with patient welfare. For example, an occupational health physician may have a primary commitment to verify that an injured or ill employee really is injured or sick; the physician's loyalty thus lies with the company, not the patient. A forensic psychiatrist may be interested in showing a patient to be sane, so that the state can prosecute. A public health physician may have the primary commitment of ensuring the health of the population as a whole, to which individual patient interests are subordinate. Instead of being committed wholeheartedly to the patient, as the professional doctor-patient ethic demands, the physician in these cases might be said to have competing or dual loyalties. Two of the most contentious areas of split loyalties arise in the context of war and capital punishment.

News reports about abusive treatment of prisoners at Abu Ghraib prison included claims that doctors had been complicit in the torture of detainees. According to government documents, army doctors not only remained silent about the abuses but allowed them to proceed by falsifying and "misplacing" medical records of prisoners who were beaten or tortured. This behavior seems clearly at odds with the professional mandate to promote the well-being of patients, and most people feel that the medical personnel involved acted unethically. Yet was their behavior wrong because of the inherent wrongness of torture per se, or was it wrong because these were medical personnel? It is not clear that prisoners are "patients" in the usual sense of the word, or that military doctors are clearly acting as doctors.

In their essay "When Doctors Go to War," **Gregg Bloche and Jonathan Marks** consider the problem of physicians involved in interrogations of suspected terrorists. In helping to draft and execute interrogation strategies, did these doctors breach medical ethics? Do doctors act as combatants or doctors? Physicians who work in interrogation tend *not* to see their role as that of physician, so they do not feel bound by the physician-patient ethic. But Bloche and Marks argue that doctors who serve social purposes do still act as physicians; they need to manage the moral conflict of dual roles, rather than deny one of the roles. In order to maintain the doctor-patient ethic, a physician's role in interrogation should not extend beyond "limit setting."

Another recent controversy has centered on physician participation in executions. In February 2006, two anesthesiologists in California refused to monitor the injection of a barbiturate that would render convicted murderer Michel Morales unconscious, in preparation for a lethal injection of drugs. The execution was postponed. The case received wide attention, and rekindled a long-standing debate about whether doctors should participate in capital punishment.

We have highlighted a few dramatic conflicts of interest for physicians, but keep in mind that the daily work of physicians is saturated with moral conflict, and physicians must constantly work to maintain their moral equilibrium in a health care environment rife with challenges to professional integrity. Even the daily setting that a physician works within can generate subtle ethical conflicts. For example, physicians working in large medical clinics often engage in "self-referral"; the clinic owns, say, an X-ray machine, and every time one of its physicians orders an X-ray on a patient, the clinic—and thus each individual doctor—makes a little extra money. Or perhaps a medical imaging company owns the X-ray equipment and offers a small kickback to the clinic for each referral. A physician working for a health maintenance organization, on the other hand, may have subtle financial incentives for offering less treatment, and ordering fewer X-rays. Furthermore, not only does a physician's work setting pose challenges, but the physician must also balance the needs of patients with his or her own personal and family needs. Should he spend an extra thirty minutes with his sick patient, or should he leave in time to catch his daughter's school play? Should she read another medical journal to stay current, or go for a game of tennis?

We might wonder whether it is realistic to say that physicians should be guided solely by the needs of the patient sitting in front of them, and whether professionalism is perhaps an outdated concept, out of touch with the reality of medical practice. On the other hand, the moral ambiguity of a doctor's work may suggest that the ethical values grounding the doctor-patient relationship need to remain ever in the foreground of attention.

REFERENCES AND FURTHER READING

Brody, Howard. *Stories of Sickness*. 2nd ed. New York: Oxford University Press, 2002.

———. *The Healer's Power*. New Haven, CT: Yale University Press, 1992.

Elliott, Carl, and Peter D. Kramer. *Better Than Well: American Medicine Meets the American Dream*. New York: W.W. Norton, 2004.

Emanuel, Ezekiel, and Linda Emanuel. "Four Models of the Physician-Patient Relationship," *JAMA* 267 no. 16 (1992): 2221–26.

Farmer, Paul. *Awakening Hippocrates: A Primer on Health, Poverty, and Global Service.* Chicago: American Medical Association Press, 2005.

Groopman, Jerome. *How Doctors Think.* New York: Mariner Books, 2008.

May, William F. *The Physician's Covenant: Images of the Healer in Medical Ethics.* Philadelphia: Westminster Press, 1983.

———. *The Patient's Ordeal.* Bloomington: Indiana University Press, 1991.

Pellegrino, Edmund D. "Toward a Reconstruction of Medical Morality." *American Journal of Bioethics* 6, no. 2 (2006): 65–71.

Phillips, W. R. "Hassle Hypertension: A Risk of Managed Care," *JAMA* 274, no. 10 (1995): 795–6.

Rodwin, Marc A. *Medicine, Money, and Morals: Physician's Conflicts of Interest.* New York: Oxford University Press, 1993.

Rothman, David J. *Strangers at the Bedside.* New York: Basic Books, 2002.

Starr, Paul. *The Social Transformation of American Medicine.* New York: Basic Books, 1984.

DISCUSSION QUESTIONS FOR THE READINGS

"'I Swear by Apollo': On Taking the Hippocratic Oath"

1. Name four of what Markel refers to as "discarded relics" of the original oath. Do you agree that these rules are no longer valid?

2. Based on your reading of the original text of the Hippocratic Oath, how would you define the professional obligations of a physician?

Hippocratic Oath, Modern Version

1. Compare the text of the modern version with the original Hippocratic Oath. What changes do you see?

2. What changes in the practice of medicine might be reflected in modern revisions of the Hippocratic Oath?

3. Which of the two versions of the Oath (old or new) do you find a more compelling statement of moral duty, and why?

Principles of Medical Ethics

1. Of the nine principles, which might be in conflict with each other? When there is conflict, how should a doctor decide which principle has priority?

2. Read the opening paragraph carefully: To whom does the doctor have primary responsibility? To whom, do you think, *should* the doctor have primary responsibility?

Medical Professionalism in Society

1. What are the three core elements of professionalism? How do these elements work together?

2. This interpretation of professionalism suggests that doctors have far more to do than simply treat patients. Do you agree with the author's expansive view of professional obligation? What might be some problems with this expansive view?

3. Based on what you read in this excerpt, what would the authors say about doctors participating in war or in executions?

Fundamental Elements of the Patient-Physician Relationship

1. Compare this document with the American Medical Association's "Principles of Medical Ethics." What is different about "Fundamental Elements"?
2. This document spells out a number of rights of patients. Are there any additional rights that patients might have? Do physicians have rights, too, in the context of the physician-patient relationship?
3. What does it mean to say that a doctor has a "fiduciary" relationship to her patient? How does this fiduciary relationship relate to professionalism?
4. How might respect for these principles by physicians improve health outcomes for patients?

Respect for Autonomy

1. What are the two basic conditions for autonomy?
2. What is the moral basis for the principle of respect for autonomy?
3. Explain the difference between respect for autonomy as a positive obligation and respect for autonomy as a negative obligation.
4. Can you identify some weaknesses in Beauchamp and Childress's concept of competence?
5. What criticisms might be leveled against their account of autonomy (e.g., from a feminist perspective)?

The Meaning and Justification of Informed Consent

1. How are the concepts of informed consent and autonomy related?
2. What are the essential elements of informed consent?
3. What are some factors that can complicate the process of obtaining informed consent?

A Framework of Standards for Surrogate Decision Making

1. In what sorts of medical situations might the need for a surrogate decision maker arise?
2. Review the three standards that a surrogate decision maker might employ. How does autonomy function in each of these standards? How are autonomy and decision making related?
3. The authors discuss a paradigm case in relation to each of the three standards of surrogate decision making. How do the particulars of these three cases differ, and how do they lead to different standards? Which standard would have been most appropriate in the case of Terri Schiavo?

Truth Telling in Medicine: The Confucian View

1. How is the Chinese ethic of hiding the truth distinguished from medical paternalism?
2. What does truthfulness in medical practice look like from a Confucian perspective?
3. What is the moral justification for deception?
4. Fan and Li discuss principles that guide practices in Chinese physicians in mainland China. What, if any, are the implications of Fan and Li's essay for American physicians in American hospitals?

Patient Confidentiality

1. What does the obligation to maintain patient confidentiality entail? Is this a legal or a moral obligation, or both? Might the legal and moral rules conflict?
2. Why is confidentiality an important element of the physician-patient relationship?
3. What are some legitimate exceptions to the obligation?

A Defense of Unqualified Medical Confidentiality

1. What happened in *Tarasoff*, and how has this case shaped the duty of confidentiality in medicine?
2. Kipnis says that questions about professional ethics cannot be answered in terms of personal values or personal morality. What does he mean?
3. Compare Kipnis's concept of a professional obligation with the definition given by Wynia et al. Would they come to different conclusions about confidentiality?
4. How does Kipnis's view of professional obligation ground his unqualified defense of confidentiality?
5. Why must the duty to protect confidentiality be (almost) absolute?

Patient Responsibilities

1. How do patient responsibilities derive from the principle of autonomy?
2. Do any of the ten responsibilities spelled out by the American Medical Association ask too much of patients? Which ones, and why?
3. Are any of these *moral* responsibilities, or are they simply practical dos and don'ts?

The Patient's Work

1. What do the authors mean by "the patient's work"? In what sense is it *moral* work?
2. Compare the paternalistic, autonomy, and mutualistic models of the doctor-patient relationship. How does the concept of the patient's work differ in each relational model? What is the physician's moral function in each model?
3. Why do the authors place each model "on an equal ethical plane"?

Limits on Patient Responsibility

1. Kelley argues that several crucial moral norms are threatened by a positive account of patient responsibility. What norms are under threat? What does she mean by a "positive" account of patient responsibility?
2. Why does Kelley argue for a forward-looking or prospective notion of patient responsibility? How does this prospective focus protect moral values in the doctor-patient relationship?
3. What relational model of the doctor-patient relationship (from Groopman, Miller, and Fins) does Kelley seem to embrace?
4. Recalling what you read in Beauchamp and Childress's excerpt "Respect for Autonomy," and in light of Kelley's essay, would you say a strong notion of patient responsibility is more likely to nurture respect for autonomy or threaten it? Why?

Cosmetic Surgery and the Internal Morality of Medicine

1. What are the four goals of medicine? How do the goals of medicine relate to the internal duties of medical practice?
2. Can you think of other medical services that might fall on the periphery of the normative domain of medicine? That might fall outside?

When Doctors Go to War

1. According to Bloche and Marks, is it ever ethically acceptable for physicians to participate in the interrogation of military prisoners? Under what conditions might it be acceptable? Do you agree with their argument?
2. What other social roles do physicians fill, and how are these in tension with professional ethics?

READINGS

"I Swear by Apollo"

On Taking the Hippocratic Oath

HOWARD MARKEL

New England Journal of Medicine 350, no. 20 (2004): 2026–29.

Every spring for almost 20 years, I have happily donned a rented robe, hood, and mortarboard to attend medical school commencement exercises. The purpose of this annual foray into pomp and circumstance goes well beyond applauding the achievements of graduates who are about to enter the medical profession. For me, commencement is the perfect opportunity to renew my vows, as it were, standing shoulder to shoulder with both newly minted doctors and like-minded colleagues as we take the Hippocratic Oath.

Although many scholars dispute the exact authorship of the writings ascribed to the ancient physician Hippocrates, who probably lived sometime between 460 and 380 B.C., the oath named for him is simultaneously one of the most revered, protean, and misunderstood documents in the history of medicine (see box). To begin with, it is often misquoted. For example, our mantra of "First, do no harm" (a phrase translated into Latin as "*Primum non nocere*") is often mistakenly ascribed to the oath, although it appears nowhere in that venerable pledge. Hippocrates came closest to issuing this directive in his treatise *Epidemics*, in an axiom that reads, "As to diseases, make a habit of two things—to help, or at least, to do no harm."

Many doctors practicing today are surprised to learn that the first recorded administration of the Hippocratic Oath in a medical school setting was at the University of Wittenberg in Germany in 1508 and that it did not become a standard part of a formal medical school graduation ceremony until 1804, when it was incorporated into the commencement exercises at Montpellier, France. The custom spread in fits and starts on both sides of the Atlantic during the 19th century, but even well into the 20th century relatively few American physicians formally took the oath. According to a survey conducted for the Association of American Medical Colleges in 1928, for example, only 19 percent of the medical schools in North America included the oath in their commencement exercises. With the discovery of the atrocities that were committed in the name of medicine during World War II and the growing interest in bioethics in the succeeding decades, oath taking began playing an increasing part in graduation ceremonies.

This spring, nearly every U.S. medical school will administer some type of professional oath to its share of about 16,000 men and women who are eager to take possession of their medical degrees. Yet it is doubtful that Hippocrates would recognize most of the pledges that are anachronistically ascribed to him. Such revisionism is hardly unique to our era. Indeed, the tinkering with Hippocrates' oath began soon after its first utterance and generally reflected the changing values, customs, and beliefs associated with the ethical practice of medicine.

Consequently, there are stark differences between the promises made in the original version and the oaths sworn today. To take the most obvious example, few if any of us now believe in the ancient Greek gods Apollo, Asclepius, Hygieia, and Panaceia, and we therefore no longer pledge allegiance to them. Indeed, the evidence indicates that spirituality in general—regardless of its form—now has a distant relationship with medical science: a "content analysis" of the oaths administered at 147 U.S. and Canadian medical schools in 1993 showed that only 11 percent of the versions invoked a deity.

In Hippocrates' day, the student made a binding vow to honor his teacher as he would his parents and to share financial and intellectual resources with his mentor and the mentor's family. Unfortunately for those of us engaged in medical education today, this pledge has long since passed into disfavor.

There are two highly controversial vows in the original Hippocratic Oath that we continue to ponder and struggle with as a profession: the pledges never to participate in euthanasia and abortion. These prohibitions applied primarily to those identified as Hippocratic physicians, a medical sect that represented only a small minority of all self-proclaimed healers. The Hippocratics' reasons for refusing to participate in euthanasia may have been based on a philosophical or moral belief in preserving the sanctity of life or simply on their wish to avoid involvement in any act of assisted suicide, murder, or manslaughter. We have fairly reliable historical documentation, however, that many ancient Greeks and Romans who were confronted with terminal illness preferred a quick, painless death by means of poison to letting nature take its course. Moreover, there were no laws in the ancient world against suicide, and it was not uncommon for physicians to recommend this option to a patient with an incurable disease. Similarly, abortion, typically effected by means of a pessary that induced premature labor, was practiced in both ancient Greece and the Roman Empire. Many Christian revisions of the Hippocratic Oath, especially those written during the Middle Ages, prohibited all abortive procedures. Not surprisingly, the contentious debate over both of these issues continues today, although the relevant sections are simply omitted in most oaths administered by U.S. medical schools. As of 1993, only 14 percent of such oaths prohibited euthanasia, and only 8 percent prohibited abortion.

Another discarded relic is the vow never to "use the knife, not even on sufferers from the stone." In an era before antiseptic and aseptic surgery, anesthesia, and the scientific management of fluids, blood loss, and surgical shock, it was wise indeed to refer sufferers of these painful concretions to persons who specialized in removing them. Many healers in the ancient world focused their work specifically on kidney and bladder stones, others on cataract removal, and still others on the treatment of external injuries such as wounds. But as recently as the end of the 19th century, most surgical operations were treacherous affairs that carried a high risk of death. Consequently, the passage about "the knife" remains difficult to interpret. Historians have debated for centuries whether this vow bans all surgical procedures by the Hippocratics because of their inherent danger, reflects the fact that these physicians considered surgery beneath their dignity, or represents a promise not to practice outside the bounds of one's abilities.

The Hippocratic physicians understood the importance of avoiding any type of sexual relationship with their patients, yet only 3 percent of the oaths administered by U.S. medical schools at the end of the 20th century specifically prohibited such contact. On the other hand, virtually all the oaths administered today include the assurances that Hippocrates insisted were touchstones of the successful patient–doctor relationship: the promises of acting in the best interest of the patient and of confidentiality.

The Hippocratic Oath

I swear by Apollo Physician and Asclepius and Hygieia and Panaceia and all the gods and goddesses, making them my witnesses, that I will fulfill according to my ability and judgment this oath and this covenant:

To hold him who has taught me this art as equal to my parents and to live my life in partnership with him, and if he is in need of money to give him a share of mine, and to regard his offspring as equal to my brothers in male lineage and to teach them this art — if they desire to learn it — without fee and covenant; to give a share of precepts and oral instruction and all the other learning to my sons and to the sons of him who has instructed me and to pupils who have signed the covenant and have taken an oath according to the medical law, but to no one else.

I will apply dietetic measures for the benefit of the sick according to my ability and judgment; I will keep them from harm and injustice.

I will neither give a deadly drug to anybody if asked for it, nor will I make a suggestion to this effect. Similarly I will not give to a woman an abortive remedy. In purity and holiness I will guard my life and my art.

I will not use the knife, not even on sufferers from stone, but will withdraw in favor of such men as are engaged in this work.

Whatever houses I may visit, I will come for the benefit of the sick, remaining free of all intentional injustice, of all mischief and in particular of sexual relations with both female and male persons, be they free or slaves.

What I may see or hear in the course of the treatment or even outside of the treatment in regard to the life of men, which on no account one must spread abroad, I will keep to myself holding such things shameful to be spoken about.

If I fulfill this oath and do not violate it, may it be granted to me to enjoy life and art, being honored with fame among all men for all time to come; if I transgress it and swear falsely, may the opposite of all this be my lot.

Translated from the Greek by L. Edelstein, in *Ancient Medicine: Selected Papers of Ludwig Edelstein* (Baltimore, MD: Johns Hopkins University Press, 1967).

Often, the additions made to the Hippocratic Oath are as historically interesting as the deletions. Many of the oaths taken this spring will include vows not to alter one's practice on the basis of the patient's race, nationality, religion, sex, socioeconomic standing, or sexual orientation. Others include assurances of the physician's accountability to his or her patients, protection of patients' autonomy, and informed consent or assistance with decision making. In a very real sense, all these changes help to make the act of oath taking eternal, a process that constantly changes to accommodate and articulate changing views of medicine and society.

But regardless of the language or provenance of the hundreds of texts collectively classified as Hippocratic, on commencement day the historian in me invariably takes a back seat to the physician. Whether I am reciting from bowdlerized or amended versions or the original Greek text, as I rise to take the oath with my peers, my heart grows full with reverence for the profession I have chosen.

Despite occasional complaints questioning the relevance or purity of the oath taking, this symbolic act is a tradition that is unlikely to become superannuated. It serves as a powerful reminder and declaration that we are all a part of something infinitely larger, older, and more important than a particular specialty or institution. Given the myriad challenges facing almost every aspect of medicine in the 21st century, the need for physicians to make a formal warrant of diligent, moral, and ethical conduct in the service of their patients may be stronger than ever.

As every experienced doctor knows, the few minutes we spend giving voice to a professional oath are far easier than the years we must devote to its faithful execution. As Hippocrates famously said, "Life is short, the art long, opportunity fleeting, experience perilous, and the crisis difficult," but the legacy of medicine suggests that we are capable of fulfilling this noble charge.

Hippocratic Oath, Modern Version

LOUIS LASAGNA

Written in 1964 by Louis Lasagna, Academic Dean of the School of Medicine at Tufts University.

I swear to fulfill, to the best of my ability and judgment, this covenant:

I will respect the hard-won scientific gains of those physicians in whose steps I walk, and gladly share such knowledge as is mine with those who are to follow.

I will apply, for the benefit of the sick, all measures [that] are required, avoiding those twin traps of overtreatment and therapeutic nihilism.

I will remember that there is art to medicine as well as science, and that warmth, sympathy, and understanding may outweigh the surgeon's knife or the chemist's drug.

I will not be ashamed to say "I know not," nor will I fail to call in my colleagues when the skills of another are needed for a patient's recovery.

I will respect the privacy of my patients, for their problems are not disclosed to me that the world may know. Most especially must I tread with care in matters of life and death. If it is given me to save a life, all thanks. But it may also be within my power to take a life; this awesome responsibility must be faced with great humbleness and awareness of my own frailty. Above all, I must not play at God.

I will remember that I do not treat a fever chart, a cancerous growth, but a sick human being, whose illness may affect the person's family and economic stability. My responsibility includes these related problems, if I am to care adequately for the sick.

I will prevent disease whenever I can, for prevention is preferable to cure.

I will remember that I remain a member of society, with special obligations to all my fellow human beings, those sound of mind and body as well as the infirm.

If I do not violate this oath, may I enjoy life and art, respected while I live and remembered with affection thereafter. May I always act so as to preserve the finest traditions of my calling and may I long experience the joy of healing those who seek my help.

Principles of Medical Ethics

AMERICAN MEDICAL ASSOCIATION

Adopted by the American Medical Association's House of Delegates, June 17, 2001.

Preamble

The medical profession has long subscribed to a body of ethical statements developed primarily for the benefit of the patient. As a member of this profession, a physician must recognize responsibility to patients first and foremost, as well as to society, to other health professionals, and to self. The following Principles adopted by the American Medical Association are not laws, but standards of conduct which define the essentials of honorable behavior for the physician.

Principles of medical ethics

I.   A physician shall be dedicated to providing competent medical care, with compassion and respect for human dignity and rights.

II. A physician shall uphold the standards of professionalism, be honest in all professional interactions, and strive to report physicians deficient in character or competence, or engaging in fraud or deception, to appropriate entities.

III. A physician shall respect the law and also recognize a responsibility to seek changes in those requirements which are contrary to the best interests of the patient.

IV. A physician shall respect the rights of patients, colleagues, and other health professionals, and shall safeguard patient confidences and privacy within the constraints of the law.

V. A physician shall continue to study, apply, and advance scientific knowledge, maintain a commitment to medical education, make relevant information available to patients, colleagues, and the public, obtain consultation, and use the talents of other health professionals when indicated.

VI. A physician shall, in the provision of appropriate patient care, except in emergencies, be free to choose whom to serve, with whom to associate, and the environment in which to provide medical care.

VII. A physician shall recognize a responsibility to participate in activities contributing to the improvement of the community and the betterment of public health.

VIII. A physician shall, while caring for a patient, regard responsibility to the patient as paramount.

IX. A physician shall support access to medical care for all people.

Medical Professionalism in Society

MATTHEW K. WYNIA, STEPHEN R. LATHAM, AUDIEY C. KAO, JESSICA W. BERG, AND LINDA L. EMANUEL

The New England Journal of Medicine 34, no. 21 (1999): 1612–16.

A Model of Professionalism

Three core elements of professionalism, each different in nature, are necessary for it to work properly. First, professionalism requires a moral commitment to the ethic of medical service, which we will call devotion to medical service and its values. This devotion leads naturally to a public, normative act: public profession of this ethic. Public profession of the ethic serves both to maintain professionals' devotion to medical service and to assert its values in societal discussions. These discussions lead naturally to engagement in a political process of negotiation, in which professionals advocate for health care values in the context of other important, perhaps competing, societal values.

Devotion to Medical Service

Physicians should cultivate in themselves and in their peers a devotion to health care values by placing the goals of individual and public health ahead of other goals. That is, physicians must be devoted to the work of providing health care.

Physicians who value individual and public health more than other social goods remain motivated to work hard even when the financial rewards for such work are not great. They criticize and police one another even when such actions have personal, social, and financial costs. They offer high-quality services whether or not patients are capable of judging their quality. They continue to provide health care even when, as during an epidemic, they risk their own health. And they maintain their obligations to care for financially disadvantaged patients. Today, the ascendance of marketplace values puts health care for the poor at particular risk. Physicians should influence the organizations in which they practice to adopt policies that address the care of impoverished persons. Similarly, physicians must resist incentives that place the trust between patient and doctor and even patient care at risk. Devotion to medical service is so important that physicians must avoid even the appearance that they are primarily devoted to their own interests rather than to the interests of others. Dramatic rises in physicians' incomes over the past four decades have fostered the trust-destroying belief, whether true or not, that physicians as a group are greedy and take advantage of patients.

Public Profession of Values

Physicians should speak out about their values. The word "profession" means, from the Latin, "speaking forth." Public avowal of values has been a distinctive feature of the professions from before medieval times.

Although acting on one's professional devotion to medical service is a form of public profession of values, it is not enough. The unique nature of the relationship between patient and physician requires an explicit and professionally protected moral base so that there can be legitimate shared expectations, even in circumstances, such as emergencies, in which individual relationships have not had time to mature. The patient–physician relationship is based on shared experiences of vulnerability and the potential for health or illness and on a resultant respect for the inestimable value of human life and health. Furthermore, health care values focus on the public as well as the individual. As Samuel Johnson noted, "A decent provision for the poor is the true test of civilization." Health care values reflect this assertion. Through public profession of health care values, patients and the public hear about these values as well as the standards that result from them. They hear

that physicians' commitment to such important standards as never exploiting patients' inherent vulnerability and not abandoning patients is timeless. They hear that other, specific aspects of health care values are delineated in a continuous dynamic process with society, to which physicians bring their training, professional virtues, interprofessional relations, and above all, experiences in caring for patients. Finally, public profession of values — for example, by participating in "white-coat ceremonies," posting ethics codes in waiting areas, and contributing to and espousing the standards of a professional association — demands commitment. A public, collective commitment to fulfill legitimate expectations implies an acceptance of accountability for one's professional actions, as well as an acceptance of the shared standards of the profession, which may sometimes conflict with personal beliefs.

Negotiation Regarding Professional Values and Other Social Values

Public profession of values inevitably requires professionals to engage with the public in negotiating social priorities that balance medical values with other societal values. This political process of negotiation should lead to what is sometimes referred to as a social contract between physicians and the public.

The process of negotiation not only clarifies legitimate public and professional expectations but can also prevent counterproductive paternalistic behavior on the part of professionals. Individually, the process fosters patient-centered care by including each patient's health goals in decision making. Collectively, it can help accommodate a suitable social disposition toward medical care. The process of negotiation can make clear professionals' obligations to meet public needs, reminding the profession that it cannot have everything its own way and simultaneously demanding appropriate advocacy. Tension may develop between what society wants of physicians and physicians' devotion to health care values. For example, portions of society today favor intense market competition among physicians as a way to lower the costs of care. But such competition encourages the development of trade secrets among physicians, such as proprietary practice guidelines, and impedes the collegial interaction and information sharing that are needed to provide high-quality care. The challenge for physicians is to be accountable to the public and its changing values while protecting core health care values.

An Archetypal Model of Professionalism

We propose that an ideal archetypal model of medical professionalism entails the three elements of devotion, profession, and negotiation. The model is ideal in that it is not descriptive of the reality today or in any other era. It is archetypal because it is intended to describe only core elements of professionalism. The purpose of the model is to provide a normative guide.

Each element may fail, may be misapplied, or may not be in balance with the other two. A failure of devotion to the ethic of medical service leads to self-protective behavior on the part of physicians, as occurred, for instance, in the difficult transition to managed care and at the start of the AIDS epidemic. Failure to profess health care values publicly may lead to uninformed, misinformed, or piecemeal public policies. And failure to negotiate an acceptable social contract leads the public to establish other contracts in order to obtain what it needs and wants. As one example, "alternative" practitioners and therapies become more attractive to the public when they provide something desirable that the profession has ignored in individual or social negotiations. Yet negotiation does not mean simply giving the public what it wants. An overemphasis on satisfying public demands, without attention to core health care values, will ultimately leave both professionals and society unprotected. In addition, professionalism may be misused if physicians become devoted, as individuals or groups, to values derived from other sources, such as business values. Finally, an exaggerated devotion to an ethic that is determined solely by professionals may lead to paternalism or to the refusal to consider other important perspectives.

A Spectrum of Professional Activism

With this model of professionalism as devotion, profession, and negotiation, exactly how, in a practical sense, should physicians act on behalf of patients, the public, and health care values? What types of activity constitute professional advocacy?

The advocacy activities of individual professionals should fall along a spectrum, with more extreme actions requiring more stringent justifications. At one end of the spectrum is routine advocacy for patients and public health. Routine advocacy constitutes physicians' regular daily activity. Physicians working in health care delivery organizations — coordinating care, working to improve practice guidelines, and so on — should advocate health care values rather than government or corporate values, speaking on behalf of patients and health care. Occasionally, this type of advocacy may be personally risky. For instance, physicians who appeal adverse coverage decisions on behalf of their patients may put at risk their standing with health plans.

If advocacy fails, physicians have an obligation to express internal dissent with regard to activities or policies that undermine core health care values. This responsibility is what distinguishes genuine professionals from "company docs." Although internal dissent is not always clearly distinct from routine advocacy, it is a negative form of activism that may go against an internal hierarchy. Internal dissent may require courage and skill to achieve a positive outcome, but it generally requires minimal moral justification.

Public dissent is next on the spectrum and should be used with more care. It may raise tensions and backfire, causing harm. For instance, the dissenter may be demoted or fired, thereby perhaps harming patients' care, or a point of dissent may become more difficult to resolve because publicity can provoke denial or defensiveness. Public dissent is warranted only when internal dissent has demonstrably failed to remedy a harmful situation, when outside pressure is likely to be required to achieve change, when public silence allows the harmful situation to continue, and when the potential harms to patients from public dissent are relatively small. For example, the proposed closing of a clinic may justify efforts to galvanize community support through public dissent.

With direct professional disobedience, the fourth form of activism on the spectrum, professionals act against authorities, publicly disobeying rules or laws that are antithetical to health care. Direct professional disobedience has a clear potential to harm patients, the profession, and professionals themselves. It should therefore be reserved for situations in which both internal and public dissent have failed, direct disobedience is likely to be effective in remedying the problem, the problem is very serious (preferably, its seriousness can be documented empirically), and the action entails as little harm as possible. Surreptitious disobedience, such as secretly "gaming" a billing code to obtain coverage for services, is not justifiable as a form of direct professional disobedience, since it is neither public nor aimed at achieving systemic change. In contrast, delivering free care despite a policy to the contrary, urging colleagues not to comply with California's Proposition 187 (which called on physicians not to treat illegal immigrants), and openly breaking a contractual "gag rule" are examples of justifiable disobedience.

Indirect professional disobedience is the disobeying of otherwise unobjectionable rules in order to call attention to a wrong. Indirect actions become appealing when it is not helpful to disobey directly. For example, physicians may not be effective in protesting a health plan's underprovision for the uninsured by directly caring for them — providing charity care is a normal part of professionalism and in an open system it may even facilitate the injustice. But an indirect action, such as collectively refusing to honor a dress code, might call attention to the situation. Although the danger of harm

from such an action may seem remote, indirect disobedience can be more harmful than direct disobedience, because in the latter the action itself preserves patient care. Protestors may also overestimate the effectiveness of their campaigns. To be justified, the disobedient act should, at a minimum, be clearly linked with the offensive situation, be seen as reasonable by the public, be unlikely to result in greater harm to patients or others, and be likely to result in lasting positive change.

Finally, a principled exit from medical practice within a health care system is justifiable in catastrophic circumstances. Patients will frequently be harmed by a physician's exit, so it must be justifiable on the following moral grounds. The harm to be prevented must be obvious and large; advocacy, dissent, and disobedience must have been tried; and there must be a good prospect that health care overall will be substantially better served if the professional makes a principled exit than if he or she continues to exert a strong voice for change within the organization. Because a principled exit is sometimes easier than disobedience, particular care should be taken to avoid distorted versions of it. A self-righteous exit helps no one in need (and actually does harm by eliminating a potential source of advocacy) and primarily serves the dissenter's self-image. This type of exit is an act of self-righteousness or even cowardice masquerading as professionalism. In the right circumstances, however, an exit may be both honorable and courageous. In one very unusual circumstance, professional disobedience and exit were chosen simultaneously by a group of physicians as the only way to maintain the moral base of medical practice: Dutch physicians in World War II turned in their licenses but continued to practice underground, to avoid practicing under Nazi rule. The extreme nature of this example illustrates the burden of proof that those who wish to exit must meet before claiming that such an action is necessary to maintain professionalism.

Fundamental Elements of the Patient-Physician Relationship

AMERICAN MEDICAL ASSOCIATION

AMA Council on Ethical and Judical Affairs, CEJA Report A — A-90.

From ancient times, physicians have recognized that the health and well-being of patients depends upon a collaborative effort between physician and patient. Patients share with physicians the responsibility for their own health care. The patient-physician relationship is of greatest benefit to patients when they bring medical problems to the attention of their physicians in a timely fashion, provide information about their medical condition to the best of their ability, and work with their physicians in a mutually respectful alliance. Physicians can best contribute to this alliance by serving as their patients' advocate and by fostering these rights:

1. The patient has the right to receive information from physicians and to discuss the benefits, risks, and costs of appropriate treatment alternatives. Patients should receive guidance from their physicians as to the optimal course of action. Patients are also entitled to obtain copies or summaries of their medical records, to have their questions answered, to be advised of potential conflicts of interest that their physicians might have, and to receive independent professional opinions.

2. The patient has the right to make decisions regarding the health care that is recommended by his or her physician. Accordingly, patients may accept or refuse any recommended medical treatment.

3. The patient has the right to courtesy, respect, dignity, responsiveness, and timely attention to his or her needs.

4. The patient has the right to confidentiality. The physician should not reveal confidential communications or information without the consent of the patient, unless provided for by law or by the need to protect the welfare of the individual or the public interest.

5. The patient has the right to continuity of health care. The physician has an obligation to cooperate in the coordination of medically indicated care with other health care providers treating the patient. The physician may not discontinue treatment of a patient as long as further treatment is medically indicated, without giving the patient sufficient opportunity to make alternative arrangements for care.

6. The patient has a basic right to have available adequate health care. Physicians, along with the rest of society, should continue to work toward this goal. Fulfillment of this right is dependent on society providing resources so that no patient is deprived of necessary care because of an inability to pay for the care. Physicians should continue their traditional assumption of a part of the responsibility for the medical care of those who cannot afford essential health care.

Respect for Autonomy

TOM L. BEAUCHAMP AND JAMES F. CHILDRESS

From *Principles of Biomedical Ethics*, 6th ed., (New York: Oxford University Press, 2009), 99–114.

The Nature of Autonomy

The word *autonomy*, derived from the Greek *autos* ("self") and *nomos* ("rule," "governance," or "law"), originally referred to the self-rule or self-governance of independent city-states. Autonomy has since been extended to individuals, but the precise meaning of the term is disputed. Personal autonomy encompasses, at a minimum, self-rule that is free from both controlling interference by others and from certain limitations such as an inadequate understanding that prevents meaningful choice. The autonomous individual acts freely in accordance with a self-chosen plan, analogous to the way an independent government manages its territories and establishes its policies. A person of diminished autonomy, by contrast, is in some respect controlled by others or incapable of deliberating or acting on the basis of his or her desires and plans. For example, cognitively challenged individuals and prisoners often have diminished autonomy. Mental incapacitation limits the autonomy of a severely retarded person, whereas coercive institutionalization constrains the autonomy of prisoners.

Virtually all theories of autonomy view two conditions as essential for autonomy: *liberty* (independence from controlling influences) and *agency* (capacity for intentional action). However, disagreement exists over the meaning of these two conditions and over whether additional conditions are required.

The Principle of Respect for Autonomy

To respect autonomous agents is to acknowledge their right to hold views, to make choices, and to take actions based on their personal values and beliefs. Such respect involves respectful *action*, not merely a respectful *attitude*. It requires more than noninterference in others' personal affairs. It includes, in some contexts, building up or maintaining others' capacities for autonomous choice while helping to allay fears and other conditions that destroy or disrupt autonomous action. Respect, in this account, involves acknowledging the value and decision-making rights of persons and enabling them to act autonomously, whereas disrespect for autonomy involves attitudes and actions that ignore, insult, demean, or are inattentive to others' rights of autonomous action.

Why is such respect owed to autonomous persons? In a later chapter, we examine the theories of two philosophers who have powerfully influenced contemporary interpretations of respect for autonomy: Immanuel Kant and John Stuart Mill. Kant argued that respect for autonomy flows from the recognition that all persons have unconditional worth, each having the capacity to determine his or her own moral destiny. To violate a person's autonomy is to treat that person merely as a means; that is, in accordance with others' goals without regard to that person's own goals. Mill concerned himself primarily with the "individuality" of autonomous agents. He argued that society should permit individuals to develop according to their own convictions, as long as they do not interfere with a like expression of freedom by others or unjustifiably harm others; but he also insisted that we sometimes have an obligation to persuade others when they have false or ill-considered views. Mill's position requires both not interfering with and actively strengthening autonomous expression, whereas Kant's position entails a moral imperative of respectful treatment of persons as ends in themselves. In their different ways, these two philosophers both support a principle of respect for autonomy (although Kant is largely concerned with *morally* correct autonomous choices).

The principle of respect for autonomy can be stated as a negative obligation and as a positive obligation. As a *negative* obligation: Autonomous actions should not be subjected to controlling constraints by others. This demand asserts a broad, abstract obligation that is free of exceptive clauses such as "We must respect individuals' views and rights so long as their thoughts and actions do not seriously harm other persons." Of course, the principle of respect for autonomy needs specification in particular contexts to function as a practical guide to conduct, and appropriate specification will incorporate valid exceptions. This process of specification will affect rights and obligations of liberty, privacy, confidentiality, truthfulness, and informed consent.

As a *positive* obligation, this principle requires both respectful treatment in disclosing information and actions that foster autonomous decision making. Many autonomous actions could not occur without others' material cooperation in making options available. Respect for autonomy obligates professionals in health care and research involving human subjects to disclose information, to probe for and ensure understanding and voluntariness, and to foster adequate decision making. As some contemporary Kantians declare, the demand that we treat others as ends requires that we assist them in achieving their ends and foster their capacities as agents, not merely that we avoid treating them solely as means to our ends.

Temptations arise in health care for physicians and other professionals to foster or perpetuate patients' dependency, rather than to promote their autonomy. But discharging the obligation to respect patients' autonomy requires enabling patients to overcome their sense of dependence and to achieve as much control as they desire. These positive obligations of respect for autonomy derive in part from the special fiduciary obligations that health care professionals have to their patients and researchers to their subjects.

These negative and positive sides of respect for autonomy are capable of supporting many more specific moral rules. (Other principles, such as beneficence and nonmaleficence, help justify some of these same rules.) Examples include the following:

1. Tell the truth.
2. Respect the privacy of others.
3. Protect confidential information.
4. Obtain consent for interventions with patients.
5. When asked, help others make important decisions.

Respect for autonomy has only prima facie standing, and competing moral considerations sometimes can override this principle. Examples include the following: If our choices endanger the public health, potentially harm innocent others, or require a scarce resource for which no funds are available, others can justifiably restrict our exercises of autonomy. The principle of respect for autonomy does not by itself determine what a person ought to be free to know or do or what counts as a valid justification for constraining autonomy. For example, a patient with an inoperable, incurable carcinoma once asked, "I don't have cancer, do I?" The physician lied, saying, "You're as good as you were ten years ago." This lie denies the patient information that he may need to determine his future course of action, thereby infringing the principle of respect for autonomy. Although the matter is controversial, the lie may be justified (by a principle of beneficence) if we posit certain major benefits to the patient.

Our obligations to respect autonomy do not extend to persons who cannot act in a sufficiently autonomous manner (and who cannot be rendered autonomous) because they are immature, incapacitated, ignorant, coerced, or exploited. Infants, irrationally suicidal individuals, and drug-dependent patients are examples.

The Capacity for Autonomous Choice

Many patients and potential subjects are not competent to give a valid consent or refusal. Inquiries about competence focus on whether patients or potential subjects are capable, psychologically or legally, of adequate decision making. Competence in decision making is closely connected to autonomous decision making, as well as to the validity of consent. Several commentators distinguish judgments of capacity from judgments of competence on the grounds that health professionals assess capacity and incapacity, whereas courts determine competence and incompetence. However, this distinction breaks down in practice. As Thomas Grisso and Paul Appelbaum note, "When clinicians determine that a patient lacks decision-making capacity, the practical consequences may be the same as those attending a legal determination of incompetence."[1]

The Gatekeeping Function of Competence Judgments

Competence judgments serve a gatekeeping role in health care by distinguishing persons whose decisions should be solicited or accepted from persons whose decisions need not or should not be solicited or accepted. (We use the terms *capacity* and *competence* interchangeably.) Health professionals' judgments of a person's incompetence may lead them to override that person's decisions, to turn to informal surrogates for decision making, to ask the court to appoint a guardian to protect his or her interests, or to seek that person's involuntary institutionalization. When a court establishes legal incompetence, it appoints a surrogate decision maker with either partial or plenary (full) authority over the incompetent individual. Physicians and other health professionals do not have the authority to declare patients incompetent as a matter of law, but, within limits, they often have the de facto power to override or constrain patients' decisions about care.

The Concept of Competence

Some commentators hold that we lack both a single acceptable *definition* of competence and a single acceptable *standard* of competence. They also contend that no nonarbitrary *test* exists to distinguish between competent and incompetent persons. We here sharply distinguish *definitions, standards*, and *tests*. We focus first on the problem of definition.

A single core meaning of the word *competence* applies in all contexts. That meaning is "the ability to perform a task." By contrast to this core meaning, the *criteria* of particular competencies vary from context to context because the criteria are relative to specific tasks. The criteria for someone's competence to stand trial, to raise dachshunds, to write checks, or to lecture to medical students are radically different. The competence to decide is therefore relative to the particular decision to be made. Rarely should we judge a person incompetent with respect to every sphere of life. We usually need to consider only some type of competence, such as the competence to decide about treatment or about participation in research. These judgments of competence and incompetence affect only a limited range of decision making. For example, a person who is incompetent to decide about financial affairs may be competent to decide to participate in medical research, or able to handle simple tasks easily while faltering before complex ones.

Competence may vary over time and may be intermittent. Many persons are incompetent to do something at one point in time but competent to perform the same task at another point in time. Judgments of competence about such persons can be complicated by the need to distinguish categories of illness that result in *chronic* changes of intellect, language, or memory from those characterized by *rapid reversibility* of these functions, as in the case of transient ischemic attack or transient global amnesia. In some of the latter cases competence varies from hour to hour. In such cases, a declaration of *specific incompetence* may prevent vague generalizations that exclude persons from all forms of decision making.

These conceptual observations have practical significance. The law has traditionally presumed that a person who is incompetent to manage his or her estate is also incompetent to vote, make medical decisions, get married, and the like. The global sweep of these laws, based on a total judgment of the person, at times has extended too far. In one classic case, a physician argued that a patient was incompetent to make decisions because of epilepsy, although in fact many persons who suffer from epilepsy are competent in most contexts. Such judgments defy much that we now know about the etiology of various forms of incompetence, even in hard cases of mentally retarded individuals, psychotic patients, and patients with uncontrollably painful afflictions. In addition, persons who are incompetent by virtue of dementia, alcoholism, immaturity, and mental retardation present radically different types and problems of incompetence.

Sometimes a competent person who can usually select appropriate means to reach his or her goals will act incompetently in a particular circumstance. Consider the following actual case of a hospitalized patient with an acute disc problem whose goal is to control back pain. The patient decided to manage the problem by wearing a brace, a method she had used successfully in the past. She believes strongly that she should return to this treatment modality. This approach conflicts, however, with her physician's unwavering and insistent advocacy of surgery. When the physician, an eminent surgeon who alone in her city is suited to treat the patient, asks her to sign the surgical permit, she is psychologically unable to refuse. Her illness increases both her hopes and her fears, and, in addition, she has a passive personality. In these circumstances, it is psychologically too risky for her to act as she desires. Even though she is competent to choose in general, she is not competent to choose on this occasion because she lacks adequate capacity.

This case indicates how close the concept of competence in decision making is to the concept of autonomy. Patients or prospective subjects are competent to make a decision if they have the capacity to understand the material information, to make a judgment about this information in light of their values, to intend a certain outcome, and to communicate freely their wishes to caregivers or investigators. Law, medicine, and, to some extent, philosophy presume a context in which the characteristics of the competent person are also the properties possessed by the autonomous person. Although *autonomy* and *competence* differ in meaning (*autonomy* meaning self-governance; *competence* meaning the ability to perform a task or range of tasks), the criteria of the autonomous person and of the competent person are strikingly similar.

Persons are more and less able to perform a specific task to the extent that they possess a certain level or range of abilities, just as persons are more and less intelligent and athletic. For example, in the emergency room an experienced and knowledgeable patient is likely to be more qualified to consent to a procedure than a frightened, inexperienced patient. This ability continuum runs from full mastery through various levels of partial proficiency to complete ineptitude. Nonetheless, it is confusing to view this *continuum* in terms of degrees of *competency*. For practical and policy reasons, we need *threshold levels* below which a person with a certain level of abilities for a particular task is incompetent. Not all competent persons are equally able, and not all incompetent persons are equally unable, but competence determinations sort persons into these two basic classes, and thus treat persons as either competent or incompetent for specific purposes. Above the threshold, we treat persons as equally competent; below the threshold we treat them as equally incompetent. Gatekeepers test to determine who is above and who is below the threshold. Where we draw the line should depend on the particular tasks involved.

Note

1. Thomas Grisso and Paul S. Appelbaum, *Assessing Competence to Consent to Treatment: A Guide for Physicians and Other Health Professionals* (New York: Oxford University Press, 1998), 11.

The Meaning and Justification of Informed Consent

TOM L. BEAUCHAMP AND JAMES F. CHILDRESS

From *Principles of Biomedical Ethics,* 6th ed., (New York: Oxford University Press, 2009), 117–124.

Since the Nuremberg trials, which exposed horrifying medical experimentation in concentration camps, biomedical ethics has placed consent at the forefront of its concerns. The term *informed consent* did not appear until a decade after these trials (held in the late 1940s). It did not receive detailed examination until the early 1970s. In recent years the focus has shifted from the physician's or researcher's obligation to *disclose* information to the quality of a patient's or subject's *understanding* and *consent*. The forces behind this shift of emphasis were autonomy driven. In this section, we treat standards of informed consent as they have evolved through the regulation of research, case law governing medical practice, changes in the patient–physician relationship, and ethical analysis.

The Meaning and Elements of Informed Consent

Some commentators have attempted to reduce the idea of informed consent to shared decision making between doctor and patient, thus rendering *informed consent* and *mutual decision making* synonymous. However, informed consent cannot be reduced to shared decision making. Professionals obtain and will continue to obtain informed consent in many contexts of research and medicine in which shared decision making is a misleading model. It is critically important to distinguish informational exchanges through which patients elect medical interventions from acts of approving and authorizing those interventions. Shared decision making is a worthy ideal in medicine, but it neither defines nor displaces informed consent.

Two Meanings of "Informed Consent"

Two different senses of "informed consent" appear in current literature and practices. In the first sense, informed consent is analyzable through the account of autonomous choice presented earlier in this chapter: An informed consent is an individual's *autonomous authorization* of a medical intervention or of participation in research. In this first sense, a person must do more than express agreement or comply with a proposal. He or she must *authorize* something through an act of informed and voluntary consent. In a classic case, *Mohr v. Williams,* a physician obtained Anna Mohr's consent to an operation on her right ear. While operating, the surgeon determined that the left ear actually needed surgery. A court found that the physician should have obtained the patient's consent to the surgery on the left ear: "If a physician advises a patient to submit to a particular operation, and the patient weighs the dangers and risks incident to its performance, and finally consents, the patient thereby, in effect, enters into a contract authorizing the physician to operate to the extent of the consent given, but no further."[1] An informed consent in this first sense occurs if and only if a patient or subject, with substantial understanding and in absence of substantial control by others, intentionally authorizes a professional to do something quite specific.

In the second sense, informed consent is analyzable in terms of *the social rules of consent* that maintain that one must obtain legally or institutionally valid consent from patients or subjects before proceeding with diagnostic, therapeutic, or research procedures. Informed consents are not necessarily autonomous acts under these rules and sometimes are not even meaningful authorizations. *Informed consent* refers here only to an institutionally or legally effective authorization, as determined by prevailing social rules. For example, if a mature minor cannot legally authorize or consent, he or she still may autonomously authorize an intervention, even if this authorization is not an effective consent under existing rules. Thus, a patient or subject can *autonomously* authorize an intervention, and so give an informed consent in the first sense, without *effectively* authorizing the intervention (because of some set of rules), and thus without giving an informed consent in the second sense.

Institutional rules of informed consent have generally not been judged by the demanding standard of autonomous authorization. Only rarely have they been so judged. As a result, institutions, laws, or courts may impose on physicians and hospitals nothing more than an obligation to warn of risks of proposed interventions. "Consent" under these circumstances is not bona fide informed consent. This problem arises from the gap between the two senses of informed consent: Physicians who obtain consent under institutional criteria can fail and often do fail to meet the more rigorous standards of an autonomy-based model.

Although it is easy to criticize institutional rules as superficial, health care professionals cannot reasonably be expected to obtain a consent that satisfies the demands of rigorous autonomy-protecting rules in all circumstances. Autonomy-protecting rules may turn out to be excessively difficult or even impossible to implement. We should evaluate institutional rules not only in terms of respect for autonomy but also in terms of the probable consequences of imposing burdensome requirements on institutions and on professionals. Policies may legitimately take account of what is fair and reasonable to require of health care professionals and researchers. Nevertheless, we take it as axiomatic that *the model of autonomous choice* (following the first sense of "informed consent") ought to serve as the benchmark for the moral adequacy of institutional rules.

The Elements of Informed Consent

Some commentators have attempted to define *informed consent* by specifying the elements of the concept, in particular by dividing the elements into an information component and a consent component. The information component refers to the disclosure of information and the comprehension of what is disclosed. The consent component refers to both a voluntary decision and an authorization to proceed. Legal, regulatory, philosophical, medical, and psychological literatures tend to favor the following elements as the components of informed consent: (1) competence, (2) disclosure, (3) understanding, (4) voluntariness, and (5) consent. Some writers present these elements as the building blocks for a definition of *informed consent*: One gives an informed consent to an intervention if (and perhaps only if) one is competent to act, receives a thorough disclosure, comprehends the disclosure, acts voluntarily, and consents to the intervention.

This five-element definition is superior to the one-element definition in terms of *disclosure* that courts and medical literature have often proposed. Many patients regard the disclosure of information as less vital in clinical medicine than a health professional's *recommendation* of one or more actions. This is typically the case in direct exchanges between physicians and patients regarding surgery, medications, and the like; but it is also true, for example, of notifications to employees after a study of hazardous chemicals.

In this chapter we accept and treat each of the following seven elements:

I. Threshold elements (preconditions)

   1. Competence (to understand and decide)
   2. Voluntariness (in deciding)

II. Information elements

   3. Disclosure (of material information)
   4. Recommendation (of a plan)
   5. Understanding (of 3 and 4)

III. Consent elements

   6. Decision (in favor of a plan)
   7. Authorization (of the chosen plan)

This list requires a brief explanation and augmentation. First, an *informed refusal* entails a modification of items under III, thereby turning the categories into refusal elements; for example, 6. "Decision (against a plan)." Whenever we use the phrase "informed consent," we always allow for the possibility of informed refusal. Second, consent for research involving human subjects does not necessarily involve a recommendation. Third, competence is more of a pre-supposition of obtaining informed consent than an element.

Having examined competence previously, we now concentrate on disclosure, understanding, and voluntariness, beginning with disclosure.

Disclosure

Disclosure is the third of our seven elements of informed consent. Some institutions or authorities have presented the obligation to disclose information to patients as the only major condition of informed consent. The legal doctrine of informed consent in the United States primarily has focused on disclosure because of a physician's general obligation to exercise reasonable care in providing information. Civil litigation has emerged over informed consent because of injury (measured in terms of monetary damages) that a physician intentionally or negligently caused by his or her failure to disclose. The term *informed consent* was born in this legal context. However, from the moral viewpoint, informed consent has less to do with the liability of professionals as agents of disclosure and more to do with the autonomous choices of patients and subjects.

Nevertheless, disclosure still plays a pivotal role. Without an adequate way for professionals to deliver information, many patients and subjects will have an inadequate basis for decision making. Professionals are generally obligated to disclose a core set of information, including (1) those facts or descriptions that patients or subjects usually consider material in deciding whether to refuse or consent to the proposed intervention or research, (2) information the professional believes to be material, (3) the professional's recommendation, (4) the purpose of

seeking consent, and (5) the nature and limits of consent as an act of authorization.

Understanding

Understanding is the fifth element of informed consent listed earlier. Clinical experience and empirical data indicate that patients and research subjects exhibit wide variation in their understanding of information about diagnoses, procedures, risks, probable benefits, and prognoses. For instance, in a study of participants in cancer clinical trials, 90% indicated they were satisfied with the informed consent process and most of them thought they were well informed. However, approximately three-fourths of them did not recognize nonstandard and unproven treatment, and approximately one-fourth did not appreciate that the primary purpose of the trials was to benefit future patients and that the benefits to them personally were uncertain.

There are many reasons for such limited understanding in the informed consent process. Some patients and subjects are calm, attentive, and eager for dialogue, whereas others are nervous or distracted in ways that impair or block understanding. Many conditions limit their understanding, including illness, irrationality, and immaturity. Furthermore, deficiencies in the communication process may hamper understanding. Some barriers to understanding can be addressed, but debate continues about how best to do so and about the level of understanding that is essential for valid consent.

The Nature of Understanding

No consensus exists about the nature of understanding, but an analysis sufficient for our purposes is that persons understand if they have acquired pertinent information and have relevant beliefs about the nature and consequences of their actions. Such understanding need not be *complete*, because a grasp of central facts is generally sufficient. Some facts are irrelevant or trivial; others are vital, perhaps decisive. In some cases, a person's lack of awareness of even a single risk or missing fact can deprive him or her of adequate understanding. Consider, for example, the case of *Bang v. Miller Hospital*, in which patient Bang did not intend to consent to a sterilization entailed in prostate surgery. Bang did, in fact, consent to prostate surgery, but without being told that sterilization was an inevitable outcome. (Although sterilization is not necessarily an outcome of prostate surgery, it is inevitable in the specific procedure recommended in this case.) Bang's failure to understand this one surgical consequence compromised what was otherwise an adequate understanding and invalidated what otherwise would have been a valid consent.

Patients and subjects usually should understand at least what an attentive health care professional or researcher believes a patient or subject needs to understand to authorize an intervention. Diagnoses, prognoses, the nature and purpose of the intervention, alternatives, risks and benefits, and recommendations typically are essential. Patients or subjects also need to share an understanding with professionals about the terms of the authorization before proceeding. Unless agreement exists about the essential features of what is authorized, there can be no assurance that a patient or subject has made an autonomous decision and provided a valid consent. Even if physician and patient both use a word such as *stroke* or *hernia*, their interpretations will be different if standard medical definitions and conceptions have no meaning for the patient.

Some argue that many patients and subjects cannot comprehend enough information or sufficiently appreciate its relevance to make decisions about medical care or participation in research. Such statements are overgeneralizations based partially on an improper ideal of full disclosure and full understanding. If we replace this ideal standard with a more acceptable account of understanding relevant information, we can thwart such skepticism. From the fact that actions are never *fully* informed, voluntary, or autonomous, it does not follow that they are never *adequately* informed, voluntary, or autonomous.

However, some patients have such limited knowledge bases that communication about alien or novel situations is exceedingly difficult, especially if physicians introduce new concepts and cognitive constructs. Studies indicate that these patients likely will have an impoverished and distorted understanding of scientific goals and procedures. But even in these difficult situations, enhanced understanding and adequate decision making are often possible. For instance, professionals may be able to communicate novel and specialized information to lay persons by drawing analogies between this information and more ordinary events familiar to the patient or subject. Similarly, professionals can express risks in both numeric and nonnumeric probabilities, while helping the patient or subject to assign meanings to the probabilities through comparison with more familiar risks and prior experiences, such as risks involved in driving automobiles or using power tools.

However, even with these strategies, enabling a patient not only to comprehend but also to appreciate risks and benefits can be a formidable task. For example, patients confronted with various forms of surgery understand that they will suffer postoperative pain. Nevertheless, their projected expectations of the pain are often inadequate. Many patients cannot, in advance, adequately appreciate the nature of the pain, and many ill patients reach a point at which they can no longer balance with clear judgment the threat of pain against the benefits of surgery. At this point, they find the benefits of surgery overwhelmingly attractive, while discounting the risks. In one respect, these patients correctly understand basic facts about procedures that involve pain, but in other respects their understanding is inadequate.

Problems of Information Processing

With the exception of a few limited studies of comprehension, studies of patients' decision making often pay too little attention to information processing. Too much information can cause just as much of a problem as too little. Information overload may prevent adequate understanding, and physicians exacerbate these problems if they use unfamiliar terms or if patients cannot meaningfully organize information. Patients and potential subjects also may rely on modes of selective perception, and it is often difficult to determine when words have special meanings for them, when preconceptions distort their processing of the information, and when other biases intrude.

Some studies have uncovered difficulties in processing information about risks, indicating that risk disclosures commonly lead subjects to distort information and promote inferential errors and disproportionate fears of some risks. Some ways of framing information are so misleading that both health professionals and patients regularly misconstrue the content. For example, choices between risky alternatives can be heavily influenced by whether the same risk information is presented as providing a gain or an opportunity for a patient, or as constituting a loss or a reduction of opportunity. One study asked radiologists, outpatients with chronic medical problems, and graduate business students to make a hypothetical choice between two alternative therapies for lung cancer: surgery and radiation therapy. Whether researchers framed the information about outcomes in terms of survival or death affected the preferences of all three groups. When faced with outcomes framed in terms of probability of *survival*, 25% chose radiation over surgery. However, when the identical outcomes were presented in terms of probability of *death*, 42% preferred radiation. The mode of presenting the risk of immediate death from surgical complications, which has no counterpart in radiation therapy, appears to have made the decisive difference.

These framing effects reduce understanding, with direct implications for autonomous choice. If a misperception prevents a person from adequately understanding the risk of death and this risk is material to the person's decision, then the person's choice of a procedure does not reflect a substantial understanding and does not qualify as an autonomous authorization. The lesson to be learned is the need for better understanding of techniques that will enable professionals to communicate both the positive and the negative sides of information—for example, both the survival and the mortality probabilities.

Voluntariness

Voluntariness is the second element of informed consent in our list of elements. We concentrate in this section on a person's voluntariness in acting. We use the term *voluntariness* more narrowly than some writers do to distinguish it from broader uses that make it synonymous with autonomy. Some have analyzed voluntariness in terms of the presence of adequate knowledge, the absence of psychological compulsion, and the absence of external constraints. If we were to adopt this broad meaning, we would be equating voluntariness with autonomous action. We therefore hold only that a person acts voluntarily if he or she wills the action without being under the control of another's influence. We consider only the condition of control by other individuals, although conditions such as debilitating disease, psychiatric disorders, and drug addiction can also diminish or void voluntariness.

Not all influences exerted on another person are controlling. If a physician orders a reluctant patient to undergo cardiac catheterization and coerces the patient into compliance through a threat of abandonment, then the physician's influence controls the patient. If, by contrast, a physician persuades the patient to undergo the procedure when the patient is at first reluctant to do so, then the physician's actions influence, but do not control, the patient. Many influences are resistible, and some are welcomed rather than resisted. The broad category of influence includes acts of love, threats, education, lies, manipulative suggestions, and emotional appeals, all of which can vary dramatically in their impact on persons.

Forms of Influence

Our analysis focuses on three categories of influence: coercion, persuasion, and manipulation. Coercion occurs if and only if one person intentionally uses a credible and severe threat of harm or force to control another. The threat of force used by some police, courts, and hospitals in acts of involuntary commitment for psychiatric treatment is coercive. Some threats will coerce virtually all persons (e.g., a credible threat to kill the person), whereas others will coerce only a few persons (e.g., an employee's threat to an employer to quit a job unless a raise is offered). Whether coercion occurs depends on the subjective responses of the coercion's intended target. However, a subjective response in which persons comply because they *feel* threatened (although no threat has been issued) does not qualify as coercion. Coercion occurs only if a credible and intended threat displaces a person's self-directed course of action. Coercion renders even intentional and well-informed behavior nonautonomous.

There is a tendency in debates in biomedical ethics for "coercion" to become an all-purpose term of ethical criticism and thus to obscure the relevant and important ethical concerns in particular cases in health care and research. For instance, it does not apply to all dire situations in which individuals have to make hard and even tragic choices. This point about the limits of the concept of coercion does not imply that it is ethically acceptable to take advantage of a person in dire straits.

In *persuasion* a person must come to believe in something through the merit of reasons another person advances. Appeal to reason—i.e., attempted persuasion—is distinguishable from influence by appeal to emotion. In health care, the problem is to distinguish emotional responses from cognitive responses and to determine which are likely to be evoked. Disclosures or approaches that might rationally persuade one patient might overwhelm another whose fear or panic would short-circuit reason.

Manipulation is a generic term for several forms of influence that are neither persuasive nor coercive. The essence of manipulation is swaying people to do what the manipulator wants by means other than coercion or persuasion. In health care, the most likely form of manipulation is informational manipulation, a deliberate act of managing information that nonpersuasively alters a person's understanding of a situation and motivates him or her to do what the agent of influence intends. Many forms of informational manipulation are incompatible with autonomous decision making. For example, lying, withholding information, and misleading exaggeration with the intent to lead persons to believe what is false all compromise autonomous choice. The manner in which a health care professional presents information—by tone of voice, by forceful gesture, and by framing information positively ("we succeed most of the time with this therapy") rather than negatively ("we fail with this therapy in 35% of the cases")—can also manipulate a patient's perception and response, thereby affecting understanding and voluntariness.

Nevertheless, it is easy to inflate the threat of control by manipulation beyond its actual significance in health care. We typically make decisions in a context of competing influences, such as personal desires, familial constraints, legal obligations, and institutional pressures. These influences usually do not control decisions to a morally worrisome degree. In biomedical ethics we need only establish general criteria for the point at which influence threatens autonomous choice, while recognizing that in many cases no sharp boundary separates controlling and non-controlling influences.

Note

1. *Mohr v. Williams*, 95 Minn. 261, 265; 104 N.W. 12, 15 (1905).

A Framework of Standards for Surrogate Decision Making

TOM L. BEAUCHAMP AND JAMES F. CHILDRESS

From *Principles of Biomedical Ethics*, 6th ed., (New York: Oxford University Press), 135–140.

We shift now from the conditions of consent to problems of consent when surrogate decision makers are involved. Surrogate decision makers are authorized to reach decisions for doubtfully autonomous or nonautonomous patients. If a patient is not competent to choose or to refuse treatment, a hospital, a physician, or a family member may justifiably exercise a decision-making role or go before a court or other authority to resolve the issues before implementing a decision. Since the Quinlan decision in New Jersey in 1976, courts and legislatures in the United States have established many procedures and standards for surrogate decision making. However, much remains unresolved. Many surrogates daily make decisions to terminate or continue treatment for incompetent patients, for example, those suffering from stroke, Alzheimer's disease, Parkinson's disease, chronic depression affecting cognitive function, senility, and psychosis.

In this section, we consider three general standards that surrogate decision makers might use: *substituted judgment*, which is sometimes presented as an autonomy-based standard; *pure autonomy*; and *the patient's best interests*. Our objective is to restructure and to integrate this set of standards for surrogate decision making into a coherent framework. Although we evaluate these standards for law and policy, our underlying argument is a moral argument that extends our earlier discussions of the value of protecting autonomy.

The Substituted Judgment Standard

The standard of substituted judgment is constructed on the premise that decisions about treatment properly belong to the incompetent or nonautonomous patient, by virtue of his or nonautonomous patient, by virtue of his or her rights of autonomy and privacy. In this conception, the patient has the right to decide and the right to have his or her values and preferences taken seriously, but is incompetent to exercise these rights, and it would be unfair to deprive such an incompetent patient of decision-making rights merely because he or she is no longer (or has never been) autonomous.

This standard is a weak standard of autonomy. It requires the surrogate decision maker to "don the mental mantle of the incompetent," as a classic court case (*Saikewicz*) put it—that is, to make the decision the incompetent person would have made if competent. In this case, the court invoked the standard of substituted judgment to decide that Joseph Saikewicz, a never-competent patient, would not have chosen treatment had he been competent. Asserting that what the majority of reasonable people would choose could differ from what a particular incompetent person would choose, the court said that,

> [T]he decision in many cases such as this should be that which would be made by the incompetent person, if that person were competent, but taking into account the present and future incompetency of the individual as one of the factors which would necessarily enter into the decision-making process of the competent person.[1]

The basic premise of the substituted judgment standard here rests on a fiction. An incompetent person cannot literally have the right to make medical decisions when other competent persons in fact exercise that right. The standard of substituted judgment should be used for once-competent patients only if reason exists to believe that the surrogate decision maker can make a judgment as the patient would have made it. In such cases, the surrogate should have such a deep and relevant familiarity with the patient that the particular judgment made reflects the patient's views and values. Merely knowing something in general about the patient's personal values is not adequate. Accordingly, if the surrogate can reliably answer the question, "What would *the patient* want in this circumstance?" substituted judgment is an appropriate standard that approximates first-person consent. But if the surrogate can only answer the question, "What do *you* want for the patient?" then this standard is inappropriate, because all connection to the patient's former autonomy has vanished. Similarly, we should reject the standard of substituted judgment for never-competent patients. No basis exists for a judgment of autonomous choice if a person has never been autonomous.

The standard of substituted judgment helps us understand what we should do for once-competent patients whose relevant prior preferences can be discerned; but, so interpreted, it collapses into a pure autonomy standard that respects previous autonomous choices.

The Pure Autonomy Standard

The second standard therefore eliminates the dubious autonomy reflected in substituted judgment and replaces it with a correct account of the role of autonomy. The pure autonomy standard applies exclusively to formerly autonomous, now-incompetent patients who expressed a relevant, autonomous treatment preference. The principle of respect for autonomy compels us to respect such preferences, even if the person can no longer express the preference for himself or herself. This standard asserts that, whether or not a formal advance directive exists, caretakers should accept prior autonomous judgments. This form of autonomy is sometimes referred to as "precedent autonomy." It has been invoked for a wide range of circumstances.

The classic Claire Conroy case, in which the New Jersey Supreme Court grappled with several standards of surrogate decision making, sheds light on some of the moral issues surrounding this standard. Conroy, an eighty-three-year-old nursing home resident, suffered from irreversible physical and mental impairments, including organic brain syndrome, arteriosclerotic heart disease, hypertension, diabetes, necrotic ulcers on her left foot, and a gangrenous left leg. She was awake enough to track persons with her eyes, but was severely demented, lay in a fetal position, and was unable to speak. She had no discernible cognitive or volitional functioning. Conroy's nephew (Thomas Whittemore), who was her guardian and only surviving blood relative, sought court permission to remove his aunt's nasogastric tube, an action that would result in her dehydration and death in about a week. He appealed to two of her expressed values and preferences: her general fear of doctors and her refusal to have her gangrenous leg amputated. He argued that his request for tube removal would conform to her wishes. Conroy's physician opposed Whittemore's petition as a violation of medical ethics. The trial court authorized removal of Conroy's feeding tube, even though she might die painfully, but a court-appointed guardian ad litem appealed the court's order. The New Jersey Supreme Court ultimately held that physicians could withhold or withdraw any medical treatment, including artificial nutrition and hydration, from an incompetent patient under certain conditions. More specifically, it held that physicians can legitimately withhold or withdraw life-sustaining treatment from an incompetent patient when a "subjective test"—meaning that there is a demonstrable basis in the patient's former autonomous choices—shows that this particular patient, when autonomous, would have preferred withdrawal. The court reasoned that a written document (such as a living will); an oral directive to family member, friend, or health care provider; a durable power of attorney; the patient's convictions about medical treatment administered to others; religious beliefs and tenets; or the "patient's consistent pattern of conduct with respect to prior decisions about medical care" can in principle, satisfy the autonomy-based standard. The court further noted that "in the absence of adequate proof of the patient's wishes, it is naive to pretend that the right to self-determination serves as the basis for substituted decision-making."

Although we too commend a pure autonomy standard, problems are evident in *Conroy* and similar legal decisions regarding satisfactory *evidence* for action under this standard. In the absence of explicit instructions, a surrogate decision maker might, for example, selectively choose from the patient's life history those values that accord with the surrogate's own values, and then use only those selected values in reaching decisions. The surrogate might also base his or her findings on values of the patient that are only distantly relevant to the immediate decision (e.g., the patient's expressed dislike of hospitals). One can reasonably ask what a decision maker could legitimately infer from Conroy's prior conduct, especially her fear and avoidance of doctors and her earlier refusal to consent to amputation of a gangrenous leg. A recurrent problem is that surrogates often assume an explicitness in a patient's directive about the future that does not directly show an autonomous preference with regard to the decision at hand.

The Best Interests Standard

Sometimes the patient's relevant preferences cannot be known. Under the best interests standard a surrogate decision maker must determine the highest net benefit among the available options, assigning different weights to interests the patient has in each option and discounting or subtracting inherent risks or costs. The term *best* is used because the surrogate's obligation is to maximize benefit through a comparative assessment that locates the highest net benefit. The best interests standard protects an incompetent person's well-being by requiring surrogates to assess the risks and benefits of various treatments and alternatives to treatment. It is therefore inescapably a quality-of-life

criterion. Those applying the best interests standard should consider the formerly autonomous patient's preferences, values, and perspectives only as far as they affect interpretations of quality of life, direct benefit, and the like.

We believe that the best interests standard can in some circumstances validly override advance directives executed by now incompetent but once autonomous patients, as well as refusals by minors and by other incompetent patients. This overriding can occur, for example, in a case in which a person has designated another by a durable power of attorney to make medical decisions on his or her behalf. If the designated surrogate makes a decision that threatens the patient's best interests, the decision should be overridden unless there is a clearly worded second document executed by the patient that specifically supports the surrogate's decision.

Problems of a person's ability to anticipate a future state often challenge reliance on advance directives. Much discussed are cases of apparently contented, nonsuffering, incompetent patients who can be expected to survive if treated against their advance directive, but who otherwise would die. Several discussions have focused on "Margo," a patient with Alzheimer's, who, according to the medical student who visited her regularly, is "one of the happiest people I have ever known." Some discussants of her situation ask us to imagine what should be done if Margo had a living will, executed just at the onset of her Alzheimer's, stating that she did not want life-sustaining treatment if she developed another life-threatening illness. In that circumstance caregivers would have to determine whether to honor her advance directive, and thereby to respect her precedent autonomy by not using antibiotics to treat her pneumonia, or to act in accord with what may appear to be her current best interests given her overall happiness.

The challenge is serious. As persons slip into incompetence, their condition can be very different from, and better than, they had anticipated. If so, it seems unfair to the now happily situated incompetent person to be bound by a prior decision that may have been ill informed. In Margo's case, not using antibiotics would arguably harm what Ronald Dworkin called, in discussing this case, "experiential interests"—her contentment with her current life. However, providing antibiotics would violate her living will, which articulates her "critical interests"—her interests in a mode of living and dying that expresses her considered values, her life story and commitments, and the like. Dworkin argues that Margo should not be treated in these circumstances. By contrast, the President's Council on Bioethics concludes that "Margo's apparent happiness would seem to make the argument for overriding the living will morally compelling in this particular case."

Except in rare cases we are obligated to respect the previously expressed autonomous wishes of the now nonautonomous person precisely because of the force of the principle of respect for the autonomy of the person who made the decision.

Finally, best interests judgments are meant to focus attention entirely on the value of the life for the person who must live it, not on the value the person's life has for others. "Quality-of-life judgments" also concern only the individual's best interests, not his or her worth to enhance another's quality of life. Unfortunately, the best interests standard has sometimes been interpreted in highly malleable ways, thereby permitting consideration of values irrelevant to the individual's benefits or burdens. For example, when parents have sought court permission for a kidney transplant from an incompetent minor child to a sibling, parental judgments about the "donor's best interests" have on occasion taken into account projected psychological trauma from the death of the sibling and the psychological benefits of the unselfish act of "donation." Such considerations should be greeted with skepticism and call attention to the need for additional procedural protections such as committee review.

In summary, it has been popular, although by no means universal, in biomedical ethics to hold that an ordered set of standards for surrogate decision making runs from (1) autonomously executed advance directives to (2) substituted judgment to (3) best interests, with the first having priority over the second and the first and second having priority over the third in a circumstance of conflict. We have argued that previously competent patients who autonomously expressed their preferences in an oral or written advance directive should be treated under the pure autonomy standard, and we have suggested an *economy of standards*; that is, we have determined that the first and second positions are essentially identical. The principle of respect for autonomy provides the only foundation, and it applies if and only if either a prior autonomous judgment itself constitutes an authorization or such a judgment supports a reasonable basis of inference for a surrogate. If the previously competent person left no reliable traces of his or her preferences, surrogate decision makers should adhere only to the best interests standard.

Note

1. *Superintendent of Belchertown State School v. Saikewicz*, Mass. 370 N.E. 2d 417 (1977).

Truth Telling in Medicine

The Confucian View

RUIPING FAN AND BENFU LI

Journal of Medicine and Philosophy 29, no. 2 (2004): 179–193.

I. Introduction: Should The Physician Directly Tell the Truth to the Patient Regardless of the Family's Wishes?

Truth-telling to competent patients is widely affirmed as a cardinal moral and biomedical obligation in contemporary Western medical practice. However, this has not always been the case. To the contrary, lying in medicine was taken for granted in the West for a long time. It is notorious that Plato did not allow any but physicians to lie, because he recognized that falsehood could be useful to people as a form of treatment (*Republic* 389b. trans. Bloom). Even a Christian theologian of the stature of St. John Chrysostom (A.D. 334–407) took for granted not only that physicians would deceive, but also that they could do so with moral justification. In a general defense of the moral obligation to lie under certain circumstances, St. John Chrysostom argues:

> To discover how useful deceit is, not only to the deceivers but to the deceived, go to any doctor and inquire how they cure their patients of diseases. You will hear them say that they do not rely on their skill alone, but sometimes they resort to deceit, and with a tincture of its help they restore the sick man to health. When the plans of doctors are hindered by the whims of their patients and the obstinacy of the complaint itself, then it is necessary to put on the mask of deception, in order to conceal the truth about what is happening – as they do on the stage.

That under certain circumstances physicians would need to deceive their patients in order to cure them was generally accepted in the West up until recently.

This traditional Western acceptance of the physician's right and even obligation to withhold truth from the patient because of the physician's judgment of the patient's best interests has largely been discredited in the dominant culture of the West. This has occurred because deception by the physician has become a paradigm example of unacceptable physician paternalism, one that undermines the autonomous choice that is now held to be core to individual dignity. As the American physician-bioethicist Pellegrino asserts, the "human capability for autonomous choices cannot function if truth is withheld, falsified, or otherwise manipulated" (1992, p. 1734). Historically, this condemnation of deceit represents a final victory in the West of a view traceable to Augustine of Hippo (A.D. 354–430) that categorically regarded lying as involving an absolute, intrinsic, wrong-making condition.

In contrast, Chinese medical ethics, even today, in theory and in practice remains committed to hiding the truth as well as to lying when necessary to achieve the family's view of the best interests of the patient. This ethics requires that, for any serious adverse diagnosis (such as cancer) or fatal prognosis, the physician must first inform a close member of the patient's family. Then it is up to the family to decide whether and how to tell the truth to the patient. If the family decides not to tell the truth to the patient, the physician must abide by that decision and hide the truth. Indeed, from time to time the physician will be obliged to lie to the patient in order to cooperate with the family.

This Chinese practice should be distinguished from traditional Western medical paternalism. In Western, physician-oriented paternalism, (1) it is up to the physician to judge whether truth-telling is beneficial to the patient, leaving (2) the physician with the final authority to decide whether to tell the truth to the patient. In contrast, in Chinese practice (1) it is up to the family, based on the information offered by the physician, to judge whether the truth will be beneficial to the patient, and (2) the family has the final authority to decide whether to tell the patient the truth. Among other things, the traditional Western practice represented an individualistic feature of physician-patient relations, while the Chinese practice embodied a familist feature. This paper explores the Chinese practice and addresses the question: should the physician tell the truth to the patient when the family decides that the truth should be hidden? Since the contemporary Chinese (ethical and legal) answer is no, it is necessary to spell out this practice in greater detail, indicate the conditions under which it can be justified, and determine what limits should be placed on family decision-making within a well-functioning Confucian ethos.

II. Confucian Truthfulness in Medical Practice

The differences separating the Confucian Chinese approach to truth-telling from that predominant in the West are stark, as the following set of observations drawn from the experience of Dr. Benfu Li in his medical practice demonstrates. These observations can be expressed as principles in the sense of chapter headings meant to bring together elements of the moral experience of Chinese physicians.

(A) First and foremost, truth-telling is set within a context of patient-centered beneficence, where the good of the patient is interpreted by a close family member under the guidance of a physician. This family member, better to be understood as a representative of the entire family, usually consults other close family members in order to make substantive decisions for the patient. As a consequence, the decision to communicate the truth about a diagnosis or prognosis to the patient depends on a consideration of

1. the patient's condition,
2. the likely impact of the communication on the patient, and
3. the family's wishes in the matter.

(B) The general justification for deception must remain the patient's best interests. In mainland China it has been observed that some hospitalized patients have either killed or attempted to kill themselves on receiving a diagnosis of cancer. Chinese physicians are of the view that, if the physician were to communicate the truth to a patient who cannot bear such a disclosure and who needs support, the result would be a constellation of harms ranging from a feeling of hopelessness to a refusal of needed treatment or even an attempt to commit suicide. Moreover, this impact on the patient would also harm the family and make further collaboration regarding treatment difficult. In mainland China, family members sometimes complain against physicians (and they have even brought physicians to court) on the grounds that the physician disclosed information directly to the patient, thus harming the patient through failing to act appropriately under the ethos of medical protection of the patient.

(C) There is an obligation to tell the truth to the family, those in authority as interpreters of the patient's best interests. As a consequence, whether or not the physician discloses the truth concerning diagnoses and prognoses to the patient, the physician is nevertheless required by Chinese cultural tradition and custom to disclose information as detailed as feasible to close family members. This is also the requirement of current Chinese law. For instance, Clause 26 of the Law of the Medical Profession of the People's Republic of China stipulates that physician should disclose the truth of an ill condition to the patient or the patient's family members and in so doing should avoid adverse effects on the patient. In practice, the treatment plan must receive approval from the family, who must consent when necessary by having a member sign the consent form. Mainland Chinese physicians can usually in this way harmoniously develop a treatment plan, given the generally good environment of mutual understanding characterizing physician-patient-family relationships in China. An overwhelming majority of patients understand and accept the physician's keeping information from the patient, as long as all information is disclosed to a family member. Because patients generally are of the view that the family member represents their best interests, patients do not usually blame physicians for non-disclosure or make claims that their rights have been violated.

The question is to determine whether the moral geography of family decision-making and physician deception can be made morally plausible. This will require both placing it within an account of the Confucian moral vision so as to decide how such practices should be evaluated and revised. But this in turn will require critically assessing the Confucian moral tradition. What will be proposed is not an attempt to remake this tradition in the image and likeness of Western moral and political assumptions, but rather to reconstruct it so as to identify its enduring commitments with a view to providing an account to guide contemporary bioethical and public policy challenges. These reflections will be used to indicate how familist virtues and responsibilities should be understood in order for the deception of the patient by the physician in service of patient care can be virtuous, not vicious.

III. Chinese Medical History and the Confucian Moral Vision

The familistic feature of the Confucian Chinese approach to medical decision making has been long-standing in Chinese history. Traditionally, the Chinese physician checked the patient at the patient's home. The medical communication was made among the physician, the patient and family

members all altogether. When a case of fatal diagnosis or prognosis occurred, the physician would manage to inform the truth to the family only, hiding it from the patient. It was up to the family to decide whether, when and how to disclose the truth to the patient. Families usually decided to conceal such information from the patient, and physicians were willing to follow such decisions and cooperate with families in deceiving patients. Directly informing the patient of a fatal diagnosis or prognosis by the physician was taken to be not only unsympathetic to the patient's unfortunate fate and causing unnecessary psychological burden on the patient, it was also taken to be disrespectful to the family, given that the patient was part of the entire family as a whole. It has been ethically improper for the Chinese physician to do so. Indeed, this has become a medical-ethics rule for all traditional Chinese physicians as clearly stated in the medical writings of a famous Han dynasty physician Chun Yuyi (ca. 215–150 B.C.): Diagnosis of a severe disease should not be told [to the patient]; instead, it should be disclosed only to the family.

The Chinese physician's abiding by the family's wishes to deceive the patient does not contradict his moral integrity as long as the family's wishes are not in conflict with his medical judgment of the patient's best interests. To the contrary, following the family's decision is in line with the essence of his role as a Confucian physician. Confucianism takes medicine as "the art of *ren* (virtue)." *Ren* is the fundamental human virtue that binds people together first in appropriate familial relations and then directs other social relations by the model of familial relations. In this regard, a Confucian physician is not an ordinary person. He is ideally a kind-parent-like master practicing the virtue of *ren* with special medical skills for pursuing the Confucian moral ideals: self-cultivation, family-regulation, state-governing, and all-under-Heaven being made peaceful. That is, he should be a *junzi*, an exemplary person of moral integrity and good character in exercising the Confucian virtues, such as filial piety to his parents, loyalty to his emperor, reverence to the old, benevolence to the young, and gradually extending his love to all-under-Heaven. The end of practicing medicine is for leading his Confucian way of life, not for treating people's diseases as a technician. Given the cardinal place of the family in decision making for the family members in the Confucian way of life, the Confucian physician's cooperation with the family in taking care of the patient's best interests is naturally derivative, even if this implies deceiving the patient in some situations.

Some would argue that directly telling the truth to the patient (rather than through the medium of the family) marks a moral progress in medical practice. For them, it is not only morally proper to overcome the physician paternalism as shown in the past of the West so as to have the patient able to control what happens to his/her body, health and life, but it is also admirable that the patient can strengthen his/her financial or psychological capacity to face his/her bad medical fate in the practice of direct informed consent. It is even more empowering to patients that by appealing to the legally approved arrangements of surrogate decision making (such as advance directives or durable power of attorney as practiced currently in America), they can extend the control of their own body to a stage when they become incompetent. However, no matter how reasonable this view appears to be, it has ignored the fact that the issue of truth telling in medicine is a function of a particular way of life. The Confucian way of life is familistic. An ill person is first and foremost a family member – a weak, uncomfortable and suffering family member that is supposed to relax and rest and be looked after by other family members. Confucians hold that family members should be interdependent, rather than independent, of each other. It is implicit in the interdependence of family members that one should not decide about one's health problem alone. It is only appropriate for one to be represented by other family members in cooperation with the physician in dealing with one's disease or disability. It is strange and even inhumane for the Chinese eyes that a suffering patient has to

sign a consent form by him/herself in order to receive a surgery. For the Confucian Chinese, the only natural and proper manner in this situation is for a family representative to sign it on the patient's behalf. In addition, there is virtually no room for the Chinese patient to prepare formal advance directives or employ durable power of attorney for preparing for his/her future health care. When the whole family makes medical decisions for the patient – even when the patient is competent – it is only logical that the family should continue to take responsibility when the patient becomes incompetent.

Even when families manage to hide fatal diagnoses or prognoses from severely sick patients, it is often the case that these patients already have tacit understanding of their true conditions. If they had wanted to push their families for the whole truth, they could have obtained it. But for the Chinese patient, it does not make much sense to push hard for knowing, e.g., that one contracts a late stage cancer and will most probably have a life of six more months. Although Confucians perfectly understand that everyone has to die, it is not positive to discuss one's forthcoming death with one's family members. It is much more comfortable to rely on one's family members to do necessary and suitable things on one's behalf. There may still be a hope for recovery, as Confucians believe that man's fate is eventually determined by the heavenly force: "Life and death have their determined appointments" (*Analects*, 12:5., trans. Legge). From the Confucian view of this situation, what is most important is not for one to know everything and make medical decisions by oneself, but to have the love and interdependence of family members. This is the true essence of Confucian truthfulness in this respect.

In this account, it is assumed that the Confucian view is not merely a cultural idiosyncrasy of China, but rather that the Confucian way of life appreciates moral realities fundamental to human life. This truth is not argued for directly, but rather through displaying the character of this way of life as an invitation to step into it and to experience its truth. The truth of the Confucian tradition and way of life can only be appreciated when one lives a life rightly ordered by virtue (*ren*) and ritual (*li*). Here one must underscore the crucial importance of traditional Chinese rituals, or *li*. *Li* was originally a sacrificial ceremony performed by family members together to memorialize the ancestors of the family. It was used metaphorically by the Zhou Chinese (3000 years ago) to refer, more broadly, to human behavior patterns and institutions established and accepted as appropriate, including what we call rites, etiquettes, and social and political systems. *Li* patterns human life, regulates familial and social relations, directs actions, and shapes institutions. Confucius (489–551 B.C.) reconstructed the *li* in terms of the fundamental human virtue, *ren*. The purpose of establishing and exercising rituals is for the virtue of *ren* (*Analects*, 3:3, trans. Legge). On the other hand, rituals constitute the substance of the virtue of *ren* – one cannot really be virtuous without learning and following the rituals (*Analects*, 12:1, trans. Legge). In short, Confucians recognize humans as ritually directed beings. It is not simply that social rituals bind humans; they also cultivate the virtue and

help open humans to the claims of the moral life. They aid one to achieve the moral vision needed to appreciate that the family constitutes the normal way of human life – a social reality necessary for the full development of cardinal human virtues and full human flourishing. The central Confucian rituals are family rituals, including the ways of meeting and cooperating with physicians by families for caring about their ill family members.

The Confucian philosophical, anthropological, and moral-epistemological claim is that by living this well-ordered, ritual-governed life one gains a possibility for moral disclosure of the truths it supports. One is invited into a domain of human experience unrecognized by many: life in a family structured by love, propriety, and virtue. It is not simply that the family allows individuals qua individuals to achieve virtue and realize their flourishing, but one encounters virtues and human flourishing understandable only within the reality of the family. The virtues and flourishing realized in and by a family cannot be reduced without loss of meaning to the virtues and flourishing realized in and by the individual members of a family.

Patient Confidentiality

AMERICAN MEDICAL ASSOCIATION

AMA Council on Ethical and Judicial Affairs, CEJA Report A—A-93.

Physicians have always had a duty to keep their patients' confidences. In essence, the physician's duty to maintain confidentiality means that a physician may not disclose any medical information revealed by a patient or discovered by a physician in connection with the treatment of a patient. In general, AMA's *Code of Medical Ethics* states that the information disclosed to a physician during the course of the patient-physician relationship is confidential to the utmost degree. As explained by the AMA's Council on Ethical

and Judicial Affairs, the purpose of a physician's ethical duty to maintain patient confidentiality is to allow the patient to feel free to make a full and frank disclosure of information to the physician with the knowledge that the physician will protect the confidential nature of the information disclosed. Full disclosure enables the physician to diagnose conditions properly and to treat the patient appropriately. In return for the patient's honesty, the physician generally should not reveal confidential communications or information without the patient's express consent unless required to disclose the information by law. There are exceptions to the rule, such as where a patient threatens bodily harm to himself or herself or to another person.

The AMA's ethical guidelines are not binding by law, although courts have used ethical obligations as the basis for imposing legal obligations. Moreover, maintaining patient confidentiality is a legal duty as well as an ethical duty. A physician's legal obligations are defined by the *US Constitution*, by federal and state laws and regulations, and by the courts. Even without applying ethical standards, courts generally allow a cause of action for a breach of confidentiality against a treating physician who divulges confidential medical information without proper authorization from the patient.

Despite these ethical and legal obligations, access to confidential patient information has become more prevalent. Electronic health information systems allow increased access to and tranmission of health data. Physicians in integrated delivery systems or networks now have access to the confidential information of all the patients within their system or network. Confidential information also is disseminated through clinical repositories and shared databases. Sharing this information allows patients to be treated more efficiently and safely. The challenge for physicians is to utilize this technology, while honoring and respecting patient confidentiality.

What Is a Breach of Confidentiality?

A breach of confidentiality is a disclosure to a third party, without patient consent or court order, of private information that the physician has learned within the patient-physician relationship. Disclosure can be oral or written, by telephone or fax, or electronically, for example, via e-mail or health information networks. The medium is irrelevant, although special security requirements may apply to the electronic transfer of information.

The legal basis for imposing liability for a breach of confidentiality is more extensive than ethical guidelines, which dictate the morally right thing to do. Although current law in this area has been referred to as "a crazy quilt of state and federal law," protecting patients' confidentiality is the law of the land. Included in the patchwork are federal and state constitutional privacy rights, federal and state legislation and regulation governing both medical records and licensing, and specific federal and state legislation designed to protect sensitive information (*e.g.*, HIV test results, genetic screening information, mental health records, and drug and alcohol abuse rehabilitation information).

Patient Consent to Release Confidential or Privileged Information

The general rule regarding release of a patient's medical record is that information contained in a patient's medical record may be released to third parties only if the patient has consented to such disclosure. The patient's express authorization is required before the medical records can be released to the following parties: patient's attorney or insurance company; patient's employer, unless a worker's compensation claim is involved; member of the patient's family, except where the family member has been appointed by the patient's attorney under a durable power of attorney for health care; government agencies; and other third parties. Some state laws expressly allow disclosure to any person upon consent of the patient. Other state laws permit release on patient consent only to specified classes of persons. Further, once the patient has given consent to release the record, the disclosure requirement may be mandatory for the holder of the medical record or merely permissive.

Who Can Consent to the Release?

Who may grant permission to release medical record information is likewise governed by state law. Generally, the authority to release medical information is granted to: (1) the patient, if a competent adult or emancipated minor; (2) a legal guardian or parent if the patient is incompetent or a minor child; and (3) the administrator or executor of the patient's estate if patient is deceased.

The patient's right to authorize release of medical records is codified in many state statutes. These statutes all state that medical records are confidential and cannot be disclosed, except in specifically provided circumstances. However, the extent of the patient's right to access varies from state to state. Some states allow the health care professional or provider to determine patient's right of access. In comparison, some states expressly grant patients access to the medical information contained in their medical records.

Failure to get the appropriate release for medical records may have serious results. Twenty-one states punish disclosure of confidential information by revoking a physician's medical license or taking other disciplinary action.

Implied Consent and Public Policy Exceptions or Required Disclosures

A patient's consent to disclosure of confidential information contained in a medical record may also be implied from the circumstances. For example, medical personnel directly involved in a patient's care or treatment generally have access to the medical record. Even if the patient has not expressly authorized disclosure of his or her medical record, such consent is implied from the patient's acceptance of treatment or hospitalization. Consent is also implied when a patient is transferred from one health care practitioner or facility to another. In such circumstances, disclosure of confidential patient information may be necessary to ensure continuation of patient care or treatment. State and federal statutes may also authorize or require disclosure of medical records to health care professionals or providers involved in the patient's treatment or upon transfer of the patient from one facility to another.

Safeguarding patient confidences also is subject to certain exceptions that are ethically and legally justified because of overriding social considerations. If there is a reasonable probability that a patient will inflict serious bodily harm on another person, for example, the physician should take precautions to protect the intended victim and notify law enforcement authorities. Communicable diseases and gunshot and knife wounds should be reported as required by applicable statutes or ordinances. Thus, the physician's duty of confidentiality at times must give way to a stronger countervailing societal interest.

A Defense of Unqualified Medical Confidentiality

KENNETH KIPNIS

The American Journal of Bioethics 6, no. 2 (2006): 7–18.

The Case of the Infected Spouse

The following fictionalized case is based on an actual incident.

1982: After moving to Honolulu, Wilma and Andrew Long visit your office and ask you to be their family physician. They have been your patients ever since.

1988: Six years later the two decide to separate. Wilma leaves for the Mainland, occasionally sending you a postcard. Though you do not see her professionally, you still think of yourself as her doctor.

1990: Andrew comes in and says that he has embarked upon a more sophisticated social life. He has been hearing about some new sexually transmitted diseases and wants to be tested. Testing reveals that he is positive for the AIDS virus, and he receives appropriate counseling.

1991: Visiting your office for a checkup, Andrew tells you Wilma is returning to Hawaii for reconciliation with him. She arrives that afternoon and will be staying at the Moana Hotel. Despite your best efforts to persuade him, Andrew leaves without giving you assurance that he will tell Wilma about his infection or protect her against becoming infected.

Do you take steps to see that Wilma is warned? If you decide to warn Wilma, what do you say to Andrew when, two days later, he shows up at your office asking how you could reveal his confidential test results?

If you decide not to warn Wilma, what do you say to her when, two years later in 1993, she shows up at your office asking how you, her doctor, could possibly stand idly by as her husband infected her with a deadly virus. She now knows she is positive for the virus, that she was infected by her husband, and that you—her doctor—knew, before they reconciled, that her husband would probably infect her.

The ethical challenges here emerge from an apparent head-on collision between medical confidentiality and the duty to protect imperiled third parties. Notwithstanding Andrew's expectation of privacy and the professional duty to remain silent, it can seem unforgivable for anyone to withhold vital assistance in such a crisis, let alone a doctor. The case for breaching confidentiality is supported by at least five considerations: First, the doctor knows, to a medical certainty, that Andrew is both infected with HIV and infectious. Second, knowing Wilma as a patient, let us suppose the doctor reasonably believes that she is not infected. (Wilma cannot be at risk of contracting the disease if she is infected already.) Third, Wilma's vulnerability is both serious and real. HIV infection is both debilitating and, during those years, invariably fatal. The couple's sexuality makes eventual infection highly likely. Fourth, assuming that preventing Wilma's death is the goal, it is probable that, were Wilma to be told of Andrew's infection, she would avoid exposing herself to the risk. This is not a trivial condition:

many people knowingly risk illness and injury out of love and other honorable motivations. Molokai's Father Damien contracted and died from Hansen's disease while caring for patients he knew might infect him. Soldiers, police, and firefighters commonly expose themselves to grave risk. It is not enough that a warning would discharge a duty to Wilma, merely so she could make an informed choice. Plainly, the paramount concern has to be to save Wilma's life. Finally, Wilma is not a mere stranger. Instead she has an important relationship with you—her doctor—that serves as a basis for special obligations: You have a special duty to look out for her health.

In the light of these five considerations, it should not be a surprise that the conventional wisdom in medical ethics overwhelmingly supports either an ethical obligation to breach confidentiality in cases like this one or, occasionally and less stringently, the ethical permissibility of doing so. Notwithstanding this consensus, it is my intention to challenge the received view. I will argue in what follows that confidentiality in clinical medicine is far closer to an absolute obligation than it has generally been taken to be; doctors should honor confidentiality even in cases like this one. Although the focus here is on the *Case of the Infected Spouse*, the background idea is that, if it can be demonstrated that confidentiality should be scrupulously honored in this one case where so many considerations support breaching it, the duty of confidentiality should be taken as unqualified in virtually all other cases as well. I shall not, however, defend that broader conclusion here.

Although this essay specifically addresses the obligations of doctors, its approach applies more broadly to all professions that take seriously the responsibility to provide distressed practitioners with authoritative guidance. With its focus narrowly on "professional obligations," the methodology used below also represents something of a challenge to much of the conventional thinking in medical ethics.

Clearing the Ground: What Professional Obligations Are Not

Among philosophers, it is commonplace that if people are not asking the same questions, they are unlikely to arrive at the same answers. It may be that the main reason doctors have difficulty reaching consensus in ethics is that, in general, systematic discussion about professional responsibility is commonly confused with at least three other types of conversation. When one asks whether one should call the hotel to warn Wilma, one can be asking: 1) what the law requires; 2) what one's personal morality requires (e.g., as an Orthodox Jew, a Roman Catholic, etc.); or 3) what is required by one's most deeply held personal values (e.g., preventing deaths or scrupulously honoring other obligations). Discussions can meander mindlessly over all three areas without attending to boundary crossings. More to the point, effective deliberation about professional obligations, as I will try to show, differs importantly from all three of these discussions. Accordingly, it is necessary to identify and bracket these other perspectives in order to mark off the intellectual space within which practitioners can productively reflect on questions of professional responsibility. Let us examine these different conversations.

Law

The conventional wisdom on the ethics of medical confidentiality has been largely shaped by a single legal case: *Tarasoff v. Regents of the University of California*. In 1969, Prosenjit Poddar, a student at U.C. Berkeley, told a university psychologist he intended to kill a Ms. Tatiana Tarasoff, a young woman who had spurned his affections. The psychologist dutifully reported him to the campus police, who held him briefly and then set him free. Shortly afterwards, Poddar did as he said he would, stabbing the young woman to death. The Tarasoff family sued the University of California for their daughter's death, finally prevailing in their contention that the psychologist (and, by implication, the University) had failed in their duty to protect, since

neither Tatiana nor those able to apprise her of danger were warned. The University was found liable and had to compensate the family for its loss. Today it is hard to find discussions of the ethics of confidentiality that do not appeal to this legal parable and, occasionally, to its California Supreme Court moral: "The protective privilege ends where the public peril begins."

Taking its cue from *Tarasoff*, the prevailing standard in medical ethics now holds that the obligation of confidentiality will give way when a doctor is aware that a patient will seriously injure some identified other person. (One might ask why disclosure is not required when a patient will seriously injure many unidentified persons. Under the narrower standard, there is no duty to alert others about an HIV-infected prostitute who neither informs nor protects a large number of anonymous at-risk clients.) We assume that the physician knows Andrew is seropositive, that Wilma is likely seronegative, that the two will likely engage in activities that transmit the virus, and that breaching confidentiality will probably result in those activities not occurring and Wilma's not becoming infected. Thus, a physician's warning in the *Case of the Infected Spouse* will mean that Wilma is very likely to remain infection-free, and a failure to warn her is very likely to result in her eventual death from AIDS.

Focusing on the legal standard, it is useful to distinguish between "special" and "general" legal duties. Special duties can apply to individuals occupying certain roles. A parent, but not a bystander, has a special duty to rescue a drowning daughter; firefighters and police officers have special duties to take certain occupational risks, and doctors have many special duties toward their patients: confidentiality is a good example. In contrast, virtually everyone has a general duty to be scrupulously careful when handling explosives, to pay taxes on income, to respect others' property, and so on. It is notable that the duty to warn in *Tarasoff* is a special duty, applicable only to those occupying special roles. So if my neighbor casually assures me he is going to kill his girlfriend tomorrow, the *Tarasoff* ruling does not require me to warn her.

It is surprising to many that the default standard in Anglo-American jurisprudence is that there is no general duty to improve the prospects of the precariously placed, no legal obligation to undertake even an easy rescue. As first-year law students discover, one can stand on a pier with a lifeline in hand and, with complete impunity, allow a stranger to drown nearby. Although we will pass over it, it is notable that, in general, the parties who are legally obligated to warn are those who are otherwise ethically obligated not to disclose. One should reflect on the absence of a general duty to warn.

The easy transition from law to ethics reflects a common error. The mistake is to move from the premise that some action is legally required (what the *Tarasoff* opinion establishes in the jurisdictions that have followed it) to the conclusion that the same action is ethically required. But ethical obligations can conflict with legal ones. Journalists, for example, are sometimes ordered by the courts to reveal the identities of their confidential sources. Although law demands disclosure, professional ethics requires silence. Reporters famously go to jail rather than betray sources. Journalists can find themselves in a quandary: while good citizens obey the law and good professionals honor their professional codes, laws requiring journalists to violate their duties to confidential sources force a tragic choice between acting illegally and acting unethically. Conscientious persons should not have to face such decisions.

Similarly in pediatrics, statutes may require doctors to report suspicions of child abuse. But where protective agencies are inept and overworked and foster care is dangerous or unavailable, a doctor's report is more likely to result in termination of therapy and further injury to the child instead of protection and care. To obey the law under these appalling, but too common, circumstances is most likely to abandon and even cause harm to the minor patient, both of which are ethically prohibited in medicine.

To assume that legal obligations always trump or settle ethical ones is to blind oneself to the possibility of conflict. Professions have to face these dilemmas head-on instead of masking them with language that conflates legal standards and ethical ones. They must conceive professional ethics as separate from the law's mandate. When law requires what professional responsibility prohibits (or prohibits what professional responsibility requires), professional organizations must press the public, legislatures, and the courts to cease demanding that conscientious practitioners dishonor the duties of their craft. This is an important responsibility of professional organizations. It is a mistake to configure professional obligations merely to mirror the law's requirements. Rather the law's requirements must be configured so that they do not conflict with well-considered professional obligations. Law is a human artifact that can be crafted well or badly. In a well-ordered society no one will have to choose between illegality and immorality. Since the law can require conduct that violates ethical standards (and ethical standards can require conduct that violates the law), it cannot be the case that legal obligations automatically create ethical obligations. As the tradition of civil disobedience shows, it can be ethically permissible or obligatory (though not legal) to violate an unjust law.

Even though laws cannot create ethical obligations by fiat, professions need to distinguish between the state's reasonable interests in the work of doctors (e.g., preventing serious harm to children) and the specific legal mandates a state imposes (e.g., requiring doctors to report suspicion of child abuse to an incompetent state agency). Just as patients can make ill-considered demands that should not be satisfied, so too can the state and its courts.

Accordingly, it is assumed that the state has a legitimate interest in preventing harm to people, and that doctors have an ethical obligation to further that important public objective. The focus in this essay is on the shape of the resulting ethical obligation as it applies narrowly to cases like those involving Wilma Long and Tatiana Tarasoff. Because they introduce complexities that will carry us far afield, we set aside cases involving: (a) children brought in by parents; (b) patients referred for independent medical evaluation; (c) mentally ill or retarded patients in the custody of health care institutions; (d) health care that is the subject of litigation; (e) gunshot, knife wounds, and the like; (f) workers' compensation cases; and a few others. While a much longer discussion could cover these areas, many readers can extend the analysis offered here to discern much of what I would want to say about those other cases.

Though I will not discuss them, institutional policies (hospital rules, for example) function very much like laws. Both involve standards that can be imposed externally upon practitioners. Both can be formulated knowledgeably and wisely or with a disregard for essential professional responsibilities.

Personal Morality

We will understand a "morality" as a set of beliefs about obligations. There are plainly many such sets of beliefs: the morality of Confucius has little in common with the moralities of George W. Bush and Thomas Aquinas. For most of us, morality is uncritically absorbed in childhood, coming to consciousness when we encounter others whose moral beliefs differ.

There are still parts of the world in which virtually all members of a community are participants in a common morality. But moral pluralism now seems a permanent part of the social order. Consider a Jehovah's Witness physician who is opposed, on religious grounds, to administering blood transfusions. If this doctor were the only physician on duty when his patient needed an immediate transfusion, a choice would have to be made between being a good Jehovah's Witness and being a good doctor. The doctor's personal moral convictions are here inconsistent with professional obligations. It follows that clarity about personal morality is not the same as clarity about medical ethics.

Professionalism can require that one set aside one's personal morality or carefully limit one's exposure to certain professional responsibilities. Here the rule has to be that doctors will not take on responsibilities that might conflict with their personal morality. Problems could be sidestepped if the Jehovah's Witness doctor specialized in a field that didn't involve transfusion (e.g., dermatology) or always worked with colleagues who could administer them. If I am morally against the death penalty, I shouldn't take on work as an executioner. If I am deeply opposed to the morning-after pill, I shouldn't counsel patients at a rape treatment center. To teach medical ethics in a pluralistic professional community is to try to create an intellectual space within which persons from varied backgrounds can agree upon responsible standards for professional conduct. Participants in such a conversation may have to leave personal morality at the door. For some, it may be a mistake to choose a career in medicine.

If ethics is a critical reflection on our moralities, then the hope implicit in the field of medical ethics is that we might some day reach a responsible consensus on doctors' obligations. While medicine has dozens of codes, it is not hard to observe commonalities: the standards for informed consent, for example. At a deeper level, there can also be consensus on the justifications for those standards. One role for the philosopher is, as in this essay, to assess carefully the soundness of those arguments. A major task for professions is to move beyond the various personal moralities embraced by practitioners and to reach a responsible consensus on common professional standards.

Personal Values

Values are commonly a part of an explanation of personal conduct. It is always reasonable to ask of any rational action: what good was it intended to promote? While some wear shoes to avoid hurting their feet (embracing the value of comfort), others think they look better in shoes (embracing aesthetic values). Where we have to make personal decisions, often we consider how each option can further or frustrate our values, and try to decide among the good and bad consequences.

This strategy can serve when the question is "What should I do?" But the question "What should a good doctor do?" calls for a different type of inquiry. For while I have many personal values, the "good doctor" is an abstraction. She is neither Protestant nor Buddhist, doesn't prefer chocolate to vanilla, and doesn't care about money more than leisure time. Questions about professional ethics cannot be answered in terms of personal values.

A second difficulty appears when we consider that one can give perfect expression to one's most deeply held personal values and still act unethically. Hannibal Lecter in *Silence of the Lambs* and Mozart's Don Giovanni are despicable villains who give vigorous effect to deeply held if contemptible personal values. While personal values can determine action, they do not guarantee that the favored actions are ethical.

Accordingly, we cannot appeal to our personal values to inquire about what physicians in general ought to do. Medicine has no personal values, only individual physicians do. When a physician must decide whether or not to resuscitate a patient, personal values should have nothing to do with the issue. Whether you like the patient or detest him, whether you are an atheist or a fundamentalist believer in a joyous hereafter, should not weigh in the balance. A key part of professionalism involves being able to set personal values aside. While medical students have much to gain by becoming clear about their personal values, that clarity is not the same as responsible certainty about professional obligations.

To summarize the argument so far, discussion about professional obligations in medicine is not the same as discussion about legal and institutional obligations, personal morality or personal values. If a responsible ethical consensus is to be achieved by a profession, it is necessary for physicians to learn to bracket their personal moral and value commitments and to set aside, at least temporarily, their consideration of legal or institutional rules and policies. The practical task is to create an intellectual space within which responsible consensus can be achieved on how physicians, as professionals, ought to act. I will now describe one way in which this might be done.

The Concept of a Professional Obligation

Professional ethics involves disciplined discussion about the obligations of professionals. One place to begin is with a distinction between personal values, already discussed, and what can be called "core professional values." A physician can prefer (1) pistachios to Brazil nuts, and (2) confidentiality to universal candor. While the preference for pistachios is merely personal, the preference for confidentiality is a value all doctors ought to possess. The distinction between personal values and "core professional values" is critical here. There is what this flesh-and-blood doctor happens to care about personally, and what the good doctor ought to care about. This idea of a "good doctor" is a social construction, an aspect of a determinate social role, an integral element of medical professionalism. Our idea of a good doctor includes a certain technical/intellectual mastery coupled with a certain commitment to specific professional values. As with the Jehovah's Witness doctor, personal and professional values may be in conflict. As part of an appreciation of the ethical claims of professionalism, physicians must be prepared to set aside their personal values and morality, to set aside what the legal system and their employers want them to care about, and to take up instead the question of what the responsible physician ought to care about. The profession's core values inform those purposes that each medical professional should have in common with colleagues. In discussing the professionally favored resolution of ethically problematic cases (the *Case of the Infected Spouse*, for example) physicians can ask—together—how medicine's core professional values ought to be respected in those circumstances.

We have alluded to some of these core professional values. Trustworthiness needs to be on the list. Beneficence toward the patient's health needs is essential. Respect for patient autonomy is a third. Others might be collegiality (duties to colleagues), and perhaps a few others: nondiscrimination and a certain deference to families are among the most commonly mentioned candidates. If we were to leave out that doctors should care about the well-being of the public, the argument for confidentiality would be easy. But it too properly goes on the list. Anyone seeing no point in furthering and securing these values would be ill-suited for the practice of medicine.

Each of these professional values has two dimensions. Along one vector, they define the shared aspiration of a profession. At any time, medicine's ability to benefit patients will be limited. But it is a part of the profession's commitment to push its envelope, to enlarge its collective competency and draw upon its knowledge and skill. Those who master and extend the profession's broadest capabilities are exemplary contributors, but practitioners do not discredit themselves by failing to serve in this estimable way.

Along the second vector, values define a bottom line beneath which practitioners shall not sink. Paraphrasing Hippocrates, although you may not always be able to benefit your patients, it is far more important that you take care not to harm them. Knowingly to harm a patient (on balance) is not merely a failure to realize the value of beneficence. It is a culpable betrayal of that value, a far more serious matter.

All the values above can be understood in this second way. Trustworthiness entails that I not lie to patients, or deliberately withhold information they have an interest in knowing. Respect for patient autonomy can require that I not use force or fraud upon them. And the concern for the well-being of the public requires that that interest somehow appear prominently upon every practitioner's radar screen, that doctors not stand idly by in the face of perils the profession can help to

avert and, as a lower limit, that they not do anything to increase public peril. Consider that the overutilization of antibiotics, resulting in drug-resistant infectious agents, is professional misconduct that increases public peril.

Ethical problems can arise, first, when core values appear to be in conflict, as with the *Case of the Infected Spouse*. At issue are trustworthiness toward Andrew on one side, and beneficence toward Wilma and a concern for the well-being of the public on the other. If the conflict is real, what is required is a priority rule. For example, the concept of decisional capacity is part of a priority rule resolving the well-studied conflict between beneficence and autonomy: when do physicians have to respect a patient's refusal of life-saving treatment? There is what the patient wants and what the patient needs. But when a patient is decisionally capacitated and informed, his or her refusal trumps the doctor's recommendation.

Second, ethical problems can also arise when it is unclear what some core professional value requires one to do. Though we can all agree that doctors should avoid harming their patients, there is no professional consensus on whether deliberately causing the deaths of certain unfortunate patients—those experiencing irremediable and intense suffering—is always a betrayal of beneficence. Likewise, although doctors may be in a position to prevent harm to third parties, it is not well understood what they must do out of respect for that value. When core values conflict, what is required is a priority rule. When they are unclear, what is required is removal of ambiguity: what philosophers call "disambiguation." These two tasks—prioritizing and disambiguating core professional values—need to be carried out with a high degree of intellectual responsibility.

The above list of medicine's core values is not controversial. Propose a toast to them at an assemblage of physicians and all can likely drink with enthusiasm. What is less clear is why such a consensus should obligate professionals. A criminal organization can celebrate its shared commitment to the oath of silence. But it doesn't follow that those who cooperate with the police are unethical. In addition to organizational "celebratability," three additional elements are required to establish a professional obligation.

The first element is that attention to core values has to be a part of professional education. Most medical education is aimed at beneficence. The procedures used in informed consent express a commitment of respect for patient autonomy and trustworthiness. If the profession wholly fails to equip its novices to further its core values, it can be argued that it is not serious about those professed values. Its public commitments will begin to look like they are intended to convey an illusion of concerned attention. In replicating itself, a profession must replicate its commitment. Students of medicine must come to care about the goods that doctors ought to care about. Because justice is rarely explored as a topic in medical education, I do not think it can be counted as a core professional value. However some parts of justice—nondiscrimination, for example—are routinely covered.

The second element is critical. The core values are not just goods that doctors care about and that doctors want other doctors to care about. They are also goods that the rest of us want our doctors to care about. I want my doctor to be trustworthy, to be intent on benefiting my health, to take my informed refusals seriously, and so on. And we want our doctors to look out for the well-being of the public. The core professional values are also social values. (Consider that it is not reasonable to want our mobsters to respect their oaths of silence.)

The third element flows from the second: an exclusive social reliance upon the profession as the means by which certain matters are to receive due attention. We mostly respect medical competence. But it is precisely because, as a community, we have also come to accept that doctors are reliably committed to their values (our values), that we have, through state legislatures, granted the medical profession an exclusive monopoly on the delivery of medical services. The unauthorized practice of medicine is a punishable crime. If, like the medical profession, one were to make a public claim that, because of unique skills and dedication, some important social concern ought to be exclusively entrusted to you, and the public believes you and entrusts those important matters to you, incidentally prohibiting all others from encroachment upon what is now your privilege, you would have thereby assumed an ethical obligation to give those important matters due attention. Collectively, the medical profession has done exactly this in securing its monopoly on the delivery of certain types of health care. Accordingly the profession has a collective obligation to organize itself so that the shared responsibilities it has assumed in the political process of professionalization are properly discharged by its membership.

A sound code of ethics consists of a set of standards that, if adhered to broadly by the profession's membership, will result in the profession as a whole discharging its responsibilities. Where physician behavior brings about a public loss of that essential trust, society may have to withdraw the monopolistic privilege and seek a better way of organizing health care. Professionalization is but one way of organizing an essential service. There are others.

In summary, the medical profession has ethical obligations toward patients, families, and the community because of its public commitment to secure and further certain critical social values and because of society's exclusive reliance on the profession as its means of delivering certain forms of health care. With the professional privilege comes a reciprocal collective responsibility. We can now turn our attention to medicine's responsibility to diminish public perils.

The Duty to Diminish Risks to Third Parties

There is an implication for the way in which we must now understand the problem in the *Case of the Infected Spouse*. The opening question "Do you take steps to warn Wilma?" has to be understood as a question about medical ethics and not about "you." We want to know what the "good doctor" should do under those circumstance? Each doctor is ethically required to do what a responsible doctor ought to do: in order to properly respect the core values of the profession. To become a doctor without a proper commitment to respect the profession's values is to be unfit for the practice of medicine. So how are trustworthiness and confidentiality to be understood in relationship to medicine's commitment to diminish risks to third parties?

In the *Case of the Infected Spouse* the ethical question is posed in 1991, after the doctor–family relationship has been in place for a decade. The dilemma arises during and immediately after a single office visit, forcing a choice between calling Wilma either you will have to explain to Andrew, in two days, why you disclosed his infection to his wife, or you will have to explain to Wilma, in two years, why you did not disclose his infection to her. Each option has a bad outcome: the betrayal of Andrew's trust or the fatal infection of Wilma. Either way, you will need to account for yourself.

Infection seems a far worse consequence for Wilma than betrayal is for Andrew. Much of the literature on confidentiality has been shaped by this fact, and perhaps the standard strategy for resolving the problem calls attention to the magnitude and probability of the bad outcomes associated with each option. While predictions of harm can sometimes be wrong, it can be evident that Tatiana Tarasoff and Wilma Long are at grave risk and, accordingly, it can seem honorable to diminish the danger to vulnerable parties like them. Justice Tobriner appeals to a version of this consequentialist argument in *Tarasoff*:

> Weighing the uncertain and conjectural character of the alleged damage done the patient by such a warning against the peril to the victim's life, we conclude that professional inaccuracy in predicting violence [or deadly infection] cannot negate the therapist's duty to protect the threatened victim.

Beauchamp and Childress, in their widely read *Principles of Biomedical Ethics*, urge clinicians to take into account "the probability that a harm will materialize and the magnitude of that harm" in any decision to breach confidentiality. (While they also urge that clinicians take into account the potential impact of disclosure on policies and laws regarding confidentiality, they are not very clear about how this assessment is to be carried out.) In brief, the very bad consequences of not disclosing risk to Wilma—disease and death and the betrayal of her trust—outweigh the not-all-that-bad consequence of breached confidentiality to Andrew. Your explanation to Andrew could cover those points.

The preferred argument would go something like this: The state's interest in preventing harm is weighty. Medicine has an obligation to protect the well-being of the community. Because the seriousness of threatened grave injury to another outweighs the damage done to a patient by breaching confidentiality, the obligation of confidentiality must give way to a duty to prevent serious harm to others. Accordingly, despite confidentiality, warning or reporting is obligatory when it will likely avert very bad outcomes in this way. Of course clinicians should try to obtain waivers of confidentiality before disclosure, thereby avoiding the need to breach a duty. But the failure to obtain a waiver does not, on this argument, affect the overriding obligation to report.

A Defense of Unqualified Confidentiality

As powerful as the above justification is, there are problems with it. Go back to 1990, when Andrew comes in to be tested for sexually transmitted diseases. Suppose he asks: "If I am infected, can I trust you not to disclose this to others?" If, following the arguments set out in the previous paragraphs, we are clear that confidentiality must be breached to protect third parties like Wilma, then the only truthful answer to Andrew's question is "No. You can't trust me." If the profession accepts that its broad promise of confidentiality must sometimes be broken, then any unqualified assurances are fraudulent and the profession should stop making them. If there are exceptions, clinicians have a duty to be forthcoming about what they are and how they work. Patients should know up front when they can trust doctors, and when they can't. To withhold this important information is to betray the value of trustworthiness.

Accordingly, the argument for breaching confidentiality has to be modified to support a qualified confidentiality rule, one that carves out an exception from the very beginning, acknowledging an overriding duty to report under defined circumstances. (In contrast, an unqualified confidentiality rule contemplates no exceptions.) Instead of undertaking duties of confidentiality and then violating them, doctors must qualify their expressed obligations so they will be able to honor them. Commentators who have walked through the issues surrounding confidentiality have long understood the ethical necessity of "Miranda warnings." A clinician would have to say early on, "Certain things that I learn from you may have to be disclosed to . . . under the following circumstances . . . ; and the following things might occur to you as a result of my disclosure: . . ." If doctors are ethically obligated to report, they need to say in advance what will be passed along, when, to whom, and what could happen then. They should never encourage or accept trust only to betray their patients afterwards. To do so is to betray the value of trustworthiness.

But now a second problem emerges. If prospective patients must understand in advance that a doctor will report evidence of a threat to others, they will only be willing to disclose such evidence to the doctor if they are willing to accept that those others will come to know. If it is important to them that the evidence not be reported, they will have a weighty reason not to disclose it to those who are obligated to report it.

Some have questioned this proposition, arguing that there is no empirical evidence that prospective patients will avoid or delay seeking medical attention or conceal medically relevant information if confidentiality is qualified in this way. Despite widespread reporting practices, waiting rooms have not emptied and no one really knows if people stop talking openly to their doctors when confidentiality is breached.

Three responses are possible regarding this claim. First, there is a serious difficulty doing empirical research in this area. How, for example, do we determine the number of abusive parents who have not brought their injured children to doctors out of a fear that they will get into trouble with the authorities? How many HIV+ patients avoid telling their doctors all about their unsafe sexual practices? How many of us would volunteer unflattering truthful answers to direct questions on these and other shameful matters? It is notoriously difficult to gather reliable data on the embarrassing, criminal, irresponsible things people do, and the steps they take to avoid exposure, especially if those are wrongful too. I don't want to suggest that these problems are insurmountable, but they are decidedly there and they often make it hard to study the effects of these betrayals.

Second, despite the problems, certain types of indirect evidence can occasionally emerge. Here are two anecdotal examples from Honolulu. There was a time, not long ago, when military enlistees who were troubled by their sexual orientation knew that military doctors and psychologists would report these problems to their officers. Many of these troubled soldiers therefore obtained the services of private psychologists and psychiatrists in Honolulu, despite the fact that free services were available in military clinics. The second example emerged from the failure of the Japanese medical system to keep diagnoses of HIV infection confidential. Many Japanese who could afford it traveled to Honolulu for diagnosis and treatment, avoiding clinics in Japan. At the same time, Japanese data on the prevalence of HIV infection were unrealistically low, especially considering the popularity of Japanese sex tours to the HIV-infected brothels of Thailand. Evidence of this sort can confirm that the failure to respect confidentiality can impair the ability of doctors to do their job.

And third, there is an argument based on the motivational principle that if one strongly desires that event E does not occur, and one knows that doing act A will bring about event E, then one has a weighty reason not to do act A. The criminal justice system is based on this idea. We attach artificial and broadly unwelcome consequences (imprisonment and other forms of punishment) to wrongful, harmful conduct with the expectation that, even if inclined, most people will decide against the conduct in order to avoid the unwelcome consequence. If I don't want to go to prison, and a career in burglary will likely result in my going to prison, then I have a weighty reason to choose a different career. Likewise, if I don't want my marriage to be destroyed by my wife's discovery that I am HIV+, and I know that telling my doctor about reconciliation will result in her discovering just that, then I have a weighty reason not to tell my doctor. The presumption must be in favor of the truth of this seemingly self-evident principle. If critics allege that it is false or otherwise unworthy of endorsement, it seems the burden of disproof belongs to them. It is their responsibility to come up with disconfirming evidence.

It can be argued, in rebuttal, that people still commit burglary and, despite reporting laws, people still go to doctors for HIV testing, even knowing that confidentiality has its limits. But no one would maintain that punishing convicted criminals totally prevents crime and that breaching confidentiality results in all people avoiding or delaying medical treatment, or concealing aspects of their lives. The situation is more complicated.

Consider that Andrew belongs to one of two groups of prospective patients. Members of the first group are willing enough to have reports made to others. Members of the second are deterred from disclosure by the fear of a report. Of course we can't know in advance which type of patient Andrew is, but if both groups are treated alike, uncertainty will not be a problem. (While this division into two groups may be oversimplified, working through the qualifications would take us too far afield.)

Consider the first group: patients who would be willing to have a report made. Recall that the physician in the *Case of the Infected Spouse* tried to obtain assurance that Wilma would be protected. Under an unqualified confidentiality rule—no exceptions—if the patient were willing to have reports made to others, the doctor should be able to obtain a waiver of confidentiality and Wilma could then be informed. Once permission to report is given, the ethical dilemma disappears. Notice that for this group of patients an exceptionless confidentiality rule works just as well as a rule requiring doctors to override confidentiality when necessary to protect endangered third parties. At-risk parties will be warned just the same, but with appropriate permission from patients. In these cases there is no need to trim back the obligation of confidentiality since patients in this first group are, by definition, willing to have a report made.

Difficulties arise with the second type of patient: those who will not want credible threats reported. Notice that these prospective patients are in control of the evidence doctors need to secure protection for parties at risk. If a patient cannot be drawn into a therapeutic alliance—a relationship of trust and confidence—then doctors will not receive the information they need to protect imperiled third parties (at least so long as patients have options). As a result, doctors will not be able to mobilize protection. When one traces out the implications of a reporting rule on what needs to be said in 1990 (when Andrew asked to be tested and the doctor disclosed the limits to confidentiality), it becomes evident that Wilma will not be protected if Andrew (a) does not want her to know, and (b) understands that disclosure to his doctor will result in her knowing. Depending on his options and the strength of his preferences, he will be careful about what he discloses to his doctor, or will go without medical advice and care, or will find another physician who can be kept in ignorance about his personal life.

We began by characterizing the *Case of the Infected Spouse* as an apparent head-on collision between the doctor's duty of confidentiality and the duty to protect imperiled third parties. But if the argument above is sound, there is no collision. The obligation to warn third parties does not provide added protection to those at-risk. In particular, a no-exceptions confidentiality rule has a better chance of getting the facts on the table, at least to the extent that honest promises of confidentiality can make it so. To be sure, clinicians would have to set aside the vexing "Should I report?" conundrum and search for creative solutions instead. These strategies will not always prevent harm, but they will sometimes. The nub of the matter is that these strategies can never work if they can't be implemented. And they can't be implemented if the fear of reporting deters patients from disclosure. Accordingly there is no justification for trimming back the obligation of confidentiality since doing so actually reduces protection to endangered third parties, increasing public peril.

The argument advanced here is that—paradoxically—ethical and legal duties to report make it less likely that endangered parties will be protected. Depending on the prospective patient, these duties are either unnecessary (when waivers can be obtained) or counterproductive (when disclosure to the doctor is deterred and interventions other than disclosure are prevented).

In part, the conventional wisdom on confidentiality errs in focusing on the decision of the individual clinician at the point when the choice has to be made to disclose or not. The decision to violate confidentiality reaches backwards to the HIV test administered years earlier and, as we shall see, even before. Perhaps little will be lost if one doctor betrays a single patient one time, or if

betrayals are extremely rare. But medical ethics is not about a single decision by an individual clinician. The consequences and implications of a rule governing professional practice may be quite different from those of a single act. Better to ask, what if every doctor did that?

While it is accepted here that doctors have an overriding obligation to prevent public peril, it has been argued that they do not honor that obligation by breaching or chipping away at confidentiality. This is because the protective purpose to be furthered by reporting is defeated by the practice of reporting. The best public protection is achieved where doctors do their best work and, there, trustworthiness is probably the most important prerequisite. Physicians damage both their professional capabilities and their communities when they compromise their trustworthiness.

It is hard enough to create therapeutic alliances that meet patients' needs. But if doctors take on the added duty to mobilize protective responses without waivers of confidentiality, their work may become impossible in too many important cases. And all of us will be the worse for that. The thinking that places the moral comfort of clinicians above the well-being of patients and their victims is in conflict with the requirements of professional responsibility, properly understood. While it will be a challenge for many honorable physicians to measure up to this standard, no one ever said it was easy to be a good doctor.

Patient Responsibilities

AMERICAN MEDICAL ASSOCIATION

AMA Council on Ethical and Judicial Affairs, CEJA Report A – A-93.

Background

It has long been recognized that successful medical care requires an ongoing collaborative effort between patients and physicians. Physician and patient are bound in a partnership that requires both individuals to take an active role in the healing process. Such a partnership does not imply that both partners have identical responsibilities or equal power. Physicians are in a position to use their training and expertise to relieve pain and suffering. While physicians have the responsibility to provide health care services to patients to the best of their ability, patients have the responsibility to communicate openly, to participate in decisions about the diagnostic and treatment recommendations, and to comply with the agreed upon therapeutic program.

Like patients' rights, patients' responsibilities are derived from the principle of autonomy. The principle of patient autonomy holds that an individual's physical, emotional, and psychological integrity should be respected and upheld. This principle also recognizes the human capacity to self-govern and choose a course of action from among reasonable options. Autonomous, competent patients assert some control over the decisions which direct their health care. With that exercise of self-governance and free choice comes a number of responsibilities.

1. Good communication is essential to a successful physician-patient relationship. To the extent possible, patients have a responsibility to express their concerns clearly to their physicians and be honest.

2. Patients have a responsibility to provide a complete medical history, to the extent possible, including information about past illnesses, medications, hospitalizations, family history of illness and other matters relating to present health.

3. In addition to explaining known medical background to their physician, patients have a responsibility to request information or clarification about their health status or treatment when they do not fully understand what has been described.

4. Once patients and physicians agree upon the goals of therapy, patients have a responsibility to cooperate with the treatment plan. Compliance with physician instructions is often essential to public and individual safety. Patients also have a responsibility to disclose whether previously agreed upon treatments are being followed and to indicate when they would like to reconsider the treatment plan.

5. Patients generally have a responsibility to meet their financial obligations with regard to medical care or to discuss financial hardships with their physicians. Patients should be cognizant of the costs associated with using a limited resource like health care and try to use medical resources judiciously.

6. Patients should discuss end of life decisions with their physicians and make their wishes known. Such a discussion might also include writing an advanced directive.

7. Patients should be committed to health maintenance through health-enhancing behavior. Illness can often be prevented by a healthy lifestyle, and patients must take personal responsibility when they are able to avert the development of disease.

8. Patients should also have an active interest in the effects of their conduct on others and refrain from behavior that unreasonably places the health of others at risk. Patients should inquire as to the means and likelihood of infectious disease transmission and act upon that information which can best prevent further transmission.
9. Patients should discuss organ donation with their physicians and make applicable provisions. Patients who are part of an organ allocation system and await needed treatment or transplant should not try to go outside or manipulate the system. A fair system of allocation should be answered with public trust and an awareness of limited resources.
10. Patients should not initiate or participate in fraudulent health care, and should report illegal or unethical behavior to the appropriate law enforcement authorities, licensing boards, or medical societies.

The Patient's Work

LEONARD C. GROOPMAN, FRANKLIN G. MILLER, AND JOSEPH J. FINS

Cambridge Quarterly of Healthcare Ethics 16 (2006): 44–52.

In *The Healer's Power*, Howard Brody placed the concept of power at the heart of medicine's moral discourse. Struck by the absence of "power" in the prevailing vocabulary of medical ethics, yet aware of peripheral allusions to power in the writings of some medical ethicists, he intuited the importance of power from the silence surrounding it. He formulated the problem of the healer's power and its responsible use as "the central ethical problem in medicine."[1] Through the prism of power he refracted a wide range of ethical problems, from informed consent to truth-telling, from confidentiality to futility, from the physician's fantasies to the physician's virtues. At times this prism shed new light on old problems, enabling us to see from an unexpected angle the elements of which the problem was composed. At other times it exposed issues of ethical significance that had been neglected in the bioethics literature.

Brody argued that without power physicians cannot heal. The healer, therefore, cannot relinquish his power—it "irreducibly remains with the physician"—so he must be aware of and acknowledge the uses he makes of it. He then is obliged to share that power with his patient by means of "transparency"—"thinking out loud"—in the service of the patient's life plans. Writing from the perspective of a primary care physician, Brody adopted the metaphor of the doctor-patient relationship as an ongoing conversation between two people who come to know and trust each other, and who construct a meaningful narrative of the patient's life through the course of their common experience and their extended conversation. Doctor and patient collaborate in the ongoing process of healing.

Yet if the healer, in order to heal, is called on to make proper use of his power, we may ask what the sufferer, the sick person, the patient—in order to be healed, cured, or treated—is called on to do. If the healing process should be collaborative, then both parties are working.

Does the concept of the patient's work make sense? The very notion of the patient's work may seem surprising if not self-contradictory. The patient, by virtue of his medical condition, generally enjoys a reduced work load, not an increased one. And it is the doctor, not the patient, who is at work when they meet. The hospital, the clinic, and the office are the workplaces of the doctor, not the patient. Medical ethics has been concerned with defining and prescribing the proper conditions of the *doctor's* work, not the patient's. Or has it? The patient's work—not unlike the healer's power—has been a subject whispered about and alluded to, but not openly and fully explored within medical ethics. Like power, work is a category that social scientists are more comfortable with than ethicists. As with power, so with work; the silence surrounding it draws our attention to it.

Work in Psychotherapy and Rehabilitation

Although in general the concept of the patient's work has been absent from the discourse of medical ethics, there are two fields within medicine in which the notion that the patient is working is not alien. In psychiatry—at least in psychotherapy—and in rehabilitation medicine, we commonly speak of the patient working. In the former the work is emotional and cognitive; in the latter it is primarily physical. In both fields the process of treatment depends fundamentally on the patient's active participation and on a collaborative interaction between therapist and patient. The patient's motivation is considered crucial to the treatment process, and resistance to the process is commonly encountered—even expected—in both fields. Engagement of the patient in the treatment process is an essential condition for both psychotherapy and rehabilitation—in a way that it may not be in other medical fields—although recognition of and respect for the need for disengagement may in some cases also be essential to maintaining a therapeutic alliance. Psychotherapy and rehabilitation medicine also share as primary goals—alongside the alleviation

of symptoms—the enhancement of the patient's functional capacity (emotional or physical functioning) and, more broadly, the enhancement of the patient's sense of autonomy—that is, his ability to direct himself either physically or psychologically. All of these goals require an active, participating—working—patient.

Psychotherapy and rehabilitation medicine occupy peripheral regions of the medical map as we currently conceive it. They can be and often are practiced by nonphysician therapists. Rehabilitation takes place after the properly medical work of surgery is done or after the acute treatment of stroke or trauma or other medical illness is complete. And although psychiatry has in recent decades become increasingly "medicalized" through psychopharmacology, psychotherapy remains ancillary to the prevailing conceptions of organicist medicine. Yet just as Brody argued that primary care is more an attitude than a specialty, and that that attitude can and should be imported into the relationship between doctor and patient, so we argue that the patient's work is a useful concept not only in psychotherapy and rehabilitation medicine, but within the doctor–patient relationship more generally.

Work in Doctor–Patient Models

Has the concept of the patient's work truly been foreign to the ethics of the doctor–patient relationship? Insofar as the patient's work has been discussed in the ethics of the doctor–patient relationship, it has been buried under other names than "work" or it has been found outside medical ethics itself. In the paternalistic paradigm of the doctor–patient relationship, the patient has had a role, most thoroughly described by the sociologist Talcott Parsons. In the autonomy paradigm the patient has had a responsibility, most strongly articulated by Jay Katz. Role and responsibility have been the disguised forms taken by the patient's work in these models.

Parsons described the sick role and the social and psychological expectations that accompanied it. He taught us that "being sick" is not simply a natural fact, but a social role, with an "institutionalized expectation system" that is "not only a right of the sick person but an obligation upon him." The exemption from normal responsibility, for example, is accompanied by the obligation to stay in bed. The sick role further relieves the sick person from responsibility for being sick—he is not to blame for his condition—but requires him to want to get well, to seek technically competent help, and to cooperate with the helper. Failure to do so would raise questions of malingering and of the "secondary gain" from illness, and would abrogate the person's exemptions from his usual responsibilities. Of the obligation to cooperate in the treatment, Parsons writes, "it is here, of course, that the role of the sick person as patient becomes articulated with that of the physician in a complementary role structure."[2] For the doctor to do his work, the patient must do his—which is to perform his socially assigned sick role.

The theorists of patient autonomy rejected this definition of the sick role, which they criticized for its dependency features. The patient in this role was deferential, compliant, and regressed. Katz writes:

It is not surprising that this model has been instinctively embraced by physicians and patients alike. Doctors embraced it because it called for unquestioning compliance, unilateral trust, and verbal silence. It appealed to patients, engulfed by pain and suffering, because surrender to powerful, wise, and soothing caretakers was strongly fostered by memories of earlier days when a parent satisfied all discomforting bodily needs. Thus, the regression to more childlike functioning that can result from illness becomes augmented by a patient's wish for caretaking by a parent–physician who, as memory informs, will immediately alleviate all suffering. The regression is also reinforced by doctors' proclivities to view patients as helpless and incompetent children.[3]

In reaction to this image of the infantilized patient, Katz painted a picture of the independent adult patient, allowed to exercise his "right to self-determination" by making well-informed decisions about his medical treatment. But this right became, in Katz's influential work, a right that the bearer had a duty to exercise:

Indeed, I take a further step and postulate a duty to reflection that cannot be easily waived. Asserting such a duty sounds strange. We are accustomed to recognizing a right to choice as an aspect of the right to self-determination, but a duty to reflection as a component of autonomy is quite another matter. Yet, if my views on psychological autonomy have merit, then respect for the right of self-determination requires respect for human beings' proclivities to exercise this right in both rational and irrational ways. Doctors are obliged to facilitate patients' opportunities for reflection to prevent ill-considered rational and irrational influences on choice.

Patients, in turn, are obligated to participate in the process of thinking about choices. In arguing that both parties make every effort to facilitate reflection in order to sort out the rational and irrational expectations that eventually can converge on choice, I express a value preference for the enhancement of individual psychological autonomy.

The patient might have to be encouraged to be autonomous and free. The exercise of choice, the making of one's own decisions, has become a duty. Informed choice is the patient's work. Moreover, it is part of the physician's moral function to lead the patient toward greater autonomy through the process of informed consent.

Behind the movement for patient autonomy lay not only reactions against dependency, distrust of authority, and an ideology of self-determination, but also an understanding of the psychology of illness. The control over bodily functions—from the regulation of excretory functions to speech and the purposive use of the limbs—is an early and significant developmental achievement, which is a source of childhood self-esteem as well as a precondition for socialization.

The loss of bodily control is a frequent, if not a universal, feature of physical illness, which, depending on the nature and severity of the illness as well as the life situation and personality of the patient, is often accompanied by feelings of shame and helplessness, and at times depression. Loss of bodily control involves a degree of loss of self-control because our sense of self is woven into our relationship to our bodies. A burgeoning psychological literature from the 1960s and 1970s based on a "learned helplesness" model of depression argued for the importance of active control over one's environment as a key to maintaining self-esteem in the face of adversity or failure.

In the face of physical illness, the patient's "taking control" became a therapeutic act. For some proponents of patient autonomy, control involved not only becoming informed—understanding one's illness and knowing what to expect—but making decisions as well. Controlling one's own treatment decisions was part and parcel of overcoming one's illness. The duty to control was simultaneously a moral duty to make one's own decisions, a therapeutic requirement for psychological health, and part of the social obligation to get well.

In retrospect, the psychological assumptions underpinning the autonomy model can seem naive. How can Katz's patient, who he describes as "engulfed by pain and suffering," be expected to exercise his right—his duty—to self-determination by making complex medical decisions? Should we condemn the dependency needs—or wishes—of sick people or assume that those needs are a form of false consciousness created by an authoritarian social structure of which the traditional doctor–patient relationship forms a part? Moreover, even if assuming active control helps many people cope with the psychological threats of illness, what of those patients to whom such control is psychologically unwelcome or emotionally detrimental? Should they be manipulated, cajoled, coerced, forced to decide? Carl Schneider, who in *The Practice of Autonomy* critically examines the vaunted benefit as well as the assumed desire of the sick to be in control of medical decision making, concludes:

> Real people are stubbornly more complicated than this model supposes. Some people may behave as autonomists imagine, but an imposing number of them act quite differently. Their desire for information is more equivocal than the model assumes; their taste for rational analysis is less pronounced; their personal beliefs are not as well developed, relevant, or strong; and their desire for control is more partial, ambivalent, and complex.[4]

Dissatisfaction with the simplifications and excesses of an individualist, autonomy-centered ethical model, and with the contractual and consumerist conception of medical treatment that usually accompanies it, has led to alternative methodological approaches to medical ethics and alternative models of the doctor–patient relationship.

Some of these newer models expand upon the concept of autonomy to encompass more than the mere exercise of control through decision making. Ezekiel and Linda Emanuel, for example, recognized that the paternalistic model of the doctor–patient relationship in which autonomy had meant patient assent had been replaced in practice by an informative model in which "the conception of patient autonomy is patient control over decision making."[5] They favored interpretive and deliberative forms of autonomy, in which patient self-understanding and moral development, rather than patient control, were the central moral ends that emerged from the doctor–patient relationship. And Brody, as we have seen, situated himself within an emerging medical ethics of collaboration and mutuality in the doctor–patient relationship, in contrast to both the medical ethics of paternalism and the medical ethics of rights-centered autonomy. This mutualist medical ethics, emphasizing the collaboration between doctor and patient, included a "renewed sense of the values of the profession of medicine as well as a more communitarian ethic generally."

Table 2.1 Comparison of Three Models of the Doctor–Patient Relationship

	Paternalism	Autonomy	Mutuality
M.D.	Diagnoses	Presents choices	Contextualizes
	Prescribes	Informs	Converses
	Protects	Leaves alone (doesn't interfere)	Empowers
		Executes/complies	Interprets
			Constructs
Patient	Defers	Questions	Collaborates
	Complies	Chooses	Converses
		Decides	Constructs
		Controls	Changes

If the patient's work in the paternalistic ethic is the performance of a sick role and in the autonomy ethic the making of decisions and taking of control, then what is the patient's work in the mutualist ethic? Brody, as we have seen, wishes the doctor–patient relationship to resemble an ongoing dialogue through which patient and physician place the patient's medical choices within the context of the patient's life plans. And Arthur Frank, a sociologist of illness and advocate for the ethical importance of illness narratives, writes of one type of illness narrative—the "quest stories"—that they "meet suffering head on; they accept illness and seek to *use* it. Illness is the occasion of a journey that becomes a quest."[6] The mutualist patient's work appears to be engagement in a conversation, construction of a meaningful life narrative, and the use of illness as a means of self-understanding and change. The hard-working mutualist patient uses his illness and suffering to create something—a narrative that bears witness to his experience or a tool in his struggle with suffering. The successful mutualist patient transforms his illness, and himself, into a "good story," as the writer Anatole Broyard wished himself—and his case of prostate cancer—to become. Although these literary products may represent exceptional results of the patient's work, it is useful to see them as examples of what the mutualist ethic calls for from the patient.

The patient's work recognizes the psychological importance for the patient of having an activity, of participating in the process of treatment, of exercising control in a situation of loss of control. The autonomy model recognizes that one way that people achieve a sense of control is by being informed and making decisions. Unfortunately, it fails to appreciate that other ways that people achieve a sense of control may include obedience or distraction or denial or telling stories. These ways are recognized by the other models.

Comparing the Models

To view these models through the prism of the concept of the patient's work, we compare them (Table 2.1) in terms of the characteristic activities of the doctor and the characteristic activities of the patient.

In many obvious ways the three models conflict: The deferential, compliant patient of the paternalistic model is incompatible with the questioning, choosing, deciding, controlling patient of the autonomy model. From another perspective, they are related dialectically—as thesis, antithesis, and synthesis, with the mutualist synthesis combining elements of the first two to produce something different from either. Yet in another respect, they are disjunctive—and therefore not in conflict—in that they apply under different medical circumstances and in different social contexts. We generally accept that in emergency situations doctors can behave paternalistically, attending first and foremost to diagnosing and treating the medical condition—serving the patient's immediate health interests—and taking the patient's autonomy rights and life plan into consideration only secondarily, unless they are clearly known ahead of time. Similarly, a consultation with a specialist unknown to the patient who recommends an invasive treatment might best fall under an autonomy model, in which the patient questions, gathers information, solicits different opinions, and decides for himself. The treatment of insulin-dependent diabetes in a primary care setting, on the other hand, might best be understood as an ongoing dialogue between doctor and patient in which an understanding of the meaning to and impact upon the patient of the illness and its treatment form the context within which choices are made and the treatment is conducted.

Yet another way of understanding these three models is that they correspond to different psychological types of patients, which we might call the dependent patient, the "take charge" patient, and the conversational or meaning-seeking patient. Different personality styles and psychological needs will fit best with each of the models. And if patient empowerment and avoidance of patient coercion by the physician are ethical aspects of all doctor–patient relationships, then adaptation of the relationship to fit patient styles and needs would place each model on an equal ethical plane. When it comes to doctor–patient relationships, one size does not fit all, and insisting that they do disrespects the individuality of the patient.

Each of these three relational models may come into play in one and the same treatment. Consider, for example, the treatment by a psychiatrist of a patient with bipolar disorder—a chronic, remitting, and recurring illness—that involves both psychopharmacology and psychotherapy. During asymptomatic periods the focus of the treatment will most resemble a conversation in which perceptions, meanings, and life plans will be explored, contextualized, interpreted, and constructed. When medications are changed, the psychiatrist is likely to present the patient with information, choices,

and a recommendation, leaving the patient to decide, although a discussion of the meaning of the medication change to the patient may be a part of the process. At times of crisis, such as an acute manic episode in which the patient has lost any insight into his illness, the psychiatrist will behave paternalistically, prescribing a treatment—hospitalization, for example—with limited if any choice or discussion.

What does this example tell us? First, it implies again that the different models apply in different clinical situations and that treatment situations are constantly evolving. Moreover, it helps us see that all three models (and perhaps others as well) are in play simultaneously in the complex reality of many treatment situations. Because these models are ideal types that are heuristically useful rather than empirical descriptions of actual relationships, it is not surprising that they are found to coexist in the "real world" of doctors and patients. The patient's "own good"—his health interests—coexists with his right to self-determination, which lives alongside his overarching life plans. At times, the patient is obeying, at times, choosing and deciding, at times, formulating, narrating, and making meaning. Or, rather, he may be doing all these things simultaneously.

The notion of the patient's work implies that the patient can fail to perform his work or work badly. Noncompliance is the best known form of the patient's failure to do his work in the paternalistic model. Passivity, dependence, and indecisiveness would represent poor work for the autonomist's patient. Resistance to conversation, narrative incoherence, or an absence of life plans would constitute poor work in the mutualist paradigm. All three paradigms therefore seem to *prescribe* the nature of the patient's work, as either compliance with doctor's orders or active control over medical decisionmaking or engagement in ongoing exploration of the meaning and place of illness in the patient's life.

In addition to prescribing forms of work to the patient, each of the three models assigns the physician a moral function alongside his technical function. The paternalistic model assigns the doctor the moral function of trustee of the patient's health interests. In the autonomy model, the physician is the facilitator of the patient's autonomy, as epitomized in the process of informed consent, through which, when properly enacted, the patient is engaged as a moral agent in his own treatment. In the mutualist model, the doctor's moral function is as interlocutor in a conversation on the meaning and living of the patient's life.

All three models, then, give both doctor and patient moral work to do with the aim of restoring the patient's health or relieving suffering. They allow the doctor to be engaged with the patient but at the same time detached from him, as in Renee Fox's classic formulation of "detached concern" and, more recently, Brody's notion of the physician's "empathic curiosity." Similarly, our concept of the patient's work allows the patient to be engaged with his illness yet not under its sway. If the patient has work to do, then the patient is not defined entirely by his illness. His illness becomes the object of his work, and he the subject. At the very least, the patient's work—whether enacting the sick role, participating in decisionmaking, or narrating his experience—provides the patient with an organizing set of responses to the condition of illness and, therefore, a framework within which to live in relation to it.

In our society, work is an important source of personal and social dignity. Conceiving of the patient as having work to do is a means of dignifying the patient's activities, of thinking about the patient as an active agent, engaged in directed, purposive activity toward an end. Seeking empathically to understand what the patient is engaged in during the process of his illness can enable those involved in treating him to see the person beneath and beyond the patient. This can help the patient maintain a sense of himself as a person during a life-altering experience such as serious illness and, therefore, maintain a sense of his dignity despite the indignities inflicted by disease.

But this requires that those treating him understand that individual psychologies can differ significantly, and that one person's way of working at maintaining his personal dignity (by making his own decisions, for example) may be quite different from another's (by obediently following doctor's orders, for example). We should not make metaphysical assumptions about the universally valid goods of life, which both the autonomy model and the mutualist model seem to make, implying that the work of making one's own decisions or of finding meaning is the proper work of humans.

Indeed, the invisibility of the patient's work—its hitherto absence from the conceptual lexicon of medical ethics—may derive in part from the fact that the healthy take health for granted and have difficulty seeing the work involved in coping with illness. Especially for people with serious or chronic illnesses, which may have a profound impact on global functioning—such as the bipolar patient we described earlier—to accept and stick with a treatment regimen despite distressing side effects and to be willing to experiment to find acceptable, if not optimal, therapy all involve work on the part of the patient.

The concept of the patient's work can serve as an organizing metaphor for physician and patient as they forge a therapeutic relationship. It reminds the physician that the patient is an active participant in the process of treatment, even if that activity may take various forms, from compliance to decisionmaking to conversing. It encourages the doctor to understand the patient's particular manner of working and to work with it himself. It can also serve as a heuristic device in educating medical students and house staff. We hope that the concept and the attendant clinical skills will help physicians integrate as part of *their* work the facilitation of the patient's work. This can enhance the doctor's ability to see beyond the patient to the person and improve the quality of medical care by rendering it both psychologically richer and morally more dignity preserving and, therefore, more humane.

Notes

1. H. Brody, *The Healer's Power* (New Haven, CT: Yale University Press, 1992), 36.

2. T. Parsons, *The Social System* (New York: Free Press, 1951), 436–7.

3. J. Katz, *The Silent World of Doctor and Patient* (New York: Free Press, 1984), 100–101.

4. C.E. Schneider, *The Practice of Autonomy: Patients, Doctors, and Medical Decisions* (New York: Oxford University Press, 1998), 229.

5. E.J. Emanuel and L.L. Emanuel, Four models of the physician-patient relationship. *JAMA* 267 (1992): 2221.

6. A. Frank, *The Wounded Storyteller*, (Chicago: University of Chicago Press, 1995), 115.

Limits on Patient Responsibility

MAUREEN KELLEY

Journal of Medicine and Philosophy 30 (2005): 189–206.

I. Introduction

Should a cardiac patient who deliberately fails to take his or her meds on time, misses appointments, and eats all meals out of a deep fryer be chided for his or her irresponsible behavior? Who should do the chiding? Can the cardiologist refuse to treat him or her? Does it make a moral difference if the patient is blocking the arteries to a newly transplanted heart versus his or her own sick heart?

Since its birth as a profession medical ethics has primarily concerned itself with defining the duties of physicians toward patients. The emphasis on protecting patients' rights provided an important corrective to a field dominated by a deeply ingrained paternalism. Questions like those above cause a certain amount of discomfort in the clinical setting, in part because many health professionals do not feel they have the moral and legal grounds to demand responsible behavior from patients and in part because such demands are out of step with the now dominant emphasis on patient choice. Holding patients responsible for adhering to treatment plans and living a healthy life, smacks of the old paternalism that much of medical culture prides itself

on rejecting. Yet health professionals are understandably frustrated with the overwhelming burden of clinical and legal responsibility for patients' well being. The emerging discussion in the clinical literature on patient compliance and recent attempts in medical ethics to offer up lists of patient responsibilities signal this frustration and an underlying desire to bring the moral pendulum back toward the middle by increasing patient accountability.

Some specific suggestions for increasing patient responsibility include the use of patient agreements whereby a patient agrees to certain terms in the physician-patient relationship, such as coming to appointments, taking prescribed medications as indicated, asking questions, and informing the physician of symptoms. Some hospitals are distributing lists of patient responsibilities, included among the admissions paperwork, with similar promises to give full histories, follow plans of care, ask questions, and report symptoms.

In 1993 the American Medical Association put forward a similar list of patient responsibilities that included a commitment to take preventive steps to maintain one's health (American Medical

Association, 1993). The standard rationale offered is: "to provide the best care possible," or "to meet your healthcare goals," and there is no mention (in print) of penalties or repercussions for failing to meet one's responsibilities as a patient.

The status of such lists and agreements remains unclear. Unlike signing a consent form, it is not yet the case that breach of a patient promise to take prescribed medications or follow dietary orders provides moral or legal grounds for firing the patient from one's service or hospital. What if patient contracts were to achieve the same moral and legal status as consent forms? There are tangible consequences for a physician who fails to meet his or her professional obligations: he or she may be reprimanded, censured by professional societies, fired, lose his or her license, be suspended, or be sued. Even if none of those things happens, he or she may, through word of mouth, lose the trust of patients. Living up to professional obligations is awarded with professional approval and a stable, trusting patient following. Such penalties and awards comprise part of an effective system of costs and benefits that encourages compliance with professional moral norms. In terms of practical morality, it is difficult to imagine any meaningful norms of responsibility that are not reinforced in some way, where there are not consequences for following or failing to follow the standards of responsible behavior. Anything else would seem to be moral window dressing.

But what would holding patients responsible for behavior affecting health and treatment mean in practice, if the lists of patient responsibilities amount to more than mere suggestions? Should patients be encouraged to behave responsibly in hopes of winning the trust and approval of physicians, or perhaps the fear of being chastised, transferred to another physician, or dropped as a patient? Should a system of patient responsibilities mirror the current norms for professional responsibility among health professionals? If so, there would be repercussions for failing in one's obligations as a patient. A patient could be fired or asked to switch physicians. A patient could

be blamed for the negative consequences of bad behavior, poor diet, or harmful habits, perhaps mitigating physician responsibility for rescuing the patient through continued treatment. Perhaps patients could even be fined or sued for wasting precious resources or a physician's time.

It is important to ask what we hope to accomplish by promoting norms of patient responsibility more forcefully and what other valuable norms governing clinical ethics might be in jeopardy if we do so. It is also not clear that we should develop a one-size-fits-all model of patient responsibility—it may be unreasonable to expect the average patient to live up to the standards of a heart transplant patient. So far, those calling for increased patient responsibility have not adequately addressed what a robust account of patient responsibility, with consequences attached to performance and failure, would mean for patients and patient choice.

As we try to focus more attention on the duties of patients we should also keep in mind the moral norms that would constrain any positive account of patient responsibility, and that is what I offer here. There are several established and valuable moral norms in clinical practice at stake in the responsibility debate, including the doctrine of informed refusals and norms encouraging nonjudgmental compassionate care.

I will defend the idea that a medical culture with a more moderate notion of patient responsibility is preferable to any system of enforced patient responsibilities (where enforcement includes the possibility of being dropped or transferred as a patient, verbally reprimanded, or penalized in other ways) because it remains compatible with these important norms.

A moderate notion of patient responsibility will remain one based on persuasion, not punishment, and will be forward-looking, that is, based on encouragement and caution regarding future consequences rather than blame for past behavior.

In arguing for a significantly constrained model of patient responsibility, I will defend two moral asymmetries in clinical ethics:

1. Even if some degree of responsible behavior from patients is called for, placing greater emphasis on professional responsibility over patient responsibility is largely correct, and

2. we have good reason to emphasize prospective rather than retrospective notions of responsibility in clinical practice.

That is, I want to defend a very limited scope for blame at the bedside.

II. The First Asymmetry: Professional Obligations Over Patient Obligations

It is true, as some have argued, that medical ethics has placed a one-sided emphasis on the ethical obligations of physicians to the exclusion of patient obligations, but not without good reason (Draper & Sorell, 2002). While there is some room to argue for increased patient responsibility, there are significant historical and moral reasons to continue emphasizing the importance of physician obligations over patient obligations.

The first reason for maintaining this imbalance of obligations in the medical profession is to heed the lessons of history. In medicine's not-so-distant past the inequality of expertise between physician and patient was systematically abused. The account of patient obligation from the 1847 American Medical Association's *Code of Ethics* reminds us of the profession's starting point: "The obedience of a patient to the prescriptions of his physician should be prompt and implicit. He should never permit his own crude opinions as to their fitness, to influence his attention to them" (AMA, 1847).

The idea of therapeutic privilege was not what it is now—a narrow and highly criticized exception to informed consent—it was an unquestioned starting point that permeated the profession. The inequality of expertise was used to justify an "ideology of professionalism," a widespread belief among physicians and patients that physicians know best and ought to be trusted to make choices on a patient's behalf (Katz, 1984). Proposing patient compliance or adherence

to a treatment plan as part of standard patient responsibilities harkens back to the old obedience model of medicine, especially if accompanied by threats of being transferred or dropped as a patient. Even physician disapproval can be a powerful incentive for going along with a treatment plan, especially for a patient who naturally defers to the authority of the physician from the start. The norms guarding against professional abuse of expertise continue to successfully protect adult patients from unwarranted interference into personal and weighty life and death decisions.

Do we really need to worry about regressing to the medical ethics of 1847? Probably not. Widespread, systematic medical paternalism is an historical phenomenon we seem to have outgrown in the health professions and it is doubtful that anyone could turn back the tide of increased patient autonomy. However, a deep fact about the structure of contemporary health professions has not changed, and will not likely ever change—and this fact motivates some vigilance over patient autonomy. There is an inherent imbalance in the relationship between patients and health experts that makes these relationships susceptible to subtler forms of paternalism. An underlying inequality characterizes any relationship that includes an expert and a layperson. Even an intelligent layperson capable of downloading and studying outside information about a disease, architectural blueprints, a critical summary of James Joyce's *Ulysses*, or a ready-made prenuptial agreement will still have to trust, respectively, the physician, architect, literature professor, or lawyer to offer honest and unbiased (or at least honestly biased) assistance in understanding these technical areas.

The need for trust in a relationship signals areas of imbalance where one person depends on another not to take advantage of a person's vulnerability or relative ignorance. In professions where the guidance sought regularly affects lives, a robust culture of professional responsibility guards against negligence, carelessness, and abuse that may cause lasting harm. More positively put, a strong role for professional responsibility engenders trust. Several late nights studying a textbook in internal medicine or perusing the Mayo Clinic's online description of a disease and its management cannot match a consultation with a person with a decade or more of training and possibly years of practical, clinical wisdom, including the very important human, non-virtual, emotional support. The conditions for a trusting relationship are built from these real-time encounters, but the encounters are also prone to the subtle forces of disapproval, withholding information, or emphasizing some information more than other information.

Despite the great strides toward real patient autonomy and an increase in the number of patients who are actively involved in their own care or care of family members, a fundamental inequality of information, expertise, and power persists in the physician-patient relationship (and arguably in relationships with other health professionals). In this sense physicians should have a greater responsibility to know the relevant technical information, ensure a patient's understanding, and support a patient's deliberation and choices.

The concern expressed here is that health professionals will be tempted to nudge patients into clinical plans favored by the health team in the name of "holding a patient responsible." That is, being a "responsible patient" will be too easily confused with the idea of being a "compliant patient," ushering in subtle, and perhaps not-so-subtle, forms of medical paternalism. Some, however, have lodged precisely the opposite worry: that a weak notion of patient responsibility encourages patients not to consider the consequences of their actions and to instead allow responsibility to fall on the shoulders of caregivers. Criticizing our current system which emphasizes patient autonomy over responsibility, Draper and Sorell have expressed concern that interpreting patient autonomy as mere participation in decisions, rather than a willingness to consider the consequences, leaves it up to physicians to protect patients from the consequences of their decisions, thereby reinforcing paternalistic behavior on the part of physicians (Draper & Sorell, 2002). This seems mistaken on empirical grounds.

First, the widely accepted practice of informed consent in this country, Europe, and the United Kingdom is not one of "mere participation." The concerted move toward more rigorous standards for informed consent and easier patient access to health information on the Internet have led to more active patient participation in decision-making. In theory, the doctrine of informed consent and refusal implies a limit on interfering in a competent adult's decision. In clinical practice it is perfectly compatible with that principled limit for a physician to try to persuade a patient by pointing out the possibly dire consequences of the patient's irresponsible behavior. As long as coercive or manipulative tactics are avoided, such discussions amount to rational persuasion, not paternalism. This gives physicians a good deal of room to discuss adverse consequences with patients and to encourage patients to take responsibility for the consequences of their actions. Substantial economic pressures also encourage patients to consider the cost-saving value of preventive health measures, including healthy behaviors, and award those patients who behave responsibly with lower insurance premiums.

The increasing transparency of clinical practice and wider availability of medical information through the Internet and advertisement give patients the tools for making active and responsible health choices. It does not, then, seem obvious that a heavier emphasis on physician responsibility over patient responsibility will encourage paternalism, in part because of prudential pressures on the patient to behave responsibly, but also as a result of a heavy emphasis on the physician's responsibility to fully inform a patient about the consequences of her decisions. Advocates of increased patient responsibility should not overlook the significant increase in patient responsibility resulting from our autonomy-driven medical ethics.

Let me then sum up the defense of the first asymmetry between professional obligations and patient obligations: The shift to a model of medical decision-making that includes patients as active participants has been driven by moral and legal arguments for the doctrine of informed consent and its derivative, the right to refuse treatment. These arguments place greater emphasis on the duties of a physician not to abuse the role of expert and to rectify the imbalance of knowledge between physicians and patients through the process of informed consent and open communication. Because the inequality of expertise is inherent in any skill-based profession, and given the past record of systemic disregard for patient choice in the history of medicine, it seems appropriate to maintain a system of professional duties that places greater responsibility on the shoulders of the ones who know.

What was wrong with the old paternalistic ideology in medicine was not so much that physicians did not really know what was best for patients—at least in a clinical sense they often *do* know what is best and that expertise carries with it greater responsibility—the mistake was to confuse greater responsibility with the notion of greater authority over a patient's choices and preferences about life and death. Old concerns about paternalism arise when we consider how patient responsibilities will be enforced. Being a good and responsible patient should not mean following a physician's orders and treatment plan without question. Unless we are willing to substantially revise the arguments against medical paternalism and our ethical standard of care regarding the choices of competent adult patients, we should not seriously consider a robust account of patient responsibility, especially one that includes penalties such as being dropped or transferred for failing to adhere to a treatment plan.

III. The Second Asymmetry: Prospective over Retrospective Responsibility

One way to assign patients responsibility without violating physicians' obligations to patients, including those implied by the doctrine of informed consent and refusal, is to assign responsibility prospectively. What we mean by responsibility depends, in large part, on whether we are facing forward or looking backward. Forward-looking, or prospective, responsibility is reflected in this public health announcement that airs on our local television channel: "Take charge of your body and your life!" The ad educates young African-American women in the community to seek family planning, education, and career training advice. The ad does not blame unmarried, pregnant teenagers for messing up lives when they should know better. The latter would involve a backward looking or retrospective notion of responsibility.

Roughly put, forward-looking responsibility encourages preventive, responsible behavior in the hopes of avoiding bad consequences for the person, third parties, and society at large. Backward looking or retrospective responsibility is about culpability, assigning blame, figuring out who caused the present state of affairs. Prospective is about taking responsibility for present actions and future consequences and retrospective is about holding someone responsible or urging someone to take responsibility for a past action and its present consequences. We can also put a more positive spin on each perspective. The causal trail backward can lead us to praise the person responsible for doing something good. And the trail forward can help guide people in taking an active role in plans for the future (rather than simply thinking of responsible behavior as avoiding mistakes). Two features of the health professions support forward-looking notions of responsibility. The complicated causal nature of health and disease and the central virtues of being a good care giver should lead us to resist a blame centered, backward looking notion of patient responsibility.

A. Factors Leading to Illness

Holding someone responsible, blaming a person, has traditionally required that two conditions be met: the person committed a wrongful act and the person could have done otherwise or can offer no excuse for his actions. In health and disease, especially, this counterfactual test is, practically speaking, useless. To a significant degree each person's state of health is determined by his or her genetic makeup and the environment he or she was exposed to during development, as well as workplace and other environmental influences. Such influences are largely outside an individual patient's control. Much of illness is a matter of bad luck, whether in the genetic lottery, social lottery, or both.

Disease is also caused by voluntary, intentional behavior on the part of many patients: patients who knew better, had a sufficiently decent lot in life to afford basic medical care and a healthy diet, and, yet, took risks that resulted in illness. A patient can certainly contribute to his or her health or illness. Genetic disposition alone is not sufficient to undercut responsibility for one's health or disease, since dispositions leave many patients room to behave responsibly in managing an inherited disorder. A family history of heart disease, breast cancer, or diabetes is a good example of dispositions for illness that need not develop into the disease with interventions taken earlier on in life. Some interventions are well known and not costly, such as dietary habits and weight maintenance. Knowledge of a genetic disposition and full information about behavioral changes that are likely to decrease one's chance of developing the disease give a patient some control over the outcome.

On one end of the spectrum are those cases of clear, genetic bad luck: Tay Sach's, Huntington's, cystic fibrosis. To the degree that such individuals could not have chosen their genes, by the "could have done otherwise" test, they should not be held responsible for their resulting illness and the hardship of managing it. Toward the other end of the spectrum are those cases that have triggered the debate about patient responsibility:

disorders associated with alcoholism, drug use, smoking, or obesity. While genetic dispositions may make some people more susceptible to the ill effects of these habits, or more prone to addiction, a significant percentage of cases could have been prevented by the individuals. Knowledge of the consequences of these behaviors is now more widely known, thanks to public health initiatives, advertisement, and education. Still, there are environmental factors like poverty and other socio-economic markers that may mitigate individual responsibility in many of these behavior-driven cases.

B. Responding to Vulnerability

Even in the cases where it can be shown that a patient had a great deal of control over a harmful, costly, devastating outcome, doling out responsibility in the backward-looking sense would violate a valuable norm and an equally valuable virtue central to the health professions: the duty to treat those in need without making treatment contingent on moral approval and the virtue of compassion toward those who are vulnerable. Even if a patient "could have done otherwise," and this causal story could be accurately traced, chastising a patient for contributing to his or her condition would show a deep lack of compassion, and failing to treat the patient or transferring the patient would violate the duty to treat. In fact, the very attempt to develop a strong notion of patient responsibility can be seen as way of motivating exceptions to the duty to treat compassionately and without moral judgment. Draper and Sorrell develop this idea in the notion of doctors as "captive helpers." They point out that physicians are permitted to end a relationship with a patient in only exceptional circumstances and even if such a relationship is broken, the system is designed in such a way that someone else (another physician or another hospital) will provide care for the patient (Draper & Sorell, 2002, pp. 347–350). They ask whether such captivity is fair and whether "it protects an interest so vital that the one-sidedness is acceptable" (p. 347).

In the account offered here, I am taking the latter position: the one-sidedness is vital. True, one of the implications of the account being offered here is a higher rate of captivity among health professionals, but I think that is to cast the issue in somewhat misleading negative terms. Put more positively, I am reinforcing a virtue of health professionals by characterizing such individuals as people who choose to enter fields wherein they are regularly called on to suspend moral judgment and help those whom few others would be willing or able to help.

Regardless of the causal factors contributing to disease, being sick is an inherently vulnerable position to be in and health care givers are often our only way out of such a predicament. As patients we find ourselves in a situation of relative dependence on our caregivers. Categorizing someone as vulnerable serves as a central signal for the moral responses of others and operates in law and policy as a signal for protection, but it is also important to understand the real consequences of the label "vulnerable." Too much emphasis on patient vulnerability can usher in paternalism. By bringing attention to a person or group it can single them out as weak, as in need of unwelcome assistance or pity. Consider, for example, the debate over the category of "vulnerable subjects" in research. Many advocates of the elderly did not want to be included alongside animals, pregnant women, children, and prisoners because they were concerned about undue protections. A similar worry motivated attempts to retract some of the protective regulations governing research on children and pregnant women. A way around this concern is not to equate patient vulnerability with incompetence or extreme weakness but as relative powerlessness and dependence on another, to think of vulnerability as characterizing the relevant relationships and appropriate responses within those relationships.

Does this relegate the average health professional to the category of martyr by virtue of their professional membership? To some degree, yes, there is an inherent element of self-sacrifice involved in these professions. This is hardly shocking news. There are many worthy professions that require a degree of self-sacrifice in exchange for other rewards, sometimes monetary, sometimes personal or moral satisfaction, fame, or a sense of making a contribution. It is a virtue found in political office, military service, social and political activism, humanitarian work, teaching, pro bono legal work or civil rights work, and first-responder professions. Those health professionals who endure extraordinary sacrifices in the course of medical practice would likely see the element of self-sacrifice in treating the enemy in war, for example, or serving in urban areas with high levels of gang-related injuries and sometimes abusive and dangerous patients, as the *call* of duty, not above and beyond. Dealing with the occasional noncompliant or irresponsible patient in the line of duty is the small price health professionals pay in order to uphold a long tradition of treating first, asking questions later, and leaving the job of moral enforcer to someone who is not at the bedside.

One way to understand the depth of this professional virtue is to think about what we mean by the virtue of forgiveness. Peter Strawson has characterized blame as withdrawing good will. Forgiveness can be understood as extending good will when we may have good reason to withdraw it. In its most generous and pure form care giving is about extending good will despite strong temptations to withdraw it. Traditionally, the threshold for withdrawing good will for a profession that is centrally about aid, rescue, and curing should be higher than a profession such as, say, music, that is about developing certain skills.

Some examples in medicine include treating an injured enemy in war, treating gunshot wounds and stab wounds (the results of gang violence) in an urban emergency room, or the duty to stabilize patients under the federal anti-dumping law, EMTALA, that prevents hospitals from refusing to accept patients who face life and death emergencies. We can certainly blame the individuals for crimes committed, hold prisoners of war accountable for their actions, and seek preventive social measures to stop gang violence, but punishing the injured person or allowing him to suffer would be inhumane. That the health professions have long cultivated this generous moral response to those society would blame for wrongdoing is a mark of moral distinction for the health professions. In choosing to be a health professional one takes on a general moral stance that goes above and beyond the call of duty for the average person. In this sense being a physician or nurse is choosing a life in relatively supererogatory professions, so too with those who choose the life of a missionary or aid worker or public servant.

One of the values of these extraordinary moral standards, in addition to reinforcing a sense of professional pride, is that the way in which compassion can foster patients' trust toward health professionals. Trust in turn becomes instrumental in changing the future behavior of patients through open lines of communication. Almost all patients are to varying degrees vulnerable in this sense and in relationships involving trust, vulnerability calls for compassion not blame. Once someone becomes sick and arrives in the clinical setting in need of help, it should cease to matter how the patient got there from the point of view of the immediate caregivers. Stronger emphasis on patient responsibility, including backward looking judgments of blame at the bedside, would seriously undermine this conception of a caregiver's virtue. Vulnerability of patients as a class of moral agent calls for limited patient responsibility, responsibility without threats of being transferred, dropped, given an ultimatum, or penalized for non-adherence.

References

American Medical Association *Code of Ethics* (1847), Chapter 1, Article II, "Obligations of Patients to their Physicians." In J. Katz, *The Silent World of Doctor and Patient* edited by J. Katz, 231–33. New York: Free Press, 1984.

American Medical Association *Code of ethics* (1993), "On Patient Responsibilities," updated June 1998, December 2000, and June 2001, Section E-10.02.

Draper, H., & Sorell, T. "Patients' Responsibilities in Medical Ethics." *Bioethics* 16, no. 4 (2002): 335–52.

Katz, J. *The Silent World of Doctor and Patient*. New York: Collier Macmillan Free Press, 1984.

Cosmetic Surgery and the Internal Morality of Medicine

FRANKLIN G. MILLER, HOWARD BRODY, AND KEVIN C. CHUNG

Cambridge Quarterly of Healthcare Ethics 9 (2000): 353–64.

Cosmetic surgery is a fast-growing medical practice. In 1997 surgeons in the United States performed the four most common cosmetic procedures—liposuction, breast augmentation, eyelid surgery, and facelift—443,728 times, an increase of 150% over the comparable total for 1992. Estimated total expenditures for cosmetic surgery range from $1 to $2 billion. As managed care cuts into physicians' income and autonomy, cosmetic surgery, which is not covered by health insurance, offers a financially attractive medical specialty.

Although increasingly popular, cosmetic surgery is a most unusual medical practice. Invasive surgical operations performed on healthy bodies for the sake of improving appearance lie far outside the core domain of medicine as a profession dedicated to saving lives, healing, and promoting health. These cosmetic procedures are not medically indicated for a diagnosable medical condition. Yet they pose risks, cause side effects, and are subject to complications, including pain, bruising, swelling, discoloration, infections, formation of scar tissue, nerve damage, hardening of implants, etc. Moreover, cosmetic surgery is a consumer oriented entrepreneurial practice, heavily promoted by advertising in newspapers, magazines, the yellow pages of the telephone directory, and by marketing on the World Wide Web. The remarkable nature of cosmetic surgery is reflected on in the following comments of a plastic surgeon: "But then on top of it all we actually operate on people who are normal. It's amazing that we're allowed to do that, the idea that we can get a permit to operate on someone who is totally normal is an unbelievable privilege."

Is cosmetic surgery a medical privilege or an abuse of medical knowledge and skill? With the exception of feminist scholarship, which focuses on the personal and social meaning and value of cosmetic surgery for the lives of women, the bioethics literature has neglected to pay attention to moral issues posed by cosmetic surgery. In this article we examine cosmetic surgery from the perspective of professional integrity and the internal morality of medicine.

The Internal Morality of Medicine

All members of our society are likely to become patients, vulnerable to life-threatening or disrupting conditions and in need of medical attention and treatment to cure, prevent, or ameliorate disease, injury, or bodily dysfunction. Owing to this vulnerability and need for professional care, medicine is not a morally neutral technique. Rather, it is a professional practice governed by a moral framework consisting of goals proper to medicine, role-specific duties, and clinical virtues. We call this framework "the internal morality of medicine." The professional integrity of physicians is constituted by loyalty and adherence to this internal morality.

A variety of formulations have been proposed for the goals of medicine. A recent report of an international group of scholars, convened by The Hastings Center, recommended a comprehensive list of four goals: (i) "the prevention of disease and injury and promotion and maintenance of health"; (ii) "the relief of pain and suffering caused by maladies"; (iii) "the care and cure of those with a malady, and the care of those who cannot be cured"; and (iv) "the avoidance of premature death and the pursuit of a peaceful death." For our inquiry into the ethics of cosmetic surgery, this list is noteworthy in two respects. The designation of multiple goals signifies that medicine is too complex and diverse in its legitimate scope to be encompassed by any single, essential goal, such as healing or promoting health. If healing is the single essential goal of medicine, then it is obvious that cosmetic surgery does not belong within legitimate medical practice. But this essentialist perspective would also rule out a variety of medical practices, such as contraception and sterilization, which prima facie are not devoted to healing or promoting health but are widely accepted as medically appropriate. The diversity of goals proper to medicine, and their openness to interpretation, makes mapping the moral domain of medicine complex and contested. Though broad in its scope, this list of goals is subject to limits. The central goal of relief of pain and suffering is confined to conditions that qualify as "maladies." What counts as a malady warranting medical attention may be subject to conflicting interpretations and may change over time. The important qualification, however, means that it is not within the purview of physicians to attempt to relieve any and all pain and suffering that may afflict human beings.

Specification of the goals of medicine is necessary but not sufficient for mapping the normative domain of medicine. In addition to being oriented to a set of proper goals, medicine is guided and constrained by a set of internal duties that pertain to the legitimacy of practices in pursuit of medical goals. We have identified four internal duties incumbent on physicians of integrity: (i) competence in the technical and humanistic skills required to practice medicine; (ii) avoiding disproportionate harms that are not balanced by the prospect of compensating medical benefits; (iii) refraining from the fraudulent misrepresentation of medicine as a scientific practice and clinical art; and (iv) fidelity to the therapeutic relationship with patients in need of care.

Mapping the Normative Domain of Medicine

One of the major purposes of a conception of the internal morality of medicine is normative evaluation of practices by physicians to determine or question whether they belong within the proper domain of medicine. Violations of the internal morality of medicine consist of practices that are not supported by the goals of medicine and/or conflict with one or more of the internal duties of physicians. Examples include physician participation in capital punishment by lethal injection and prescribing anabolic steroids for athletes. Since these practices have nothing to do with treating or preventing a disease, injury, or malady, they do not serve the goals of medicine. Both involve causing or risking harms that are not compensated by medical benefits. Their performance by physicians fraudulently misrepresents medical practice by suggesting that it is proper for a physician to execute criminals or prescribe drugs to enhance athletic prowess. In addition, capital punishment is inconsistent with the context of a therapeutic relationship between physician and patient. Surgical procedures performed by a physician on close family members offer another example of a violation of the internal morality of medicine. Here the violation does not concern the goals of medicine, assuming that the procedure is medically indicated. However, the close family relationship has the potential to interfere substantially with competence (by impairing objectivity, clinical judgment, and thoroughness of medical inquiry) and with the therapeutic relationship between physician and patient.

In a previous essay we discussed a number of "borderline" medical practices, which belong within the legitimate domain of medicine but are not clearly supported by the goals of medicine and seem to conflict to some extent with one or more of the internal duties. Examples include contraception and sterilization. On further reflection, we suggest that it is preferable to describe such procedures and practices as "peripheral" rather than borderline, since there are no precise, specifiable borders circumscribing unqualifiedly legitimate medical practices and defining violations. Among the definitions of "periphery" is "a zone constituting an imprecise boundary," which we think aptly characterizes the normative terrain. Thus we suggest a normative mapping of medicine that encompasses a core of legitimate medical practice, consistent with the goals and internal duties of medicine, a periphery of more or less acceptable procedures and practices outside the core, and a range of violations beyond the pale of medical legitimacy. Designating the zone within which a procedure or practice belongs is a matter of judgment based on coherence or fit with the internal morality of medicine.

Reasonable differences of opinion are likely with respect to mapping practices and procedures as within the core or the periphery. Consider the case of contraception and sterilization. Although not a disease or a malady, pregnancy is a condition that in our society brings women under medical attention. Unwanted pregnancy can be understood as a disability, which interferes with the ability of women to function normally in social life. This suggests the conclusion that contraception promotes the health of women. The health promotion rationale for contraception or sterilization is stronger in the case of women who are likely to experience serious health risks from becoming pregnant, which would support including these procedures within the core of medicine in these circumstances. Male sterilization via vascctomy, in contrast, would seem to lie more clearly in the periphery. If undertaken to prevent unwanted pregnancy, the pregnancy it prevents belongs to another person, not to the one sterilized. Unwanted paternity, unlike unwanted pregnancy, does not qualify as a medical condition to be prevented. Vasectomy, then, appears more like a "life-style" procedure than tubal ligation—a medical means of permitting sexual intercourse without risking pregnancy and paternity. This surgical procedure does pose some risks and complications not compensated by medical benefits. Yet we consider it an acceptable peripheral medical practice that does not threaten or violate professional integrity.

Is Cosmetic Surgery Compatible with the Internal Morality of Medicine?

From the perspective of the ethics of the marketplace, governed by consumer sovereignty and honesty and fair play on the part of providers of commercial services, there appears to be nothing wrong with cosmetic surgery. It falls within the vast domain of commercial and consumer activity devoted to enhancing appearance. Cosmetic surgery involves certain risks and complications, but so does a range of other legitimate consumer activities, such as driving cars and engaging in recreational sports. In a "free society" what grounds are there for restricting the freedom of adults to purchase, and of medical practitioners to sell, cosmetic surgery? According to business ethics there are no ethical objections to cosmetic surgery as long as patients are adequately informed about risks and complications and are not subject to fraudulent marketing, and practitioners are technically competent. "Shaping up" by liposuction, for example, would seem to be an ethically acceptable, though less virtuous, alternative to jogging and working out, which are not without risks and potential complications.

Outside the minimalist ethics of the marketplace, a variety of value considerations are relevant to ethical appraisal of cosmetic surgery. The practice of cosmetic surgery may be criticized on the grounds that it is fueled by vanity and narcissistic fixation on bodily appearance. It reinforces intense concern with body image

and culturally prescribed standards of beauty, especially among women, who are the major "consumers" of cosmetic surgery. It contributes to a youth culture that disdains and stigmatizes aging and the elderly. Cosmetic surgery upholds culturally specific standards of beauty—Caucasian, Anglo-Saxon, or Northern European—that stigmatize the appearance of ethnic groups that deviate from this standard. Finally, it promotes inequality between those who have and those who lack the resources to purchase the marketplace advantages of enhanced appearance via cosmetic surgery. None of these considerations, however, is relevant to the internal morality of medicine.

How, then, does cosmetic surgery stand with respect to the internal morality of medicine and professional integrity? It is difficult to find any solid support for cosmetic surgery within the goals of medicine. Those who seek to enhance their appearance by cosmetic surgery do not suffer from a diagnosable disease or injury. The qualifier "cosmetic" signifies that the surgery is not medically indicated or needed to promote health.

It might be objected that the description of cosmetic surgery as an appearance enhancement fails to do justice to the real, often prolonged, suffering from a negative body image that typically precedes choice of cosmetic surgery. The point is well taken, but it does not follow that the suffering involved belongs within the purview of medicine. As discussed above, the goals of medicine concern not all human suffering, but only that suffering connected with a malady. "Malady" in the medical context suggests an objectively diagnosable condition calling for medical treatment; and this is precisely what is lacking in the case of cosmetic surgery. The "need" for cosmetic surgery is a function entirely of subjective preference.

Kathy Davis conducted fieldwork in the Netherlands to study individuals who sought cosmetic surgery during a time in which it was covered by national health insurance. She observed 55 individuals who were examined by an official medical inspector to determine eligibility for cosmetic surgery. Davis observes,

> With one exception, a man with a cauliflower nose, I was never able to guess what the person had come in for. In some cases, I had a suspicion, as, for example, when a woman with a rather prominent nose appeared, only to have them dashed when she explained that she wanted an eyelid correction because her five-year-old son was always asking her 'why she had been crying.' My first impression confirmed that applicants for cosmetic surgery looked no different than the run-of-the-mill woman (or man) on the street and some were even decidedly attractive. Their appearance did not seem to warrant corrective measures as drastic as cosmetic surgery.

Davis's inability to perceive the deficit in appearance prompting a request for cosmetic surgery was matched by a similar inability on the part of the responsible medical inspector. "Despite attempts to develop objective criteria for appearance, my observations of the Inspector's difficulties in actually making decisions about who should have cosmetic surgery presented a different picture. In practice, he routinely complained that he was unable to see why the applicant wanted cosmetic surgery."

Whether all cosmetic surgery falls outside the core domain of medicine may be subject to conflicting interpretations. Reconstructive plastic surgery to correct ravages of disease and injuries as well as gross physical abnormalities constitutes a core medical practice. Reconstructive procedures, however, lie along a continuum, without any clear boundary between therapeutic reconstructive surgery for a diagnosable problem and purely cosmetic surgery. In addition, reconstructive surgery in response to deformity is guided by aesthetic considerations. Yet compare, for example, plastic surgery to remove a port-wine stain causing severe facial disfigurement, but without any functional impairment, with liposuction to produce a trimmer appearance or a facelift to "rejuvenate" facial features. The for-

mer appearance problem qualifies as a malady that is objectively discernable by all observers, and it is reasonable to describe corrective surgery as medically indicated. In the latter cases the appearance problems giving rise to a request for cosmetic surgery are a matter entirely of subjective judgment. If surgery to remove a disfiguring port-wine stain is regarded as in part cosmetic, then at least some cosmetic procedures belong within the core of medical practice. This conclusion has no bearing, however, on the vast majority of purely cosmetic surgery procedures performed on normal bodies, which are not supported by the goals of medicine.

To give an aura of standard medical legitimacy to cosmetic surgery, cosmetic surgeons have concocted diagnostic categories warranting cosmetic surgical intervention, most notably, the "inferiority complex." The extent to which this disposition to construct diagnostic categories can be taken is exemplified by Davis's account of a case conference by an eminent Dutch plastic surgeon, who described a rhinoplasty for a 15-year-old Moroccan girl. The rationale for surgery was explained in terms of a new syndrome: "inferiority complex due to racial characteristics." Although on critical reflection such a medical diagnosis is apt to appear blatantly bogus, the felt need to invoke some diagnostic category to warrant cosmetic surgery testifies to the point that objective diagnosis underlies legitimate medical treatment.

Let us imagine for a moment what would be required of cosmetic surgery if we really believed that dissatisfaction with one's bodily appearance was a legitimate medical diagnosis. We have a model for such a state of affairs in the surgical treatment of transsexuals, who find their body appearance totally at odds with their perceived gender identity, and suffer considerable anguish as a result. It is considered a legitimate surgical practice to operate on such persons to change their secondary sexual characteristics. But it is important to note how this is done in centers that can claim to be competent and comprehensive in their care. In particular, it is common to have sex change surgeons working very closely with teams of psychiatrists and other mental health workers, who do intensive screening of each applicant before the team decides that surgery should be performed. If the mental health assessment uncovers any evidence of psychological problems, so that managing those problems might relieve the gender dysphoria without doing surgery, then surgery is withheld and the appropriate psychotherapy is recommended instead.

This model suggests that if cosmetic surgeons truly believed that they were treating "real" psychiatric "maladies," then in order to provide minimally competent care, they ought to be working in tandem with mental health teams of this sort, and offering nonsurgical options to at least some of their patients. To our knowledge, very few if any cosmetic surgery offices and clinics are run in this fashion, which tends to suggest that cosmetic surgeons themselves do not take very seriously the claim that their practices are legitimated by the reality of psychiatric disease.

In addition to lacking support by the goals of medicine, cosmetic surgery is also ethically questionable with respect to the internal medical duties. These procedures pose risks of harm and have the potential for complications that are not compensated by any medical benefits. Furthermore, it is arguable that the willingness of physicians to perform cosmetic surgery on bodies that are not diseased, injured, or grossly abnormal fraudulently misrepresents medicine. This practice suggests a medical need and rationale for intervention, when in fact there is no diagnosable condition warranting medical treatment.

These considerations lead to the hardly surprising conclusion that cosmetic surgery lies outside the core of normative medical practice. But they leave open the question whether cosmetic surgery is a legitimate practice within the periphery of medicine or should be considered a violation of the internal morality of medicine. It is interesting to note that some of the early leaders of plastic surgery in the 1920s and 1930s expressed ethical concerns about cosmetic surgery. They distinguished ethically appropriate reconstructive surgery in response to deformity and injury from purely cosmetic surgery, which they saw as the province of unprofessional "beauty doctors." For example, in an influential 1926 article published in *Annals of Surgery,* John Staige Davis wrote: "What is the ethical difference between doing an abdominal operation and removing wrinkles from a sagging face? The abdominal operation is necessary to the health of the patient, the operation for removal of wrinkles is unessential and is simply decorative surgery. True plastic surgery without question...is absolutely distinct and separate from what is known as cosmetic or decorative surgery." Although a persuasive argument might be advanced that purely cosmetic surgery, not associated with any diagnosable deformity, violates the internal morality of medicine, we do not take this position. The continuum between reconstructive and cosmetic surgery, which makes it difficult to determine where the former ends and the latter begins, casts doubt on a blanket judgment that cosmetic surgery lies outside the domain of legitimate medical practice.

Professional integrity concerns the fit between commitment to the norms of the internal morality of medicine and medical practice. All peripheral medical procedures and practices challenge professional integrity, since they are at best weakly supported by the goals of medicine, and they are apt to conflict with one or more of the internal duties. We submit that professional integrity is threatened, and potentially compromised, when peripheral procedures are not isolated or occasional occurrences within practice dedicated to core medical activities but are the predominant or exclusive focus of medical practice, as commonly characterizes cosmetic surgery. Moreover, the consumer-oriented, business context of cosmetic surgery risks compromising professional integrity, particularly insofar as it makes use of demand-stimulating marketing.

When Doctors Go to War

M. GREGG BLOCHE AND JONATHAN H. MARKS

New England Journal of Medicine 352, no. 1 (2005): 3–6.

When military forces go into combat, they are typically accompanied by medical personnel (physicians, physician assistants, nurses, and medics) who serve in noncombat roles. These professionals are bound by international law to treat wounded combatants from all sides and to care for injured civilians. They are also required to care for enemy prisoners and to report any evidence of abuse of detainees. In exchange, the Geneva Conventions protect them from direct attack, so long as they themselves do not become combatants.

Recently, there have been accounts of failure by U.S. medical personnel to report evidence of detainee abuse, even murder, in Iraq and Afghanistan. There have also been claims, less well supported, that medics and others neglected the clinical needs of some detainees. The department of Defense says it is investigating these allegations, though no charges have been brought against caregivers.

But Pentagon officials deny another set of allegations: that physicians and other medical professionals breached their professional ethics and the laws of war by participating in abusive interrogation practices. The International Committee of the Red Cross (ICRC) has concluded that medical personnel at Guantanamo Bay shared health information, including patient records, with army units that planned interrogations. The ICRC called this "a flagrant violation of medical ethics" and said some of the interrogation methods used were "tantamount to torture." The Pentagon answered that its detention operations are "safe, humane, and professional" and that "the allegation that detainee medical files were used to harm detainees is false."

Our own inquiry into medical involvement in military intelligence gathering in Iraq and Guantanamo Bay has revealed a more trouble-some picture. Recently released documents and interviews with military sources point to a pattern of such involvement, including participation in interrogation procedures that violate the laws of war. Not only did caregivers pass health information to military intelligence personnel; physicians assisted in the design of interrogation strategies, including sleep deprivation and other coercive methods tailored to detainees' medical conditions. Medical personnel also coached interrogators on questioning technique.

Physicians who did such work tend not to see these practices as unethical. On the contrary, a common understanding among those who helped to plan interrogations is that physicians serving in these roles do not act as physicians and are therefore not bound by patient-oriented ethics. In an interview, Dr. David Tornberg, Deputy Assistant Secretary of Defense for Health Affairs, endorsed this view. Physicians assigned to military intelligence, he contended, have no doctor–patient relationship with detainees and, in the absence of life-threatening emergency, have no obligation to offer medical aid.

Most people we interviewed who had served or spent time in detention facilities in Iraq or Guantanamo Bay reported being told not to talk about their experiences and impressions. Dr. David Auch, commander of the medical unit that staffed Abu Ghraib during the time of the abuses made notorious by soldiers' photographs, said military intelligence personnel told his medics and physician assistants not to discuss deaths that occurred in detention. Physicians who cared for so-called high-value detainees were especially hesitant to share their observations.

Yet available documents, the consistency of multiple confidential accounts, and confirmation of key facts by persons who spoke on the record make possible an understanding of the medical role in military intelligence in Iraq and Guantanamo. They also shed light on how those involved tried to justify this role in ethical terms.

In testimony taken in February 2004, as part of an inquiry into abuses at Abu Ghraib (and recently made public under the Freedom of Information Act and posted on the Web site of the American Civil Liberties Union [ACLU] at www.aclu.org), Colonel Thomas M. Pappas, chief of military intelligence at the prison, described physicians' systematic role in developing and executing interrogation strategies. Military intelligence teams, Pappas said, prepared individualized "interrogation plans" for detainees that included a "sleep plan" and medical standards. "A physician and a psychiatrist," he added, "are on hand to monitor what we are doing."

What was in these interrogation plans? None have become public, though Pappas's testimony indicates that he showed army investigators a sample, including a sleep deprivation schedule. However, a January 2004 "Memorandum for Record" (also available on the ACLU Web site) lays out an "Interrogation and Counter-Resistance Policy" calling for aggressive measures. Among these approaches are "dietary manipulation — minimum bread and water, monitored by medics"; "environmental manipulation — i.e., reducing A.C. [air conditioning] in summer, lower[ing] heat in winter"; "sleep management — for 72-hour time period maximum, monitored by medics"; "sensory deprivation — for 72-hour time period maximum, monitored by medics"; "isolation — for longer than 30 days"; "stress positions"; and "presence of working dogs."

Physicians collaborated with prison guards and military interrogators to put such approaches into practice. "Typically," said Pappas, military intelligence personnel give guards "a copy of the interrogation plan and a written note as to how to execute [it]....The doctor and psychiatrist also look at the files to see what the interrogation plan recommends; they have the final say as to what is implemented." The psychiatrist would accompany interrogators to the prison and

"review all those people under a management plan and provide feedback as to whether they were being medically and physically taken care of," said Pappas. These practices, he conceded, were without precedent. "The execution of this type of operation...is not codified in doctrine," he said. "Except for Guantanamo Bay, this sort of thing was a first."

At both Abu Ghraib and Guantanamo, "behavioral science consultation teams" advised military intelligence personnel on interrogation tactics. These teams, each of which included psychologists and a psychiatrist, functioned more formally at Guantanamo; staff shortages and other administrative difficulties reduced their role at Abu Ghraib.

A slide presentation prepared by medical ethics advisors to the military as a starting point for internal discussion poses a hypothetical case that, we were told, is a "thinly veiled" account of actual events. A physician newly deployed to "Irakistan" must decide whether to post physician assistants and medics behind a one-way mirror during interrogations. A military police commander tells the doctor that "the way this worked with the unit here before you was: We'd capture a guy; the medic would screen him and ensure he was fit for interrogation. If he had questions he'd check with the supervising doctor. The medic would get his screening signed by the doc. After that, the medic would watch over the interrogation from behind the glass."

Interrogation facilities at Abu Ghraib included a one-way mirror, according to internal FBI documents obtained and made public by the ACLU in December. Draft rules of conduct, now under review, would permit army medical personnel to attend interrogations but would give them a right to refuse on ethical grounds.

Military intelligence interrogation units also had access to detainees' medical records and to clinical caregivers in both Iraq and Guantanamo Bay. "They couldn't conduct their job without that info," Tornberg told us. Caregivers, he said, have only a limited doctor–patient relationship with detainees and "make it very clear to the individuals that their medical information will not be protected... To the extent it is military-relevant..., that information can be used."

In helping to plan and execute interrogation strategies, did doctors breach medical ethics? Military physicians and Pentagon officials make a case to the contrary. Doctors, they argue, act as combatants, not physicians, when they put their knowledge to use for military ends. A medical degree, Tornberg said, is not a "sacramental vow"—it is a certification of skill. When a doctor participates in interrogation, "he's not functioning as a physician," and the Hippocratic ethic of commitment to patient welfare does not apply. According to this view, as long as the military maintains a separation of roles between clinical caregivers and physicians with intelligence-gathering responsibilities, assisting interrogators is legitimate.

Military physicians point to civilian parallels, including forensic psychiatry and occupational health, in arguing that the medical profession sometimes serves purposes at odds with patient welfare. They argue, persuasively in our view, that the Hippocratic ideal of undivided loyalty to patients fails to capture the breadth of the profession's social role. This role encompasses the legitimate needs of the criminal and civil justice systems, employers' concerns about workers' fitness for duty, allocation of limited medical resources, and protection of the public's health.

But the proposition that doctors who serve these social purposes don't act as physicians is self-contradictory. Their "physicianhood" — encompassing technical skill, scientific understanding, a caring ethos, and cultural authority — is the reason they are called on to assume these roles. The forensic psychiatrist's judgments about personal responsibility and competence rest on his or her moral sensibility and grasp of mental illness. And the military physician's contributions to interrogation — to its effectiveness, lawfulness, and social acceptance in a rights-respecting society — arise from his or her psychological insight, clinical knowledge, and perceived humanistic commitment.

In denying their status as physicians, military doctors divert attention from an urgent moral challenge — the need to manage conflict between the medical profession's therapeutic and social purposes. The Hippocratic ethical tradition offers no road map for resolving this conflict, but it provides a starting point. The therapeutic mission is the profession's primary role and the core of physicians' professional identity. If this mission and identity are to be preserved, there are some things doctors must not do. Consensus holds, for example, that physicians should not administer the death penalty, even in countries where capital punishment is lawful. Similarly, when physicians are involved in war, some simple rules should apply.

Physicians should not use drugs or other biologic means to subdue enemy combatants or extract information from detainees, nor should they aid others in doing so. They should not be party to interrogation practices contrary to human rights law or the laws of war, and their role in legitimate interrogation should not extend beyond limit setting, as guardians of detainees' health. This role does not carry patient care responsibilities, but it requires physicians to tell detainees about health problems they find and to make treatment available. It also demands that physicians document abuses and report them to chains of command. By these standards, military medicine has fallen short.

The conclusion that doctors participated in torture is premature, but there is probable cause for suspecting it. Follow-up investigation is essential to determine whether they helped to craft and carry out the counter-resistance strategies — e.g., prolonged isolation and exposure to temperature extremes — that rise to the level of torture.

But, clearly, the medical personnel who helped to develop and execute aggressive counter-resistance plans thereby breached the laws of war. The Third Geneva Convention states that "[n]o physical or mental torture, nor any other form of coercion, may be inflicted on prisoners of war to secure from them information of any kind whatever." It adds that "prisoners of war who refuse to answer [questions] may not be threatened, insulted, or exposed to any unpleasant or disadvantageous treatment of any kind." The tactics used at Abu Ghraib and Guantanamo were transparently coercive, threatening, unpleasant, and disadvantageous. Although the Bush administration took the position (rejected by the ICRC) that none of the Guantanamo detainees were "prisoners of war," entitled to the full protections of the Third Geneva Convention, it has acknowledged that combatants detained in Iraq are indeed prisoners of war, fully protected under this Convention.

The Surgeon General of the U.S. Army has begun a confidential effort to develop rules for health care professionals who work with detainees. Such an initiative is much needed, but it ought not to happen behind a veil of secrecy. Ethicists, legal scholars, and civilian professional leaders should participate, and the process should address role conflict in medicine more generally. An Institute of Medicine study committee, broadly representative of competing concerns (including the military's), would be a more suitable venue. To their credit, some military physicians in leadership roles have tried to involve outside ethicists in discussion of duties toward detainees. The Pentagon's civilian leadership has blocked these efforts.

Military physicians, nurses, and other health care professionals have served with courage in Iraq and other theatres of war since September 11, 2001. Some have received serious wounds, and some have died in the line of duty. By most accounts, they have delivered superb care to U.S. soldiers, enemy combatants, and wounded civilians alike. We owe them our gratitude and respect. We would affirm their honor, not besmirch it, by acknowledging the tensions between their Hippocratic and national service commitments and by working with them to map a course between the two.

CASES

The White Coat

Medical oaths are typically recited as part of a so-called "white coat ceremony." The white coat ceremony began in 1993 at Columbia University's medical school. It marks the transition of medical students into the clinical stage of studies (usually the beginning of their third year), or is performed when they first enter medical school. It is the time when students are first allowed to don the white coat and take on the role of real doctor. Some say the white coat ceremony marks a kind of "conversion" of a layperson into membership in the medical profession. Ethicist Roy Branson even likens the ceremony to a kind of ordination, as to the priesthood.

Medical student Joe Wright provided this white coat commentary on the radio program *All Things Considered*.

> The equation of doctor equals white coat began in the 19th century when a set of doctors decided they should ditch older traditions and embrace the new world of science. They put on lab scientist drag to help convince their patients and themselves of the transformation. The lab outfit became an icon of doctordom; a symbol for the knowledge and the authority of the physician....

The white coat is still a cherished icon.... A doctor named Arnold Gold wanted to add to its meaning values [of] care and compassion.

These days future doctors seem to want to embrace long-held ideals of nursing: care, concern, knowing patients as whole people. I hold those ideals dear, and I thought about becoming a nurse. But I wanted to be an expert and I wanted to be in charge, at least as much as I wanted to be kind.

When I was a teenager, I thought I should get some kind of award every time I did the dishes. I think doctors sometimes act the same way about being compassionate: "Look at me. Aren't I good?" There are doctors worth praising. On the other hand, in the United States, health care is still a product to be purchased. Seen in that light, "compassion" is just another word for "customer service."

Discussion Questions

1. What do you think of Wright's suggestion that compassion is "just another word for 'customer service'"?
2. Some people are critical of white coat ceremonies because they underline the power of the white coat and thus the power of the physician. Is power necessary or useful to the profession of medicine? Why or why not?

Sources

Branson, Roy. "The Secularization of American Medicine." *Hastings Center Studies* 1, no. 2 (1973): 17–28.

Wright, Joe. "The New White Coat." Interview by Jacki Lyden. *All Things Considered*, NPR, November 29, 2002. http://studentweb.med.harvard.edu/jmw16/html/whitecoat.html.

Can a Killer Be a Doctor?

The Karolinska Institute in Stockholm, Sweden, is one of the most prestigious medical schools in the world, and has an extremely competitive admissions process. Among the students admitted to their 2007 freshman class was a man named Karl Helge Hampus Svensson.

Sometime during the fall 2007, several anonymous letters arrived at the Institute, claiming that Karl Svensson was a criminal. The letters claimed that Mr. Svensson had been convicted in 2000 of murder, that he was a Nazi sympathizer, and that police had called the murder a hate crime. The Institute checked into things, and found that the claims were true. Svensson had only recently been paroled from a maximum security prison.

Never having faced such a situation, school officials had no policy to guide their response. The only established grounds for expelling a student were psychiatric illness or posing a threat to others. The Institute finally expelled Svensson, not on principle but on a technicality: Svensson had changed his name after being convicted of murder and had falsified his high school transcripts to reflect this name change.

Many doctors and medical students, both at Karolinska and elsewhere, agreed with the decision to expel Mr. Svensson. Some argued that trust is an essential component of medicine, and that people would not be able to trust someone with a history of murder. Others said that they themselves felt unsafe having Svensson as a classmate and colleague. Yet Mr. Svensson also had a number of supporters who felt that because he had served his time, he should be permitted to study medicine.

For a related case about a rehabilitated drug-runner who trained to be a surgeon but was denied licensure by the state of Pennsylvania, see "Convict-Turned-Doctor Provokes Pennsylvania License Battle," *New York Times*, December 8, 1985.

Discussion Question

1. Are the private lives of doctors relevant in any way to their work as professionals?
2. Do you agree with the decision to expel Svensson?

Source

Altman, Lawrence K. "Swedes Ponder Whether Killer Can Be a Doctor." *New York Times*, January 25, 2008.

Vaccine Skeptics Refuse to Inoculate Children

In March 2008, twelve children in San Diego, California, fell ill with measles. None of the children were immunized against the disease. Public health experts expect that more outbreaks of measles and other communicable diseases are on the way, the result of what they consider a disturbing trend: more and more parents are refusing to inoculate their children.

Parents are legally required to have their children vaccinated against a small number of highly contagious and serious diseases: measles, mumps, rubella, varicella, polio, and meningitis. Not only are unvaccinated children at risk of contracting these diseases, but they pose a risk to other children—those who have had their shots (the vaccinations are not one hundred percent effective), and those too young to have been inoculated. Nonetheless, the health laws requiring vaccination allow for exemptions. Most permit exemptions based on religious belief and practice—and some of the parents refusing vaccines fall into this group. More and more parents, however, are refusing based on what are called "personal health beliefs." Most states allow these exemptions based on personal, but not distinctly religious, beliefs. Public health officials call these parents "vaccine skeptics." Vaccine skeptics believe that the shots may be harmful to children. In particular, there is a widespread fear that vaccinations can cause autism. Fear of vaccinations is driven by word of mouth, and by Internet sites warning parents about the dangers of vaccinations. In particular, the fear of vaccines has been fueled by the widely reported case of Hannah Poling. Poling's parents believe that their daughter, who is now nine, developed autism after receiving vaccinations as a nineteen-month old baby. The Polings sued the Department of Health and Human Services for compensation. Claims about the dangers of vaccinations remain scientifically unverified. Although studies have thus far failed to find a link between vaccinations and autism, the National Vaccine Advisory Committee has agreed to conduct further research.

Some parents feel that the risk of vaccines outweighs any potential benefits. After all, the diseases against which children are vaccinated are rare; you almost never hear of a child with measles or polio (in the United States, at any rate). Public health officials, on the other hand, argue that the very reason these diseases are rare is successful vaccination programs. If substantial numbers of parents continue to opt out of these programs, communicable diseases like measles will become more common.

Discussion Questions

1. Should parents have the option to opt out of vaccination programs? Why or why not?
2. How is vaccine skepticism like and unlike religious belief?
3. How do you think a doctor should best respond to a parent who refuses to inoculate his or her child?

Sources

Offit, Paul A. "Vaccines and Autism Revisited—The Hannah Poling Case." *New England Journal of Medicine* 358, no. 20 (2008): 2089–91.
Steinhauer, Jennifer. "Rising Public Health Risk Seen as More Parents Reject Vaccines." *New York Times*, March 21, 2008.

Should Medical Students Believe in Evolution? The Case of Professor Dini

The faculty website of Professor Michael Dini of Texas Tech University states:

> If you set up an appointment to discuss the writing of a letter of recommendation, I will ask you: "How do you account for the scientific origin of the human species?" If you will not give a scientific answer to this question, then you should not seek my recommendation.
>
> Why do I ask this question? Let's consider the situation of one wishing to enter medical school. Whereas medicine is historically

rooted first in the practice of magic and later in religion, modern medicine is an endeavor that springs from the sciences, biology prominent among these. The central, unifying principle of biology is the theory of evolution, which includes both micro- and macro-evolution, and which extends to ALL species. Someone who ignores the most important theory in biology cannot expect to properly practice in a field that is now so heavily based on biology. It is easy to imagine how physicians who ignore or neglect the Darwinian aspects of medicine or the evolutionary origin of humans can make poor clinical decisions. The current crisis in antibiotic resistance may partly be the result of such decisions.

Good medicine, like good biology, is based on the collection and evaluation of physical evidence. So much physical evidence supports the evolution of humans from non-human ancestors that one can validly refer to the "fact" of human evolution, even if all of the details are not yet known; just as one can refer to the "fact" of gravity, even if all of the details of gravitational theory are not yet known. One can ignore this evidence only at the risk of calling into question one's understanding of science and the scientific method. Scientists do not ignore logical conclusions based on abundant scientific evidence and experimentation because these conclusions do not conform to expectations or beliefs. Modern medicine relies heavily on the method of science. In my opinion, modern physicians do best when their practice is scientifically based.

The designated criteria for a letter of recommendation should not be misconstrued as discriminatory against anyone's personal beliefs. Rather, the goals of these requirements are to help insure that a student who wishes my recommendation uses scientific thinking to answer scientific questions.

Discussion Questions

1. Dini says, "Someone who ignores the most important theory in biology cannot expect to

properly practice in a field that is now so heavily based on biology." Do you agree with his claim?
2. Is his recommendation policy problematic or justified?

Source

Dini, Michael. Texas Tech Biology: Faculty home page http://www.biol.ttu.edu/faculty_detail.aspx?id=michael.dini@ttu.edu (accessed May 19, 2008).

Pillow Angel

"Ashley" was born with static encephalopathy. At age nine, she had reached her full developmental potential—the level of a three-month-old infant. She was unable to stand, walk, speak, sit up, or eat.

Ashley's parents, working with her doctors at Seattle's Children's Hospital, developed what they called the "Ashley treatment." They gave Ashley a high-dose estrogen therapy, and removed her uterus and her breast buds. The treatment will keep her at her current size, about seventy-five pounds, and will prevent her from entering puberty.

Her parents care for her at home, and say that keeping her small and light will make it possible for them to move her more easily from her bed to her wheelchair. This will allow them to include her in more family activities. Being able to move her frequently will also help keep bedsores from developing. Preventing her from going through puberty will spare her the "inconvenience and discomfort" of menstrual periods. Removal of her breast buds will prevent growth of breasts, which the parents argue could "sexualize" Ashley. In response to harsh criticism, Ashley's parents have defended their "Ashley treatment," arguing that they devised the treatment in her best interests, in order to improve Ashley's quality of life and alleviate her "discomfort and boredom."

Discussion Questions

1. What might be the main objections to Ashley's treatment?

2. Should the medical team have performed the surgeries?

3. What ethical principles might be offered in support of the parent's decision?

4. Recall the best interests standard of decision making discussed by Beauchamp and Childress. What problems with the best interests standard of decision making may exist in a case like this?

Sources

Liao, S. Matthew, Julian Savulescu, and Mark Sheehan. "The Ashley Treatment: Best Interests, Convenience, and Parental Decision-Making." *Hastings Center Report* 37, no. 2 (2007): 16–20.

Verhovek, S. "Parents Defend Decision to Keep Disabled Girl Small." *Los Angeles Times*, January 3, 2007.

College Student Requests Modafinil

Grete is a senior at a prestigious university. She is home for the Thanksgiving holiday and has come in to see her family doctor, Dr. Beckwith, for a routine yearly exam. When the doctor asks if she has any concerns or problems, she explains that she is preparing for the LSATs, taking an extra course so that she can complete her double major, and serving on the student council. The workload is pretty heavy, and she has heard from several friends that a drug called modafinil will increase her stamina and concentration. She asks Dr. Beckwith for a prescription for just a few pills, enough to help her through this tough semester. She tells him that some people she knows obtain the drug illegally, but that she does not feel comfortable doing this, and does not see the point. It is much better to simply ask up front, and to obtain a legitimate prescription. She did a little bit of research on the drug, and feels that it is safe. She also learned that about ninety percent of all prescriptions for modafinil are "off-label," so she figures that her request is not unusual.

Discussion Questions

1. Should Dr. Beckwith write the prescription?

2. What ethical concerns might Dr. Beckwith have?

3. What else might you want to know about modafinil in deciding about this case?

CHAPTER 3

At the End of Life

INTRODUCTION

This book begins with the Terri Schiavo case, which garnered worldwide attention and fueled an already heated discussion of bioethics at the end of life. People who had perhaps only occasionally thought about such issues, if ever, were now discussing them explicitly, and were even writing living wills so that there would be no confusion regarding their wishes if they ever had a similar misfortune.

The Schiavo case was not, however, the first to tackle the issue of discontinuing life-sustaining medical treatment. There were two cases in the 1970s that were groundbreaking for bioethics. In 1973, Donald "Dax" Cowart was critically injured in a propane gas explosion that caused severe burns over sixty-five percent of his body. For more than a year, he objected to the painful treatments that he was receiving. Cowart was physically incapable of ending his own life, since his hands had been severely damaged in the accident, but he made repeated verbal requests that he be allowed to die, or that someone help him end his own life. Despite his protestations, his doctors and his mother continued to provide treatment, including a number of painful skin graft surgeries. Cowart's plight was documented in a 1974 video entitled *Please Let Me Die*, and his case has been instrumental in upholding patient autonomy and decision making, even regarding the withholding and withdrawing of life-sustaining treatment. (Cowart survived the ordeal and is still alive today, but insists that he should have been allowed to die.)

The second case involved a young woman named Karen Ann Quinlan. Like Schiavo, Quinlan was in a persistent vegetative state. In 1975, the twenty-one-year-old Quinlan fell unconscious after a night out with some friends. She suffered an extended period of respiratory failure (perhaps as long as fifteen to twenty minutes), and her brain was irreversibly damaged. She remained in a coma. After watching her condition in the hospital deteriorate over a period of several months, Quinlan's parents decided to remove their daughter's respirator and allow her to die. The hospital refused. Her parents took the case to the New Jersey Supreme Court, and eventually won their legal battle to remove her respirator. This case established the precedent that life-sustaining treatment could be removed if the care were futile (no hope for recovery) and if there were proxy consent. Quinlan shocked her family and physicians, however, by breathing on her own after the ventilator was shut off. Her father approved the continuation of artificial nutrition and hydration (ANH), and Quinlan survived in a nursing home for another ten years before dying of pneumonia. Subsequent cases involving Paul Brophy (1986) and Nancy Cruzan (1990), specifically regarding the removal of ANH, established further legal guidelines regarding proxy consent in such cases.

What makes end-of-life cases so important and controversial? No doubt it has to do with the widespread belief that life is precious, and because death is final it must be avoided whenever possible. Historically, humanity has had strong prohibitions not only on murder, but also on suicide in many traditions and cultures, and has praised life-saving attempts to rescue. In the medical context, the goals of medicine include the treatment of disease and injury and the preservation of life, supported by the ethical principles of nonmaleficence and beneficence. End-of-life cases run counter to the imperatives embodied in these goals and principles.

Arguably, the majority of famous cases in bioethics concern end-of-life care, and some of the most contentious issues are in this area. This chapter covers some of the central questions with which bioethics has grappled: When is someone dead? When is treatment no longer appropriate? Who may reject treatment, under what conditions, and for what reasons? May medical professionals assist in a patient's death, or even directly cause it, and if so, under what circumstances?

Defining Death

It's not that I'm afraid to die. I just don't want to be there when it happens.
—Woody Allen, *Love and Death*

Most people eschew discussions of death. Even obituaries in the United States tend to avoid the word, instead saying that the person has "passed away" or "gone home to the Lord." Still, we know that people die. And at first glance, it may not seem that declaring someone dead should be ethically problematic. Intuitively, we think that someone is either alive or dead and that it should be easy to discern the difference. Nevertheless, diagnosing death has historically been a challenge, with many documented cases of mistake. Occasionally an exhumed coffin would show signs that the person had revived after interment (claw marks on the coffin lid) and sometimes people were fortunate enough to revive before burial, including during their own funerals. Even today with our superior technology, there have been documented errors. In a 1992 Seattle case, sixty-eight-year-old Roberta Jones was found unconscious and declared dead when medical examiners could not detect a pulse. Later at the funeral home, an employee noticed that she was breathing. The county medical examiner suspected that Jones was suffering from extreme hypothermia, which can cause a coma that resembles death. He speculated that she may have revived when placed in a body bag and her core body temperature rose.

Jones's mistaken diagnosis might have been avoided through the use of additional technology, but that assumes we have agreement on what counts as death, short of physical decay. Terri Schiavo's tombstone reflects some of the contemporary disagreement regarding the definition of death. It reads: "Born December 3, 1963; Departed this Earth February 25, 1990; At Peace March 31, 2005."

When did Schiavo die? That depends on how we define death. As prominent philosopher and bioethicist Robert Veatch notes, the concept is not strictly medical and scientific, but also philosophical and religious. Historically, death was considered to occur when the soul left the body, which might be determined by the cessation of breath and heartbeat. Regardless of religious persuasion, the traditional definition of death was cardiopulmonary—when the heart and lungs ceased to function. This definition became increasingly problematic with the development of medical technology that enabled physicians to prolong heartbeat and respiration after a person's brain was no longer capable of doing so. Advances in organ transplantation also fueled the controversy, because of increased interest in cadaveric organ procurement.

In 1968, a Harvard Medical School ad hoc committee recommended that when the brain of a person on life support has irreversibly lost the ability to function, then that person should be removed from the respirator because he or she is dead. Death occurs before the body is removed from the medical technology, not after. The 1970s was a transitional period in the United States and internationally, as medical practice and law began shifting toward what is often called the *whole-brain standard* of death. In 1981, the President's Commission for the Study of Ethical Problems in Medicine and Biomedical and Behavioral Research recommended that all jurisdictions in the United States adopt the Universal Determination of Death Act, which incorporated both brain and cardiopulmonary standards. Today, the whole-brain standard has become the most widely accepted definition of death in the industrialized world, with death determined by neurological criteria.

Acceptance is not universal, however. Japan, for example, permits its citizens to choose between the brain standard and the traditional cardiopulmonary model. In the United States, New Jersey state law provides an exemption from the brain standard in order to accommodate religious objections. Furthermore, scholars continue to debate the validity of the whole-brain standard. Alan Shewmon, for example, claims that the brain is not unique in integrating bodily functions and does not direct the entire organism, so brain death is not equivalent to the death of the organism. Amir Halevy takes another approach, arguing that some brain function may remain even after the most of the organ, including the brain stem, irreversibly ceases to function and direct bodily processes. He concludes that death is a process, rather than an isolable event. Finally, Veatch for many years has advocated the *higher-brain standard* of determining death, necessarily linking a functioning mind and bodily existence with life. He thinks that the loss of cognitive capacity, sometimes called the loss of personhood, should be understood as death.

Despite these objections and others that he admits have not been adequately addressed, **James Bernat** contends that the whole-brain standard remains conceptually coherent, "most accurately maps our consensual implicit concept of death," and remains the best one for public policy purposes. The scientific, philosophical, and religious disagreements regarding death push **Robert Veatch**, however, to claim that public policy should reflect this lack of consensus. He would like the law to include a "conscience clause" that allows people to choose for themselves a definition of death among a limited range of standards. A default option would apply to anyone who neglects to choose a standard by which he would be declared dead.

How Much Treatment?

> Whoever has lived long enough to find out what life is, knows how deep a debt of gratitude we owe to Adam, the first great benefactor of our race. He brought death into the world.
>
> —Mark Twain, *Pudd'nhead Wilson*

One of the goals of medicine is to preserve life, but what are the limits, if any, in the pursuit of that goal? Can we not only avoid discussion of death, but evade death altogether? Should medicine seek to defeat death and provide humanity with virtual immortality, or at least further extend the average life span? **Leon Kass** addresses these issues in his article "The Case for Mortality," defending the notion of limits with an interesting blend of arguments (philosophical, religious, and biological) and with various types of ethical reasoning (deontological, utilitarian, virtue, and relational).

Patient mortality and the limits of medical care are at the forefront in cases of *medical futility*—when a patient's condition is untreatable other than by palliative measures. Not all futility cases arise at the end of life (e.g., when a patient suffers from the common cold or arthritis), but those that do are cases of special concern, because withholding or withdrawing treatment may hasten a patient's death. The moral legitimacy of medical futility is recognized and accepted not only by professional guidelines, but also by the major religious traditions. Catholicism, for example, does not insist that treatment always be provided, even if it may afford some benefit to the patient. It does not advocate vitalism, the preservation of life at any cost. According to Pope John Paul II: "It needs to be determined whether the means of treatment available are objectively proportionate to the *prospects for improvement*. To forego extraordinary or disproportionate means is not the equivalent of suicide or euthanasia; it rather expresses acceptance of the human condition in the face of death."

The language of "extraordinary or disproportionate" is important here, because traditionally many people have utilized terminology commonly employed in Catholic thought—the distinction between *ordinary* and *extraordinary* means of treatment. While conceptually important, the terms themselves have proven confusing, because ordinary has often been understood as usual, customary, well-established medical practice, while extraordinary has been understood as unusual, experimental, even "heroic" procedures. The focus tended to be on particular forms of treatment, and confusion ensued when some of those forms went from being experimental to being established medical practice, such as organ transplantation. Today, many scholars prefer the terms *obligatory* and *optional* care, which ideally will focus on the context of the patient's condition and less on the medical procedures themselves. The Vatican, as evidenced from the preceding quotation, uses the language of *proportionate* and *disproportionate* for the same reasons. The standard for treatment apparently is subjective, based upon the concrete circumstances of a particular patient, rather than objective in terms of types of treatment used. Obligatory/proportionate/ordinary care, then, has a reasonable chance for success, and the benefits to the patient outweigh the burdens to the patient. Optional/disproportionate/extraordinary care has no reasonable chance for success, and/or the burdens to the patient outweigh the benefits to the patient. For example, surgery to repair torn knee cartilage for an otherwise healthy twenty-year-old would certainly be appropriate and expected as part of ordinary care. That same surgery on a ninety-year-old dying from bone cancer and who had just had a massive stroke would be extraordinary.

Who should make medical futility judgments? Based on their expertise, physicians are in a good position to make an empirical judgment regarding a patient's prognosis and the likely effectiveness of various treatment options. A patient or the patient's family, however, may reject a futility diagnosis and insist that the physician continue the present treatment or attempt something else. As discussed in chapter 2, a doctor owes many things to a patient, including a duty to respect the patient's autonomy. Should the doctor abide by the patient's wishes, or refuse because he or she believes that further treatment is futile? It is generally accepted that professional autonomy gives doctors the right to refuse requests to provide treatment that they find objectionable. These objections might have a moral basis—perhaps the doctor is unwilling to prescribe contraception to teenage children—or they may have an empirical basis—the doctor may believe that the patient would not benefit from the drug he or she saw advertised on television. **Eric Gampel** argues that professional autonomy ought not to govern end-of-life medical futility cases, however, because they are quite different from other types of cases. For example, to deny treatment in futility cases would mean certain death for the patient, and patient values in futility cases are among their most important values, intimately tied to religious and philosophical outlooks. Gampel contends that because determinations of futility involve value judgments, they are best made by patients and/or their families or surrogate decision makers.

Rejecting Treatment

It is now well-established in contemporary Western medical practice that the principle of respect for autonomy requires doctors to respect the wishes of competent patients who decline treatment. This principle holds even in end-of-life cases, such as when a patient with cancer decides against another round of chemotherapy because the treatment is quite unpleasant and would only be marginally effective, although it probably would extend his or her life.

But what if a patient refuses nonfutile, life-sustaining treatment when there is a good prognosis for recovery? The principle of respect for autonomy still seems to support the patient in such cases, but does the term "obligatory" in the earlier distinction between obligatory and optional care mean that such treatment is absolutely required? Is there an obligation to accept the care, or only an obligation to provide it if it is desired? The Catholic tradition clearly sees the obligations both for patients and health care providers. According to John Paul II: "Certainly there is a moral obligation to care for oneself and to allow oneself to be cared for." Respect for human dignity in ourselves as well as others creates both obligations. Such a position is not strictly a religious one. In contrast to Tom Beauchamp and James Childress's view of autonomy in the previous chapter, **Jukka Varelius** provides a Kantian-style argument, claiming that respect for autonomy actually demands that refusing patients be treated in such cases.

Proxy Decision Making

Perhaps the two most contentious issues regarding end-of-life care are who should make decisions in cases when the patient is incompetent, and the standards that ought to be used when making these decisions. As Beauchamp and Childress note in chapter 2, competent patients can "understand a therapeutic or research procedure, deliberate regarding its major risks and benefits, and make a decision in light of this deliberation." Incompetent patients cannot do one or more of these things. When a patient is incompetent, the closest next of kin typically decides, such as a spouse, a parent for minor children, or an adult child for a widowed parent. They do so in consultation with the patient's physicians, and perhaps also with a hospital ethics committee.

If *a patient is institutionalized* or there is no next of kin, then there may be a court-appointed guardian. Adults may also designate a decision maker in the event that they become incompetent, and may choose a close friend or sibling, whom they trust more than others. Disputes often arise within families regarding treatment decisions and who should make them, as we see in the Schiavo case, and laws provide a preference order. Because Terri Schiavo was married and had not designated someone else as her decision maker, her husband rather than her parents had the legal authority to make her health care decisions. His authority, like that of any proxy decision maker, was not absolute, and he could be removed from his role as proxy if he were incompetent or made decisions contrary to Terri's wishes or interests. It was on this latter basis that the Schindlers sought to impeach him and take on the proxy role.

On what basis should proxies make their decisions? Two distinct standards have emerged regarding treatment for incompetent patients: *substituted judgment* and *best interests*. Substituted judgment is based on the principle of respect for autonomy, and is suitable for adults who had previously been sufficiently competent to make their own decisions regarding medical treatment. Because such decisions properly belong to the patient, the substituted judgment standard mandates that medical treatment should proceed, or not proceed, according to the choices the now-incompetent person would make if he or she were still competent. The best sources for making a substituted judgment are advance directives or living wills. Ideally, these documents or oral statements provide clear guidance about the patient's wishes in particular scenarios (e.g., persistent vegetative state), particular treatments (e.g., a ventilator to assist with breathing), and a preferred order of decision makers. Without an advance directive, a proxy may then refer to the patient's values, both implicit and explicit, regarding worldview (including religious beliefs), lifestyle, and health care. At issue in the Schiavo case was the nature of Terri's values, and who could best represent them.

In many cases, a proxy may not have any information about a patient's values. These situations most often occur for patients who have never been competent to develop and express values, such as infants, young children, and mentally disabled adults. They also occur when a previously competent adult's wishes and values are unclear or unknown. The substituted judgment standard is obviously not applicable in these cases, and so proxies must use the best interests standard. The best interests standard is based on the principles of nonmaleficence and beneficence, and considers what would be best for the patient. Generally, this standard assumes that health is preferable to illness, and life is preferable to death, so there is a presumption in favor of treatment, whether or not it is life sustaining. This presumption is rebuttable, however, if the treatment options are futile or overly burdensome to the patient, and so contrary to an assessment of the patient's best interests.

Three readings in this chapter address the difficult issues of proxy decision making. **John Arras** analyzes the case of Mrs. Smith, an eighty-five-year-old nursing home resident who is severely demented and "minimally functional." He explores how the substituted judgment and best interests standards apply to Mrs. Smith's case. If Mrs. Smith's wishes and best interests are unclear, however, then neither standard would resolve the matter. It would fall into an ethically ambiguous "gray area." Arras thinks that gray area cases should be left to the discretion of "involved and well-intentioned family members . . . to decide as they see fit."

Turning from adult patients to extremely premature infants, **John Robertson** observes that the federal child abuse laws have led hospitals to treat "all conscious, viable premature newborns . . . even if they are likely to have severe physical and mental disabilities," and to do so despite parental objection. How might the general principle of treating equally all children born alive coexist with respecting the decision-making authority of parents? Robertson suggests that cases of extreme disability, when children completely lack "the capacity for meaningful symbolic interaction," constitute legitimate exceptions to the principle of equal treatment regardless of disability. Decision-making authority should reside with the parents and the burden of proof should lie with others to override it.

John Paris and colleagues consider the scenario in which continued care for premature infants is futile. They develop a narrative ethics perspective, drawing upon Dostoevsky's famous novel, *The Brothers Karamazov*. Contrary to Robertson's emphasis on parental decision making and Gampel's view that families ought to make futility judgments, Paris and his coauthors contend that parents tend not to want such an awful burden placed on them. Instead, they claim that a merciful physician would offer no choices, but rather would paternalistically make the difficult decision for the parents.

Artificial Nutrition and Hydration

As we said previously, judgments regarding what constitutes obligatory and optional care must be decided in particular cases, but are there any particular treatments that are always warranted, regardless of a patient's condition? One candidate that has emerged is ANH. This is the type of care at issue in the Terri Schiavo case, and sometimes is seen as qualitatively different from medical care because it involves basic sustenance. Not providing it is viewed as the equivalent of starving someone to death, and a violation of human dignity.

John Paul II made such claims in a 2004 speech. **Thomas Shannon and James Walter** argue that the pope's words reflect a developing perspective in the Catholic tradition regarding ANH. In their article, they maintain that a "revisionist" movement in the Catholic tradition shifts from the ethical framework of proportionality and teleology to that of deontology regarding this particular form of care. Interestingly, James Bretzke provides an alternative framework for interpreting John Paul II's statement in a way that avoids making this shift. According to Bretzke, the context of the Pope's statement indicates that he did not intend to overturn the ordinary/extraordinary distinction, nor did he intend to put ANH into an entirely separate category from other medical care, but instead was discussing the Church's continued opposition to euthanasia.

David Casarett, Jennifer Kapo, and Arthur Caplan agree with the general consensus among doctors, bioethicists, and courts that ANH should be understood as medical treatment, and contend that decisions about its use should be subject to the same benefits/burdens analysis as any other form of treatment. They emphasize that ANH does not always benefit patients and also involves risks. While some states demand a higher standard of evidence to show that a patient would reject ANH than they do for other life-sustaining therapies, Casarett, Kapo, and Caplan reject the higher standard as illogical and unrealistic. They find it critically important that clinicians engage patients and families in meaningful discussion about ANH.

Hastening Death

In 2002, the Netherlands became the first country to legally permit euthanasia, limiting it to situations in which patients face terminal illness or unbearable, interminable suffering. Belgium quickly followed suit, but, internationally, supporters of legalized euthanasia are clearly in the minority. *Euthanasia* means easy death or good death, but there is no consensus regarding what would count as a good death. In his song "The Gambler," Kenny Rogers says that "the best you can hope for is to die in your sleep," while others, such as Japan's Samurai, would prefer to die in battle. Polling data shows that doctors and patients define "good death" very differently. Patients associate being treated as a "whole person" with a good death. For example, a study published in 2000 by *JAMA* showed the following: ninety-two percent of patients want to be mentally aware when facing death, while only sixty-five percent of doctors think that is important; eighty-nine percent of patients do not want to be a burden on others when facing death, while only fifty-eight percent of doctors think that is important; and eighty-five percent of patients want to be able to pray when facing death, while only fifty-five percent of doctors think that is important.

Euthanasia is a broad concept, and its acceptability often rests on how it is defined above and beyond "good death." Some moral philosophers and bioethicists, such as **Peter Singer**, find euthanasia morally acceptable if the patient chooses it. Singer provides a utilitarian defense of voluntary euthanasia, claiming that individuals are the best judges of their interests, including judgments about whether it would be better to die than to continue living. "The right act is the one that will, in the long run, satisfy more preferences than it will thwart, when we weigh the preferences according to their importance for the person holding them." Euthanasia is most often acceptable, however, only through making certain distinctions that separate "good" euthanasia from "bad," and in some cases, the term euthanasia itself is rejected, even though some version of hastening death is accepted.

The most common distinction is between *active* and *passive* euthanasia—directly killing the patient or allowing the patient to die by withholding or withdrawing life-sustaining treatment. Contrary to Singer, most bioethicists reject active euthanasia, but find passive euthanasia ethically acceptable in futile cases. But is this distinction between active and passive forms of euthanasia a morally meaningful one? After all, omissions can be as morally culpable as actions if we intentionally fail to do what we should, such as provide nonfutile, life-sustaining treatment when the patient desires it, and some actions, such as removing a respirator, are required to allow a patient to die. In a famous article, philosopher James Rachels argues that the distinction between active and passive euthanasia fails, because he finds the purpose to be the same in both cases—relief of patient suffering through the patient's death. He sees no clear logical distinction between the two. If passive euthanasia is acceptable, so is active euthanasia. In fact, Rachels argues that passive euthanasia is morally worse than active in cases where the patient suffers unnecessarily while awaiting death. (Rachels does not actually advocate active euthanasia, but rejects the view that passive euthanasia is morally superior.)

Interestingly, while the Catholic tradition explicitly rejects both active and passive forms of euthanasia, it apparently does so in the context of ordinary or proportionate care, which is morally obligatory. We have already noted that Catholicism accepts the omission of treatment in the instance of medical futility. If treatment would only provide a "burdensome prolongation of life" and there are no prospects for improvement, then the patient or the patient's proxy can reject it. Death must not be the purpose of the omission, but instead is the indirect result of omitting optional care. Indirectly causing a patient's death through one's actions is also permissible in some cases. If a patient is suffering tremendously, and the only way to relieve pain is to provide a large dose of medication that the physician knows could also hasten death, the physician may nevertheless provide it. In this conflict between relieving pain and the duty not to kill, *terminal sedation* is permitted as long as the patient's death is not intended, but instead is a foreseen, indirect effect of the attempt to alleviate pain. Behind this justification is the so-called *principle of double effect*, which provides moral legitimacy for actions that can satisfy four conditions. First, the action must be good or indifferent, and not wrong in itself (e.g., providing morphine). Second, the actor must intend only the good effect (e.g., pain relief, rather than death). Third, the evil effect cannot be a means to the good effect (e.g., pain is relieved before death occurs). And fourth, the good effect must outweigh the evil effect (e.g., relief of the patient's suffering in this instance outweighs the risk of death). (The rule of double effect is also important in relation to the Catholic view of abortion, which we discuss in chapter 4.) As outlined by **Damien Keown**, the Buddhist view of these end-of-life issues closely resembles the Catholic view in terms of their positions, but they employ different reasons to support their position.

Whether double effect provides sufficient moral grounding for terminal sedation remains a matter of contention, even among supporters of the practice. **Roger Magnusson** argues for an alternate moral framework, using the metaphor of "the devil's choice," for situations "where choice itself is perverse and not choosing is not an option." He contends that physicians really do intend to hasten the patient's death when they recognize that death will be the likely consequence of providing adequate pain relief. Such intention does not mean that the doctor actually desires the patient to die, but only that he or she does what is necessary under the circumstances.

Physician-Assisted Suicide

Although active euthanasia remains illegal in the United States, another practice that permits the direct taking of a patient's life—physician-assisted suicide (PAS)—is legal in Oregon and Washington, and perhaps also in Montana. PAS differs from active euthanasia in that the patient, rather than the physician, administers the lethal medication. The physician assists by approving the procedure and writing the prescription. Oregon's "Death with Dignity Act" (DWDA) became law via public referendum. It originally was approved in 1994 by a fifty-one to forty-nine percent vote, but its implementation was delayed in the courts. In 1997, the DWDA was affirmed by a sixty percent majority of the largest voter turnout in thirty-four years. It also has survived a challenge by the federal government. Former U.S. Attorney General John Ashcroft directed the Drug Enforcement Agency to enforce the Controlled Substances Act in Oregon even against physicians in compliance with the DWDA. In April 2002, a federal judge backed the state law, declaring that Ashcroft lacked the authority to decide "what constitutes the legitimate practice of medicine." Ashcroft and his successor, Alberto Gonzales, unsuccessfully continued to pursue the case through the appeals process. In 2006, the U.S. Supreme Court upheld the DWDA, with Justice Anthony

Kennedy writing that the attorney general may not declare illegitimate "a medical standard for care and treatment of patients that is specifically authorized under state law." Washington's DWDA became law in 2008 when the ballot initiative passed with fifty-nine percent of the vote, and was implemented in 2009. Montana's situation is less clear. In December 2008, a state judge ruled that mentally competent, terminally ill patients have a right to PAS. As of this writing, that ruling is being appealed.

Between 1998 and 2007, 341 patients died after ingesting a lethal dose of prescribed medication under Oregon's DWDA. Eighty-two percent of the patients had some form of cancer, eighty-six percent were under hospice care, and ninety-nine percent had some form of medical insurance. Over eighty percent listed such reasons as "losing autonomy," being "less able to engage in activities that make life enjoyable," and "loss of dignity" as why they wanted to die. It is important to note that not just anyone can gain access to PAS under the DWDA. Patients must meet several criteria, such as being a competent adult resident of Oregon and having a diagnosis of terminal illness.

In contrast to Oregon and Washington, Switzerland permits assisted suicide without requiring that the person be terminally ill, and also allows foreigners to receive assistance in what is sometimes called "suicide tourism." The Swiss medical profession does not condone physician participation in suicide; thus, the practice occurs outside of the medical context. Any citizen may assist someone else to commit suicide, as long as he or she does not act out of selfish motives (e.g., a desire to inherit money sooner), but assisted suicide is often coordinated by nonprofit organizations dedicated to the practice. In their role as citizen rather than as physician, doctors may provide assistance, and many of them do write prescriptions for lethal medication.

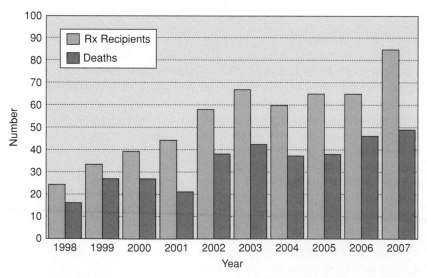

■ **Number of DWDA Prescription Recipients and Deaths, by Year, Oregon, 1998–2007**
Oregon Department of Human Services, http://egov.oregon.gov/DHS/ph/pas/docs/year10.pdf

Oregon DWDA Eligibility Conditions

- An adult (18 years of age or older).
- A resident of Oregon.
- Capable (defined as able to make and communicate health care decisions), and
- Diagnosed with a terminal illness that will lead to death within six months.
- The patient must make two oral requests to his or her physician, separated by at least fifteen days.
- The patient must provide a written request to his or her physician, signed in the presence of two witnesses.
- The prescribing physician and a consulting physician must confirm the diagnosis and prognosis of terminal illness (less than six months to live).
- The prescribing physician and a consulting physician must determine whether the patient is competent.
- If either physician believes the patient's judgment is impaired by a psychiatric or psychological disorder, the patient must be referred for a psychological examination.
- The prescribing physician must inform the patient of feasible alternatives to assisted suicide including comfort care, hospice care, and pain control.
- The prescribing physician must request, but may not require, the patient to notify his or her next-of-kin of the prescription request.

PAS has divided physicians and bioethicists. The American Medical Association (AMA) officially opposes PAS in its Code of Ethics: "Physician-assisted suicide is fundamentally incompatible with the physician's role as healer, would be difficult or impossible to control, and would pose serious societal risks." Obviously, various physicians in Oregon and elsewhere disagree with the AMA. Also disagreeing is **Michael Gill**, who defends an autonomy-based justification for allowing PAS, defining autonomy primarily as the ability to make the "big decisions" in life. Big decisions are about the things that matter most, like getting married, while little decisions are relatively inconsequential, like what to have for dinner. Not only are the big decisions properly made by people for themselves, but in the case of terminally ill people, deciding upon PAS may be the only big decision that they can make in their limited time to live. In contrast, **Susan Wolf** finds arguments for PAS based upon patient autonomy to be problematic, contending that women in particular are vulnerable patients, more likely to suffer from depression and less likely to have adequate pain management and access to quality health care. Furthermore, she notes that because female gender roles tend to require self-sacrifice, they undermine notions of autonomous choice. Several bioethicists have voiced concern for various other vulnerable patient groups, such as the disabled, the elderly, and minorities, who, for various reasons including cultural biases, also may lack access to adequate pain management and quality health care. Surveys show that African-Americans in particular are wary of PAS—and also of withholding and withdrawing end-of-life care—because of actual and perceived racial bias in the health care system. Analyses of noted "suicide doctor" Jack Kevorkian's patients clearly show a preponderance of women, but data from the Netherlands and Oregon thus far do not indicate that vulnerable groups like women, racial and ethnic minorities, and the elderly are at risk from the practice of PAS.

The discussion in this chapter primarily concerns whether and how patients should control the end of life when this end takes place within the health care system (which it very often does). It involves whether and when they may claim rights, such as the right to die and the right to assistance in dying. It also involves the changing nature of a physician's role in relation to patients at the end of life. When may physicians discontinue patient care? May a physician participate in euthanasia or PAS? Does respect for patient autonomy extend to abiding by request for death?

REFERENCES AND FURTHER READING

Battin, Margaret P., Agnes Vander Heide, Linda Garzini, Gerrit van der Licel, and Bregíe D. Onwateaku-Philipsan "Legal Physician-Assisted Dying in Oregon and the Netherlands: Evidence Concerning the Impact on Patients in 'Vulnerable' Groups." *Journal of Medical Ethics* 33, no. 10 (2007): 591–97.

Bretzke, James. "A Burden of Means: Interpreting Recent Catholic Magisterial Teaching on End-of-Life Issues." *Journal of the Society of Christian Ethics* 60, no. 2 (2006): 183–200.

Council on Ethical and Judicial Affairs, American Medical Association. "Physician-assisted Suicide." 1996. http://www.ama-assn.org/apps/pf_new/pf_online?f_n=browse&doc=policyfiles/HnE/E-2.211. HTM&&s_t=&st_p=&nth=1&prev_pol=policyfiles/HnE/E-1.02.HTM&nxt_pol=policyfiles/HnE/E-2.01.HTM& (accessed August 5, 2007).

Dula, Annette, and September Williams. "When Race Matters." *Clinics in Geriatric Medicine* 21, no. 1 (2005): 239–53.

Halevy, Amir. "Beyond Brain Death." *Journal of Medicine and Philosophy* 26, no. 5 (2001): 493–501.

Henderson, Diedtra, and Dee Norton. "Life Still Flickered in 'Dead' Woman—Mortuary Worker Noticed Vague Sign She Was Breathing." *Seattle Times,* November 2, 1992.

John Paul II. *Evangelium Vitae.* 1995. http://www.vatican.va/holy_father/john_paul_ii/encyclicals/documents/hf_jp-ii_enc_25031995_evangelium-vitae_en.html (accessed January 30, 2005).

——"To the Participants in The International Congress on Life-Sustaining Treatments and Vegetative State: Scientific Advances and Ethical Dilemmas." 2004. http://www.vatican.va/holy_father/john_paul_ii/speeches/2004/march/documents/hf_jp-ii_spe_20040320_congress-fiamc_en.html (accessed January 30, 2005).

President's Commission for the Study of Ethical Problems in Medicine and Biomedical and Behavioral Research. *Defining Death: Medical, Legal and Ethical Issues in the Determination of Death.* Washington, DC: U.S. Government Printing Office, 1981.

Quill, Timothy E., and Margaret Battin. *Physician-Assisted Dying: The Case for Palliative Care and Patient Choice.* Baltimore, MD: Johns Hopkins University Press, 2004.

Rachels, James. "Active and Passive Euthanasia." *New England Journal of Medicine* 292 (1975): 78–80.

Shewmon, Alan. "The Brain and Somatic Integration: Insights into the Standard Biological Rationale for Equating 'Brain Death' with Death." *Journal of Medicine and Philosophy* 26, no. 5 (2001): 457–78.

Solomon, Louis M., and Rebekka C. Noll. "Physician-Assisted Suicide and Euthanasia: Disproportionate Prevalence of Women Among Kevorkian's Patients." *Gender Medicine* 5, no. 2 (2008): 110–14.

State of Oregon. *Death with Dignity Act*. http://egov.oregon.gov/DHS/ph/pas/ (accessed June 3, 2008).

Steinhauser, Karen E., Nicholas A. Christakis, Elizabeth C. Clipp, Maya McNeilly, Lauren, McIntyre, and James A. Tulsky "Factors Considered Important at the End of Life by Patients, Family, Physicians, and Other Care Providers." *JAMA* 284, no. 19 (2000): 2476–82.

United States Supreme Court. *Gonzales v. Oregon*. 546 U.S. 243 (2006).

Veatch, Robert M. *Death, Dying, and the Biological Revolution: Our Last Quest for Responsibility*. Rev. ed. New Haven, CT: Yale University Press, 1989.

Veatch, Robert M. "The Death of Whole-Brain Death: The Plague of the Disaggregators, Somaticists, and Mentalists." *Journal of Medicine and Philosophy* 30, no. 4 (2005): 353–78.

DISCUSSION QUESTIONS FOR THE READINGS

The Whole-Brain Concept of Death Remains Optimum Public Policy

1. How does Bernat define death?
2. Distinguish the whole-brain, higher-brain, and brain-stem criteria of death. Do you find Bernat's support for the whole-brain formulation over the other two criteria persuasive?
3. In the final analysis, Bernat's support for the whole-brain formulation rests on its public policy success, in spite of its biological and philosophical shortcomings. Is Bernat's position ethically justified?

The Conscience Clause: How Much Individual Choice in Defining Death Can Our Society Tolerate?

1. Should people have the right to choose their own definition of death?
2. Veatch claims that death is a religious, philosophical, ethical, and public policy question, not a scientific one. Do you find his argument persuasive?
3. Who should determine the definition of death when a person's wishes are unknown or unknowable?

The Case for Mortality

1. How much longer life is an unqualified good for people?
2. Kass outlines several possible problems for an increased life span. How serious are these problems? Can they be sufficiently addressed?
3. Is our finitude good for us?

Does Professional Autonomy Protect Medical Futility Judgments?

1. How does Gampel distinguish quantitative, qualitative, and physiological futility?
2. Should professional autonomy permit physicians to make medical futility judgments?
3. How are futility cases similar and dissimilar to other medical cases?

Autonomy, Wellbeing, and the Case of the Refusing Patient

1. How do the subjective and objective theories of wellbeing differ?
2. If a patient refuses life-sustaining treatment, what response would truly respect the patient's autonomy?

3. Is autonomy intrinsically valuable, or only instrumentally valuable insofar as it contributes to a person's wellbeing?

The Severely Demented, Minimally Functional Patient

1. Do you agree with Arras that "Mrs. Smith" is no longer a "person?"
2. When, if ever, should patients no longer be considered persons?
3. When patients whose best interests regarding medical treatment are unclear, what standards should guide treatment decisions?

Extreme Prematurity and Parental Rights After Baby Doe

1. When should doctors seek to override parents' wishes regarding life-sustaining treatment for newborns?
2. Should the CAA apply to extremely premature newborns?
3. How much weight should the probability for severe disability have in deciding whether to require treatment for extremely premature newborns?

Has the Emphasis on Autonomy Gone Too Far? Insights from Dostoevsky on Parental Decisionmaking in the NICU

1. Should doctors spare parents from the difficult decisions associated with life-sustaining treatments for dying infants? Would that be legitimate paternalism?
2. Is Dostoevky's novel a good guide for doctors in this situation?
3. How important is literature for bioethics and medical practice?
4. What novels, stories, and films might be good guides for medical practice?

Appropriate Use of Artificial Nutrition and Hydration: Fundamental Principles and Recommendations

1. Should decisions about ANH be made in the same way as other medical treatment decisions?
2. Should decisions about ANH for incompetent patients be held to a higher standard of evidence?

Assisted Nutrition and Hydration and the Catholic Tradition

1. How do you understand the term "revisionist?" Do you consider it to be an appropriate term to describe the new Catholic position on ANH?
2. How does the meaning of the term "ordinary" impact the ANH debate?
3. Should there be a presumption in favor of ANH before considering particular patients?

The Devil's Choice: Re-Thinking Law, Ethics, and Symptom Relief in Palliative Care

1. Does "the devil's choice" metaphor provide a better way to explain palliative sedation than does the principle of double effect?
2. Does the legal defense of "necessity" clearly distinguish between palliative sedation and unlawful killing?
3. Is it possible to intend a patient's death without desiring it?

Voluntary Euthanasia: A Utilitarian Perspective

1. Should the rule against killing apply to the competent person who determines that it would be better to die?
2. From a utilitarian perspective, does it make sense to limit euthanasia to terminally or incurably ill patients?
3. Is the slippery slope argument against euthanasia convincing?

End of Life: The Buddhist View

1. Because Buddhism lacks a central authority, could Buddhist values be used by individual Buddhists to justify euthanasia?
2. Would it be possible to aim at death while also being compassionate?

Gender, Feminism, and Death: Physician-Assisted Suicide and Euthanasia

1. How might gender dynamics impact PAS and euthanasia?
2. Are women more vulnerable than are men for nonvoluntary PAS and euthanasia?
3. Is a rights framework an appropriate way to approach PAS and euthanasia?
4. What does feminist analysis add to the ethical debate?

A Moral Defense of Oregon's Physician-Assisted Suicide Law

1. Do autonomy-based arguments provide a strong defense of PAS?
2. If the only "big decision" available to a person is how and when to die, does respect for autonomy require permitting that person to engage in PAS?
3. Even if suicide is morally acceptable in certain cases, is it ethical for a physician to assist in a patient's death?
4. Because withdrawal of life-sustaining treatment is morally permissible for physicians, should PAS also be morally permissible?

READINGS

The Whole-Brain Concept of Death Remains Optimum Public Policy

JAMES L. BERNAT

Journal of Law, Medicine and Ethics 34, no. 1 (2006): 35–43.

The definition of death is one of the oldest and most enduring problems in biophilosophy and bioethics. Serious controversies over formally defining death began with the invention of the positive-pressure mechanical ventilator in the 1950s. For the first time, physicians could maintain ventilation and, hence, circulation on patients who had sustained what had been previously lethal brain damage. Prior to the development of mechanical ventilators, brain injuries severe enough to induce apnea quickly progressed to cardiac arrest from hypoxemia. Before the 1950s, the loss of spontaneous breathing and heartbeat ("vital functions") were perfect predictors of death because the functioning of the brain and of all other organs ceased rapidly and nearly simultaneously thereafter, producing a unitary death phenomenon.

With the advent of mechanical support of ventilation, (permitting maintenance of circulation) the previous unitary determination of death became ambiguous. Now patients were encountered in whom some vital organ functions (brain) had ceased totally and irreversibly, while other vital organ functions (such as ventilation and circulation) could be maintained, albeit mechanically. Their life status was ambiguous and debatable because they had features of both dead and living patients. They resembled dead patients in that they could not move or breathe, were utterly unresponsive to any stimuli, and had lost brain stem reflex activity. But they also resembled living patients in that they had maintained heartbeat, circulation and intact visceral organ functioning. Were these unfortunate patients in fact alive or dead?

In a series of scientific articles addressing this unprecedented state, several authors made the bold claim that patients who had totally and irreversibly lost brain functions were dead, despite their continued heartbeat and circulation. In the 1960s, they popularized the concept they called "brain death" to acknowledge this idea.[1] The intuitive attractiveness of the concept of "brain death" led to its rapid acceptance by the medical and scientific community, and to legislators expeditiously drafting public laws permitting physicians to determine death on the basis of loss of brain functioning. Medical historians have emphasized utilitarian factors in this rapid acceptance, because a determination of brain death permitted the desired societal goals of cessation of medical treatment and organ procurement.

The practice of determining human death using brain death tests has become worldwide over the past several decades. The practice is enshrined in law in all 50 states in the United States and in approximately 80 other countries, including nearly all of the developed world and much of the undeveloped world.

Yet despite this consensus, from its beginning, a persistent group of critics have attacked the concept and practice of brain death as being conceptually invalid or a violation of religious beliefs. Recently, through the intellectual leadership of Alan Shewmon, additional critics have concluded that the concept of brain death is incoherent, anachronistic, unnecessary, a legal fiction, and should be abandoned. In this essay I show that, despite admitted shortcomings, the classical formulation of whole-brain death remains both conceptually coherent and forms a solid foundation for public policy surrounding human death determination and organ transplantation.

An Analysis of Death

Defining death is a formidable task. In their rigorous, thoughtful, and highly influential book *Defining Death*, the President's Commission for the Study of Ethical Problems in Medicine and Biomedical and Behavioral Research chose as their conceptual foundation the analysis of death that I published with my Dartmouth colleagues Charles Culver and Bernard Gert. Our analysis was conducted in three sequential phases: (1) the philosophical task of determining the definition of death by making explicit the consensual concept of death that has been confounded by technology; (2) the philosophical and medical task of determining the best criterion of death, a measurable condition that shows that the definition has been fulfilled by being both necessary and sufficient for death; and (3) the medical-scientific task of determining the tests of death for physicians to employ at the patient's bedside to demonstrate that the criterion of death has been fulfilled with no false positive and minimal false negative determinations. Most subsequent scholars have accepted this method of analysis, if not our conclusions, with two recent exceptions.[2]

Following a series of published critiques and rebuttals of our position over the past two decades, I concluded that much of the disagreement over our account of death resulted from the lack of acceptance by dissenting scholars of the "paradigm of death." By "paradigm of death" I refer specifically to a set of conditions and assumptions that frame the discussion of the topic of death by identifying the nature of the topic, the class of phenomena to which it belongs, how it should be discussed, and its conceptual boundaries. Accepting a paradigm of death permits scholars to rationally analyze and discuss death without falling victim to the fallacy of category noncongruence and consequently talking past each other. But the paradigm remains useful even if scholars do not agree on all its elements, because it can help clarify the root of their disagreement.

My paradigm of death comprises seven sequential elements. First, the word "death" is a common, nontechnical word that we all use correctly to refer to the cessation of a human being's life. The philosophical task of defining death seeks not to redefine it by contriving a new meaning, but rather to divine and make explicit the implicit meaning of death that we all accept but that has been made ambiguous by technological advances.

Second, death is fundamentally a biological phenomenon. We all agree that life is a biological entity; thus also should be its cessation. Accepting that death is a biological phenomenon neither denigrates the richness and beauty of various cultural and religious practices surrounding death and dying, nor denies societies their proper authority to govern practices and establish laws regulating the determination and time of death. But death is an immutable and objective biological fact and not fundamentally a social contrivance.

Third, we restrict our analysis to the death of higher vertebrate species for which death is univocal. That is, we mean the same phenomenon of "death" when we say our cousin died as we do when we say our dog died. Although individual cells within organisms and single celled organisms also die, our analysis of defining human death is simplified by restricting our purview to the death of related higher vertebrate species.

Fourth, the term "death" can be applied directly and categorically only to organisms. All living organisms must die and only living organisms can die. Our use of language may seem to confuse this point, for example, when we say "a person died." But by this usage we are referring directly to the death of the living organism that embodied the person, not to a living organism ceasing to be a person.

Fifth, a higher vertebrate organism can reside in only one of two states, alive or dead:

no organism can be in both states or in neither. Simply because we currently lack the technical ability to always accurately identify an organism's state does not necessitate postulating an in-between state.

Sixth, and inevitably following from the preceding premise, death must be an event and not a process. If there are only two exclusive underlying states of an organism, the transition from one state to the other, at least in theory, must be sudden and instantaneous, because of the absence of an intervening state. To an observer, it may appear that death is an ineluctable process within which it is arbitrary to stipulate the moment of death, but such an observation simply underscores our current technical limitations. For technical reasons, the event of death may be determinable with confidence only in retrospect.

Seventh and finally, death is irreversible. By its nature, if the event of death were reversible it would not be death but rather part of the process of dying that was interrupted and reversed. Advances in technology permit physicians to interrupt the dying process in some cases and postpone the event of death.

The Definition of Death

Given the set of assumptions and conditions comprising the paradigm of death, we can now explore the definition, criterion, and tests of death. Defining death is the conceptual task of making explicit our understanding of it. It poses an essential question: what does it mean for an organism to die, particularly in our contemporary circumstance in which technology can compensate for the failure of certain vital organs?

We all agree that by "death" we do not require the cessation of functioning of every cell in the body, because some integument cells that require little oxygen or blood flow continue to function temporarily after death is customarily declared. We also do not simply mean the cessation of heartbeat and respiration, though this circumstance will lead to death if untreated. Although some religious believers assert that the soul

departs the body at the moment of death, this is not an adequate definition of death because it is not what religious believers fundamentally mean by "death."

Beginning early in the brain-death debate, Robert Veatch advocated a position that became known as the "higher-brain formulation of death." He claimed that death should be defined formally as "the irreversible loss of that which is considered to be essentially significant to the nature of man." He expressly rejected the idea that death should be related to an organism's "loss of the capacity to integrate bodily function" asserting that "man is, after all, something more than a sophisticated computer." His project attempted not to reject brain death, but to refine the intuitive thinking underlying the brain death concept by emphasizing that it was the cerebral cortex that counted in a brain death concept and not the more primitive integrating brain structures.

Irrespective of the attractiveness of this idea, the higher-brain formulation contains a fatal flaw as a candidate for a definition of death: it is not what we mean when we say "death." Its logical criterion of death would be the irreversible loss of consciousness and cognition, such as that which occurs in patients in an irreversible persistent vegetative state (PVS). Thus a higher-brain formulation of death would count PVS patients as dead. However, despite their profound and tragic disability, all societies, cultures, and laws consider PVS patients as alive. Thus, despite its potential merits, the higher-brain formulation fails the first condition of the paradigm: to make explicit our underlying consensual concept of death and not to contrive a new definition of death.

In 1981, my colleagues and I strove to capture the essence of the concept of human death that formed the intuitive foundation of the brain-based criterion of death. We defined death as "the cessation of functioning of the organism as a whole." This definition utilized a biological concept proposed by Jacques Loeb in 1916. Loeb explained that organisms are not simply composites of cells, tissues, and organs, but possess overarching functions that regulate and integrate all systems to maintain the unity and interrelatedness of the organism to promote its optimal functioning and health. The organism as a whole comprises that set of functions that are greater than the mere sum of the organism's parts.

More recently, biophilosophers have advanced the concept of "emergent functions" to explain this type of phenomenon with greater conceptual clarity. An emergent function is a property of a whole that is not possessed by any of its component parts, and that cannot be reduced to one or more of its component parts. The physiological correlate of the organism as a whole is the set of emergent functions of the organism. The irretrievable loss of the organism's emergent functions produces loss of the critical functioning of the organism as a whole and therefore is the death of the organism.

Examples of critical functions of the organism as a whole include: (1) consciousness, which is necessary for the organism to respond to requirements for hydration and nutrition; (2) control of circulation, respiration, and temperature control, which are necessary for all cellular metabolism; and (3) integrating and control systems involving chemoreceptors, baroreceptors, and neuroendocrine feedback loops to maintain homeostasis. Death is the irreversible and permanent loss of the critical functions of the organism as a whole.

The Criterion of Death

The next task is to identify the criterion of death, the general measurable condition that satisfies the definition of death by being both necessary and sufficient for death. There are several plausible candidates for a criterion of death. Among brain death advocates, three separate criteria have been proposed: (1) the whole-brain formulation, the criterion recommended by the Harvard Committee and the President's Commission, and accepted throughout the United States and in most parts of the world; (2) the higher-brain formulation, popular in the academy but accepted in no jurisdictions anywhere; and (3) the brain stem formulation accepted in the United Kingdom.

The whole-brain criterion requires cessation of all brain clinical functions including those of the cerebral hemispheres, diencephalon (thalamus and hypothalamus), and brain stem. Whole-brain theorists require widespread cessation of neuronal functions because each part of the brain serves the critical functions of the organism as a whole. The brain stem initiates and controls breathing, regulates circulation, and serves as the generator of conscious awareness through the ascending reticular activating system. The diencephalon provides the center for bodily homeostasis, regulating and coordinating numerous neuroendocrine control systems such as those regulating body temperature, salt and water regulation, feeding behavior, and memory. The cerebral hemispheres have an indispensable role in awareness that provides the conditions for all conscious behavior that serves the health and survival of the organism.

All clinical brain functions measurable at the bedside must be lost and the absence must be shown to be irreversible. But the whole-brain criterion does not require the loss of all neuronal activities. Some neurons may survive and contribute to recordable brain activities (by an electroencephalogram, for example) but not to clinical functions. The precise number, location, and configuration of the minimum number of critical neuron arrays remain unknown.

Despite the fact that the whole-brain criterion does not require the cessation of functioning of every brain neuron, it does rely on a pathophysiological process known as brain herniation to assure widespread destruction of the neuron systems responsible for the brain's clinical functions. When the brain is injured diffusely by trauma, hypoxicischemic damage during cardiorespiratory arrest or asphyxia, meningoencephalitis, or enlarging intracranial mass lesions such as neoplasms, brain edema causes intracranial pressure to rise to levels exceeding mean arterial blood pressure. At this point, intracranial circulation ceases and nearly all brain neurons that were not destroyed by the initial brain injury are secondarily destroyed by lack of intracranial circulation.

Thus the whole-brain formulation provides a fail-safe mechanism to eliminate false-positive brain death determinations and assure the loss of the critical functions of the organism as a whole. Showing the absence of all intracranial circulation is sufficient to prove widespread destruction of all critical neuronal systems.

The higher-brain formulation fails to provide an adequate criterion of death because its conditions are insufficient for the loss of the critical functions of the organism as a whole. Its criterion is the irreversible loss of consciousness and cognition. The most common clinical manifestation of this condition is the PVS, caused by diffuse damage to the cerebral hemispheres, thalami, or disconnections between those structures. In most cases of PVS, brain stem neurons and their functions remain intact, so PVS patients, although unaware, have retained wakefulness and sleep-wake cycles (through the function of the intact ascending reticular activating system), have continued control of respiration and circulation by the intact medulla, and retain other brain stem mediated regulatory functions. The higher-brain formulation, thus, serves as neither an adequate definition nor criterion of death.

The criterion of the brain stem formulation is the loss of consciousness and the capacity for breathing. Diffuse damage to the brain stem that is sufficient to destroy the ascending reticular activating system and the medullary breathing center satisfies this criterion. But the brain stem formulation does not require commensurate damage to the diencephalon or cerebral hemispheres. It therefore leaves open the possibility of misdiagnosis of death because of a pathological process that appears to destroy brain stem activities but that permits some form of residual conscious awareness that cannot be easily detected. It thus lacks the fail-safe feature of whole-brain death to test for and guarantee the irreversible loss of these critical systems.

As a criterion of death, the circulation formulation fails for precisely the opposite reason of the higher-brain and brain stem formulations. Whereas the higher-brain and brain stem criteria both fail because they are necessary but not sufficient for death, the circulation criterion fails because it is sufficient but not necessary for death. The loss of all systemic circulation produces the destruction of all bodily organs and tissues so it is clearly a sufficient condition for death. But it is unnecessary to require the cessation of functions of organs that do not serve the critical functions of the organism as a whole.

The Tests of Death

Brain death tests must be used to determine death only in the unusual case in which a patient's ventilation is being supported. If positive-pressure ventilation is neither employed nor entertained, the traditional tests of death – prolonged absence of breathing and heartbeat – can be used successfully. These traditional tests are absolutely predictive that the brain will be rapidly destroyed by lack of blood flow and oxygen, at which time death will have occurred. Traditional examinations for death, in addition to testing for heartbeat and breathing, always included tests for responsiveness and pupillary reflexes that directly measure brain function.

The bedside tests satisfying the whole-brain criterion of death have been designed with a sufficiently high degree of concordance to permit the drafting of widely accepted clinical practice guidelines on the determination of brain death. The tests require demonstrating the loss of all clinical brain functions, irreversibility, and a known structural process sufficient to produce the clinical findings. Laboratory tests showing the absence of intracranial blood flow or the absence of electrical activity in the hemispheres and brain stem can be used to confirm the clinical diagnosis to expedite the determination.

Irreversibility is an indispensable requirement for brain death. There is general belief that irreversibility can be adequately demonstrated by conducting serial neurological examinations, excluding potentially reversible factors, and demonstrating a structural cause that is sufficient to account for the clinical signs. But, while highly plausible, these conditions have never been proved to assure irreversibility. Two recent factors prompted me to reassess my previous position that irreversibility could be proved solely by clinical factors and to suggest that a laboratory test showing cessation of all intracranial blood flow should become mandatory in brain death determination.

There are several published studies documenting the alarming frequency of physician variations and errors in performing brain death tests, despite clear guidelines for performing and recording the tests. Patients with "chronic brain death" have been reported who were diagnosed as brain dead but whose circulation and visceral organ functioning were successfully physiologically maintained for months or longer. Eelco Wijdicks and I questioned whether all of the reported patients were correctly diagnosed, and if some brain-damaged but not brain dead patients were included because of inadequate examinations and resultant incorrect brain death determinations. Reacting to both these findings, I proposed that the mere assertion of irreversibility may no longer be sufficient to diagnose brain death and that a test showing cessation of all intracranial blood flow, such as transcranial Doppler ultrasonography, radionuclide angiography, or computed tomographic angiography, should become mandatory, at least if there is any question about the diagnosis or if the examiner is inexperienced.

Public Policy on Death

Brain death is widely regarded as the prime example of a formerly contentious bioethical and biophilosophical issue that has been resolved to the point of widespread public consensus. Evidence for this consensus is the enactment of effective and well-accepted brain death laws and policies throughout the world. In the United States, the Uniform Determination of Death Act, recommended by the President's Commission and the National Conference of Commissioners on Uniform State Laws, has been enacted in most states, and others have enacted statutes with similar language. Contemporaneously, the Law Reform Commission of Canada produced a similar statute.

But an observer unaware of this consensus and public acceptance, who relied solely on reading the output of scholarly articles and university conferences on brain death, would reach a far different conclusion. The publication of anti-brain death articles has never been greater than during the past decade. Yet, despite those arguments, the 1995 Institute of Medicine conference on brain death recommended no changes in public laws in the United States, no jurisdiction has abandoned its brain death statute, and there is evidence that many additional countries have embraced the practice of determining brain death during the past decade of scholarly dissention. What accounts for the mismatch between public acceptance and scholarly agitation?

Higher-brain proponents continue to accept brain death but argue that the criterion of death should be changed to the higher-brain formulation. Brain stem death proponents also accept the conceptual validity of brain death but hold that the criterion of death should be the brain stem formulation. Religious authorities continue a debate that has raged for 40 years about whether brain death is compatible with the doctrines of the world's principal religious traditions. Protestantism, including fundamentalism, has accepted brain death. The debate in Roman Catholicism was largely settled by Pope John Paul's 2000 pronouncement embracing brain death as consistent with Catholic teachings. In Judaism, brain death is accepted by Reform and Conservative authorities, but an Orthodox rabbinic debate continues between those who declare brain death compatible with Jewish law and those who do not. Brain death determination is also practiced in several Islamic societies, Hindi societies, and in Confucian-Shinto Japan.

The principal active opponents within the academy are those who reject the concept of brain death outright and promote the concept that a human being is not dead until the systemic circulation ceases and all organs are destroyed. The circulation proponents see no special role for brain functions in a determination of death.

Alan Shewmon, the intellectual leader of the circulationists, has written eloquently on the conceptual problems inherent within the whole-brain (or any brain criterion) formulation.

Another critic, Robert Taylor, has called the brain death concept a "legal fiction" that is accepted by society in a manner analogous to the concept of legal blindness. We all know that most people who are declared legally blind are not truly blind. But we employ a legal fiction and use the term "blindness" in a biologically incorrect way for its socially beneficial purpose. Taylor argues that, by analogy, we know that people we declare "brain dead" are not truly dead, but we consider them dead for the socially beneficial goal of organ procurement.

As a longstanding proponent of whole-brain death, I acknowledge that the whole-brain formulation, although coherent, is imperfect, and that my attempts to defend it have not adequately addressed all valid criticisms. But my inadequacies must be viewed within the larger context of the relationship of biology to public policy.

In the real world of public policy on biological issues, we must frequently make compromises or approximations to achieve acceptable practices and laws. For these compromises to be tolerable, generally they should be minor and not affect outcomes. For example, in the current practice of organ donation after cardiac death (formerly known as non-heart-beating organ donation), I and others raised the question of whether the organ donor patients were truly dead after only five minutes of asystole. The five-minute rule was accepted by the Institute of Medicine as the point at which death could be declared and the organs procured. Ours was a biologically valid criticism because, at least in theory, some such patients could be resuscitated after five minutes of asystole and still retain measurable brain function. If that was true, they were not yet dead at that point so their death declaration was premature.

But thereafter I changed my position to support programs of organ donation after cardiac death. I decided that it was justified to accept a compromise on this biological point when

I realized that donor patients, if not already dead at five minutes of asystole, were incipiently and irreversibly dying because they could not auto-resuscitate and no one would attempt their resuscitation. Because their loss of circulatory and respiratory functions was permanent if not yet irreversible, there would be no difference whatsoever in their outcomes if their death were declared after five minutes of asystole or after 60 minutes of asystole. I concluded that, from a public policy perspective, accepting the permanent loss of circulatory and respiratory functions rather than requiring their irreversible loss was justified. The good accruing to the organ recipient, the donor patient, and the donor family resulting from organ donation justified overlooking the biological shortcoming because, although the difference in the death criteria was real, it was inconsequential.

Of course Alan Shewmon is correct that not all bodily system integration and functions of the organism as a whole are conducted by the brain (though most are) and that the spinal cord and other structures serve relevant roles. And Robert Taylor is correct that many people view brain death as a legal fiction and regard such patients "as good as dead" but not biologically dead. But despite its shortcomings, the whole-brain death formulation comprises a concept and public policy that make intuitive and practical sense and have been well accepted by the public throughout many societies. Therefore, while I am willing to acknowledge that whole-brain death formulation remains imperfect, I continue to support it because on the public policy level its shortcomings are relatively inconsequential.

References

1. "Brain death" is the colloquial term for human death determination using tests of absent brain functions. But it is an unfortunate term because it is inherently misleading. It falsely implies that there are two types of death: brain death and ordinary death, instead of unitary death tested using two sets of tests. It also wrongly suggests that only the brain is dead in such patients. Robert Veatch

stated that because of these shortcomings he uses the term only in quotation marks (personal communication, November 4, 1995).

2. Alan and Elisabeth Shewmon recently claimed that my approach is futile because language constrains our capacity to conceptualize life and death. They regard death as an "ur-phenomenon" that is "…conceptually fundamental in its class; no more basic concepts exist to which it can be reduced. It can only be intuited from our experience of it…."

See D. A. Shewmon and E. S. Shewmon, "The Semiotics of Death and its Medical Implications," *Advances in Experimental Medicine and Biology* 550 (2004): 89–114. Winston Chiong also rejected my analytic approach, claiming that there can be no unified definition of death. Yet, he agreed that the whole-brain criterion of death is the most coherent concept of death. See W. Chiong, "Brain Death Without Definitions," *Hastings Center Report* 35 (2005): 20–30.

The Conscience Clause

How Much Individual Choice in Defining Death Can Our Society Tolerate?

ROBERT M. VEATCH

From *The Definition of Death*: Contemporary Controversies, edited by S. J. Younger, R. M. Arnold, and R. Shapiro. (Baltimore, MD: Johns Hopkins University Press), 137-160.

On the morning of March 1, 1994, a blue 1978 Chevrolet Impala pulled next to a van as it began to cross the Brooklyn Bridge. The van was carrying 15 students from the Lubavitch Hasidic Jewish sect returning from a prayer vigil in Manhattan. As the car neared the van, a lone gunman fired at least five rounds of bullets from two separate semiautomatic weapons into the side of the van while reportedly yelling, "Kill the Jews." Four students were injured, two critically. One, 15-year-old Aaron Halberstam, was "declared brain dead, but he remained on life support."

New York has adopted a brain-oriented definition of death through administrative regulation of the State Hospital and Planning Council and with the endorsement of the State Health Commissioner, which reads, "Both the individual standard of heart and lung activity and the standard of total and irreversible cessation of brain function should be recognized as the legal definition of death in New York." That would seem to imply that Mr. Halberstam was dead once the diagnosis of the death of the brain was confirmed. However, the parents, following widely held Jewish beliefs, insisted that the individual does not die when the brain dies. They would accept only a criterion based on respiratory function. The rabbis for the Halberstam family were reported to have said that Mr. Halberstam should be kept on support systems as long as his heart could beat on its own. The physician, honoring the parents' wishes, refused to pronounce the death. Depending on interpretation, this may have been legal. A sentence in the regulation permits (but does not require) physicians to accommodate family views on the definition of death.

One can hardly imagine what the result would have been had the family placed their ventilator-dependent, brain-dead, but not legally pronounced dead son in an ambulance and driven him through the Holland Tunnel to New Jersey. When they arrive in New Jersey, they are in a jurisdiction with an even more complex legal situation. New Jersey has a whole-brain-oriented criterion of death, but the law explicitly permits religious objectors to object to the use of that criterion in their own cases, thus making the patient alive until cardiac function ceases irreversibly. Had Mr. Halberstam been known to hold such views, he would clearly be alive in New Jersey, assuming the law applies to minors. The present law, however, does not explicitly permit family members to choose a cardiac criterion of death based on their own religious beliefs. Thus, unless his own views were known or the law were extended to permit surrogate decision making, he could not have been treated as alive.

The Present State of the Law

The New Jersey law is unique in the world. A few countries have not yet adopted a whole-brain criterion of death. They continue to use the traditional cardiac definition. All other jurisdictions except New Jersey have adopted a whole-brain-oriented definition without any provision for individuals to conscientiously object for religious or other reasons. The New York regulation appears to introduce some discretion, based on family objections to a brain-oriented definition, but actually gives the discretion to the physician who is contemplating death pronouncement based on a brain-oriented concept of death. A family could express dissent to one physician who is willing to accommodate, but, if they happen to be dealing with another physician, that physician could refuse the request to refrain from pronouncing death.

The law in most American jurisdictions specifies that if the criteria for measuring the irreversible loss of all functions of the entire brain are met, "death shall be pronounced." In other jurisdictions, the law actually reads "death may be pronounced." This seems to imply that the physician has the discretion, as in New York, except that the discretion is actually broader.

The physician could refuse to pronounce based on his or her own personal values, economic considerations, or other factors in addition to family wishes. Clearly, these laws seem defective if they give the physician the opportunity legally to choose whether to pronounce death based on the physician's values.

The common wisdom has been that such discretion makes no sense. After all, being dead seems to be an objective matter to be determined by good science (or perhaps good metaphysics) rather than by individual conscientious choice. Concern is often expressed that such discretion not only makes no sense but would produce public chaos leading to situations in which some patients are dead while medically identical patients are alive. I will make the case for the legitimacy of a conscientious objection to a uniform definition of death, a conscientious objection that permits patients to choose, while competent, an alternative definition of death provided that it is within reason and does not pose serious public health or other societal concerns. In cases in which the patient has not spoken while competent (in cases of infants, children, and adults who simply have not expressed themselves), I will argue that the next of kin should have this discretion within certain limits.

Concepts, Criteria, and the Role of Value Pluralism

The Early Fact-Value Distinction

Early in the debate over the definition of death, commentators insisted that a basic distinction be made between two elements of the discussion. What at first appeared to be one question turned out to include at least two separate issues. First, there was a question that seemed primarily scientific: How can we measure that the brain has been irreversibly destroyed (that it has "died")? That seems like the kind of question that those skilled in neurology could answer. The neurological community, sometimes aided by others, has offered many sets of criteria with associated tests and measures for determining that the brain will never again be able to conduct any of its functions. We have come to understand this as primarily a question for competent medical scientists.

The second question is quite different in character. It asks whether we as a society or as individuals ought to treat an individual with a dead brain as a dead person. This question is clearly not something about which the neurological community can claim expertise. No amount of neurological study could possibly determine whether those with dead brains should be considered dead people. This is a religious, philosophical, ethical, or public policy question, not one of neurological science.

When society determines that someone is dead, many social behavioral changes occur. The medical team may stop treating the patient if previously a decision had been made to treat aggressively to the very end of life; health insurance coverage will cease, while life insurance will pay off; if the patient is married, the spouse becomes a widow or widower; grieving can begin in a way that was not appropriate previously; and, if the deceased was president of the United States, the vice president automatically assumes the presidency. A great deal is at stake in determining exactly when someone dies. Wills will be read, assets distributed, and the timing of the occurrence of the death, which may be critical for determining inheritance, prosecution of crimes, and other things, will be established. These are not neurological issues; they are social, normative issues about which all citizens may reasonably voice a position relying on their personal religious, philosophical, and ethical view of the world. I have been pressing for this distinction between concept and criteria and some critical implications that follow since the late 1960s.

Democratic Pluralism and Value Variation

In a democratic, pluralistic culture, we have great insight into how to deal with religious, philosophical, and ethical issues about which there are strongly held views and unresolvable controversy. At the level of morality, we agree to tolerate diverse opinion, and we even let a person

act on those opinions, at least until the effects on the lives of others become intolerable. This is the position we take regarding religious dissent.

Religious and Other Positions

To the extent that the disagreement is a religious or quasi-religious disagreement, toleration of pluralism seems the appropriate course. It permits people with differences to live together in harmony. And at least one major source of division over the definition of death is surely theological. The case with which this chapter opened seems not only to have been caused by tensions between Jewish people and Muslims; the moral disagreement about whether to declare Mr. Halberstam dead also has religious roots. Judaism has long been known to include persons who oppose brain criteria for death pronouncement. Not that all Jews oppose it. Rabbi Moses Tendler, a well-known moral commentator, has supported it. But many Orthodox rabbinical scholars strongly oppose it, maintaining that where there is breath there is life. Japanese, influenced by Buddhist and Shinto belief systems, see the presence of life in the whole body, not just in the brain. Native Americans reportedly sometimes hold religious beliefs that oppose a brain-oriented definition of death. Fundamentalist Christians, sometimes associated with the right-to-life movement, and some Catholics focusing on pro-life issues press for a consistent pro-life position by opposing death pronouncement of brain-dead individuals.

On the other hand, mainstream Christians, both Protestant and Catholic, support a brain-oriented definition, claiming that being prolife does not foreclose being clear on when life ends. One Christian theological argument supporting brain-oriented definitions starts with the ancient Christian theological anthropology that sees the human as the integration of body and mind or spirit. When the two are irreversibly separated, then the human is gone. This view, as we shall see, places many Christian theologians in the higher-brain camp.

There are, of course, also many secular persons who support a cardiac definition of death. One, now somewhat dated, survey found that about a third continued to support a cardiac definition. The only plausible conclusion is that the definition of death is heavily influenced by theological and metaphysical beliefs, along with theories of value. We have learned that, in a pluralistic society, it is unrealistic to expect unanimity on such questions. Hence, a tolerance of pluralism may be the only way to resolve the public policy debate.

This conclusion seems even more inevitable when one realizes that there are not just two or three plausible definitions (cardiac, whole-brain, and higher-brain definitions); there are literally hundreds of possible variants. Some insist on irreversible loss of anatomical brain structure at the cellular level; others only on irreversible loss of function. Some insist on loss of function at the cellular level, while others insist only on irreversible loss of supercellular functions or integration of bodily function. Some might insist on loss of all central nervous system functions, including spinal cord function (an early position of Henry Beecher, the chair of the Harvard ad hoc committee), while others draw a line between spinal cord and brain. Among defenders of the higher-brain concept, there are countless variations on what counts as "higher": everything above the brainstem, the cerebrum, the cerebral cortex, the neocortex, the sensory cortex, and so forth. Some, insisting on loss of all brain functions, ignore electrical functions, limiting their attention to clinical functions. Some are even willing to ignore functions of "nests of cells," claiming they may be "insignificant."

When all the possible variants are combined, there will be a large number of positions; no group is likely to gain the support of more than a small minority of the population. The only way to have a single definition of death is for those with power to coerce others to use their preferred definition. If that single definition were the current "whole brain" one with a requirement that literally all functions of the brain must be gone before death is pronounced, the result could be disastrous. No one really believes that every last function of the entire brain must be irreversibly

lost for a brain to be dead. That would include all electrical functions, all neurohumoral functions, and cellular functions. Since clinicians would necessarily have to exercise discretion in deciding which functions are to be ignored, patients would be at the mercy of the discretion of the clinician who happens to be present when the question of pronouncing death arises. Even if we were willing to let some ride roughshod over others, it is very unlikely that any one position could gain majority support; in fact, it is unlikely that any single position could come close to a majority. There may be no alternative but to tolerate multiple views.

Problems Limiting Conscientious Objection to Religious Objectors

A state limiting conscientious objection to religious objectors, as New Jersey has done, is likely to face potentially difficult constitutional challenges. We learned from laws permitting religious conscientious objection to service in the military that restricting objection to certain types may be legally indefensible. During the Vietnam war era, some objectors had views that were clearly moral or philosophical, but they had a hard time accepting or demonstrating to others that they were religious. Especially if *religious* is defined as involving belief in a Supreme Being, many individuals whose objections seemed very similar to religious objections could not qualify. Even members of certain groups often classified as *religions* could not meet the belief in a Supreme Being test: Buddhism, Confucianism, Native American belief systems, all look much like religions but fail the Supreme Being test. Gradually, the restriction of conscientious objection to religions objection was challenged and was found to be discriminatory. The concept of religious objection was gradually broadened to include many belief systems that may not, at first, appear to be overtly religious.

Some scholars who have studied the New Jersey criterion of death law (including some most closely involved with the drafting of the law) believe that restriction of the beliefs supporting objection to the brain-oriented definition of death to those that were narrowly religious would be interpreted to include more broadly moral objections as well.

There are enormous practical as well as moral problems with attempts to limit the law to religion narrowly construed. At a practical level, enforcement officials would have to establish mechanisms for verifying whether an objection was truly religious. A nonpracticing Jew who had a nonreligious objection to a brain-oriented definition of death could cite his religious background, and it would be almost impossible for the state to establish whether his objection was religious. Morally, the principle of equal respect would seem to require that, if religious objections were permitted, equally sincere and equally deeply held nonreligious philosophical objections would be equally acceptable. If little is at stake in terms of public interest, little is lost by accepting both on equal terms.

Assuming that the case is made that individuals should be able to exercise religiously or nonreligiously based conscientious choice of an alternative definition of death, should that discretion be extended to surrogate decision makers in the manner of decisions to refuse treatment by patients with terminal illness? I see no reason to limit the choice to competent and formerly competent persons who have executed advance directives.

Consider a formerly competent adult or adolescent who has never formally written a document choosing an alternative definition of death, but who has left an oral record or a life-style pattern that appears to the surrogate to favor an alternative. Mr. Halberstam was returning from an Orthodox Jewish prayer service when he was shot. Assuming that he has not written an instruction stating a preference for a cardiac-oriented definition of death, should parents (or other next of kin) be permitted formally to choose it for Mr. Halberstam (as, in fact, Mr. Halberstam's did through the informal decisions in New York)? It appears that he had continued to live

the religious life of his parents, and I see no reason to doubt that he would choose as they did. Just as the next of kin can presently exercise substituted judgment in decisions to forgo treatment, his parents likewise should be permitted to choose on his behalf based on the values he is most likely to have held.

But suppose we had no idea what Mr. Halberstam's wishes were about which definition of death should be used in his case. Or suppose he suffered his injury when he was 1 year old rather than 15 or 21. Clearly, in these cases respecting autonomy is out of the question. The only moral alternative is to use what is considered the best concept of death. But should it be the concept of death considered best by the society—perhaps some version of a whole-brain-oriented death, assuming that is the law of the state—or should it be the concept considered best by his next of kin? In the context of decisions to forgo treatment, I have long argued that the discretion should go to the next of kin under the doctrine of what I have called *limited familial autonomy*. Just as the individual has an autonomous right to choose a definition of death (or a treatment plan), so likewise families are given a range of discretion in deciding what is best for their wards. They select the schooling and religious education that so dramatically shapes the system of values and beliefs of the child. They are expected to socialize the child into some value system. In a liberal pluralistic society, we do not insist that the familial surrogate choose the best possible value system for their wards; we expect them to exercise discretion, drawing on their own beliefs and values. As long as the ward's interests are not jeopardized too substantially and the interests of the society are not threatened, parents should not only be permitted, but actually be expected to make a choice of a definition of death for their wards.

Limits on the Range of Discretion

In my early writing on the subject of individual choice of a definition of death, I assumed without stating it that the range of choice would be limited among a range of tolerable alternatives. If the risks to the society became too great, surely a limit would have to be placed. Hence, probably, no one should be able to decide that he or she should be treated as alive if cardiac, respiratory, and brain function have all completely and irreversibly ceased. At least such choice should be foreclosed if it would pose public health problems or be grossly unfair to spouse and beneficiaries. Likewise, I believe no one should be able to choose to be considered dead when he or she retains all of these functions. Also, for pragmatic reasons a state should choose a default definition, leaving it up to individuals to exercise conscientious objection if they disagree with the default. What I now make explicit is that the choice must be within a range of reasonable or tolerable alternatives.

The Inclusion of Higher-Brain Concepts of Death

For over 20 years I and many other people have argued that it is no longer plausible to hold to a literal whole-brain definition in which every last function of the entire brain must be dead before death can be pronounced. A case can be made that some versions of higher-brain formulations of a definition of death should be among the choices permitted. Under such an arrangement, a whole-brain definition might be viewed as the centrist view that would serve as the default definition, permitting those with more conservative views to opt for cardiac-oriented definitions and those with more liberal views to opt for certain higher-brain formulations. Of course, this would permit people with brainstem function including spontaneous respiration to be treated as dead. Organs could be procured that otherwise would not be available (assuming the dead-donor rule is retained), bodies could be used for research (assuming proper consent is obtained), and life insurance would pay off.

Some might be concerned that this would give surrogates the authority to have their wards treated as dead while some brain and cardiac functions remain. They see this as posing risks for unacceptable choices, for ending a lingering state of disability, for example. Assuming that the only cases that could be classified as dead by surrogates would be those who have lost all capacity for consciousness (i.e., who have lost all higher-brain functions), the risks to the individual classified as deceased would be minimal. We must keep in mind that surrogates are already presumed to have the authority to terminate all life support on these people. Often such decisions by surrogates to terminate life support would mean that the patient would soon be dead by the most traditional definitions of death. Death by traditional cardiac and whole-brain criteria would occur within minutes in many cases if the surrogate exercised his or her authority to forgo life support. The effect on inheritance and insurance would be trivial if these cases were simply called dead before stopping medical support rather than stopping prior to pronouncing death. Even for those vegetative or comatose patients who had sufficient lower-brain function to breathe on their own, a suspension of all medical treatment would lead to death fairly soon.

Adding a higher-brain option to the range of discretion would have only minimal effect on practical matters and would be a sign that we can show the same respect to the religious and philosophical convictions of those favoring the higher-brain position as we do now in New Jersey for the holders of the cardiac position. If there are actually scores of potential definitions of death within the range from higher-brain to cardiac positions, then only a relatively small minority is likely to be in agreement with the default position. The wise thing to do seems to be to pick some intermediary position and permit people to deviate to both somewhat more liberal and somewhat more conservative positions. The choices would probably have to be limited to this range. Both public health and moral problems become severe if the scope of choice is expanded much further.

The Problem of Order: Objections to a Conscience Clause

All of this, of course, depends on my as-yet-undefended claim that there are no significant societal or third-party harms from permitting conscientious objection to a default definition within the range I have specified. The President's Commission for the Study of Ethical Problems in Medicine and Biomedical and Behavioral Research prepared an important report in 1981 reviewing the debate on the definition of death. In that report the commission examined the cardiac, whole-brain, and higher-brain options. In spite of the fact that their two philosophical consultants on the issue endorsed versions of a higher-brain formulation, the commission endorsed the whole-brain position. They gave serious consideration to the higher-brain position before rejecting it for a number of reasons, most of which can be summarized under the heading of the problems that would be created for social order.

Death as a Biological Fact

One preliminary objection that was not dwelt on by the commission but that arises in many discussions of the issue is the claim that death is not a matter of religious or philosophical or policy choice, but rather a matter of biological fact. It is now generally recognized that the choice of a concept of death (as opposed to formulation of criteria and tests) is really normative or ontological. We are debating when as a matter of social policy ought we to treat someone as dead. No amount of biological research can answer that question at the conceptual level. Of course, many people could still hold that, although the definition of death is a normative or ontological question, there is still only one single correct formulation. That seems to me to be a very plausible position, but we are not discussing the issue of whether there can be only one true definition of death; we are discussing whether society can function for public policy purposes while tolerating differences in beliefs about the true definition. Tolerating a Jew's or Native American's belief in a definition that is perceived as wrong is no different from having a society tolerate more than one belief about whether abortion or forgoing life support in the living is morally correct. We are asking whether society can treat people as dead based on their own beliefs rather than whether people are really dead, really conform to some metaphysically correct conception of what it means to be dead, in such circumstances. (It is possible to hold that there is one and only one metaphysically correct concept of death, but that society can treat some people who conform to this meaning of death as if they were alive.)

Policy Chaos

One of the consistent themes in the criticism of higher-brain definitions, especially with the conscience clause I am defending, is that its adoption would lead to policy chaos. Presumably critics have in mind stress of health professionals, insurers, family members, and public policy processes, such as succession of the presidency. But a very similar substituted-judgment and best-interest discretion is already granted surrogates regarding decisions to forgo life support on still-living patients. One would think that the potential for abuse and for chaos would be much greater granting this discretion. It remains to be seen what chaos would be created from conscientious objection to a default definition of death. If each of the envisioned policy problems can be addressed successfully, then we are left with a religious/philosophical/policy choice for which we should be tolerant of variation if possible and no good social reasons to reject individual discretion. Some of the rebuttal against the charge of policy chaos has already been suggested.

Problems with the Stoppage of Treatment

One concern is that life-sustaining medical treatment would be stopped on different people with medically identical conditions at different times if conscientious choice among definitions of death is permitted. That assumes, however, that decisions to stop treatment are always linked to pronouncement of death. We now know that normally it is appropriate to consider suspension of treatments in a manner that is decoupled from the question of whether the patient is dead. A large percentage of in-hospital deaths now occur as a result of a decision to stop treatment and let the patient die. Presumably any valid surrogate who was contemplating opting for a higher-brain definition of death would, if told that option were not available, immediately contemplate choosing to forgo treatment, letting the patient die. In either case the patient will be dead within a short period.

Health Insurance

I have already mentioned the potential impact on health insurance if someone chooses a definition of death that would have the effect of making someone alive longer—if, for instance, a cardiac definition were chosen. (If some version of a higher-brain definition were chosen, the effect would more likely be a savings in health insurance.) There is good reason to believe that the effect on health insurance would be minimal. A relatively small number of people would actively make a pro-treatment choice based on their preference for a cardiac definition or any alternative that would require longer treatment. The small costs would probably be justified to preserve respect for individual freedom on religious or philosophical matters. If an insurer were worried about unfair impact on the subscriber pool if its funds were used to provide care for patients without brain function who had selected a cardiac definition of death, they could simply exclude care for living patients with dead brains.

Life Insurance

The concern by life insurance companies is exactly the opposite. Insisting on a cardiac definition would simply delay payment, which would be in the insurer's interest; however, selecting a higher-brain definition would make the individual dead sooner, potentially quite a bit sooner. However, most living persons with dead brains die fairly soon either because such patients are hard to maintain or because an advance directive or surrogate opts for termination of treatment.

Inheritance

As in the case of pensions and life insurance, some surrogate might be inclined to manipulate the timing of death to gain an inheritance more quickly. This could lead to choosing a higher-brain definition. However, the same surrogate already has the power to decline medical treatment, which would theoretically expose the patient to similar risks, and such cases are exceedingly rare. If a surrogate is suspected of abusing a patient by choosing an inappropriate concept of death, such a surrogate can always be challenged and removed. If one compares the risk of abuse from surrogate discretion in deciding to forgo treatment with that from deciding on a variant definition of death, surely the discretion in forgoing treatment is more controversial and more subject to abuse. Yet that has not proved to be a significant problem.

Spousal or Marital Status

Another social practice that can be affected directly by the timing of a death is the marital status of the spouse. Spouses may want to retain their status as spouses rather than become widows or widowers for various psychological and financial reasons. Or they may want to become widows or widowers so that they can get on with their lives. Conceivably, some may be ready to remarry. For example, a spouse who had been caring for a PVS patient for years may have already separated psychologically from his or her mate even though that mate was not actually dead. This person could be ready to remarry, which could be done legally once the spouse were deceased. This problem seems quite farfetched, but it could happen. Such spouses would probably already have contemplated refusing life support and could be removed as inappropriate surrogates if it is clear that they are motivated for non-patient-centered reasons.

The Effect on Health Professionals

A final potential problem with authorizing conscientious choice is the possible effect on health professionals providing care for the patient. Nurses will be required to suffer potential emotional stress at having to continue care or cease care at a time they believe inappropriate. Physicians will face similar problems. But this is hardly a problem unique to a choice of a definition of death. Some living patients or their surrogates refuse life-supporting therapy before the nurse or physician believes appropriate. The health professional is simply obliged to stop according to laws about informed consent and the right to refuse treatment. More recently, health professionals have been disturbed about requests for care the clinicians deem futile. Patients who insisted on not being pronounced dead until their heart stopped potentially could insist on hospital-based treatment even though their brains were dead. That is potentially the situation in New Jersey now. But the responsibility of the health professional to deliver care deemed futile against his or her will is already a matter of considerable controversy. It will have to be resolved whether or not other states adopt the New Jersey conscience clause. Most patients demanding such care are clearly not dead by any definition. The resolution could be the same for patients with dead brains as it is for terminally ill or vegetative patients, or it could be different. The law could determine, for instance, that conscious patients would have a right of access to normatively futile care (perhaps with the proviso that they have independent funding), but that permanently unconscious patients or those with dead brains would have no right of access. In any case, the effect on care givers is not a problem unique to patients who might exercise an option for an alternative definition of death.

The Implementation of a Conscience Clause

The procedural implementation of a conscience clause would require some additional planning, but the problems would not be novel. Most are addressed in the existing Patient Self-Determination Act and required response laws. The former requires that someone inquire about the existence of an advance directive upon admission to a hospital and provide assistance in executing an advance directive if the patient desires. The latter requires that the next of kin be notified of the opportunity to donate organs in suitable cases. The most plausible way to record a choice of something other than a default concept of death would be in one's advance directive. That is the kind of document that ought to be on the minds of those caring for a patient who is near death. An addition specifying a choice of an alternative concept of death would be easy; it would be crucial in the case of those who are writing an advance directive demanding that life support continue even though the brain is dead. It would be a simple clarification in the case of one asking that support be forgone when the patient is permanently unconscious. A sentence choosing a higher-brain concept of death (and perhaps donating organs at that point) would be a modest addition.

Whether the new definition-of-death laws authorizing a conscience clause should also impose a duty on health professionals to notify patients or their surrogates of alternative concepts of death is a pragmatic question that would have to be addressed. I do not think that would be necessary. Just as Orthodox Jews presently carry the burden of notifying others of their requirements for a kosher diet and Jehovah's Witnesses carry the burden of notifying about refusal of blood transfusions, so those with alternative concepts of death would plausibly carry that burden. Something akin to the subjective standard for informed consent would apply. According to that standard, health professionals, when they negotiate a consent, are required to inform the patient of what the patient would reasonably want to know, but they are not expected to surmise all unusual views and interests of the patient. According to this approach, they would be expected to initiate discussions on alternative definitions of death only when they knew or had reason to know that the patient plausibly would have an interest in such a discussion. A clinician who knew his patient was an Orthodox Jew and knew that many Orthodox Jews prefer a more traditional concept of death would have such an obligation, but there would be no obligation if he or she had no reason to believe the patient might be inclined toward an alternative concept.

Some might claim that adding a conscience clause is unnecessary because only a small group of people would favor an alternative. In fact, a not insignificant number seem to prefer a more traditional cardiac or respiratory concept of death (Jews, Native Americans, Japanese, and others who are still committed to the importance of the heart or lungs). If a higher-brain-oriented concept of death were among the options, a much larger minority would have an interest in exercising the conscience clause. In fact, there have been court cases and anecdotal reports of families objecting to the use of whole-brain-based concepts. It seems reasonable to assume that these represent only a fraction of the total number of cases in which patients or families would prefer either a more traditional or a more innovative concept of death.

Even if it could be shown that few people would care enough about the concept and criteria of death used to pronounce them or their loved ones dead, this is still an important issue to clarify. It is important if only the rights of a small minority are violated. It is also important as a matter of conceptual clarity and of principle. Getting people to think why a conscience clause is appropriate for this issue has an important teaching function and serves to respect the rights of minorities on deeply held religious and philosophical convictions.

Conclusion

Once one grasps that the choice of a definition of death at the conceptual level is a religious/philosophical/policy choice rather than a question of medical science, the case for granting discretion within limits in a liberal pluralistic society is very powerful. There seems to be no basis for imposing a unilateral normative judgment on the entire population when the members of the society are clearly divided. When one realizes that there are many variants and that no one is likely to receive the support of a majority, pluralism seems to be the only answer. Having a state choose a default definition (probably the whole-brain, middle-of-the-road position) and then granting individuals a limited range of discretion within the limits of reason seems to be the only defensible option. There is no reason to limit this discretion to religiously based reasons and no reason why familial surrogates should not be empowered to use substituted judgment or best-interest standards for making such choices, just as they presently do for forgoing treatment decisions that determine even more dramatically the timing of death. A default with an authorization for conscientious objection seems the humane, respectful, fair, and pragmatic solution.

The Case for Mortality

LEON R. KASS

The American Scholar 52, no. 2 (1983): 173–191.

Why should we die? Why should we, the flower of the living kingdom, lose our youthful bloom and go to seed? Why should we grow old in body and in mind, losing our various powers—first gradually, then altogether in death? Until now, the answer has been simple: We should because we must. Aging, decay, and death have been inevitable, as necessary for us as for other animals and plants, from whom we are distinguished in this matter only by our awareness of this necessity. We *know* that we are, as the poet says, like the leaves, the leaves that the wind scatters to the ground.

Recently, this necessity seems to have become something of a question, thanks to research into the phenomena of aging. Senescence, decay, and even our species-specific life span are now thought to be the result of biological processes that are, at least in part, genetically controlled, open to investigation, and in principle subject to human intervention and possible control. Slowing the processes of aging could yield powers to retard senescence, to preserve youthfulness, and to prolong life greatly, perhaps indefinitely. Should these powers become available, "Whether to wither and why?" will become questions of the utmost seriousness.

But there is a more far-reaching reason for looking at the project to control aging, inasmuch as its objectives are, in many respects, continuous with the aspirations of modern medicine for longer life and better health. Indeed, prolongation of healthy and vigorous life—and ultimately, a victory over mortality—is perhaps the central goal and meaning of the modern scientific project, associated in its founding with men like Bacon and Descartes. Bacon it was who first called mankind to "the conquest of nature for the relief of man's estate," and there is ample suggestion in

Bacon's writings that he regarded mortality itself as that part of man's estate from which he most needs relief.

Descartes, in a famous passage in Part VI of the *Discourse on Method*, rejects the speculative philosophy of his predecessors in favor of a new practical philosophy that would "render ourselves as masters and possessors of nature." Descartes prophesied "that we could be free of an infinitude of maladies both of body and mind, and even also possibly of the infirmities of age, if we had sufficient knowledge of their causes, and of all the remedies with which nature has provided us."

Examining the campaign against aging might therefore shed some light on our entire scientific and technological project—its promise and its danger, its benefits and its costs. Thought about this future—albeit somewhat futuristic—prospect may along the way illuminate current practice and belief. At a minimum it will cause us to re-examine some of the basic assumptions on which we have been proceeding—for example, that everything possible should be done to make us healthier and more vigorous, that life should be prolonged and death postponed as long as possible, and that the ultimate goal of medical research is to help us live in health and vigor, indefinitely. Most important, we might become more thoughtful about the meaning of mortality and its implications for how to live.

II

Aging research is pursued and supported by those who aspire to longer life for man, recognizing as they do that medicine's contributions to longevity have nearly reached their natural limit. As more fatal diseases and other causes of death are brought under control, more and more people are living out the natural human life span. But aging research is also pursued and encouraged by many more who hope that it will help to prevent or treat the infirmities, degenerations, and general loss of vigor that afflict the growing number of old people. These ailments are, in large part, the hitherto necessary price for the gift of longevity, a gift made possible by previous advances in hygiene, sanitation, medicine, and general living conditions. The benefits of success for individuals are obvious—who would not like to avoid or minimize for himself or his loved ones the burdens of weakness, immobility, memory loss, and progressive blindness, deafness, and dementia? These burdens to individuals are also costly for the society: there is loss of productivity and expensive medical and social services. By reducing these losses and these costs, the community, too, would presumably benefit from alleviating the handicaps and dependencies of the aged.

Yet this is but a narrow view of the social implications of retarding aging and contains a rather shrunken view of the old. The elderly are related to us not only as non-producing objects of care and expenditure. They are, it should go without saying, in the first instance human beings—now our ancestors, soon ourselves—most of whom do not think of themselves as belonging to a separated class, insultingly called "senior citizens." Especially as they are fit and able, they participate as individuals in the complex network of functions, institutions, customs, and rituals that bind us all together. Yet for some purposes it is useful to recognize what each of the age groups has in common and to notice as well the interdependence of these groups. It should then be clear that one cannot change the lot of one segment of the population without affecting the entire network of relations.

To begin with, if life were extended ten to twenty years, what would be the effects on the size and distribution of the population? The percentages and number of people over age sixty-five continues to increase. How would the growing numbers of nonagenarians and centenarians affect work opportunities, retirement plans, new hiring and promotion, social security, housing patterns, cultural and social attitudes and beliefs, the status of traditions, the rate and acceptability of social change, the structure of family life, relations between the generations, or the locus of rule and authority in government, business, and the professions? Clearly these are very complex issues, affected not only by changing demographic patterns, but also by social attitudes and practices relating these various matters to perceived stages of the life cycle, and also by our ability to anticipate and plan for, or at least to respond flexibly to, dislocations and strains. Still, even the most cursory examination of any of these matters suggests that the cumulative effect of the result of aggregated individual decisions for longer and more vigorous life could be highly disruptive and undesirable, even to the point that many individuals would be *sufficiently worse off* through most of their lives as to offset the benefits of better health afforded them near the end of life.

Let me illustrate with one example. Consider employment. How will the large numbers of seventy- and eighty- and ninety-year-olds occupy themselves? Less infirm, more vigorous, they will be less likely to accept being cut off from power, work, money, and a place in society, and it would seem, at first glance, to be even more reprehensible than it now is to push them out of the way. New opportunities and patterns for work or leisure would appear to be needed. Mandatory retirement could be delayed, permitting the old to remain active and permitting society to gain from the continued use of their accumulated skills. But what about the numerous tedious, unrewarding, or degrading jobs? Would delaying retirement be desirable or attractive? Also, would not delayed retirement clog the promotional ladders and block opportunities for young people just starting out, raising obstacles to the ambitions and hopes of all—save for longer job security for those who have made it aboard?

The planned undertaking of second and third careers could provide alternatives to later retirement, but with few exceptions such opportunities would require re-education during mid-career, especially now that knowledge and skills needed for work are increasingly sophisticated and require more and more specialized education. These same educational requirements render difficult the development of new and rewarding uses of post-retirement leisure, and it is far from clear that leisure is most fruitfully used when stacked up at the end of a life in which work is regarded as the main source of dignity. And, in any case, if the old are to be at leisure, the middle-aged will have to pay—a task they are unlikely to want to undertake, strapped as they are by the mounting costs of caring for their young. A basic question we are already struggling with, and not very well, is how to accommodate our growing elderly population in a society whose young people are greatly troubled by feelings of powerlessness, frustration, and alienation. If people lived healthily to 100 or 120, if institutions were altered to meet their needs, we would likely have traded our problems of the aged for problems of youth. Retardation of aging could really mean prolongation of functional immaturity. Consider the young: isolated not only from the top of the ladders of power but also from some of their lower rungs, supported by or even living with parents into their thirties or beyond, kept in a protracted sexually mature "adolescence," frustrated, disaffected, rebellious or apathetic—the picture is not difficult to complete.

Against all these concerns about social consequences, it will be argued that we will soon enough adjust to a world of longevity. We will figure out a way. This confidence rests on what seems to be good evidence: we have always adjusted in the past. Let us grant this point. Let us accept the optimist's view: longer life for individuals is an unqualified good; we will, in due time, figure out a way to cope with the social consequences.

III

Conceding all this, how *much* longer life is an unqualified good for an individual? Ignoring

now the possible harms flowing back to individuals from adverse social consequences, let us consider only the question "How much more life is good for us as individuals, other things being equal?" How much more life do we want, assuming it to be healthy and vigorous? Assuming that it were up to us to set the human life span, where would or should we set the limit and why?

The simple answer is that no limit should be set. Life is good, and death is bad. Therefore, the more life the better, provided, of course, that we remain fit and our friends do, too.

This answer has the virtues of clarity and honesty. But most public advocates of prolonging life through slowing aging deny such greediness. Immortality, or rather indefinite prolongation, is not their goal—it is, they say, out of the question (one wonders whether this is only because they deem it impossible). They hope instead for something reasonable; just a few more years.

How many years is reasonably few? Let us start with ten. Which of us would find unreasonable or unwelcome the addition of ten healthy and vigorous years to his or her life, years like those between ages thirty and forty? We could learn more, earn more, see more, do more. Maybe we should ask for five additional years? Or ten more? Why not fifteen, or twenty, or more?

If we can't immediately land on the reasonable number of added years, perhaps we can locate the principle. What is the principle of reasonableness? Time needed for our plans and projects yet to be completed? Some multiple of the age of a generation, say, that we might live to see great grandchildren fully grown? Some notion—traditional, natural, revealed—of the proper life span for a being such as man? We have no answer to this question. We do not know even how to choose among the principles for setting our new life span. The number of years chosen will have to be arbitrary, barring some revelation or discovery.

Under such circumstances, lacking a standard of reasonableness, we fall back on our wants and desires. Under liberal democracy, this means on the desires of the majority. Though what we desire is an empirical question, I suspect we know the answer: the attachment to life—or the fear of death—knows no limits, certainly not for most human beings. It turns out that the simple answer is the best: we want to live and live and not to wither and not to die. For most of us, especially under modern secular conditions in which more and more people believe that this is the only life they have, the desire to prolong the life span (even modestly) must be seen as expressing a desire *never* to grow old and die. However naive their counsel, those who propose immortality deserve credit: they honestly and shamelessly expose this desire.

Some, of course, eschew any desire for longer life. They profess still more modest aims: not adding years to life, but life to years. No increased life span, but only increased health, increased vigor, no decay. For them, the ideal life span would be our natural fourscore and ten, or if by reason of strength, fivescore, lived with full powers to the end, which end would come rather suddenly, painlessly, at the maximal age.

This has much to recommend it. Who would not want to avoid senility, crippling arthritis, the need for hearing aids and dentures, and the degrading dependencies of old age? Yet leaving aside whether such goals are attainable without simultaneously pushing far back the midnight hour, one must wonder whether, in the absence of these degenerations, we could remain content to spurn longer life, whether we would not become still more disinclined to exit. Would not death become even more of an affront? Would not the fear and loathing of death increase, in the absence of its antecedent harbingers? We could no longer comfort the widow by pointing out that her husband was delivered from his suffering. Death would always be untimely, unprepared for, shocking.

Withering is nature's preparation for death, for the one who dies and for those who look upon him. We may wish to flee from it, perhaps, or seek to cover it over, but we must be cognizant of the costs of doing so.

By the way, it is well worth pausing to ask, of *what* will we die in that golden age of prolonged vigor? Perhaps there will be a new spate of diseases, as yet unknown. More likely, the unnatural or violent causes will get us, as they increasingly do: some by auto, some by pistol, some by fire and some by drowning, some by lightning and some by bombing, some through anger and some through mercy, and some by poison from their own hand.

But to return from these macabre speculations to the main point: It is highly likely that either a modest prolongation of life with vigor or even only a preservation of youthfulness with no increase in longevity would make death even less acceptable, and would exacerbate the desire to keep pushing it further away—unless, for some reason, such life should also prove to be less satisfying.

Could longer, healthier life be less satisfying? How could it be, if life is good and death is bad? Perhaps the simple view is in error. Perhaps mortality is not simply an evil, perhaps it is even a blessing—not only for the welfare of the community, but even for us as individuals. How could this be?

IV

It goes without saying that there is no virtue in the death of a child or a young adult—or the untimely or premature death of anyone—before they have attained to the measure of man's days. I do not mean to imply that there is virtue in the particular *event* of death for anyone. Nor am I suggesting that separation through death is ever anything but pain for the survivors, those for whom the deceased was an integral part of their lives. Nor have I forgotten that, at whatever age, the process of dying can be painful and degrading, smelly and mean—though we now have powerful means to reduce much of, at least, the physical agony. Instead my question concerns the fact of our finitude, the fact of our mortality—that is, the fact that we must die, the fact that a full life for human beings has a biological, built-in limit, one that has evolved as part of our nature. Does this fact also have value? Is our finitude good for us—as individuals? (I intend this question entirely in the realm of natural reason and apart from any question about a life after death.)

To praise mortality must seem to be madness. If mortality is a blessing, it surely is not widely regarded as such. Life seeks to live, and rightly suspects all counsels of finitude. "Better to be a slave on earth than the king over all the dead," says Achilles in Hades to the visiting Odysseus, in apparent regret for his prior choice of the short but glorious life (*Odyssey*, Book XI, 489). Moreover, though some cultures—like the Eskimo—can instruct and moderate somewhat the lust for life, ours gives it free rein, beginning with a political philosophy founded on the fear of violent death and on the mastery of nature for the relief of man's estate, and reaching to our current cults of youth and novelty, the cosmetic replastering of the wrinkles of age, and the widespread, and not wholly irrational, anxiety about disease and survival. Finally, the virtues of finitude—if there are any—may never be widely appreciated in any age or culture, if appreciation depends on a certain wisdom, if wisdom requires a certain detachment from the love of oneself and one's own, and if the possibility of such detachment is given only to the few.

Let us, then, consider the problem of *boredom* and *tedium*. If the life span were increased—say by twenty years—would the pleasures of life increase proportionately? Would professional tennis players really enjoy playing 25 percent more games of tennis? Would the Don Juans of our world feel better for having seduced 1,250 women rather than 1,000? Having experienced the joys and tribulations of bringing up a family until the last left for college, how many parents would like to extend the experience by another ten years? Similarly, those who derive their satisfaction from progressing up the career ladder might well ask what there would be to do for fifteen years after one had become president of General Motors or after one had been chairman of the House Ways and Means Committee for a quarter of a century. Even less clear are the additions to personal happiness from more-of-the-same of the less pleasant and fulfilling activities that so many of us engage in so much of the time.

The problem of boredom is worse for us than it once might have been because of how we have come to understand it. For us, with our self-centered views, the fear of boredom is the fear that sooner or later the world and its objects will fail us. For the medievals, boredom meant that we will fail the world. They regarded boredom as a defect within oneself. It was an aspect of sloth—one of the seven deadly sins, according to Thomas Aquinas—a sin against the Sabbath, that is, against the created order, not, as we might think, against the workweek.

The question of boredom leads directly to the second and more serious question, the question of *seriousness*. Could life be serious or meaningful without the limit of mortality? Is not the limit on our time the ground of our taking life seriously and living it passionately? To know and to feel that one goes around only once, and that the deadline is not out of sight, is for many people the necessary spur to the pursuit of something worthwhile. To number our days is the condition for making them count and for treasuring and appreciating all that life brings. Homer's immortals, for all their eternal beauty and youthfulness, live shallow and rather frivolous lives, their passions only transiently engaged, in first this and then that. They live as spectators of the mortals, who by comparison have depth, aspiration, genuine feeling, and hence a real center to their lives. Mortality makes life matter—not only in the chemist's sense.

A third matter: *Beauty*. Death, says the poet, is the mother of beauty. What he means is not easy to say. Perhaps he means that only a mortal being, aware of his mortality and the transience and vulnerability of all natural things, is moved to make beautiful artifacts, objects that will last, objects whose order will be immune to decay as their maker is not, beautiful objects that will bespeak and beautify a world that needs beautification, beautiful objects for other mortal beings who can appreciate what they themselves cannot make, because of a taste for the beautiful, a taste perhaps connected to awareness of the ugliness of decay.

Perhaps the poet means to speak of natural beauty as well, which beauty—unlike that of objects of art—depends on its impermanence. Does the beauty of flowers depend on the fact that they will soon wither? Does the beauty of spring warblers depend upon the fall drabness that precedes and follows? What about the fading, late afternoon winter light or the spreading sunset? In general, is change necessary to the beautiful? Is the beautiful necessarily fleeting, a peak that cannot be sustained? Or does the poet perhaps mean not that the beautiful is beautiful because mortal, but that our appreciation of its beauty depends on our appreciation of mortality—in us and in the beautiful? Does not love swell before the beautiful precisely on recognition that it (and we) will not always be? It seems too much to say that mortality is the cause of beauty and the worth of things, but not at all much to suggest that it may be the cause of our enhanced appreciation of the beautiful and the worthy and of our treasuring and loving them.

Finally there is the matter of that peculiarly human beauty, the beauty of *character*, of *virtue*, of *moral excellence*. To be mortal means that it is possible to give one's life, not only in one moment, say, on the field of battle—though that excellence is nowadays improperly despised— but also in the many other ways in which we are able in action to rise above attachment to survival. Through moral courage, endurance, greatness of soul, generosity, devotion to justice—in acts great and small—we rise above our mere creatureliness for the sake of the noble and the good. We free ourselves from fear, from bodily pleasures, or from attachments to wealth—all largely connected with survival—and in doing virtuous deeds overcome the weight of our neediness; yet for this nobility, vulnerability and mortality are the necessary conditions. The immortals cannot be noble.

V

What is the meaning of this concern with immortality? We are interested here not in the theological question but in the anthropological one: Why do human beings seek immortality? Why do we want to live longer or forever? Is it really first, and most, because we do not want to die, because we do not want to leave this embodied life on earth or give up our earthly pastimes, because we want to see more and do more? I do not think so. This may be what we say, but it is not what we mean. Mortality as such is not our defect, nor is bodily immortality our goal. Rather mortality is at most a pointer, a derivative manifestation, or an accompaniment of some deeper deficiency. That so many cultures speak of a promise of immortality and eternity suggests, first of all, a certain truth about the human soul: the human soul yearns for, longs for, aspires to some condition, some state, some goal toward which our earthly activities are directed but which cannot be attained during earthly life. Our soul's reach exceeds our grasp; it seeks more than continuance; it reaches for something beyond us, something that for the most part eludes us. True happiness, a genuine fulfillment of these deepest longings of our soul, is not in our power and cannot be fully attained, much less commanded. Our distress with mortality is the derivative manifestation of the conflict between the transcendent longings of the soul and the all-too-finite powers and fleshly concerns of the body.

What is it that we lack and long for? Notwithstanding their differences, many of our poets and philosophers have tried to tell us. One possibility is completion in another person. In Plato's *Symposium*, the comic poet Aristophanes speaks of the tragedy of human love and its unfulfillable aspiration. You may recall how we are said to spend our lives searching for our own complement, our own other half, from whom we have been separated since Zeus cleaved our original nature in half.

Plato's Socrates both agrees and disagrees with Aristophanes. He agrees that we long for wholeness, completeness, but not in bodily or psychic union with a unique beloved. Rather, *eros* is the soul's longing for the noetic vision—that is, for the sight of the beautiful truth about the whole: our soul aspires most to be completed by knowledge, by understanding, by wisdom; for only by possessing such wisdom about the whole could we truly come to ourselves, could we be truly happy.

The Bible also teaches about human aspiration. Once we dwelled in the presence of God, the source of all goodness and righteousness; now we are estranged. That separation from God's presence occurs as the immediate result of eating of the tree of knowledge of good and evil, itself an act of autonomy (since all choice is non-obedience) and hence of separation. The expulsion from the garden merely ratifies our estrangement from God and testifies to our insufficiency, of which our accompanying mortality is but a visible sign—or perhaps even God's gift to put an end to our sad awareness of deficiency.

The decisive facts about all these—and many other—accounts of human aspiration, notwithstanding their differences, are the following:

1. Man longs not so much for deathlessness as for wholeness, wisdom, goodness.
2. This longing cannot be satisfied fully in our embodied earthly life—the only life, by natural reason, we know we have. Hence the attractiveness of any prospect or promise of a different and thereby fulfilling life hereafter. We are, in principle, unfulfilled and unfulfillable in earthly life, though human happiness—that semblance of complete happiness of which we are capable—lies in pursuing that completion to the full extent of our powers.
3. Death itself, mortality, is not the defect, but a mark of that defect.

From these facts, the decisive inference is this:

This longing—any of these longings—cannot be answered by prolonging earthly life. No amount of more-of-the-same will satisfy our own deepest aspirations.

If this is correct, then the proper meaning of the taste for immortality, for the imperishable and eternal, is not a taste that the conquest of aging would satisfy: we would still be incomplete; we would still lack wisdom; we would still lack God's presence; we would still lack purity. Mere continuance will not buy happiness. Worse, its pursuit threatens human happiness by distracting us from the goal(s) toward which our souls naturally point. By diverting our aim, by misdirecting so much individual and social energy toward the goal of bodily immortality, we may seriously undermine our chances for living as well as we can and for satisfying to some extent, however incompletely, our deepest longings for what is best.

VI

But perhaps this is all a mistake. Perhaps there is no such longing of the soul. Perhaps there is no soul. Certainly modern biology doesn't speak about the soul; neither does medicine or even our healers of the soul, our psychiatrists. Perhaps we are just animals, complex ones to be sure, but animals nonetheless, content just to be here, frightened in the face of danger, avoiding pain, seeking pleasure.

Curiously, however, biology has its own view of our nature and its inclinations. Biology also teaches about transcendence, though it eschews talk about the soul. Much as it acknowledges and delineates our capacities and instincts for self-preservation and our remarkable powers to restore and maintain our wholeness, biology, too, teaches us how our life points beyond itself—to our offspring, to our community, to our species. Man, like the other animals, is built for reproduction. Man, more than other animals, is also built for sociality. And, man, alone among the animals, is built for culture—not only through capacities to transmit and receive skills and techniques, but also through capacities for shared beliefs, opinions, rituals, traditions. The origins of these powers for culture and their significance are matters of dispute, but their existence is not.

To be sure, the present orthodoxy in sociobiology treats our sociality as but a fancy mechanism geared to the sole end of the survival of the human gene pool. A richer sociobiology might come to understand that it is not just *survival*, but survival of *what*, that matters. It might again remember that sociality and culture, admittedly part of the means of preservation, are also part of the end for which we seek to preserve ourselves, and that only in community and through culture do we come into our own as that most special animal. But however this may be, biology does teach that we must see ourselves as species-directed, and not merely self-directed. We are built with leanings toward and capacities for perpetuation.

Is it not possible that aging and mortality are part of this construction, and that life span and the rate of aging have been selected for their usefulness to the task of perpetuation? Could not overturning the process of aging place a great strain on our nature, jeopardizing our project and depriving us of success? For, interestingly, perpetuation is a goal that is attainable. Here is transcendence of self that is largely realizable. Here is a form of participation in the enduring that is open to us, without qualification—provided, that is, that we remain open to it.

Biological consequences aside, simply to covet a prolonged life span for ourselves is both a sign and a cause of our failure to open ourselves to this—or any higher—purpose. It is probably no accident that it is a generation whose intelligentsia proclaim the meaninglessness of life that embarks on its indefinite prolongation and that seeks to cure the emptiness of life by extending it. For the desire to prolong youthfulness is not only a childish desire to eat one's life and keep it; it is also an expression of a childish and narcissistic wish incompatible with devotion to posterity. It seeks an endless present, isolated from anything truly eternal, and severed from any true continuity with past and future. It is in principle hostile to children, because children, those who come after, are those who will take one's place;

they are life's answer to mortality, and their presence in one's house is a constant reminder that one no longer belongs to the frontier generation. One cannot pursue youthfulness for oneself and remain faithful to the spirit and meaning of perpetuation.

In perpetuation, we send forth not just the seed of our bodies, but also a bearer of our hopes, our truths, and those of our tradition. If our children are to flower, we need to sow them well and nurture them, cultivate them in rich and wholesome soil, clothe them in fine and decent opinions and mores, and direct them toward the highest light, to stand straight and tall—that they may take our place as we took that of those who planted us and who made way for us, so that in time they, too, may make way and plant. But if they are truly to flower, we must go to seed; we must wither and give ground.

Those who look primarily at the aging of the body and those who look upon the social and cultural aspects of aging forget a crucial third aspect: the psychological effects simply of the passage of time—that is, of experiencing and learning about the way things are. After a while, no matter how healthy we are, no matter how respected and well-placed we are socially, most of us cease to look upon the world with fresh eyes. Little surprises us, nothing shocks us, righteous indignation at injustice dies out. We have seen it all already, seen it all. We have often been deceived, we have made many mistakes of our own. Many of us become small-souled, having been humbled not by bodily decline and not by "the system" but by life itself. So our ambition also begins to flag, or at least our noblest ambitions. In many ways, perhaps in the most profound ways, most of us go to sleep long before our deaths. In the young, aspiration, hope, freshness, boldness, openness spring anew—even if and when it takes the form of overturning our monuments. Immortality for oneself through children may be a delusion, but participating in the natural and eternal renewal of human possibility through children is not—not even in today's world.

Does Professional Autonomy Protect Medical Futility Judgments?

ERIC GAMPEL

Bioethics 20, no. 2 (2006): 92–104.

Introduction

Over the past decade there has been a lively debate over whether HCPs must provide treatments they judge to be futile, when the patients involved, or their surrogate decision-makers, are insisting on those treatments. In the midst of this debate, a number of professional associations and hospitals have adopted policies on medical futility, to help define the category and to specify procedures for resolving disputes over whether a treatment is genuinely futile. Though there are important differences amongst the futility policies, they all reflect what proponents have called an 'overwhelming consensus' amongst clinicians and health administrators that genuinely futile treatments need not be provided. There has been somewhat less agreement in the bioethics literature, however, with critics insisting that futility determinations be left to patients and family, and evidence that many members of the general public agree. What seems to have convinced so many HCPs and policymakers is an argument grounded in professional autonomy: physicians, nurses, and other HCPs should not be forced to provide treatments they consider futile, for that would make them slaves to patients or family who may make inappropriate demands. Though influential, this line of argument has not received much critical scrutiny, so my task is to clarify and evaluate that argument.

The significance of this issue is not that there is a large number of cases where HCPs find themselves at loggerheads with patients or families. Studies suggest it is reasonably rare for an irreconcilable conflict to arise over the matter of medical futility. That is why futility policies emphasize procedures of discussion, counseling, review by an ethics committee, and other means of arriving at an agreement amongst patients, family members, and caregivers. Such procedures are likely to resolve an initial dispute, since patients or family members who demand questionable treatments are often acting out of denial, misunderstandings, an inability to let go, irrational hope, guilt, or linguistic barriers. But while intractable disagreement may be relatively rare, the issue of who may ultimately decide the question of futility has a significant impact on the early stages of the decision-making process.

If it were widely accepted that physicians and other health professionals have the ultimate authority in cases of conflict over whether a treatment is futile, there would be support for the routine use of the concept of futility in shaping the options and advice offered by HCPs, and pressure on patients to accept the point of view of the HCP in charge. In addition, it would allow health administrators to rely on clinical judgments of futility in their goal of preserving medical resources, whether in the environment of managed care in the US, or in the contexts of national health insurance and socialized medicine elsewhere. Of course, the word 'futile' may not be widely used, but clinicians and health administrators commonly express a judgment of medical futility in other words, such as 'there is nothing we can do for' a patient, or 'there would be no point to CPR at this stage', or 'all we can do now is keep her comfortable'. The existence of a publicly acknowledged norm on which physicians may refuse to provide treatments they judge futile would encourage the use of such phrases, even in borderline cases. On the other hand, if it were widely agreed that the final decision-making authority rested with patients and family, clinicians and health administrators would need to be far more cautious in judging a treatment to be futile. Instead, there would be pressure on HCPs to play the role of informing the patient or family about the specific odds and outcomes involved, letting the patient or surrogate judge as to whether a marginal treatment 'makes sense' in light of such factors. So the ethics of cases where agreement cannot be reached makes a significant difference to the basic framework governing end-of-life care.

Defining Futility

Much of the early controversy over medical futility concerned how to define the category. In ordinary contexts, an act is futile if it cannot achieve the desired result. According to the *Oxford English Dictionary*, 'futile' means '1. Incapable of producing any results; useless, ineffectual, vain. 2. Lacking in purpose.' The controversy was over how to understand the terms 'incapable' and 'lacking in purpose'.

The first problem is that a treatment may be 'capable' of producing a result but extremely unlikely to do so (what Lawrence Schneiderman and Nancy Jecker have called 'quantitative futility'). In some such cases, clinicians and health administrators may speak of recovery as 'impossible' or 'virtually impossible', but certainty is rare in the art of medicine. Indeed, if clinical certainty of a zero chance of success were required, there would be little if any room for the use of the concept of futility in medical practice. As a result, most proposals about how to define medical futility indicate that a treatment can be considered futile if it has a very low chance of producing a desired effect. But then controversy arises: how low must the probabilities be to make a treatment futile, and how are the probabilities to be determined? It is rare in clinical practice to have reliable numbers based on scholarly studies – Baruch Brody and Amir Halevy have recently argued that it is extremely rare to be able to identify patients who have less than a 5% chance of survival to discharge, based on an evidence-based standard of evaluation. So assessments are usually made by reference to the individual HCP's experience with similar patients. One practical measure that has been proposed is that

if a treatment has failed for 100 'similar' cases, it should be considered futile (statistically, this means 'the clinician can be 95% confident that no more than three successes would occur in each 100 comparable trials'). On some views, this is sufficient ground for saying to the family that recovery is 'virtually impossible' or that there is 'nothing that can be done'. Quantitative futility, then, arises in cases where there is a nonzero chance that a treatment in question will produce a result that all parties grant to be beneficial, but the HCP judges that the chances are so slim as to not justify attempting the treatment.

A second kind of futility, 'qualitative futility', arises when the problem lies not in the low probabilities, but when there are questions about the value of the end result ('lacking in purpose'). In the bioethics literature, as well as in clinical practice, the most common cases where qualitative futility is in question are ones where life can be sustained, but only for a short period of time (because of terminal illness or system failures), and only in the form of a persistent vegetative state. In such situations, when there is a medical consensus that there is no chance for recovery, clinicians and health administrators overwhelmingly consider medical intervention to be futile – no meaningful purpose can be achieved. This applies of course to aggressive measures such as CPR and major surgery, but is sometimes thought to apply to continued life support, including artificial nutrition and hydration. Should this be an occasion for clinicians and health administrators to refuse requests to sustain life on futility grounds, as some have maintained? The sticky problem is that some family members of such patients, as well as some ethicists and theologians, think the medical interventions in such cases would not be futile, because they believe the continuation of life under such circumstances to be of value. This is true for a vitalist, for instance, who considers human life as such to be extremely valuable, even life in a comatose state. And it is true for a skeptic about medical predictions of the possibility of recovery (which makes it a dispute over quantitative futility).

The problem of medical futility, then, is what to do when there is a disagreement between HCPs and the patients or family over whether a treatment really is futile – i.e. over whether its chance of success is high enough ('quantitative futility'), or whether the possible results are worthwhile ('qualitative futility'). If discussion and negotiation cannot produce agreement, even after extensive education, counseling, and perhaps a meeting with an ethics committee, should the medical staff be able to refuse to provide the treatments they judge to be futile? Should health administrators be permitted to rely on the futility judgments of the medical staff, or higher-level health managers, in deciding whether to authorize care? One answer, grounded in the patient autonomy model that has come to dominate medical ethics, is that in all such cases the patient or surrogate should be the judge: whether low odds of benefit justify taking action, or whether an effect counts as a genuine benefit, involve questions of value, and respect for patient autonomy requires letting the patient's own values reign. In the face of this argument, and its reflection in court decisions and public opinion, a number of authors and policies have retreated to a more restrictive and less controversial definition.

Physiological Futility

The cautious proposal that seems to be gaining ground in some contexts is to consider a treatment futile only when it cannot produce the physiological effect desired by the patient or designated surrogate. This definition, usually referred to under the label 'physiological futility', would allow the patient or surrogate to define the goal of treatment, restricting the HCP to judging whether the therapy can produce the desired result. This strategy appears to avoid the most controversial cases, which involve qualitative futility, restricting futility judgments to quantitative cases where there is a clear consensus of medical opinion that a given therapy cannot succeed. In this sort of case, there is far less controversy over whether HCPs should be able to refuse the treatment, since it cannot produce the very result desired by the patient or surrogate. As the proponents of this approach have noted, this would mean that most cases usually considered matters of futility would not count as such at all, and that brings out three serious problems with this proposal.

First, the proposal goes against a widespread practice, in medicine and elsewhere, of using the concept of futility more loosely, i.e. despite lack of prognostic certainty, and in a way that appeals to one's own concept of what counts as a legitimate purpose. In most areas of decision-making, certainty about whether an endeavor will succeed is rare, and it is common for parties to disagree over whether a limited result, short of the ideal, would count as a success or a failure. Is it futile to drop bombs in Afghanistan to eliminate terrorism? Is it futile to send your children to extensive after-school programs to keep them away from drugs and violence? These are commonsense uses of the term 'futile', but making the judgment is not hostage to gaining certainty of the result, or knowing what would be agreed to by all parties as counting as success in the endeavor. The same goes for medical contexts: studies have found 'wide variation and lack of agreement' on when the concept of futility applies to a treatment, but also that HCPs use the concept of futility quite frequently in clinical practice. So the proposal to restrict HCPs to determinations of physiological futility, where certainty or 'near certainty' can be ascertained, is fighting a widespread and natural tendency to use the term more loosely.

Second, there is therefore a danger that policies and procedures appealing to physiological futility will operate, in practice, as a means for supporting the application of the looser, more ordinary concept. Once an HCP or committee begins asking whether a treatment is futile, it will be difficult to enforce a strict physiological conception. Certainty is hard to come by, as is any well-grounded estimate of very low probabilities, so the decision is likely to come down in practice to whether a group of HCPs take themselves to be 'virtually certain' the treatment will not be effective. This criterion provides plenty of room for moving away from the intent of the stricter definition.

Finally, and most importantly, the strategy of restricting futility to physiological futility does not help with the fundamental issue of whether HCPs may refuse to provide the kinds of treatments that have led to the futility debate, whether we call those treatments 'futile' or simply 'inappropriate' on some other grounds. Even if we restrict futility to physiological futility, an HCP may refuse to provide a treatment as 'inappropriate' because the risks outweigh the potential benefits, or because the patient's request is irrational or ill-considered given the low odds or limited benefit involved.

So the futility debate cannot be resolved by attempting to legislate a strict, physiological concept of futility. That strategy is unlikely to succeed in changing the concept of futility used in clinical practice, and it begs the larger question of whether HCPs must provide treatments they judge to be pointless, either because of the low odds of success or because the results would not be what they consider a genuine medical benefit.

Physician Autonomy

An influential argument that HCPs need not provide treatments they judge to be futile, in this wider sense of 'pointless', is that like patients, physicians have a right to autonomy, and should not be forced to provide treatments they do not consider to be medically beneficial. As Lawrence Schneiderman and Alexander Capron have said, 'patients have a right to refuse any treatment; they do not have a right to demand any treatment'. The objection can be put in the form of a *reductio*: unless HCPs have the authority to refuse some patient demands, there would be no end to what HCPs would be required to do, making them slaves to whatever patients want. And there is widespread agreement that this is not the way medicine should operate: there are many situations in which HCPs may and indeed must refuse patient requests. If a patient demands a coronary artery graft to eliminate chest pain

from an inflamed sternum, no physician need acquiesce. Moreover, HCPs regularly depend on their own judgments about acceptable levels of risk and degrees of benefit in offering patients treatment options. This is part of the expertise and autonomy involved in being a medical professional; so why shouldn't it protect the HCP's judgments about whether a given course of treatment would be futile?

The first point to note is that it is not simply the HCP's individual autonomy that lies behind their authority to control a course of treatment. If an HCP were to impose idiosyncratic values, or act from financial self-interest, in a manner that clearly conflicted with standards of practice in the medical community, the HCP would be vulnerable to civil suits and a risk of losing the license to practice medicine. HCPs need to follow norms established in the medical community regarding appropriate care: norms defined by a combination of actual medical practice, expert opinion, laws, and explicit guidelines promulgated by professional societies. So if there is an argument for HCPs' refusals of futile treatment, it is grounded not in the self-governance of individuals, but in the self-governance of the medical community.

Professional Autonomy

The stronger argument is that an HCP may refuse treatments which the medical profession gauges to be inappropriate, i.e. as being inconsistent with the basic goals and values of medicine. This would mean that each HCP 'inherits' a right of refusal from the right of the medical profession to be a self-governing body, one which defines its own standards of professional practice. There are existing standards of care in medicine, given deference in legal as well as clinical contexts, which concern not only the medical effectiveness of treatments, but also questions of value such as how to balance risks and burdens, or when confidentiality may be set aside to protect third parties. For instance, if a patient wants a high-risk heart bypass so she can continue golfing, where there is little threat to her life or other activities without the bypass, there are grounds for refusal in an appeal to standards of practice, so long as it can be shown that few if any HCPs would be willing to subject the patient to the surgical risk.

Perhaps we can say the same about futility cases, if a standard of practice defining when a treatment is futile were established in the medical community. For then it would arguably be within currently accepted principles of professional autonomy that HCPs follow that standard of practice in deciding whether to offer treatments. Indeed, this has more than theoretical relevance: it is arguable that a standard of practice for futility cases has been developing for a number of years. Thus, in 1996 the American Medical Association advised US healthcare institutions to adopt futility policies; many have done so, and there is evidence that the policies are being used in practice to guide clinical decision-making. Although it has turned out to be difficult to define medical futility explicitly so as to provide clear or mechanical guidelines, that is true for many risk/benefit standards in medicine, where appeal to expert opinion and common practice define the standard. So if the use of futility judgments to guide treatment decisions continues in accord with procedures specified by hospital policies and under something approaching a consensus in the medical community, there would be grounds in professional autonomy for denying care even when patients or surrogates are demanding it.

Note that the category of futility promises to bring together sometimes conflicting goals: the desire of HCPs for autonomy in their professional decisions, and the imperative for health administrators to minimize financial outlays. Direct, everyday managerial oversight of physicians has increased in recent years, mostly driven by financial concerns – in the US, through managed care insurance, and elsewhere through governmental rules and financial accounting procedures. Physicians are increasingly losing autonomy in medical decision-making, in ways that many HCPs have lamented, finding themselves forced to go against what they consider best for the patient because of the high costs objected to by health administrators. If the professional autonomy argument protects HCPs in their futility determinations, that may (for a change) fit well with the financial goals of health administrators. However, it is important to note that this could easily turn around: one could imagine managerial pressures on HCPs to use and extend the category of futility beyond what they feel comfortable with, thus actually working *against* professional autonomy. So the professional autonomy argument can only be understood as protecting futility judgments if it is the clinical end of the profession making the futility determinations, not if non-clinical managers are doing so.

Note, however, that the professional autonomy enjoyed by medicine is far from complete or unrestricted, and must be informed by ethical and political standards, as well as medical ones. Physicians have a state-endorsed monopoly on many forms of health care, and the medical field has received substantial government funds over the years for research, development, and delivery of services, even in the 'free market' context of the US. With the monopoly and funding come certain responsibilities, e.g., not to turn away patients in an emergency, to secure informed consent, not to discriminate, to treat contagious patients, and so on. These responsibilities are formalized in various ways, politically and legally, and by reference to various socially-endorsed values (e.g., fairness, equality, autonomy). Moreover, medicine is also what some have called a 'moral enterprise', shaped by internal values such as nonmaleficence, beneficence, and patient autonomy. Those internal values also constrain what the profession can define as appropriate standards of care. So the professional autonomy of HCPs is limited, and decisions of the medical profession about standards of practice can be constrained and guided both by values internal to the profession, and by external constraints imposed by the community.

This opens the door to an important line of objection to developing a standard of practice governing medical futility cases. For futility cases are, in important respects, quite unlike the other cases in which HCPs have a long-sanctioned power to act according to professional standards defining appropriate care. There are three differences that matter crucially here.

First, in futility cases the treatment in question is usually the *only* one which has any chance of bringing about the hoped-for improvement, so that to deny the treatment is to consign the patient to certain death. In contrast, the uncontroversial cases where a professional standard of practice supports HCP refusals either do not involve certain death as a result, or allow for alternative methods of treatment. For instance, the patient who wants a bypass to golf is not being consigned to death if refused, and the patient seeking surgery for a brain tumor too risky to remove can be offered chemotherapy as another means of fighting the cancer. But when an HCP withholds a treatment on futility grounds, that HCP is taking away the patient's last chance for achieving his or her ends.

A second significant difference is that it is far less plausible in futility cases that the medical professional has a special expertise in making the relevant risk assessment. In futility cases, the options and their potential consequences are reasonably easy to understand: treat, with some small chance of producing a desired effect (e.g., resuscitation, improvement of condition, or continuation of a comatose state); or don't treat, and face no chance of producing the desired effect, typically resulting shortly in death. Contrast this with the standard, uncontroversial situations in which HCPs may refuse to provide a treatment based on standards of practice. For instance, in the case of the heart bypass for the golfer, the risk assessment involves a complex balancing of potential harms and benefits, since both the bypass and non-surgical treatments involve the risk of death, as well as some chance of improvement. For the bypass, the claim that HCPs are the better judges is plausible, since the decision involves a subtle assessment of probabilities and outcomes, and HCPs can draw from the accumulated wisdom imparted in their training and

reflected in customary practice. Not so for futility cases, where the factors involved in the decision are comparatively clear-cut.

Finally, notice that futility cases involve the overriding of values which are more tied up with deep matters of religion and philosophical outlook. This is especially evident for qualitative futility cases, when a health care professional judges that a potential result (e.g., continuation of a comatose state, or permanent dependence on ICU care) does not involve a benefit. For in these cases the HCP is rejecting the patient's (or surrogate's) own judgments regarding what is important in life, and what kind of life is worth living. Consider the vitalist patient who seeks CPR, despite low odds and likely harms, valuing life whatever its condition. Such a request can be grounded in mainstream religious traditions, ones endorsed by some HCPs. Refusing CPR or other life-sustaining measures under this circumstance is paternalism of an extreme sort, denying a patient's assessment of what matters most in his or her life. Contrast this with the case of the golfer: even if she would try to claim golfing as her only reason for living, this judgment would not be grounded in philosophical or religious traditions, is a fairly idiosyncratic view, is likely being overstated in order to make the case for the surgery and, even if heartfelt, is likely to be modified if circumstances demand it. Not so for futility contexts: the treatment is the only chance for continued existence, and the patient is judging the kind of existence involved to be worthwhile. As for quantitative futility, note that whether the low odds are worth taking depends both on the valuation of the hoped-for outcome (the importance of continued life in such a condition), and on the disvaluation of the injuries, pain, and indignities risked by the treatment. All of this can be made fairly clear to the patient (or surrogate), and depends on highly personal views about when life is worthwhile despite the disabilities, injuries, indignities, and pain involved in sustaining it.

So there is a high burden of argument to be met: what could justify the profession of medicine in developing a standard of practice that routinely leads to refusing treatments which 1) are the only chance for continued life, 2) do not involve special expertise to understand, and 3) involve fundamental value judgments about when life is worth living? I do not believe this challenge can be met, at least on the grounds of the professional autonomy of HCPs.

Some have attempted to appeal to the goals of medicine as providing an objective, unimpeachable stance for medical professionals. But this just shifts the dispute to the issue of what counts as a *legitimate* goal of medicine.

Moreover, it is far from clear that an appeal to medicine's traditional goals would rule out treatments with extremely low odds or poor outcomes. For appeal can always be made to the traditional goal of preserving life. There are certainly precedents in the history of medical practice for using low probability procedures to save a life. This is especially clear in the case of experimental treatments: when there are no other treatments and life is at stake, it is common to permit highly experimental, low-probability treatments, both in the hopes of helping the patient, and in the pursuit of new knowledge to help future patients. Why not do the same in apparent futility cases, where there are also no other alternatives for preserving life, and where patients or family are desperate for some kind of assistance? Even if the HCP sees the odds as extremely low, or the outcome as not worthwhile, why not provide the treatment with the aim not of furthering medical knowledge, but of respecting the patient's wishes, a newer but still well-embedded element in the modern practice of medicine?

Moral Integrity

A different kind of argument attempts to ground professional autonomy in the deeper value of respect for moral integrity. The kinds of treatments at issue in the futility debate typically impose various burdens on the patient and risks of harm, and have little or no chance of producing what the HCP or medical community counts as a medical benefit. To require HCPs to provide such treatments may therefore be asking them to act against the dictates of their own consciences, a violation of their moral integrity. As Tom Tomlinson and Howard Brody have argued, 'A principle that denied the HCP any power to act on his or her professional values, rather than the patient's, would leave the HCP powerless to refuse to perform actions that harm patients.' Thus unless HCPs have a sufficient degree of professional autonomy, protecting decisions which are based on moral considerations, the moral integrity of those HCPs is at risk, leaving them forced to perform actions that may conflict with their own moral judgments. In addition to the potential damage to moral integrity, this would show a failure to respect HCPs as moral agents.

The general principle that HCPs should be able to refuse to engage in practices they deem immoral is highly plausible, and has a backing in medical history and professional guidelines. But the claim of moral integrity, like that of HCP autonomy, cannot serve as a trump card in the dispute over medical futility, though it is sometimes offered as such. For there are limits to the right of conscientious refusal, in medicine as well as in other fields. An HCP who believes it immoral to cease artificial respiration, even at the patient's request, cannot simply force that patient to stay alive. Nor can an HCP refuse to treat a patient on the grounds that the patient is a criminal, a drug addict, a member of the Aryan Nation, or a racial minority. As argued above, the political and legal context of medicine puts conditions on its practice, as do the values internal to the medical tradition. So an argument based on moral integrity needs to be examined in light of those factors.

When a physician has not yet accepted someone as a patient, or when a transfer to another HCP would be easily managed, there is fairly wide scope for a physician's individual conscience to reign. Even idiosyncratic values or prejudices might be the basis of such decisions, without facing legal or professional sanction in many countries and contexts of care. The problem emerges when a patient has no other choice, being already under a physician's care without the possibility of transfer. For then the physician's moral integrity may provide an absolute barrier to the patient's receiving the care at issue. In such situations, the value of respecting moral integrity comes up against the other values at stake. Futility cases are typically like that: by the time the matter of futility arises, and the parties have gone through the steps of speaking with other medical staff and perhaps an ethics committee, it is unlikely that other physicians feel differently or would accept a transfer. Instead, a typical dispute over futility will pitch patients and family on one side, against all medical staff on the other. Transfer then is not a realistic option. But this means that when a physician, clinic, or hospital is seeking to refuse a therapy on futility grounds, it is usually the patient's last chance for continued survival, and this affects the force of the appeal to moral integrity.

On the one hand, the consensus amongst medical staff provides support for the claim that the HCP's moral integrity is genuinely at stake, and some reason to think the HCP's judgment should be respected. For the consensus indicates that the futility judgment is not ill-considered, or based merely on personal interests (e.g., exhaustion with the case), but rather is grounded in professional norms and standards of treatment that deserve consideration. In general, as Mark Wicclair has recently argued, conscientious objection by an HCP is stronger if grounded in professional norms, rather than in idiosyncratic values.[1] But as Wicclair himself points out, that is not a decisive consideration, since there are other factors important to deciding whether a conscientious objection is sufficient ground for a refusal to provide care.

Wicclair identifies the following five factors in evaluating a conscientious objection in a medical context:

1. centrality to the physician's core ethical values;
2. basis in professional norms, and relevance to the moral integrity of the medical profession;
3. grounding in the physician's conception of herself as an ethical physician (rather than an ethical person generally);
4. impact on patient's rights and interests;
5. recognition of competing rights and interests by law or by norms of medical ethics.

Applying Wicclair's framework to the case of futility, the conscientious objection argument can be seen to have little force. Consider 1–3, which concern the issue of the moral integrity of the HCP. Even when there is a consensus amongst medical staff that a treatment is futile, the values at stake in that judgment are unlikely to be as central to an individual HCP, or to the medical profession, as the values that tell against acts such as assisted suicide or abortion. Treatments judged futile are typically standard medical procedures in themselves, employed to provide at least some chance of sustaining biological life. The controversy is over whether the treatment provides *sufficient chance* of producing a benefit (quantitative futility), or whether the end result is *worthwhile* (qualitative). But these are value questions about the risks and benefits for the individual patient. Indeed, to refuse to let the patient or surrogate weigh the risks and benefits is itself a moral failing, viz. a failure to respect patient autonomy.

This raises the issue of the impact on the rights and interests of the patient, factor 4 on Wicclair's list. In futility cases the treatments in question provide the only chance, however slim, for continued survival. The patient's life is most likely to be at its end, but there are no guarantees. In addition, being able to have control over the last stages before death is of great importance to many patients, and widely recognized as such (5). Many popular books and patients' rights groups have emphasized this ideal, and it has been recognized in law under the form of the right of patients to refuse unwanted medical treatments. So given the relative stakes for the patient and for the HCP, these considerations tell against the argument from moral integrity, and in favor of requiring HCPs to provide medical interventions even when by their own judgment that would not be advisable. For it is the patient's life that is at stake, and it should be the patient who decides the kinds of questions at issue.

Conclusion

Despite its influence, the professional autonomy argument does not provide support for the widespread use of futility rationales. Whether a treatment is futile involves evaluating its chances of producing a given result, and judging whether that result would be worthwhile. This decision should be in the patient's hands, or in the surrogate's, since the treatment in question is typically the only chance for continued life, the options are not difficult to understand, and the decision depends on personal views regarding when life is worth living. Of course, this completely ignores the tremendous financial and resource pressures on the medical system, which provide strong reasons for resisting the sorts of treatments in question. But it would be highly misleading to use a futility rationale, implying that a goal cannot be achieved, when the real thought is that it would be a waste of resources to attempt to achieve the goal.

None of this tells against extensive discussions amongst clinicians and health administrators, patients, and family about whether treatments are futile or make sense. The claim is only that the basic model for decision-making should put the patient and his or her values at center stage. This is true even though there are other situations where paternalistic considerations, or the values and goals of the medical profession, should override patient choice. But in futility cases, short of certainty that a result desired by the patient cannot be achieved, the question of futility is not one for which HCPs should be the ultimate judge.

Note

1. M. R. Wicclair, "Conscientious Objection in Medicine," *Bioethics* 14, no. 3 (2000): 205–227.

Autonomy, Wellbeing, and the Case of the Refusing Patient

J. VARELIUS

Medicine, Health Care and Philosophy 9 (2006): 117–125.

Introduction

Consider the case in which a person has a disease that, untreated, will cause her to die in the near future. There is a treatment available for this disease and if this patient is given it, she will be able to continue her life. However, the patient competently refuses the treatment. This gives rise to a moral problem. Should the patient's life be saved even though it would be against her will? An influential approach to questions of biomedical ethics sees certain considerations pertaining to individual autonomy as providing a solution to this problem. According to this line of thinking, we should respect the patient's autonomy and, since she has made an autonomous decision against accepting the treatment, the person in our example should not be treated. In this article, I will argue against this view and maintain that our answer to the question of whether or not this patient should be treated should be determined on the basis of whether we accept a subjective or an objective conception of individual wellbeing. I will begin by considering the options of treating and not treating the refusing patient from the point of view of her autonomy. Then I will reformulate this patient's case in terms of subjective and objective theories of individual wellbeing. Since I expect that my approach to the case of the refusing patient will give rise to a number of objections, a major part of this article consists of replies to possible criticisms of my way of conceiving and dealing with this case.

Defining the Terms

I will be talking about individual autonomy and subjective and objective theories of wellbeing. Although the notion of autonomy has been used in many distinct senses in different connections, it seems that in biomedical ethics there is a common core understanding of the meaning of this notion. According to this idea, autonomy means self-government. As an actual condition of an individual agent, autonomy means, roughly, that an agent uses her capacity to make her own decisions concerning her own life, and lives by these decisions. Of course, what exactly this means is controversial. I would however argue that all plausible theories of individual autonomy accept at least the following requirements of autonomy. If a person's decisions, beliefs, desires, etc. are due to such external influences as unreflected socialization, manipulation, coercion, brainwash, etc., they are not autonomous but heteronomous. And if a person's beliefs concerning some matter are false, inconsistent with each other, or she is uninformed about that matter without her realizing this, then she is not autonomous with respect to that matter. Similarly, if a person's behaviour results from such things as compulsion and weakness of will, then it is not autonomous but heteronomous.

This procedural conception of the nature of personal autonomy contrasts with the theories of autonomy that take there to be substantive views that all autonomous persons must accept. These substantive theories of autonomy may hold, for example, that an autonomous person cannot want to become a subservient housewife, that an autonomous agent will never want an abortion or request for euthanasia, etc. Here it is not possible to go into the pros and cons of these two kinds of conception of autonomy in detail. Instead, I will just present two reasons for my referring to the procedural conception of personal autonomy in this connection.

First, the procedural view on autonomy is commonly, but not universally, accepted in biomedical ethics. Indeed, problems like that of the refusing patient would not arise at all if a substantive conception of personal autonomy were adopted, since then there would not usually be any reason to consult the patient herself in making decisions about her treatment. Assuming that the health care personnel would qualify as autonomous, they would know the right answer to the substantive question of whether or not the patient should be treated and, consequently, there would be no need to ask the patient's own opinion on that matter. [The] second reason is that the substantive theories of autonomy face the overwhelming problem of explaining exactly what substantive views qualify as autonomous and why. Although there have been many attempts, this far no one has been able to present a satisfactory solution to this problem. Consequently, of these two types of autonomy theory, the procedural conception is the more plausible one.

According to the commonly accepted understanding of what the distinction between subjective and objective theories of wellbeing, or prudential value, is about, subjective theories make prudential value dependent on individuals' attitudes of favor and disfavor. Objective theories of value deny this dependency. Thus, when our task is to determine whether or not some particular thing, activity, or state of affairs is valuable for a person, the subjective theories of value advise us to consult that person's preferences and attitudes of favor and disfavor. Usually subjective theories require that the preferences that determine prudential value must be informed or rational. Objective theories, in their pure forms, maintain that what is good and bad for individuals is not determined by their own attitudes of favor and disfavor. Instead of these kinds of subjective states, objective theories usually make prudential value dependent on such purportedly objective issues as whether a thing or an activity satisfies human needs, realizes the human nature, etc. This distinction between subjective and objective theories of value is put in terms of prudential value, but it applies to the case of other values as well. Thus, when I talk about subjective and objective evaluative views in general, I mean the terms 'subjective' and 'objective' to be understood as in the case of prudential value. With this understanding of the notions of individual autonomy and subjective and objective theories of (prudential) value, I turn to considering the case of the refusing patient.

Reconsidering the Role of Autonomy

According to the approach now under consideration, respecting a patient's autonomy implies that we must allow a patient whose life is in danger to refuse a treatment that would save her life if she autonomously decides against accepting that treatment. However, it could equally well be maintained that by obeying this patient's decision not to be treated we fail to give sufficient weight to her autonomy. Since the treatment now in question would save this patient's life, treating her would allow her to continue her existence as an autonomous agent. And obeying her decision not to be treated would undermine the autonomy that this treatment would allow her to have in the future.

It is thus possible to maintain that, although treating her goes against a decision she has made, giving her the treatment is the only way of truly respecting her autonomy, for it is only by being cured that she is able to go on living as an autonomous agent. Thus, respecting the patient's autonomy does not necessarily commit us to accepting her decision not to be treated. However, since treating the patient would be against

her autonomous decision, neither does respect for autonomy univocally imply that this patient should be treated. Since it can be said that the patient's autonomy is being respected whether or not she is treated, commitment to autonomy as such does not answer the problem that is faced in the case of this patient.

It could be taken that this problem can be solved simply by weighing the options of treating and not treating the patient from the point of view of autonomy and choosing the option with superior weight. It could, for example, be maintained that since the autonomy that the patient is able to have if she continues living is greater than the autonomy expressed in her decision not to accept the treatment, the patient should be treated against her will. But the problem we are facing here is not as simple as this way of answering it suggests it to be. First, before we could in this way determine which of the options of treating and not treating the patient would be more in line with respect for her autonomy, we would need to know how exactly this kind of weighing is to be done. And then it is necessary to know whether there is an objective method for determining the weights of the options of treating and not treating the patient from the point of view of autonomy or whether these weights are based on the attitudes and desires that the patient has towards these options.

Second, it seems plausible that the question we are now facing ultimately concerns the patient's wellbeing, not the value of autonomy as such. Two main reasons for valuing individual autonomy have been presented in the bioethics literature. First, it has been maintained that autonomy is valuable as an instrument of promoting the patient's wellbeing. Secondly, it has been claimed that, in addition to whatever instrumental value autonomy has in enhancing the patient's wellbeing, autonomy is also valuable for the patient independent of its role in promoting her good. Let us briefly consider the latter view.

If autonomy's value for a patient is not exhausted by its role in promoting her wellbeing, then the patient's autonomy should be respected even if the courses of action she is considering taking were harmful to her. But how should this be understood? Since it is commonly accepted that medicine should be looking at things from the point of view of the patient's best interest, it is plausible that the view that a patient's autonomy should be respected even if the courses of action she is considering taking were harmful to her should be interpreted to be saying that we must allow a patient, acting from self-interested reasons, to perform actions that are harmful to her. But whose conception of harm is at use here? It rationally cannot be that of the patient herself, since an autonomous person acting from self-interested reasons will not want to perform actions that she herself considers as harmful to her and, consequently, there is no good reason to require that the patient should be allowed to perform such actions. So, it seems that the conception of what is harmful to the patient would have to be that of someone else.

Since other persons' subjective determinations of what is and what is not prudentially valuable may not apply to the patient's case at all, the question here rationally must be about an objective conception of what harms persons. And it would seem that we could have reason to think that a person's autonomy has value for her over and beyond its role in promoting her wellbeing only if objectivism about what harms and benefits patients is true, for it appears that only then we could have any grounds to require that patients should be allowed to perform actions that are harmful to them. This is because then a patient's conception of what is harmful to her could differ from the standard of harm adopted by the proponents of the view that a patient's autonomy should be respected even if the courses of action she is considering taking were harmful to her and, consequently, the patient acting from self-interested reasons could be willing to perform actions that are harmful to her according to that standard. However, even if what is and what is not prudentially valuable were determined objectively, the patient as an autonomous agent would

be aware of what is good and bad for her, or at least could appreciate it when it was presented to her, and, consequently, she would not insist on performing objectively self-harming actions from self-interested reasons. Again, we have no good reason to require that autonomous patients acting from self-interested reasons should be allowed to perform self-harming actions, since they are not willing to perform such actions.

Thus, the only reason for insisting that autonomy has value for patients beyond its instrumental value in promoting their wellbeing would be that it would guarantee that heteronomous patients are allowed to hurt themselves if that is what they happen to want. But since we are now considering the case of autonomous patients, this reason does not apply here at all and, consequently, we have no good reason to hold on to the view that autonomy's value for patients is not exhausted by its worth in enhancing their wellbeing. But if this view is rejected, then the patients' autonomy should be valued only when, and to the extent that, it enhances their wellbeing. In other words, the primary value here is wellbeing, not autonomy. These considerations suggest that in order to reach a reasonable decision in the case of the refusing patient, we must redirect our attention and aim to determine how the value of the options of treating and not treating the patient should be determined from the point of view of her wellbeing.

Reformulating the Issue in Terms of Theories of Wellbeing

Our question is whether or not the refusing patient should be treated, and the answer to this question is to be determined from the point of view of her wellbeing. Since the distinction between subjective and objective theories of individual wellbeing concerns the issue of whether or not what is prudentially valuable is determined by individuals' own decisions, it is consequential to see the question we are facing with the refusing patient as the problem of whether we should accept a subjective or an objective theory of individual wellbeing.

If we accept a subjective theory of wellbeing, we see a person's good as being determined by her own decisions. Then the patient herself is entitled to determine the weights that the options of treating and not treating her have from the point of view of her wellbeing. Thus, if we accept prudential subjectivism, we are committed to obeying the patient's autonomous decision not to be treated. But if we accept an objective theory of wellbeing, we allow that the patient herself need not be the ultimate judge of what is good and bad for her and thus may decide that the person in our example should be treated after all. If the autonomy this person had if she continued living is objectively good for the person to the extent that it overweighs other competing values, then the patient's decision not to be treated should not be obeyed.

Possible Objections Considered

Since I expect that my approach to the case of the refusing patient will give rise to many objections, I will now consider a number of possible criticisms of the argument presented above. My purpose is both to present replies to possible objections and to further clarify my approach to the case of the refusing patient.

Is Autonomy Independent of Wellbeing?

Another possible objection to my view is this. Instead of assuming that the value of autonomy in health care is dependent on its role in promoting individual wellbeing, autonomy should be seen as an independent value that constrains what is done in the name of persons' wellbeing. Thus, this objection would proceed, reformulating the case of the refusing patient in terms of prudential subjectivism versus prudential objectivism badly distorts the issues at stake here.

There are two points I would like to make concerning this possible criticism. First, if autonomy were conceived of as this kind of a constraining value, it seems to me implausible to hold that in the context of health care it should constrain in the name of some other thing than what is good for the patient. And if its role is to secure that the

patient's good is promoted, we face the questions pertaining to prudential value I have discussed above. Second, even if autonomy itself were seen as the ultimate end here, we would face questions pertaining to subjectivism and objectivism about value. For even in this case, if we are to reach a plausible decision in the case of the refusing patient, we should be able to determine the weights that the options of treating and not treating this patient would have from the point of view of promoting her autonomy. Thus, we should be able to decide whether these weights are to be determined subjectively or objectively, and it is arguable that in other spheres of value the notions of subjectivity and objectivity should be defined in the same way as in the prudential sphere.

It could be objected to this that in spheres other than the prudential objective should be defined in terms of what is real and only mind-independent entities have real existence. Thus, since my definition of objective may allow that things existing merely intersubjectively qualify as objective, it is implausible. However, even if we accepted the view that the subjective versus objective controversy is essentially similar to, if not the same as, the realism versus anti-realism controversy, this need not imply that my definition of objective is implausible. The question of realism versus anti-realism arises in many different subject areas and it is not clear that reference to mind-independence is a reasonable way to define realism in all of them. Whereas it seems, for example, reasonable to define realism about macrophysical objects in terms of independence of the mental, it sounds implausible to characterize psychological realism in this particular way. Since it is currently common to define realist theories of value in terms of opinion-independence, response-dependence, and other such features that make values mind-dependent, it would beg the question to assume that real existence in the evaluative sphere necessarily means mind-independent existence. So, I take it that the questions we would be facing if autonomy instead of wellbeing were considered to be the ultimate end in biomedical ethics would be quite similar to those concerning the issue of subjectivism versus objectivism about wellbeing discussed above.

Can the Refusing Patient's Autonomy Be Respected by Treating Her?

It could also be objected that my argument here is implausible, since my characterisation of the case of the refusing patient is suspect. According to this possible objection, it would be counterintuitive to maintain that the refusing patient's autonomy could be respected by treating her, since she does not want the life that she would have if she were cured. It is just implausible, this objection would proceed, to accept that we could respect a person's autonomy by forcing her to live a life that she does not want to live. So, since it assumes that treating the patient would be a way of respecting her autonomy, the case of the refusing patient as it is presented here is misconceived to begin with.

Above I argued that whether we should treat the refusing patient or not depends on whether we accept a subjective or an objective conception of individual wellbeing. Our decision to treat the patient is reasonable only if we can show prudential objectivism to be true, or at least more plausible than its rivals, and the objective value gained by treating her overweighs other competing values. But if we can show that continuing life as an autonomous agent is objectively good for the refusing patient and this patient is a reasonable person, then she will accept our objective reasons for treating her when we present them to her. In other words, if objectivism about prudential value is true and giving the treatment is objectively more valuable than not giving it, this patient's decision to refuse the treatment must be based on an error and we can expect that, having considered all relevant issues, she will herself come to see her refusal as confused and change her decision about accepting the treatment.

But, the critic could continue, if objectivism about prudential value, is true, how can it be said that there could be autonomous agents

at all? If there are objective evaluative facts that determine how we should live, our life is not ultimately based on our own autonomous decisions. In other words, the critic would accept that autonomy is possible only if subjectivism about value is true. There are two points I would like to make concerning this possible criticism. First, it seems to be compatible with objectivism about value that, although there are evaluative questions that have answers uniquely determined by objective evaluative facts, there are also spheres in which there is room for exercises of autonomy in (something quite like) the sense that the present possible objector seems to understand it. The most obvious example would be the case in which all options open to an agent are of equal objective value. In a case like this, the agent is free to choose whichever option she likes.

Second, and more importantly, the conception of autonomy on which this objection is based is implausible. Why should we accept that one is autonomous with respect to some facts only if one is able to determine the nature of these facts? It seems to me that the possibility of living in contact with the objective evaluative facts that existed if objectivism about value were true would be sufficient for the possibility of individual autonomy. Admittedly, this kind of autonomy would not be as radical as what the present critic is after, but this is not a sufficient reason for disqualifying it as autonomy altogether. If objective evaluative facts existed, it would be unreasonable to define our conception of individual autonomy in a way that is incompatible with their existence.

Conclusion

In this article I have discussed the case of a patient who refuses a treatment that would save her life. I argued against the view that certain considerations pertaining to individual autonomy allow us to reach an acceptable decision concerning what should be done in this person's case. More precisely, I argued against the view that respecting this patient's autonomy commits us to obeying her decision not to be treated. Instead, I maintain that treating this patient may also be conceived as a way of respecting her autonomy and that, in order to reach a plausible answer to the moral question concerning what we should do in this person's case, we must determine the significance of the options of treating and not treating her from the point of view of her wellbeing. If we accept a subjective theory of individual wellbeing, we are committed to accepting this patient's autonomous decision and will not treat her. But if we see more reason to accept an objective conception of individual wellbeing than a subjective one and come to the conclusion that the autonomy this person would have if she continued living is objectively more valuable than the other values competing with it in this case, we will decide against obeying this patient's decision not to be treated.

Of course, the applicability of this result is not limited to the case of a dying patient. Whenever a patient's refusal from appropriate treatment is defended by saying that we must respect the patient's autonomy, it should be noticed that giving the treatment may be more conducive to the patient's autonomy than not giving it and that what ultimately should be done in such a case depends on whether we have reason to choose a subjective or an objective theory of individual wellbeing.

The Severely Demented, Minimally Functional Patient
An Ethical Analysis

JOHN D. ARRAS

Journal of the American Geriatrics Society 36, no. 10 (1988): 938–44.

Mrs. Smith, an 85-year-old resident of a nursing home, was transferred to the hospital for treatment of pneumonia. Although she has responded well to antibiotic therapy, her overall condition and prognosis remain grim. For the past 3 years her mental state has been steadily deteriorating due to a series of strokes which have finally rendered her severely demented. She is now nonambulatory, incapable of sitting up in bed, and uncommunicative most of the time. When she does talk, her speech is completely incoherent and repetitive. Mrs. Smith shows no signs of recognizing or remembering her family and primary caregivers. The nurses in charge of her care assert that she appears to experience pleasure only when her hair is combed or her back rubbed.

During her recovery from the pneumonia, Mrs. Smith began to have problems with swallowing food. Following a precipitous decline in her caloric intake, her son and daughter (the only involved family members) consented to the placement of a nasogastric tube. Mrs. Smith continually pulled out the tube, however, and continues to resist efforts to reinsert it.

The health care team faces difficult choices regarding Mrs. Smith's care. Foremost among them is whether her physicians should surgically insert a gastrostomy tube in spite of her aversive behavior. Mrs. Smith has neither left behind a living will nor has she indicated to family or friends at the nursing home what her preferences would be regarding life-sustaining care in this sort of circumstance. Both her son and daughter have stated that she would nevertheless not have wanted a gastrostomy tube inserted and would, if she could presently decide, prefer an earlier death to being sustained indefinitely in the twilight of her minimally functional condition. In defense of this claim, they note that she has always been a very active, independent person who avoided doctors whenever possible.

Probing the Patient's Subjectivity

The first order of business in deciding for incompetent patients is to inquire, whenever possible, what the patient would want were she presently able to communicate. In the absence of a designated proxy or living will that speaks with rare precision about which modes of treatment are to be forgone under which circumstances, this task is more difficult than many commentators and jurists would have us think. The case before us yields two distinct sources of revelation bearing on the patient's putative subjective wishes regarding the present decision. As we shall see, neither provides evidence sufficiently compelling for us to conclude with moral certitude that she would not allow the insertion of a G-tube.

Extrapolating from the Patient's Prior Values

First, we have the testimony of family members who claim that the patient's character traits of independence and aloofness from physicians point to the conclusion that she would not want to be sustained by a G-tube. Although this claim may well be *plausible* and at least *consistent* with Mrs. Smith's previously held attitudes and behaviors, it would require a great leap of both faith and logic to conclude that evidence of this sort *entails* a negative decision on life-sustaining treatment. As several commentators have pointed out, there is a great difference between the degree of respect owed to a patient's *actual choices*, even choices made prior to the advent of incompetency, and to his or her preferences or

tastes. It is one thing to have negative attitudes towards aggressive life support, but it is quite another to actually refuse it in your own case. By doing so, a person *commits* himself or herself to a particular course of action and it is this commitment, rather than mere attitudes or generalized preferences abstracted from the particular details of choosing situations, that commands especially stringent respect.

Even if someone's generalized views about life, dependency, and doctors deserved the status of right claims, which they do not, they usually do not yield unequivocal answers to treatment dilemmas. Supposing that Mrs. Smith was indeed fiercely independent and skeptical of the medical profession, does this necessarily mean that she would prefer death to her present "twilight state" sustained by tube feedings? Conversely, if Mrs. Smith were an exceptionally dependent sort of person who actively sought and followed the advice of physicians, would that mean that she would presently prefer an indefinite extension of her barely conscious existence to an early death? Although such character traits indisputably have *some* evidentiary value, they appear to be compatible with a range of possible responses. In Mrs. Smith's case, it is certainly *plausible* that she would decline the insertion of a G-tube, but that is not the only plausible interpretation. For all we know, she might have been content, were she miraculously lucid and communicative for an instant, to accede to the operation rather than go peacefully into that dark night. The question for Mrs. Smith's caregivers, then—and we shall explore this point more fully later on—is not whether her loved ones have provided a uniquely correct extrapolation of her previous values to her present situation, for in most cases that will simply be an unattainable goal; rather, the question is whether their plausible invocations of her values and character traits should be given the benefit of the doubt.

The Evidentiary Value of Aversive Behavior

Mrs. Smith has been constantly pulling out her nasogastric tube and waiving off the attentions of her caregivers. What are we to make of this behavior? In contrast to the patient's previous preferences and attitudes, which are ill-matched in their generality to the concreteness of the present situation, Mrs. Smith's aversive behavior at least has the advantage of being contemporaneous. She is extubating herself right here and now. According to Daniel Callahan, a philosopher who generally sees no justification for terminating food and fluids in severely demented patients, such behavior constitutes a "clear signal" mandating withdrawal of the tube.

But a clear signal of what? It is crucial to remember at this juncture that Mrs. Smith is severely demented and completely incompetent. Even though her aversive behavior occurs in the present, it is the behavior of a woman who has completely lost her rational capacity. She cannot even recognize her family, let alone engage in sophisticated deliberations bearing on the respective benefits and burdens of continued tube feeding in her minimally functional state versus an earlier death.

It is possible that her tube-pulling represents a firm and fixed present desire to forgo aggressive life-sustaining treatments in favor of an early death. It is also possible that it signals some kind of deeply sedimented personal desire manifested in spite of her present incompetence. But it is equally possible that her aversive behavior is nothing more than an elemental reflex signalling only her transient irritation from the tube.

Mrs. Smith's "signal" is thus anything but clear, and this is a significant fact for her caregivers to ponder. The real problem facing Mrs. Smith's physicians is that they have no reliable way of discerning the "real meaning" behind her ongoing resistance to feeding tubes. It would certainly help if Mrs. Smith had been known to shun tube feeding even while she was competent, for that would at least provide some plausible evidence connecting her presently aversive behavior to sedimented preferences. But in the absence of such a record, the meaning of her "rejection" remains profoundly unclear.

Given the inconclusiveness of this inquiry into the patient's previous attitudes and present behavior, her caregivers might reasonably shift their focus of attention away from the patient's elusive subjectivity and toward a more objective assessment of her "best interest."

The Best Interest Standard

In the absence of reliable indicators of the patient's actual or hypothetical preferences, courts and commentators recommend an inquiry into the best interests of the patient. What course of action (or inaction) will bring about the best overall result for the patient? Rather than finding this "objective" path an easier route to the correct decision, caregivers attempting to apply such a test to the case of a severely demented, minimally functional patient such as Mrs. Smith will immediately confront a series of equally perplexing questions. What will be the actual impact of placing a G-tube on Mrs. Smith's well being? What definition of the good will ground their assessments of her best interests? And, given her low level of functioning, is it quite accurate even to describe Mrs. Smith as a full-fledged "person" with actual, discernable interests? Since these exceedingly difficult questions lack intuitively obvious answers, perhaps the best way to proceed is to examine categories of patients on either side of Mrs. Smith on the continuum of incompetency, categories that do yield fairly firm moral intuitions, and then attempt to locate a proper response to her case by means of "moral triangulation."

Patients in Persistent Vegetative States

What if, instead of being minimally functional, Mrs. Smith were completely non-functional? (We shall call this hypothetical patient, Mrs. Jones.) What if, instead of slowly declining into a twilight of consciousness, she were to have experienced a protracted period of anoxia that consigned her to a persistently vegetative condition? Although still alive, Mrs. Jones would subsist on brainstem activity alone, her neo-cortex—the physical substratum of her capacity for consciousness—having been completely destroyed. What rights, if any, would Mrs. Jones have, and what duties would be owed her by caregivers?

If we were to apply straightforwardly the best interests test to the case of Mrs. Jones, we would be hard pressed to discover actual interests that could be meaningfully imputed to her. Lacking consciousness, she lacks a conception of herself as a moral agent with real interests in continued life and in the pursuit of her own vision of the good. Lacking the ability to experience pleasure and pain, she cannot be physically benefitted or harmed.

If we seek a solution to the problem of Mrs. Jones in an examination of her best interest, we discover the paradoxical result that her best interest will probably be served by further treatment. True, except for the possibility of misdiagnosis, she cannot be benefitted in any way by continued existence, but her lack of capacity for conscious experience renders her equally incapable of being harmed by further treatments and the extension of her life. Thus, we cannot say, as the best interest test would appear to require, that Mrs. Jones is being excessively burdened by her treatments or that she would be "better off dead." This result is indeed paradoxical, because if anyone's life need not be maintained, one would think that patients in persistently vegetative conditions must be at the top of the list.

Given the vanishingly small likelihood of misdiagnosis, especially after the passage of several weeks, I would argue that it is ethically appropriate to treat all PVS patients as though they had no interests either for or against treatment. Since continued medical interventions cannot realistically be thought to benefit them in any way, since caregivers cannot realistically be thought to have duties towards patients who cannot be helped or harmed, and since such treatments entail considerable costs—including the expenditure of huge sums of money, the time and energy of caregivers, and emotional strains on survivors—they may be ethically forgone.

The important lesson here is that although a rigorously patient-centered best interest test

might be ethically appropriate in most cases involving incompetent patients, it cannot be meaningfully applied when the patient under consideration lacks all fundamentally human capacities. In cases such as this, a judgment in favor of nontreatment must be based, not on an objective weighing of benefits and burdens to the patient—for such patients are capable of neither benefit nor burden—but rather upon a judgment that the patient has ceased to be a "person" in any meaningful moral sense. Once this determination has been made, it is then ethically permissible to consider the financial and emotional impact of continued treatment upon other interested parties. Certainly some families will, for religious or other personal reasons, continue to request life-sustaining treatments for their persistently vegetative relations; but others would be acting ethically to request the termination of all medical care, including artifically administered food and fluids.

Marginally Functional Patients

On the other side of Mrs. Smith are those patients who might usefully be described as "marginally functional." Mr. Black, for example, is a 90-year-old man presenting with rectal bleeding and suspected colon cancer who refuses a laparotomy to confirm the diagnosis. "I have lived a good life," he says, "and I don't want any surgery." His daughter, to whom he appears very close, concurs with his decision. Although Mr. Black appears on the surface to be sufficiently competent to make this decision, subsequent examinations by liaison psychiatrists reveal a glaring absence of short term memory and significant confusion about his medical diagnosis and surroundings. He is described as "pleasantly demented."

Although patients like Mr. Black are strictly speaking incapable of rational decision-making most or all of the time, they differ from Mrs. Jones in their ability to reason, albeit rather poorly, in their ability to relate to other persons, and in their capacities to experience emotions, pain and pleasure. Notwithstanding their inability to make most health care decisions, these patients are clearly "persons" with a multitude of interests that can be advanced or frustrated by their caregivers. In spite of their deficits and relatively low quality of life, such moderately functional patients have every right to a patient-centered best interests analysis. While invasive, painful and risky surgery may or may not eventually be deemed to be in Mr. Black's best interests, his capacities for experiencing the world are sufficiently intact to rule out any thought of forgoing other sorts of life-sustaining therapies, such as artificial nutrition and hydration.

The Minimally Functional Patient

Returning now to the example of Mrs. Smith, we find her to fall squarely between the permanently vegetative and moderately functional patient. Like the totally nonfunctional, vegetative patient, she is so demented that she lacks most of the criteria of "moral personhood." Unfortunately, she appears to have been reduced to a mere shell of her former self. She can no longer reason, communicate (except in the most rudimentary, reflexive manner), relate to her family, or experience manifestations of love. Indeed, it is doubtful that she can be accurately described as a self-conscious, moral agent whose identity through time is cemented by the bonds of memory. There is, in cases such as this where the psychological glue of memory has given out, simply no enduring "self" there.

On the other hand, Mrs. Smith resembles Mr. Black at least in her possession of some conscious life, albeit on a very low level, and in her ability to experience pleasure, pain, and perhaps some rudimentary emotions. Although she is not a "person" in the strict sense, she does have some interests. Insofar as she is open to pleasure and pain, she has a definite interest in experiencing the former and avoiding the latter. How might a "best interests" test be applied to someone like Mrs. Smith?

Better Off Dead?

In order to justify the termination of food and fluids under a best interests test, decision-makers would have to show that the burdens of a patient's life with the proposed treatment would clearly and markedly outweigh whatever benefits she might derive from continued life. In other words, they would have to show that the patient would be "better off dead."

The most influential formulation of this best interests test, the majority opinion in the Conroy case, requires not merely that the burdens of life clearly outweigh the benefits, but also that further treatment would be inhumane due to the presence of severe and uncontrollable pain. The court's motivation in establishing such a strict standard is not hard to grasp. While people might disagree about the desirability of persisting in a minimally functional condition, severe and intractable pain is presumably something that just about everyone would prefer to avoid. It is this nearly universal sentiment that death would be preferable to a life of unmitigated pain and suffering that gives this test an air of "objectivity," as opposed to the subjectivity of tests based upon the patient's past preferences.

How then would this strict formula apply to Mrs. Smith? As we have seen, there isn't much to place in the "benefits" column. No longer able to take food by mouth or to interact meaningfully with her family and caregivers, it appears that Mrs. Smith experiences few pleasures apart from an occasional rub or combing. The only possible benefit to be derived from further treatment would appear to be the indefinite continuation of this twilight existence. And although the patient might conceivably derive some pleasure merely from lying in bed and dwelling in her alien world, it is highly doubtful that such a patient—bereft of memory, a sense of continuing selfhood, hopes and plans—could possibly have an interest in, or be benefitted by, *continued* existence.

Given Mrs. Smith's low level of existence, it is equally difficult to discern the burdens of continued treatment. To be sure, she will experience some degree of pain and discomfort from the surgical insertion of a G-tube, but this pain will not approximate the kind of prolonged, severe and intractable pain required by the Conroy best interests formula.

Another possible source of pain and suffering would be the forcible imposition of medical treatment against the wishes of the incompetent patient. Even incompetent patients can have strong preferences for or against treatment or diagnostic procedures, and even if these preferences are not well grounded in medical reality or in the patient's previously authentic value system, forcible treatment will often be experienced as a painful and humiliating violation.

In Mrs. Smith's case, however, the side effects of coercive treatment are likely to be nonexistent. As we have already seen, her aversive reaction to NG tube feeding could just as easily be ascribed to immediate physical discomfort as to some deep-seated desire to die through the refusal of life-sustaining treatment. Mrs. Smith is probably too demented at this point to have preferences about tube feedings or to acknowledge the forcible imposition of surgery over against her aversive behavior. It is highly unlikely, then, that she would experience the insertion of a G-tube as a violation of her wishes (no matter how distorted) or as a painful humiliation.

In the absence of any persistent and severe pain underlying her condition, it would appear highly doubtful that the burdens of Mrs. Smith's continued existence clearly and markedly outweigh the benefits, even when the benefits approach zero. A literal reading and application of the Conroy formula would thus lead to the conclusion that the G-tube should be surgically implanted and that she should be maintained indefinitely with artificial nutrition and hydration.

Limitations of the Best Interest Standard

Not everyone will be satisfied with this result. Those who believe that quality of life should never affect treatment decisions will no doubt applaud this conclusion, but others might well think that something important has been left out of our deliberations. Judge Handler, the lone dissenter in *Conroy* identifies this missing factor as a legitimate concern for the patient's probable feelings about broader issues, such as privacy, dependency, dignity and bodily integrity. By focusing the entire best interests discussion upon the narrow issue of pain, we tend to reduce the patient from the full-fledged person that she once was to the status of a mere physical repository of pleasures and pains. Is this crudely hedonistic notion of the good an adequate or desirable measure of humane treatment decisions for minimally functional patients? Should we simply ignore the patient's probable responses to such abject dependency and daily violations of dignity?

The obvious problem for Judge Handler's proposed enlargement of this formula is that severely demented, minimally functional patients like Mrs. Smith are presently incapable of experiencing what more functional patients would describe as insults to their privacy, dignity and physical integrity. Although it is quite possible that the formerly competent Mrs. Smith would have been appalled at the loss of dignity entailed by her present situation, the present Mrs. Smith knows nothing of dignitary insults or violations of privacy. She is so demented that she cannot be affected, one way or the other, by solicitude for her present responses to these larger, humanistic issues.

In order to vindicate Judge Handler's concerns, we will have to reintroduce them at the stage of our inquiry into the patient's prior preferences (ie, the substituted judgment test). Under that test, we would have to show that Mrs. Smith would have clearly viewed continued treatment under these circumstances as an indignity, and that she would have preferred an early death to the insertion of a G-tube. The problem with this move is that, as we have already seen, Mrs. Smith left behind neither a precise advance directive nor a pattern of analogous choices that clearly demonstrate what she would have wanted under present circumstances. Indeed, our earlier failure to provide this sort of clear evidence mandated our present effort to find a solution in terms of Mrs. Smith's best interests.

So we have come full circle. Our inability to satisfy a rigorous substituted judgment test required us to search for a solution in terms of

Mrs. Smith's best interests. But the best interest test, at least as articulated in *Conroy*, led to an unacceptably narrow focus on pain that excluded important values. Mrs. Smith's present lack of capacity to appreciate such values finally led us back again to the substituted judgment test. Clearly, something has gone wrong here.

A Procedural Solution

According to lawyer-bioethicist Nancy Rhoden, the problem lies not in our inability to come up with better evidence of a patient's wishes or level of pain and suffering, but rather in the questions we are asking. She argues convincingly that both the substituted judgment and best interests tests set the standard of evidence far too high. By requiring *clear and convincing* evidence either that a patient's prior values would dictate the withdrawal of life-sustaining treatment or that the burdens of a patient's life outweigh the benefits, these tests establish a standard that cannot realistically be met by the kinds of evidence we are likely to have at our disposal. As we have seen, in the absence of a carefully drafted living will, a durable power of attorney, or severe and intractable pain, it will rarely be *clear* either that a patient would have refused treatment or that death is in her best interests. Given the usual evidentiary materials at hand, in most cases the best we can do is conclude that forgoing treatment is *probably* what the patient would have wanted, or that death is *likely* to be in the patient's best interest, although we will never know for sure in either case.

To be sure, there are some easy cases where a patient's best interests are clearly and perceptibly being violated. For example, greedy relatives might request the termination of treatment that could realistically return the patient to a good quality of life; or guilt-ridden relatives might press for full resuscitative measures on a moribund patient riddled with metastatic cancer. But apart from such clear-cut cases of unmistakable undertreatment and overtreatment, most of the truly problematical cases (like Mrs. Smith's) fall

into a vast gray area between these extremes where the patient's best interests will remain unclear and largely inscrutable. Our problem, then, is that we have been asking questions for which there exist, in most of the hard cases at least, no clearly correct answers.

Rhoden's solution, in which I concur, is to bypass this substantive impasse with a procedural solution. Taking her cue from the President's Commission report addressed to the problem of severely impaired newborns, she argues that when a proposed course of action falls into the gray area of uncertainty, involved and well-intentioned family members should have discretion to decide as they see fit. Presumably, they will invoke precisely the same kinds of evidence bearing on the patient's value system, religious affiliation, quality of life, and the potential benefits and burdens of treatment, but they would not be held to a standard of evidence requiring that their choice by uniquely correct.

To be sure, many caring and well-meaning family members will also want to weigh the impact of continued treatment upon themselves and the family unit. Sometimes the ongoing provision of care and treatment to severely demented patients like Mrs. Smith can impose great burdens, both financial and emotional, upon families. I believe that such concerns are for the most part inevitable and that they often subtly color treatment decisions even when officially banished under the auspices of the usual ethical-legal standards. This is to be expected and should not give us grounds for concern so long as the case originally falls within the gray area of ethical ambiguity, and so long as the interests of family do not *clearly* violate the best interests of the patient.

The correct question for us, then, is not whether forgoing treatment is clearly the right answer, but rather whether Mrs. Smith's case falls into the problematical gray area. If it does, then the decision of a trustworthy surrogate should prevail over objections from caregivers, unless the latter can show a clear violation of best interests. Since a case must exhibit considerable ethical ambiguity to fall into this gray zone in the first place, we should expect that well-meaning and ethically sensitive people will reach different conclusions about the care of such patients. The opinions of trustworthy surrogates should be given priority simply because they are usually in the best position to assess the prior wishes and best interests of incompetent patients, and because their familial and emotional bonding to patients usually gives them a greater claim than members of the health care team.

What, then, are the boundaries of the gray area? When is a case sufficiently ambiguous to warrant our trust in surrogate decision-making? We can begin with a reassertion of the *Conroy* best interest formula. If a patient's capacity for benefitting from continued life appears to be eclipsed by the constant presence of severe and intractable pain, then the case falls either in the gray area or the clear-cut zone of nontreatment. I would add that this imbalance of burdens over benefits need not be conclusively proven by clear and convincing evidence. It should be sufficient merely for the surrogate to make a strong case that the burdens are disproportionate to the benefits. In Mrs. Smith's case, however, no such claim can be made.

In the absence of severe pain, we must ask whether the patient is genuinely capable of benefitting from continued existence. Does she recognize and interact with other persons, including her family and caregivers? Does she have a sufficiently intact self to conceive of the future and to care about what happens in it? If the answers to these questions are negative, even if the patient is capable of some rudimentary physical pleasures, I would argue that the patient has no real interest in continued life or the administration of life-sustaining treatments and thus falls squarely into the gray area.

Mrs. Smith fits this profile. She is so demented that she cannot recognize family or caregivers. Her memory is so depleted, and her sense of self so fractured, that she cannot be said to have genuinely human interests.

Since the boundaries of this morally ambiguous zone will inevitably correspond to the limits of societal toleration, it will often be helpful to ask what most reasonable people would want for themselves in this circumstance. Although this question is generally not allowed in more patient-centered inquiries into the patient's prior preferences or best interests, it should be allowable here, where we are merely trying to determine whether a case is sufficiently morally problematic to fit into the gray zone. If we ask the question with regard to Mrs. Smith, I think that the overwhelming majority of persons would say that they would rather die than continue to live in such a physically, emotionally and socially impoverished state.

Another useful clue is to ask how we would have responded to Mrs. Smith's death from lack of adequate nutrition had it occurred prior to the advent of artificial feeding. No doubt there would have been the inevitable sadness associated with the death of any human being, but there would have been no shock, no outrage, no sense of tragedy, nor even any feeling that death had deprived her of any real benefits. The predominant response to such a death would most likely have been relief, both for the sake of the patient and for her loved ones.

In such cases, the only apparent rationale for the imposition of life-sustaining technologies is that since they exist, they must be used. And the more they are used, the more pervasive their presence in hospital and longterm care facilities, the more their expanded use assumes the necessity of a moral imperative. But it is precisely here, in cases such as Mrs. Smith's, that we must pause to ask about the proper uses of such technologies. If they do nothing to further the real interests of patients, if all they do is to prolong the biological existence of patients whose biographical lives have long since come to an end, then biomedical technologies assume the status of idols—ie, inanimate objects worshipped by the human beings who created them, objects that return to dominate us rather than serving our purposes.

Extreme Prematurity and Parental Rights After *Baby Doe*

JOHN A. ROBERTSON

Hastings Center Report 34, no. 4 (2004): 32–39.

Contemporary ethical and legal norms hold that all human beings born alive should be treated equally, regardless of disability. Yet there is a strong sense that some lives are so diminished in capacity for interaction or experience that little good is achieved by providing medical treatments necessary to keep them alive. In addition, many persons believe that the parents who have the chief responsibility to provide care should have a dominant say in whether their children are treated.

Before 1970, the question of whether to withhold treatment from such newborns was rarely contested. The ancient Spartan practice of exposing babies on hillsides and keeping those that survived had a contemporary counterpart in the common medical practice of simply not treating those born with major handicaps. As late as 1972, some doctors and parents thought it appropriate to withhold from children with Down syndrome or spina bifida surgery necessary for their survival. Noted pediatricians published articles in major medical journals reporting the withholding of life-saving treatment from infants with many kinds of disabilities. Surveys of doctors showed that these practices were not exceptions.

In the mid-1970s, the emerging discipline of bioethics began to question the ethics and legality of these practices even as they were publicized. Courts became more willing to order treatment over parental wishes, though neither a uniform response nor clear guidelines emerged. It took the Baby Doe controversy of 1981 and the federal Child Abuse Amendments (CAA) of 1984 to produce a rough consensus about the norms and practices that would govern this area. Since passage of the CAA, ethical and legal controversy over parental authority to withhold treatment from handicapped or disabled newborns, although still featured in bioethics courses and texts, has largely ceased.

Yet one aspect of the controversy was never directly resolved. Because the Baby Doe controversy had focused on infants with genetic and chromosomal anomalies, the extent to which the CAA norms might require changes in practices with very premature and low birth weight infants remained open, even though it was occasionally mentioned in articles. As a result, physicians and hospitals that insisted on treating premature newborns over parental objections were vulnerable to tort actions by parents. This article reviews the controversy and assesses the extent to which parents should have the right to decide not to treat severely premature newborns.

The Baby Doe Controversy

The Baby Doe controversy, which played such a key role in clarifying norms and practices in this area, arose in 1981 in Bloomington, Indiana. Parents of a newborn child with Down Syndrome and a trachealesophageal fistula refused to consent to a standard operation that would enable the child to take food and water by mouth. The hospital and doctors sought approval from a family court to perform surgery against the parents' wishes. A probate court denied the request on the ground that the parents had the right to make the decision. The child's guardian *ad litem* appealed the case unsuccessfully to the Indiana and then to the United States Supreme Court. While the case was pending, it drew wide media coverage and the attention of right-to-life and disability rights groups. Before the United States Supreme Court could rule on the guardian's appeal, Baby Doe died.

Groups opposed to the outcome in the Baby Doe case sought relief from federal officials in the Reagan administration sympathetic to right to life concerns. Soon after, the Department of Health and Human Services issued regulations that required newborn nurseries and neonatal intensive care units receiving federal funds to post notice of a hotline number to report cases of discrimination in treatment based on handicap. When reports came in, "Baby Doe squads" of doctors, nurses, and social workers were dispatched to hospitals, demanding medical records to determine whether treatment was inappropriately denied.

Greatly disturbed by these interventions, the pediatric and hospital community sued to invalidate them on the ground that they were beyond federal regulatory authority. A federal district court enjoined enforcement because of the government's failure to follow legal requirements for new regulations. The administration then complied with those requirements and issued slightly less intrusive regulations. Further litigation ensued. The United States Supreme Court eventually ruled, in *Bowen v. American Hospital Association*, that Congress had not authorized federal agencies to regulate nontreatment decisions in hospitals and newborn nurseries.

The battleground shifted to Congress. The resulting tussle among the administration, right to life, disability, hospital and physician groups produced a compromise bill, the Child Abuse Amendments of 1984. Under this legislation, direct federal intervention in newborn nurseries and neonatal intensive care units would cease. Instead, states, as a condition of receiving federal child abuse prevention funds, would agree to set up systems, including infant care review committees, to make sure that all newborn children were protected against discrimination on the basis of disability. The only exceptions recognized to equal treatment of children with handicaps were for children who were permanently comatose, near death, or for whom treatment would be inhumane because futile or virtually futile.

A Consensus of Sorts

The Child Abuse Amendments of 1984 ended the political controversy over the federal role in decisions to withhold treatment from handi-capped newborns. In terms of substantive norms, right to life and disability groups could claim victory. The substantive provisions of the CAA were strongly protective of the rights and interests of those with disabilities and left little room for nontreatment decisions to be based on expected low quality of life or the interests of parents. All children, whatever the extent of their disabilities, were to be provided medical treatment unless they met the narrowly defined exceptions.

Procedurally, however, physician and hospital groups could also claim victory. As a legal matter, the CAA substantive provisions were not directly imposed on any individual or institution, nor did they directly amend federal or state substantive law. They did not, for example, make it a federal crime or a civil wrong for a doctor, parent, or hospital not to treat a child who did not meet the narrow exceptions. Nor did the CAA require hospitals to comply with its standards in order to receive Medicare and Medicaid funds. Instead, it obligated the states to set up protective procedures in order to receive child abuse funds. Any regulatory action would thus be the responsibility of individual states, which were less well equipped than the federal government for strong enforcement action. This was a far cry from federal hotlines and intrusive Baby Doe squads.

But while the CAA imposed no legal duties directly on doctors and hospitals, many doctors, hospital administrators, and even lawyers perceived its passage as creating a legal presumption in favor of treating children likely to have disabilities. Technically this was inaccurate, but it was not an unreasonable conclusion. At the very least, the CAA could be perceived as setting the standard of care to which hospitals and doctors would be held, both by accrediting bodies and by courts hearing challenges to nontreatment decisions. In addition, the ethical controversy over nontreatment decisions had convincingly shown the importance of respecting the life and interests of disabled children and recognizing limits on parental rights. The values incorporated in the CAA showed a deep ethical commitment to respecting human life regardless of disability.

Whatever its actual legal reach, passage of the CAA awakened pediatricians, neonatologists, and hospitals to the problem of discrimination against handicapped newborns. The norms of practice shifted: most physicians and hospitals were now more reluctant to defer automatically to parental wishes. Parents could no longer deny needed surgery to children with Down syndrome or spina bifida, as had occurred in the much publicized Baby Jane Doe case at Stony Brook. If treatment were to be denied, a parent would have to show that the child was comatose, terminally ill, or that treatment would be futile or virtually futile. In borderline cases, some quality of life judgments might unavoidably occur, but overall a high degree of compliance followed passage of the CAA. Indeed, both the American Academy of Pediatrics and the American Medical Association, which had fought the Baby Doe rules, issued policies calling for equal treatment of newborns regardless of disability and low quality of life and recommended the use of institutional ethics committees to review contested cases.

The Problem of Prematurity and Very Low Birth Weight Infants

The area with the least consensus and the most uncertainty about the reach of the CAA was that of extreme prematurity. Due to a large investment of public resources, regionalization of perinatal intensive care units, and growing technical abilities, treatment of premature newborns had shown great success. The line for viability and successful survival has been continuously pushed back to earlier and earlier ages. Before 1980, few babies born in the 1000-1500 gram range before twenty-eight weeks would do well. Now they are routinely saved and restored to a relatively normal life. Great success is also occurring with smaller babies. It is now routine to save babies as young as twenty-five weeks and as little as 750 grams. Under twenty-five weeks, however, results are much more mixed. At the margins of viability, twenty-three to twenty-four weeks' gestation, mortality occurs in half or more of the cases, and survivors often have significant physi-

cal and mental handicaps, including blindness, hydrocephalus, cerebral palsy, limited use of language, and learning disabilities.

Newborns born under 750 grams and before twenty-five weeks pose a major problem under the CAA. On their face, the CAA standards leave no room for discretion. All conscious, viable premature newborns must be treated, even if they are likely to have severe physical and mental disabilities. Not to treat them would be to discriminate against them on the ground of expected disability.

In effect, the CAA supplied an ethical and legal justification for the intense efforts of neonatologists to push back the limits of viability. Most hospitals and neonatal programs treated premature newborns in conformity with the CAA, with neonatologists present at all premature deliveries and likely to resuscitate newborns born alive, regardless of parental wishes.

Not all neonatal programs complied equally strictly with the CAA standards in cases of very low birth weight, however. In more marginal cases, under twenty-five weeks or where Grade IV intraventricular hemorrhaging or other major problems had occurred, some programs would provide "compassionate care" or nontreatment only if parents requested it (usually without ethics committee or legal review of the decision). A 1991 *New York Times* survey found that two programs in the same New York county had completely different attitudes toward treatment in marginal cases, one treating aggressively, the other deferring to parental wishes. A 1994 *Chicago Tribune Sunday Magazine* survey showed similar disparities. In most cases the disparity in approach was due to the personal philosophy of the NICU director or perceptions of legal risk.

The aggressive approach to treatment of low birth weight infants in some programs has led to conflicts between parents and doctors and hospitals. Many parents reported being given little choice about treatment of their premature newborns, with the result that infants born at twenty-three to twenty-six weeks' gestation were resuscitated and vigorously treated, in some cases over parental wishes. While half or more of these children survived, many survivors were likely to have serious disabilities, including cerebral palsy, blindness, mental retardation, and learning disabilities. Increasingly, parents have requested that no resuscitation or treatment occur in these cases, thus pitting parental wishes against the neonatology ethic of trying to save all premature newborns and the no-discrimination requirements of the CAA.

Miller v. HCA as the Catalyst for Reexamination

In a litigation-oriented society, it is no surprise that this conflict is now played out in lawsuits brought by parents claiming violation of their rights to control the medical care provided to their children. Such suits shift the forum for defining treatment norms from Congress and the federal judiciary, which played a major role in the Baby Doe controversy, to state juries and trial and appellate judges. The jury award in the recent case of *Miller v. HCA* suggests that there is popular support for recognizing some parental right to have treatment withheld in low birth weight cases. Although the award was eventually overturned, the question remains whether parents should have a right to deny life-saving medical treatment to low birth weight newborns because of the high probability that they will have severe mental or physical disabilities.

The parents sued the hospital and its corporate owners, but not the physicians, for treating the child at birth without their consent. After a two-week trial in January 1998, a jury awarded the family $30 million in compensatory and $13 million in punitive damages. The compensatory damages were based in part on the cost of providing care to Sidney until age seventy.

In finding for the parents, the jury was necessarily finding that they had not consented to treatment, and that their consent was essential to the treatment, thus squarely posing the question of whether they had a right to deny treatment to a viable newborn who was likely to have substantial disabilities.

Modifying the Substantive Standard

Some persons might argue that the jury verdict in *Miller* in favor of the parents was appropriate because of the great burdens that treatment against their wishes imposed on them. According to this view, the substantive norms for treatment reflected in the CAA and the law of many states (including Texas, as clarified on appeal) are too strict; they should be modified to privilege the parents' reluctance to take on those burdens. The parents' wishes should trump arguments that focus narrowly on the interests of a severely impaired child with little chance of a normal life. Because parents (and other children) will bear the burdens of caring for the child with severe impairments, they should have the right to refuse resuscitation or treatment in such cases.

Few would not have deep sympathy for a family faced with an extremely premature child and the great burdens that rearing the child could impose. In addition, many would find that the CAA standards are too demanding, given the realities that families face in these situations and the importance of respecting family autonomy. Yet modifying the equal treatment standards of the CAA and the law of most states to allow parental choices to trump the severely impaired child's interest in treatment would deviate from the principle that all persons who are conscious and not imminently dying should have equal access to needed medical services.

Given these competing concerns, the ethical and legal challenge is to uphold the general principle that all children born alive are to be treated equally regardless of disability while also recognizing the importance of parental decisional authority. The problem is that any modification of the equal treatment standards may be seen as opening the door to full-scale quality-of-life-based decisions, yet anything that clearly does not permit some quality-of-life decisions may still seem to improperly restrain the rightful sphere of parental choice.

One way to try to reconcile these competing concerns is to declare that treatment against the parents' wishes is required only if the child possesses some threshold level of cognitive ability. A second strategy would be to clarify the burden of proof so that parents are recognized as the primary decisionmakers, with the burden of proof on caregivers or others to establish that the child has the required level of cognitive ability. Finally, a decision is needed as to whether parental choices made *before* birth should have the same presumptive weight as those made after birth (the issue in the *Miller* case).

How, then, to think about the threshold level of cognitive ability? One route would be to adopt a change that recognizes that some states of consciousness rest on such limited cognitive ability as to call into question whether the child's putative interest in continued life is substantial enough to warrant protection. In that case, denial of treatment could be justified under a patient-centered approach as not harming the child because the child simply lacks strong interests in continued life. Some threshold of cognitive ability beyond mere consciousness—such as the capacity for language or meaningful symbolic interaction—is needed to endow a person with interests in living and thus a duty to treat.

A standard based on relational ability is consistent with mainstream ethical writing on the subject. Father Richard McCormick, the highly regarded Catholic bioethicist, recognized in 1974 that treatment need not be provided if the child lacks the ability for interaction or human relationship. Professor Nancy Rhoden argued in 1986 that there should be an additional category for withholding treatment under the CAA when the infant or child "lacks potential *for human interaction* as a result of profound retardation." The President's Commission for the Study of Ethical Problems in Medicine and Biomedical Research and many bioethicists also supported such a standard. Indeed, even authors who have strongly supported the right of handicapped newborns to be treated at birth have recognized that an exception in cases of extreme prematurity or lack of meaningful interests should also exist.

None of these commentators, however, has specified more precisely what lack of "interaction or relationship" means. Under such a standard, treatment would still be required for premature infants who have suffered or might suffer intraventricular hemorrhaging and severe brain damage because such infants are still capable of some interaction with others. Despite their severe physical and mental disabilities, such children do respond to stimuli and appear to experience pleasure when touched or rubbed—arguably a form of "interaction or relationship" because it leads to further touching or rubbing. In the *Miller* case, for example, there was evidence that Sidney smiled and responded favorably to physical contact.

If interaction or relationship is taken to mean the human capacity for meaningful symbolic interaction or communication, then some greater mental capacity would be required than such severely damaged children have. If one lacks altogether the capacity for meaningful symbolic interaction, then one lacks the characteristics that make humans the object of moral duties beyond that of not imposing gratuitous suffering on them. We value humans in large part because of the capacity to have conscious interests and experiences, including meaningful symbolic interaction with others.

A modification in the CAA's substantive standards and in similar state laws to permit nontreatment in extreme cases would necessarily rest on quality of life assessments based on disability. But the mental disability in such cases is so extreme, so far from those cases in which children may be said to have valid interests in living, that they arguably do not threaten or harm the important values underlying the injunction against quality of life assessments in cases of disability. We could adopt such a standard without encouraging discrimination against disabled persons who have the capacity for symbolic thought and interaction.

Process Solutions and the Burden of Proof

Substantive norms are not easily separated in practice from the procedures by which they are implemented. Another way to give greater deference to parental interests while upholding the norm of equal treatment would be to devise a procedural approach that better balances the interests of each. Both the American Academy of Pediatrics and the President's Commission for the Study of Bioethical Problems in Medicine recommended that institutional ethics committees review such decisions, particularly when there was disagreement or uncertainty about whether the child's interests required treatment.

In future cases, the burden of proof that must be met to have a child treated over the parents' wishes should be clarified. Parents should have a presumptive right to have their decisions about the child's welfare respected unless a clear need to protect the child is shown. The burden would lie with physicians, hospitals, and other caregivers to challenge the parents' decision against treatment. If the "symbolic capacity" standard were employed, then the caregivers would have the burden of establishing, by at least a preponderance of the evidence, that the child is likely to have the minimum cognitive ability for symbolic interactions. In less certain cases, the parents' wishes would control.

Deciding After Birth

Any modification of the CAA's non-treatment standard and clarification of the burden of proof should also specify the point at which increased deference to the parents is appropriate. Parental autonomy is important, but it is not so robust that parents have the right to deny a disabled child the medical resources necessary for life regardless of the child's interests in living or ability to interact with others.

To determine whether a particular infant lacks or is reasonably certain to lack the mental capacity for symbolic interaction or relationship one must first assess the child and its condition. But this can be known only after birth, when a full assessment of the child's situation and likely capacity is possible. Doing so will require immediate treatment to stabilize the situation and a full work-up by neonatologists to determine the child's condition and prospects.

As a result, parents' directions not to resuscitate at birth should not be given effect until a medical assessment of the child's condition and prognosis justifying nontreatment has been made. Doctors and hospitals should be legally free to have neonatologists resuscitate and treat for a limited period after birth to assess the child's capacity regardless of parental consent or orders not to resuscitate. Under this standard, the initial medical response in the *Miller* case—resuscitation at birth if the child is alive—was reasonable. If medical evaluation after resuscitation shows that the child is likely to develop the capacity for meaningful symbolic interaction and the parents continue to refuse life-sustaining treatment, then ethics committee and judicial review should be sought to determine whether to treat the child over the parents' wishes.

A rule that permits initial treatment pending assessment admittedly carries burdens for parents. It means that closure on a difficult and trying event in their lives may be postponed for a few days. Also, it is easier to say no to treatment for an abstract child than for one that has a personal presence for them. The parents may find themselves bonding with the child during the assessment period, making it harder for them to refuse treatment later, even if doing so would be justified. Unless resuscitation and initial treatment occurs, however, there will be no firm basis for finding that the child lacks the relevant capacity that must be shown to justify denying treatment. Allowing parents to refuse resuscitation at birth based on prebirth estimates of age and size risks denying infants who are unexpectedly large or vigorous the chance for life.

Has the Emphasis on Autonomy Gone Too Far?

Insights from Dostoevsky on Parental Decisionmaking in the NICU

JOHN J. PARIS, NEIL GRAHAM, MICHAEL D. SCHREIBER, AND MICHELE GOODWIN

Cambridge Quarterly of Healthcare Ethics 15 (2006): 147–151.

In a recent essay, George Annas, the legal columnist for *The New England Journal of Medicine*, observed that the resuscitation of extremely premature infants, even over parental objection, is not problematic because "once the child's medical status has been determined, the parents have the legal authority to make all subsequent decisions." Annas himself is quick to concede that treatment in a high-technology neonatal intensive care unit (NICU) frequently takes on a life of its own. He also acknowledges that although bioethicists and courts agree that there is no ethical or legal difference between withholding or withdrawing a respirator from a patient, parents and physicians find the withdrawal much more emotionally troubling.

Stopping a treatment that is sustaining the life of their child is, for many parents, psychologically or morally impossible. Even if assured that the cause of death would be the underlying disease and not the withdrawal, these parents continue to believe that turning off the respirator would "cause" their child's death. They could never agree to such an action.

Other parents, and they are numerous and well known in neonatal medicine, insist that a decision to end a life can only be made by God. Once the discussion moves into the theological realm, the medical team is defenseless. How does a physician argue against the position that "Doctors don't have the right to play God"? For these religiously oriented parents, once their infant is resuscitated, there is no turning back. Moral arguments on the proportionate burden and benefit to the patient, the classical approach for evaluation of the usefulness of medical interventions, prove unpersuasive. As a result, the child is trapped in the technology from which the only exit is death. When death does occur,

those involved in the infant's care can assure themselves, "We did everything possible. It was God's decision, not ours, that ended the life."

The desire of parents and sometimes of physicians to avoid responsibility for the death of a patient, particularly a newborn infant, can be overwhelming. An insight into that reality is found in Dostoevsky's novel *The Brothers Karamazov*. There we learn the novelist's understanding of human nature is fundamentally at odds with the emphasis in contemporary American bioethics on rationality, autonomy, and individual self-determination. For Dostoevsky, individual choice or freedom is not a "right" to be exercised, but a burden to be shunned.

Montello and Lantos explored these differing perceptions of human psychology in an intriguing essay entitled "The Karamazov Complex: Dostoevsky and DNR Orders."[1] They observed that although most legal and philosophical discussions on medical decisionmaking stress patient autonomy as the overriding moral principle, in practice, many patients and families do not want the responsibility philosophers thrust upon them. The wide gulf between the pronouncements of bioethicists on responsibility for termination of treatment decisions and the actual practices of doctors led Montello and Lantos to seek a rationale for this disparity. Do patients need more empowerment and legal authority or is the present focus on personal autonomy a misplaced emphasis, one at odds with how we as humans really behave?

Montello and her colleague argued for the latter position. They held that families may not want the empowerment that the prevailing bioethics doctrine insists belongs to them. The authors found support for their position in *The Brothers*

Karamazov, where families take collective rather than personal responsibility for the choices and actions of each family member. In the novel, three of the four brothers want their father dead. He is an evil, nasty man, a drunk, a child abuser, a rapist, and a cheat. Although each wishes him dead for different reasons, it remains uncertain through most of the novel whether any of them will actually kill him. The sons are ambivalent. They have misgivings and moral qualms. None wants to be the one to take direct responsibility for the death, though each desires that outcome.

The authors believe that a similar pattern is prevalent in many end-of-life medical decisions, particularly those made in the NICU. Family members may want the treatment to be withdrawn, but no one wants to be the one to give the directive to do so. As evidence, they cite the experience of a neonatal intensive care doctor, who, when asked to describe the process of decision-making in the NICU, recalled the following case:

> I talked to the parents about this [withdrawing treatment]. I told them we can't make their baby better and that we wanted to withdraw support. Dad said, "You can't. That's murder." And then he clenched both hands and started to come towards me. I thought he might hit me, but he walked past me and hit the wall. It was a strange moment. It's like time stood still. I watched him come towards me and I just stood there—I didn't want to flinch, because I didn't want him to think that I didn't trust him. And I wanted them to trust me. But I thought he might hit me. But fortunately he didn't and he didn't hurt anybody. He went out the door. A few minutes later, I saw him in the hall and he asked me if I had done it yet. I said I was on my way now. I turned off the O_2 and went up on the fentanyl to keep her comfortable. The father saw me and smiled. He was tearful and he left, smiling at me. It was a big turnaround for him.

It is apparent in both the novel and the medical narrative that people are not eager to take responsibility for tragic decisions. Instead, they try to avoid that role even to the point of adamantly denying their involvement in a choice they desperately want implemented. In such circumstances, the best outcome, from the perspective of those participating in the decision, is one in which it is not clear who really made the decision or even if one were being made.

Dostoevsky's genius was uncovering the primal psychological forces at work in coming to a decision. For him, once there is agreement on a goal, the focus is not, as in the canons of bioethics, on identifying a specific decisionmaker and assigning responsibility. Rather, it is to disguise the decision and to diffuse and submerge responsibility for it.

Dostoevsky expounded on that insight in great detail in his chapter on "The Grand Inquisitor." There, in the guise of a poem about the return of Christ to 16th century Seville, we discover the novelist's perspective on human nature. Jesus has returned to Spain where He witnesses the daily ritual of the splendid *auto de fé* in which the wicked heretics are burned. The crowds recognize Him, as does the withered old Cardinal of Seville, The Grand Inquisitor, who condemns Jesus to be burned at the stake. And His crime? Christ holds too lofty a view of mankind. Christ came to proclaim love and freedom. But, as the Grand Inquisitor observes, men do not want freedom. Freedom involves responsibility. Responsibility, in turn, is fraught with ambiguity, anxiety, doubt, and guilt. Mankind, too weak and too vile for such a realm, cringes from the task.

Far from freedom, what men seek are miracles, mystery, and authority. They desire someone to take responsibility from them, someone to make their decisions, someone who will simply give them bread. Gladly then will they come and lay their freedom at that individual's feet. By substituting authority for freedom, the Grand Inquisitor claims to have lifted suffering from men's hearts and thereby saved them from the terrible agony they must endure in making free decisions.

This work says Alyosha, the kind and saintly Karamazov brother, is only a senseless poem, a fantasy. And so it is. Why then should we take it seriously? Why has the poem endured? What insight does it give us into human nature? How useful a guide is it to understanding the difficult and trying decisions faced by parents in the NICU, particularly when the prognosis for their child shifts from "hopeful" to "dim" to "dismal"?

For the philosopher, the lawyer, or the judge who looks at end-of-life decisionmaking in the abstract, the issue is eminently clear. Once the physician concludes that there is no realistic expectation of survival, the parents should be informed and given the option of withdrawing the life-sustaining interventions. For the parents that choice is not so easy. They look at the physician and ask, "Doctor, do you mean you want our permission to kill our baby?" How could a parent agree to that? Or endure the guilt of having given up on their own child?

Dostoevsky's use of literature to probe into the recesses of the human psyche helps us understand that a parental decision to terminate treatment on a child is not the rational calculus of balancing burdens and benefits proposed by the philosophers. Nor is it simply the logical conclusion of legal precedents cited by a lawyer. These decisions are tormented situations, situations fraught with anguish, ambiguity, and doubt. Such situations—overlaid with feelings of guilt, rage, and inadequacy—are not readily subjected to rational analysis. Nor are they seen as an opportunity to exercise personal values and individual choice. They are, at best, an awful and unwelcomed burden.

Literature, unlike philosophy, pays exquisite attention to the truths of lived experience. Philosophy speaks to the way things ought to be. Its demands, however, may be too daunting and too devastating to be embraced in individual circumstances. The novel or the poem capture life as lived—with its emotions, conflicts, and contradictions exposed. The novelist or the poet portray a far more nuanced understanding of our limitations and inadequacies than does philosophy, bioethics, or the law.

If, as Dostoevsky indicated and our experience in dealing with parents facing the difficult and try-

ing decision in the NICU confirms, human nature balks at making a decision to end the life of one's child, we might want to reconsider our approach to termination of treatment decisions. Rather than laying out the medical facts, providing the possible options, and then confronting the parents with the stark reality that, "It is your child, your decision: choose," we might acknowledge parental reluctance to make such a decision and accept parents' desire to avoid being forced to do so.

A first step might be to change our approach to these decisions. A typical scenario might be as follows. Talk to parents from the outset about how fragile, precarious, and vulnerable a 23-week, 614-g infant is. Even in the face of the daunting prospects for such infants, many parents remain hopeful and ask the doctors to do "everything possible" for the baby. If so, intensive treatment will be initiated. On the second day of life, an intracranial ultrasound shows a left sided grade III intraventricular hemorrhage. Despite treatment with dopamine, hydrocortisone, and fluid boluses, by day of life 4 (DOL 4) hypotension is a significant problem. High ventilator settings of 80% FIO_2 are needed to keep adequate oxygenation. The hematocrit and platelets remain consistently low despite blood product replacement. A severe metabolic acidosis remains unresolved. The skin turns gray and incurs significant breakdown. An ultrasound on DOL 6 shows a massive grade IV intraventricular hemorrhage on the left and a large grade III on the right.

At this point, rather than asking the parents to, in effect, sign a death warrant for this baby, the physician's approach might be: "We have known from the start that your baby's chances were really very, very small. We began a trial of therapy, but despite our best efforts, your child is being overwhelmed with problems, problems we are unable to reverse. The best we can do now is to keep your baby comfortable and allow you to be with him and hold him."

Do not ask the parents, "If your baby suffers a cardiac arrest, do you want us to try to save him?" Such a question gives parents false hopes and unrealistic expectations, expectations that inevitably lead to demands for more and more interventions and the risk of further complications. More importantly, as Singh and colleagues noted in a recent article on death in a neonatal intensive care unit, "CPR is ineffective in preventing death of moribund NICU patients."

Once you have explained that additional aggressive interventions or escalation of treatment will be unavailing, emphasize that their baby's care should now be directed to assuring the child's comfort. If the parents agree, the physician should then write in the chart: "I have discussed the infant's condition with the parents. They understand further aggressive measures are not medically warranted and that our goal has shifted from attempts to reverse the disease process to providing comfort and company for their child. In light of this care plan, I am entering a DNR order in the chart so that when the patient's heart stops, cardiopulmonary resuscitation will not be attempted."

Left unasked, but not unaddressed, in this approach is any question about letting the child die. Nor is there any seeking of parental permission to adjust the dopamine level or to omit a vasopressin drip. These are discussions that are painful for parents and unnecessary.

Also left unasked is authorization to shut off the ventilator. Unless the parents indicate they would like everything removed so they can hold their child unimpeded by lines or tubes, that step might not be necessary. Without other aggressive responses to the infant's rapidly deteriorating condition, the extremely preterm infant assaulted with the sequelae of marked prematurity will not survive long.

Once the parents understand and accept that further aggressive measures are not warranted, the appropriate care of their child changes from intensive interventions to what Paul Ramsey, in an essay entitled "On (Only) Caring for the Dying," called "comfort and company." This is the most the physician or parent can provide for the infant whose physical status has slipped beyond the reach of medicine. Such an approach is not one that ignores the right of a parent to make the treatment decisions for a child. It is one that recognizes that there comes a point when further medical interventions serve only to prolong an inevitable death. Such efforts produce no benefit to the patient, but do result in increased pain and suffering for both the infant and parents. There is no need to compound the suffering of the patient by prolonging it, nor of the parents by insisting that they must agree to what nature has already decreed.

Our approach to end-of-life care is not new. The treatise entitled *The Art* in the Hippocratic Corpus defines medicine as having three roles: "To do away with the suffering of the sick, to lessen the violence of their diseases, and to refuse to treat those who are overmastered by their diseases, realizing that in such cases medicine is powerless." If there is no realistic choice to be made, Hippocrates advised, *no choice should be offered.* When, despite our best efforts, medical interventions on the extremely premature infant do not succeed in reversing disease processes, we need not compound the grief of parents by asking their permission to withdraw the failed therapies. It is enough for the parents to agree that in light of their baby's condition, the focus should be on keeping the child's final moments as comfortable as possible. Then the most the physician can do is to support the parents as they keep company with their baby in the last stages of its brief life.

Note

1. M. Montello and J. Lantos, "The Karamazov complex: Dostoevsky and DNR orders," *Perspectives in Biology and Medicine* 45 (2002): 190–9.

Appropriate Use of Artificial Nutrition and Hydration

Fundamental Principles and Recommendations

DAVID CASARETT, JENNIFER KAPO, AND ARTHUR CAPLAN

New England Journal of Medicine 353 (2005): 2607–12.

For two decades, clinicians have been guided by an agreement about the appropriate use of artificial nutrition and hydration (ANH). In general, ANH has been seen as a medical treatment that patients or their surrogates may accept or refuse on the basis of the same considerations that guide all other treatment decisions: the potential benefits, risks, and discomfort of the treatment and the religious and cultural beliefs of the patients or surrogates. Although this agreement has never been universal, it is well established among ethicists, clinicians, and the courts. For instance, the 1990 Supreme Court decision in the well-known case of Nancy Cruzan specifically stated that the administration of ANH without consent is an intrusion on personal liberty.

However, this agreement has faced recent challenges to its legitimacy. For instance, even though the cases of Terri Schiavo and Robert Wendland were complicated by disagreements among family members, the cases also involved public questioning of the premise that decisions about ANH should be made in the same way in which decisions about other treatments are made. Similarly, a recent papal statement that strongly discourages the withdrawal of ANH from patients in a permanent vegetative state will have a profound effect on decisions about ANH if it is accepted into Catholic doctrine. Several states have made the withdrawal of ANH more difficult than the withdrawal of other forms of life-sustaining treatment.

Clinicians also face substantial obstacles that prevent them from applying sound, ethical reasoning when discussing ANH with patients and families. For instance, patients and families are often not fully informed of the relevant risks and potential benefits of ANH. In addition, financial incentives and regulatory concerns promote the use of ANH in a manner that may be inconsistent with medical evidence and with the preferences of patients and their families. Finally, preferences about ANH may not be honored after a patient is moved from one care setting to another.

It is not possible to prevent all disagreements about the use of ANH. But it is possible, and indeed it is essential, to clarify the principles that should underlie decisions about ANH and to ensure that these principles guide decisions in clinical practice. Therefore, in this article we examine the ethical principles that have guided the appropriate use of ANH during the past 20 years and recommend steps to promote clinical practices that are more consistent with these principles.

Clinical Decisions and Medical Evidence

ANH may improve survival among patients who are in a permanent vegetative state. These patients may live for 10 years or more with ANH but will die within weeks without nutritional support. Parenteral ANH can also prolong the lives of patients with extreme short-bowel syndrome, and tube feeding can improve the survival and quality of life of patients with bulbar amyotrophic lateral sclerosis. Finally, ANH may improve the survival of patients in the acute phase of a stroke or head injury and among patients receiving short-term critical care, and it may improve the nutritional status of patients with advanced cancer who are undergoing intensive radiation therapy or who have proximal obstruction of the bowel.

There is less evidence of benefit when ANH is used for other indications. For instance, some studies suggest that ANH improves the survival rate among patients receiving chemotherapy, but other studies do not support this finding. Studies of the effect of ANH on complication rates after cancer surgery have also produced conflicting results. The bulk of the available evidence suggests that ANH does not improve the survival rate among patients with dementia.

ANH is associated with considerable risks. For instance, patients with advanced dementia who receive ANH through a gastrostomy tube are likely to be physically restrained and are at increased risk of aspiration pneumonia, diarrhea, gastrointestinal discomfort, and problems associated with feeding-tube removal by the patient. In addition, when a patient's renal function declines in the last days of life, ANH may cause choking due to increased oral and pulmonary secretions, dyspnea due to pulmonary edema, and abdominal discomfort due to ascites.

Ethical Principles for Decision Making

Decisions about the use of ANH should be made in the same way in which decisions about other medical treatment are made. Many people believe that nutrition must always be offered, just as pain management, shelter, and basic personal care must be. This view is deeply rooted in cultural and religious beliefs. It is often expressed with the use of the word "starvation" to describe the condition of a patient who does not receive ANH. Patients, families, and physicians are entitled to hold these beliefs, which are not easily set aside. However, to help patients and families make decisions about ANH, physicians should present the contrary view by emphasizing three key points.

First, physicians should emphasize that ANH is not a basic intervention that can be administered by anyone, as food is. ANH is a medical therapy administered for a medical indication (e.g., dysphagia) with the use of devices that are placed by trained personnel using technical procedures. ANH therefore has more in common with other surgical and medical procedures that require technical expertise than with measures such as simple feeding. Second, physicians should explain that unlike the provision of food

or other forms of comfort (such as warmth or shelter), the procedures required for ANH and the subsequent administration of ANH are associated with uncertain benefits and considerable risks and discomfort. These factors need to be considered carefully before ANH is initiated. Finally, physicians should clarify that the goal of ANH is not to increase the patient's comfort. In fact, during the administration of high-quality palliative care, symptoms of hunger or thirst generally resolve in a short time or can be managed effectively (e.g., mouth dryness can be alleviated with ice chips) without the provision of ANH. Throughout the comprehensive informed-consent process for patients and families, physicians should explain the potential benefits of ANH for a patient, as well as its risks and discomfort and all relevant alternatives, just as they would for other health care decisions.

After this discussion, patients and families may remain convinced that ANH differs from other treatments. Beliefs about food and the associations concerning food are deep-seated, and in some cohorts and communities they are linked to historical or personal experiences with starvation (e.g., during the Holocaust or the Great Depression). Patients and families may decide to accept or refuse ANH on the basis of these beliefs. When physicians have beliefs about ANH that prevent, them from supporting the decisionmaking process of a patient and his or her family in an unbiased way, they should consider transferring the patient's care to another physician. Hospitals and health care facilities should support physicians in doing so.

Withholding or Withdrawal of Treatment

Many people believe it is more acceptable to withhold a treatment than to withdraw it, and one cannot discount the emotional burden that families in particular may feel when they believe that the withdrawal of treatment will allow a patient to die. This distinction is not supported, however, by currently accepted ethical and legal reasoning. In fact, a more cogent argument can usually be made for the withdrawal of ANH after it has been administered for a trial period if it has proved to be ineffective or if experience has provided more information about its risks and discomfort.

Evidence of Patient Preference

When a patient lacks the capacity to make decisions, a single surrogate (usually defined in a state law according to a hierarchy) should make choices on that patient's behalf on the basis of available evidence of the patient's preferences and values. These decisions may be based on previous statements (either oral or written) by the patient or on a surrogate's knowledge of the patient. This standard of surrogate decision making has been widely supported in the law and among ethicists. In some states, however, a patient's advance directive must include a statement that the patient would not want ANH. This higher standard of evidence is inappropriate for two reasons.

First, decisions about ANH should not be held to a higher standard of evidence, because the balance of risks and potential benefits is, in most situations, no different for ANH than for many other medical treatments. For many patients, such as those with dementia, the balance may favor other interventions over ANH. Therefore, it is illogical to require a higher level of evidence in order to withhold or withdraw ANH than would be required for other medical treatments or procedures that offer a similar risk–benefit balance.

Second, a higher standard that requires specific evidence of a patient's preferences regarding ANH is not realistic. Although in its decision in the Cruzan case, the Supreme Court upheld the constitutionality of requiring clear and convincing evidence of a patient's preferences, any higher standard has proved to be very difficult to satisfy. Despite moderate increases in the prevalence of advance directives as a result of the Patient Self-Determination Act, most adults have not executed a written advance directive, and even those who have may not have specified their preferences about ANH. Therefore, a higher evidentiary standard makes it harder for surrogates to make decisions that reflect a patient's goals and preferences. Furthermore, a higher standard is illogical because it would permit certain restraints on liberty — the imposition of ANH without consent — whereas impositions of other treatments are prohibited.

Lack of Advance Directive

Although surrogates should make decisions on the basis of a patient's preferences, sometimes an advance directive is not available. In this situation, the patient cannot be assumed to want ANH. Indeed, there are a variety of reasons why patients do not complete advance directives, including cultural concerns, lack of information, and reluctance to initiate discussions about advance directives. When a patient's preferences are unknown, surrogates must consider how a reasonable person with a cultural background, life experience, and worldview similar to the patient's would weigh the risks and potential benefits of ANH. This "reasonable person" standard often may be easier to apply than the related "best interest" standard, which requires surrogates to consider the difficult philosophical question of whether a decision that could result in death is in a patient's best interest.

Although only a minority of states explicitly permit the reasonable-person standard, reasonable people often choose to forgo life-sustaining treatment if its discomfort outweighs its benefits or if those people perceive a health condition to be worse than death. The balance of risks and potential benefits for ANH may be less favorable than the balance for other treatments that surrogates refuse on a patient's behalf. Therefore, states that allow surrogates to make other health care decisions on the basis of a reasonable-person standard also should permit this standard for decisions about ANH.

Provision of Palliative Care

When ANH is withheld or withdrawn, physicians should reassure patients and families that most of the resulting discomfort can be managed effectively. All patients who forgo ANH should be offered comprehensive palliative care, including hospice. A comprehensive palliative care or hospice plan should address physical and psychological symptoms and should include emotional and spiritual support as well as bereavement support for the family after the patient's death.

Obstacles to Ethical Decision Making

Despite general agreement about these ethical principles, their application to decisions about ANH at the bedside may encounter numerous obstacles. We propose the following five recommendations to help ensure that patients and their families retain the right to make decisions about ANH and that these decisions are supported at the bedside by health care providers, by the law, and by the health care system.

First, given the inadequacies in the typical informed-consent process for ANH, all clinicians need to be better able to engage patients and families in meaningful discussions. Medical educators should better prepare clinicians to engage in these and other difficult end-of-life discussions by emphasizing both the ethical principles that underlie decisions about ANH and effective communication techniques.

Second, decision making about ANH in nursing homes should be shielded from financial and regulatory pressures. Although the loss of the ability to eat is an expected part of dementia, one third of cognitively impaired nursing-home residents have a feeding tube. Nursing homes should not be reimbursed at a higher rate for residents who are receiving ANH than for those not receiving ANH, since providing ANH costs less than feeding by hand. In addition, staff and surveyors should be informed that nursing homes should not be cited when a patient loses weight after a decision to forgo ANH.

Third, state laws should allow the same standard of evidence of a patient's preferences for decisions about ANH as they do for other decisions. These laws should allow families to make reasoned and caring decisions on the patient's behalf if they are based on knowledge of the patient's values and preferences. If a patient's preferences are unknown, surrogates should be allowed to make decisions, in close collaboration with the patient's health care providers, that are guided by thoughtful judgments about what a reasonable person would choose.

Fourth, attorneys, physicians, and other health care providers should encourage and help patients to complete advance directives and to include preferences about ANH. Because decisions about ANH are often complicated by disagreements among family members, advance directives should also identify a decision maker. More generally, state laws should specify a hierarchy of decision makers to reduce the possibility of ambiguity and conflict among family members.

Fifth, health care facilities should ensure that preferences are respected in all health care settings. Problems with information transfer between institutions can affect all patients and are particularly common when nursing-home residents are transferred to a short-term care setting. Nursing homes and hospitals should develop effective documentation strategies, such as Physician Orders for Life-Sustaining Treatment forms, which ensure that a patient's preferences are clearly documented and readily available to guide the patient's care.

Conclusions

Patients and families should be allowed to make decisions about ANH in an informed-consent process that is guided by well-established principles. Moreover, the right of the patients and their families to make independent decisions about ANH and other medical treatment should be defended against legal, financial, and administrative challenges at the bedside. A variety of stakeholders — including organizations of medical professionals, legal associations, and other health care organizations — will be needed to ensure this defense. Through advocacy activities, disease-based organizations can also help guarantee that all patients who forgo ANH receive high-quality, compassionate care near the end of life.

But efforts by individual organizations will not be enough. In order to ensure that patients' preferences are respected and that obstacles to high-quality care are removed, these organizations will need to work together closely.

Moreover, they will need to form partnerships with legislators, payers, and regulatory agencies to promote the five recommendations. More generally, efforts to facilitate decisions about ANH that are compassionate, ethically sound, and clinically reasonable need to be part of a larger agenda to improve care for all patients with serious illness.

Assisted Nutrition and Hydration and the Catholic Tradition

THOMAS A. SHANNON AND JAMES J. WALTER

Theological Studies 66 (2005), 651–62.

The Terri Schiavo case in Florida focused attention on a variety of issues related to the end of life: who is the decision maker, the status of advanced directives, the role of family members with respect to married adult children, and issues related to the removal of life support systems, particularly assisted nutrition and hydration. Terri Schiavo is now linked to two other young women who played a critical role in helping us to think through ethical issues at the end of life. Karen Ann Quinlan and her family raised the issue of the removal of a ventilator. In her case the physicians were reluctant to do this because they feared legal repercussions. The legal and ethical analysis concurred that such removal was justified because it constituted extraordinary means of treatment. Nancy Cruzan and her family focused attention on the removal of artificial nutrition and hydration (ANH). Again law and ethics concurred that such removal was justified, particularly because people testified that being maintained in such circumstances were not her wishes.

On February 25, 1990, Terri Schiavo had suffered a heart attack, possibly brought on as a result of chemical imbalances from an eating disorder. She suffered loss of oxygen to her brain and was eventually diagnosed as being in a persistent vegetative state. A decade later, in February 2000, her husband Michael Schiavo requested that her feeding tube be removed. After a five-year legal battle, the feeding tube was removed, and Terri Schiavo died on March 31, 2005, at the age of 41.

A critical element in the debate was the ethics of the use of feeding tubes for patients in a persistent vegetative state. Several bishops, particularly in light of the papal allocution on feeding tubes in March 2004, argued that their use was morally obligatory. Thus Bishop Vaga of Baker, Oregon: "She may well die in the future from an inability to digest food but it would be murder to cause her death by denying her the food she still has the ability to digest and which continues to provide for her a definite benefit—life itself." That sentiment was echoed by Representative Thomas DeLay of Texas who said: "That act of barbarism can be and must be prevented." A comment on the ethical issue underlying the provision of ANH was offered by Bishop Loverde of Arlington, Virginia, who said: "If Mrs. Schiavo were facing imminent death, or were unable to receive food and water without harm, then removing nutrition and hydration would be morally permissible. It is however never permissible to remove food and water to *cause* death. Food and water are basic human needs, and therefore basic human rights." And Richard Doerflinger of the United States Catholic Conference of Bishops was reported to have articulated the normative nature of this position in an interview with the *Washington Post*:

> Before the pope made his statement about feeding-tube cases at a conference last year there was enough uncertainty about the church's position that Catholics could remove feeding tubes without fear of committing a sin. No one could fairly have said to you that you were dissenting from clear Catholic teaching. Now you would have to say, "Yes, you are."

The issue on which we focus in this note is the state of the question in the Catholic tradition regarding the use of assisted nutrition and hydration, an issue that became central in the media and in public debate.

Our position is that there have been four unacknowledged shifts within the last 25 years from the traditional method of analyzing our moral obligations during illness and the dying process. The first of these is a shift in the very method itself: from proportionate reasoning as in the "Declaration on Euthanasia" from the Congregation for the Doctrine of the Faith in 1980 to a deontological reasoning as in the March 2004 papal allocution "Care for Patients in a 'Permanent' Vegetative State." Second, there is a shift in applying the ordinary-extraordinary distinction from the general context of obligations to oneself while ill to restricting the application to the context of imminent dying. Third, there has been a shift from making a determination of whether or not to use an intervention such as chemotherapy or assisted nutrition and hydration to a presumption in favor of using such interventions. Finally, following John Paul II's allocution, there is a shift

from a presumption to use to an obligation to use. Thus, in a series of statements from various ecclesial commissions and magisterial authorities, the tradition has been moved recently from both a patient-centered focus and obligations determined through the use of proportionate reason to a technology and intervention-centered focus with obligations being determined by deontological principles. We call this more recent position the revisionist position.

The Development of the Revisionist Position

Methodological Shift

Many moral theologians argue that there are two different ethical methodologies operating in Roman Catholicism. The first is deontological or a principle-based ethic and is used primarily in the areas of sexual morality and in medical morality where sexual morality is the content, e.g., assisted reproduction. The resolutions of ethical issues are deducted from the principles and there are no exceptions to the principles and no parvity of matter in sexual issues. The principles bind absolutely and are not qualified by circumstances. The other method is the one used in the area of social justice, for example in the analysis of the morality of war or economic policy. The conclusions drawn are recognized to be provisional in that new data can reshape the conclusion, and there is a recognition that one can come to different conclusions that are in harmony with one's starting principles.

Historically, the method of analysis of issues related to end-of-life issues has mostly utilized the second method. This ethic has traditionally been patient-centered and focused on an evaluation of benefits and burdens or on whether the intervention was proportionate or disproportionate. This is the method of, for example, the 1980 "Declaration on Euthanasia" from the Congregation for the Doctrine of the Faith.

First the Congregation notes that it "pertains to the conscience either of the sick person, or of those qualified to speak in the sick person's name, or of the doctors, to decide, in the light of moral obligation and of the various aspects of the case" (IV). The "Declaration" says that the patient can make a correct decision about whether a treatment is proportionate or disproportionate by "studying the type of treatment to be used, its degree of complexity or risk, its cost and the possibilities of using it, and comparing these elements with the result that can be expected, taking into account the state of the sick person and his or her physical and moral resources." (IV). Finally, the "Declaration" notes that one can refuse treatments based on a "desire not to impose excessive expense on the family or the community" (IV).

The "Declaration on Euthanasia" is a clear and articulate summary of the moral teaching of the Catholic Church on end-of-life issues from about the 16th century to the present. The constant theme of the moralists is that the patient needs to determine what is extraordinary in light of his or her medical circumstances, financial situation, and values. If the effects of the intervention are disproportionate to the desired outcome, they need not be used.

However, a shift seems to be occurring in this tradition and in the method over the past two and half decades. When one reads the 2004 allocution by John Paul II on assisted nutrition and hydration, there is a methodological shift to deontology and determination of principles by definition or stipulation. Briefly, the pope stated that such tubes were "not a medical act" and their use "always represents a natural means of preserving life" and is part of "normal care." Therefore, their use is to be considered in principle ordinary and obligatory. "If done knowingly and willingly" the removal of such feeding tubes is "euthanasia by omission." The person's medical condition is not really relevant in making a determination about the use of feeding tubes, except if the body cannot assimilate the fluids or the intervention does not alleviate the suffering of the patient, because the food and water delivered through such tubes is ordinary care and provides a benefit—"nourishment to the patient and alleviation of his suffering."[1]

What is interesting about this papal allocution is that it seems to represent a significant departure from the Roman Catholic bioethical tradition with respect to both the method and the basis upon which such decisions are made. Historically, the method for making a determination about the use of a medical intervention was the proportion between the benefits of the intervention and its harms or burdens to the individual, family, and community. The method is a teleological balancing of the impact of the intervention. This has been the central teaching of the tradition from the mid-1600s through Pope Pius XII and the 1980 "Declaration on Euthanasia" by the Congregation for the Doctrine of the Faith. The method announced by Pope John Paul II appears to be deontological in nature. The use of feeding tubes to deliver artificial nutrition and hydration is stipulated as in principle ordinary, and such an intervention apparently must not be forgone or withdrawn unless or until the body cannot assimilate the nutrients or they do not alleviate the suffering of the patient.

The Shift from Illness to Imminent Dying

When one reads the manualist tradition on this question, the general framing of the question is in terms of preserving one's life during an illness. Historically, particularly up to about 1950, there was a coincidence of becoming ill and dying but that was because of the general lack of any genuinely useful medical interventions. Typically when one got seriously ill, one died. However, the moralists did not cast the teaching as applicable only in the context of dying. The obligation is cast in terms of the general context of illness and the prolongation of life.

Pius XII, in his 1957 address on "The Prolongation of Life," discusses the possibility of terminating attempts at resuscitation by not placing a patient on a mechanical ventilator. In this address the discussion of termination of life support occurs within the context of deep unconsciousness and hopelessness but not within the context of dying or of terminal illness. Additionally, Pius does not posit a presumption to resuscitate but rather uses the traditional burden-benefit method to determine whether or not there is an obligation to resuscitate.

Finally, the "Declaration on Euthanasia" speaks in this vein as well. Section IV, as noted above, discusses the issue under the rubric of caring for one's health and how to determine what remedies to use. The last six sentences of section IV refer to the dying process but only in that one can refuse "means of treatment that would only secure a precarious and burdensome prolongation of life…." (IV). The condition of dying or being terminally ill is not the general context for the application of the decision making process, but rather one more situation in which one can apply the method of analysis.

A shift in analysis seems to stem from *Evangelium vitae* in which John Paul II, in talking about aggressive medical therapies that are disproportionate or too burdensome, says "in such situations, when death is clearly imminent and inevitable, one can in conscience" (65) refuse treatments. The footnote for this section is to the CDF "Declaration on Euthanasia," but this seems to misrepresent what the document says. The "Declaration" does talk about imminent death in section IV, but it does not do it in the manner that *Evangelium vitae* suggests. *Evangelium vitae* restricts the application of the criteria of proportionality and burden to the situation of imminent and inevitable death. But this is not what the CDF document says. Rather the analysis of section IV is to identify the method of decision making and what is to be included in it as the patient makes decisions about his or her treatment. The context of dying is yet another time when this method can be brought to bear on the situations. The restriction of the application of the ordinary-extraordinary distinction to imminent death is new and has not been part of the general moral tradition nor of the CDF document.

From the Appropriateness of a Therapy to the Presumption of Its Use

Imbedded in the distinction between ordinary and extraordinary means of medical technology is the possibility of an equivocation on the term "ordinary." When we discuss medical interventions, we frequently discuss some of them as routine, standard, the treatment of choice, standard of care, or ordinary. What is meant in this discussion is that for this particular situation, this is what is usually or ordinarily done. Such interventions can range from a blood transfusion, to chemotherapy, to cardiac bypass surgery, to dialysis, to the insertion of a feeding tube, etc. However, no determination has yet been made on the effect of such an intervention on the patient or on others. From the perspective of the tradition, this is where the moral evaluation begins. What is the impact on the patient, what benefits or burdens will it bring him or her, what is the likely outcome of the intervention, what is the cost, both psychological and economic for the patient and his or her family? The patient must determine whether there is a proportion between what is done ordinarily in medicine and the expected benefits, both short term and long term. What may be *medically* ordinary or routine may not in fact be *morally* ordinary because of a disproportion of the benefit-burden ratio for the patient. We must avoid the common equivocation on the word ordinary.

Another version of this equivocation concerns the distinction as a means of categorizing interventions. When one categorizes medical interventions in the abstract apart from the concrete circumstances of the patient, the basis of the classification itself determines the moral status of the intervention, not the effects of the intervention on the patient. Thus we look at the intervention and ask if this is routinely done. If the answer is yes, then we must use it. Again the assumption is that, because an intervention is customarily used, it must be morally obligatory. And again the moral analysis is short-circuited because of the equivocation, and one attempts to draw an "ought" or moral obligation directly from an "is" or what is routinely done.

Another problem this equivocation sets up is that the terms ordinary and extraordinary are used as methods of classification or categorizations of interventions. If an intervention is categorized as ordinary—based on the observation that this is customary or ordinary medical practice—then it is morally obligatory. Fortunately, the tradition does not use the terms ordinary and extraordinary as a means of abstract classification but as the conclusion of an argument about the proportion or disproportion of benefits and burdens, as the CDF phrases it. This point was also nicely made by the founder of American Catholic bioethics, Gerald Kelly, S.J., who noted in 1950 that sometimes even "ordinary artificial means are not obligatory when relatively useless."

The equivocation on the term ordinary and the use of the terms as means of categorizing interventions set the context for the presumption of use of assisted nutrition and hydration. For example, in 1986, the Committee for Pro-Life Activities of the then NCCB noted that food and water are necessities of life. And since they can be provided without risks and burdens associated with more aggressive life-supporting interventions, there should be a presumption in favor of their use. This position was repeated in the *Ethical and Religious Directives for Catholic Health Care Services* issued in 1994 by the NCCB/USCC. After repeating the traditional means of determining burden and benefit, the document states:

> There should be a presumption in favor of providing nutrition and hydration to all patients, including patients who require medically assisted nutrition and hydration, as long as this is of sufficient benefit to outweigh the burdens involved to the patient.[2]

What is interesting is the structure of the sentence. The tradition would usually begin with an analysis of whether there is burden or benefit and then determine whether ANH is required or not. The revisionist position begins with a presumption and then moves to disprove the presumption. The problem with this comes from either an equivocation on the term ordinary or from using the term as a method of classification. The position of the long-standing tradition has been to evaluate the proposed intervention and then come to a moral conclusion.

A final difficulty with this shift concerns determining to what we have presumptive or prima facie obligations. In the tradition, one had a presumptive obligation to preserve one's life, not a presumptive obligation to accept or take any particular medical technology, e.g., mechanical ventilators, heart transplants, or assisted nutrition and hydration. In recent statements, however, patients have a presumptive obligation to take artificial nutrition and hydration. This presumptive obligation can be overridden if and when it can be shown from the circumstances, e.g., the body cannot assimilate the nutrients or the patient is imminently dying or they do not alleviate the suffering of the patient, that this obligation is not one's actual moral obligation.

From Presumption of Use to the Necessity of Use of Assisted Nutrition and Hydration

The first note of a shift away from considering the context of the sick person as morally relevant to decision making at any stage of the illness is in the Cor Unum document of 1981. This document states that:

> There remains the strict obligation to apply under all circumstances those *therapeutic measures* which are called "minimal": that is, those which are normally and customarily used for the maintenance of life (*alimentation*, blood transfusions, injections, etc.). To interrupt these minimal measure would in practice, be equivalent to wishing to put an end to the patient's life.

Note here that feeding is defined as a medical intervention and that there is the presumption of benefit of this intervention.

The Pontifical Academy of Sciences in 1985 noted: "If the patient is in a permanent irreversible coma, as far as can be foreseen, treatment is not required, but all *care* should be lavished on him, *including feeding*." Note here that "feeding" is not placed within the category of "medical treatment" but is defined as "care," which indicates that such interventions are not subject to the normal moral criterion of proportionality between benefits and burdens.

This position is repeated in John Paul II's allocution on assisted nutrition and hydration in which the pope stated in March 2004 that such tubes were "not a medical act" and their use "always represents a natural means of preserving life" and is part of "normal care." Therefore, their use is to be morally considered in principle as ordinary and obligatory. "If done knowingly and willingly" the removal of such feeding tubes is "euthanasia by omission." Other than the inability of the body to absorb the nutrients or that the patient is imminently dying or that the patient's suffering cannot be alleviated, the person's medical condition is not relevant in making a determination about the use of feeding tubes because the food and water delivered through such tubes is ordinary care and provides a benefit—"nourishment to the patient and alleviation of his suffering." Such a shift to the requirement that assisted nutrition and hydration must be used essentially takes the decision about this intervention out of the patient-centered approach that has so characterized the historical tradition of the past.

Conclusions

The Terri Schiavo case provides an interesting insight into a major change in the methodology to determine whether or not an intervention is a benefit or a burden, whether or not it is proportionate or disproportionate. To our knowledge, no one in any of the discussions has argued that there is no moral obligation to provide cures or care for those who are ill or in medically compromised positions. At issue is how one determines that obligation. Our observation is that the tradition from at least the 16th century through Pius XII, the Congregation for the Doctrine of the Faith in 1980, and the vast majority of moral theologians has determined this obligation by having the patient consider the benefits and burdens of the intervention to determine if they were proportionate or disproportionate. The tradition did not start with assumptions about interventions, nor did it categorize interventions.

Since the early- to mid-1980s, though, a revisionist position has been emerging in the statements from the pope, Pontifical Academies, Commissions, and Committees that radically change the methodology. These statements categorize interventions and stipulate obligations. The method shifts from proportionality of effects on the patient (teleology) to deontology.

The shift seems to be motivated by two moves: one ethical and the other political. The ethical move seems to emerge out of an eliding of two distinct but related elements that make up a moral judgment. The axiological element, which is concerned with the determination of value, affirms the value or sanctity of life of the patient. This assessment opposes, correctly, efforts to devalue life lived under difficult circumstances or problematic medical conditions, such as permanent coma. Thus the axiological element of the moral judgment in the Catholic tradition opposes any use of the phrase "quality of life" as a shorthand way of arguing that a patient's life is not worth preserving. The second and distinct element, the normative, is a determination of what obligations I have in the concrete to maintaining this *valued* life. This normative element has traditionally been resolved by determining the burden-benefit ratio of the proposed intervention. Failure to make this important and traditional ethical distinction between axiology and normativity leads one to affirm wrongly that the affirmation of the value or sanctity of life of the patient in and of itself imposes normative obligations with respect to medical interventions. In addition to being the fallacy of deriving an "ought" from an "is," the failure also implicitly may signify a form of vitalism that affirms that biological life is the only or most important value. Finally, the failure to make the distinction leads to a form of a "medical indications policy" as the moral criterion that mandates that particular interventions necessarily must follow from the diagnosis.

The political move both incorporates the failure to make the distinction between the axiological and the normative and incorporates this into the rhetoric of the right to life movement. Thus the rhetoric of the right to life movement focuses on the obligation to maintain biological life under virtually any and all conditions and in the more excessive strands of the movement comes close to committing idolatry by making biological life the only value to be considered. This is certainly not the traditional Catholic "sanctity of life" position, and, in fact, it begins to move this rhetoric into materialism in that biological life is the only or most important value under consideration. There is no doubt that recent magisterial attempts to protect the dignity of unconscious patients are important and utterly necessary, but the movement to require the use of technologies that sustain biological life may in fact have the opposite effect on a society that is prone to devaluing life.

In an earlier article we developed the following position, and we continue to argue that it will serve as an appropriate basis on which to make decisions about the morality of the use of assisted nutrition and hydration.

> [W]hen a proposed intervention cannot offer the patient any reasonable hope of pursuing life's purposes at all or can offer the patient a condition where the pursuit of life's purposes will be filled with profound frustration or with utter neglect of these purposes because of the energy needed merely to sustain physical life, then any medical intervention (1) can only offer burden to the life treated, (2) is contrary to the best interests of the patient, (3) can cause iatrogenic harm or risk of such harm, and (4) has reached its limit based on medicine's own principal reason for existence, and thus treatment should not be given except to palliate or to comfort.[3]

The more recent revisionist perspective approaches end-of-life judgments by defining and categorizing particular interventions in the abstract as ordinary, and, on the basis of this maneuver, mandating these interventions. This method that appears to have entered magisterial statements by stipulation undercuts the traditional benefit-burden method and risks imposing great hardship on patients and families at a time of great crisis. We can think of no greater burden to impose on people at this time than to have them feel abandoned by the Church when they are in greatest need of its benefits. Bluntly stated, the Catholic tradition on end-of-life issues has never mandated doing useless or inane things to people in the name of morality. We should not start doing this now.

Notes

1. John Paul II, "Care for Patients in a 'Permanent' Vegetative State." This allocution can be found on the Vatican website: http://www.vatican.va/holy_father/john_paul_ii/speeches/2004/march/documents/hf_jp-ii_spe 20040320_congress-fiamc_en.html (accessed April 13, 2005); also in *Origins* 33 (April 8, 2004) 737 and 739–40.

2. USCC, *Ethical and Religious Directives for Catholic Health Care Services*, (Washington: USCC, 1994), Directive # 58. Interestingly, in the latest version of the ERDs (2001), the introduction to Part V, in which directive # 58 is found, states: "These statements agree that hydration and nutrition are not morally obligatory either when they bring no comfort to a person who is imminently dying or when they cannot be assimilated by the person's body." Note here that a proportion between benefit and burden is not the criterion used.

3. Thomas A. Shannon and James J. Walter, "The PVS Patient and the Forgoing/Withdrawing of Medical Nutrition and Hydration," *Theological Studies* 49 (1988): 645.

The Devil's Choice

Re-Thinking Law, Ethics, and Symptom Relief in Palliative Care

ROGER S. MAGNUSSON

Journal of Law, Medicine, and Ethics 34, no. 3 (2006): 559–69.

In 1982, cinemas around the world screened *Sophie's Choice*, a film starring Meryl Streep and Kevin Kline, adapted from the book by William Styron. The film opens with Stingo, a young journalist from the South, who arrives in New York in 1947 and rents a room in Brooklyn. Stingo is drawn into a relationship with Sophie and Nathan, the couple who live upstairs. Sophie is a Polish concentration camp survivor; Nathan is the man who saved her when she arrived in America. Nathan is charismatic, schizophrenic, and violent.

In one of the film's flashbacks, a German soldier imposes a terrible choice on Sophie, a young mother who arrives at Auschwitz with other prisoners from Krakow. Sophie is ordered to choose which of her two children will be sent to the ovens, and which will live. She *must* choose, or the soldier will take them both. It is the devil's choice. Sophie finally cries out, "Take my daughter!" In the film, she never recovers from the guilt and trauma of her decision.

Sophie's choice is an archetype of what I will call "the devil's choice": a choice coerced by circumstances beyond one's control, and made all the more terrible by the conviction that tragedy will follow, whichever option is taken. In so far as morality and ethics are useful when facing the devil's choice, it cannot be to point out the "right choice," because circumstantial constraints mean that all options are perverse.

It is often assumed, explicitly or implicitly, that the role of medical ethics and of law is to guide us towards the "right choice." In this paper, however, I argue that some of medicine's most painful decisions are, in fact, the devil's choices. I will focus in particular on the provision of pain relief and the administration of palliative sedation in end-of-life care, arguing that the devil's choice provides a better model for explaining these practices than the traditional account found in law and medical ethics. The benefit of applying the devil's choice to palliative care is that it permits empathy with the dilemmas physicians face, while still acknowledging the extraordinary power that physicians have over the lives of patients at what is perhaps the most vulnerable time of their lives.

While this paper will focus on palliative care, the devil's choice is equally applicable where life-supporting technologies are withdrawn from suffering, severely damaged neonates, from permanently unconscious patients and from others for whom curative (as distinct from palliative) interventions, are futile. The performance of late-term abortions may also illustrate the devil's choice.

The Devil's Choice in Medical Law: Britain's Conjoined Twins

Professor Ian Kennedy has argued that in the future, law will become increasingly enmeshed with medicine, and the most difficult issues in bioethics will continue to be addressed by courts "the one institution which, once asked, cannot refuse to supply a response." Before turning to the context of palliative care, it is worth pointing out that courts have on many occasions been forced to grapple with the devil's choice: *Re A*, a case that came before the English Court of Appeal in 2000, provides a well-known, but nonetheless spectacular and instructive example.

Jodie and Mary were conjoined twins whose devout Catholic parents had traveled from Malta to Britain for assistance, but who opposed surgical separation. With no functioning heart or lungs, little Mary's life depended on her ailing sister. Without an operation, both would die; with an operation, at best, one would live. Under English law, the Court was obliged to determine whether or not the operation was in the twins' best interests. After some soul-searching, the Court authorized the operation. Lord Justice Ward began by comparing the advantages and disadvantages that would flow from the operation for each twin. Since the operation would kill Mary and for that reason could not be said to be in her interests, the surgery was nevertheless "the lesser of the two evils" and the "least detrimental choice," because it gave Jodie the chance of a life that both would otherwise be denied.

Re A provides a helpful example of a court forced to justify a choice that no one involved in the case wished to make (the need to choose arose from the growing threat to Jodie's life), where the available alternatives could only be described as bad, or worse. The court's approach has been influential in other cases. Significantly, the court's decision to absolve the surgeons from liability for hastening Mary's death depended neither on the doctrine of double effect, nor on the distinction between acts and omissions. The doctrine of double effect has been used by courts, lawyers and ethicists in other end-of-life scenarios to exempt a doctor from having any intention of causing death, whereas the distinction between acts and omissions has been applied to ensure that the patient's underlying illness, rather than the doctor's clinical intervention, is treated as the legal cause of death. The operation to separate Jodie and Mary took twenty hours and, as expected, Mary died during the course of it.

As illustrated by *Sophie's Choice* and *Re A*, the "devil's choice" exhibits two critical features. First of all, the ethical parameters within which the choice takes place are not of the chooser's making, and are *perversely constrained or limited*. All the available options are not only unwanted, but are morally perverse, to a greater or lesser degree. Secondly, avoiding evil by opting out or failing to choose, is itself a choice. It is not possible *not to choose*, since the physician is morally

and legally charged with the care of the patient, and doing nothing ensures its own tragic consequences. In a very real sense, the physician is trapped within a narrow set of more or less perverse alternatives.

Foresight, Intention, and the Devil's Choice in Palliative Care

Although conjoined twins are rare, I would argue that the devil's choice is a metaphor that rings true for many health professionals who provide palliative care at the end-of-life. It may arise, firstly, with the provision of opioid analgesics for the relief of pain and symptoms, in circumstances where the physician foresees that these drugs may suppress the patient's breathing or cough reflex and allow fluids to accumulate in the lungs in a way that contributes to an earlier death. Nurses may also face this issue when administering the dosages charted by the physician, often in the physician's absence, based on their own experience of the effects of analgesics and sedating agents on distressed patients who are in a severely weakened state. One nurse comments, "It's an unspoken thing that happens between health care professionals: you know that the four o'clock dose of morphine is going to be the last dose that anybody's ever going to give that patient…*it's just done.*"

Secondly, the devil's choice may arise when the strategy for pain management or symptom relief in a terminally ill patient is, in fact, sedation: intractable pain or distress is controlled by rendering the patient unconscious, with or without the continued administration of hydration and nutrition. Palliative sedation (occasionally called "terminal sedation" or "pharmacological oblivion") is ethically controversial and continues to generate debate. In a survey of internists' attitudes, Kaldjian and colleagues reported that seventy-eight percent favored using terminal sedation as a treatment for refractory pain, while ninety-seven percent favored aggressive use of analgesia even if it risked hastening death. Given that a hastened death may be the foreseeable result of some symptom relief practices, the dividing line between palliative care and unlawful killing is crucially important, both ethically and legally. Public confidence in the medical profession, and in the specialty of palliative medicine, demands that we can distinguish between doctors and killers, and doctors themselves deserve the clearest advice on what separates lawful from unlawful conduct.

The traditional ethical justification for the provision of life-shortening analgesics in palliative care relies upon the principle of double effect. This principle holds that clinical interventions that foreseeably shorten life may nonetheless be justified by the physician's intention to pursue a separate (noble) end, provided that other key conditions are also satisfied. Sulmasy and Pellegrino point out that treating patients with morphine satisfies the principle of double effect because: it is not immoral to administer morphine; the morphine is administered with the intention of relieving pain (not with the intention of killing the patient); the morphine does not need to first kill the patient in order to relieve pain; and the relief of pain is a sufficiently noble end to justify the risk of hastening death. Keown provides a helpful description of double effect as the principle of "unintended bad side-effects."

What does the principle of double effect achieve? It acknowledges that end-of-life care imposes hard choices, and permits doctors both to limit suffering and to hasten death in circumstances where high-dose opioids incidentally shorten the patient's life. Moreover, it enables the doctor to avoid describing their act as killing: something that may bring comfort not only to them, but to the patient and the patient's family as well. However, whether the distinction between foreseeing and intending death is strictly applied by physicians involved in palliative care is dabatable. In one Australian survey (admittedly, of surgeons), Douglas and colleagues reported that while few had ever administered a bolus lethal injection, a large proportion (36.2%) had given drugs with the intention of hastening death, presumably by

infusion, in ways that would be difficult to distinguish from accepted palliative care other than by the doctor's self-reported intention.

It is difficult to believe that courts would find the compassionate provision of analgesia in hospitals and hospices to be unlawful. Although the issue has been considered only infrequently, court decisions in the United States and, to an extent, in Britain, provide support for a legal distinction between foresight and intention as a basis for upholding the lawfulness of aggressive palliative care. In the United States, analysis surrounds comments made by members of the United States Supreme Court in two cases, *Vacco v. Quill*, and *Washington v. Glucksberg*. In each case, the Supreme Court rejected argument by a coalition of patients and doctors that the laws prohibiting physician-assisted suicide in New York State, and in Washington State, respectively, were unconstitutional.

In upholding state law in *Vacco*, the majority opinion confirmed the distinction between foresight and intention, noting that the law distinguishes actions taken "'because of' a given end from actions taken 'in spite of' their unintended but foreseen consequences." A physician who provides aggressive palliative care, therefore, acts lawfully since their "purpose and intent is, or may be, only to ease [the] patient's pain." Justice O'Connor's opinion, filed in both cases, went even further, endorsing sedation that alleviates suffering "even to the point of causing unconsciousness and hastening death." Her Honor reiterated: "There is no dispute that dying patients in Washington and New York can obtain palliative care, even when doing so would hasten their deaths."

The lawfulness of pain-relieving practices has also been considered by English courts, most famously in the 1957 murder trial of a family practitioner, Dr. Bodkin Adams, who had injected 2.6 grams of heroin and 2.6 grams of morphine into his eighty-one-year-old stroke patient. Justice Devlin, the presiding judge, famously stated that while the criminal law carved out no special defenses for doctors:

that did not mean that a doctor who was aiding the sick and dying had to calculate in minutes or even hours, perhaps not in days or weeks, the effect on a patient's life of the medicine which he would administer. If the first purpose of medicine – the restoration of health – could no longer be achieved, there was still much for a doctor to do, and he was entitled to do all that was proper and necessary to relieve pain and suffering, even if the measures he took might incidentally shorten life by hours or perhaps even longer.[1]

The distinction between foreseen consequences, and intended consequences, lies at the heart of the principle of double effect. Where analgesia is sufficiently aggressive to shorten life, it is the absence of intention to do so that distinguishes this practice from euthanasia. The foresight/intention distinction is more tenuous in the context of palliative sedation, particularly when the patient is denied artificial hydration or nourishment. The distinction is downright absurd when life-supporting treatment, including hydration and nourishment, is withdrawn from a patient in a persistent vegetative state. This is because death is the logical and certain consequence of the intervention. In so far as there is an overwhelming moral imperative never to intentionally cause death, therefore, moral responsibility can only be avoided by asserting an intention not to bring about consequences that are the certain outcome of one's actions.

Doctors respond to this dilemma in different ways. While intentions may be ambiguous and inscrutable, some doctors clearly regard hastening death as part of the spectrum of palliative care. One comments, "dying patients are given larger and larger doses of morphine. We talk about the 'double effect,' and know jolly well we are sedating them into oblivion, providing pain relief but also providing permanent relief, and we don't tell them." "This stuff goes on in general hospitals all the time, you know," one palliative care nurse told me in interview: "give the little old lady with the 'fracky neck' who's going to die in a week a little bit extra Brompton's cocktail."

Another palliative care physician, explaining why only intravenous morphine (but not water or food) was administered to patients who could not eat or drink for themselves, remarked meaningfully: "If you gave intravenous fluids, at the same time as giving morphia for breathlessness or pain, *you could keep the patient alive for weeks.*" In Loewy's view:

> Terminal sedation is done with the full knowledge that no further active treatment will be done and that patients, as rapidly as possible, will now die as a result of their underlying disease process....Patients are intentionally kept asleep, their vital functions are deliberately not artificially supported, and they are allowed to die in comfort. That they should die in comfort is clearly the goal...of terminal sedation.... These goals do not differ from those of physician assisted suicide, or, for that matter, voluntary euthanasia.[2]

Despite all this, there are strong legal, ethical and emotional reasons why many doctors – palliative care physicians in particular – would not wish their actions in providing symptom relief to be seen as *killing.* Even where a hastened death is the certain consequence of the physician's action, some would vigorously defend the sincerity and meaningfulness of their belief that they did not *intend* to hasten the patient's death, regardless of the certainty of that result.

How should law and ethics resolve this standoff? It seems that the best that law and professional ethics can do is to cordon off palliative care from euthanasia by distinguishing, as the principle of double effect does, between foresight of death, and intention to cause death. Where this strategy fails, as it may where palliative sedation is administered, and as it must where the doctor removes a ventilator from an incurably comatose patient, ethics and law retreat to a fall-back position that manipulates the concept of causation by distinguishing between acts and omissions. This enables the doctor to claim that where – and only where – further treatment would be futile, the removal of the ventilator is an omission, with the result that the patient's underlying disease, rather than the doctor's intervention, is the cause of death. This is hardly convincing, for there is "nothing psychologically or physically passive about taking someone off a mechanical ventilator who is incapable of breathing on his or her own." For the same reason, it strains common sense to regard the administration of sedating agents in palliative care as a failure to act, when it is clearly the opposite.

The Devil at the Bedside

The devil's choice is a moral dilemma that arises in circumstances where choice itself is perverse and not choosing is not an option. It provides a helpful metaphor for re-interpreting some – but not all – of the decisions that physicians are called on to make.

"Therapeutic Optimism"

In the scenario of the risky operation, the surgeon may foresee the possibility, even the likelihood, that the patient will die. The surgeon's conviction, however, is that while they intend to cut into the patient's body, they do not intend to kill or harm the patient. This conviction reflects the doctor's *therapeutic optimism*: the hope that the surgery will be successful, even if there is but a slim chance of achieving this. Hope plays an important role in medicine: the physician, as much as the patient, clings to hope. Not surprisingly, the surgeon's language fastens onto the (possibly) small chance that the patient might not die, that treatment will be beneficial. It is meaningful for the surgeon to argue that they have no intention of hastening the patient's death, given the altruistic aims of the surgeon, and their rational assessment that the patient *might survive the surgery*. On the other hand, if the patient were so weak that they would inevitably die in surgery, the surgery would amount to unlawful killing unless, as in *Re A*, some legal excuse could be found. A surgeon who went ahead with surgery in the knowledge that it would kill the patient would rightly be imputed with the intention to bring about that result.

In palliative care, the distinction between foresight and intention holds true much of the time because in most circumstances where pain relief is administered, the denial of intention reflects therapeutic optimism: the considered assessment that the morphine will relieve pain but without killing or hastening death. Pain management is a moving field, and mercifully so. The extent to which the skilful provision of analgesics and adjuvants can successfully manage pain is a clinical and empirical question. Similarly, whether or not particular pharmacological practices do, in fact, hasten death, is an empirical issue. In hard cases, however, the metaphor of the devil's choice may provide a more appropriate model for interpreting the doctor's choice than the principle of double effect.

Beyond the "Devil's Threshold"

Beyond the devil's threshold, medical interventions that are reasonably certain to hasten death but which do not, in fact, do so, might be called miracles. A doctor might shrink from the prospect of causing death, but in turning away they face another perverse alternative: to abandon the patient to their suffering. What characterizes the devil's threshold is that, beyond it, all the choices available to the doctor are perverse, to a greater or lesser degree. In an environment where no "right choice" is available, the role of medical ethics becomes one of assisting the physician to choose the least perverse alternative.

Beyond the devil's threshold, physicians face what are literally life or death decisions. Especially at the end of life, when patients are weak or suffering, it is appropriate for both law and ethics to acknowledge the vulnerability of patients and the power of the medical profession over them. Unfortunately, the principle of double effect has the opposite effect: by downplaying the moral significance of foresight, it exempts the physician from moral responsibility for their actions at the time when moral responsibility is most needed.

The importance of this point was brought home to me by Liz, a palliative care nurse, who met secretly with me in a department-store coffee shop and who proceeded to give an anguished account of non-consensual euthanasia upon a patient with AIDS. The patient "had about a hundred T-cells," so he "wasn't close to the end of his life," although he had lost control of his bodily functions, required a catheter, and could no longer move his arms. On the other hand, his body was not wasted, and nurses were able to control his pain with oral medication. "This man was determined to live," said Liz, "he was determined to get better, but the physician didn't see it this way. It got to the point that one Thursday, the physician came into the unit and said 'This has got to stop, send mum home to have a shower.'" As soon as the mother had left the ward, the physician charted an infusion of midazolam, morphine and Tegratol (carbamazepine) which he instructed Liz to hook up. Liz remembers the physician's words clearly: "Get it up and get him out of here by sundown."

"I actually went out to the ladies," Liz recalls. "I was sitting there and I was crying and I was thinking 'what can I do?' I wanted to run down to...the Director of Nursing, but I thought, my God, if I do that, this is going to open up a hornet's nest." Liz approached two registrars working on the unit. "What are we doing to this man?" she asked. "We're *killing* him," but the registrars said "no, it's come to the point that he's going to die, and if we don't step in he's going to have a very bad death. He's going to fit."

Remarkably, Liz alleged that the unit where she worked had, on occasion, accepted patients who had "booked [themselves] in" to receive a lethal infusion of drugs, and Liz had willingly participated in voluntary euthanasia on prior occasions. On this occasion, however, she felt the procedure was involuntary. She was frightened and felt coerced into participating. "[I]t was like I was the only person there that could see clearly what was happening," she said. "It was murder."

"He had a little dog and, you know, that was his life, he lived with his mum...he didn't want to die, no way at all. They were such a close

family...just working class people...they just thought...'this doctor knows what he's doing.'"

The infusion was administered and the patient died that night. Predictably, the procedure was rationalized as being necessary to relieve distress and suffering. Liz admitted to being an inexperienced nurse at the time this incident took place. Was it involuntary euthanasia, or symptom relief causing death as an unintended, incidental consequence? Liz has little doubt: "The doctor played God, he thought he was God...he'd decided this was the time for this patient."

The Devil's Choice: Implications for Legal and Ethical Accounts of Palliative Care

Given the vulnerability of patients at the end of their lives, I would argue that law and medical ethics ought to regard a physician as intending to hasten the patient's death in circumstances where this is the highly likely or inevitable consequence of providing adequate symptom relief. While the effect was intended, it does not follow that the doctor desired the patient's death. The doctor was, after all, faced with the devil's choice.

How, then, might we separate lawful palliative care, from unlawful killing or euthanasia? To be helpful, the distinction needs to institutionalize good symptom-relief practices, while also immunizing the doctor from a charge of unlawful killing. It would be tragic if, by recognizing the dilemma the physician faces, the law created an incentive for doctors to under-treat, to chart inadequate dosages for symptom relief, thereby ensuring that patients suffered more than if the ambiguity of the foresight/intention distinction had never been challenged.

As seen above, there are three ways of justifying the doctor's actions. The first is to apply the foresight/intention distinction criticized throughout this paper. The second is to apply a theory of legal causation that simply states, as a matter of positive law, that the doctor was not legally responsible, or incurs no civil or criminal liability, for causing the patient's death (despite foreseeing that this was an incidental consequence of treatment), provided that certain criteria are satisfied. This carries the same disadvantages of the first approach: it fails to recognize the power that physicians wield over patients.

A third and more satisfactory way of resolving the problem is to recognize through common law doctrine, or through legislation, a defense of "necessity" that applies in circumstances where physicians face the devil's choice. Such a defense accurately recognizes the nature of the choice the physician made in providing adequate palliative care. Furthermore, the presumption that the physician should only proceed to shorten a patient's life in circumstances when the criteria for the defense are satisfied is an important protection for patients. These criteria draw a bright line between palliative care and unlawful killing in circumstances beyond the devil's threshold where adequate symptom relief is highly likely to hasten the patient's death. Two conditions would need to be satisfied. Firstly, the physician's desire to help the patient without causing death ("therapeutic optimism") will be reflected in the choice of sedatives and analgesics that have established therapeutic properties: the defense would clearly be inappropriate where the doctor administers a lethal injection of, say, potassium chloride. Secondly, the defense should also require that the dosages administered be proportionate to the degree of suffering the patient was enduring. This condition would not be satisfied, for example, if the doctor administered a massive bolus dose in order to kill the patient, thereby incidentally reducing their suffering in the process. The defense of necessity, within the context of palliative care, ought not to exempt doctors who set out to kill the patient, as distinct from *risking the patient's life* through measures reasonably considered to be proportionate to the patient's suffering.

Some may feel that necessity opens the door to a utilitarian calculus that may undermine the sanctity of life principle in other areas. What would be worse, however, is to continue to undermine the sanctity of life principle while obscuring and denying that this is even happening. This is worse because it precludes scrutiny of life and death decisions and the values underlying them. Despite the professed commitment of conservative ethicists to sanctity of life, patients' best interests are hardly protected when death by palliative care comes, in the words of one interviewee, "packed in this sort of soggy cotton wool of evasion so that we don't know what other people's motives are."

The Devil's Choice and the *Crie De Coeur*

What, then, should we make of the doctor who, while administering pain relief, or sedating a dying patient, or removing life-support from a suffering and gravely damaged neonate, foresees the certainty of a hastened death, yet resolutely and sincerely insists that causing death was never their intention? A doctor in these circumstances faced a perverse choice between relieving distress and hastening death, or giving inadequate symptom relief in order not to shorten life. In circumstances where there are no grounds for therapeutic optimism, there is no third alternative.

The physician's denial, made in these circumstances, is best understood as a *crie de coeur* that conveys a complex set of meanings. Moral clarity and patient safety require, however, that the denial should not be accepted at face value. In exploring the meanings that arise, we can put to one side those cases where the physician privately admits that they did intend to kill the patient, but preferred to disguise their intent for legal reasons, or to avoid institutional scrutiny of their clinical decisions.

The physician's denial must be understood, firstly, against the external constraints that characterize the devil's choice. In the palliative care ward it is the patient's ill health, rather than German guards or a shared heart, that limits the clinical choices and their likely outcomes. Secondly, the physician's denial takes place against the background norms of law and clinical ethics that prohibit intentional killing. The physician's denial reflects the abhorrence of killing that the physician genuinely feels. Closely associated with this, the physician's denial is an implicit claim for moral approval: a claim that the physician is innocent and justified, even if the patient does die as a result of the physician's attempt to relieve suffering. The clearer view, I would argue, is that the physician is morally responsible for hastening the patient's death, but that they were faced with the devil's choice, and in the circumstances, hastening death was necessary and justified as the least perverse option. For those who believe that intentional killing is always wrong, however, this is no answer at all. In fact, this is what drives the doctor to deny having any intention to kill.

Fourthly, while the physician's denial cannot reasonably be explained in terms of therapeutic optimism (because the doctor's intervention is certain to hasten death), it may nevertheless reflect the doctor's emotions and wishes. Faced with the prohibition on killing embodied in law and ethics, the physician's desire to relieve suffering, and the constraints imposed by the patient's failing health, the doctor recoils and their denial of intention expresses what they wish were the case. The *crie de coeur* is a wish for a miracle, a wish so common at the bedside at the end-of-life.

Conclusion

The conventional construction of palliative care relies upon the principle of double effect to exempt physicians from moral and legal responsibility for hastening death, in circumstances where this is the unintended consequence of symptom relief practices. However, if intentionally assisting patients to die is as morally and legally unacceptable as opponents of physician-assisted dying contend, then the line between palliative care and unlawful killing ought to be clearer. Moving beyond the principle of double effect is a good first step, since although this principle recognizes the doctor's dilemma, it fudges the moral significance of clinical interventions

and leaves the patient at the mercy of motivations and intentions that can rarely, if ever, be questioned.

In circumstances where the provision of symptom relief is highly likely or indeed certain to shorten a patient's life, it is appropriate to impute to the physician an intention to hasten death. This does not mean that law or medical ethics is committed to acknowledging euthanasia as a routine part of palliative care: it is the surreptitious, undeclared practice of euthanasia that justifies the critique of conventional accounts of palliative care. It is, however, to recognize that physicians must sometimes face the devil's choice: a choice, that is, between relieving suffering and hastening death in circumstances where there is no third alternative and where it is not possible not to choose.

Finally, in accordance with the defense of necessity proposed above, the physician's action in hastening death will be justified where the physician has administered recognized, analgesic drugs in dosages that were a proportionate response to the patient's suffering. These two criteria provide a clearer evidentiary basis for defending compassionately motivated interventions than the "illusory" language of what the doctor says they intended. The defense of necessity immunizes palliative care practices that accord with accepted and responsible professional practice, while permitting law and ethics to better acknowledge the gravity and consequences of these end-of-life decisions.

Notes

1. H. Palmer, "Dr. Adams' Trial for Murder," *Criminal Law Review* (1957) 365–77, at 375.
2. E. Loewy, "Terminal Sedation, Self-Starvation, and Orchestrating the End of Life," *Archives of Internal Medicine* 161 (2001) 329–32, at 331; see also R. Syme, "Pharmacological Oblivion Contributes to and Hastens Patients' Deaths," *Monash Bioethics Review* 18 (1999): 40–43.

Voluntary Euthanasia

A Utilitarian Perspective

PETER SINGER

Bioethics 17, nos. 5–6 (2003): 526–41.

Utilitarianism

There is, of course, no single 'utilitarian perspective', for there are several versions of utilitarianism and they differ on some aspects of euthanasia. Utilitarianism is a form of consequentialism.

What consequences do we take into account? Here there are two possible views. Classical, or hedonistic, utilitarianism counts only pleasure and pain, or happiness and suffering, as intrinsically significant. Other goods are, for the hedonistic utilitarian, significant only in so far as they affect the happiness and suffering of sentient beings. That pleasure or happiness are good things and much desired, while pain and suffering are bad things that we want to avoid, is generally accepted. But are these the *only* things that are of intrinsic value? That is a more difficult claim to defend. Many people prefer to live a life with less happiness or pleasure in it, and perhaps even more pain and suffering, if they can thereby fulfil other important preferences. For example, they may choose to strive for excellence in art, or literature, or sport, even though they know that they are unlikely to achieve it, and may experience pain and suffering in the attempt. We could simply say that these people are making a mistake, if there is an alternative future open to them that would be likely to bring them a happier life. But on what grounds can we tell another person that her considered, well-informed, reflective choice is mistaken, even when she is in possession of all the same facts as we are? The difficulty of satisfactorily answering this question is one reason why I favour preference utilitarianism, rather than hedonistic utilitarianism. The right act is the one that will, in the long run, satisfy more preferences than it will thwart, when we weigh the preferences according to their importance for the person holding them.

When Killing Is, and Is Not, Wrong

Undoubtedly, the major objection to voluntary euthanasia is the rule that it is always wrong to kill an innocent human being. Anyone interested in an ethics that is free of religious commitments should be ready to ask sceptical questions about this view.

The idea that it is always wrong to kill an innocent human being gains its strongest support from religious doctrines that draw a sharp distinction between human beings and other sentient beings. Without such religious ideas, it is difficult to think of any morally relevant properties that separate human beings with severe brain damage or other major intellectual disabilities from other beings at a similar mental level. For why should the fact that a being is a member of *our* species make it worse to kill that being than it is to kill a member of another species, if the two individuals have similar intellectual abilities, or if the non-human has superior intellectual abilities?

I can think of only one non-religious reason that has any plausibility at all, as a defence of the view that the boundary of our species also marks the boundary of those who it is wrong to kill. This is a utilitarian argument, to the effect that the species boundary is sharp and clear, and if we allow it to be transgressed, we will slide down a slippery slope to widespread and unjustified killing. I will consider slippery slope arguments against allowing voluntary euthanasia towards the end of this paper. Here it is sufficient to note that this argument effectively admits that there is no intrinsic reason against attributing similar rights to life to humans and non-humans with similar intellectual capacities, but warns against the likely consequences of doing so. For our present inquiry into the underlying reasons against killing human beings, this is enough to show that one cannot simply assume that to be human is to give one a right to life. We need to ask, not: what is wrong with killing a human being; but rather, what makes it wrong to kill any being? A consequentialist might initially answer: whatever goods life holds, killing ends them. So if happiness is a good, as classical hedonistic utilitarians hold, then killing is bad because when one is dead one is no longer happy. Or if it is the satisfaction of preferences that is good, as modern preference utilitarians hold, then when one is dead, one's preferences can no longer be satisfied.

These answers suggest their own limits. First, if the future life of the being killed would hold more negative elements than positive ones – more unhappiness than happiness, more frustration of preferences than satisfaction of them – then we have a reason for killing, rather than against killing. Needless to say, this is highly relevant to the question of euthanasia.

At this point, however, some further questions arise that suggest the relevance of higher intellectual capacities. Among these questions are: who is to decide when a being's life contains, or is likely to contain, more positive characteristics than negative ones? And what further impact will the killing of a being have on the lives of others?

Regarding the first of these questions, the nineteenth century utilitarian John Stuart Mill argued that individuals are, ultimately, the best judges and guardians of their own interests. So, in a famous example, he said that if you see people about to cross a bridge you know to be unsafe, you may forcibly stop them in order to inform them of the risk that the bridge may collapse under them, but if they decide to continue, you must stand aside and let them cross, for only they know the importance to them of crossing, and only they know how to balance that against

the possible loss of their lives. Mill's example presupposes, of course, that we are dealing with beings who are capable of taking in information, reflecting and choosing. So here is the first point on which intellectual abilities are relevant. If beings are capable of making choices, we should, other things being equal, allow them to decide whether or not their lives are worth living. If they are not capable of making such choices, then someone else must make the decision for them, if the question should arise.

The conclusion we can draw from this is as follows: if the goods that life holds are, in general, reasons against killing, those reasons lose all their force when it is clear that those killed will not have such goods, or that the goods they have will be outweighed by bad things that will happen to them. When we apply this reasoning to the case of someone who is capable of judging the matter, and we add Mill's view that individuals are the best judges of their own interests, we can conclude that this reason against killing does not apply to a person who, with unimpaired capacities for judgement, comes to the conclusion that his or her future is so clouded that it would be better to die than to continue to live. Indeed, the reason against killing is turned into its opposite, a reason for acceding to that person's request.

Now let us consider the second question: what impact does killing a being have on the lives of other beings? The answer will range from 'none' to 'devastating', depending on the particular circumstances. Even in the case of beings who are unable to comprehend the concept of death, there can be a great sense of loss, when a child or a parent, for example, is killed. But putting aside such cases of close relationship, there will be a difference between beings who are capable of feeling threatened by the deaths of others in circumstances similar to their own, and those who are not. This will provide an additional reason to think it wrong – normally – to kill those who can understand when their lives are at risk, that is, beings with higher intellectual capacities.

Once again, however, the fact that killing can lead to fear and insecurity in those who learn of the risk to their own lives, is transformed into a reason in favour of permitting killing, when people are killed only on their request. For then killing poses no threat. On the contrary, the possibility of receiving expert assistance when one wants to die relieves the fear that many elderly and ill people have, of dying in unrelieved pain and distress, or in circumstances that they regard as undignified and do not wish to live through.

Thus the usual utilitarian reasons against killing are turned around in the case of killing in the circumstances that apply in the case of voluntary euthanasia.

What of an argument based on a right to life? Here everything will depend on whether the right is treated as most other rights are, that is, as an option that one can choose to exercise or to give up, or if it is seen as 'inalienable', as something that cannot be given up. I suggest that all rights should be seen as options. An 'inalienable right' is not a right at all, but a duty. Hence the idea of a right to life does not provide a basis for opposing voluntary euthanasia. Just as my right to give you a book I own is the flip side of my right to keep my property if I choose to retain it, so here too, the right to end one's life, or to seek assistance in doing so, is the flip side of the right to life, or to seek assistance in doing so, is the flip side of the right to life, that is, my right not to have my life taken against my will.

Against this, it will be said that we do not allow people to sell themselves into slavery. If, in a free society, people are not allowed to give up their freedom, why should they be able to give up their lives, which of course also ends their freedom?

It is true that the denial of the right of competent adults to sell themselves, after full consideration, into slavery creates a paradox for liberal theory. Can this denial be justified? There are two possible ways of justifying it, neither of which implies a denial of voluntary euthanasia. First, we might believe that to sell oneself into slavery – irrevocably to hand over control of your life to someone else – is such a crazy thing to do that the intention to do it creates an irrebutable presumption that the person wishing to do it is not a competent rational

being. In contrast, ending one's life when one is terminally or incurably ill is not crazy at all.

A second distinction between selling yourself into slavery and committing suicide can be appreciated by considering another apparently irrational distinction in a different situation. International law recognises a duty on nations to give asylum to genuine refugees who reach the nation's territory and claim asylum. Although the recent increase in asylum seekers has strained this duty, as yet no nation has openly rejected it. Instead, they seek to prevent refugees crossing their borders or landing on their shores. Yet since the plight of the refugees is likely to be equally desperate, whether they succeed in setting foot on the nation's territory or not, this distinction seems arbitrary and morally untenable. The most plausible explanation is that it is abhorrent to forcibly send refugees back to a country that will persecute them. Preventing them from entering is slightly less abhorrent. Similarly, a law recognising a right to sell oneself into slavery would require an equivalent of America's notorious fugitive slave law; that is, those who sold themselves into slavery, and later, regretting their decision, ran away, would have to be forced to return to their 'owners'. The repugnance of doing this may be enough explanation for the refusal to permit people to sell themselves into slavery. Obviously, since no one changes their mind after voluntary euthanasia has been carried out, it could not lead to the state becoming involved in any similarly repugnant enforcement procedures.

Some will think that the fact that one cannot change one's mind after voluntary euthanasia is precisely the problem: if people might make mistakes about selling themselves into slavery, then they might also make mistakes about ending their lives. That has to be admitted. If voluntary euthanasia is permitted then some people will die who, if they had not opted for euthanasia, might have come to consider the remainder of their life worthwhile. But this has to be balanced against the presumably much larger number of people who, had voluntary euthanasia not been permitted, would have remained alive, in pain or distress and wishing that they had been able to die earlier. In such matters, there is no course of action that entirely excludes the possibility of a serious mistake. But should competent patients not be able to make their own judgements and decide what risks they prefer to take?

Competence, Mental Illness, and Other Grounds for Taking Life

We have seen that Mill thought that individuals are the best judges and guardians of their own interests, and that this underlies his insistence that the state should not interfere with individuals for their own good, but only to prevent them harming others. This claim is not an implication of utilitarianism, and a utilitarian might disagree with it. But those who, whether for utilitarian or other reasons, support individual liberty, will be reluctant to interfere with individual freedom unless the case for doing so is very clear.

It is sometimes claimed that patients who are terminally ill cannot rationally or autonomously choose euthanasia, because they are liable to be depressed. The American writer Nat Hentoff, for example, has claimed that many physicians 'are unable to recognize clinical depression, which, when treated successfully, removes the wish for death.' Even if this statement is true, it is not an argument against legalising voluntary euthanasia, but an argument for including in any legislation authorising voluntary euthanasia, a requirement that a psychiatrist, or someone else trained in recognising clinical depression, should examine any patient requesting voluntary euthanasia and certify that the patient is not suffering from a treatable form of clinical depression.

In any case, not all clinical depression is susceptible to treatment. This leads to a different question, whether doctors should act on requests for euthanasia from patients who wish to die because they are suffering from clinical depression that has, over many years, proven unresponsive to treatment. This issue was raised in the Netherlands in 1991, when a psychiatrist, Dr Boudewijn Chabot, provided assistance in dying to a 50-year-old woman who was severely

depressed, but suffered from no physical illness. When prosecuted, Chabot contended that the woman was suffering intolerably, and that several years of treatment had failed to alleviate her distress. He thus sought to bring the case under the then-accepted guidelines for voluntary euthanasia in the Netherlands. He was convicted, but only because no other doctor had examined the patient, as the guidelines required. The Supreme Court of the Netherlands accepted the more important claim that unbearable mental suffering could, if it was impossible to relieve by any other means, constitute a ground for acceptable voluntary euthanasia, and that a person suffering from this condition could be competent.

From a utilitarian perspective, Chabot and the Dutch courts were correct. For the hedonistic utilitarian, what matters is not whether the suffering is physical or psychological, but how bad it is, whether it can be relieved, and – so that others will not be fearful of being killed when they want to live – whether the patient has clearly expressed a desire to die. Whether preference utilitarians would reach the same conclusion would depend on whether they are concerned with the satisfaction of actual preferences, or with the satisfaction of those preferences that people would have if they were thinking rationally and in a psychologically normal state of mind. It is easy to say: 'If you were not depressed, you would not want to die.' But why should we base our decision on the preferences a person would have if in a psychologically normal state of mind, even when it is extremely unlikely that the person in question will ever be in a psychologically normal state of mind?

Some cases of depression are episodic. A person can be depressed at times, and at other times normal. But if, having experienced many periods of depression, she knows how bad these periods are, and knows that they are very likely to recur, she may, while in a normal state of mind, desire to die rather than go through another period of depression. That could be a rational choice and one that a preference utilitarian should accept as providing a basis for assisted suicide or voluntary euthanasia. Given this, it seems possible to be rational about one's choice to die, even when depressed. The problem for the physician lies in recognising that the choice is one that would persist, even if the person were, temporarily, not depressed, but able to see that he would again become depressed. If this can be ascertained, a preference utilitarian should not dismiss such a preference.

Richard Doerflinger has argued that those who invoke autonomy in order to argue for voluntary euthanasia or physician-assisted suicide are not being entirely straightforward, because they defend the autonomy of terminally ill or incurably ill patients, but not of people who are just bored with life. A recent Dutch case raised that issue. Edward Brongersma, an 86-year-old former senator in the Dutch parliament, committed suicide with the assistance of a doctor, simply because he was elderly and tired of life. The doctor who assisted him was initially acquitted, but the Dutch Ministry of Justice appealed against the acquittal. This led to the doctor's conviction, on the grounds that what he did was outside the existing rules. Nevertheless, since the court recognised that the doctor had acted out of compassion, it did not impose any penalty. A utilitarian should not find anything wrong in the doctor's action, either because the desire to die was Brongersma's considered preference, or because no one was in a better position than Brongersma to decide whether his life contains a positive or negative balance of experiences. Of course, it is relevant that Brongersma was 86-years old, and his life was unlikely to improve. We do not have to say the same about the situation of the love-sick teenager who thinks that without the girl he loves life can never again be worth living. Such cases are more akin to a temporary mental illness, or period of delusion. Neither a preference nor a hedonistic utilitarian would justify assisting a person in that state to end his life.

The reason that the focus of debate has been on people who are terminally or incurably ill, rather than on people who are simply tired of life, may just be political. Advocates of voluntary euthanasia and physician-assisted suicide find it difficult enough to persuade legislators or the public to change the law to allow doctors to help people who are terminally or incurably ill. To broaden the conditions still further would make the task impossible, in the present climate of opinion. Moreover, where terminally or incurably ill patients who want to die are concerned, both respect for the autonomy of the patients and a more objective standard of rational decision-making point in the same direction. If permissible assistance in dying is extended beyond this group it becomes more difficult to say whether a person's choice is persistent and based on good reasons, or would change over time. From a utilitarian perspective, this is a ground for saying, not that it is necessarily wrong to help those who are not terminally or incurably ill and yet want to die, but that it is more difficult to decide when the circumstances justify such assistance. This may be a ground against changing the law to allow assistance in those cases.

Palliative Care

I return now to another of Nat Hentoff's objections to the legalisation of voluntary euthanasia and physician-assisted suicide. Hentoff thinks that many physicians are not only unable to recognise depression, but also not good at treating pain, and that sometimes good pain relief can remove the desire for euthanasia. That is also true, but most specialists in palliative care admit that there is a small number of cases in which pain cannot be adequately relieved, short of making patients unconscious and keeping them that way until death ensues a few days later. That alternative – known as 'terminal sedation' – is sometimes practised. Some ethicists, even non-religious ones, do not consider it equivalent to euthanasia, despite the fact that, since terminally sedated patients are not tube-fed, death always does ensue within a few days.

From a utilitarian perspective, it is hard to see that terminal sedation offers any advantages over euthanasia. Since the unconscious patient has no experiences at all, and does not recover consciousness before dying, the hedonistic utilitarian will judge terminal sedation as identical, from the point of view of the patient, to euthanasia at the moment when the patient becomes unconscious. Nor will the preference utilitarian be able to find a difference between the two states, unless the patient has, while still conscious, a preference for one rather than the other. Since additional resources are involved in caring for the terminally sedated patient, and the family is unable to begin the grieving process until death finally takes place, it seems that, other things being equal, voluntary euthanasia is better than voluntary terminal sedation.

But to return to the issue of whether better pain relief would eliminate the desire for euthanasia, there is again an obvious solution: ensure that candidates for euthanasia see a palliative care specialist. If every patient then ceases to ask for euthanasia, both proponents and opponents of voluntary euthanasia will be pleased. But that seems unlikely. Some patients who want euthanasia are not in pain at all. They want to die because they are weak, constantly tired, nauseous, or breathless. Or perhaps they just find the whole process of slowly wasting away undignified. These are reasonable grounds for wanting to die.

It is curious that those who argue against voluntary euthanasia on the grounds that terminally ill patients are often depressed, or have not received good palliative care, do not also argue against the right of terminally ill patients to refuse life-sustaining treatment or to receive pain relief that is liable to shorten life. Generally, they go out of their way to stress that they do not wish to interfere with the rights of patients to refuse life-sustaining treatment or to receive pain relief that is liable to shorten life. But the patients who make these decisions are also terminally ill, and are making choices that will, or may, end their lives earlier than they would have ended if the patient had chosen differently. To support the right of patients to make these decisions, but deny they should be allowed to choose physician-assisted suicide or voluntary euthanasia, is to assume that a patient can rationally refuse treatment (and that doctors ought, other things being equal, to co-operate with this decision) but that the patient cannot rationally choose voluntary euthanasia. This is implausible. There is no reason to believe that patients refusing life-sustaining treatment or receiving pain relief that will foreseeably shorten their lives, are less likely to be depressed, or clouded by medication, or receiving poor treatment for their pain, than patients who choose physician-assisted suicide or voluntary euthanasia. The question is whether a patient can rationally choose an earlier death over a later one (and whether doctors ought to co-operate with these kinds of end-of-life decisions), and that choice is made in either case. If patients can rationally opt for an earlier death by refusing life-supporting treatment or by accepting life-shortening palliative care, they must also be rational enough to opt for an earlier death by physician-assisted suicide or voluntary euthanasia.

The Slippery Slope Argument

Undoubtedly the most widely invoked secular argument against the legalisation of voluntary euthanasia is the slippery slope argument that legalising physician-assisted suicide or voluntary euthanasia will lead to vulnerable patients being pressured into consenting to physician-assisted suicide or voluntary euthanasia when they do not really want it. Or perhaps, as another version of the argument goes, they will simply be killed without their consent because they are a nuisance to their families, or because their healthcare provider wants to save money.

What evidence is there to support or oppose the slippery slope argument when applied to voluntary euthanasia? A decade ago, this argument was largely speculative. Now, however, we can draw on evidence from two jurisdictions where for several years it has been possible for doctors to practice voluntary euthanasia or physician-assisted suicide without fear of prosecution. These jurisdictions are Oregon and the Netherlands. According to Oregon officials, between 1997, when a law permitting physician-assisted suicide took effect, and 2001, 141 lethal prescriptions were issued, according to state records, and 91 patients used their prescriptions to end their lives. There are about 30 000 deaths in Oregon annually. There have been no reports of the law being used to coerce patients to commit suicide against their will, and from all the evidence that is available, this does not appear to be a situation in which the law is being abused.

Opponents of voluntary euthanasia do contend, on the other hand, that the open practice of voluntary euthanasia in the Netherlands has led to abuse. In the early days of non-prosecution of doctors who carried out voluntary euthanasia, before full legalisation, a government-initiated study known as the Remmelink Report indicated that physicians occasionally – in roughly 1000 cases a year, or about 0.8% of all deaths – terminated the lives of their patients without their consent. This was, almost invariably, when the patients were very close to death and no longer capable of giving consent. Nevertheless, the report gave some grounds for concern. What it did not, and could not, have shown, however, is that the introduction of voluntary euthanasia has *led to* abuse. To show this one would need *either* two studies of the Netherlands, made some years apart and showing an increase in unjustified killings, *or* a comparison between the Netherlands and a similar country in which doctors practising voluntary euthanasia are liable to be prosecuted.

Such studies have become available since the publication of the Remmelink report. First, there was a second Dutch survey, carried out five years after the original one. It did not show any significant increase in the amount of non-voluntary euthanasia happening in the Netherlands, and thus dispelled fears that that country was sliding down a slippery slope.[1]

In addition, studies have been carried out in Australia and in Belgium to discover whether there was more abuse in the Netherlands than in other comparable countries where euthanasia was illegal and could not be practised openly. The Australian study used English translations of the survey questions in the Dutch studies to ask doctors about decisions involving both direct euthanasia and foregoing medical treatment (for example, withholding antibiotics or withdrawing artificial ventilation).[2] Its findings suggest that while the rate of active voluntary euthanasia in Australia is slightly lower than that shown in the most recent Dutch study (1.8% as against 2.3%), the rate of explicit *non*-voluntary euthanasia in Australia is, at 3.5%, much higher than the Dutch rate of 0.8%. Rates of other end-of-life decisions, such as withdrawing life-support or giving pain relief that was foreseen to be life shortening, were also higher than in the Netherlands.

The Belgian study, which examined deaths in the country's northern, Flemish-speaking region, came to broadly similar conclusions. The rate of voluntary euthanasia was, at 1.3% of all deaths, again lower than in the Netharlands, but the proportion of patients given a lethal injection without having requested it was, at 3% of all deaths, similar to the Australian rate and like it, much higher than the rate in the Netherlands. The authors of the Belgian study, reflecting on their own findings and those of the Australian and Dutch study, concluded:

> Perhaps less attention is given to the requirements of careful end-of-life practice in a society with a restrictive approach than in one with an open approach that tolerates and regulates euthanasia and PAS (Physician Assisted Suicide).[3]

These two studies discredit assertions that the open practice of active voluntary euthanasia in the Netherlands had led to an increase in non-voluntary euthanasia. There is no evidence to support the claim that laws against physician-assisted suicide or voluntary euthanasia prevent harm to vulnerable people. It is equally possible that legalising physician-assisted suicide or voluntary euthanasia will bring the issue out into the open, and thus make it easier to scrutinise what is actually happening, and to prevent harm to the vulnerable. If the burden of proof lies on those who defend a law that restricts individual liberty, then in the case of laws against physician-assisted suicide or voluntary euthanasia, that burden has not been discharged.

Conclusion

The utilitarian case for allowing patients to choose euthanasia, under specified conditions and safeguards, is strong. The slippery slope argument attempts to combat this case on utilitarian grounds. The outcomes of the open practice of voluntary euthanasia in the Netherlands, and of physician-assisted suicide in Oregon, do not, however, support the idea that allowing patients to choose euthanasia or physician-assisted suicide leads to a slippery slope. Hence it seems that, on utilitarian grounds, the legalisation of voluntary euthanasia or physician-assisted suicide would be a desirable reform.

Notes

1. P.J. van der Maas, G. van der Wall, et al. "Euthanasia, Physician-Assisted Suicide, and other Medical Practices Involving the End of Life in the Netherlands, 1990–1995," *New England Journal of Medicine*, 335 (1996): 1699–1705.
2. Helga Kuhse, Peter Singer, Maurice Richard, Malcolm Clark, and Peter Baume, "End-of-Life Decisions in Australian Medical Practice," *Medical Journal of Australia* 166 (1997): 191–96.
3. L. Deliens, E. Mortier, et al., "End of Life Decisions in Medical Practice in Flanders, Belgium: A Nationwide Survey," *The Lancet* 356 (2000): 1806–11; see also: http://europe.cnn.com/2000/WORLD/europe/11/24/brussels.euthanasia

End of Life

The Buddhist View

DAMIEN KEOWN

The Lancet 366 (2005): 952–55.

In many Asian cultures, Buddhism is acknowledged as the religion that has most to say about death and the afterlife. Buddhist teachings emphasise the ubiquity and inevitability of death, and for this reason. Buddhists tend to be psychologically prepared to accept impending death with calmness and dignity.

Buddhism imposes few special requirements on patients or physicians, and there is no reason why the terminal care of Buddhist patients should pose any specific problems. The only exception would be that if the patient is a monk or nun, it would not be appropriate for them to be on a mixed ward, and preferable for them to be treated by a physician of the same sex. Attitudes in this respect vary with the age and cultural background of patients, but nowadays there is increasing acceptance of treatment by physicians and nurses of the opposite sex, especially where medical resources are limited.

Buddhism is a flexible and moderate religion that has little time for rigid formalities. Concepts of taboo and religious purity have little, if any, part to play and religious law imposes no special requirements or limitations on medical treatment. There are no special hygiene, purification, or dietary requirements (many Buddhists are vegetarians but not all). Cremation is the most common way of disposing of the dead.

In practice, local custom will have a greater bearing on the physician-patient relationship than Buddhist doctrine. It is difficult to generalise about local customs, but provided the conventions of normal medical etiquette are respected, there is no reason why difficulties should arise. This is particularly so in the case of the many people from the developed world who have converted to Buddhism and who are unlikely to have any problems with the conventions of modern medical practice.

One point to note is that mindfulness and mental clarity are important values for Buddhists, hence the importance placed on meditation. Buddhism emphasises the importance of death with an unclouded mind wherever possible, because it is believed that this can lead to a better rebirth. Some Buddhists may therefore be unwilling to take pain-relieving drugs or strong sedatives, and even those who are not in a terminal condition might prefer to remain as alert as possible, rather than take analgesics that would impair their mental or sensory capacities.

Buddhist Values

In Buddhism, there is no central authority competent to pronounce on matters of doctrine or ethics, nor is there a college or other body of Buddhist medical practitioners that exists to provide guidelines or codes of conduct for the health-care professional. Instead, individuals must follow their consciences, which should be informed by reflection on scriptural teachings, custom and tradition, and the opinions of distinguished teachers. Despite the absence of central authority, there are fundamental moral values and principles that virtually all schools of Buddhism accept. Chief among these are compassion and respect for life, which underpin the Buddhist approach to medical ethics and have a considerable bearing on end-of-life issues.

Euthanasia

Euthanasia is the intentional causing of the death of a patient by act or omission in the context of medical care. Here, we are concerned only with voluntary euthanasia, which is when a mentally competent patient freely requests medical help in ending his life. No terms are synonymous with euthanasia in early Buddhist sources, nor is the morality of the practice discussed in a systematic way. However, given that monks were active as medical practitioners, circumstances occasionally arose when the value of life was called into question. These circumstances are outlined in certain case histories preserved in the Monastic Rule (*Vinaya*), a corpus of canonical literature whose main purpose is to lay down the regulations governing monastic life.

The cases relevant to euthanasia are recounted under the rubric of the precept against the destruction of human life (the third parajika; one of the four most serious offences in the monastic code that are punished by lifetime expulsion from the monastic community). In the 60 or so cases reported under this rubric, about a third are concerned with deaths that took place following medical intervention of one kind or another by monks. In some of these instances, the death of a patient was thought desirable for quality of life considerations, such as the avoidance of protracted terminal care or to minimise the suffering of patients with serious disabilities.

The Buddha included this precept in the monastic code to prohibit conduct of this kind on discovering that several monks had either killed themselves or asked others to kill them after developing disgust for their bodies, an attitude not unknown in ascetic traditions. After some monks convinced a patient that death was a better option for him than life, the Buddha expanded the definition of the precept to include incitement to death:

> Should any monk intentionally deprive a human being of life, or look about for a knife-bringer [to help him end his life], or eulogise death, or incite [anyone] to death saying 'My good man,

what need have you of this evil, difficult life? Death would be better for you than life,'—or who should deliberately and purposefully in various ways eulogise death or incite [anyone] to death: he is also one who is defeated [in the religious life], he is not in communion.

Vinaya, volume 3, p. 72[1]

This amplification of the scope of the precept is particularly important in the context of euthanasia, since the weight of the case for allowing euthanasia rests on the postulate that death would be better than life, especially when, to quote the precept, life seems "evil and difficult". The prohibition on taking life would therefore seem to extend to both the assistance of suicide (including physician-assisted suicide) and euthanasia.

Compassion

However, as noted earlier, compassion is also an important Buddhist moral value. This is particularly so when linked to the concept of the Bodhisattva, a Buddhist saint distinguished by self-sacrificing compassion for others. Some sources reveal an increasing awareness of how a commitment to the alleviation of suffering can create conflict with the principle of the inviolability of life. Compassion, for example, might lead a person to take life in order to alleviate suffering, and is one of the main grounds on which euthanasia is commonly advocated.

The question of mercy killing arises in the Monastic Rule, in the first of the cases to be reported after the precept against killing was declared.[1] In this case, the motive for bringing about the death of the patient is stated to have been compassion (karuna) for the suffering of a dying monk. According to the influential fifth-century commentator Buddhaghosa, those found guilty in this situation took no direct action to terminate life, but merely suggested to a dying monk that death would be preferable to his present condition.[2]

Despite this apparently benevolent motive—ie, to spare a dying person unnecessary pain—the judgment of the Buddha was that those involved

were guilty of a breach of the precept. What had they done wrong? In Buddhaghosa's analysis, the essence of their wrongdoing was that they "made death their aim" (marana-atthika). It would therefore appear immoral, from a Buddhist perspective, to embark on any course of action whose aim is to destroy human life, irrespective of the quality of the individual's motive. We may therefore conclude that while compassion is always a morally good motive, it does not by itself justify whatever is done in its name.

Must Life Be Preserved at All Costs?

Does the foregoing mean that Buddhism teaches that life must be preserved at all costs? At one point in his commentary, Buddhaghosa has a brief but interesting discussion about the situation of terminally ill patients, in which two contrasting scenarios are mentioned:

> If one who is sick ceases to take food with the intention of dying when medicine and nursing care are at hand, he commits a minor offence (dukkata). But in the case of a patient who has suffered a long time with a serious illness the nursing monks may become weary and turn away in despair thinking 'when will we ever cure him of this illness?' Here it is legitimate to decline food and medical care if the patient sees that the monks are worn out and his life cannot be prolonged even with intensive care.
>
> *Samantapasadika*, volume 2, p 467[2]

The contrast in Buddhaghosa's discussion appears to be between the person who rejects medical care with the express purpose of ending his life, and the person who resigns himself to the inevitability of death after treatment has failed and the medical resources have been exhausted. The moral distinction is that the first patient seeks death or "makes death his aim", to use Buddhaghosa's phrase, whereas the second simply accepts the inevitability and proximity of death and rejects further treatment or nourishment as pointless. The first patient wishes to die; the second wishes to live. However, the second patient is resigned to the fact that he is beyond medical help.

This example suggests that Buddhism does not believe there is a moral obligation to preserve life at all costs. Recognising the inevitability of death, of course, is a central element in Buddhist teachings. Death cannot be postponed forever, and Buddhists are encouraged to be mindful and prepared for the evil hour when it comes. To seek to prolong life beyond its natural span by recourse to increasingly elaborate technology when no cure or recovery is in sight is a denial of the reality of human mortality, and would be seen by Buddhism as arising from delusion (moha) and excessive attachment (tanha).

In terminal care, and in cases where persistent vegetative states have been conclusively diagnosed, there is no need to go to extreme lengths to provide treatment if there is little or no prospect of recovery. Thus, there would be no requirement to treat subsequent complications—eg, pneumonia or other infections—by administering antibiotics. Although an untreated infection might be seen to lead to the patient's death, it would also be recognised that any course of treatment that is contemplated must be assessed against the background of the prognosis for overall recovery. Rather than embarking on a series of piecemeal treatments, none of which would produce a net improvement in the patient's overall condition, it would often be appropriate to reach the conclusion that the patient was beyond medical help, and allow events to take their course. In such cases, it is justifiable to refuse or withdraw treatment that is either futile or too burdensome in light of the overall prognosis for recovery.

Conclusion

The care of Buddhist patients in the end-of-life phase should pose few special problems for the physician. Buddhism teaches that death is an integral part of life, and by virtue of their belief in rebirth, Buddhists believe that death is an experience they will undergo many times. The paradigm example of meeting death is that of the Buddha, who died in a serene and mindful state aged 80 years. However, the definition of death is problematic, and physicians should not assume that the criterion of brain death will be accepted by all Buddhists. Japanese patients, in particular, are likely to reject it, along with the practice of cadaver transplants (transplants from living donors should not pose a problem). Nutrition and hydration should presumptively be continued for patients in persistent vegetative states, but there is no requirement to treat secondary complications.

Euthanasia is rejected by most Buddhists as contrary to the First Precept, which prohibits intentional killing. This applies even when motivated by a compassionate desire to relieve suffering. However, in this respect, Buddhism adheres to the principle of the middle way (majjhima patipada), and the prohibition on euthanasia does not imply a commitment to vitalism, namely the doctrine that life should be prolonged at all costs. The withdrawal of medical intervention when the end is nigh is accordingly not seen as immoral.

Notes

1. H. Oldenberg, ed., *The Vinaya Pitakam*, translated by I. B. Horner (Oxford: Pali Text Society, 1964). *The Book of the Discipline* (Oxford: Pali Text Society, 1992).
2. J. Takakusu and M. Nagai, eds., *Samantapasadika* (Oxford: Pali Text Society, 1975).

Gender, Feminism, and Death

Physician-Assisted Suicide and Euthanasia

SUSAN M. WOLF

From *Feminism and Bioethics: Beyond Reproduction*, edited by Susan M. Wolf.
(New York: Oxford University Press, 1996), 282–317.

The debate in the United States over whether to legitimate physician-assisted suicide and active euthanasia has reached new levels of intensity.

Yet the debate over whether to legitimate physician-assisted suicide and euthanasia (by which I mean active euthanasia, as opposed to the termination of life-sustaining treatment) is most often about a patient who does not exist—a patient with no gender, race, or insurance status. This is the same generic patient featured in most bioethics debates. Little discussion has focused on how differences between patients might alter the equation.

Even though the debate has largely ignored this question, there is ample reason to suspect that gender, among other factors, deserves analysis. The cases prominent in the American debate mostly feature women patients. This occurs against a backdrop of a long history of cultural images revering women's sacrifice and self-sacrifice. Moreover, dimensions of health status and health care that may affect a patient's vulnerability to considering physician-assisted suicide and euthanasia—including depression, poor pain relief, and difficulty obtaining good health care—differentially plague women. And suicide patterns themselves show a strong gender effect: women less often complete suicide, but more often attempt it. These and other factors raise the question of whether the dynamics surrounding physician-assisted suicide and euthanasia may vary by gender.

Indeed, it would be surprising if gender had no influence. Women in America still live in a society marred by sexism, a society that particularly disvalues women with illness, disability, or merely advanced age. It would be hard to explain if health care, suicide, and fundamental dimensions of American society showed marked differences by gender, but gender suddenly dropped out of the equation when people became desperate enough to seek a physician's help in ending their lives.

Gender in Cases, Images, and Practice

The tremendous upsurge in American debate over whether to legitimate physician-assisted suicide and euthanasia in recent years has been fueled by a series of cases featuring women. The case that seems to have begun this series is that of Debbie, published in 1988 by the *Journal of the American Medical Association* (*JAMA*).

The narrator of the piece tells us that Debbie is a young woman suffering from ovarian cancer. The resident has no prior relationship with her, but is called to her bedside late one night while on call and exhausted. Entering Debbie's room, the resident finds an older woman with her, but never pauses to find out who that second woman is and what relational context Debbie acts within. Instead, the resident responds to the patient's clear discomfort and to her words. Debbie says only one sentence, "Let's get this over with." It is unclear whether she thinks the resident is there to draw blood and wants that over with, or means something else. But on the strength of that one sentence, the resident retreats to the nursing station, prepares a lethal injection, returns to the room, and administers it. The story relates this as an act of mercy under the title "It's Over, Debbie," as if in caring response to the patient's words.

The lack of relationship to the patient; the failure to attend to her own history, relationships, and resources; the failure to explore beyond the patient's presented words and engage her in conversation; the sense that the cancer diagnosis plus the patient's words demand death; and the construal of that response as an act of mercy are all themes that recur in the later cases. The equally infamous Dr. Jack Kevorkian has provided a slew of them.

They begin with Janet Adkins, a 54-year-old Oregon woman diagnosed with Alzheimer's disease. Again, on the basis of almost no relationship with Ms. Adkins, on the basis of a diagnosis by exclusion that Kevorkian could not verify, prompted by a professed desire to die that is a predictable stage in response to a number of dire diagnoses, Kevorkian rigs her up to his "Mercitron" machine in a parking lot outside Detroit in what he presents as an act of mercy.

Then there is Marjorie Wantz, a 58-year-old woman without even a diagnosis. Instead, she has pelvic pain whose source remains undetermined. By the time Kevorkian reaches Ms. Wantz, he is making little pretense of focusing on her needs in the context of a therapeutic relationship. Instead, he tells the press that he is determined to create a new medical specialty of "obitiatry."

The subsequent cases reiterate the basic themes. And it is not until the ninth "patient" that Kevorkian finally presides over the death of a man. By this time, published criticism of the predominance of women had begun to appear.

Kevorkian's actions might be dismissed as the bizarre behavior of one man. But the public and press response has been enormous, attesting to the power of these accounts. Many people have treated these cases as important to the debate over physician-assisted suicide and euthanasia. Nor are Kevorkian's cases so aberrant—they pick up all the themes that emerge in "Debbie."

But we cannot proceed without analysis of Diane. This is the respectable version of what Kevorkian makes strange. I refer to the story published by Dr. Timothy Quill in the *New England Journal of Medicine*, recounting his assisting the suicide of his patient Diane.[1] She is a woman in her forties diagnosed with leukemia, who seeks and obtains from Dr. Quill a prescription for

drugs to take her life. Dr. Quill cures some of the problems with the prior cases. He does have a real relationship with her, he knows her history, and he obtains a psychiatric consult on her mental state. He is a caring, empathetic person. Yet once again we are left wondering about the broader context of Diane's life—why even the history of other problems that Quill describes has so drastically depleted her resources to deal with this one, and whether there were any alternatives. And we are once again left wondering about the physician's role—why he responded to her as he did, what self-scrutiny he brought to bear on his own urge to comply, and how he reconciled this with the arguments that physicians who are moved to so respond should nonetheless resist.

This collection of early cases involving women cries out for analysis. It cannot be taken as significant evidence predicting that more women may die through physician-assisted suicide and euthanasia; these individual cases are no substitute for systematic data. But to understand what they suggest about the role of gender, we need to place them in context.

The images in these cases have a cultural lineage. We could trace a long history of portrayals of women as victims of sacrifice and self-sacrifice. In Greek tragedy, that ancient source of still reverberating images, "suicide . . . [is] a woman's solution." Almost no men die in this way. Specifically, suicide is a wife's solution; it is one of the few acts of autonomy open to her. Wives use suicide in these tragedies often to join their husbands in death. Men, in contrast, die by the sword or spear in battle.[2]

The connection between societal gender roles and modes of death persists through history. "By the mid-nineteenth century characterizations of women's suicides meshed with the ideology described by Barbara Welter as that of 'True Womanhood . . . .' Adherence to the virtues of 'piety, purity, submissiveness and domesticity' translated into the belief that 'a "fallen woman" was a "fallen angel." . . .[3] Even after statistics emerged showing that women completed suicide less often than men, the explanations offered centered on women's supposedly greater willingness to suffer misfortune, their lack of courage, and less arduous social role.

Given this history of images and the valorization of women's self-sacrifice, it should come as no surprise that the early cases dominating the debate about self-sacrifice through physician-assisted suicide and euthanasia have been cases of women. In Greek tragedy only women were candidates for sacrifice and self-sacrifice, and to this day self-sacrifice is usually regarded as a feminine not masculine virtue.

This lineage has implications. It means that even while we debate physician-assisted suicide and euthanasia rationally, we may be animated by unacknowledged images that give the practices a certain gendered logic and felt correctness. In some deep way it makes sense to us to see these women dying, it seems right. It fits an old piece into a familiar, ancient puzzle. Moreover, these acts seem good; they are born of virtue. We may not recognize that the virtues in question—female sacrifice and self-sacrifice—are ones now widely questioned and deliberately rejected. Instead, our subconscious may harken back to older forms, reembracing those ancient virtues, and thus lauding these women's deaths.

Analyzing the early cases against the background of this history also suggests hidden gender dynamics to be discovered by attending to the facts found in the accounts of these cases, or more properly the facts not found. What is most important in these accounts is what is left out, how truncated they are. We see a failure to attend to the patient's context, a readiness on the part of these physicians to facilitate death, a seeming lack of concern over why these women turn to these doctors for deliverance. A clue about why we should be concerned about each of these omissions is telegraphed by data from exit polls on the day Californians defeated a referendum measure to legalize active euthanasia. Those polls showed support for the measure lowest among women, older people, Asians, and African Americans, and highest among younger

men with postgraduate education and incomes over $75,000 per year. The *New York Times* analysis was that people from more vulnerable groups were more worried about allowing physicians actively to take life. This may suggest concern not only that physicians may be too ready to take their lives, but also that these patients may be markedly vulnerable to seeking such relief. Why would women, in particular, feel this?

Women are at greater risk for inadequate pain relief. Indeed, fear of pain is one of the reasons most frequently cited by Americans for supporting legislation to legalize euthanasia. Women are also at greater risk for depression. And depression appears to underlie numerous requests for physician-assisted suicide and euthanasia. These factors suggest that women may be differentially driven to consider requesting both practices.

That possibility is further supported by data showing systematic problems for women in relationship to physicians. As an American Medical Association report on gender disparities recounts, women receive more care even for the same illness, but the care is generally worse. Women are less likely to receive dialysis, kidney transplants, cardiac catheterization, and diagnostic testing for lung cancer. The report urges physicians to uproot "social or cultural biases that could affect medical care" and "presumptions about the relative worth of certain social roles."[4]

This all occurs against the background of a deeply flawed health care system that ties health insurance to employment. Men are differentially represented in the ranks of those with private health insurance, women in the ranks of the others—those either on government entitlement programs or uninsured. In the U.S. two-tier health care system, men dominate in the higher-quality tier, women in the lower.

Moreover, women are differentially represented among the ranks of the poor. Many may feel they lack the resources to cope with disability and disease. To cope with Alzheimer's, breast cancer, multiple sclerosis, ALS, and a host of other diseases takes resources. It takes not only the financial resource of health insurance, but also access to stable working relationships with clinicians expert in these conditions, in the psychological issues involved, and in palliative care and pain relief. It may take access to home care, eventually residential care, and rehabilitation services. These are services often hard to get even for those with adequate resources, and almost impossible for those without. And who are those without in this country? Disproportionately they are women, people of color, the elderly, and children.

Women may also be driven to consider physician-assisted suicide or euthanasia out of fear of otherwise burdening their families. The dynamic at work in a family in which an ill member chooses suicide or active euthanasia is worrisome. This worry should increase when it is a woman who seeks to "avoid being a burden," or otherwise solve the problem she feels she poses, by opting for her own sacrifice. The history and persistence of family patterns in this country in which women are expected to adopt self-sacrificing behavior for the sake of the family may pave the way too for the patient's request for death. Women requesting death may also be sometimes seeking something other than death. The dominance of women among those attempting but not completing suicide in this country suggests that women may differentially engage in death-seeking behavior with a goal other than death. Instead, they may be seeking to change their relationships or circumstances.

What I am suggesting is that there are issues relating to gender left out of the accounts of the early prominent cases of physician-assisted suicide and euthanasia or left unexplored that may well be driving or limiting the choices of these women. I am not suggesting that we should denigrate these choices or regard them as irrational. Rather, it is the opposite—that we should assume these decisions to be rational and grounded in a context. That forces us to attend to the background failures in that context.

Important analogies are offered by domestic violence. Such violence has been increasingly recognized as a widespread problem. It presents some structural similarities to physician-assisted suicide and especially active euthanasia. All three can be fatal. All three are typically acts performed behind closed doors. In the United States, all three are illegal in most jurisdictions, though the record of law enforcement on each is extremely inconsistent. Though men may be the victims and women the perpetrators of all three, in the case of domestic violence there are some conceptions of traditional values and virtues that endorse the notion that a husband may beat his wife. As I have suggested above, there are similarly traditional conceptions of feminine self-sacrifice that might bless a physician's assisting a woman's suicide or performing euthanasia.

Clearly, there are limits to the analogy. But my point is that questions of choice and consent have been raised in the analysis of domestic violence against women, much as they have in the case of physician-assisted suicide and active euthanasia. If a woman chooses to remain in a battering relationship, do we regard that as a choice to be respected and reason not to intervene? While choosing to remain is not consent to battery, what if a woman says that she "deserves" to be beaten—do we take that as reason to condone the battering? The answers that have been developed to these questions are instructive, because they combine respect for the rationality of women's choices with a refusal to go the further step of excusing the batterer. We appreciate now that a woman hesitating to leave a battering relationship may have ample and rational reasons: well-grounded fear for her safety and that of her children, a justified expectation of economic distress, and warranted concern that the legal system will not effectively come to her aid. We further see mental health professionals now uncovering some of the deeper reasons why some women might say at some point they "deserve" violence. Taking all of these insights seriously has led to development of a host of new legal, psychotherapeutic, and other interventions meant to address the actual experiences and concerns that might lead women to "choose" to stay in a violent relationship or "choose" violence against them. Yet none of this condones the choice of the partner to batter or, worse yet, kill the woman. Indeed, the victim's consent, we should recall, is no legal defense to murder.

All of this should suggest that in analyzing why women may request physician-assisted suicide and euthanasia, and why indeed the California polls indicate that women may feel more vulnerable to and wary of making that request, we have insights to bring to bear from other realms. Those insights render suspect an analysis that merely asserts women are choosing physician-assisted suicide and active euthanasia, without asking why they make that choice. The analogy to other forms of violence against women behind closed doors demands that we ask why the woman is there, what features of her context brought her there, and why she may feel there is no better place to be. Finally, the analogy counsels us that the patient's consent does not resolve the question of whether the physician acts properly in deliberately taking her life through physician-assisted suicide or active euthanasia. The two people are separate moral and legal agents.

This leads us from consideration of why women patients may feel vulnerable to these practices, to the question of whether physicians may be vulnerable to regarding women's requests for physician-assisted suicide and euthanasia somewhat differently from men's. There may indeed be gender-linked reasons for physicians in this country to say "yes" to women seeking assistance in suicide or active euthanasia. In assessing whether the patient's life has become "meaningless," or a "burden," or otherwise what some might regard as suitable for extinguishing at her request, it would be remarkable if the physician's background views did not come into play on what makes a woman's life meaningful or how much of a burden on her family is too much.

Second, there is a dynamic many have written about operating between the powerful expert physician and the woman surrendering to his care. It is no accident that bioethics has focused on the problem of physician paternalism. Instead of an egalitarianism or what Susan Sherwin calls "amicalism," we see a vertically hierarchical arrangement built on domination and subordination. When the patient is female and the doctor male, as is true in most medical encounters, the problem is likely to be exacerbated by the background realities and history of male dominance and female subjugation in the broader society.

This brief examination of the vulnerability of women patients and their physicians to collaboration on actively ending the woman's life in a way reflecting gender roles suggests the need to examine the woman's context and where her request for death comes from, the physician's context and where his accession comes from, and the relationship between the two. We need to do that in a way that uses rather than ignores all we know about the issues plaguing the relations between women and men, especially suffering women and powerful expert men. The question, then, is whether we want to bless deaths driven by those dynamics.

All of this suggests that physician-assisted suicide and euthanasia, as well as the debate about them, may be gendered. I have shown ways in which this may be true even if women do not die in greater numbers.

Feminism and the Arguments

Shifting from the images and stories that animate debate and the dynamics operating in practice to analysis of the arguments over physician-assisted suicide and euthanasia takes us further into the concerns of feminist theory. Arguments in favor of these practices have often depended on rights claims. More recently, some authors have grounded their arguments instead on ethical concepts of caring. Yet both argumentative strategies have been flawed in ways that feminist work can illuminate. What is missing is an analysis that integrates notions of physician caring with principled boundaries to physician action, while also attending to the patient's broader context and the community's wider concerns. Such an analysis would pay careful attention to the dangers posed by these practices to the historically most vulnerable populations, including women.

Such a rights approach raises a number of problems that feminist theory has illuminated. In particular, feminist critiques suggest three different sorts of problems with the rights equation offered to justify physician-assisted suicide and euthanasia. First, it ignores context, both the patient's present context and her history. The prior and surrounding failures in her intimate relationships, in her resources to cope with illness and pain, and even in the adequacy of care being offered by the very same physician fade into invisibility next to the bright light of a rights bearer and her demand. In fact, her choices may be severely constrained. Some of those constraints may even be alterable or removable. Yet attention to those dimensions of decision is discouraged by the absolutism of the equation: either she is an eligible rights bearer or not; either she has asserted her right or not. There is no room for conceding her competence and request, yet querying whether under all the circumstances her choices are so constrained and alternatives so unexplored that acceding to the request may not be the proper course. Stark examples are provided by cases in which pain or symptomatic discomfort drives a person to request assisted suicide or euthanasia, yet the pain or discomfort are treatable. In circumstances in which women and others who have traditionally lacked resources and experienced oppression are likely to have fewer options and a tougher time getting good care, mechanical application of the rights equation will authorize their deaths even when less drastic alternatives are or should be available. It will wrongly assume that all face serious illness and disability with the resources of the idealized rights bearer—a person of means untroubled by oppression. The realities of women and others whose circumstances are far from that abstraction's will be ignored.

Second, in ignoring context and relationship, the rights equation extols the vision of a rights bearer as an isolated monad and deni-grates actual dependencies. Thus it may be seen as improper to ask what family, social, economic, and medical supports she is or is not getting; this insults her individual self-governance. Nor may it be seen as proper to investigate alternatives to acceding to her request for death; this too dilutes self-rule. Yet feminists have reminded us of the actual embeddedness of persons and the descriptive falseness of a vision of each as an isolated individual. In addition, they have argued normatively that a society comprised of isolated individuals, without the pervasive connections and dependencies that we see, would be undesirable. Indeed, the very meaning of the patient's request for death is socially constructed; that is the point of the prior section's review of the images animating the debate. If we construe the patient's request as a rights bearer's assertion of a right and deem that sufficient grounds on which the physician may proceed, it is because we choose to regard background failures as irrelevant even if they are differentially motivating the requests of the most vulnerable. We thereby avoid real scrutiny of the social arrangements, governmental failures, and health coverage exclusions that may underlie these requests. We also ignore the fact that these patients may be seeking improved circumstances more than death. We elect a myopia that makes the patient's request and death seem proper. We construct a story that clothes the patient's terrible despair in the glorious mantle of "rights."

In fact, there are substantial problems with grounding advocacy for the specific practices of physician-assisted suicide and euthanasia in a rights analysis, even if one accepts the general importance of rights and self-determination. I have elsewhere argued repeatedly for an absolute or near-absolute moral and legal right to be free of unwanted life-sustaining treatment. Yet the negative right to be free of unwanted bodily invasion does not imply an affirmative right to obtain bodily invasion (or assistance with bodily invasion) for the purpose of ending your own life.

Moreover, the former right is clearly grounded in fundamental entitlements to liberty, bodily privacy, and freedom from unconsented touching; in contrast there is no clear "right" to kill yourself or be killed. Suicide has been widely decriminalized, but decriminalizing an act does not mean that you have a positive right to do it and to command the help of others. Indeed, if a friend were to tell me that she wished to kill herself, I would not be lauded for giving her the tools. In fact, that act of assistance has *not* been decriminalized. That continued condemnation shows that whatever my friend's relation to the act of suicide (a "liberty," "right," or neither), it does not create a right in her sufficient to command or even permit my aid.

Finally, the rights argument in favor of physician-assisted suicide and euthanasia confuses two separate questions: what the patient may do, and what the physician may do. After all, the real question in these debates is not what patients may request or even do. It is not at all infrequent for patients to talk about suicide and request assurance that the physician will help or actively bring on death when the patient wants; that is an expected part of reaction to serious disease and discomfort. The real question is what the doctor may do in response to this predictable occurrence. That question is not answered by talk of what patients may ask; patients may and should be encouraged to reveal everything on their minds. Nor is it answered by the fact that decriminalization of suicide permits the patient to take her own life. The physician and patient are separate moral agents. Those who assert that what a patient may say or do determines the same for the physician, ignore the physician's separate moral and legal agency. They also ignore the fact that she is a professional, bound to act in keeping with a professional role and obligations. They thereby avoid a necessary argument over whether the historic obligations of the physician to "do no harm" and "give no deadly drug even if asked" should be abandoned. Assertion of what the patient may do does not resolve that argument.

The inadequacy of rights arguments to legitimate physician-assisted suicide and euthanasia has led to a different approach, grounded on physicians' duties of beneficence. This might seem to be quite in keeping with feminists' development of an ethics of care. Yet the beneficence argument in the euthanasia context is a strange one, because it asserts that the physician's obligation to relieve suffering permits or even commands her to annihilate the person who is experiencing the suffering. Indeed, at the end of this act of beneficence, no patient is left to experience its supposed benefits. Moreover, this argument ignores widespread agreement that fears of patient addiction in these cases should be discarded, physicians may sedate to unconsciousness, and the principle of double effect permits giving pain relief and palliative care in doses that risk inducing respiratory depression and thereby hastening death. Given all of that, it is far from clear what patients remain in the category of those whose pain or discomfort can only be relieved by killing them.

What does feminism have to offer these debates? Feminists too have struggled extensively with the question of method, with how to integrate detailed attention to individual cases with rights, justice, and principles. Thus in criticizing Kohlberg and going beyond his vision of moral development, Carol Gilligan argued that human beings should be able to utilize both an ethics of justice and an ethics of care. What was less clear was precisely how the two should fit together. And unfortunately for our purposes, Gilligan never took up Kohlberg's mercy killing case to illuminate a care perspective or even more importantly, how the two perspectives might properly be interwoven in that case.

That finally, I would suggest, is the question. Here we must look to those feminist scholars who have struggled directly with how the two perspectives might fit. Lawrence Blum has distinguished eight different positions that one might take, and that scholars have taken, on "the relation between impartial morality and a morality of care:"[5] (1) acting on care is just acting on complicated moral principles; (2) care is not moral but personal; (3) care is moral but secondary to principle and generally adds mere refinements or supererogatory opportunities; (4) principle supplies a superior basis for moral action by ensuring consistency; (5) care morality concerns evaluation of persons while principles concern evaluation of acts; (6) principles set outer boundaries within which care can operate; (7) the preferability of a care perspective in some circumstances must be justified by reasoning from principles; and (8) care and justice must be integrated. Many others have struggled with the relationship between the two perspectives as well.

Despite this complexity, the core insight is forth rightly stated by Owen Flanagan and Kathryn Jackson: "[T]he most defensible specification of the moral domain will include issues of both right and good."[6] Martha Minow and Elizabeth Spelman go further. Exploring the axis of abstraction versus context, they argue against dichotomizing the two and in favor of recognizing their "constant interactions."[7]

Here we find the beginning of an answer to our dilemma. It appears that we must attend to both context and abstraction, peering through the lenses of both care and justice. Yet our approach to each will be affected by its mate. Our apprehension and understanding of context or cases inevitably involves categories, while our categories and principles should be refined over time to apply to some contexts and not others. Similarly, our understanding of what caring requires in a particular case will grow in part from our understanding of what sort of case this is and what limits principles set to our expressions of caring; while our principles should be scrutinized and amended according to their impact on real lives, especially the lives of those historically excluded from the process of generating principles.

This last point is crucial and a distinctive feminist contribution to the debate over abstraction versus context, or in bioethics, principles versus cases. Various voices in the bioethics debate over method—be they advocating casuistry, specified principlism, principlism itself, or some other position—present various solutions to the question of how cases and principles or other higher-order abstractions should interconnect. Feminist writers too have substantive solutions to offer, as I have suggested. But feminists also urge something that the mainstream writers on bioethics method have overlooked altogether, namely, the need to use cases and context to reveal the systematic biases such as sexism and racism built into the principles or other abstractions themselves. Those biases will rarely be explicit in a principle. Instead, we will frequently have to look at how the principle operates in actual cases, what it presupposes (such as wealth or life options), and what it ignores (such as preexisting sexism or racism among the very health care professionals meant to apply it).

What, then, does all of this counsel in application to the debate over physician-assisted suicide and euthanasia? This debate cannot demand a choice between abstract rules or principles and physician caring. Although the debate has sometimes been framed that way, it is difficult to imagine a practice of medicine founded on one to the exclusion of the other. Few would deny that physician beneficence and caring for the individual patient are essential. Indeed, they are constitutive parts of the practice of medicine as it has come to us through the centuries and aims to function today. Yet that caring cannot be unbounded. A physician cannot be free to do whatever caring for or empathy with the patient seems to urge in the moment. Physicians practice a profession with standards and limits, in the context of a democratic polity that itself imposes further limits. These considerations have led the few who have begun to explore an ethics of care for physicians to argue that the notion of care in that context must be carefully delimited and distinct from the more general caring of a parent for a child (although there are limits, too, on what a caring parent may do). Physicians must pursue what I will call "principled caring."

This notion of principled caring captures the need for limits and standards, whether technically stated as principles or some other form of generalization. Those principles or generalizations will articulate limits and obligations in a provisional way, subject to reconsideration and possible amendment in light of actual cases. Both individual cases and patterns of cases may specifically reveal that generalizations we have embraced are infected by sexism or other bias, either as those generalizations are formulated or as they function in the world. Indeed, given that both medicine and bioethics are cultural practices in a society riddled by such bias and that we have only begun to look carefully for such bias in our bioethical principles and practices, we should expect to find it.

Against this background, arguments for physician-assisted suicide and euthanasia—whether grounded on rights or beneficence—are automatically suspect when they fail to attend to the vulnerability of women and other groups. If our cases, cultural images, and perhaps practice differentially feature the deaths of women, we cannot ignore that. It is one thing to argue for these practices for the patient who is not so vulnerable, the wealthy white male living on Park Avenue in Manhattan who wants to add yet another means of control to his arsenal. It is quite another to suggest that the woman of color with no health care coverage or continuous physician relationship, who is given a dire diagnosis in the city hospital's emergency room, needs then to be offered direct killing.

To institute physician-assisted suicide and euthanasia at this point in this country—in which many millions are denied the resources to cope with serious illness, in which pain relief and palliative care are by all accounts woefully mishandled, and in which we have a long way to go to make proclaimed rights to refuse life-sustaining treatment and to use advance direc-

tives working realities in clinical settings—seems, at the very least, to be premature. Were we actually to fix those other problems, we have no idea what demand would remain for these more drastic practices and in what category of patients. We know, for example, that the remaining category is likely to include very few, if any, patients in pain, once inappropriate fears of addiction, reluctance to sedate to unconsciousness, and confusion over the principle of double effect are overcome.

Yet against those background conditions, legitimating the practices is more than just premature. It is a danger to women. Those background conditions pose special problems for them. Women in this country are differentially poorer, more likely to be either uninsured or on government entitlement programs, more likely to be alone in their old age, and more susceptible to depression. Those facts alone would spell danger. But when you combine them with the long (indeed, ancient) history of legitimating the sacrifice and self-sacrifice of women, the danger intensifies. That history suggests that a woman requesting assisted suicide or euthanasia is likely to be seen as doing the "right" thing. She will fit into unspoken cultural stereotypes. She may even be valorized for appropriate feminine self-sacrificing behavior, such as sparing her family further burden or the sight of an unaesthetic deterioration. Thus she may be subtly encouraged to seek death. At the least, her physician may have a difficult time seeing past the legitimating stereotypes and valorization to explore what is really going on with this particular patient, why she is so desperate, and what can be done about it.

The required interweaving of principles and caring, combined with attention to the heightened vulnerability of women and others, suggests that the right answer to the debate over legitimating these practices is at least "not yet" in this grossly imperfect society and perhaps a flat "no." Beneficence and caring indeed impose positive duties upon physicians, especially with patients who are suffering, despairing, or in pain. Physicians must work with these patients intensively; provide first-rate pain relief, palliative care, and symptomatic relief; and honor patients' exercise of their rights to refuse life-sustaining treatment and use advance directives. Never should the patient's illness, deterioration, or despair occasion physician abandonment. Whatever concerns the patient has should be heard and explored, including thoughts of suicide, or requests for aid or euthanasia.

Such requests should redouble the physician's efforts, prompt consultation with those more expert in pain relief or supportive care, suggest exploration of the details of the patient's circumstance, and a host of other efforts. What such requests should not do is prompt our collective legitimation of the physician's saying "yes" and actively taking the patient's life. The mandates of caring fail to bless killing the person for whom one cares. Any such practice in the United States will inevitably reflect enormous background inequities and persisting societal biases. And there are special reasons to expect gender bias to play a role.

We cannot ignore that such practice would allow what for now remains an elite and predominantly male profession to take the lives of the "other." We cannot explain how we will train the young physician both to care for the patient through difficult straits and to kill. We cannot protect the most vulnerable.

Notes

1. See Timothy E. Quill, "Death and Dignity—A Case of Individualized Decision Making," *New England Journal of Medicine* 324 (1991): 691–94.
2. Nicole Loraux, *Tragic Ways of Killing a Woman*, Anthony Forster, trans. (Cambridge, MA: Harvard University Press, 1987), 11.
3. Howard I. Kushner, "Women and Suicidal Behavior: Epidemiology, Gender, and Lethality in Historical Perspective," in Silvia Sara Canetto and David Lester, eds., *Women and Suicidal Behavior* (New York: Springer, 1995), 195, citing Barbara Welter, "The Cult of True Womanhood: 1820–1860," *American Quarterly* 18 (1960): 151–55.
4. Council on Ethical and Judicial Affairs, American Medical Association, "Gender Disparities in Clinical Decision Making," *Journal of the American Medical Association* 266 (1991): 559–62, 561–62.
5. See Lawrence A. Blum, "Gilligan and Kohlberg: Implications for Moral Theory," *Ethics* 98 (1988): 477.
6. Owen Flanagan and Kathryn Jackson, "Justice, Care, and Gender: The Kohlberg-Gilligan Debate Revisited," in Larrabee, ed., *An Ethic of Care*, 69–84, 71.
7. Martha Minow and Elizabeth V. Spelman, "In Context," *Southern California Law Review* 63 (1990): 1597–652, 1625.

A Moral Defense of Oregon's Physician-Assisted Suicide Law

MICHAEL B. GILL

Mortality 10, no. 1 (2005): 53–67.

Introduction

Since 1998, physician-assisted suicide (PAS) has been legal in the state of Oregon. If an Oregon resident has less than six months to live and is mentally competent, she can request that a physician prescribe her drugs that will cause a quick and painless death.

Most of the objections to the Oregon law fall into one of three categories. In the first category is the claim that it is intrinsically wrong for someone to kill herself. In the second category is the claim that it is intrinsically wrong for physicians to assist someone in killing herself. In the third category is the claim that legalizing PAS will lead to very bad consequences for the sick, the elderly and other vulnerable elements of our population.

In this article, I address the first and second categories of objections. In the first part of the article, I try to show that it is not intrinsically wrong for someone with a terminal disease to kill herself. In the second part, I try to show that it is not intrinsically wrong for physicians to assist someone with a terminal disease who has reasonable grounds for wanting to kill herself.

I do not discuss the consequentialist arguments that occupy the third category of objections to the Oregon law. These consequentialist arguments are important, and they need to be addressed. But they fall outside my current purview.

Why It Is Not Intrinsically Wrong for a Terminal Patient to Commit Suicide

Arguments Against the Autonomy-Based Justification for Allowing Suicide

Leon Kass has provided one of the most influential statements of the belief that someone using the Oregon law to kill herself is doing something intrinsically wrong. Kass uses the concept of tragedy to frame his opposition. Something is tragic, Kass tells us, if it is necessarily self-contradictory. "In tragedy the failure is imbedded in the hero's success, the defeats in his victories, the miseries in his glory" (2002a). Kass claims that many of the recent developments in health care are tragic in the way that he defines it, or necessarily self-contradictory. PAS under the Oregon law is one of his prime examples. PAS, Kass argues, inevitably destroys the thing of value that it is intended to promote.

The value the Oregon law is intended to promote is the autonomy of human beings. In the following, I say more about how we ought to conceive of what is valuable about autonomy, but for now we can think of it simply as a person's ability to make decisions for herself, to decide for herself what will happen to her own body. According to its proponents, the Oregon law promotes autonomy because it expands the range of decisions a person can make. When PAS is legal, a person has the choice of deciding whether or not to end her life by taking a pill. But when PAS is illegal, a person does not have that choice. And a state of affairs that gives a person more choices is, from the standpoint of trying to promote autonomy, better than a state of affairs that offers a person fewer choices.

According to Kass, however, this way of thinking is tragically simplistic, shallow and short-sighted. For in fact the legalization of PAS does not promote autonomy but encourages its destruction. Far from giving people more choices, PAS brings about a state of affairs in which a person has lost the ability to make choices altogether. For the person who engages in PAS will, obviously, be dead, and someone who is dead can no longer exercise her autonomy. It is thus *self-contradictory* to argue for PAS by claiming that it promotes autonomy, as PAS destroys a person's ability to make decisions. As Kass puts it, there can be "no ground at all" for claiming that "autonomy licenses an act that puts our autonomy permanently out of business" (2002a).

Opponents of PAS often color in this charge of self-contradiction by contending that the autonomy-based justification of PAS leads to obvious absurdities. One such absurdity is the legalization of a certain kind of slavery. It is illegal to sell yourself into slavery. Even if you want to contract with someone to become her slave, you are not allowed to do so. The contract would be null and void. According to PAS opponents, however, the autonomy-based justification of PAS implies that forbidding someone from selling herself into slavery restricts her range of self-determining choices, and that as a result we should give everyone the option of deciding whether or not to become a slave. So the autonomy-based justification of PAS implies that we should legalize self-slavery contracts. But the idea of legalizing slavery of any kind is absurd. And so, PAS opponents conclude, the autonomy-based justification of PAS is fundamentally flawed.

Another absurdity PAS opponents try to foist on the attempted justification of the Oregon law is the legalization of PAS for people who are healthy and non-terminal. Oregon's law allows PAS only for people who have six months or less to live. But the autonomy-based justification of PAS implies that we ought to expand the range of self-regarding decisions every competent individual can make. The autonomy-based justification implies, then, that we should give even healthy and non-terminal people the option of deciding whether or not to commit suicide. But, opponents of PAS argue, the idea of legalizing PAS for healthy and non-terminal people is absurd. So we have, once again, a clear reason to reject the autonomy-based justification for PAS.

Defense of the Oregon Law's Autonomy-Based Justification for Allowing Suicide

Proponents of PAS can respond to these criticisms of their autonomy-based justification in one of two ways. First, they can take the hard-line libertarian route, which consists of biting the bullet and embracing the implications that PAS opponents say are absurd. Hard-line libertarian supporters of PAS will agree that their justification of PAS implies that we should legalize self-slavery and assisted suicide for healthy, non-terminal individuals, but then go on to argue that people *should* be allowed to sell themselves into slavery if they freely choose to do so, and that healthy, non-terminal individuals should be allowed to seek assisted suicide. According to this hard-line libertarian approach, everyone really should be given the legal option to make whatever self-regarding decisions she wants. Whether we think a decision is moral or immoral is legally irrelevant. As long as no one else is harmed, the moral status of a person's justificatory principles is none of the law's business. So even if we come to believe that there is some kind of "self-contradiction" involved in a person's choosing to undertake some course of action, that would not justify using the law to prevent a person from undertaking that course of action, so long as no other person is hurt. This hard-line libertarian position has an internal consistency that shields it from any quick and simple refutation.

The reason the Oregon law conflicts with the hard-line libertarian position is that it does not allow healthy, non-terminal individuals to choose PAS. And this feature of the Oregon law points towards the second way in which one can try to defend the autonomy-based justification of PAS against the charge of self-contradiction. Those proposing this second kind of defense will agree that self-slavery and assisted suicide for healthy, non-terminal individuals ought to remain illegal, but then go on to argue that their autonomy-based justification of the Oregon law does not imply that those other things ought to be legal. They will argue, rather, that there is a clear and morally significant difference between what the Oregon law provides for, on the one hand, and self-slavery and assisted suicide for healthy, non-terminal individuals, on the other.

The Oregon law has provisions to ensure that the people who engage in PAS are competent, and that their decision to commit suicide is a result of autonomous decision making. But, crucially, it also has provisions to ensure that the people who engage in PAS have terminal illnesses. Specifically, the Oregon law allows a person to receive lethal drugs only if two doctors have verified that she has six months or less to live. And what defenders of the Oregon law can argue is that the suicide of a person who is about to die does not violate the value of autonomy because the person's decision-making ability is going to disappear whether she commits suicide or not. The person with a terminal disease who decides to commit suicide is not changing the universe from a place in which she would have been able to exercise her autonomy in the future into a place in which she will not be able to exercise her autonomy in the future. For she will not be able to exercise her autonomy in the future no matter what she does. Hers is not a decision to prevent herself from being able to make future decisions, because future decisions will not be hers to make regardless. The ending of her decision-making ability is a foregone conclusion. She is simply choosing that it end in one way rather than another.

This autonomy-based defense of the Oregon law gains strength through a consideration of how the final stages of a terminal disease can corrode a person's autonomous nature. Progressive bodily deterioration can limit and ultimately eliminate one's ability to undertake physical action, and mental deterioration can limit and ultimately eliminate one's ability to make any kind of decision at all. In the end, one may be barely conscious and maintained by machines, bereft of the autonomous nature that gives human beings dignity and inestimable moral worth. It is this lingering half-life that persons who use the Oregon law may seek to prevent. And such a decision does not necessarily contradict the value of autonomy because during such a half-life autonomy does not exist anyway. Indeed, defenders of the Oregon law can argue that the decision to commit suicide in the final stages of a terminal illness can proceed from a great respect for autonomy, as such a decision can reveal that what a person values about herself is not simply her physical existence but the ability to decide what happens to her.

The fact that the Oregon law allows only terminal patients to commit suicide also gives PAS proponents the conceptual resources for repelling the absurd consequences PAS opponents try to foist on them. Someone who makes herself into a slave or commits suicide while healthy is throwing away the capacity for self-determination. If she does not make herself a slave or commit suicide, she will be able to make her own decisions for years to come; but if she does either of those things, she will not be able to make her own future decisions. But a person who is about to die is not going to be able to make decisions for years to come, whether she commits suicide or not. She is not throwing away her ability to determine her future because that ability no longer exists. So the autonomy-based justification of assisted suicide for terminal individuals is completely compatible with the prohibitions on self-slavery and assisted suicide for healthy, non-terminal individuals. PAS proponents can consistently condemn actions that destroy the ability to make future decisions, because the suicide of a terminal individual is not a case of such destruction.

Autonomy as the Ability to Make "Big Decisions"

Many ethical discussions that invoke the value of autonomy equate autonomy with the ability to make one's own decisions. To this point, I too have accepted this equation. But if we want to be clear about what the value of autonomy in end-of-life issues really involves, we need to draw a distinction between the kinds of decisions a person may make. The distinction I want to draw is between what I will call "big decisions" and "little decisions."

Big decisions are decisions that shape your destiny and determine the course of your life. Big decisions call on you to make a choice in light of things that matter most to you, in light of the things that give your life whatever meaning it has. Big decisions proceed from your deepest values. Little decisions, by contrast, concern matters that are momentary or insignificant. They do not proceed from your deepest values, but draw only on preferences that rest on the surface of your character. Big decisions are momentous, in that making one big decision rather than another will change in some non-negligible way the course of your life. But little decisions don't matter that much. Regardless of whether you make one little decision or another, your life will continue in much the same way. Little decisions don't shape your destiny. So an example of a big decision would be deciding to get married, while an example of a little decision would be deciding to eat the blue jello instead of the red jello.[1]

I maintain that to respect autonomy is, first and foremost, to respect a person's ability to make big decisions. It is to respect a person's ability to determine her own fate, to shape her own life. The capacity to make little decisions matters less. That's not to say that the freedom to make little decisions doesn't matter at all. We should let people make as many of the little decisions that affect them as is possible. But it is the ability to make big decisions that is of inestimable value. That is where the great moral weight of the value of autonomy lies.

A person who meets the Oregon law's criteria of competence and terminality will probably have the capacity to make little decisions for weeks or months to come. She will, that is, probably be able to continue to make decisions about many of the details of her daily routine. But she may very well not have the same ability to make big decisions. Her ability to determine her own destiny, to shape her own life, may be all but gone. There are two reasons for this. First, the limited amount of time a person with a terminal disease has left to live eliminates many of the options that constitute big decision making. Long-range planning of a life is impossible when the life will end in a few months. Second, the nature of many terminal diseases can preclude big decision making in a manner that is distinct

even from the amount of time a person has left to live. Terminal diseases can consume the mind as well as the body. And all too often, the only decisions a person ends up making at the end-stage are those that concern pain management and the most basic of bodily functions. The kinds of concerns that involve big decision making, the kind that call on one's deepest values and create the opportunity to shape a life, are crowded out by the immediacy of disease.

There is, however, one big decision a person who meets Oregon's criteria will still be able to make, one choice about her destiny that will still be open to her. She can still decide how and when to die. She can still choose the shape of the end of her life, the concluding words of her final chapter. This may, in fact, be the only big decision that her limited time left affords her. Thus, giving a person with a terminal disease the option of PAS can promote the thing of value that we have in mind when we talk of respect of autonomy. For the option of PAS can enhance such a person's ability to make a big decision for herself. When, by contrast, we make it more difficult for a person with a terminal disease to commit suicide, we restrict her ability to make a big decision. And this restriction cannot be justified by claiming that we are respecting her autonomy, unless what we mean by autonomy is simply the capacity to make little decisions for a few more weeks or months. For besides the choice of how she wants her life to end, ever littler decisions may be all that such a person has any prospect of making.

Once again, then, we can see the clear difference between PAS for people with terminal diseases, on the one hand, and the suicide of healthy people, on the other. A typical healthy person possesses the ability to make big decisions in the future. Such a person, typically, can control her own destiny and shape her own life for years to come. So by killing herself, a healthy person does violate what is most important about autonomy: she has before her the choice between a future in which she can make big decisions and a future in which she cannot make big decisions, and she opts for the latter. But a person with a terminal disease may not be able to make big decisions in the future, no matter what decision she makes now. So it is not necessarily the case that a person with a terminal disease will be choosing between a future in which she can make big decisions and a future in which she cannot make big decisions. It may be the case, rather, that such a person's ability to make big decisions will be nonexistent in all the futures between which she must choose.

The difference between PAS for people with diseases and self-slavery is even more clear and instructive. A slave may very well be able to make numerous little decisions throughout her life. She may be in control of the details of fulfilling her basic bodily needs, and she could have some degree of choice about how to go about completing her assigned tasks. But even if a slave possesses the capacity to make little decisions, we will still believe that her slavery violates autonomy in a fundamental way. And that is because the slave lacks the ability to make big decisions. She lacks the ability to control her own destiny, to shape her own life. It is the ability to make big decisions that is of profound moral importance. The fact that the slave may be able to make little decisions is, by comparison, morally insignificant. It is the ability to make big decisions that ought not to be tossed away. But a person with a terminal disease who chooses PAS will not necessarily be tossing away her ability to make big decisions; she may, rather, be exercising it in the only way she can. For the ability of such a person to make big decisions may already be all but gone, the only big decision left to her being that of deciding how her life will end.

Opponents of PAS may object that I have underestimated the extent to which a person with a terminal disease can be able to make big decisions. They may argue that even a person whose physical abilities are severely limited and who will die within a few months may still be able to do many things to affect the shape of her life. Such a person may, for instance, use the time she has left to change her will or to make vital arrangements for the care of her loved ones. She may reconcile with people from whom she has

long been estranged. Through the experience of suffering and dying, she may learn profound truths about herself and the human condition. She may forge a new relationship with God. All of these things are of the utmost importance to the shape of a life. None of them is little or insignificant. But by availing herself of PAS, a person destroys her ability to do any of these things.

In response to this objection, let me say first of all that it is true that *some* people may have profound, life-changing experiences at the very end of life. The very end of life may be the time when *some* people achieve a new awareness or forge new relationships that cast all their previous years in an entirely different light. What is crucial to realize, however, is that this may not be true for *all* people. There may also be people who have settled all their worldly and spiritual affairs a month or two before they are expected to die. Some people may have no need to make financial arrangements or pursue any sort of interpersonal reconciliation in the final months of life because they may already have done all the work on their wills and their relationships that they believe they need to do. Some people may not need to experience any more suffering and dying because they may believe that they have learned all the lessons about themselves and the human condition that they are ever going to learn. Some people may have already achieved exactly the relationship with God to which they aspire. So while PAS may be the wrong thing for *some* people, it is not necessarily the wrong thing for *all* people. Proponents of the Oregon law do not claim, of course, that everyone with a terminal disease should commit suicide. They claim, rather, that because suicide may be right for some people, it should be an option. It should be available to all people who are terminal and competent to make their own decisions.

Opponents of PAS seem to believe, however, that it is wrong for *anyone* with a terminal disease to commit suicide. They seem to believe that there are morally significant reasons against suicide in every situation, that everyone should live for as long as she can so that she can learn for herself, and teach others, profound lessons about the meaning of life. Thus, Kass maintains that "what humanity needs most" are people who "continue to live and work and love as much as they can for as long as they can," and that such people are worthy of admiration in a way that suicides are not (2002b). And Callahan implies that people who live for as long as they can in the face of suffering and a lack of control are more "noble and heroic" than those who choose suicide, that the former fulfill the "duty to bear suffering as a form of mutual human support" in a way that the latter do not.

But some people may believe that the very end of their lives will *not* produce any profound and meaningful insights, for them or anyone else, into "the point or purpose or end of human existence." And this belief of theirs may follow from their own fundamental values. It may proceed from their own deepest views of what is profound and meaningful about life. To respect autonomy is to promote their ability to act on these fundamental values. Suicide may be an unreasonable end to the lives of some people with terminal diseases. But it may not be an unreasonable end for the lives of others. And everyone should be allowed to decide for herself whether she is the first sort of person or the second. It is a big decision, deciding what sort of ending is for you the fundamentally right one, maybe one of the biggest decisions of all. That is why everyone whose end is imminent should be allowed to make it for herself.

Why It Is Not Intrinsically Wrong for a Physician to Participate in PAS

Physicians and the Decision of Whether Life Is Worth Living

Let us now turn to the second objection to PAS as it occurs under the Oregon law. This objection is based on the role of a physician. Even if it is in some cases morally acceptable for a person to commit suicide, PAS opponents maintain, it still will always be wrong for a physician to assist her. Those who defend PAS "misunderstand the moral foundations of medical practice," failing to appreciate that medicine "is intrinsically a moral profession, with *its own* immanent principles and standards of conduct that set limits on what physicians may properly do" (Kass, 2002b).

Opponents of the Oregon law contend that, in requesting PAS, a person is asking her physician to make a decision that is inappropriate for a physician to make. This is because a physician who must decide whether to assist in a person's suicide is forced to make a judgment about moral and spiritual matters that have nothing to do with medicine. Thus Kass contends that to comply with a request for PAS, "the physician must, willy-nilly, play the part of judge, and his judgments will be decidedly nonmedical and nonprofessional, based on personal standards" (2002b). And Pellegrino maintains that in prescribing a lethal dose a physician is making the non-medical judgment that her patient's "life is unworthy of living." Callahan makes the same point when he writes, "The purpose of medicine is not to relieve all the problems of human mortality, the most central and difficult of which is why we have to die at all or die in ways that seem pointless to us... This is not the role of medicine because it has no competence to manage the meaning of life and death, only the physical and psychological manifestations of those problems. Medicine's role must be limited to what it can appropriately do, and it has neither the expertise nor the wisdom necessary to respond to the deepest and oldest human questions."

This criticism seems to me to miss entirely the provisions of the Oregon law. For the Oregon law makes very clear the role physicians are to play in requests for PAS. It says that physicians are to determine if the patient requesting PAS has a terminal disease and if the patient is competent. These are both medical judgments. In order to make them, a physician does not need to make any judgments about "fundamental philosophical and religious matters" pertaining to the meaning of life. The physician is not asked to decide for the patient whether or not life is worth living. The patient makes that decision for herself. Indeed, it is Kass, Pellegrino and Callahan who would take the decision about whether life is worth living out of the hands of the patient. For they are the ones who contend that suicide is always the morally inferior option. It is their view that passes a substantive "philosophical and religious" judgment on how one should cope with terminal disease. The Oregon law, by contrast, asks physicians to make two medical judgments, and then (if the patient meets the relevant criteria) to assist the patient in doing whatever the patient herself has decided about how best to cope with suffering and loss of control at the end of life.

Of course, there may be some physicians who are personally morally opposed to all forms of suicide (just as there are some physicians who are personally morally opposed to abortion), and such physicians should have the option of refusing to participate in any requests for PAS. But there may also be some physicians who believe that an individual should be allowed to make up her own mind about how she wants her life to end, and those physicians' participation in requests for PAS will consist entirely of their making medical judgments about individuals' mental competence and life expectancy, and then facilitating the patient's own decision.

The Duty to Promote Health and the Duty to Reduce Suffering

Kass, Pellegrino and Callahan go on to argue, however, that so long as the physician is knowingly involved in a process that leads to suicide, she is doing something wrong. For, according to Kass, Pellegrino and Callahan, to participate in such a process is to violate the essential moral duty of the medical profession: it is to violate the medical duty to promote health.

Kass, Pellegrino and Callahan are certainly correct in saying that physicians have a moral duty to promote health. But there is an obvious problem with claiming that trying to make patients healthy is a physician's *only* moral duty. The problem is that people with terminal diseases cannot be made healthy. A physician cannot heal someone whose disease is lethal and untreatable. So if trying to make patients healthy were their *only* duty, physicians would have no role to play in the care of

dying patients. It is clear, however, that physicians do have a role to play in the care of the dying. No one advocates that physicians are obligated by their professional ethic to abandon their patients upon making a terminal diagnosis. On the contrary, it is well recognized that physicians have especially pressing obligations to such patients' care.

In caring for dying patients, one of a physician's principal roles is to reduce suffering. When healing is no longer possible, the reduction of suffering takes center stage.

This duty to reduce the suffering of dying patients is limited in at least one crucial respect. If the dying patient is competent, then physicians should reduce her suffering only in ways to which the patient consents. This limitation on the duty to reduce suffering also applies to the physician's duty to promote health. It is just as wrong for a physician to try to cure a competent patient by undertaking a course of action to which the patient does not agree as it is for a physician to try to reduce the suffering of a competent patient by undertaking a course of action to which the patient does not agree.

Kass, Pellegrino and Callahan acknowledge this role of the physician. They agree that a physician has a moral duty to help to reduce the suffering of a patient with a terminal disease. I presume they would also agree with the limitation on the duty to reduce pain that I have described—that is, that they would agree that physicians should undertake courses of action to reduce the suffering of competent patients with terminal diseases only if the patients have consented to those courses of action. But Kass, Pellegrino and Callahan place another limitation on this duty as well. They argue that a physician's duty to reduce the suffering of patients with terminal diseases can never include assistance in suicide.

Kass argues that the second limitation on the duty to reduce suffering is warranted because it is impossible to benefit a patient by helping to bring about her death. Thus, the idea that we can make a patient better off by helping to kill must be morally incoherent. As Kass puts it, " 'Better off dead' is logical nonsense—unless, of course, death is not death indeed but instead a gateway to a new and better life beyond. Despite loose talk to the contrary, it is in fact impossible to compare the goodness or badness of one's existence with the goodness or badness of one's 'nonexistence', because it nonsensically requires treating 'nonexistence' as a condition one is nonetheless able to experience and enjoy . . . [T]o intend and to act for someone's good requires that person's continued existence for the benefit to be received . . . This must be the starting point in discussing all medical benefits: no benefit without a beneficiary" (2002b).

Kass claims, then, that it is logically impossible and morally incoherent to try to justify assisted suicide by saying that a person may be better off dead than alive. And perhaps there is some peculiarly literal reading of the words "person" and "better off" that makes Kass's claim true. But there is nothing at all incoherent about a person's preferring a state of affairs in which she is dead to a state of affairs in which she is alive. Throughout human history, many people have believed death is preferable to life under intolerable conditions. And some of the people who have acted on those preferences—people who have sacrificed their lives—have been deemed morally heroic. Even if we refrain from saying that these people are "better off" dead, we can still make perfect sense of the idea that they had morally impeccable reasons for their actions. But what of others who assisted those who sacrificed their lives? What should we say about those who have helped another person undertake a course of action that leads to her death? Again, we might refrain from saying that these others made the person who sacrificed her life "better off." But that does not mean that what those others did is morally incoherent. If a person has morally impeccable reasons to sacrifice her life, then a person who helps her may have reasons that are equally morally impeccable. Just as assisting someone in carrying out the ultimate sacrifice can be morally coherent, so too may helping a dying patient carry out suicide be morally coherent. The fact that the person will not be able to "experience and enjoy" the results of this course of action does not vitiate any attempted justification to help her.

The Principle of Double Effect

The idea that physicians must always place morally conclusive value on life itself fits well with Kass, Pellegrino and Callahan's suggestion that all people ought "to live . . . for as long as they can." But this devotion to life seems *not* to fit with a practice that is common to the medical profession today—the practice of participating in the withdrawal of life-sustaining treatment, including food and water, which Kass, Pellegrino and Callahan all explicitly endorse. A physician who participates in the withdrawal of life-sustaining treatment undertakes a course of action that does not promote life itself. Such a physician is participating in a course of action that will lead to less life rather than more. So how do Kass, Pellegrino and Callahan justify physician participation in the withdrawal of life-sustaining treatment without committing themselves to the justifiability of assisted suicide? How do they fit the withdrawal of life-sustaining treatment into their conception of the moral role of physicians while at the same time keeping PAS out? They do so by deploying the principle of double effect.

So the argument that the Oregon law conflicts with physicians' moral duty presupposes the principle of double effect. Indeed, the principle of double effects seems to be doing more work in this argument than the duty to heal or promote life. For Kass, Pellegrino and Callahan's endorsement of the withdrawal of life-sustaining treatment shows that they accept physician participation in courses of action that are intended neither to heal nor to promote life, which seems to imply (in contrast to some of their other comments) that they do not take the duty to heal or promote life to be always applicable to medical practice.

Now the principle of double effect is a general moral principle. It is not unique to the world of medical ethics. This is worth noting because opponents of the Oregon law sometimes contend that their arguments against PAS are based on the special moral status of physicians. Callahan, for instance, often relies on claims about the "purpose of medicine" or "medicine's role" and Kass maintains that his "argument rests on understanding the special moral character of the medical profession and the ethical obligations it entails" (2002b). If a person really understands the intrinsic moral character of medicine, opponents of the Oregon law suggest, she will never accept PAS. We now find, however, that their arguments against PAS depend on the principle of double effect. And a defense of that principle cannot be grounded in the "special moral character of the medical profession." The anti-PAS position is based, in other words, not on the unique moral role of medicine but on a contentious non-medical moral principle.

This raises the question of whether there are in fact decisive grounds for accepting the principle of double effect. I myself think that the principle is extremely problematic. It relies on the drawing of a very sharp distinction between, on the one hand, the intentions and goals of all the physicians who engage in terminal sedation or withdraw food and water and, on the other hand, the intentions and goals of all the physicians who would prescribe a lethal dose of drugs. It seems to me, however, that there is no principled way of distinguishing the morally relevant features of the intentions and goals of these two groups of physicians, no non-question-begging reason to think that there is some feature of the actions of all those who would prescribe lethal doses that is inconsistent with the practice of medicine but is also absent from the actions of all those who engage in terminal sedation or withdraw food and water. Unfortunately, an extensive treatment of the principle of double effect is beyond the scope of this article. Note, however, that even if the principle is generally defensible, that on its own will not vindicate Kass, Pellegrino and Callahan's argument against the Oregon law. For not all defensible moral principles ought to be enforced by law. Some moral questions are so difficult, profound or personal that the law rightly allows each person the opportunity to answer them for herself. If reasonable people can disagree about the soundness of a moral principle, the best public policy might be one that is neutral between a person's living in accord with it or not. And it seems that the principle of double effect is something with which reasonable people can disagree.

Kass's claim that the principle of double effect is a "well-established rule of medical ethics" does not help to make the case. For not all medical ethicists or physicians agree that the essential moral duty of physicians implies that the principle of double effect should be used to forbid PAS. Miller, Brody and Quill, for instance, have argued that assisting in suicide can be entirely consistent with the integrity of the medical profession.

But the greatest weakness of the attempt to use the principle of double effect to defeat the Oregon law is that the principle will imply the wrongness of PAS only on the assumption that it is bad that a person with a terminal disease die sooner rather than later. The only business the principle of double effect is in is telling us when it is permissible to perform an action that has foreseeable bad consequences and when it is impermissible. If an action's consequences are not bad, the principle is completely inapplicable. Now the opponents of PAS believe that it is bad if a terminal patient dies sooner rather than later, and it is on the basis of the badness of such a death that they deploy the principle of double effect. But many proponents of PAS disagree, holding that in certain circumstances it is not bad if a terminal patient dies sooner rather than later. Of course, there is a great deal of dispute about which side is correct—about whether it is necessarily bad that a terminal patient dies sooner rather than later (this was one of the topics of the first part of this article). But unless that issue is resolved in their favor, opponents of PAS cannot use the principle of double effect to argue against the Oregon law.

The final point I want to make about the principle of double effect is that it cannot be used to bolster another significant criticism of PAS that Kass, Pellegrino and Callahan present. This other criticism is that although it may seem as though the Oregon law leaves the decision of whether or not to request PAS entirely up to the patient, in fact the law leads her physician to make that decision for her. In theory, the Oregon law restricts the physician's role simply to medical judgments. But in practice (according to Kass, Pellegrino and Callahan's criticism), the physician's own values will pressure the patient into whatever decision finally gets made. The patient's thinking will be "easily and subtly manipulated" by the physician. The physician will exercise "subtle coercion" that will undermine "the patient autonomy that assisted suicide and euthanasia presume to protect."

Now in claiming that the legalization of PAS will increase the chance of manipulation and coercion, Kass, Pellegrino and Callahan are making an essentially consequentialist argument. They are contending not that PAS is intrinsically morally wrong but that it will lead to morally unacceptable consequences. This consequentialist argument against PAS has to be taken very seriously. If it turns out that the Oregon law increases manipulation and coercion, then there will be at least one consequentialist but still extremely important reason to reject the law.

It seems to me, however, that the fact that physicians can ethically participate in the withdrawal of life-sustaining treatment gives us at least some reason for doubting that the legalization of PAS will necessarily lead to increased manipulation and coercion. For if allowing physicians to participate in the withdrawal of food and water does not necessarily increase manipulation and coercion, why think that allowing physicians to participate in PAS will do so? If it is possible for the option of withdrawing life-sustaining treatment to exist without an increase in manipulation and coercion, why should it not also be possible for the option of PAS to exist with an increase in manipulation and coercion?

We have seen, of course, that opponents of the Oregon law believe that there is an intrinsic moral difference between assisting in suicide and withdrawing life-support, a difference explained by the principle of double effect. But they cannot rely on that putative intrinsic difference when they are making the consequentialist argument that the Oregon law will lead physicians to manipulate and coerce patients into choosing PAS. For this consequentialist argument is based on claims about the real-world effects of the Oregon law. And we cannot determine what those effects will be simply through an examination of the morally contentious principle of double effect.

Conclusion

I have presented reasons for thinking that there is nothing intrinsically morally wrong with PAS as it is currently practiced in Oregon. In the first part of this article, I have tried to show that there are morally reasonable grounds to restrict PAS to individuals who are competent and have less than six months to live. In the second part, I have tried to show that participation in PAS does not necessarily violate physicians' professional integrity. The value of autonomy and physicians' duty to reduce the suffering of dying patients together imply that PAS can sometimes be a morally acceptable option.

Note

1. Of course this distinction is far from sharp. For one thing, the combination of all of your little decisions does affect in a non-negligible way the shape of your overall life. For another thing, there are many decisions that fall somewhere between the big and the little, decisions that are not as momentous as deciding to get married but are nonetheless more important than deciding to eat the blue jello. There is a continuum between big decisions and little ones, not an absolute cut-off. Still, some decisions are clearly closer to one end of the continuum rather than the other, and we often find it natural and easy enough to draw such a distinction.

References

Callahan, D. "Reason, Self-Determination, and Physician-Assisted Suicide." In *The Case Against Assisted Suicide*. edited by K. Foley and H. Hendin. Baltimore, MD: Johns Hopkins University Press, 2002.

Kass, L. *Life, Liberty and the Defense of Dignity*. San Francisco: Encounter Books, 2002a.

——"'I Will Give No Deadly Drug': Why Doctors Must Not Kill." In *The Case Against Assisted Suicide*, edited by K. Foley and H. Hendin. Baltimore, MD: Johns Hopkins University Press, 2002b.

Miller, F. G., and H. Brody "Professional Integrity and Physician-Assisted Death." *Hastings Center Report* 25 (1995): 8–17.

Pellegrino, E. "Compassion Is Not Enough." In *The Case Against Assisted Suicide*, edited by K. Foley and H. Hendin. Baltimore, MD: Johns Hopkins University Press, 2002.

Quill, T. E. "Death and Dignity: A Case of Individualized Decision Making." *New England Journal of Medicine* 324 (1991): 691–94.

——, R. Dresser, and D. W. Brock. "The Rule of Double Effect—A Critique of Its Role in End-of-Life Decision Making." *New England Journal of Medicine*, 337 (1997): 1768–71.

Sade, R. M., and M. F. Marshall. "Legistrothanatry: A New Specialty for Assisting in Death." *Perspectives in Biology and Medicine*, 39 (1996): 222–24.

CASES

Not Dead Yet—Part I

Fifteen-year-old Teresa Hamilton slipped into a diabetic coma at Sarasota (Florida) Memorial Hospital, and within days doctors declared her to be brain dead. Teresa's parents, however, refused to accept the diagnosis, insisting that she was still alive. They declined to give the hospital permission to discontinue treatment, and insisted that they be allowed to bring Teresa home. After six weeks of contentious discussion and nearly two months after Teresa was declared brain dead, she returned home in an ambulance, still connected to a ventilator and an IV. Nurses would provide twenty-four-hour, in-home care.

According to hospital spokesman Mike Vizvary, "It's been brutal. We've been trying to do the compassionate thing and go with what the family wants, and also honor the professional judgment of the doctors involved."

It is the doctors' professional judgment that Teresa's parents rejected. Sharon and Frederick Hamilton believed that Teresa merely was in a deep coma, and in the comfortable surroundings of home she would get better. In fact, they said that Teresa would respond to requests, such as moving her leg or fluttering her eyelashes when asked. "If you love someone, you don't give up on them," said Sharon.

Dr. James Orlowski of the University Community Hospital in Tampa said that the more compassionate thing to do would have been to discontinue treatment. Instead, the parents have been confused by the hospital's actions. "We know for absolute certainty that she's brain dead and she's never going to wake up. She's really a corpse."

Two months after her negotiated release from the hospital, Teresa suffered a heart attack. Paramedics were initially able to revive her, but gave up when her heart failed again. This time, her parents believed she was dead.

Discussion Questions

1. When did Teresa die? At the hospital or at home four months later?

2. What do you think the hospital should have done in this case?

3. How would Robert Veatch's "conscience clause" apply to this case? Do you think that Teresa's parents should have the authority to decide whether she is dead?

4. How does Eric Gampel's claim that families not doctors should make medical futility judgments apply to this case?

Sources

Associated Press. "Girl on Life Support Taken Home." *St. Petersburg Times*, March 4, 1994.

——. "Teresa Hamilton, 15, in Coma Four Months." *St. Petersburg Times*, May 13, 1994.

Croft, Jay. "Parents Keep Hope Alive for Brain-dead Girl; Move Home Hasn't Helped." *New Orleans Times-Picayune*, March 18, 1994.

Not Dead Yet—Part II (or There *Is* Cryonics in Baseball)

In 2002, baseball legend Ted Williams died and his body was shipped to the Alcor Life Extension Foundation in Scottsdale, Arizona, for cryonic preservation. Alcor claims to be the world leader in cryonics, which they define as "the science of using ultra-cold temperature to preserve human life with the intent of restoring good health when technology becomes available to do so." Alcor stores its clients' heads and bodies separately, and Williams's head is in a nitrogen-filled steel can while his body is in a steel tank. The separate storage of the heads and bodies reflects Alcor's understanding of the body's incidental nature in relation to the brain.

Alcor claims that it does not engage in preserving dead tissue; its purpose is not to reverse death, but to suspend life until it can be revived. Are Alcor's patients then still alive? Legally, no; they are dead by the cardiopulmonary standard. The brain, though, retains viability for some time after the heart stops beating, and Alcor strives to preserve a viable brain for resuscitation. Alcor admits that its program will not work for anyone who is brain dead. But for those who are not, then cryonics, like baseball, does not use a clock; it takes as much time as is necessary for the game to end, and remains hopeful for a positive outcome. As Yogi Berra would say, "It ain't over 'til it's over."

While the whole process may seem ghoulish, Alcor claims the moral high ground for attempting to extend the human life span.

> The moral argument for an unfixed life span is rooted in the dignity and worth of human life. Medicine recognizes the worth of human life by seeking to treat and cure fatal disease, religion recognizes the worth of human life by praying for the sick to get better, and law recognizes the worth of human life by the illegality of murder. The operating principle in all cases is that no one should die against their will. In other words, the moral argument for an unfixed life span is the immorality of advocating the alternative: conditions in which people are forced to die by a specific time whether they are ready or not.

Alcor also claims religious support for its services, citing contemporary pastors regarding cryonics and historic Christian doctrine regarding life and death. Orthodox Christian belief, as articulated by C. S. Lewis and others, is that death is not really natural, and not originally part of God's creation. Death enters the world only after the Fall, when Adam and Eve are banished from the Garden of Eden. Extending life is not blasphemous, but rather an acknowledgment of God's original plan for humanity.

If Ted Williams is only legally dead, but not really dead, what happens to his soul while he is in storage? Alcor notes that we already have a precedent of freezing and reviving humans—we do it with embryos, which are thawed and implanted in women, resulting in live births. The souls of its patients, like those of frozen embryos, are in a state of "quiescent waiting." "If resuscitation is still possible (even with technology not immediately available) then the correct theological status is coma, not death, and the soul remains."

How much does it cost? Alcor charges a minimum fee of $150,000 for whole body preservation and a minimum $80,000 for "neuropreservation" (head only). The fee is usually paid via life insurance, although Alcor is happy to accept cash or other forms of payment.

Discussion Questions

1. Was Ted Williams dead or alive when he was shipped to Alcor's facility in Arizona?
2. What do you think Leon Kass would say about Alcor and its plan to extend human life?
3. How does your own view compare with that of Kass?

Sources

Cryonics: Alcor Life Extension Foundation. http://www.alcor.org. (accessed February 8, 2008).

"What Happened to Ted?" SI.com (August 12, 2003). http://sportsillustrated.cnn.com/baseball/news/2003/08/12/williams_si (accessed June 3, 2008).

Slow Medicine

Retirement often is considered a time to slow down, especially when people enter their eighties. But because health problems tend to increase as people get older, medicine speeds up. Dr. Dennis McCullough and some of his colleagues at Dartmouth Medical School want to put on the brakes, and encourage a new approach to caring for older patients, called "slow medicine." According to McCullough: "American medicine is best at managing acute crises and supplying specialized elective procedures, such as joint replacements, organ transplants, eye surgeries, cosmetic changes—all of them modern technological wonders. As for the more ordinary and common management and support of elders and families dealing with the chronic problems of aging and slow-moving diseases, our medical-care system has not done so well."

Many elderly patients do not fare well with "modern technological wonders," which create additional problems that require more medical attention. Even CPR for patients in their eighties and nineties rarely extends their lives for more than a month. According to McCullough, ninety percent of patients who live into their eighties will eventually be unable to care for themselves because of frailty or dementia.

Slow medicine means going "back to the future," replacing high-tech medicine with old-fashioned methods. Modern diagnostic tests should be used only rarely, and medications should begin at low dosages, increasing only gradually, if necessary. Slow medicine involves attending to chronic care and the daily needs of the patient "by offering emotional support and social stimulation, supplying better nutrition, and making sleeping, moving, bathing, dressing, and voiding easier. [It]...is not a plan for getting ready to die. It is a plan for caring, and for living well, in the time that an elder has left."

Discussion Questions

1. If a ninety-year-old patient has not indicated her preferences regarding medical treatment and is currently unable to communicate, do you think slow medicine would be in her best interests?
2. Do you think that you might choose slow medicine for yourself when you get older?
3. What do you think John Arras and Leon Kass would say about slow medicine?
4. How does your own view compare with those of Arras and Kass?

Sources

Gross, Jane. "For the Elderly, Being Heard About Life's End." *New York Times*, May 5, 2008. http://www.nytimes.com/2008/05/05/health/05slow.html (accessed May 20, 2008).

McCullough, Dennis. "Slow Medicine." *Dartmouth Medicine* 32, no. 3 (2008): 62.

Zuger, Abigail. "For the Very Old, a Dose of 'Slow Medicine.'" *New York Times*, February 26, 2008. http://www.nytimes.com/2008/02/26/health/views/26books.html (accessed June 5, 2008).

Is There Anybody in There?

Among the several points of contention in the Terri Schiavo case were Terri's medical diagnosis and prognosis. Was Terri really in a persistent vegetative state (PVS)? Was Terri, who had suffered brain damage because of oxygen deprivation, really beyond any hope of recovery? Tests showed almost no activity in Terri's brain, and, after she died, an autopsy showed that she had extensive brain damage and atrophy. The diagnosis and prognosis were confirmed.

PVS patients, unlike those in a coma, have periods of wakefulness, but show no awareness of their surroundings and make no purposeful movements. Scientist Adrian Owen has demonstrated, however, that not all PVS patients are completely without conscious awareness, and retain some cognitive ability. While there are cases of misdiagnoses, even some patients who are correctly diagnosed as PVS still retain limited conscious awareness. The criteria for diagnosing PVS apparently are incomplete.

Owen uses functional magnetic resonance imaging (fMRI) to measure neural responses to spoken sentences and requests to perform mental imagery. In one experiment, he asked a twenty-three-year-old patient, who had suffered a traumatic brain injury in a traffic accident and had been unresponsive for five months, to imagine playing tennis and to imagine visiting all of the rooms in her house. Her brain showed significant motor activity in response to the request to imagine playing tennis, and it showed activity in other areas when asked to imagine walking through her house. The responses were the same as the fMRI scans of healthy volunteers in the control group. She obviously possessed some conscious awareness, and could respond through brain activity, even if not through speech or movement.

Kate Bainbridge was Owen's first PVS patient in 1997, and he discovered similar brain activity in her case. Since then, she has made considerable progress, both mentally and physically. She has regained much of her mental functioning, and can use her arms, although she still cannot walk and has difficulty talking. Owen cautions, though, that there are limits both to his method of detection and the ability of PVS patients to recover. He estimates that the probability of recovering consciousness following traumatic brain injury is twenty percent, and far worse for patients with nontraumatic brain injury (e.g., anoxia, or loss of oxygen). Likelihood of recovery is also far worse for patients who meet the diagnostic criteria for *permanent* vegetative state—nonresponsive for twelve months after traumatic brain injury and six months for anoxic brain injury.

Discussion Questions

1. If the treatment preferences of PVS patients are unknown, what kind of treatment, if any, would be justified by the best interests standard?
2. Do PVS cases fall into Arras's "gray area"?
3. In cases that even Owen would diagnose as hopeless, but the patient nevertheless would want to be kept alive regardless of physical condition, should the patient's wishes be followed?

4. In writing your own living will, how would Owen's findings influence your instructions to others regarding your treatment should you be diagnosed with PVS?

Sources

Groopman, Jerome. "Silent Minds." *New Yorker*, October 15, 2008, 38–43.

Owen, Adrian M. "Disorders of Consciousness." *Annals of the New York Academy of Sciences* 1124 (2008): 225–38.

Owen, Adrian M., Martin R. Coleman, Melanie Boly, Matthew H. Davis, Steven Caureys, and John D. Pickard. "Detecting Awareness in the Vegetative State." *Science* 313 (2006): 1402.

A Patient's *Rights* Act? The Limits of Patient Autonomy in Israel

Israel is a democratic nation, but unlike most Western democracies, Israel ranks life above liberty and dignity. People on hunger strikes may be force-fed and terrorists will not be executed. When it comes to patients, they may be kept alive against their will. The Israel Patient's Rights Act (IPRA) of 1996 contains provisions about the right to receive health care, informed consent, privacy, and confidentiality, but it also permits physicians to forcibly treat competent patients against their will when they think that patients are making the wrong decision.

IPRA stipulates three conditions that must be met for a physician to treat a competent patient without that patient's informed consent: (1) "The patient has received information as required to make an informed choice"; (2) "The treatment is anticipated to significantly improve the patient's medical condition"; and (3) "There are reasonable grounds to suppose that, after receiving treatment, the patient will give his retroactive consent." What constitutes "significant improvement?" Israeli law states that a patient must face "grave danger" before a physician may forcibly treat a patient, meaning that the patient's life is in danger without intervention.

Discussion Questions

1. How do you think Beauchamp and Childress (from chapter 2), Varelius, and Gampel would evaluate IPRA?
2. Do you think that IPRA is ethically justifiable?
3. If IPRA had a provision regarding quality of life such that physicians may intervene only if they could preserve a high quality of life, what difference would that make in your evaluation?

Sources

Gross, Michael L. "Treating Competent Patients by Force: The Limits and Lessons of Israel's Patient's Rights Act." *Journal of Medical Ethics* 31, no. 1 (2005): 29–34.

Patient's Rights Act, 1996. http://waml.haifa.ac.il/ index/reference/legislation/israel/israel1.htm (accessed June 5, 2008).

The Texas Advance Directives Act

In 1999, Texas combined three existing laws regulating end-of-life treatment into a single law called the Texas Advance Directives Act (TADA). TADA establishes a procedure for resolving end-of-life disputes, which may be used in response to requests to "do everything" or "stop all treatments" when physicians feel the opposite course of action is more appropriate. Fine and Mayo summarize its provisions:

1. The family must be given written information about hospital policy on the ethics consultation process.
2. The family must be given 48 hours' notice and be invited to participate in the consultation process.
3. The ethics consultation committee must provide a written report detailing its findings to the family.
4. If the ethics consultation process fails to resolve the dispute, the hospital, working with the family, must try to arrange transfer of the patient to another physician or institution willing to give the treatment requested by the family.
5. If after 10 days (measured from the time the family receives the written summary from the ethics consultation committee) no such provider can be found, the hospital and physician may unilaterally withhold or withdraw therapy that has been determined to be futile.
6. The patient or surrogate may ask a state court judge to grant an extension of time before treatment is withdrawn. This extension is to be granted only if the judge determines that there is a reasonable likelihood of finding a willing provider of the disputed treatment if more time is granted.
7. If the family does not seek an extension or the judge fails to grant one, futile treatment may be unilaterally withdrawn by the treatment team with immunity from civil and criminal prosecution.

Although TADA was designed to reduce conflict, it has had its share of controversial cases and has increasingly received harsh criticism. In spring 2007, seventeen-month-old Emilio Gonzales gained national attention when Children's Hospital of Austin sought to discontinue his care in spite of his mother's desire for treatment. Emilio was diagnosed with Leigh's disease, a rare disorder that causes the central nervous system to collapse. He could not breathe on his own, and required artificial nutrition and hydration. Doctors determined and the hospital ethics committee concurred that the treatment was futile, causing suffering without providing any medical benefit. Catarina Gonzales understood that Emilio was terminally ill, but disagreed that it was already time to let him go. Children's Hospital voluntarily extended the deadline, but could not find another hospital willing to take Emilio. A court order temporarily prevented Children's Hospital from withdrawing treatment, but Emilio died before the judge could issue a final ruling. He was at Children's Hospital for five months, including two months after doctors initiated the TADA procedure.

Discussion Questions

1. Was it in Emilio's best interests to continue treatment?
2. How would Gampel and Paris et al. evaluate TADA? How does your view compare with theirs?
3. Do you find TADA ethically justifiable?
4. Do you think the ten-day waiting period is too short, too long, or about right? If ten days is not the right length of time, what would be?
5. TADA failed to eliminate conflict in Emilio's case, as well as many others. How could it be improved?

Sources

Dexheimer, Eric. "Ill Boy's Fight Ends in Death." *Austin American-Statesman*, May 20, 2007.

Fine, Robert L., and Thomas W. Mayo. "Resolution of Futility by Due Process: Early Experience with the Texas Advance Directives Act." *Annals of Internal Medicine* 138, no. 9 (2003): 743–46.

Shannon, Kelley. "Unusual Texas Law at Center of Fight over Baby's Life." *Dallas Morning News*. http://www.dallasnews.com/sharedcontent/APStories/stories/D8OD95K80.html# (accessed June 5, 2008).

Truog, Robert D. "Tackling Medical Futility in Texas." *New England Journal of Medicine* 357, no. 1 (2007): 1–3.

Don't Mess with Texas: Cancer, Custody, and Katie

Katie Wernecke was twelve years old when she was diagnosed with Hodgkin's disease in January 2005. After four cycles of chemotherapy, her oncologist, Dr. Alter, wanted Katie to receive radiation treatment. Katie's parents objected to the radiation treatment; her cancer was now in remission, and they were worried about the harmful effects that the radiation might have on her. Dr. Alter said that treatment was the only option and her condition was life-threatening.

Mrs. Wernecke hid with Katie on a relative's property, and Dr. Alter complained to the Texas Department of Family and Protective Services.

In June, child protection authorities won a court order to place the now thirteen-year-old Katie with a foster family. Social workers, saying that the Wernecke house was unsafe, then removed their three sons to a children's home, but the judge ordered their return within two weeks. When an exam showed that Katie's cancer had returned, the judge also required Katie to undergo a cycle of high-dose chemotherapy over her parents' objections.

Katie herself also objected to her court-ordered treatment. She pulled out catheters, refused to allow her pulse to be taken, and drank a soda, all of which delayed her treatment. The Child Protective Services lawyers blamed Katie's defiance on her father, and asked the judge to cut off all communication between Katie and her family. The judge declined.

In November, after Katie had received her cycle of high-dose chemotherapy, a new judge returned Katie to her family. Her parents promised to seek the best cancer treatment possible, and had already made contact with the Center for the Improvement of Human Functioning in Wichita, Kansas. The Center integrates nutritional therapies with traditional medicine. Mr. Wernecke said that he would consider radiation therapy, but only as a last resort.

Did the Werneckes' endanger their daughter by rejecting the radiation treatment? Not necessarily. Dr. James Nachman, a Hodgkin's expert and professor of pediatrics at the University of Chicago said it is controversial whether children who show a complete response to chemotherapy get any added benefit from radiation. "I would not hesitate to bring in child services to insist on cancer treatment that parents are resisting if it's a matter of life or death, but radiation for this situation is not one of them."

Discussion Questions

1. Did Katie's parents make medical decisions against her best interests?
2. Do you think that Dr. Alter did the right thing, given that he sincerely thought Katie would die without radiation treatment?

3. Why is it important for parents to make the medical decisions for their children?

4. Under what circumstances, if any, do you think parents should lose the right to make medical decisions for their children, and even lose custody of them? Do Katie's parents meet your criteria?

5. Katie also objected to her continued treatment. Is it necessary to get her informed consent?

Sources

Associated Press. "Case of Texas Girl with Cancer Gets Review." September 6, 2005. http://start.earthlink.net/channel/news/ (accessed September 6, 2005).

———. "Texas Judge Orders Treatment for a 13-Year-Old with Cancer." *New York Times*, September 10, 2005. http://www.nytimes.com/2005/09/10/national/10texas.html (accessed June 5, 2008).

Blumenthal, Ralph. "Girl with Cancer Reunites with Family as State Gives Up Custody." *New York Times*, November 4, 2005. http://www.nytimes.com/2005/11/04/national/04katie.html (accessed June 5, 2008).

Healy, Bernadine. "The Tyranny of Experts." *U.S. News and World Report*. http://www.usnews.com/usnews/opinion/articles/050627/27healy.htm (accessed June 5, 2008).

Not Dead Yet—Part III

Joe, age fifty-five, had been diagnosed with pulmonary fibrosis, a disease that involves scarring of the lungs and fibrotic tissue gradually replacing the lungs' air sacs. As the scar forms, lung tissue thickens and loses the ability to transfer oxygen into the bloodstream. There are currently no known treatments for the scarring or cure for the disease. Joe's condition got progressively worse, and he eventually collapsed at home. An ambulance rushed him to St. Clair's Hospital, but Joe had suffered a severe brain injury because of oxygen deprivation, leaving him extremely debilitated. After consultation with Joe's physician, his family requested discontinuation of all treatment, including artificial nutrition and hydration (ANH). Dr. Goldstein put Joe on a morphine IV to relieve any discomfort. The nurses in Joe's area of the hospital were quite unhappy with the situation. Many of the nurses at St. Clair's are Catholic, and frequently express their disapproval when life-sustaining care is withheld or withdrawn, especially ANH. In particular, they think that Catholic hospitals like St. Clair's should follow Catholic teaching, which they understand to mandate providing ANH to all patients who cannot eat or drink on their own.

Two weeks later, Joe was still alive, and quite mysteriously, was producing normal amounts of urine despite discontinuation of ANH. Dr. Goldstein ordered a change in morphine delivery, reducing fluids to the bare minimum needed to administer the drug. A few days later, Joe's urine output had dropped slightly, but was still incredibly high for someone receiving no fluids. Dr. Goldstein again changed Joe's medication; this time he ordered a morphine patch, which would entirely eliminate all fluid intake. Suspecting that the nurses were providing ANH at night, or allowing someone else access to Joe for that purpose, Dr. Goldstein also ordered Joe to be weighed daily, reasoning that a patient who received no nourishment or hydration should be losing weight. The nurses refused to weigh Joe.

Discussion Questions

1. Do you think that the family's decision was in Joe's best interests?

2. How do you think Arras would analyze Joe's case? Would you agree with Arras?

3. How would you evaluate the nurses' actions?

4. Do you think that the nurses are following Catholic teaching on ANH?

5. Was the decision to remove ANH consistent with guidelines articulated by Casarett, Kapo, and Caplan?

Source

Pulmonary Fibrosis Foundation. http://www.pulmonaryfibrosis.org (accessed June 5, 2008).

The Groningen Protocol—Euthanasia for Newborns

In the Netherlands, competent patients age sixteen and older may request euthanasia. We know that some severely impaired newborns experience tremendous suffering with no hope of recovery, yet they cannot request euthanasia. Must they be kept alive when their suffering cannot be reduced?

Drs. Eduard Verhagen and Pieter Sauer developed a procedure called the Groningen protocol to handle cases when a decision needs to be made regarding whether to end the life of a newborn. They divide newborns for whom such decisions might need to made into three categories: (1) infants with no chance of survival, and who will die shortly after birth; (2) infants with very poor prognosis who require intensive care, such as those with severe brain abnormalities or extensive organ damage, and who would likely have a poor quality of life even if they were able to leave intensive care; and (3) infants with a prognosis of poor quality of life and extended suffering.

The Groningen Protocol for Euthanasia in Newborns

Requirements that must be fulfilled

The diagnosis and prognosis must be certain
Hopeless and unbearable suffering must be present
The diagnosis, prognosis, and unbearable suffering must be confirmed by at least one independent doctor
Both parents must give informed consent
The procedure must be performed in accordance with the accepted medical standards

Information needed to support and clarify the decision about euthanasia

Diagnosis and prognosis

Describe all relevant medical data and the results of diagnostic investigations used to establish the diagnosis

List all the participants in the decision-making process, all opinions expressed, and the final consensus
Describe how the prognosis regarding long-term health was assessed
Describe how the degree of suffering and life expectancy were assessed
Describe the availability of alternative treatments, alternative means of alleviating suffering, or both
Describe treatments and the results of treatment preceding the decision about euthanasia

Euthanasia decision

Describe who initiated the discussion about possible euthanasia and at what moment
List the considerations that prompted the decision
List all the participants in the decision-making process, all opinions expressed, and the final consensus
Describe the way in which the parents were informed and their opinions

Consultation

Describe the physician or physicians who gave a second opinion (name and qualifications)
List the results of the examinations and the recommendations made by the consulting physician or physicians

Implementation

Describe the actual euthanasia procedure (time, place, participants, and administration of drugs)
Describe the reasons for the chosen method of euthanasia

Steps taken after death

Describe the findings of the coroner
Describe how the euthanasia was reported to the prosecuting authority
Describe how the parents are being supported and counseled
Describe planned follow-up, including case review, postmortem examination, and genetic counseling

Discussion Questions

1. Do you think that it can ever be in a newborn's best interests to discontinue treatment and be allowed to die?
2. Do you think that euthanasia can ever be in a newborn's best interest?
3. Assuming that euthanasia for children is legal, do you think that the Groningen Protocol provides an ethical procedure?
4. What impact do you think legalizing euthanasia would have on public trust of physicians?

Source

Verhagen, Eduard, and Pieter J.J. Sauer. "The Groningen Protocol—Euthanasia in Severely Ill Newborns." *New England Journal of Medicine* 352, no. 10 (2005). 959–61.

A Friend in Need

The British General Medical Council (GMC) determined that Michael Irwin, seventy-four, a retired physician and former chairman of the Voluntary Euthanasia Society, was unfit to practice medicine, because he had agreed to help a terminally ill friend commit suicide. A GMC panel criticized Dr. Irwin for stockpiling medications for "an act of deception." It also accused him of a criminal offence for writing false prescriptions for himself, when he intended to use the pills to assist in his friend's suicide. Dr. Irwin said the drugs were to relieve jet lag, but the GMC panel found the number of pills "excessive."

Dr. Irwin agreed to help fellow euthanasia campaigner Patrick Kneen, who was dying of prostate cancer, commit suicide. But when he arrived, Kneen was too ill to take the pills. Kneen's doctor put him on morphine drip, and he died a few days later.

In his testimony, Dr. Irwin told the panel that he knew of several doctors who had "twinning" arrangements with fellow doctors to help each other commit suicide if a painful death threatened. He thought it would be a "double standard" if these same doctors would not have the same compassion for a friend or long-term patient who is terminally ill and suffering. In a statement to the GMC, he said:

> I believe passionately that in this apparently enlightened 21st century, terminally ill patients should have the right to obtain medical assistance to die, if this is their wish: to be able to pick a time for their death, preferably in their own familiar home environment. Although our British society is in principle just, I strongly believe that the existing law on assisted suicide is unjust and that sometimes a compassionate physician has a greater duty to a patient or a close friend than his or her duty to the state.

Dr. Irwin might have escaped sanction if he had taken Kneen to Switzerland. Swiss law not only permits assisted suicide (as long as it does not proceed from selfish motives), but also permits foreigners to receive assistance. During the past decade, about one hundred Britons have committed suicide at Dignitas, a Swiss nonprofit organization dedicated to the practice.

Discussion Questions

1. Do you agree with the GMC that Dr. Irwin is unfit to practice medicine?
2. Dr. Irwin claims that he has a greater duty to a friend or patient than to the state, apparently meaning that he should be willing to break the law in order to help them. Do you agree with Dr. Irwin?
3. Do you think that the law should be changed, so that Dr. Irwin could legally help his friend?
4. If assisted suicide becomes legal, what rules should govern its practice?

Sources

Dyer, Clare. "GP Is Disciplined for Willingness to Help Friend Commit Suicide." *British Medical Journal* 331 (2005): 717.

Lyall, Sarah. "TV Broadcast of an Assisted Suicide Intensifies a Contentious Debate in Britain." *New York Times*, December 11; 2008. http://www.nytimes.com/2008/12/11/world/europe/11suicide.html (accessed Dec. 14, 2008).

At the Beginnings of Life

INTRODUCTION

In chapter 3, we noted that most of the famous cases in bioethics have centered around the end of life, and that some of the most contentious issues are in that area. Chapter 3, however, did not cover what has been possibly the most divisive issue in the United States for over thirty years: abortion. Perhaps what makes abortion so problematic is the controversy over whether it, too, is an end-of-life issue, and, if so, to what degree. Also embedded in the debate are people's views about sexuality and contraception.

The beginning of life is the focal point for chapter 4. Besides abortion, this chapter covers maternal-fetal relations and reproductive technologies, including human cloning. The various questions it addresses include the following: When does human life begin, biologically and morally? What obligations exist for women in relation to their fetuses? Are the new reproductive technologies oppressive or liberating? What is the moral status of human embryos when they exist outside of a woman's body? Furthermore, why does it matter how humans reproduce?

Abortion

Passions clearly run high regarding abortion. There are peaceful protests both supporting and opposing abortion rights. There also have been intimidation campaigns against abortion seekers and providers, bombings at abortion clinics, and even murders of doctors who provide abortions. It is easy to characterize the abortion debate as a clash of absolutes—life versus liberty—such that moral conversation is impossible. Even more extreme, the debate is sometimes viewed as one of good versus evil, with each side demonizing the other. Yet the landscape is, in reality, much more complex. These radical and polarizing positions exist alongside of moderate ones (e.g., "pro-life," but willing to allow abortion in special circumstances, like rape or severe fetal abnormality, and "pro-choice," but willing to make moral distinctions among reasons for abortion, like rejecting sex selection as morally invalid). Furthermore, many values are widely shared on both sides (e.g., a commitment to children and a desire to alleviate situations that lead women to seek abortions, like extreme poverty or a lack of birth control). Even feminism contains its own pro-life wing, featuring an emphasis on the importance of relationships and inclusivity, along with the emphasis on women's autonomy and well-being.

As we noted in chapter 1, most people's ethics are a composite rather than emerging from one distinct source, and perhaps that is most obvious concerning beliefs about abortion. Religion, philosophy, law, biology, medicine, and the social sciences all influence personal and social views about abortion. The critical questions of whether abortion should be permitted, and, if so, under what circumstances, draw on all of these sources in addressing them. These sources also represent logically distinct facets of the abortion issue. For example, the morality of abortion and its legal status are separate questions. While a negative moral judgment about abortion often leads someone to also desire abortion to be illegal, other moral and legal considerations may lead some to conclude that abortion law should be less restrictive than their moral judgments about it. As a practical matter, people may also decline to focus on restrictive laws, viewing them as less effective in reducing abortions than are things like health care and economic support for prospective mothers.

The Legal Landscape

More than any other issue in bioethics, the moral controversy over abortion has played out in the public forum of law, and understanding the complexity of the abortion debate requires some understanding of the ongoing legal skirmishes over what will be permitted, when, and by whom. The modern abortion debate in the United States begins with the Supreme Court's controversial decision to strike down anti-abortion laws. The history behind *Roe v. Wade* (1973) is, of course, much longer and reflects changing and conflicting attitudes regarding abortion.

The common law tradition in the United States (case-based rulings by judges) did not view abortion as a moral problem until "quickening," which is when the fetus begins to move independently, about four to five months after pregnancy begins. At that point, the common law took an interest in protecting the fetus. Late-term abortions, however, were rarely prosecuted. Statutory laws initially codified the common law approach, but gradually became more restrictive. By 1900, every jurisdiction had laws prohibiting abortion, and they were in effect until the 1970s in most states.

Roe struck down the laws proscribing abortion, establishing abortion rights at the national level. But the decision was a compromise—the Court refused to endorse an unqualified right to privacy that would permit abortion on demand, instead opting for a trimester framework that permits restrictions to increase during pregnancy. During the first trimester of pregnancy, a woman's privacy and liberty interests are primary, with the abortion decision left between her and her physician. After the first trimester but before *viability* (when the fetus can survive outside of the mother's womb), states may regulate abortion procedures, but not the decision itself, to protect maternal health. After the fetus reaches viability, the state may regulate and even prohibit abortion, except insofar as it would be required to save the life or health of the mother. (With the medical technology available in 1973, a fetus reached viability after about twenty-eight weeks of gestation.)

Roe is one of the Supreme Court's most controversial decisions, causing both celebration and resentment. It has been celebrated because it gives women control over their own bodies, respects their autonomy to choose if and when they want to bear children, and maintains the safety of abortion by allowing it to be part of medical practice. The pro-life movement emerged from the resentment to the decision, and many conservative politicians pledged to do what they could to restrict abortion and get the case overturned, resulting in many legal challenges to *Roe*. The nominating process for Supreme Court justices now includes close scrutiny of the candidates' views about abortion and whether they would support *Roe* or seek to overturn it. As Court membership has changed—and the Court as a whole has become more conservative—the *Roe* doctrine has been modified, but never explicitly overturned. No justices remain from the group that decided *Roe*.

Among the most important abortion cases since *Roe* are *Webster v. Reproductive Health Services* (1989), *Planned Parenthood v. Casey* (1992), *Stenberg v. Carhart* (2000), and *Gonzales v. Carhart* (2007). In *Webster*, the Court upheld a Missouri law that required viability tests after twenty weeks of pregnancy. While the Missouri law violated *Roe*'s trimester framework, the Court reasoned that viability could occur before the twenty-fifth week. The Court also upheld the provision that prohibited abortions at public hospitals or on state-owned property, contending that the restriction did not unduly interfere with a woman's rights, because she could still obtain an abortion from private facilities. These two justifications—concern for fetal viability and holding that the restriction in question did not unduly interfere with a woman's right to seek an abortion—have been grounds for permitting many state restrictions on abortion, but also overturning others that did not meet those standards. *Casey* struck down one Pennsylvania regulation (spousal notification), but upheld four others: an "informed consent" provision that required doctors to provide women with information about the health risks of abortion, parental notification for minors seeking abortion, a twenty-four-hour waiting period, and some facility reporting requirements. None of these four rules, the Court said, placed an undue burden on women seeking abortion, although spousal notification did. The Court also specifically rejected *Roe*'s trimester formula on the grounds that improved medical technology had pushed viability earlier.

The *Stenberg* and *Carhart* cases both concern "partial-birth abortion" laws, and show how the change in personnel can be crucial in the Court's decisions—Sandra Day O'Connor, part of the five to four majority in *Stenberg* retired in 2006, and her replacement, Samuel Alito, took the other side in *Carhart*. Partial-birth is an ambiguous term that is used to refer to particular methods of abortion employed during the second and third trimesters of pregnancy. (Although the methods have important differences, and the feasibility of their use depends upon the extent of fetal development, they all involve dilation of the cervix, and involve at least some destruction of the fetus as it is removed. For intact dilation and extraction, the fetus is partially removed from the woman's vagina before it is destroyed.) The *Stenberg* decision struck down a Nebraska law prohibiting partial-birth abortion, arguing that the law placed an undue burden on a woman's right to have an abortion and did not allow for exceptions when the woman's health was threatened by the pregnancy. The *Carhart* decision, written by Anthony Kennedy, one of the dissenters in *Stenberg*, also claims to follow both *Roe* and *Casey*, but upholds the federal Partial-Birth Abortion Ban Act of 2003. The Court concluded that the federal law did not impose an undue burden on women's right to abortion; other abortion procedures are still available. The decision apparently does conflict with *Roe*, however, because the law was not enacted for the reason that the method is unsafe for women, and the only exception it provides is for preserving a woman's life, but not her health. The Court's ruling does permit women to challenge the Act on that point in special cases.

Overview of State Abortion Laws

- *Physician and Hospital Requirements:* Thirty-nine states require an abortion to be performed by a licensed physician. Nineteen states require an abortion to be performed in a hospital after a specified point in the pregnancy, and eighteen states require the involvement of a second physician after a specified point.

- *Gestational Limits:* Thirty-six states prohibit abortions, generally except when necessary to protect the woman's life or health, after a specified point in pregnancy, most often fetal viability.

- *"Partial-Birth" Abortion:* Fourteen states have laws in effect that prohibit "partial-birth" abortion. Four of these laws apply only to postviability abortions.

- *Public Funding:* Seventeen states use their own funds to pay for all or most medically necessary abortions for Medicaid enrollees in the state. Thirty-two states and the District of Columbia prohibit the use of state funds except in those cases when federal funds are available: where the woman's life is in danger or the pregnancy is the result of rape or incest. In defiance of federal requirements, South Dakota limits funding to cases of life endangerment only.

- *Coverage by Private Insurance:* Four states restrict coverage of abortion in private insurance plans to cases in which the woman's life would be endangered if the pregnancy were carried to term. Additional abortion coverage is permitted only if the woman purchases it at her own expense.

- *Refusal:* Forty-six states allow individual health care providers to refuse to participate in an abortion. Forty-three states allow institutions to refuse to perform abortions, sixteen of which limit refusal to private or religious institutions.

- *State-Mandated Counseling:* Seventeen states mandate that women be given counseling before an abortion that includes information on at least one of the following: the purported link between abortion and breast cancer (six states), the ability of a fetus to feel pain (eight states), long-term mental health consequences for the woman (seven states) or information on the availability of ultrasound (six states).

- *Waiting Periods:* Twenty-four states require a woman seeking an abortion to wait a specified period of time, usually twenty-four hours, between when she receives counseling and the procedure is performed. Six of these states have laws that effectively require the woman to make two separate trips to the clinic to obtain the procedure.

- *Parental Involvement:* Thirty-five states require some type of parental involvement in a minor's decision to have an abortion. Twenty-two states require one or both parents to consent to the procedure, while eleven require that one or both parents be notified, and two states require both parental consent and notification.

Source: The Guttmacher Institute

"Personhood," The Beginning of Life, and Abortion

As a matter of ethics, it is important to determine who and what counts as a "person," that is, who is a member of the human moral community and so deserving respect and possessing rights. Today, all human beings are typically considered members of the moral community, although historically many societies have excluded some human groups from membership. Regarding abortion, two important questions are whether and when a fetus should be considered a *moral person*. If a fetus is a person, then a fetus has moral standing, separate from its mother, possessing all of the same rights.

Some people equate moral personhood with the biological beginning of human life. Historically, the question of when life begins focused on when humans received their souls (or some analogous concept of life's essence). The mirror image of the traditional understanding of death—the moment when the soul leaves the body—human life was considered to begin with ensoulment. Abortion before ensoulment might be permitted, but not afterward, except perhaps in exceptional circumstances. While we typically understand soul as a religious concept today, that has not always been the case. In ancient Greece, for example, soul was simultaneously a religious, philosophical, and scientific concept. Abortion and infanticide were common practices in that society, including participation by Hippocratic physicians and others, but the strong Pythagorean influence on the Hippocratic Oath was crucial to its rejection of abortion. As part of their religious beliefs, the Pythagoreans believed that ensoulment occurred at conception, and so fetuses had full moral worth, the same as any living human.

While ensoulment may remain an important concept for religious discussions of the beginning of life and abortion, it has no place in contemporary biological discussions, and rarely receives attention in philosophy except by religious philosophers and their critics. The focus now is on particular stages of fetal development. (Religious and some philosophical accounts may then link ensoulment to some particular biological indicator.) There are several possible markers in fetal development that could be claimed as the beginning of life. Among them are the following:

- *Conception*. The formation of a new biological entity is the earliest commonly held point at which life could be said to begin. The term "moment of conception" is scientifically problematic, however, because contemporary embryology holds that conception is a process rather than a single event. It does not occur all at once.
- *Implantation*. While conception does result in new genetic material different from the providers of the gametes, pregnancy does not actually occur until the fertilized egg implants in the woman's uterus, which typically happens six to seven days later. If implantation does not occur—and it fails to occur more than half of the time—the fertilized egg will die.
- *Uniqueness and/or unity*. Implantation of a fertilized egg does not necessarily signify an individual life. Twinning may occur up to four weeks after conception, although usually only during the first two weeks, and materials from different fertilized eggs could fuse into a single entity. Formation of the primitive streak, which occurs at about fourteen days following fertilization, typically indicates that an individual embryo has been formed, and fetal development can begin.
- *Brain life*. Under the whole-brain standard of death, life is associated with the existence of measurable neurological activity. Its absence means the person is dead. The outset of human life could also be equated with brain activity, which begins about eight weeks after conception.
- *Quickening*. As noted earlier, this was considered the key moment in common law when the fetus now deserved legal protection. It could also be used to mark the beginning of life, because it is when the fetus begins to move independently of its mother. This occurs when the fetus is four to five months old.

- *Viability*. This occurs when the fetus could survive outside of the womb; before that, it lacks independence. The obvious difficulty with this marker is that it is elastic and can change depending upon the sophistication of medical technology.
- *Birth*.

Others view the *potentiality* of personhood as sufficiently important to provide strict moral limits on when abortion may be procured. Actual personhood need not yet be achieved in order for the fetus to have some moral standing. In his article "Abortion and the Beginning and End of Human Life," **Don Marquis** reviews many of these markers for the beginning of human life, and finds them all problematic. He thinks that none of them provide a clear and convincing point at which to say human life begins. Marquis contends that a better pro-life strategy is available: the "future of value" view of why killing is wrong. This view claims that killing is wrong because it deprives victims of their futures of value, "whatever they will or would regard as making their lives worth living." Abortion thus is wrong because it deprives an entity—whether or not it yet qualifies as a moral person—of its future of value. An exception to this rule would be badly damaged fetuses, which would have no future of value. They could be aborted.

A consensus regarding what counts as personhood, independent moral status, or when life has begun, would not necessarily resolve the issue of abortion. Some instances of abortion may be morally problematic, even if a fetus is not considered a moral person or even a potential person. Bonnie Steinbock recognizes some moral limits on abortion, even though she believes that fetuses lack sentience and thus have no interests to consider. She argues that abortion for trivial reasons—like wanting to look good in a bikini for your St. Tropez vacation—is morally unacceptable. There may also be justifiable reasons for abortion even after a fetus attains moral standing. For example, many people who believe that life begins at conception would nevertheless permit abortion if pregnancy is the result of rape, or if the pregnancy endangered the woman's life or health. Others might permit it in a case of severe fetal abnormality or selectively in the instance of a multiple pregnancy that threatens the survival of all fetuses. Still others might claim that a woman's autonomy over her own body is morally weightier than another being's claims on it, and so in many cases would permit abortion regardless of moral standing. In perhaps the most famous article about abortion, **Judith Jarvis Thomson** does just that, utilizing several imaginative scenarios to make her case. Thomson's argument supports a woman's right to be free from the burdens of pregnancy, which she sees as distinct from a right to destroy a fetus.

Fetal personhood is beside the point according to **Farhat Moazam**, who examines the social context in India, where the preference for sons leads to abortion of female fetuses. She supports a ban on prenatal gender determination in order to reduce, if not eliminate, abortion based on sex selection. The practice does not stem from women exercising their autonomy, so much as a cultural context that constrains women's choices. Moazam thinks that in this case, having more choices is harmful to women, and so feminists ought to support restrictions.

Although the abortion debate may seem intractable, **Christopher Kaczor** proposes a possible resolution. Kaczor suggests that if artificial wombs could be developed, and if it were possible to remove a fetus without destroying it or harming the mother, then women could be free of their pregnancies without destroying nascent life. In support of his position, he cites pro-choice advocates like Thomson, who understand abortion as a right of evacuation rather than a right of termination. Kaczor then turns to specific objections to abortion and reproductive technology made by the Catholic Church. He ultimately finds no basis for condemning artificial wombs.

Modern Religious Perspectives

Major religious traditions, while generally condemning abortion, offer a range of views regarding the conditions when it might be permitted. There are variations within these traditions as well, including pro-choice outlooks in traditions known for their restrictive positions.

Christianity, particularly its Protestant denominations, reflects both pro-life and pro-choice perspectives. The pro-life standpoint of the Roman Catholic Church, however, is the most widely known Christian view of abortion. According to church doctrine, full human life begins at the moment of conception; even the earliest embryo deserves respect and the full protection of morality and law. Destroying an embryo is murder. (The Church has held this position since the nineteenth century. Previously, the Church had rejected abortion, but considered it murder only after ensoulment had occurred, which was a matter of contention. During the Middle Ages, the Church settled on Thomas Aquinas's position that ensoulment occurred when the body was sufficiently formed to receive it—at forty days for males and ninety days for females.) Direct abortion is always immoral, even to save the mother's life, or if the pregnancy resulted from rape.

Catholicism does, however, provide some exceptions to this rigid deontological position. Indirect abortion is permitted under the principle of double effect (the four elements of this principle are listed in the introduction to chapter 3). If the pregnant woman has uterine cancer or an ectopic pregnancy (implantation in a fallopian tube rather than the uterus), life-sustaining surgery to remove the cancer or the fallopian tube would also result in an abortion. The abortion would be the indirect result of the procedure, rather than the purpose of it.

Unlike Catholicism, Judaism does not consider the fetus to be a person until birth. It is considered to be part of the mother's body, not a separate entity, until its head or the greater part of its body has emerged during the birthing process. Despite this view, Judaism holds a restrictive view regarding abortion, albeit less restrictive than Catholicism. A woman may have a very early abortion for any reason, because the fertilized egg is considered to be "mere fluid" until forty days after conception, thus having no status at all until that point. After that the fetus is considered to be a potential person, deserving respect, and so abortion is permitted only in select circumstances. In situations of conflict between mother and fetus, priority goes to the mother, with abortion not merely permitted but required in order to save her life. An exception to the woman's priority is when the fetus's head or greater part has emerged; then physicians must treat them equally. Many rabbinic authorities also permit abortion to protect the physical and even mental health of the mother. Although Judaism does not permit abortion for infant abnormality per se, it may be permitted if such a birth would be mentally traumatic for the mother.

The third Abrahamic tradition, Islam, holds that ensoulment occurs after four months of gestation. Abortion is forbidden after that point, except if necessary to save the life of the mother. Abortion is also strongly discouraged before that point. In recent years, several scholars in both the Sunni and Shi'a branches of Islam have permitted abortions before the end of the fourth month if the pregnancy endangers the woman's health, if the fetus has a severe disorder, or if having a child would result in severe social or economic hardship.

Another interesting religious perspective comes from Buddhism. Historically, most Buddhists have held that the transmigration of consciousness necessary for reincarnation occurs at conception. Abortion thus is killing, and so is forbidden, bringing negative karma to anyone who engages in it. Many contemporary Buddhists still reject abortion, holding that life begins at our current biological notion of conception, but others, such as Michael Barnhardt, question whether the fetus can embody all five *skandhas* (life components: body, sensations, thoughts, feelings, consciousness), and so qualify as a person. "A human life, in the moral sense, starts unambiguously when all the *skandhas* are in place, and the Buddha as well as the early Buddhist scriptures leave room for a rather large number of interpretations as to exactly when such a condition occurs in the process of embryonic development." Barnhardt suggests that the correct approach to the morality of abortion is to make analogies between the fetus at its present state of development and living persons. Early abortions thus would be more readily justifiable, and later term abortions more difficult. Helen Tworkov contends that while all abortions would bring negative karma, the reasons for abortion would have karmic significance. Good reasons will diminish bad karma; bad reasons enhance it. A woman would receive worse karma for not using contraception than if she had. The negativity of karma would increase during pregnancy, so there is a sliding scale.

Health Care Professionals and Abortion

The original Hippocratic Oath called for physicians to swear, "I will not give to a woman an abortive remedy." Based on the Greek term it uses, the Oath rejects a particular method of abortion (a pessary that induced premature labor), but arguably also prohibits the entire practice. As we noted above, the Hippocratic group was influenced by the Pythagoreans, who believed that life begins at conception. The Hippocratic group also likely made this decision because pessaries were unsafe for the pregnant women.

Abortion is much safer if performed in the health care setting than if is performed by others elsewhere. Health care professionals, however, may have moral and/or religious concerns about abortion that lead them to reject performing this service. After the *Roe* decision in 1973, states began to enact "conscience clause" legislation that permitted doctors to refuse to provide abortion services. Now forty-six states have such laws for doctors, and forty-three states have a similar provision for health care institutions. Some conscience laws pertain to contraception, with eight states allowing physicians to refuse to provide contraception to patients, and four explicitly permitting pharmacists to refuse to dispense them. While these laws reflect some people's general rejection of contraception, they are primarily aimed at emergency contraception like Plan B, which is taken after intercourse. Plan B works primarily by preventing ovulation and fertilization, although it may also prevent implantation of a fertilized egg. It is not an abortifacient in that it will not end a pregnancy. (As noted earlier, pregnancy does not occur until implantation.) Nevertheless, because of ignorance regarding how Plan B works, or because of a special concern for fertilized eggs as full human life, some doctors and pharmacists oppose it. Moving in the other direction, New Jersey enacted a law in 2007 that prohibits pharmacists from refusing to fill prescriptions on religious, philosophical, or moral grounds. **Julie Cantor and Ken Baum** discuss conscientious objection by pharmacists in relation to emergency contraception. They provide an overview of arguments that support and oppose a pharmacist's right to object, and then argue for the middle ground of a limited right of refusal. They also outline duties that objecting pharmacists have to patients.

Abortion Worldwide

Abortion is illegal in many countries. But laws seem to have no impact on women seeking abortion, especially in the absence of reliable contraception. For example, the abortion rate is approximately the same in Africa (twenty-nine per thousand women ages fifteen to forty-four), where abortion is generally illegal, as it is in Europe (twenty-eight), where it is generally legal. According to the World Health Organization (2007), each year "there are 65,000 to 70,000 deaths and close to five million women with temporary or permanent disability due to unsafe abortion." The vast majority of deaths and health problems occur in developing countries where abortion is illegal.

Maternal-Fetal Relations

Most women who become pregnant do not seek abortions. Whether or not they intended to become pregnant, these women often undergo profound lifestyle changes to accommodate their pregnancy, and not strictly out of physical necessity. They often will change personal habits that they enjoy, such as diet, drinking, smoking, and physical activities in order to protect and benefit their fetuses. They seek medical care, not only for themselves, but to ensure that they will deliver a healthy baby. Are these actions moral obligations for women who choose to carry their pregnancies to term, or strictly praiseworthy? Do they mark the beginnings of a relationship, or does this notion of a "maternal-fetal relationship" make no sense because there can be no mutuality between the two?

The moral status of the fetus plays a crucial role in determining the nature and extent of the responsibilities a pregnant woman may have. If a fetus is a moral person, then it would have certain rights against others, including the mother. If a fetus is not a moral person, it still may have some moral standing as a potential person, and so the mother may have some limited duties to benefit and not harm it. Another key issue is whether these maternal responsibilities are strictly moral, or also legal, and so could be coercively enforced. Also important is determining how stringent the obligations of a pregnant woman might be. How much risk and sacrifice must a mother undertake for the sake of her fetus? Must she live for her fetus, rather than for herself?

The starkest ethical challenges arise not in relation to the millions of women who nurture and protect their fetuses, but from the rare exceptions. What do we make of the pregnant women who, through ignorance, negligence, or even malice, place their fetuses at risk? Women who do not make socially expected accommodations for their fetuses have in recent years not only found themselves subject to social pressure, but also criminal prosecution. Pregnant women have faced charges of "fetal neglect," child endangerment, drug delivery (to the fetus via umbilical cord), homicide, and vehicular homicide (when reckless driving under the influence of alcohol caused miscarriage). For example, in 1999 Regina McKnight of South Carolina was convicted of homicide by child abuse when her baby was stillborn. The prosecution charged that McKnight's cocaine use caused the stillbirth. (After she spent several years in prison, her conviction was overturned in 2008.) Some pregnant women have even been preemptively jailed to protect fetuses from potential harm caused by drug abuse or the lack of prenatal care.

Women have also faced criminal charges after refusing a doctor's recommendation for a caesarian section. In 2004, Melissa Rowland of Utah was charged with murder when one of her twins was stillborn. Prosecutors claimed that her refusal to have a C-section showed "depraved indifference to human life." (In a plea bargain, charges were reduced to two counts of child endangerment, and Rowland was to serve eighteen months probation and complete a drug treatment program.)

In her essay in this chapter, **Mary Briody Mahowald** discusses the unique situation of pregnant patients, and the notion of fetal patients. Although some commentators are willing to view the fetus as a patient, even if it not a person, Mahowald insists that the pregnant woman be viewed as one patient, not two, even when she seeks treatment for her fetus. Mahowald rejects the notion that physicians have duties to care for a fetus that are distinct from their duties to care for the pregnant woman. **Deborah Hornstra** rejects the notion of fetal rights, such as the right to be born healthy. Such rights would be difficult to define and enforce, and intrude too much on the lives of women. Furthermore, Hornstra claims that fetal rights would destroy the maternal-fetal relationship by casting them as adversaries.

Reproductive Technology

Humanity's concern with reproduction is not only about how to avoid it (contraception and abortion), but also how to achieve it when children are desired but not forthcoming. The standard medical definition of infertility is the inability of a heterosexual couple to conceive after one year of vaginal intercourse without contraception. Under this definition, about 2.1 million couples in the United States are affected. Historically, humanity has engaged in a range of rituals, potions, and practices in order to combat infertility. The book of Genesis in the Hebrew Bible (or Christian Old Testament) provides an account of three cases of matriarchs using *surrogate motherhood* (a woman bearing a child for another woman) when they were unable to become pregnant. Sarah had a child with Abraham via her handmaid Hagar, while Rachel and Leah had children with Jacob via their handmaids Bilhah and Zolpah. The ancient Hebrews also had a surrogate fatherhood practice, known as the levirate, which was used when a man died childless. One male member of his family, usually a brother, would father a child for him with his widow. (Versions of levirate marriage were also practiced in other cultures.) It is interesting to note that infertility treatments have focused on women, but research is increasingly showing that the male is often the one with the problem. Unfortunately, there are cultural taboos or fears for men—for example, low sperm count as a sign of insufficiency and lack of manhood—which often lead couples and doctors to focus on women alone.

While infertility is clearly a misfortune for people who desire children, how should it be conceptualized? If infertility is viewed as a medical problem, then it is readily understood as an illness that needs treatment. Alternatively, infertility could be viewed as a frustrated desire to have a child of one's own. In that case, there may be medical solutions, but they would exist alongside other nonmedical options, including adoption and merely accepting one's fate. In this framework, artificial reproduction might be viewed in the same light as elective, cosmetic surgery.

One's understanding of infertility will lead to different ethical evaluations. The President's Council on Bioethics apparently views infertility as a medical problem, calling it an "ailment," and the medical means for addressing it "therapeutic." The Council raises ethical concerns regarding such things as the safety of reproductive technology for women and the resulting children, informed consent, equitable access to the procedures, and various potential developments at the margins of reproductive medicine, such as implanting human embryos into other species, producing embryos from more than two parents, and creating cross-species hybrids. Nevertheless, it embraces rather than rejects reproductive technology, calling it established medical practice for the sake of "relieving the suffering and sorrow" of childless couples who want to participate in the "deep biological and anthropological significance" of pro-creation. **Thomas Murray** is more skeptical. He claims that the standard approach to the ethics of reproductive technologies is procreative liberty, and that this framework is insufficient and "morally confused." Procreative liberty emphasizes the personal autonomy of adults, and disregards the interests of the children it seeks to create. A better ethics of reproductive technology would focus on important relationships, including the parent-child relationship, and their significance to human flourishing. It would begin with the question, what are families for?

While some religious traditions accept the use of reproductive technologies and might find common ground with the President's Council or with Murray, the Roman Catholic tradition rejects nearly all forms of artificial reproduction as unnatural. The Vatican claims that sexual intercourse and reproduction ought to be inseparable. Just as every act of sexual intercourse ought to be open to the possibility of procreation, which forbids artificial means of contraception and nonvaginal heterosexual acts, procreation must stem from sexual intercourse. The integrity or completeness of sexual activity includes both the unitive (love-making) and procreative (child-making) aspects of intercourse. Thus, there should be no sex without potential for babies, and no babies without sex. The integrity of sexual intercourse also requires that it not be "dominated" by outsiders, including physicians. According to the

Vatican, most forms of reproductive technology involve this type of dominance. The Vatican does, however, accept the use of fertility drugs, because they do not intrude upon sexual activity or intimacy.

Paul Lauritzen engages in an interesting comparative analysis of the Vatican's view and contemporary feminist opposition to reproductive technology. Although there are crucial differences between the Catholic and feminist frameworks, he notes that there is clear overlap in their arguments against reproductive technologies in that both make appeals to the importance of embodiment. Within these appeals to embodiment, Lauritzen finds both striking similarities and striking differences. He contends that the similarities provide great insight, while the differences point to shortcomings in both groups' understanding of embodiment.

Less Invasive Methods

There are various methods of reproductive technology. Many of the ethical issues are common to all of them, but some of the methods raise unique concerns. The least physically invasive and least costly form is artificial insemination, where sperm from the husband or donor is injected into the woman's vagina. The technique is old, with documented cases going back as early as 1790. Today, sperm is obtained not only from anonymous donors, but also can be retrieved from recently deceased cadavers, as in the 2008 case of an army widow seeking to obtain sperm from her husband's body after he was killed in Iraq. Whatever the sperm's source, it can be preserved and used at a later date. In 2004, sperm that had been frozen for twenty-one years was used to produce a child. Artificial insemination thus can occur long after the donor's death and raise interesting issues regarding inheritance rights and dispositional authority.

Fertility drugs are not physically invasive, but are chemically so. They stimulate ovulation in women—sometimes called hyperovulation—and are used to increase the likelihood of conception during sexual intercourse. These drugs raise ethical concerns regarding their safety for women and the resulting children, not because they do not work, but because they may work too well. The most famous case of working too well may be the septuplets born to Kenny and Bobbi McCaughey in 1997. The McCaughey story is mostly a happy one, because the mother and all seven septuplets survived. The children were born premature, however, which is often the case in multiple pregnancies, and suffered various health problems. Although generally healthy now, two of the children have cerebral palsy, a common problem of premature birth.

In Vitro Fertilization

In vitro fertilization (IVF) is clearly the most physically invasive of the common artificial reproductive techniques. A woman's eggs are harvested by inducing hyperovulation and removed via a surgical method called laparoscopy. Eggs are fertilized in the lab, and then either implanted in the woman or frozen for later use (cryopreservation). The first human baby born via IVF was Louise Brown in 1978. Now, nearly one percent of all babies born in the United States are conceived via IVF (35,000 babies each year). There are a host of ethical issues surrounding IVF. Safety concerns exist for the women, the resulting extra-corporeal (outside of the body) embryos, and the resulting children. For women, the egg harvesting procedure imposes risks, as does the possibility of a multiple pregnancy. For embryos, implanting too many may result in selective abortion in the case of multiple pregnancy. For children, the safety concerns are related to disabilities caused by damage to their embryos or by complications from a multiple pregnancy.

Besides concerns about safety, moral debate has focused on the question of who should be allowed to use reproductive technologies such as IVF. Should IVF be available only to married couples or also to unmarried couples and single women? Should gay and lesbian couples be able to use reproductive technology? Should there be any age limits for using IVF? As of this writing, the world's oldest mothers were Omraki Panwar and Rajo Devi of India, who both gave birth at age seventy in 2008. Devi would like to have another child—this time a boy to go with her daughter.

Surrogacy

A surrogate is someone who acts in another's place. A surrogate mother agrees to become pregnant and give the baby to someone else. The contemporary version of surrogate motherhood does not involve actual intercourse, as it did in Biblical times, but uses reproductive technology, either artificial insemination of the surrogate with sperm from the husband or a donor, or IVF using an egg from the wife or a donor, and then implantation into the surrogate. New Jersey's 1986 Baby M case is the most famous involving surrogacy, because of the custody dispute between the contracting couple (William and Elizabeth Stern) and the surrogate mother (Mary Beth Whitehead). The surrogacy agreement was ruled illegal by New Jersey's Supreme Court, and the case was determined utilizing family law standards. William Stern was awarded custody of Baby M, and as the birth mother Whitehead received visitation rights. California was the first state to uphold and enforce a surrogacy contract as legally binding in 1993. Among the ethical issues related to surrogacy is a consideration of what is paid for. Is the agreement a personal services contract, like you would have with someone you hire to perform a job, or is it baby selling? Are children now commodities? Surrogacy also raises concerns about the exploitation of poor women, who take on the risks of pregnancy and childbirth for the wealthy out of desperation.

A tension exists among feminists in this regard, whether surrogacy should be considered an autonomous decision that women are capable of making, or if it is a matter of exploitation. **Janice Raymond** contends that concerns about exploitation of women exist in all surrogacy arrangements, not just in commercial surrogacy. Noncommercial surrogacy should not be viewed as altruistic, because even within families there can be exploitation and coercion. Inducements do not have to be monetary, and gifts can be linked to obligations. "Altruism cannot be separated from the history, the values, and the political structures reinforcing women's reproductive inequality in our society." She claims that altruistic reproductive exchanges maintain women as a "breeder class."

In contrast to Raymond, **Alan Wertheimer** contends that even if all surrogacy is exploitative, it is not necessarily unethical. If the exploitation is harmful to the surrogate, or if the exploitation is "moralistic"—involving incommensurable values or wrongful commodification—then it would be unethical. However, exploitation may be voluntary and mutually advantageous to both parties, in which case surrogacy agreements ought to be permitted and even enforced.

Human Cloning

Another type of reproduction is sufficiently different from the others that it deserves separate mention: cloning. Cloning is often viewed through the lens of Aldous Huxley's novel, *Brave New World* (1932). The novel serves as a metaphor, connoting a negative future brought about through the use of technology. In Huxley's fictional world, cloning is used as part of a reproduction process that generates particular kinds of people to fill particular slots in society. They lack the freedom to determine their own futures. *Brave New World* is a powerful story, and such stories tend to have a strong impact, even among people who do not typically employ narrative ethics. **Leon Kass** probably should not be classified as a narrative ethicist, but he does find certain stories particularly insightful, and they shape his thinking. *Brave New World* is one such story, and Kass claims that it provides a profound warning regarding reproductive technology. We need to seize control over where this technology is taking us. Why should we oppose human cloning? Kass provides two kinds of reasons. The first is emotional; we feel repugnance to human cloning, much like John Savage felt toward the clones in *Brave New World*, and we should heed the wisdom of this emotion. He also lists a range of problems that cloning would bring.

Real-life cloning would not necessarily resemble that of *Brave New World*, and the technique used in the book—embryo splitting—differs from the type that Scottish scientist Ian Wilmut used to create Dolly (a cloned sheep) in 1996. (Embryo splitting is commonly used in agriculture, such as with cattle, to produce identical offspring from different mothers.) Wilmut's creation of Dolly was a scientific breakthrough, because the technique—somatic-cell nuclear transfer (SCNT)—had never been successfully used with mammals. SCNT involves removing the nucleus of an egg, and using electricity to fuse the nucleus of an adult cell into the egg, creating a zygote. This fusion sparks cell division, just as fertilization of a standard egg would. The clone thus is a delayed genetic twin that arrives as an infant, not an adult. Dolly was born after 276 failures. Since the creation of Dolly, the success rate has improved, and many other mammals have been cloned, such as dogs, cats, cows, and horses. Cloned animals have also been re-cloned, and clones have reproduced sexually, although many cloned males are sterile (the earliest successful clones were all female). K. C., a cow cloned at the University of Georgia from the cells of a dead cow, gave birth in December 2004 to Sunshine, a calf who seems normal in every way.

Thus far, SCNT has not been used for human reproduction, although there have been a few unsubstantiated claims of attempts and success. In 1997, Wilmut expressed strong opposition to using the technique on humans, saying that he would find it "absolutely offensive." At least fourteen countries, including the United Kingdom, Australia, and Israel, have laws prohibiting human reproductive cloning. In 2001, a Council of Europe protocol prohibiting cloning human beings went into effect, and the United Nations passed a nonbinding resolution against human cloning in 2005. The United States has opposed reproductive cloning at the federal level since 1997, when President Bill Clinton issued a moratorium against the use of federal funds for human cloning research. Federal law does not prohibit privately funded research. At least fifteen states have proceeded to pass their own legislation regarding human cloning. All fifteen ban reproductive cloning, while some support, or are silent about, therapeutic cloning (cloning for the purpose of research or therapy, such as producing stem cells). In 2002, the President's Council on Bioethics recommended that reproductive cloning be banned, because it is unsafe and for five additional reasons. First, cloned humans may face problems of identity and individuality, because they are genetically identical to people who have already lived, and there may be expectations to be like their predecessors (e.g., a Michael Jordan clone would be under pressure to have a stellar basketball career). Second, cloning could contribute to the commodification of children and the commercialization of reproduction. Third, cloning could lead to eugenics, favoring particular genetic traits. Fourth, family relations might be confused, such as if a father and son were genetic twins, thus also "brothers." Finally, there might be a slippery slope impact on society, leading to such things as genetic enhancement and genetic control over the next generation.

Although Kass and many other bioethicists and scientists have made their opposition to human cloning clear, especially during the immediate aftermath of Dolly, several bioethicists and scientists have taken a neutral or more permissive position. In this volume, **Raanan Gillon** explores the large range of arguments against human cloning, among them Kass's notion of repugnance and invocation of *Brave New World*, and others grouped according to the four bioethics principles. Gillon finds most of the arguments to be unconvincing, except for those regarding safety and distributive justice. He argues for a temporary moratorium so that we can have a better-informed discussion before making such an important social decision.

REFERENCES AND FURTHER READING

Annas, George J. "The Supreme Court and Abortion Rights." *New England Journal of Medicine* 356, no. 21 (2007): 2201–7.

Barnhardt, Michael G. "Buddhism and the Morality of Abortion." *Journal of Buddhist Ethics* 5 (1998): 276–97.

Carrick, Paul. *Medical Ethics in the Ancient World*. Washington, DC: Georgetown University Press, 2001.

Cates, Willard, Jr., David A. Grimes, and Kenneth F. Schulz. "The Public Health Impact of Legal Abortion: 30 Years Later." *Perspectives on Sexual and Reproductive Health* 35, no. 1 (2003): 25–28.

Downs, Karen M. "Embryological Origins of the Human Individual." *DNA and Cell Biology* 27, no. 1 (2008): 3–7.

Guttmacher Institute. "State Policies in Brief: An Overview of Abortion Laws." June 1, 2008. http://www.guttmacher.org/statecenter/spibs/spib/_OAL.pdf (accessed June 7, 2008).

———. "State Policies in Brief: Refusing to Provide Health Services." June 1, 2008. http://www.guttmacher.org/statecenter/spibs/spib_RPHS.pdf (accessed June 9, 2008).

Hedayat, K.M., P. Shooshtarizadeh, and M. Raza. "Therapeutic Abortion in Islam: Contemporary Views of Muslim Scholars and Effect of Recent Iranian Legislation." *Journal of Medical Ethics* 32, no. 11 (2006): 652–57.

Huxley, Aldous. *Brave New World*. New York: Harper, 1932.

Little, Margaret. "Abortion, Intimacy, and the Duty to Gestate." *Ethical Theory and Moral Practice* 2, no. 3 (1999): 295–312.

Maguire, Daniel. *Sacred Rights: The Case for Contraception and Abortion in World Religions*. New York: Oxford University Press, 2003.

National Conference of State Legislatures. "Pharmacist Conscience Clauses: Laws and Legislation" 2007. http://www.ncsl.org/programs/health/ConscienceClauses.htm (accessed June 10, 2008).

Mohr, James C. *Abortion in America: The Origins and Evolution of National Policy, 1800–1900*. New York: Oxford University Press, 1978.

Noonan, John T. "An Almost Absolute Value in History." In *The Morality of Abortion: Legal and Historical Perspectives*. Cambridge, MA: Harvard University Press, 1970: 51–59.

Pence, Gregory. *Cloning After Dolly: Who's Still Afraid?* Totowa, NJ: Rowman & Littlefield, 2005.

President's Council on Bioethics. *Human Cloning and Human Dignity: An Ethical Inquiry.* 2007. www.bioethics.gov.

———. *Reproduction and Responsibility: The Regulation of New Biotechnologies*. 2004. www.bioethics.gov.

Reagan, Leslie J. *When Abortion Was a Crime: Women, Medicine, and Law in the United States, 1867–1973*. Berkeley: University of California Press, 1996.

Rosner, Fred. "Abortion." In *Biomedical Ethics and Jewish Law,* edited by Fred Rosner, 175–96. Hoboken, NJ: Ktav Publishing, 2001.

United States Supreme Court. *Roe v. Wade*. 410 U.S. 113 (1973).

———. *Webster v. Reproductive Health Services*. 492 U.S. 490 (1989).

———. *Planned Parenthood v. Casey*. 505 U.S. 833 (1992).

———. *Stenberg v. Carhart*. 530 U.S. 914 (2000).

———. *Gonzales v. Carhart*. 550 U.S. 124 (2007).

Virk, Jasveer, Jun Zhang, and Jørn Olsen. "Medical Abortion and the Risk of Subsequent Adverse Pregnancy Outcomes." *New England Journal of Medicine* 357, no. 7 (2007): 648–53.

Warren, Mary Anne. "On the Moral and Legal Status of Abortion." *The Monist* 57, no. 1 (1973): 43–61.

World Health Organization. *Unsafe Abortion: Global and Regional Estimates Of Incidence of Unsafe Abortion and Associated Mortality in 2003*. 5th ed. 2007. http://www.who .int/reproductive-health/publications/unsafeabortion_2003/ua_estimates03.pdf (accessed June 9, 2008).

DISCUSSION QUESTIONS FOR THE READINGS

A Defense of Abortion

1. Would it be morally acceptable to unplug yourself from the violinist? Does his right to life create an obligation on your part?

2. What difference would it make if the duration of time was one hour, nine months, or nine years?

3. Are Thomson's cases (unconscious violinist, box of chocolates, and open windows) sufficiently analogous to pregnancy?

4. Should the focus regarding abortion be on what mothers may do or what third parties may do?

5. Is continuing a pregnancy like being a Good Samaritan?

Abortion and the Beginning and End of Human Life

1. Does Marquis provide a persuasive argument against the "standard view"?

2. Do you find the "future of value" view superior to the standard view regarding the wrongness of killing and beginning of life issues?

3. Do you think that abortion opponents would be better served by adopting the future of value view?

4. Would the future of value view prohibit all abortions? Might abortions still be permitted, as per Thomson's article?

Feminist Discourse on Sex Screening and Selective Abortion of Female Foetuses

1. Is feminism culturally relative?

2. Is the consent given by Indian women for prenatal gender screening truly voluntary?

3. Is the limitation on Indian women's autonomy to make decisions regarding prenatal gender screening ethically justifiable? Is it a dangerous state intrusion into the procreative rights of women?

Could Artificial Wombs End the Abortion Debate?

1. Should ethical abortion involve the right to terminate the fetus, or only the right to terminate the pregnancy (i.e., evacuation)?

2. Are there reasons to believe that artificial wombs would not end the abortion debate for supporters of choice?

3. Does Kaczor successfully address Catholic concerns regarding partial ectogenesis?

The Limits of Conscientious Objection: May Pharmacists Refuse to Fill Prescriptions for Emergency Contraception?

1. Why should an objecting pharmacist refer a patient elsewhere for emergency contraception?

2. Would the pharmacist still be participating in an immoral action by providing the referral?

3. If no reasonable alternatives exist for a patient, is a pharmacist obligated to provide emergency contraception in spite of moral objections?

4. Cantor and Baum claim that health professionals have a right to object, but not a right to obstruct. What do you understand this claim to mean?

Distinguishing Features of Women's Health Care

1. Should a pregnant woman and her fetus be considered as separate and separable patients?

2. Should a fetus be considered a patient independent of its presentation by the pregnant woman, or in spite of her objections?

3. Is the moral status of the fetus determined by the decisions of the pregnant woman?

A Realistic Approach to Maternal-Fetal Conflict

1. Is the maternal-fetal relationship contingent upon the pregnant woman's attitude toward her pregnancy?
2. Does a fetus have the right to be born healthy? Does a pregnant woman have a duty to refrain from activities that could damage a fetus's health?
3. Has technology like ultrasound led to viewing a fetus as a person, separate from its mother?

What Are Families For? Getting to an Ethics of Reproductive Technology

1. Are the claims of procreative liberty (autonomy and control) necessarily divorced from the values of families and relationships (love, loyalty, intimacy)?
2. Might not a desire to experience parenthood along with its associated values lead someone to make a liberty-based appeal in order to achieve it?
3. How would a flourishing-centered approach to reproductive technology discern who may use it and who may not?

Whose Bodies? Which Selves? Appeals to Embodiment in Assessments of Reproductive Technology

1. Do the problems that Corea identifies with reproductive technology mean that it should be banned? Can these problems be avoided?
2. Do you think that reproductive technology violates the purpose of sexuality, marriage and family, as understood by the Catholic Church?
3. Do you think that there are more similarities or differences between the feminist and Catholic opposition to reproductive technology?
4. Is Lauritzen correct when he says that feminists who discount the value to women of pregnancy and parenthood have not taken embodiment seriously enough?

Reproductive Gifts and Gift Giving: The Altruistic Woman

1. Is altruistic surrogacy morally superior to commercial surrogacy?
2. Is altruistic surrogacy truly voluntary?
3. Does altruistic surrogacy exploit women any less than does commercial surrogacy?
4. Does surrogacy reinforce gender inequality?

Two Questions About Surrogacy and Exploitation

1. Is surrogacy necessarily harmful exploitation of women?
2. Is the commodification of pregnancy necessarily harmful to women?
3. Is surrogacy an inherently immoral activity, thus harmful to women who participate in it?
4. Can a mutually advantageous surrogacy arrangement still involve morally unacceptable exploitation?

Preventing a *Brave New World*: Why We Should Ban Cloning Now

1. Is human cloning a gateway to a *Brave New World* society?
2. Does the prospect of human cloning cause you to feel revulsion?

3. Would cloning necessarily create serious issues of identity and individuality?

4. Would cloning negatively impact the meaning of having children and the parent-child relationship?

5. Should laws be enacted to prohibit human cloning?

Human Reproductive Cloning: A Look at the Arguments Against It and a Rejection of Most of Them

1. How can a person discern which gut feelings should be followed and which should not?

2. Does the novel *Brave New World* provide reasons to oppose human cloning?

3. Is human cloning unnatural?

4. Does reproductive cloning violate human dignity?

5. Would human cloning likely cause harm to the resulting children or to society?

READINGS

A Defense of Abortion

JUDITH JARVIS THOMSON

Philosophy and Public Affairs 1, no. 1 (1971): 47–66.

Most opposition to abortion relies on the premise that the fetus is a human being, a person, from the moment of conception. The premise is argued for, but, as I think, not well. Take, for example, the most common argument. We are asked to notice that the development of a human being from conception through birth into childhood is continuous; then it is said that to draw a line, to choose a point in this development and say "before this point the thing is not a person, after this point it is a person" is to make an arbitrary choice, a choice for which in the nature of things no good reason can be given. It is concluded that the fetus is, or anyway that we had better say it is, a person from the moment of conception. But this conclusion does not follow. Similar things might be said about the development of an acorn into an oak tree, and it does not follow that acorns are oak trees, or that we had better say they are.

I am inclined to agree, however, that the prospects for "drawing a line" in the development of the fetus look dim. I am inclined to think also that we shall probably have to agree that the fetus has already become a human person well before birth. Indeed, it comes as a surprise when one first learns how early in its life it begins to acquire human characteristics. By the tenth week, for example, it already has a face, arms and legs, fingers and toes; it has internal organs, and brain activity is detectable. On the other hand, I think that the premise is false, that the fetus is not a person from the moment of conception. A newly fertilized ovum, a newly implanted clump of cells, is no more a person than an acorn is an oak tree. But I shall not discuss any of this. For it seems to me to be of great interest to ask what happens if, for the sake of argument, we allow the premise. How, precisely, are we supposed to get from there to the conclusion that abortion is morally impermissible? Opponents of abortion commonly spend most of their time establishing that the fetus is a person, and hardly any time explaining the step from there to the impermissibility of abortion. Perhaps they think the step too simple and obvious to require much comment. Or perhaps instead they are simply being economical in argument. Many of those who defend abortion rely on the premise that the fetus is not a person, but only a bit of tissue that will become a person at birth; and why pay out more arguments than you have to? Whatever the explanation, I suggest that the step they take is neither easy nor obvious, that it calls for closer examination than it is commonly given, and that when we do give it this closer examination we shall feel inclined to reject it.

I propose, then, that we grant that the fetus is a person from the moment of conception. How does the argument go from here? Something like this, I take it. Every person has a right to life. So the fetus has a right to life. No doubt the mother has a right to decide what shall happen in and to her body; everyone would grant that. But surely a person's right to life is stronger and more stringent than the mother's right to decide what happens in and to her body, and so outweighs it. So the fetus may not be killed; an abortion may not be performed.

It sounds plausible. But now let me ask you to imagine this. You wake up in the morning and find yourself back to back in bed with an unconscious violinist. A famous unconscious violinist. He has been found to have a fatal kidney ailment, and the Society of Music Lovers has canvassed all the available medical records and found that you alone have the right blood type to help. They have therefore kidnapped you, and last night the violinist's circulatory system was plugged into yours, so that your kidneys can be used to extract poisons from his blood as well as your own. The

director of the hospital now tells you, "Look, we're sorry the Society of Music Lovers did this to you—we would never have permitted it if we had known. But still, they did it, and the violinist now is plugged into you. To unplug you would be to kill him. But never mind, it's only for nine months. By then he will have recovered from his ailment, and can safely be unplugged from you." Is it morally incumbent on you to accede to this situation? No doubt it would be very nice of you if you did, a great kindness. But do you *have* to accede to it? What if it were not nine months, but nine years? Or longer still? What if the director of the hospital says, "Tough luck, I agree, but you've now got to stay in bed, with the violinist plugged into you, for the rest of your life. Because remember this. All persons have a right to life, and violinists are persons. Granted you have a right to decide what happens in and to your body, but a person's right to life outweighs your right to decide what happens in and to your body. So you cannot ever be unplugged from him." I imagine you would regard this as outrageous, which suggests that something really is wrong with that plausible-sounding argument I mentioned a moment ago.

In this case, of course, you were kidnapped; you didn't volunteer for the operation that plugged the violinist into your kidneys. Can those who oppose abortion on the ground I mentioned make an exception for a pregnancy due to rape? Certainly. They can say that persons have a right to life only if they didn't come into existence because of rape; or they can say that all persons have a right to life, but that some have less of a right to life than others, in particular, that those who came into existence because of rape have less. But these statements have a rather unpleasant sound. Surely the question of whether you have a right to life at all, or how much of it you have, shouldn't turn on the question of whether or not you are the product of a rape. And in fact the people who oppose abortion on the ground I mentioned do not make this distinction, and hence do not make an exception in case of rape.

Nor do they make an exception for a case in which the mother has to spend the nine months of her pregnancy in bed. They would agree that would be a great pity, and hard on the mother; but all the same, all persons have a right to life, the fetus is a person, and so on. I suspect, in fact, that they would not make an exception for a case in which, miraculously enough, the pregnancy went on for nine years, or even the rest of the mother's life.

Some won't even make an exception for a case in which continuation of the pregnancy is likely to shorten the mother's life; they regard abortion as impermissible even to save the mother's life. Such cases are nowadays very rare, and many opponents of abortion do not accept this extreme view. All the same, it is a good place to begin: a number of points of interest come out in respect to it.

I. Let us call the view that abortion is impermissible even to save the mother's life "the extreme view." I want to suggest first that it does not issue from the argument I mentioned earlier without the addition of some fairly powerful premises. Suppose a woman has become pregnant, and now learns that she has a cardiac condition such that she will die if she carries the baby to term. What may be done for her? The fetus, being a person, has a right to life, but as the mother is a person too, so has she a right to life. Presumably they have an equal right to life. How is it supposed to come out that an abortion may not be performed? If mother and child have an equal right to life, shouldn't we perhaps flip a coin? Or should we add to the mother's right to life her right to decide what happens in and to her body, which everybody seems to be ready to grant—the sum of her rights now outweighing the fetus' right to life?

The most familiar argument here is the following. We are told that performing the abortion would be directly killing the child, whereas doing nothing would not be killing the mother, but only letting her die. Moreover, in killing the child, one would be killing an innocent person, for the child has committed no crime, and is not aiming at his mother's death.

If directly killing an innocent person is murder, and thus is impermissible, then the mother's directly killing the innocent person inside her is murder, and thus is impermissible. But it cannot seriously be thought to be murder if the mother performs an abortion on herself to save her life. It cannot seriously be said that she *must* refrain, that she *must* sit passively by and wait for her death. Let us look again at the case of you and the violinist. There you are, in bed with the violinist, and the director of the hospital says to you, "It's all most distressing, and I deeply sympathize, but you see this is putting an additional strain on your kidneys, and you'll be dead within the month. But you *have* to stay where you are all the same. Because unplugging you would be directly killing an innocent violinist, and that's murder, and that's impermissible." If anything in the world is true, it is that you do not commit murder, you do not do what is impermissible, if you reach around to your back and unplug yourself from that violinist to save your life.

The main focus of attention in writings on abortion has been on what a third party may or may not do in answer to a request from a woman for an abortion. This is in a way understandable. Things being as they are, there isn't much a woman can safely do to abort herself. So the question asked is what a third party may do, and what the mother may do, if it is mentioned at all, is deduced, almost as an after-thought, from what it is concluded that third parties may do. But it seems to me that to treat the matter in this way is to refuse to grant to the mother that very status of person which is so firmly insisted on for the fetus. For we cannot simply read off what a person may do from what a third party may do.

I should perhaps stop to say explicitly that I am not claiming that people have a right to do anything whatever to save their lives. I think, rather, that there are drastic limits to the right of self-defense. If someone threatens you with death unless you torture someone else to death, I think you have not the right, even to save your life, to do so. But the case under consideration here is very different. In our case there are only two people involved, one whose life is threatened, and one who threatens it. Both are innocent: the one who is threatened is not threatened because of any fault, the one who threatens does not threaten because of any fault. For this reason we may feel that we bystanders cannot intervene. But the person threatened can.

In sum, a woman surely can defend her life against the threat to it posed by the unborn child, even if doing so involves its death. And this shows that the extreme view of abortion is false.

2. The extreme view could of course be weakened to say that while abortion is permissible to save the mother's life, it may not be performed by a third party, but only by the mother herself. But this cannot be right either. For what we have to keep in mind is that the mother and the unborn child are not like two tenants in a small house which has, by an unfortunate mistake, been rented to both: the mother *owns* the house. The fact that she does adds to the offensiveness of deducing that the mother can do nothing from the supposition that third parties can do nothing. But it does more than this: it casts a bright light on the supposition that third parties can do nothing. Certainly it lets us see that a third party who says "I cannot choose between you" is fooling himself if he thinks this is impartiality. If Jones has found and fastened on a certain coat, which he needs to keep him from freezing, but which Smith also needs to keep him from freezing, then it is not impartiality that says "I cannot choose between you" when Smith owns the coat. Women have said again and again "This body is *my* body!" and they have reason to feel angry, reason to feel that it has been like shouting into the wind.

We should really ask what it is that says "no one may choose" in the face of the fact that the body that houses the child is the mother's body. It may be simply a failure to appreciate this

fact. But it may be something more interesting, namely the sense that one has a right to refuse to lay hands on people, even where it would be just and fair to do so, even where justice seems to require that somebody do so. Thus justice might call for somebody to get Smith's coat back from Jones, and yet you have a right to refuse to be the one to lay hands on Jones, a right to refuse to do physical violence to him. This, I think, must be granted. But then what should be said is not "no one may choose," but only "*I* cannot choose," and indeed not even this, but "*I* will not *act*," leaving it open that somebody else can or should, and in particular that anyone in a position of authority, with the job of securing people's rights, both can and should. So this is no difficulty. I have not been arguing that any given third party must accede to the mother's request that he perform an abortion to save her life, but only that he may.

3. Where the mother's life is not at stake, the argument I mentioned at the outset seems to have a much stronger pull. "Everyone has a right to life, so the unborn person has a right to life." And isn't the child's right to life weightier than anything other than the mother's own right to life, which she might put forward as ground for an abortion?

This argument treats the right to life as if it were unproblematic. It is not, and this seems to me to be precisely the source of the mistake.

For we should now, at long last, ask what it comes to, to have a right to life. In some views having a right to life includes having a right to be given at least the bare minimum one needs for continued life. But suppose that what in fact *is* the bare minimum a man needs for continued life is something he has no right at all to be given? If I am sick unto death, and the only thing that will save my life is the touch of Henry Fonda's cool hand on my fevered brow, then all the same, I have no right to be given the touch of Henry Fonda's cool hand on my fevered brow. It would be frightfully nice of him to fly in from the West Coast to provide it. It would be less nice, though no doubt well meant, if my friends flew out to the West Coast and carried Henry Fonda back with them. But I have no right at all against anybody that he should do this for me. Or again, to return to the story I told earlier, the fact that for continued life that violinist needs the continued use of your kidneys does not establish that he has a right to be given the continued use of your kidneys. He certainly has no right against you that *you* should give him continued use of your kidneys. For nobody has any right to use your kidneys unless you give him such a right; and nobody has the right against you that you shall give him this right—if you do allow him to go on using your kidneys, this is a kindness on your part, and not something he can claim from you as his due. Nor has he any right against anybody else that *they* should give him continued use of your kidneys. Certainly he had no right against the Society of Music Lovers that they should plug him into you in the first place. And if you now start to unplug yourself, having learned that you will otherwise have to spend nine years in bed with him, there is nobody in the world who must try to prevent you, in order to see to it that he is given something he has a right to be given.

Some people are rather stricter about the right to life. In their view, it does not include the right to be given anything, but amounts to, and only to, the right not to be killed by anybody. But here a related difficulty arises. If everybody is to refrain from killing that violinist, then everybody must refrain from doing a great many different sorts of things. Everybody must refrain from slitting his throat, everybody must refrain from shooting him—and everybody must refrain from unplugging you from him. But does he have a right against everybody that they shall refrain from unplugging you from him? I shall come back to third-party interventions later. But certainly the violinist has no right against you that *you* shall allow him to continue to use your kidneys. As I said, if you do allow him to use them, it is a kindness on your part, and not something you owe him.

I would stress that I am not arguing that people do not have a right to life—quite to the contrary, it seems to me that the primary control we must place on the acceptability of an account of rights is that it should turn out in that account to be a truth that all persons have a right to life. I am arguing only that having a right to life does not guarantee having either a right to be given the use of or a right to be allowed continued use of another person's body—even if one needs it for life itself. So the right to life will not serve the opponents of abortion in the very simple and clear way in which they seem to have thought it would.

4. There is another way to bring out the difficulty. In the most ordinary sort of case, to deprive someone of what he has a right to is to treat him unjustly. Suppose a boy and his small brother are jointly given a box of chocolates for Christmas. If the older boy takes the box and refuses to give his brother any of the chocolates, he is unjust to him, for the brother has been given a right to half of them. But suppose that, having learned that otherwise it means nine years in bed with that violinist, you unplug yourself from him. You surely are not being unjust to him, for you gave him no right to use your kidneys, and no one else can have given him any such right. But we have to notice that in unplugging yourself, you are killing him; and violinists, like everybody else, have a right to life, but you do not act unjustly to him in doing it.

The emendation which may be made at this point is this: the right to life consists not in the right not to be killed, but rather in the right not to be killed unjustly.

But if this emendation is accepted, the gap in the argument against abortion stares us plainly in the face: it is by no means enough to show that the fetus is a person, and to remind us that all persons have a right to life—we need to be shown also that killing the fetus violates its right to life, i.e., that abortion is unjust killing. And is it?

I suppose we may take it as a datum that in a case of pregnancy due to rape the mother has not given the unborn person a right to the use of her body for food and shelter. Indeed, in what pregnancy could it be supposed that the mother has given the unborn person such a right? It is not as if there were unborn persons drifting about the world, to whom a woman who wants a child says "I invite you in."

But it might be argued that there are other ways one can have acquired a right to the use of another person's body than by having been invited to use it by that person. Suppose a woman voluntarily indulges in intercourse, knowing of the chance it will issue in pregnancy, and then she does become pregnant; is she not in part responsible for the presence, in fact the very existence, of the unborn person inside her? No doubt she did not invite it in. But doesn't her partial responsibility for its being there itself give it a right to the use of her body? If so, then her aborting it would be more like the boy's taking away the chocolates, and less like your unplugging yourself from the violinist—doing so would be depriving it of what it does have a right to, and thus would be doing it an injustice.

And then, too, it might be asked whether or not she can kill it even to save her own life: If she voluntarily called it into existence, how can she now kill it, even in self-defense?

The first thing to be said about this is that it is something new. Opponents of abortion have been so concerned to make out the independence of the fetus, in order to establish that it has a right to life, just as its mother does, that they have tended to overlook the possible support they might gain from making out that the fetus is *dependent* on the mother, in order to establish that she has a special kind of responsibility for it, a responsibility that gives it rights against her which are not possessed by any independent person—such as an ailing violinist who is a stranger to her.

On the other hand, this argument would give the unborn person a right to its mother's body only if her pregnancy resulted from a voluntary act, undertaken in full knowledge of the chance a pregnancy might result from it. It would leave out entirely the unborn person whose existence is due to rape. Pending the availability of some further argument, then, we would be left with the conclusion that unborn persons whose existence is due to rape have no right to the use of their mothers' bodies, and thus that aborting them is not depriving them of anything they have a right to and hence is not unjust killing.

And we should also notice that it is not at all plain that this argument really does go even as far as it purports to. For there are cases and cases, and the details make a difference. If the room is stuffy, and I therefore open a window to air it, and a burglar climbs in, it would be absurd to say, "Ah, now he can stay, she's given him a right to the use of her house—for she is partially responsible for his presence there, having voluntarily done what enabled him to get in, in full knowledge that there are such things as burglars, and that burglars burgle." It would be still more absurd to say this if I had had bars installed outside my windows, precisely to prevent burglars from getting in, and a burglar got in only because of a defect in the bars. It remains equally absurd if we imagine it is not a burglar who climbs in, but an innocent person who blunders or falls in. Again, suppose it were like this: people-seeds drift about in the air like pollen, and if you open your windows, one may drift in and take root in your carpets or upholstery. You don't want children, so you fix up your windows with fine mesh screens, the very best you can buy. As can happen, however, and on very, very rare occasions does happen, one of the screens is defective; and a seed drifts in and takes root. Does the person-plant who now develops have a right to the use of your house? Surely not—despite the fact that you voluntarily opened your windows, you knowingly kept carpets and upholstered furniture, and you knew that screens were sometimes defective. Someone may argue that you are responsible for its rooting, that it does have a right to your house, because after all you *could* have lived out your life with bare floors and furniture, or with sealed windows and doors. But this won't do—for by the same token anyone can avoid a pregnancy due to rape by having a hysterectomy, or anyway by never leaving home without a (reliable!) army.

It seems to me that the argument we are looking at can establish at most that there are *some* cases in which the unborn person has a right to the use of its mother's body, and therefore *some* cases in which abortion is unjust killing. There is room for much discussion and argument as to precisely which, if any. But I think we should sidestep this issue and leave it open, for at any rate the argument certainly does not establish that all abortion is unjust killing.

5. There is room for yet another argument here, however. We surely must all grant that there may be cases in which it would be morally indecent to detach a person from your body at the cost of his life. Suppose you learn that what the violinist needs is not nine years of your life, but only one hour: all you need do to save his life is to spend one hour in that bed with him. Suppose also that letting him use your kidneys for that one hour would not affect your health in the slightest. Admittedly you were kidnapped. Admittedly you did not give anyone permission to plug him into you. Nevertheless it seems to me plain you *ought* to allow him to use your kidneys for that hour—it would be indecent to refuse.

Again, suppose pregnancy lasted only an hour, and constituted no threat to life or health. And suppose that a woman becomes pregnant as a result of rape. Admittedly she did not voluntarily do anything to bring about the existence of a child. Admittedly she did nothing at all which would give the unborn person a right to the use of her body. All the same it might well be said, as in the newly emended violinist story, that she *ought* to allow it to remain for that hour—that it would be indecent in her to refuse.

Now some people are inclined to use the term "right" in such a way that it follows from the fact that you ought to allow a person to use your body for the hour he needs, that he has a right to use your body for the hour he needs, even though he has not been given that right by any person or act. They may say that it follows also that if you refuse, you act unjustly toward him. This use of the term is perhaps so common that it cannot be called wrong; nevertheless it seems to me to be an unfortunate loosening of what we would do better to keep a tight rein on. Suppose that box of chocolates I mentioned earlier had not been given to both boys jointly, but was given only to the older boy. There he sits, stolidly eating his way through the box, his small brother watching enviously. Here we are likely to say "You ought not to be so mean. You ought to give your brother some of those chocolates." My own view is that it just does not follow from the truth of this that the brother has any right to any of the chocolates. If the boy refuses to give his brother any, he is greedy, stingy, callous—but not unjust. I suppose that the people I have in mind will say it does follow that the brother has a right to some of the chocolates, and thus that the boy does act unjustly if he refuses to give his brother any. But the effect of saying this is to obscure what we should keep distinct, namely the difference between the boy's refusal in this case and the boy's refusal in the earlier case, in which the box was given to both boys jointly, and in which the small brother thus had what was from any point of view clear title to half.

A further objection to so using the term "right" that from the fact that A ought to do a thing for B, it follows that B has a right against A that A do it for him, is that it is going to make the question of whether or not a man has a right to a thing turn on how easy it is to provide him with it; and this seems not merely unfortunate, but morally unacceptable. Take the case of Henry Fonda again. I said earlier that I had no right to the touch of his cool hand on my fevered brow, even though I needed it to save my life. I said it would be frightfully nice of him to fly in from the West Coast to provide me with it, but that I had no right against him that he should do so. But suppose he isn't on the West Coast. Suppose he has only to walk across the room, place a hand briefly on my brow—and lo, my life is saved. Then surely he ought to do it, it would be indecent to refuse. Is it to be said "Ah, well, it follows that in this case she has a right to the touch of his hand on her brow, and so it would be an injustice in him to refuse"? So that I have a right to it when it is easy for him to provide it, though no right when it's hard? It's rather a shocking idea that anyone's rights should fade away and disappear as it gets harder and harder to accord them to him.

So my own view is that even though you ought to let the violinist use your kidneys for the one hour he needs, we should not conclude that he has a right to do so—we should say that if you refuse, you are, like the boy who owns all the chocolates and will give none away, self-centered and callous, indecent in fact, but not unjust. And similarly, that even supposing a case in which a woman pregnant due to rape ought to allow the unborn person to use her body for the hour he needs, we should not conclude that he has a right to do so; we should conclude that she is self-centered, callous, indecent, but not unjust, if she refuses. The complaints are no less grave; they are just different. However, there is no need to insist on this point. If anyone does wish to deduce "he has a right" from "you ought," then all the same he must surely grant that there are cases in which it is not morally required of you that you allow that violinist to use your kidneys, and in which he does not have a right to use them, and in which you do not do him an injustice if you refuse. And so also for mother and unborn child. Except in such cases as the unborn person has a right to demand it—and we were leaving open the possibility that there may be such cases—nobody is morally *required* to make large sacrifices, of health, of all other interests and concerns, of all other duties and commitments, for nine years, or even for

nine months, in order to keep another person alive.

6. We have in fact to distinguish between two kinds of Samaritan: the Good Samaritan and what we might call the Minimally Decent Samaritan. The story of the Good Samaritan, you will remember, goes like this:

> A certain man went down from Jerusalem to Jericho, and fell among thieves, which stripped him of his raiment, and wounded him, and departed, leaving him half dead.
>
> And by chance there came down a certain priest that way; and when he saw him, he passed by on the other side.
>
> And likewise a Levite, when he was at the place, came and looked on him, and passed by on the other side.
>
> But a certain Samaritan, as he journeyed, came where he was; and when he saw him he had compassion on him.
>
> And went to him, and bound up his wounds, pouring in oil and wine, and set him on his own beast, and brought him to an inn, and took care of him.
>
> And on the morrow, when he departed, he took out two pence, and gave them to the host, and said unto him, "Take care of him; and whatsoever thou spendest more, when I come again, I will repay thee."
>
> (Luke 10:30–35)

The Good Samaritan went out of his way, at some cost to himself, to help one in need of it. We are not told what the options were, that is, whether or not the priest and the Levite could have helped by doing less than the Good Samaritan did, but assuming they could have, then the fact they did nothing at all shows they were not even Minimally Decent Samaritans, not because they were not Samaritans, but because they were not even minimally decent.

These things are a matter of degree, of course, but there is a difference, and it comes out perhaps most clearly in the story of Kitty Genovese, who, as you will remember, was murdered while thirty-eight people watched or listened, and did nothing at all to help her. A Good Samaritan would have rushed out to give direct assistance against the murderer. Or perhaps we had better allow that it would have been a Splendid Samaritan who did this, on the ground that it would have involved a risk of death for himself. But the thirty-eight not only did not do this, they did not even trouble to pick up a phone to call the police. Minimally Decent Samaritanism would call for doing at least that, and their not having done it was monstrous.

After telling the story of the Good Samaritan, Jesus said "Go, and do thou likewise." Perhaps he meant that we are morally required to act as the Good Samaritan did. Perhaps he was urging people to do more than is morally required of them. At all events it seems plain that it was not morally required of any of the thirty-eight that he rush out to give direct assistance at the risk of his own life, and that it is not morally required of anyone that he give long stretches of his life—nine years or nine months—to sustaining the life of a person who has no special right (we were leaving open the possibility of this) to demand it.

Indeed, with one rather striking class of exceptions, no one in any country in the world is *legally* required to do anywhere near as much as this for anyone else. The class of exceptions is obvious. My main concern here is not the state of the law in respect to abortion, but it is worth drawing attention to the fact that in no state in this country is any man compelled by law to be even a Minimally Decent Samaritan to any person; there is no law under which charges could be brought against the thirty-eight who stood by while Kitty Genovese died. By contrast, in most states in this country women are compelled by law to be not merely Minimally Decent Samaritans, but Good Samaritans to unborn persons inside them.

But we are not here concerned with the law. What we should ask is not whether anybody should be compelled by law to be a Good Samaritan, but whether we must accede to a situation in which somebody is being compelled—by nature, perhaps—to be a Good Samaritan. We have, in other words, to look now at third-party interventions. I have been arguing that no person is morally required to make large sacrifices to sustain the life of another who has no right to demand them, and this even where the sacrifices do not include life itself; we are not morally required to be Good Samaritans or anyway Very Good Samaritans to one another. But what if a man cannot extricate himself from such a situation? What if he appeals to us to extricate him? It seems to me plain that there are cases in which we can, cases in which a Good Samaritan would extricate him. There you are, you were kidnapped, and nine years in bed with that violinist lie ahead of you. You have your own life to lead. You are sorry, but you simply cannot see giving up so much of your life to the sustaining of his. You cannot extricate yourself, and ask us to do so. I should have thought that—in light of his having no right to the use of your body—it was obvious that we do not have to accede to your being forced to give up so much. We can do what you ask. There is no injustice to the violinist in our doing so.

7. Following the lead of the opponents of abortion, I have throughout been speaking of the fetus merely as a person, and what I have been asking is whether or not the argument we began with, which proceeds only from the fetus' being a person, really does establish its conclusion. I have argued that it does not.

But of course there are arguments and arguments, and it may be said that I have simply fastened on the wrong one. It may be said that what is important is not merely the fact that the fetus is a person, but that it is a person for whom the woman has a special kind of responsibility issuing from the fact that she is its mother. And it might be argued that all my analogies are therefore irrelevant—for you do not have that special kind of responsibility for that violinist, Henry Fonda does not have that special kind of responsibility for me. And our attention might be drawn to the fact that men and women both *are* compelled by law to provide support for their children.

I have in effect dealt (briefly) with this argument in section 4 above; but a (still briefer) recapitulation now may be in order. Surely we do not have any such "special responsibility" for a person unless we have assumed it, explicitly or implicitly. If a set of parents do not try to prevent pregnancy, do not obtain an abortion, and then at the time of birth of the child do not put it out for adoption, but rather take it home with them, then they have assumed responsibility for it, they have given it rights, and they cannot *now* withdraw support from it at the cost of its life because they now find it difficult to go on providing for it. But if they have taken all reasonable precautions against having a child, they do not simply by virtue of their biological relationship to the child who comes into existence have a special responsibility for it. They may wish to assume responsibility for it, or they may not wish to. And I am suggesting that if assuming responsibility for it would require large sacrifices, then they may refuse. A Good Samaritan would not refuse—or anyway, a Splendid Samaritan, if the sacrifices that had to be made were enormous. But then so would a Good Samaritan assume responsibility for that violinist; so would Henry Fonda, if he is a Good Samaritan, fly in from the West Coast and assume responsibility for me.

8. My argument will be found unsatisfactory on two counts by many of those who want to regard abortion as morally permissible. First, while I do argue that abortion is not impermissible, I do not argue that it is always permissible. I am inclined to think it a merit of my account precisely that it does *not* give a general yes or a general no. It allows for and supports our sense that, for example, a sick and desperately frightened fourteen-year-old schoolgirl, pregnant due to rape, may *of course* choose abortion, and that any law which rules this out is an insane law. And it also allows for and supports our sense that in other cases resort to abortion is even positively indecent. It would be indecent in the woman to request an abortion, and indecent in a doctor to perform it, if she is in her seventh month, and wants the abortion just to avoid the nuisance of postponing a trip abroad.

Secondly, while I am arguing for the permissibility of abortion in some cases, I am not arguing for the right to secure the death of the unborn child. It is easy to confuse these two things in that up to a certain point in the life of the fetus it is not able to survive outside the mother's body; hence removing it from her body guarantees its death. But they are importantly different. I have argued that you are not morally required to spend nine months in bed, sustaining the life of that violinist; but to say this is by no means to say that if, when you unplug yourself, there is a miracle and he survives, you then have a right to turn round and slit his throat. You may detach yourself even if this costs him his life; you have no right to be guaranteed his death, by some other means, if unplugging yourself does not kill him. There are some people who will feel dissatisfied by this feature of my argument. A woman may be utterly devastated by the thought of a child, a bit of herself, put out for adoption and never seen or heard of again. She may therefore want not merely that the child be detached from her, but more, that it die. All the same, I agree that the desire for the child's death is not one which anybody may gratify, should it turn out to be possible to detach the child alive.

At this place, however, it should be remembered that we have only been pretending throughout that the fetus is a human being from the moment of conception. A very early abortion is surely not the killing of a person, and so is not dealt with by anything I have said here.

Abortion and the Beginning and End of Human Life

DON MARQUIS

Journal of Law, Medicine and Ethics 34, no. 1 (2006): 16–25.

How can the abortion issue be resolved? Many believe that the issue can be resolved if, and only if, we can determine when human life begins. Those opposed to abortion choice typically say that human life begins at conception. Many who favor abortion choice say that we will never know when human life begins. The importance of the when-does-human-life-begin issue is not so much argued for as it is taken to be self-evident. Furthermore, belief that this issue is fundamental is taken for granted – at least outside of philosophy – by many of the people who seem to disagree about almost everything else concerning abortion. It has been my experience that – with rare exceptions – even those who insist that the issue of abortion should focus on the interests of pregnant women believe that this focus is warranted because fetuses are either not yet fully alive or not yet fully human.

This assumption is not unreasonable. It has been taken for granted at the highest levels. Consider, for example, the most famous legal opinions concerning abortion, the majority opinions in *Roe v. Wade* and *Planned Parenthood v. Casey.*

Justice Harry Blackmun, writing for the majority in *Roe,* said:

> We need not resolve the difficult question of when life begins. When those trained in the respective disciplines of medicine, philosophy, and theology are unable to arrive at any consensus, the judiciary, at this point in the development of man's knowledge, is not in a position to speculate as to the answer.

Blackmun went on to defend this view. First, he claimed that according to many religions and philosophies, life does not begin before live birth.

Second, Blackmun went on to defend the view that "In areas other than criminal abortion, the law has been reluctant to endorse any theory that life, as we recognize it, begins before live birth or to accord legal rights to the unborn...." He concluded that the court had neither judicial precedent nor philosophical or theological authority for making a decision based on the judgment that life begins before live birth. It is not hard to understand how this conclusion, when combined with women's liberty rights or privacy rights, leads to the permissibility of abortion.

Blackmun's view deserves discussion. Suppose it is true that life does not begin before live birth. Given this, what is the appropriate way to think of fetuses? It follows from our supposition that we should not think of fetuses as *now* actually alive. Since life presumably begins at the time of live birth, these fetuses will become alive at a later date under favorable environmental conditions. This explains, at least in part, why, when thinking of fetuses, Blackmun spoke of the state's legitimate interest in "protecting the *potentiality* of human life" (my emphasis).

This same language turns up often in *Planned Parenthood v. Casey.* In this opinion the State's interest in potential life, or the State's interest in the *protection* of potential life is repeatedly mentioned. What is the nature and extent of this interest? One would naturally suppose the Court to be claiming that the State has *some* interest in the protection of a fetus in virtue of its interest in potential life. There is, however, a problem with this supposition. If the State has an interest in fetuses because they are potential lives, then the State should also have an interest in gametes because they are potential lives.

Reflection on Blackmun's view suggests another question. Just what is the nature of this potential life in which the State is supposed to have an interest? Potential life talk seems to result from the denial that there is good reason for believing that fetuses are actually alive, and the acknowledgement that under the appropriate conditions the individuals in the fetal phase of existence would later be actually alive. Neither of these characterizations are of the present nature of fetuses. Certainly it is legitimate to ask what about a fetus, *when it is a fetus*, makes it potentially alive? If one considers what it is about fetuses that distinguishes them from other things that one would not dream of characterizing as potentially alive, such as rocks, one thinks of features such as metabolism, cell division, growth, and development into something that we might call a mature human being. The trouble with paying much attention to these features is that they seem to be signs of *actual* life. But the point of the talk about *potential* life was to deny this. This suggests that the Court's claim about the State's interest in potential life is incoherent.

There is absolutely no doubt, of course, that the Court in both *Roe* and *Casey* was concerned with the question of fetal moral status. However, it does not follow from this that the Court was not concerned with the question of when life begins. It seems clear that the issues of whether the fetus has moral status and when life begins were considered to be equivalent by the Court. They simply took for granted what I shall call in this essay "the standard view." The standard view is the common view that all living human beings have the right to life *because* they are living human beings (although there may be, of course, special circumstances in which that right may be overridden or waived).

There are obvious rhetorical advantages to using the standard view to argue against the conclusion of the majority. There are also obvious rhetorical advantages to arguing from the assumptions of pro-choice Constitutional law to an anti-choice conclusion, and advantages to arguing from the standard view to claim that abortion is wrong. Nevertheless, I want to argue that these advantages should be foregone. In the final analysis this apparently attractive argument strategy is unsound. I want to argue this not on the ground that there is a different, superior argument strategy that is either pro- or anti- choice (although I think that there is), but on the ground that the standard view common to *Roe, Casey*, and the pro-choice and anti-choice movements simply cannot withstand serious analysis.

Readers of this essay should beware. You will find it easy to assume as you read that I am criticizing the assumptions common to *Roe, Casey*, and the popular anti-choice movement in order to support the platform of abortion choice. Nothing could be further from the truth. My analysis of the standard view will constitute the bulk of this essay. After that I shall offer a brief account of a replacement for the standard view that underwrites the prohibition of abortion choice. I shall contend that this replacement view remedies the deficiencies of the standard view. I shall also suggest that this replacement is far more plausible than the standard view for other reasons.

I

Let me make explicit the cluster of views with which this essay is concerned. According to what I have called "the standard view," what makes ending an individual's life wrong is, with rare exceptions, that her life is a *human* life. Of course, there may be exceptions for killing in time of war or in self-defense, or for state sanctioned killing of those who commit horrendous crimes. But these exceptions are rare, and require careful justification. Since these exceptions are not within the province of the issues discussed in this essay, they shall be neglected here. If ending a human life is wrong *because* the life ended is human, then it is important to establish the boundaries of human life. An action that would be wrong after life has begun would not be wrong before actual life has started. Apparently, given the standard view, if one wishes to discuss the wrongness of abortion, one must say something about the question of when life begins.

One argument against the view that human life begins at birth has already been presented. Here is another version of that argument. The characteristics in virtue of which we would say that an infant is alive, such as cellular metabolism, growth, the capacity to develop into a mature human being, and biological integration are all characteristics of the fetuses these infants were before birth. Therefore, human life could not have begun at birth. Another argument, that human life begins at birth because a human being becomes independent when she is separated from her mother, is also unsound for two reasons. The first is that independence is not a necessary condition of being alive. Many living adult human beings are dependent for their life functions, sometimes on machines, sometimes on insulin, and sometimes, as in the case of conjoined twins, on other biological entities. The second is that independence is not one of those characteristics, like metabolism, that *makes* one alive. It is a different *kind* of characteristic.

This argument that life does not begin at birth can be pushed backward through pregnancy. For each week of gestation in which it is clear that a fetus exhibits signs of life, we can find an earlier week of gestation in which a fetus exhibits at least some of the same signs. Opponents of choice who take the standard view for granted will thus claim that human life can be traced back all the way to conception; they then argue that, since life begins at conception, abortion is immoral.

There is a problem with this argument. It does not follow from the fact that we can trace life back to conception that life begins at conception. It is quite compatible with the "trickle back" argument that there was life before conception. Indeed, there was. The sperm and unfertilized ovum (hereafter UFO) that were your precursors had to have been alive or your conception would not have taken place. Fertilization is a biological process. Life does not *begin* at conception because there is life *before* conception. Therefore, the standard claim of abortion opponents is demonstrably false.

This argument shows not only a serious problem with the anti-choice arguments based on the standard view, but also a problem with the standard view itself. The reasoning that leads from the standard view to a rejection of abortion choice also leads from the standard view to a rejection of contraception. This "contraception problem" suggests that there is something wrong with the standard view.

II

A "brain death strategy" for rescuing the standard view is more promising. This strategy requires adopting a conception of human life richer than a bare metabolic notion.

A number of authors have argued that our understanding of when life begins should be based on our understanding of when life ends. Here is one way of working out this plausible suggestion. According to the orthodox legal definition of death in this country, a human being is dead if and only if she has sustained either irreversible cessation of circulatory and respiratory functions, or irreversible cessation of all functions of the entire brain, including the brain stem. This definition is unnecessarily complicated for most purposes because all mammals who have sustained irreversible cessation of circulatory and respiratory functions will sustain irreversible cessation of all functions of the brain within a few minutes. Therefore, the orthodox legal definition of death can be simplified: an individual is dead if and only if that individual has sustained total and irreversible cessation of all brain function.

Now the argument can proceed as follows. Because the total loss of brain function is the mark of no longer being alive, a human is not yet alive until she manifests some brain function. Plainly a zygote does not manifest brain function. Therefore, human life does not begin until after conception.

Here is a first cousin of the above argument. We are essentially living human beings. Brain function is essential to life. Therefore, someone who has sustained irreversible loss of all brain function has gone out of existence. It also follows that we did not come into existence until we first manifested brain function. Notice that this brain death strategy appears to rescue the standard view from the contraception difficulty. Notice also that this way of understanding the standard view may open the door to some abortion choice.

If the end of life is understood in terms of the *totality* of the loss of brain function, it seems reasonable to locate the beginning of life at the time at which anything remotely describable as function in the cells of the developing brain is present. The cephalic end of the embryonic neural tube differentiates itself from the remainder of the neural tube even before the sixth week. It does not seem wrong to locate the beginning of life, using the brain death strategy, as early as the fourth week of gestation. Accordingly, the standard view, when combined with the orthodox brain death definition of death, permits few abortions.

III

The argument in the previous section suggested that if the orthodox legal account of the end of life is correct, then one can make an inference concerning when life begins. In addition, if the standard view is correct, then one can make an inference concerning the moral permissibility of abortion and indeed, make an inference to a view that supports the anti-choice view. In addition, one can avoid the contraception problem. But is the orthodox legal account of the end of life correct?

It has been criticized because many of the humans who are pronounced dead on the basis of death of the entire brain do in fact manifest signs of brain life. The criticism is based on the fact that the typical criteria for brain death are fixed dilated pupils, lack of awareness or purposive movement, and ventilator dependency.

Some patients who meet such criteria exhibit increased heart rate and blood pressure when incisions are made to remove their organs for transplant. In some cases their EEGs are not flat. These criticisms are not compelling. They are not objections, strictly speaking, to the brain death definition of death. Rather, they are objections to how the brain death definition is applied in clinical situations.

There is a better objection to the brain death definition of death. In the case of brain dead bodies maintained on a ventilator, virtually all of the capacity to integrate the body's remaining organ systems is indeed lost. However, continuing circulatory and respiratory functions integrate the digestive system, urinary system, respiratory system, reproductive organs and circulatory system. This is, by the standards of a well-functioning human body, extremely low-level integration, of course. But it is integration, nonetheless. It follows that it is not the case that when all brain function is lost irreversibly – that is, when there is brain death – the body ceases to function as an integrated whole. Accordingly, a crucial premise of the argument for the orthodox brain death definition of death is false.

A proponent of the brain death definition might reply to this criticism by pointing out that the remaining integration in a brain dead, but otherwise functioning, body is merely artificially maintained by a machine. Such a human is not integrating her own remaining vital functions. A machine is doing it. Therefore, because she is not the integrator of her vital functions, she is dead. The trouble with this reply is that it is not quite true. The systems supplying oxygen and food to the body, eliminating metabolic waste products, and preserving electrolyte balance continue in a brain dead body supported by a ventilator. Of course, it is true that in the absence of a ventilator this integration would no longer continue. However, it is also true that in the absence of artificially supplied insulin, physiological integration will no longer continue in an insulin-dependent diabetic. Accordingly, the "must do it without help" criterion of life must be rejected. The orthodox legal definition of death is indefensible. This being the case, the account of the beginning of life that is based upon it should be rejected. The brain death strategy for rescuing the standard view from the contraception problem fails. Thus the standard view remains subject to the contraception problem.

IV

The standard view is subject to even more serious problems. Recall that according to the standard view, the wrong-making feature of ending a life like ours is that the life in question is a *human* life. This wrong-making feature is used to generate our right to life. Our right to life is used to generate the obligations of others not to kill us, and the obligations of some medical personnel to preserve our lives. It is permissible for competent adults to *waive* this right under some, but not all, circumstances. Advance directives and oral refusals of medical care are based upon this right of waiver. However, it is not permissible now in this country for you to waive your right to life, even if you are a competent adult, to make it permissible for your physician (or anyone else) to kill you.

Suppose that when a patient in PVS had been a competent adult, she had not clearly waived her right to the medical care necessary to preserve her life. Courts have famously struggled with cases like this, as the familiarity of the names of Karen Anne Quinlan, Nancy Cruzan, and Terri Schiavo remind us. Keeping such patients alive seems pointless because we do not believe that withdrawing medical care from such patients would harm them. It would not deprive them of any future experience that they would value, *whatever* their values may be now or in the future. The trouble with the standard view, with its right of waiver exception, is that in the absence of an advance directive, evidence that a patient did indeed waive her right to life sustaining care may be less than compelling. Legal battles in these cases utilize a conceptual framework of surrogate decision-making and substituted judgment, a frame-work based on the right of waiver. This conceptual framework, based ultimately upon the standard view, makes these cases far more difficult than they should be. They should be simple, for withdrawing medical care from such patients cannot harm them.

A similar problem arises for individuals with circulatory function and respiratory function, but who have suffered whole brain death, or whose brains are so severely damaged that they will never recover awareness or the capacity to breathe on their own. I have already argued that there are good reasons for regarding such patients as alive. Because the removal of their vital organs for transplantation does not deprive them of any future experience valuable to them (whatever their values might be now or in the future), removing their vital organs *cannot* harm them. Nevertheless, the standard view, combined with the present ban on euthanasia, prevents this. Bioethicists have dealt with this problem by giving bad arguments for the view that such patients are dead in order to permit transplantation. Accordingly, analysis of an issue concerning transplantation ethics reveals another problem with the standard view. The standard view makes killing wrong even when killing could not harm the victim – it makes killing wrong when it really is not.

The standard view is so called because it is the generally accepted common sense view of the wrongness of killing. Because this is so, one would expect it to give the correct answers concerning the wrongness of killing in virtually all cases. It does. It yields the incorrect answer in only a few cases. But that is enough to suggest that the standard view is not quite right. In addition, the standard view is indefensible. For many the need for justification of the standard view will not be obvious, so a bit of explanation is in order.

Is the standard view true because it is the consensus view? There are two reasons that it is not. In the first place, moral views that at one time represented a consensus have later been realized to be unsound. (Think of attitudes toward racial or sexual equality.) In the second place, the standard view is not really as standard as many believe. One reason for this is because the standard view seems to imply that abortion is seriously wrong. Accordingly, defenders of abortion choice have tried to give accounts of the wrongness of killing that are different from the standard view, that account for the wrongness of killing in all situations in which there is consensus that killing is wrong, and that allow abortion choice. Some have suggested our having interests of a sort that many fetuses lack is what makes killing us wrong. Others have argued that it is wrong to kill us because we are owed respect, and fetuses are not. Still others have suggested our being persons with certain psychological properties makes it wrong to kill us. But fetuses don't yet have these psychological properties. And still others have argued that the wrongness of killing adults and children is based upon our desire to live. But fetuses lack that desire. It follows that the standard view cannot be based on an appeal to consensus. There is – in academic circles, at least – no consensus at all.

Sometimes an argument by elimination is used to attempt to justify the standard view. In such an argument one attempts to show that all the alternative accounts of the wrongness of killing are unsatisfactory because they do not show that it is wrong to kill in all of the cases in which the wrongness of killing is uncontroversial. Having eliminated all of the alternatives to the standard view, proponents of this argument conclude that the standard view must be correct. However, such an argument for the standard view has two weaknesses. In the first place, the standard view, as we have already seen, also handles some cases in an implausible manner. Accordingly, the criterion used for eliminating alternative accounts of the wrongness of killing also leads to the elimination of the standard view. In the second place, the argument from elimination works only if *all* of the possible alternatives to the standard view have been considered and rejected. One can never be certain that this condition obtains, for there may be some alternative to the standard view that has not yet been proposed. Hence, the argument by elimination for the standard view suffers from two fatal flaws.

A Biblical defense of the standard view is more directly relevant to the anti-choice view of abortion, especially because it is the defense the standard view proponents often offer. According to one argument, of all accounts of the wrongness of killing, only the standard view prohibits abortion. The Bible prohibits abortion. Therefore, the standard view must be correct.

But does the Bible actually prohibit abortion? The following passage from Jeremiah seems to be cited as much as any other:

> Then the word of the Lord came unto me, saying. Before I formed thee in the belly, I knew thee: and before thou camest forth out of the womb I sanctified thee, *and* I ordained thee a prophet unto the nations. (Jer 1:5)

This passage certainly seems to show that God had Her eye on Jeremiah prior to his birth and that She had great things in mind for him. It is reasonable to infer that aborting Jeremiah would have been contrary to God's will. Perhaps we can even permit the inference that aborting any of the prophets would have been contrary to God's will. However, because virtually everyone is not a prophet, the inference to the proposition that abortion is in general wrong is unsound. Perhaps God had plans for all of us. Perhaps She had them when we were in the womb. But God would not have plans for any humans who were aborted. After all, She is omniscient, and She would not be unwise enough to make plans for anyone who would not exist after birth. The implications of this analysis for the standard view are worth notice. The truth of the above passage from Jeremiah is quite compatible with abortion choice. All we are permitted validly to infer in the case of Jeremiah is that the abortion of Jeremiah would have been wrong *because* God had plans for him, not *because* he was human and alive. There is no aid and comfort for the standard view here.

Opponents of abortion choice cite other Biblical passages in support of their views. Such persons seem to think that a prohibition of abortion is entailed by any passage in which the word "womb" and some word referring to children are found together. Surely this is an unduly broad reading of sacred texts.

Another problem with Biblically based anti-abortion arguments is that they require the assumption that the Bible provides an infallible guide to right conduct. Deuteronomy 21: 18–21 recommends stoning to death one's repeatedly rebellious son. This strongly suggests that the assumption that the Bible is an infallible guide is not true. Therefore, neither does the Bible provide an infallible guide to conduct, nor, if it did, would it, in general, prohibit abortion or support the standard view.

Another problem besets the standard view. Suppose that a space ship lands on your front lawn and something that bears no resemblance to anything you have ever seen before emerges. This individual has learned your language, can converse with you and seems very person-like. Suppose further that you, being a sophisticated biologist, take a sample of this person's body and can find nothing resembling human DNA. Would it be permissible to kill this individual because she is not biologically human?

Most of us would say "no." Presumably the reason we would offer for the wrongness of killing this extra-terrestrial individual would be a reason that would apply also to human beings. This suggests that being human and alive is not quite the *reason* why it is wrong to kill us; there is some deeper consideration.

In sum, we can conclude that the standard view lacks an adequate defense, makes too many instances of ending a life wrong, leads its proponents into making false claims regarding the beginning of life, and probably is merely a surrogate for a deeper reason why killing is wrong when it is wrong. Although the standard view offers anti-choicers obvious rhetorical advantages, there are excellent reasons for rejecting it.

V

Recall that this essay is a critique of an anti-choice argument strategy, not a critique of the anti-choice conclusion. A much better anti-choice argument strategy is available. Consider human adults and already born children, about whom a consensus exists that killing them is wrong. How does killing victimize them? It harms them. Killing harms its victims by depriving them of all of the goods of life that they otherwise would have experienced. In other words, killing them deprives them of their futures of value. Their futures of value consist of whatever they will or would regard as making their lives worth living.

The implications of this account of the wrongness of killing for the ethics of abortion are straightforward. Fetuses have futures very much like ours; indeed, their futures contain whatever ours contain and more. Therefore, (given certain defensible assumptions and a few qualifications) abortion is immoral.

The future of value account of the wrongness of killing is superior to the standard account because it appeals to what we actually do believe makes life valuable and what makes premature death a misfortune. In addition, the future of value account handles end of life issues better than the standard account. For example, because individuals in PVS are both human and alive, the standard view entails that they have the right to life and medical personnel have an obligation to keep them alive unless these patients have waived their right to treatment. Problems arise if it is unclear that they have waived that right. Because the future of value view bases the wrong of ending someone's life on the harm of death and because terminating medical treatment cannot harm PVS patients, withdrawing medical treatment from PVS patients is morally unproblematic in the absence of special circumstances.

Consider now a brain dead patient in whom, with ventilator support, respiratory and circulatory functions continue. Because she is still a (minimally) integrated biological organism, she is still alive. Because to remove her vital organs for transplantation is to kill her, bioethicists have endorsed bad arguments for the view that such individuals are dead, in order to justify transplantation. Notice how much better the future of value argument handles these cases. Since such a patient will never have, in the future, experiences she will value, removing her vital organs does not harm her. Assuming, therefore, that permission was obtained from the donor or her family, removing her vital organs neither harms nor wrongs her, even though removing her organs is indeed killing her.

Does the future of value view permit euthanasia? It could. Consider a patient who suffers from severe pain that cannot be relieved and who wants to die. Such a patient lacks a future of value. Because killing him does not harm him, euthanasia is morally permissible. Of course, there may be no such cases in this country because of modern methods of pain control. However, one can imagine individuals with severe battlefield injuries or individuals in underdeveloped countries in which the future of value framework would open the door to euthanasia.

The future of value account also handles beginning of life issues better than the standard account. The standard view is subject to the contraception problem. The future of value account is not, because the issue of when life begins is irrelevant in the future of value account. What is important is that fetuses have futures of value. They have futures of value because they are earlier stages of the very same individuals who later will (or would) have valuable experiences. A simple argument shows that sperm and UFOs are not earlier stages of the very same individuals who later will (or would) have valuable experiences. Suppose they were. Consider your own case. If the sperm and the UFO that were your precursors were each an earlier stage of the same individual you are now, then, because identity is transitive, that sperm and UFO would be the same individual. That is false. Therefore, neither the sperm nor the UFO that was the precursor of any of us had a future of value. Although it is false that life begins at conception, it is true that the same individual that we are now began either at conception or implantation.

Finally consider our visitor from another planet whom it would be wrong to kill. The standard view cannot account for this. The future of value view can, for it would be wrong to kill that visitor for the same reason it is wrong to kill ordinary humans and fetuses: they have futures like ours.

VI

Let us conclude with an overview of the analysis of this essay. What I have called "the standard view" has been taken for granted by most people on both sides of the abortion controversy. According to this view there are certain basic rights that all humans have in virtue of being human and alive. We call these "human rights." The right to life is, perhaps, the most basic human right. Thus, if fetuses are fully human and alive, then abortion violates a basic fetal right. And because abortion violates a basic fetal right, it is wrong. Those who are pro-choice often deal with this assumption by supposing that a fetus is not fully human, or that a fetus is merely a potential life, or that we will never know when life begins. Because they make these suppositions, those who are pro-choice argue that the abortion issue should be about women's rights. Given these suppositions, of course, they are absolutely correct.

And why shouldn't those who are pro-choice feel justified in making these suppositions? They have also been made by the highest court in the land.

The trouble is that this way of thinking about the abortion issue opens the door to the arguments of the anti-choice movement. There are, as we have seen, good arguments that life does not begin at any time during pregnancy and that fetuses are actually – not merely potentially – alive. Furthermore, there are obvious arguments that human fetuses are, well, fully human; they are not partially members of another species during their intrauterine existence! Accordingly, those opposed to choice can use the standard view – which is, after all, accepted by most of those who are pro-choice – to argue against the permissibility of abortion.

I have argued in this essay that those who are anti-choice should forego this compelling rhetorical strategy. The claim that life begins at conception is false. The end of biological life does not have implications for abortion via the determination of the beginning of biological life. The standard view is implausible in other respects. Nevertheless, one should not conclude from this that the anti-choice view is indefensible.

There is a replacement for the standard view. The future of value view provides us with a better account of what makes it wrong to kill us. This replacement view is not subject to the deficiencies in the standard view, is more intuitively plausible than the standard view, and underwrites the wrongness of abortion. Therefore, opponents of abortion are better served by adopting the future of value view.

Feminist Discourse on Sex Screening and Selective Abortion of Female Foetuses

FARHAT MOAZAM

Bioethics 18, no. 3 (2004): 205–220.

The age of reproductive technology has brought with it an extraordinary capability for the prenatal screening of the foetus, and increasingly the embryo itself, for genetic disorders. With this has also come the possibility of determining with certainty the gender of the foetus. Although a preference for sons is reportedly a universal phenomenon, in some Asian societies daughters are considered financial and cultural liabilities. Increasing availability of ultrasonography and amniocentesis has led to widespread gender screening and selective abortion of normal female foetuses in many countries where there is a strong cultural preference for sons. This practice in India has perhaps received the maximum attention in bioethical and sociological literature.

Feminists have taken widely divergent positions, oftentimes in a vitriolic manner, on the morality of foetal sex determination leading to selective abortion of female foetuses. Feminists from India have strongly opposed screening and selective abortion of female foetuses, considering this as leading to further disenfranchisement of females in their patriarchal, male-dominated society, and have agitated successfully for legislative prohibitions. Various state laws and the Medical Termination of Pregnancy Act of India passed in the last decade prohibit foetal sex screening, with violators liable to fines and imprisonment. Libertarian feminists on the other hand, primarily from industrialised countries like the United States, while uncomfortable with selective abortion of female foetuses, have nevertheless seen any prohibition of the use of this technology as a curtailment of a woman's choice and a violation of her right to make autonomous decisions regarding her procreation. Indian feminists who support legal prohibition of prenatal sex selection have been characterised as radical feminists who are willing to ride roughshod over basic ethical principles in their fight against male dominion. Others have argued that it is not possible to know in advance the long-term social consequences of sex pre-selection, and therefore a wholesale condemnation of the practice cannot be justified. But above all, the Indian Act has been seen as a dangerous state intrusion into the procreative liberty rights of women.

What is evident is that feminists have brought their own perspectives and cultural hues, their own life experiences to this debate. They understandably speak not in one moral voice but from the vantage-points of their own local moral worlds. This is not surprising since to suppose that there is *a* feminist position on this, or many other issues, is a utopian concept. As Fox-Genovese, a historian and professor of humanities, states, 'an assumption that any "orthodox" feminism can embody the aspirations of all women', in other words a 'totalitarianism', would in many ways negate the very point of feminist revolt against a uniform, 'male' moral philosophy of this world.[1] For even as gender may unite women, class, culture and ethnicity divide them. In the case of the Indian versus the libertarian disagreement on this issue, one must also take into account a growing criticism in developing countries against what is perceived as the increasing hegemony of the 'West' (in economics, but also culture and values) over the 'East.' The female experience (and thus the responses to it) is socially and culturally constructed.

This paper will limit itself to reflections on the issue of antenatal screening specifically for gender determination and abortion when the foetus is a *normal* female, one without a genetic predisposition to any disease. The discussion will be formulated in the context of countries in which the social and cultural mores place the female at a significant, overt disadvantage in relationship to the male. I will use the 'Indian case' as a paradigm both because selective abortion of female foetuses has been widely reported in that country, but also because legal criminalisation of this practice by the Indian government has been the focus of a lively debate among bioethicists and feminists. I shall argue that within the *context* of what prevails in such societies, resorting to an ethical argument that hinges largely on the principle of individual autonomy as understood in the west can be problematic. Furthermore, I will propose that a liberal *theoretical* assumption that it is always better to have more rather than fewer choices may not hold up well against the *realities* of life for such women. I will also review the basis of the uniformly negative response of liberal feminists to the Indian legislature prohibiting antenatal sex screening, a move supported and lauded by Indian feminists.

The Autonomy Argument

Autonomy and the right of autonomous agents to make their own choices in shaping their lives is a cornerstone of bioethics as it has evolved in the Western hemisphere. Respect for autonomy has undoubtedly played a major, and generally successful, role in the struggle of women towards achieving the ideal of moral equality of all humans, irrespective of their gender and race. This importance of autonomy has been extended to women's reproductive rights. Any action, therefore, that may have any possible negative implications for this right, any suspected interference with one's autonomy, is viewed with considerable concern. Liberal feminists particularly from the United States, although considering sex selection as 'undesirable', have argued that limiting Asian women's autonomy to make decisions for prenatal gender screening cannot be ethically justified. In their opinion, under cultural mores that make it imperative for females to be the bearer of sons, a legal prohibition of the use of a technology that provides this option with its obvious advantages to them, is curtailing the woman's autonomy and 'probably causing more harm than good to the very people it seeks to protect.'

This argument relies on an understanding of the autonomy of a woman to make reproductive choices freely and as *she* sees fit. This remains one of the most cherished rights in Western cultures. However, in my opinion, the issue of autonomy of women in India must be examined within the context of a different culture, one in which women are still largely powerless and subjugated to men, with little recourse to fight this oppression. Technology exported from the West has found fertile soil within developing countries, but this is not the case for many Western values, particularly those that emphasise individual rights and liberty.

Ultrasonography and amniocentesis are relatively simple, and the latter particularly effective, modes of determining foetal gender. These technologies are widely available both in the public and private sectors in India, and the simplicity of these procedures has made a burgeoning, lucrative business possible. It is estimated that almost 85% of all gynaecologists now offer these services, and a majority is willing to comply with the request for abortion if the foetus is female. (It is not known whether these statistics have changed since Indian legislation made gender screening and selection a criminal offence.) In 1986, of 8000 abortions that were preceded by amniocentesis in six clinics in Mumbai alone, 7999 involved female foetuses. One can only speculate on the cumulative numbers of female feticides in a country with a population of a billion people.

In the hierarchical and strongly patriarchal culture of India, daughters are considered a liability on many fronts. The accepted norm is that daughters are reared only to be eventually married — an event that necessitates payment of a large dowry to the groom and his family. A woman's role is thus primarily seen as that of a wife and the bearer of children (preferably sons) for her husband and her family by marriage. A son on the other hand carries on the lineage, the 'name', of the family, and is also seen as a means of economic support for ageing parents with whom he will often continue to reside following marriage. This role of the male offspring is not uncommon in many Asian cultures where kinship systems involve extended families, but among Hindus in addition, it is only the son who can undertake essential rites connected to the death and cremation of parents. Therefore, a woman who cannot provide sons is liable to repercussions that can range from abuse to divorce. It is against this background that one must struggle to make sense of the pregnant woman's 'autonomy' when she chooses to undergo prenatal gender screening.

One of the prerequisites for making an autonomous decision is that the individual arrives at it freely and rationally without undue influence or external pressures. The consent for any intervention can be truly voluntary (as opposed to merely informed) only if given without being threatened, forced or manipulated. In the case of a woman married into a family that sees her worth as a bearer of sons with repercussions for her if she does not meet this standard, it is difficult to see her as a free agent exercising her right to autonomy. In effect, childbearing is something that she owes to her husband and society regardless of her own feelings. She is a hostage to a situation in which if she fails to bring forth male offspring, she is liable to significant negative repercussions including divorce, a catastrophic event for a woman in such societies. It would thus be reasonable to argue that in many instances her 'consent' to proceed with the screening and subsequent abortion is in fact coerced, forcibly or subtly, and thus morally unjustifiable. As coercion is a term that is often used, and sometimes rhetorically abused, it may be helpful to test this against Wertheimer's definition.

Wertheimer proposes a two-prong theory, both of which prongs must be met, to establish if an action is truly coerced.[2] The first requirement is that the individual has no other *reasonable* option available to choose. One could argue in this case that perhaps the woman does have another option, namely to bear and give birth to a female child. But in view of the significantly negative implications for her if she were to do so, it is difficult to consider this as a choice she arrives at autonomously. Furthermore, Wertheimer's theory and its application involve a reference point of what can be considered as morally right or wrong. In this background, these women begin from a *baseline situation*; one that involves subjugation based on their gender, which is difficult to defend on moral grounds.

The second prong of his theory is that the 'proposer' (in this case the husband and/or his family) does not have a right to make such a proposal. The illustrative examples that Wertheimer utilises for his theory include such a right within a legal framework. It can be argued therefore that with the passage of the Indian Act prohibiting foetal sex screening, the proposer(s) therefore no longer have a right to propose this action to the pregnant woman. Based on this analysis then, a woman's 'decision' to utilise this technology would appear to be coerced rather than one that represents a genuine exercise of an autonomous decision. This conclusion is further supported by the fact that the Indian Act includes no penalty for the woman, reserving punishment only for the husband and the gynaecologist, a tacit acknowledgement that she may not have undergone the procedure willingly.

The Argument for Choices

Liberal feminists have argued that, especially in misogynist societies where the ideal of individual equality irrespective of gender is yet to be achieved, the best course of action is to increase women's choices and options in life. This argument has also been used to defend prenatal gender screening. Medical technology that makes this possible in effect provides additional choices to women and this can help to improve their overall situation. The assumption that for rational individuals more choices are always preferable to fewer originated from economists, but has now been widely embraced by many sectors in the industrialised world. There is also an assumption that reasonable people also always *prefer* to be permitted to choose as well as be offered expanded choices.

Gerald Dworkin argues that a theory 'that more choices is always preferable to less is false.'[3] He also notes that perhaps insufficient attention has been paid to another feature of having more choices: the costs that this 'benefit' may carry with it. In his opinion, making choices 'is not a costless activity.' It involves trade-offs that must be included in the equation when assessing the net benefit of having more rather than fewer choices.

Dworkin identifies one of the costs as 'bearing the responsibility' for the choice one makes. Amniocentesis provides a choice to the woman to ascertain the female gender of her foetus and proceed with an abortion. Abortion for any reason is a tragic choice, one that can have a substantial emotional impact on the woman involved. In this case, it is the abortion of what would have been a healthy child belonging to one's own gender, perhaps a daughter that the woman may have desired to rear. Shouldering the responsibility of making the choice to proceed with aborting her (particularly if done to protect one's own interest) must inevitably carry tremendous psychological and emotional burdens for many women. This cost would be compounded if this were a choice that must be made on more than one occasion, with cycles of screening, abortion of the female foetus, and screening again with the next pregnancy. To serve as the instrument for the destruction of a potential member of one's own gender must surely carry a significant toll for many women. Instead of enhancing a sense of control, this additional choice may in fact serve to heighten a sense of powerlessness and reinforce the belief that the worth of females, and therefore herself, lies primarily in a capacity to bear sons.

The physical cost of recurrent abortions in view of the general poor health of women in developing countries is another factor that cannot be overlooked in this equation. Amniocentesis is generally performed around 14 to 16 weeks of pregnancy when there is sufficient amniotic fluid to aspirate and examine. It may take as much as a week to get confirmed results. (It may be possible to get these faster as technology advances.) The abortion, a medical 'intervention', is therefore generally done in the second trimester, carrying significant risks for the mother that generally outweigh those related to a normal pregnancy followed by a term delivery. Repeated abortions would of course magnify these risks.

The second cost of having additional choices, according to Dworkin, is that of a subtle 'coercion that comes into play to conform to societal pressures.' As an example, prenatal genetic testing now makes it possible to check for genetic disabilities. There can be subtle pressures on a woman to make use of this technology with an in-built assumption that if she rejects amniocentesis, she must bear the responsibility of bringing a handicapped child into the world. The issue of societal pressures is equally relevant when it comes to prenatal gender determination. In societies that value a woman for her success in bearing sons and not daughters, the availability of technology that makes this possible inevitably carries pressures, both subtle and perhaps not so subtle, on the woman to avail herself of this choice. In the guise of having more choices, for many women this technology may in fact enslave them further. Reproductive technology has replaced the natural lottery of offspring with human choices. It can be argued

that many women would have been better off with a baseline of *no* choice between having a girl or a boy.

The value of choices lies in increasing the probability that they will lead to enhancing an individual's self-satisfaction, a satisfaction derived from contemplating options, reflecting on one's preferences and then exercising a choice. It is difficult to see how this would apply to women in India in the context of the ground realities of their lives. As Dworkin states, the value of more choices must be grounded within and be a part 'of a larger complex that is itself valued.' Thus the value of having choices resides neither in the causal effects nor in any *intrinsic* value of choices. The value lies in the idea of 'what it is to be a person and a moral agent equally worthy of respect by all.' In the case of India, choices would be meaningful only if women could freely choose between alternative options and shape their lives as they see fit. Instead, the choice for prenatal gender determination in reality only perpetuates the woman's position as a baby-making machine that can be manipulated and controlled to bring forth a product that society has deemed superior. Under these circumstances, the argument offered by some feminists that sex pre-selection provides some women 'with a new means of resistance to patriarchy', or an opportunity to 'resist patriarchy by refusing to add to the female underclass', appears meaningless.

The State Interference Argument

Intense lobbying in the last two decades by many women's organisations in India as well as national feminists has been successful in forcing the Indian legislature to pass state laws and the Medical Termination of Pregnancy Act of India prohibiting prenatal gender determination. Husbands and healthcare professionals (but not, as noted, the pregnant women themselves) who violate this law are liable to fines and imprisonment.

This legislation has been widely criticised by liberal feminists who see this as state interference and the curtailment of individual procreative liberty rights of women. Their language primarily emphasises individual rights pitted against a paternalistic policy of the government. Although troubled by selective abortion of female foetuses, most have felt that legally prohibiting women from using relevant technology is the thin edge of the wedge, a cost that is too high to pay.

Liberal feminists opposing the Indian legislation have also expressed their concerns using 'the slippery slope' argument. According to this argument, once the state gets a toehold in controlling reproductive decisions, this will inevitably lead to a nibbling away of hard-won reproductive control. A possible fallout could be increasing limitation of a woman's choices through legal definition of acceptable and unacceptable reasons for abortions. More so than any other, it is this argument offered by feminists in the United States that is deeply coloured by their own experience with the loud and polarising debate about abortions that continues in this country. This is the prism through which the circumstances in India are being viewed. The ongoing debate in the United States is occurring within the context of a pluralistic society with strong opposing religious and secular strands and mutual mistrust among the protagonists. Abortion has been legal in India for many years and, without the benefit of a divisive Roe vs. Wade, it has never been a riveting call for feminists. Pro-life and pro-choice are charged terms that are a product of the particularities of this debate within the cultural context of the West, particularly the United States. Therefore, although Western liberal concerns around the issue of abortion itself are understandable, these are not automatically transplantable into another country that may have vastly different priorities and concerns and where abortion is not one of the rallying cries for women.

Perhaps a more constructive approach may be to move the argument against state interference from criticism of a policy that is seen as paternalistic over to whether there is a *wrongness* of the policy. Individual rights and freedoms are of tremendous value, yet they are not considered absolute in any society. States and governments encroach upon them if the long term good of the wider community or society is at stake. Common examples of this are policies for mandatory vaccinations in most countries, including India. Similarly, the rights of property owners have been restricted to prevent environmental hazards.

While analysing 'liberty-limiting principles', Feinberg, a liberal himself, nevertheless argues that state interference in a citizen's behaviour 'can be morally justified' when there is 'the need to prevent harm (public or private) to parties other than the person interfered with.'[4] Under the 'harm principle' penal legislation is justifiable to prevent harm to others. Although the extreme liberal position holds that only the harm principle can be considered a good enough reason to curtail individual liberty, Feinberg argues that in certain instances state intervention can also be morally justifiable under what he terms the '(profound) offense principle.'

While elaborating on profound offences, Feinberg is careful to differentiate them from 'offensive nuisances', such as pornography, that are usually 'shallow', personal grievances that may not justify state intervention against individual rights.[5] Profound offences in contrast are those that result in 'an affront to standards of propriety and higher-order sensibilities.' They impact on moral sensibilities of people even in the absence of their personal involvement or direct harm to them. Profound offences 'alter public environment to the detriment of public interest' and can serve to 'tarnish the image' of a community or the nation itself. It can be argued that such offences injure public good and collective community welfare and ultimately harm the interest of individual members. According to Feinberg, individual fulfilment is undoubtedly good for people and personal autonomy is its essential pre-requisite, but 'government invasion of liberty to protect others' if ever 'legitimate', must surely include instances 'when the offense is of a profound variety.'

It would seem reasonable to argue that exercising reproductive choices that lead to the destruction of thousands of normal female foetuses would qualify as an example of profound offence to the deepest moral sensibilities of rational human beings. Such practice legitimises discrimination based on gender, is an affront to human rights and weakens the moral fabric of the entire society. In addition, it tarnishes the image of the country among other nations. It would seem that a liberal view that espouses the importance of individual choices must be ready to accept that there can be genuine collective harms and grave offences to a society that justifies state intrusion into individual interests and rights.

The move of the Indian government, a form of legal moralism, can be construed as an action directed towards the welfare of the larger community through prohibition of the denigration of half of its members. Reproduction has a social dimension that extends beyond the individual. Reproductive choices made over time by many individuals eventually form societal norms, shaping, altering or re-enforcing societal attitudes and presumptions. These can have a profound impact, both real and symbolic, on the larger community. General acceptance of sex screening with the primary aim of selectively aborting female foetuses, if seen merely as one more right that must be respected, strengthens the degrading *status quo* for women and defeats the universal moral ideal that human worth must not be related to gender. Admittedly, it takes more than legal action to change basic attitudes and beliefs, but it would seem that a legally sanctioned discriminatory practice would be far more difficult to eradicate. The Indian Act sends a symbolic message by removing at least the legal legitimacy of gender selection, making it more difficult for husbands and in-laws to expect that screening and aborting female foetuses is no more than another routine event in any pregnancy. It also provides a check to a burgeoning business of aborting normal female foetuses.

Having said all this, one of the concerns expressed by liberal feminists related to the legal prohibition of sex screening in India remains valid. This is the possibility that this legislation will do nothing to control these practices from continuing in the hands of charlatan screeners and abortionists willing to ply their trade illegally for sufficient compensation. Until the social norms regarding the status of women change, many women, particularly the poor, will continue to be exploited financially and perhaps under riskier medical conditions. But this reality of life (risky, backdoor abortions) has existed for years for countless women in impoverished countries even prior to the advent of sex screening. This is not a moral justification for it, but the solution for this can be neither simple nor immediate. What can be argued, however, is that an absence of societal measures to stem the mass elimination of female foetuses in which, sadly, women themselves are made accomplices to the act, does not seem conducive to achieving an already difficult task of achieving gender equality within communities.

Conclusions

There are universal themes that unite feminist thought. These include recognition that females are oppressed and that this is morally and politically wrong, together with a commitment to address these issues and transform society. How to achieve this objective (not yet a reality even in many industrialised countries) will, however, require varying strategies. And although feminists may have little disagreement concerning substantive matters, it is in the area of strategy where most differences of opinion have arisen. This is not surprising as 'womanhood' may be a universal condition but women differ substantially in the cultural, social and economic realities of their lives. Inevitably the culture, ethnicity, class and race to which women belong give them their identities and shape their moral reasoning and responses. Strategies undertaken are sometimes best understood within the *context* of culturally based realities that characterise a society. The issue of sex screening and selective abortion of female foetuses in India is an illustrative case.

Liberal feminists have emphasised individual autonomy and choice as their primary values. According to Tong, in their caution that women not emphasise their differences from men, they have tended to 'adopt the male ontology of the self's separation from others.'[6] The notion of extreme individualism, that individual freedom and rights could, and indeed must, be absolute runs the risk of non-recognition and rejection of differences among women and the diversity of mechanisms necessary to cope with the negative repercussions on women of a still over-whelmingly man's world. Such a 'totalitarianism', a radical individualism that overrides the claims of society itself also negates the very point of feminist revolt. A view that a single 'orthodox' feminism of *any* variety can embody the aspiration of all women reverts back to some of the problematic issues in the evolution of the rationalistic, individualistic, 'male' ethics against which women have consistently raised objections.

Within the context of cultural norms and gender relationships in India, and other societies that share them, a focus on principles of individual autonomy and a right to make reproductive choices may not be the only, or the most effective, way to address the problem of societal subjugation of women. A strategy on the other hand that looks towards a wider goal of public welfare, and utilises the power of the state to do so, may have a more realistic chance of achieving this goal eventually.

Notes

1. Elizabeth Fox-Genoveso, *Feminism Without Illusions*, 229–230. (Chapel Hill: University of North Carolina Press, 1991).
2. Alan Wertheimer, *Coercion*, 64–80 (Princeton, NJ: Princeton University Press, 1987).
3. Gerald Dworkin, "Is More Choice Better Than Less? The Theory and Practice of Autonomy," in *Studies in Philosophy*, edited by Sydney Shoemaker, 62–81. (Cambridge: Cambridge University Press, 1988).
4. Joel Feinberg, *Harm to Others*, 10–13, 95–103 (New York: Oxford University Press, 1984).
5. Joel Feinberg. *Offense to Others*, 57–60. (New York: Oxford University Press, 1985).
6. Rosemarie Tong, "Feminist Approaches to Bioethics", in *Feminism and Bioethics*, edited by Susan M. Wolf, 67–89. (New York: Oxford University Press, 1996).

Could Artificial Wombs End the Abortion Debate?

CHRISTOPHER KACZOR

National Catholic Bioethics Quarterly 5, no. 2 (2005): 283–301.

Although artificial wombs may seem fanciful when first considered, certain trends suggest they may become reality. Between 1945 and the 1970s, the weight at which premature infants could survive dropped dramatically, moving from 1000 grams to around 400 grams. In 1973, the U.S. Supreme Court, in deciding *Roe v. Wade*, considered viability to begin around twenty-eight weeks. In 2000, premature babies were reported to have survived at eighteen weeks. Advanced incubators already in existence save thousands of children born prematurely each year. It is highly likely that such incubators will become even more advanced as technology progresses.

If artificial wombs were made available and relatively affordable, and the procedure was no more intrusive than present-day abortion, would abortion defenders be satisfied with extractive abortion (removing the living human fetus for implantation into an artificial womb) or would they insist on the right to terminative abortion (ending human fetal life)? Would the use of an artificial womb in lieu of abortion be morally permissible for consistent critics, especially Catholic critics, of abortion? Or, has magisterial teaching or Catholic tradition excluded, if only implicitly, this practice? Depending on how these questions are answered, it could be the case that most consistent critics of abortion and most consistent defenders of abortion could both be satisfied, and the abortion debate among intellectuals, at least as we know it now, would change profoundly, if not altogether be ended. Needless to say, my remarks here are necessarily "exploratory" insofar as they apply traditional moral reasoning to an as yet nonexistent technology. It would be extremely difficult, if not impossible, beforehand to explore in depth the political, social, economic, and theological ramifications of an artificial uterus, and yet an admittedly incomplete consideration of the ethical dimensions of this possibility may better prepare us, if and when this possibility becomes a reality.

Artificial Wombs and Consistent Defenders of Abortion

Consistent defenders of abortion believe that abortion is morally permissible in all circumstances throughout all nine months of pregnancy. In moral and usually also legal terms, consistent defenders of abortion assert an absolute right to abortion, even as consistent critics of abortion defend an exceptionless norm against intentionally killing the human fetus. But what exactly is meant by the "right to abortion"?

One should distinguish two aspects of abortion that are currently but not necessarily linked—extraction and termination. Abortion rights might be understood as the right not to be pregnant, the right not to have the human fetus in the womb, the right of extraction. On the other hand, abortion rights might be defined as the right to end the life of the human fetus in utero, the right to terminate not just the pregnancy, but also the life of the fetus. These two understandings of abor-

tion, although distinct, are at least for the present linked, since one cannot currently accomplish evacuation of the human fetus from the uterus at an early stage of pregnancy without also terminating the life of the human fetus. Accordingly, one could advocate the right of evacuation or extraction, that is, the right to have the fetus removed from the woman's body, and yet not advocate a right of termination, that is, the right to have the fetus killed within the woman's body. The question can then be asked, When someone defends the right to an abortion, does this include only evacuation or also termination?

Most defenders of abortion in fact only advocate a right to evacuation and not a right to termination. For example, the American College of Obstetricians and Gynecologists in 1977 wrote:

> The College affirms that the resolution of such conflict (between woman and fetus) by inducing abortion in no way implies that the physician has an adversary relationship towards the fetus and therefore, the physician does not view the destruction of the fetus as the primary purpose of abortion. The College consequently recognizes a continuing obligation on the part of the physician towards the survival of a possibly viable fetus where this can be discharged without additional hazard to the health of the mother.

If methods of nonlethal evacuation were available and safe for maternal health, then this statement would require that doctors use these means. Artificial wombs as envisioned are precisely the means that would enable the survival of a viable fetus without additional hazard to the health of the mother. If all physicians abided by this statement, this alone would dramatically change the abortion debate, for if the medical community refused to perform terminative abortions and would only perform evacuative abortions, then the abortion debate as we know it today would be over.

Among philosophers defending abortion, the most prominent, such as Mary Ann Warren, Judith Jarvis Thomson, and David Boonin, understand the right to abortion as a *right of evacuation* and *not a right of termination*.

Mary Anne Warren writes, "If and when a late-term abortion could be safely performed without killing the fetus, [the mother] would have no absolute right to insist on its death (e.g., if others wish to adopt it or pay for its care), for the same reason that she does not have a right to insist that a viable infant be killed."[1] Warren believes that the rights of the fetus to be in the womb do not trump the woman's right of freedom, which is violated by the pregnancy. However, if the fetus were removed and placed in an artificial womb, the rights of the woman would no longer be violated.

So these philosophers, the most prominent defenders of abortion, defend only a right of evacuation, not a right of termination. Safe, practical artificial wombs should therefore end the abortion debate for them. An added advantage, from their perspective, would be that the right to evacuation abortion would be relatively, if not absolutely, uncontested, unlike the present heavily contested abortions—heavily contested because they include termination of the life of the human fetus.

The 1977 statement from the American College of Obstetricians and Gynecologists implicitly raises an important objection, namely, that partial ectogenesis (development of a baby outside the maternal womb for part of the gestational period) could be more dangerous for the woman and therefore abortion as termination would be preferable. In the words of David N. James:

A foetal transplant would be an elaborate surgical procedure aimed at the delicate removal of the foetus from the mother's placenta and its transfer and attachment to the external artificial womb. Unlike an early abortion, foetal transplantation would thus require general anesthesia as well as a surgical incision through the abdominal wall and uterus, with all the risks of medical complications which accompany these more invasive procedures.[2]

James also notes that intensive care for such children could be massively expensive and lead to many new orphanages, foster care homes, and related services.

These possible difficulties may or may not be realized. If these difficulties were to take place, they would be technological, economic, or social difficulties and not per se moral difficulties. Ex hypothesis, partial ectogenesis, as imagined in the future, would not be dangerous for women. Many procedures that were dangerous and invasive forty years ago are now safe and noninvasive. Many surgeries formerly requiring days in the hospital have become outpatient surgeries. The choice between termination and extraction would not be the choice between no danger and danger, but between two choices both risking dangers. As medical care advances, it is highly likely that the differences in danger among the various procedures will be negligible, and the cost for such treatments less expensive—as is seen, for example, in the cheap, fast, and powerful computers of today, compared with the expensive, slow, and not very powerful computers of the 1970s.

The foreseen social cost of extraction rather than termination may also prove to be mistaken. The countries most likely to use partial ectogenesis in lieu of abortion are the same countries that will encounter *underpopulation* problems in the near future—Western Europe and, to a lesser extent (due to immigration), the United States. These countries will face severe financial difficulties in the future, with fewer and fewer workers to support a growing class of retirees. For them, an increase in the number of children and future workers may be a social boon, securing social support for seniors. Social considerations are not decisive arguments against evacuation and the use of artificial wombs.

Of course, not all doctors, philosophers, or activists defending abortion understand abortion rights in terms of evacuation rather than termination. For some, "abortion rights" includes the right to secure the death of the human fetus.

However, even among advocates of infanticide, there is a recognition that insisting on fetal death in the context of the availability of artificial wombs might be going too far. As Peter Singer and Deane Wells wrote:

> Freedom to choose what is to happen to one's body is one thing; freedom to insist on the death of a being that is capable of living outside of one's body is another. . . . [Even if there is no fetal right to life,] it is difficult to see why a healthy foetus should die if there is someone who wishes to adopt it and will give it the opportunity of a worthwhile life. We do not allow a mother to kill her newborn baby because she does not wish either to keep it or to hand it over for adoption.[3]

If consistent advocates of abortion and even infanticide such as Peter Singer can embrace the use of advanced incubators in lieu of abortion, then it is likely that there will be few advocates of abortion who will disagree. If advocates of abortion such as these are consistent, and really meant what they have said about not desiring the death of the human fetus, for at least these defenders of abortion, artificial wombs would end the abortion debate.

Artificial Wombs and Consistent Critics of Abortion

The most consistent and forceful critic of abortion in the modern world is the Roman Catholic Church, so in accessing the acceptability of the use of artificial wombs in lieu of abortion, I will make special reference to the Church's official teaching on matters relevant to this question, especially *Donum vitae*. The Catholic teaching on abortion is quite clear. In the words of John Paul II,

> *I declare that direct abortion, that is, abortion willed as an end or as a means, always constitutes a grave moral disorder*, since it is the deliberate killing of an innocent human being.[4]

What I believe is not clear (indeed, has never to my knowledge been explicitly addressed) is the Catholic answer to the question of the moral permissibility of artificial wombs in lieu of abortion. However, Catholic teaching does provide principles that could be applied to this case. Indeed, although the magisterium may at some point in the future explicitly address this situation, several important arguments against artificial wombs from magisterial teaching should be acknowledged, namely, (1) the artificiality objection, (2) the IVF objection, (3) the embryo transfer objection, (4) the deprivation of maternal shelter objection, (5) the birth-within-marriage objection, (6) the integrative parenthood objection, (7) the surrogate motherhood objection, and finally, (8) the wrongful experimentation objection. Each objection to artificial wombs arises from the Catholic tradition and has some plausibility. However, I believe that each objection fails and that there are compelling reasons to conclude that the use of artificial wombs in lieu of abortion is morally permissible.

I should first clarify a number of key terms in the discussion. By complete ectogenesis, I mean the generation and development of a human being outside the womb from the beginning of embryonic existence until the equivalent of forty weeks' gestation. By partial ectogenesis, I mean the development of a human being during the typical gestational period outside the maternal womb for part of (but not the entire) gestational period. An artificial womb might be used for complete or partial ectogenesis; i.e, it could be used to generate and sustain development of an embryo or fetus during the entire period of gestation, or it might be used to sustain development after partial development within the maternal womb. Embryo transfer moves the human embryo, having never been planted in a womb, to another location, such as an artificial womb or maternal womb. Fetal transfer moves the fetus from a maternal womb to another maternal womb or to an artificial womb. So, let us now consider some of the likely objections to artificial wombs.

(1) *The artificiality objection.* This possible objection against artificial wombs arises precisely because these wombs are *artificial*. As utilizing an artificial, man-made product for the purpose of gestation, ectogenesis of any kind would be against nature. Since human beings should act in accordance with nature, artificial wombs are impermissible.

However, the "artificiality" of such wombs is not sufficient grounds for rejecting their use. In speaking of various technologies used to create human life, such as IVF, *Donum vitae* indicates that

> [t]hese interventions are not to be rejected on the grounds that they are artificial. As such, they bear witness to the possibilities of the art of medicine. But they must be given a moral evaluation in reference to the dignity of the human person, who is called to realize his vocation from God to the gift of love and the gift of life.

Indeed, current advanced incubators are highly "artificial," making use of cutting-edge technology of all kinds, but they are not ethically impermissible. Indeed, the artificial wombs envisioned by researchers are nothing more than extremely advanced versions of incubators routinely used today.

(2) *The IVF objection.* This objection against artificial wombs arises from the Catholic opposition to IVF. The Catholic Church, it would seem, must oppose ectogenesis because it would seem to presuppose the use of cloning, parthenogenesis, or IVF in creating an embryo.

However, this objection fails to distinguish between partial ectogenesis and complete ectogenesis. Catholic teaching as expressed in *Donum vitae* clearly excludes complete ectogenesis (because the document forbids fertilization outside the human body), but a condemnation of complete ectogenesis is not decisive for the question at issue, since the use of artificial wombs in lieu of abortion would be considered partial ectogenesis. A woman tempted to seek abortion

already has a human fetus within her. Complete ectogenesis is already excluded. Partial ectogenesis is the continued development of an already generated human being in an artificial womb after transfer from a maternal womb. By definition, partial ectogenesis does not involve generation and development *entirely outside* the womb. So although the Catholic Church opposes IVF, twin fission, cloning, and parthenogenesis, and must therefore oppose complete ectogenesis, it does not necessarily follow that it would oppose partial ectogenesis.

(3) *The embryo transfer objection.* This possible objection arises from the belief of impermissibility of *embryo transfer* (ET). If embryo transfer is impermissible, fetal transfer (FT) from a maternal womb to an artificial womb would also seem to be impermissible. Partial ectogenesis necessarily involves FT, the transfer of the human fetus from the maternal womb to an artificial womb, and so partial ectogenesis would seem to be impermissible.

It is important to note that embryo transfer has not been explicitly condemned by the Catholic Church. Indeed, the previous issue of the *National Catholic Bioethics Quarterly* (Spring 2005) devoted several articles to the topic, which were written from various perspectives and came to different conclusions. In the condemnation of embryo transfer in *Donum vitae*, the problematic nature of embryo transfer is always spoken of in connection with IVF. It could be that IVF and ET are objectionable *as a combination*, and yet ET alone is not wrong *ex objecto*. Indeed, many authors argue that the "rescue" of abandoned frozen embryos via implantation, even into adoptive mothers, is permissible, indeed heroic.

A final case may make clear the acceptability of embryo transfer. In treating ectopic pregnancy, some doctors have removed the embryo from the fallopian tube and implanted the embryo in the mother's uterus. There have been reports of successful pregnancies resulting. Surely, such efforts to preserve the health of the mother and secure the life of the embryo are not only permissible but laudable. At least in such cases, the moving of the embryo to avoid potentially lethal harm to the mother and certainly lethal harm to the child is clearly permissible. If ET is not wrong *ex objecto*, then it would seem that transfer of a human being prior to full term from one location to another is not in itself impermissible—which is what is required for partial ectogenesis.

However, even if ET were unacceptable *ex objecto*, it does not necessarily follow that FT is problematic. Indeed, fetal transfer is already widely practiced and accepted. The emergency cesarean delivery of a preterm baby in danger of dying is not morally problematic, and may, in some cases, even be morally obligatory. As incubator technology progresses, some premature babies who now are seriously injured or who die because of preterm delivery will instead become viable and healthy.

(4) *The deprivation of maternal shelter objection*. This objection is more difficult. In the words of *Donum vitae*,

> The freezing of embryos, even when carried out in order to preserve the life of an embryo—cryopreservation—constitutes an offense against the respect due to human beings by exposing them to grave risks of death or harm to their physical integrity, and *depriving them, at least temporarily, of maternal shelter and gestation*, thus placing them in a situation in which further offenses and manipulation are possible.

It is possible, however, that deprivation of maternal shelter and gestation is prima facie wrong, but nevertheless may be justified in certain circumstances. Consider the case of a viable baby whose mother begins to die, or actually dies. Surgeons on-hand rush to remove the premature baby from the mother, depriving him or her of maternal gestation—but of course this removal is not in itself morally objectionable. One can imagine other situations in which a preborn child must be removed from the uterus or else he or she will die, such as a case of a mother who has an incompetent uterus, or a situation in which the mother has been poisoned, and the poison will kill the child unless it is immediately removed from the womb. In these cases, removing the child from the maternal womb does no offense to the dignity of the child. Maternal gestation and shelter are important to the human being in utero to the extent that they aid and support the well-being of the human fetus. In cases in which it endangers the life of a human being to remain in utero, depriving a human fetus of maternal gestation is not morally objectionable, but may be morally praiseworthy.

Of course, all the cases appealed to in the previous paragraph involve medical pathology threatening fetal life rather than a free choice of the will. If natural causes endanger the life of the human fetus, then removal is permissible and deprivation of maternal gestation does not offend the dignity of the human being in utero. On the other hand, if the life of the human fetus is threatened by the choice of abortion, deprivation of maternal gestation is blameworthy. Depriving the human being in utero of care and shelter may be permissible in the first case of natural causes, but not permissible in the second case, in which the danger to the child is voluntarily caused and could be voluntarily removed.

Does the voluntary or involuntary nature of the danger mark a morally decisive difference between the two cases? Whether the danger is voluntarily or nonvoluntarily caused makes no difference from the perspective of the preborn who are threatened with death. Death is just as final from a voluntary cause as from a nonvoluntary cause. Indeed, many causes of danger to the human fetus which could be considered "natural" can be originally caused by voluntary actions. For example, one can imagine a case in which a pregnant woman is dying because she was in a car accident that she caused by her irresponsible driving, or perhaps a case in which a woman is dying from lung cancer because she smoked too many cigarettes. The details of a causal chain which ends with a human fetus being in danger of death unless removed from the womb do not, therefore, appear to be morally decisive in determining the permissibility of the use of highly advanced incubators.

Another important distinction between the two cases (partial ectogenesis instead of abortion on the one hand, and on the other hand, fetal removal on account of a maternal pathology threatening fetal well-being) is that in the first case, the removal is motivated by the (perceived) well-being of the mother, but in the second, the removal is motivated by the well-being of the child. Perhaps this difference could account for the impermissibility of the first act but the clear permissibility of the second.

However, there are other cases, not normally viewed as problematic, in which the removal of the child takes place for the well-being of the woman. In the case of a gravid cancerous uterus, the removal of uterus and child takes place to preserve the mother's, not the child's, well-being. According to widely accepted understandings of double effect reasoning, the removal of the gravid cancerous uterus is morally permissible even if the premature child would die. If fetal viability has already been achieved, the removal is even easier to justify. For a variety of reasons, many women choose to have labor induced so as to deliver their babies before their due date. It seems that there is tacit agreement that such practices are morally unproblematic so long as the safety of the mother and child is not endangered. If ectogenesis can function in the future as currently envisioned, then induction of labor or surgical removal of the human fetus at any stage of pregnancy could become no less dangerous than induction of labor is now with contemporary technology a few days before the due date. In such circumstances, whatever would justify delivering a child a few days earlier would also justify ectogenesis.

This arguably proves too much, for even if partial ectogenesis might be permissible in lieu of abortion, it seems prima facie morally problematic to choose partial ectogenesis for trivial reasons. One might then carve out a "middle position" such that partial ectogenesis ought *not* to be used for utterly trivial reasons, and yet *may* be chosen in circumstances in which

a person might otherwise be tempted to choose abortion.

(5) *The birth-within-marriage objection.* The right of a child to be born within marriage is another objection that could be raised to the use of highly advanced incubators in the context of possible abortion. In the words of *Donum vitae,*

> Techniques of fertilization *in vitro* can open the way to other forms of biological and genetic manipulation of human embryos, such as attempts or plans for fertilization between human and animal gametes and the gestation of human embryos in the uterus of animals, or the hypothesis or project of constructing artificial uteruses for the human embryo. *These procedures are contrary to the human dignity proper to the embryo, and at the same time they are contrary to the right of every person to be conceived and to be born within marriage and from marriage.*

This passage is particularly noteworthy in that it explicitly mentions the possibility of constructing artificial uteruses and seems to condemn ectogenesis.

Indeed, this passage of *Donum vitae* clearly indicates the moral impermissibility of complete ectogenesis, but it does not necessarily exclude partial ectogenesis. Whenever the human fetus leaves his or her mother's womb, whether by surgical intervention or naturally, whether at full term or earlier, a human being can rightly be said to be born. Unlike complete ectogenesis, condemned by this passage, partial ectogenesis takes place after human birth, albeit a preterm, surgically initiated human birth. Hence, partial ectogenesis is simply not within the scope of this passage from *Donum vitae,* which discusses the right to be born within marriage.

(6) *The integrative parenthood objection.* *Donum vitae* does, however, clarify the meaning of the right to be born within marriage in the following passage, in ways that would seem to also exclude partial ectogenesis. Call this the *integrative parenthood* objection to partial ectogenesis. "The child has the right to be conceived, *carried*

in the womb, brought into the world and brought up within marriage: it is through the secure and recognized relationship to his own parents that the child can discover his own identity and achieve his own proper human development." Artificial insemination using egg or sperm from someone outside the marriage is also impermissible for the same reason.

At first glance, these passages seem to clearly exclude partial ectogenesis as undermining *gestational parenthood*, which is important in securing the well-being of the child. Integrative parenthood involves not separating genetic parenthood, gestational parenthood, and what might be called social parenthood, namely, the responsibility for raising and rearing the child. A child has a right to *integrative parenthood*, and even partial ectogenesis violates this right by depriving the human fetus of gestational parenthood.

However, this interpretation of the importance of integrative parenthood cannot be maintained. If a right to be conceived, gestated, and raised within marriage were understood to mean that every child *once conceived* must be brought up within marriage, it would follow that all women who find themselves pregnant outside of marriage (even by rape) must marry the father. In many cases of extramarital pregnancy, marriage of the father and mother constitutes the best response to the situation. However, marriage following pregnancy is not always advisable, let alone a moral duty. Indeed, in at least some cases of extramarital pregnancy, marriage not only would be gravely imprudent but indeed is not permissible or even possible, such as when a pregnancy occurs as the result of incest, when a prior valid marriage exists for one or both parties, or when a pregnancy involves a party of very young age.

In addition, if the right to integrative parenthood were interpreted as the right of every existing child to be nurtured in his or her mother's womb until full-term birth and then raised in a marriage, then every birth mother placing a child for adoption and every couple accepting a child

for adoption would be acting impermissibly. Of course, given appropriate circumstances, birth parents and adoptive parents do nothing wrong in their acts of giving and receiving a child. Indeed, a birth mother acts generously and bravely in placing her child in another family through adoption. When adoption is in the child's best interest, the birth mother performs a loving and heroic act and those who adopt the child likewise perform a generous act. A child's right to integrative parenthood is misinterpreted if this right would lead to a condemnation of adoption.

Although it would be wrong to conceive a child simply in order to place him or her for adoption, the Catholic Church's teaching and ongoing support of adoption makes it clear that it is not wrong to choose adoption following the conception of a child. Whether this adoption takes place at a few weeks after birth, at forty weeks of full gestation, at twenty-five weeks following conception on account of premature birth, or at seven weeks following conception does not, in itself, seem morally relevant, so long as the well-being of the child is not endangered. The right to integrative parenthood does not exclude adoption and would seem also not to exclude partial ectogenesis.

(7) *The surrogate motherhood objection.* This objection would describe ectogenesis as a form of surrogate motherhood. *Donum vitae* clearly teaches that surrogate motherhood is ethically impermissible.

If surrogate motherhood is wrong, and if ectogenesis is a form of surrogate motherhood, indeed an artificial surrogate motherhood, then ectogenesis would also be wrong. This might be called the *surrogate motherhood objection* to the use of highly advanced incubators in lieu of abortion.

In response, one should recall the very precise definition of surrogate motherhood given in *Donum vitae*:

By "surrogate mother," the instruction means:

(a) The woman who carries in pregnancy an embryo implanted in her uterus and who is genetically a stranger to the embryo because it has been obtained through the union of the gametes of "donors." She carries the pregnancy with a pledge to surrender the baby once it is born to the party who commissioned or made the agreement for the pregnancy.

(b) The woman who carries in pregnancy an embryo to whose procreation she has contributed the donation of her own ovum, fertilized through insemination with the sperm of a man other than her husband. She carries the pregnancy with a pledge to surrender the child once it is born to the party who commissioned or made the agreement for the pregnancy.

By neither of these definitions would partial ectogenesis be a form of surrogate motherhood. Both definitions of surrogate motherhood involve promises made by the surrogate mother to give up the baby once it is born to whomever commissioned or made the agreement for pregnancy. Obviously, an artificial womb cannot pledge or agree to anything, nor must partial ectogenesis involve giving the baby to those who initiated creation of the baby. Indeed, in cases where partial ectogenesis is chosen instead of abortion, the woman who otherwise would have chosen abortion does not want to raise the baby. In sum, one can reject the permissibility of surrogate motherhood as understood in *Donum vitae* without rejecting the permissibility of using highly advanced incubators in lieu of abortion.

(8) *The wrongful experimentation objection.* Finally, that this solution to the abortion problem might involve *wrongful experimentation* is perhaps the most powerful objection to partial ectogenesis.

If scientific experimentation on human beings before birth is only permissible when directed to the healing or sustaining of the well-being of the individual not yet born, then to attempt partial ectogenesis would be wrong. The use of artificial wombs in lieu of abortion subjects the human fetus to risks, not for the sake of the human fetus's own welfare, but for the sake of the mother being free from pregnancy. Although some day techniques of partial ectogenesis may be made eventually routine and no more risky than normal pregnancy, all early attempts at partial ectogenesis would be wrongful experimentation.

However, as others have pointed out, ectogenesis could be developed as an extension of saving premature babies. Experimental procedures undertaken to save the life of premature infants are fully acceptable given the principles suggested by John Paul II, since they would be directed towards the individual survival of the human beings in question. If these techniques were improved over time by means of this type of acceptable experimentation, the sustaining of very young human fetuses outside the womb would eventually no longer be experimental but could become a common procedure, exposing its human subjects to no disproportionate risks. Partial ectogenesis may someday become *less risky* than normal gestation, since an artificial womb would not, presumably, get into car crashes, slip and fall, or be assaulted. Accepting that experimentation should only be undertaken for the good of the one experimented upon does not exclude the legitimate development of artificial wombs, if these artificial wombs are developed in the process of trying to save premature infants who would otherwise die. For the many couples experiencing painful premature deliveries due to an incompetent uterus, such technology would be a great blessing.

Having examined the artificiality objection, the IVF objection, the embryo transfer objection, the deprivation of maternal shelter objection, the birth-within-marriage objection, the integrative parenthood objection, the surrogate motherhood objection, and finally the wrongful experimentation objection, I can find no basis in Catholic magisterial teaching as presently articulated for the condemnation of the use of artificial wombs in lieu of abortion.

Doubtless there are objections and sources that could be brought to bear on this question that could lead to a different conclusion. However, even if it were to turn out that

Catholic principles did lead to the moral impermissibility of highly advanced incubators in place of abortion, partial ectogenesis still might be counselled as the lesser of two evils in situations in which a woman is determined to end her pregnancy. In cases in which an agent is determined to do wrong, it is permissible to counsel him or her to do the lesser of two evils. If an agent is intent on harming an innocent person as an act of "revenge," and will not be deterred despite one's best efforts, one can counsel the agent to do less harm rather than more. When comparing abortion to the use of artificial wombs, an extermination to an extraction, it is clear that abortion involves a more serious evil, since abortion involves a more serious harm to the preborn, the intentional taking of human life, and partial ectogenesis, even if morally problematic, does not involve harms that are as serious. Thus, even if artificial wombs are morally impermissible considered in themselves, their use might still be urged in lieu of abortion, if a woman was determined to terminate her pregnancy in one way or another, as it seems is often the case.

Thus far, I have sought to remove reasonable but ultimately, I believe, mistaken objections to partial ectogenesis based on magisterial Catholic teaching. I have not addressed the positive case for limited use of partial ectogenesis. The most obvious answer is that artificial wombs could save innocent human lives. In the year 2000 alone, there were approximately 1.31 million abortions in the United States and in 1995, it is estimated that there were approximately 46 million abortions worldwide. If only a small percentage of abortions were eliminated by the use of artificial wombs, this would be a great service to the human community. Like orphanages long sponsored by the Church, support of highly advanced incubators would help preserve the well-being of innocent preborn human persons who otherwise would be lost.

Artificial wombs could also be a great aid to couples facing infertility problems. Even aside from the abortion issue, such advanced incubators could help married couples who experience repeated miscarriages, due to maternal health problems, various kinds of maternal-fetal incompatibility, or other pathologies. A woman whose uterus had to be removed because of cancer could have an artificial womb constructed from those cancer-free sections of her own uterine lining and then have this artificial uterus transplanted in her body, facilitating "normal" conception, gestation, and birth. Like heart or kidney transplants, such medical advances would be welcomed by the Church as morally unproblematic. If an artificial womb could permissibly be used within a woman's body, it is difficult to see why it could not permissibly be used outside a woman's body.

An End to the Abortion Debate?

Important public debates do not end when there is not a single person left on a given side of an issue, but rather when the vast majority of both sides comes to a consensus. As noted in the first section of this article, the vast majority of defenders of abortion who have written about the topic in scholarly journals and books do not defend a right of extermination but rather the right of extraction. The termination of pregnancy, and not the termination of human life, is their stated goal. If they are consistent with what they have written, it would seem that the vast majority of these people could accept the use of artificial wombs in lieu of abortion. It was then argued that the foremost opponent of abortion in the modern world, the Catholic Church, has not condemned artificial wombs in lieu of abortion and has strong reason to support their use. If this is correct, then both consistent defenders and consistent critics of abortion could accept the permissibility of using artificial wombs in lieu of abortion. Of course, in this article, I have considered only a relatively small aspect of the "abortion debate," namely, the intellectual debate, without taking into consideration its social, legal, and political aspects. Nevertheless, although many scientific, social, legal, and economic hurdles remain, the day may come when, thanks to the use of artificial wombs, the abortion debate is as settled and distant as debates over slavery are today.

Notes

1. Mary Anne Warren, "The Personhood Argument in Favor of Abortion," in *Life and Death: A Reader in Moral Problems*, edited by Louis P. Pojman (Belmont, CA: Wadsworth Publishing Company, 2000), 267.

2. David N. James, "Ectogenesis: A Reply to Singer and Wells," *Bioethics* 1, no. 1 (1987): 87.

3. Peter Singer and Deane Wells, *The Reproduction Revolution: New Ways of Making Babies* (Oxford: Oxford University Press, 1984), 135–36.

4. John Paul II, *Evangelium vitae*, March 25, 1995, n. 62.

The Limits of Conscientious Objection

May Pharmacists Refuse to Fill Prescriptions for Emergency Contraception?

JULIE CANTOR AND KEN BAUM

New England Journal of Medicine 351, no. 19 (2004): 2008–2012.

Health policy decisions are often controversial, and the recent determination by the Food and Drug Administration (FDA) not to grant over-the-counter status to the emergency contraceptive Plan B was no exception. Some physicians decried the decision as a troubling clash of science, politics, and morality. Other practitioners, citing safety, heralded the agency's prudence. Public sentiment mirrored both views. Regardless, the decision preserved a major barrier to the acquisition of emergency contraception — the need to obtain and fill a prescription within a narrow window of efficacy. Six states have lowered that hurdle by allowing pharmacists to dispense emergency contraception without a prescription. In those states, patients can simply bypass physicians. But the FDA's decision means that patients cannot avoid pharmacists. Because emergency contraception remains behind the counter, pharmacists can block access to it. And some have done just that.

Across the country, some pharmacists have refused to honor valid prescriptions for emergency contraception. In Texas, a pharmacist, citing personal moral grounds, rejected a rape survivor's prescription for emergency contraception. This fall, a New Hampshire pharmacist refused to fill a prescription for emergency contraception or to direct the patron elsewhere for help. Instead, he berated the 21-year-old single mother, who then, in her words, "pulled the car over in the parking lot and just cried." Although the total number of incidents is unknown, reports of pharmacists who refused to dispense emergency contraception date back to 1991 and show no sign of abating.

Though nearly all states offer some level of legal protection for health care professionals who refuse to provide certain reproductive services, only Arkansas, Mississippi, and South Dakota explicitly protect pharmacists who refuse to dispense emergency and other contraception. But that list may grow. In past years, legislators from nearly two dozen states have taken "conscientious objection" — an idea that grew out of wartime tension between religious freedom and national obligation and was co-opted into the reproductive-rights debate of the 1970s — and applied it to pharmacists.

This issue raises important questions about individual rights and public health. Who prevails when the needs of patients and the morals of providers collide? Should pharmacists have a right to reject prescriptions for emergency contraception? The contours of conscientious objection remain unclear. This article elucidates those boundaries and offers a balanced solution to a complex problem. Because the future of over-the-counter emergency contraception is in flux, this issue remains salient for physicians and their patients.

Arguments in Favor of a Pharmacist's Right to Object

Pharmacists Can and Should Exercise Independent Judgment

Pharmacists, like physicians, are professionals. They complete a graduate program to gain expertise, obtain a state license to practice, and join a professional organization with its own code of ethics. Society relies on pharmacists to instruct patients on the appropriate use of medications and to ensure the safety of drugs prescribed in combination. Courts have held that pharmacists, like other professionals, owe their customers a duty of care. In short, pharmacists are not automatons completing tasks; they are integral members of the health care team. Thus, it seems inappropriate and condescending to question a pharmacist's right to exercise personal judgment in refusing to fill certain prescriptions.

Professionals Should Not Forsake Their Morals as a Condition of Employment

Society does not require professionals to abandon their morals. Lawyers, for example, choose clients and issues to represent. Choice is also the norm in the health care setting. Except in emergency departments, physicians may select their patients and procedures. Ethics and law allow physicians, nurses, and physician assistants to refuse to participate in abortions and other reproductive services. Although some observers argue that active participation in an abortion is distinct from passively dispensing emergency contraception, others believe that making such a distinction between active and passive participation is meaningless, because both forms link the provider to the final outcome in the chain of causation.

Conscientious Objection Is Integral to Democracy

More generally, the right to refuse to participate in acts that conflict with personal ethical, moral, or religious convictions is accepted as an essential element of a democratic society. Indeed, Oregon acknowledged this freedom in its Death with Dignity Act, which allows health care providers, including pharmacists, who are disquieted by physician-assisted suicide to refuse involvement without fear of retribution. Also, like the draftee who conscientiously objects to perpetrating acts of death and violence, a pharmacist should have the right not to be complicit in what they believe to be a morally ambiguous endeavor, whether others agree with that position or not.

Arguments Against a Pharmacist's Right to Object

Pharmacists Choose to Enter a Profession Bound by Fiduciary Duties

Although pharmacists are professionals, professional autonomy has its limits. As experts on the profession of pharmacy explain, "Professionals are expected to exercise special skill and care to place the interests of their clients above their own immediate interests." When a pharmacist's objection directly and detrimentally affects a patient's health, it follows that the patient should come first. Similarly, principles in the pharmacists' code of ethics weigh against conscientious objection. Given the effect on the patient if a pharmacist refuses to fill a prescription, the code undermines the right to object with such broadly stated objectives as "a pharmacist promotes the good of every patient in a caring, compassionate, and confidential manner," "a pharmacist respects the autonomy and dignity of each patient," and "a pharmacist serves individual, community, and societal needs." Finally, pharmacists understand these fiduciary obligations when they choose their profession. Unlike conscientious objectors to a military draft, for whom choice is limited by definition, pharmacists willingly enter their field and adopt its corresponding obligations.

Emergency Contraception Is Not an Abortifacient

Although the subject of emergency contraception is controversial, medical associations, government agencies, and many religious groups agree that it is not akin to abortion. Plan B and similar hormones have no effect on an established pregnancy, and they may operate by more than one physiological mechanism, such as by inhibiting ovulation or creating an unfavorable environment for implantation of a blastocyst. This duality allowed the Catholic Health Association to reconcile its religious beliefs with a mandate adopted by Washington State that emergency contraception must be provided to rape survivors. According to the association, a patient and a provider who aim only to prevent conception follow Catholic teachings and state law. Also, whether one believes that pregnancy begins with fertilization or implantation, emergency contraception cannot fit squarely within the concept of abortion because one cannot be sure that conception has occurred.

Pharmacists' Objections Significantly Affect Patients' Health

Although religious and moral freedom is considered sacrosanct, that right should yield when it hinders a patient's ability to obtain timely medical treatment. Courts have held that religious freedom does not give health care providers an unfettered right to object to anything involving birth control, an embryo, or a fetus. Even though the Constitution protects people's beliefs, their actions may be regulated. An objection must be balanced with the burden it imposes on others. In some cases, a pharmacist's objection imposes his or her religious beliefs on a patient. Pharmacists may decline to fill

prescriptions for emergency contraception because they believe that the drug ends a life. Although the patient may disapprove of abortion, she may not share the pharmacist's beliefs about contraception. If she becomes pregnant, she may then face the question of abortion — a dilemma she might have avoided with the morning-after pill.

Furthermore, the refusal of a pharmacist to fill a prescription may place a disproportionately heavy burden on those with few options, such as a poor teenager living in a rural area that has a lone pharmacy. Whereas the savvy urbanite can drive to another pharmacy, a refusal to fill a prescription for a less advantaged patient may completely bar her access to medication. Plan B is most effective when used within 12 to 24 hours after unprotected intercourse. An unconditional right to refuse is less compelling when the patient requests an intervention that is urgent.

Refusal Has Great Potential for Abuse and Discrimination

The limits to conscientious objection remain unclear. Pharmacists are privy to personal information through prescriptions. For instance, a customer who fills prescriptions for zidovudine, didanosine, and indinavir is logically assumed to be infected with the human immunodeficiency virus (HIV). If pharmacists can reject prescriptions that conflict with their morals, someone who believes that HIV-positive people must have engaged in immoral behavior could refuse to fill those prescriptions. Similarly, a pharmacist who does not condone extramarital sex might refuse to fill a sildenafil prescription for an unmarried man. Such objections go beyond "conscientious" to become invasive. Furthermore, because a pharmacist does not know a patient's history on the basis of a given prescription, judgments regarding the acceptability of a prescription may be medically inappropriate. To a woman with Eisenmenger's syndrome, for example, pregnancy may mean death. The potential for abuse by pharmacists underscores the need for policies ensuring that patients receive unbiased care.

Toward Balance

Compelling arguments can be made both for and against a pharmacist's right to refuse to fill prescriptions for emergency contraception. But even cogent ideas falter when confronted by a dissident moral code. Such is the nature of belief. Even so, most people can agree that we must find a workable and respectful balance between the needs of patients and the morals of pharmacists.

Three possible solutions exist: an absolute right to object, no right to object, or a limited right to object. On balance, the first two options are untenable. An absolute right to conscientious objection respects the autonomy of pharmacists but diminishes their professional obligation to serve patients. It may also greatly affect the health of patients, especially vulnerable ones, and inappropriately brings politics into the pharmacy. Even pharmacists who believe that emergency contraception represents murder and feel compelled to obstruct patients' access to it must recognize that contraception and abortion before fetal viability remain legal nationwide. In our view, state efforts to provide blanket immunity to objecting pharmacists are misguided.

Complete restriction of a right to conscientious objection is also problematic. Though pharmacists voluntarily enter their profession and have an obligation to serve patients without judgment, forcing them to abandon their morals imposes a heavy toll. Ethics and law demand that a professional's morality not interfere with the provision of care in life-or-death situations, such as a ruptured ectopic pregnancy. Whereas the hours that elapse between intercourse and the intervention of emergency contraception are crucial, they do not meet that strict test. Also, patients who face an objecting pharmacist do have options, even if they are less preferable than having the prescription immediately filled. Because of these caveats, it is difficult to demand by law that pharmacists relinquish individual morality to stock and fill prescriptions for emergency contraception.

We are left, then, with the vast middle ground. Although we believe that the most ethical course is to treat patients compassionately — that is, to stock emergency contraception and fill prescriptions for it — the totality of the arguments makes us stop short of advocating a legal duty to do so as a first resort. We stop short for three reasons: because emergency contraception is not an absolute emergency, because other options exist, and because, when possible, the moral beliefs of those delivering care should be considered. However, in a profession that is bound by fiduciary obligations and strives to respect and care for patients, it is unacceptable to leave patients to fend for themselves. As a general rule, pharmacists who cannot or will not dispense a drug have an obligation to meet the needs of their customers by referring them elsewhere. This idea is uncontroversial when it is applied to common medications such as antibiotics and statins; it becomes contentious, but is equally valid, when it is applied to emergency contraception. Therefore, pharmacists who object should, as a matter of ethics and law, provide alternatives for patients.

Pharmacists who object to filling prescriptions for emergency contraception should arrange for another pharmacist to provide this service to customers promptly. Pharmacies that stock emergency contraception should ensure, to the extent possible, that at least one nonobjecting pharmacist is on duty at all times. Pharmacies that do not stock emergency contraception should give clear notice and refer patients elsewhere. At the very least, there should be a prominently displayed sign that says, "We do not provide emergency contraception. Please call Planned Parenthood at 800-230-PLAN (7526) or visit the Emergency Contraception Web site at www.not-2-late.com for assistance." However, a direct referral to a local pharmacy or pharmacist who is willing to fill the prescription is preferable. Objecting pharmacists should also redirect prescriptions for emergency contraception that are received by telephone to another pharmacy known to fill such prescriptions. In rural areas, objecting pharmacists should provide referrals within a reasonable radius.

Notably, the American Pharmacists Association has endorsed referrals, explaining that "providing alternative mechanisms for patients . . . ensures patient access to drug products, without requiring the pharmacist or the patient to abide by personal decisions other than their own." A referral may also represent a break in causation between the pharmacist and distributing emergency contraception, a separation that the objecting pharmacist presumably seeks. And, in deference to the law's normative value, the rule of referral also conveys the importance of professional responsibility to patients. In areas of the country where referrals are logistically impractical, professional obligation may dictate providing emergency contraception, and a legal mandate may be appropriate if ethical obligations are unpersuasive.

Inevitably, some pharmacists will disregard our guidelines, and physicians — all physicians — should be prepared to fill gaps in care. They should identify pharmacies that will fill patients' prescriptions and encourage patients to keep emergency contraception at home. They should be prepared to dispense emergency contraception or instruct patients to mimic it with other birth-control pills. In Wisconsin, family-planning clinics recently began dispensing emergency contraception, and the state set up a toll-free hotline to help patients find physicians who will prescribe it. Emergency departments should stock emergency contraception and make it available to rape survivors, if not all patients.

In the final analysis, education remains critical. Pharmacists may have misconceptions about emergency contraception. In one survey, a majority of pharmacists mistakenly agreed with the statement that repeated use of emergency contraception is medically risky. Medical misunderstandings that lead pharmacists to refuse to fill prescriptions for emergency contraception are unacceptable. Patients, too, may misunderstand or be unaware of emergency contraception. Physicians should teach patients about this option before the need arises, since patients may understand their choices better when they are not under stress. Physicians should discuss emergency contraception during office visits, offer prescriptions in advance of need, and provide education through pamphlets or the Internet.

Our principle of a compassionate duty of care should apply to all health care professionals. In a secular society, they must be prepared to limit the reach of their personal objection. Objecting pharmacists may choose to find employment opportunities that comport with their morals — in a religious community, for example — but when they pledge to serve the public, it is unreasonable to expect those in need of health care to acquiesce to their personal convictions. Similarly, physicians who refuse to write prescriptions for emergency contraception should follow the rules of notice and referral for the reason previously articulated: the beliefs of health care providers should not trump patient care. It is difficult enough to be faced with the consequences of rape or of an unplanned pregnancy; health care providers should not make the situation measurably worse.

As patients understand their birth-control options, conflicts at the pharmacy counter and in the clinic may become more common. When professionals' definitions of liberty infringe on those they choose to serve, a respectful balance must be struck. We offer one solution. Even those who challenge this division of burdens and benefits should agree with our touchstone — although health professionals may have a right to object, they should not have a right to obstruct.

Distinguishing Features of Women's Health Care

MARY BRIODY MAHOWALD

From *Bioethics and Women: Across the Life Span*, (New York: Oxford University Press, 2006), 30–49.

The most salient distinguishing feature of women's health care is the fact that most women are capable during a considerable portion of their lives of conceiving and bearing children. Although this sex-based characteristic is often relevant to treatment of women, it also has many gender-based or social implications. Ethically relevant variables that arise from these implications include (but are not limited to) the circumstances in which a pregnancy is initiated, continued, or terminated; the costs and availability of medical assistance during pregnancy; the impact of pregnancy on women's lifestyles; societal supports (or lack of support) for pregnant women; and social attitudes and laws about decisions to continue or terminate pregnancy. In addition, the ethical complexity of health care of pregnant women and research involving women of reproductive age is inseparable from diverse positions about the moral status of the fetus.

Possible Modifications of Principlist and Casuistic Methods

Proponents of principlism and casuistry do not adequately address issues involving pregnant women because they neither identify nor defend a position on the moral status of the fetus, which inevitably affects decisions on these issues. The most recent edition of *Clinical Ethics*, for example, fails even to consider pregnancy, abortion, or infertility treatment as topics relevant to the field.[1] This omission virtually excludes pregnant women from the domain of clinical ethics, violating the authors' own version of casuistry, which calls for attention to the particularities of cases.

A schematic by which to incorporate concerns about the fetus into their interpretation of the principles of Beauchamp and Childress was proposed by Frank Chervenak, an obstetrician and gynecologist, and Laurence McCullough, a philosopher, in 1985. Presumably assuming that beneficence encompasses nonmaleficence, their modification of the Georgetown mantra is the following:[2]

Table 4.1 Best Interests of Mother vs. Fetus

Best Interests of Mother		Best Interests of Fetus	
Maternal autonomy-based obligations of physician	Maternal beneficence-based obligations of physician	Fetal beneficence-based obligations of mother	Fetal beneficence-based obligations of physician

Although the authors thus identify obligations applicable to physicians who care for pregnant women, their schematic offers no clues on how to prioritize these obligations in cases of conflict. In their arguments for specific positions, however, they implicitly invoke justice as a relevant principle for cases of conflict by arguing that one set of interests outweighs the other. This accords with the balancing function that Beauchamp and Childress propose as a means of settling conflicts that arise in applications of their principles. On the issue of coercive treatment of pregnant women, for example, Chervenak and McCullough weigh "fetal beneficence-based obligations" and "maternal beneficence-based obligations" against "maternal autonomy-based obligations" and conclude that the former outweigh the latter. Their positions on different ethical issues faced by pregnant women rely on their consideration of women and their fetuses as separate or separable patients.

By distinguishing between the interests of the woman and her fetus, Chervenak and McCullough apply the principle of beneficence differently to each; the autonomy-based obligations are obviously only applicable to the woman. The authors' consideration of the fetus as if it is separable from the pregnant woman is another illustration of the fallacy of abstraction. Neither conceptually nor practically is it true that fetuses as such are separable from pregnant women. Embryos are occasionally separate or separable from women (e.g., when they are formed through in vitro fertilization or flushed from the woman's body after in vivo fertilization), but fetuses, once separated from women, are no longer fetuses but newborns or abortuses or stillborns. Scholars taking different positions on "maternal-fetal conflict" seem to ignore this inseparability when they argue for the priority of either the fetus's or the woman's interests.

As already indicated, the casuistic framework of Jonsen, Siegler, and Winslade fails to take account of the uniqueness of pregnant patients. If they were to amend their method so that it incorporates recognition of the fact that some patients are pregnant, two of their topics, medical indications and quality of life, would need to be subdivided into those applicable to the fetus and those applicable to the woman. However, this modification would again exemplify the prevalent but misguided tendency to construe the fetus and the pregnant woman as separate or separable, and it offers no guidance on how to prioritize fetal and maternal interests.

The topic of "contextual factors" in the casuistic method allows inclusion of others' interests, including those of the potential father, as morally relevant, whereas the framework proposed by Chervenak and McCullough only identifies "maternal interests" and "fetal interests" as morally relevant. However, their method as well as an amended method of casuistry are both preferable to methods of analyses that totally ignore the unique status of pregnant patients, and the prioritizing guidelines or maxims proposed earlier may be used to resolve or reduce conflicts that

arise between the interests of fetus and pregnant woman if these are treated as if they were separate. The application of the proposed maxims to specific cases depends crucially on the extent, if any, to which embryos or fetuses are regarded as separate patients.

An obvious weakness of Jonsen and Toulmin's casuistry relates to the selection of paradigmatic cases. Descriptive personhood, for example, serves as a relevant paradigm for those who believe that its achievement entails obligations that lack of it do not entail. Those for whom genetic humanity alone entails equal obligations toward all who possess it, regardless of their developmental stage, embrace a different paradigm. Because of their different views about the moral status of the fetus, practitioners and patients alike may utilize different paradigms on issues involving pregnancy. An egalitarian approach recognizes the relevance of different paradigms for different people. It does not imply, however, that any paradigm is acceptable; acceptable paradigms must meet a minimal standard of egalitarian justice by requiring respect for individuals who hold positions that are at odds with each other but consistent with defensible starting points.

Another weakness of casuistry, is that it fails to provide adequate guidance for prioritizing the values or principles at stake.

Many scholars who write about issues involving pregnant woman attempt to bypass the question of fetal moral status because they consider the abortion issue, to which it is obviously related, interminably controversial and irresolvable. Chervenak and McCullough attempt to avoid the issue by distinguishing between concepts of patienthood and personhood, and they are hardly alone in considering pregnant women as two patients rather than one. In the literature of obstetrics, for example, fetuses are described as "a whole new patient population," and books such as *Fetology* and *The Unborn Patient* have become commonplace in the libraries of physicians who treat pregnant women. But treating a gestating woman as two patients suggests what is impossible: that she and the fetus exist or are able to exist apart from each other. As Margaret Little puts it, the *essential* tie between them is "left out of the conceptual paradigm." In the next section, I explain more fully why this omission is both conceptually and practically problematic.

Who Is the Patient?

The question "Who is the patient?" is relevant not only to pregnant women and the practitioners who treat them but also to infertility specialists and their patients, including fertile partners of infertile patients and those who may provide gametes or agree to gestate a child for another. Note, however, that the term "patient" does not apply exclusively to persons or potential persons: veterinarians treat patients that fit neither characterization. Attribution of moral status is thus a separable question from determination of patienthood. Some practitioners who treat human patients view those in persistent vegetative state as patients but not persons, despite the fact that they are legally persons. It is plausible, therefore, to consider fetuses patients even if they are not persons, as Chervenak and McCullough propose.

Competent adults choose to be patients by seeking or consenting to diagnosis or treatment for themselves; those who choose otherwise—for example, by leaving the hospital against medical advice—are no longer patients, even though they may have conditions that deserve treatment. Those who refuse life-saving treatment while remaining in the hospital are no longer patients with regard to their life-threatening condition; they may then become patients as recipients of palliative care to ease their dying. Similarly, women who leave the hospital after free and informed refusal of medically recommended surgical delivery are no longer patients. If they remain in the hospital, however, they may then become patients as recipients of comfort care or measures that facilitate vaginal delivery.

Choosing to be patients is obviously not possible for those who are decisionally incapacitated; their patienthood status is necessarily determined by others. Infants and profoundly impaired adults, for example, become patients when parents or guardians seek treatment in their behalf. If fetuses are considered patients, they can only become so by being presented for care by others. Individuals unrelated to fetuses may attempt to secure care for them, but the only person who is indispensable to presentation of a particular fetus as patient is the pregnant woman herself. Regardless of who seeks treatment on its behalf, the patienthood of the fetus is thus dependent on others and on the patienthood status of the pregnant woman.

As already indicated, Chervenak and McCullough consider the controversy regarding personhood (or lack thereof) in fetuses avoidable through their focus on the fetus as a patient. Determining whether the fetus is a patient, they claim, allows practitioners to treat it as such, even, at times, over the objection of the pregnant woman. Accordingly, they identify variables by which clinicians may make this determination. The criteria they propose are morally relevant but inadequate for determination of patienthood if the woman decides not to present her fetus for care. Even if some fetuses are patients, this does not imply that they are separate or separable patients. Perhaps the most compelling support for the view that fetuses are separable or separate patients occurs in the context of maternal-fetal surgery, when the woman's uterus is opened and the fetus is removed from it for treatment. But the fetus is still not a separate or separable patient because its physical connection to the pregnant woman is maintained through the umbilical cord. As long as this connection remains, even if the fetus is considered a person, it is never treatable as a patient without the pregnant woman being treated as a patient. This inseparable entwinement cannot justifiably be ignored.

Determining whether the fetus is a patient does not settle moral questions regarding its treatment because answers may still differ on grounds of whether the fetus is or is not a person. If there are two patients with conflicting interests, and one is a person but the other is not, the interests of the patient who is clearly a person may trump those of the patient who is not a person. Persons as such have a legal and moral right to life, which may not be claimed for nonpersons to whom lesser, or no, moral status is imputed. With regard to other rights or goods, the verities apply more compellingly to patients who are uncontroversially persons than to those whose personhood is disputed or denied. Regardless of whether agreement can be reached on whether fetuses are persons, then, the issue is not ultimately separable from that of patienthood. The moral status of the fetus remains an unavoidable and crucial variable in addressing ethical questions involving pregnant women. Chervenak and McCullough implicitly acknowledge this when they attribute "dependent moral status" to some fetuses.

Beyond moral status, another variable with regard to fetuses is that they cannot all be considered patients even if, for the sake of argument, patienthood is imputed to them. Most patients seek medical assistance because they need it, but some seek it for nonmedical reasons, and physicians would be remiss if they treated these individuals as patients by providing medically unnecessary treatment solely on grounds of their requests. When physicians provide unnecessary treatment such as cosmetic surgery for enhancement of appearance or infertility treatment for healthy postmenopausal women, they still must weigh the hazards of the treatment against the expected (nonmedical) benefit to the patient, and they must decline to provide it if the medical risks are high. Pregnant women are encouraged to seek prenatal care on the grounds that this will promote their health and that of their potential children. Whether all pregnant women need or benefit by the care of physicians has nonetheless been questioned. One high-risk obstetrician, for example, has argued that healthy pregnant women do not need obstetricians because prenatal care and assistance in childbirth by physicians does not generally improve the outcome for the woman or the newborn.[3] According to studies he cites, pregnant women are not only well cared for but also tend to be more satisfied with the care they receive from nonphysicians such as midwives than with the care they receive from obstetricians.

On Chervenak and McCullough's understanding of "patient," a fetus may become one when it needs medical assistance and the pregnant woman seeks such assistance on its behalf. The analogy that supports this view is that of an adult who brings a minor for needed health care; the minor thus becomes a patient. If parents of children or guardians of decisionally incapacitated individuals fail to present them for necessary care, they may be accused (and convicted) of neglect; others in society will then be required to assume this responsibility, through either court-ordered hospitalization or treatment. The requirement that anyone in need of medical assistance *should* be considered a patient implies that such an individual has an independent claim or positive right to care. Such individuals are thus regarded not only as patients but also as persons who, as such, have independent, not dependent, moral status. In contrast, nonpersons, such as pets, may not become patients when they need care. Whether they become patients depends on their being presented for care by those responsible for them or others who choose, but are not obliged, to fill that role (e.g., members of an animal humane society).

Admittedly, an ethically relevant difference between human fetuses and non-humans whose patienthood status depends on others is that the former are uncontroversially regarded as having at least the potential for independent and full moral status or personhood. Arguments based on potential personhood are unnecessary to those whose starting premise is that (actual) personhood begins with human fertilization. To others, the status of potential personhood is legally and morally significant and, in some cases, compelling. If the interests being compared are proportionate, however, the interests of potential persons cannot override those of actual persons. Indeed, it may be argued that the interests of potential beings can never override those of actual beings of any kind.

A child or pet in need of care may be physically presented to a physician or veterinarian by someone other than a parent or owner. Regardless of who "presents" an individual in need of care, however, the patient is then left in the hands of the appropriate practitioner, and the "presenter" may then turn to other tasks or interests. In contrast, when fetuses are "presented" for care, the crucial "presenter" cannot leave the facility to resume other activities. More significantly, she cannot consent to testing or treatment of the fetus apart from herself. Any intervention on behalf of the fetus can only be provided through her body, often with risks or harms to her. Empirically, then, the pregnant woman is the only presenting patient when care of a fetus is contemplated or undertaken. As *pregnant* woman, she is one patient, not two, albeit one whose choices and welfare importantly and inevitably affect her potential offspring even as they may also affect the choices or welfare of those already born.

Chervenak and McCullough consider the pregnant woman as more than one patient, but not in all situations. An individual is a patient, they maintain, "when the *individual* is (1) presented to a physician (2) for the purpose of applying clinical interventions that are reliably expected to protect and promote the interests of that individual." In light of the fact that some women present their fetuses for abortion, the second requirement is crucial. With regard to the first requirement, the term "individual" is problematic. Webster's dictionary defines "individual" as "separate and distinct from others of the same kind." Because of the essential physical connection between fetuses and the women in whom they develop, fetuses do not fit this understanding of the term. As already mentioned, the meaning and reality of a human fetus is accurately understood as contained within the meaning and reality of any pregnant woman. Recognizing the genetic distinctness and potential for personhood of the fetus is entirely compatible with this position.

Pregnant women occasionally present themselves as patients for care of conditions unrelated to their fetuses or potential children. Even then, they necessarily present the fetuses within them. Except when abortion is desired, women usually want and expect the clinician to do what is medically best not only for themselves but also for their potential children. Arguments for treating fetuses as distinct patients are consistent with the latter goal insofar as fetuses are destined or intended to become indisputably persons after birth. However, this rationale is based on the potential rather than the actual status of an existing being. In situations of conflict, proportionate obligations to existing persons generally override obligations to possible or potential persons. Because decisions intended to benefit the potential child can only be implemented through the woman, fetuses are not patients in their own right—that is, apart from the patients on whom they depend for survival or treatment—unless their status as patients is determined on grounds that they are already persons.

The variables that Chervenak and McCullough propose for determining whether fetuses are patients (regardless of whether they are persons) are based on two distinctions, one biological and the other psychological. The first distinction is between viable and previable fetuses; the second, which applies only to previable fetuses, distinguishes between those that the pregnant woman has decided to abort and those she has chosen to carry to viability or term. On grounds of these distinctions, they argue that either of two criteria identifies a fetus as a patient: its viability, or the decision of the woman to continue her pregnancy. For these authors, a fetus that satisfies either criterion is a patient, that is, an individual "presented to a physician for the purpose of applying clinical interventions, etc." By becoming a patient, they argue, the fetus acquires "dependent moral status." As discussed in the next section, this view is at odds with their attempt to bypass the moral controversiality of abortion.

Patients and "Dependent Moral Status"

While acknowledging that persons as such have "independent moral status," Chervenak and McCullough attribute "dependent moral status" to all viable fetuses and some previable fetuses on grounds that they are patients. A viable fetus, they argue, has dependent moral status because its ongoing development is "reliably linked to later achievement of independent moral status." A previable fetus, however, has dependent moral status if and only if the pregnant woman "presents the previable fetus to the physician, that is, when she elects to continue her pregnancy to viability." The latter criterion seems to ignore the fact that a fetus as such is not presented to the physician; instead, a woman presents herself as a pregnant person who in many but not all cases desires care for herself and her potential child. It also ignores the fact that a woman's decision to continue her pregnancy is not necessarily accompanied by presentation of herself to a physician. By Chervenak and McCullough's account, some fetuses that women have elected to carry to term are not patients until and unless they become viable. At that point, the authors apparently consider them patients even if the pregnant woman does not seek health care.

Although dependent persons (e.g., children) as well as nonpersons (e.g., pets) become patients when presented to practitioners for diagnosis or treatment, this does not imply that they thereby acquire "dependent moral status." Children and incompetent adults have independent moral status despite their dependence on others; they thus have a right to life and health care, and practitioners have duties to them as patients independently of their parents or others on whom they depend for care. By arguing that physicians have similar duties to fetuses that meet their criteria for patienthood, Chervenak and McCullough in effect regard these fetuses as having the same moral status as children and incompetent adults who have independent moral status.

The difference between the criteria for patienthood that Chervenak and McCullough propose for viable versus previable fetuses is morally significant in its own right. For viable fetuses, moral status depends on achievement of a specific developmental milestone; for previable fetuses, it depends on the subjective decision of the pregnant woman, which may be made at any point after the woman knows she is pregnant, until the viability criterion is applicable. Although the authors deny that fetuses in either category have "independent moral status," they argue that the pregnant woman's wishes may be overridden for the sake of the viable fetus if her refusal is likely to harm her and her fetus, or when the apparent urgency of the situation prevents recourse to the courts. In these cases at least, the moral status of the fetus is obviously not dependent on the autonomy of the pregnant woman, who is indisputably a person with independent moral status.

As is the case with infants for whom parents are unable or unwilling to care, it may be argued that others are obliged to present viable fetuses for care if the pregnant woman does not do so. This implies that the pregnant woman herself may be coercively presented and treated involuntarily for the sake of the fetus. Chervenak and McCullough do not argue in favor of such coercion outside of the health care setting, but their position supports this conclusion. If the decision of a pregnant patient is overridable by the interests of the fetus-as-patient, the alleged moral status of the fetus is obviously not dependent on the woman's. In effect, the right of the fetus to treatment is as independently established as is that of any child or adult.

With regard to previable fetuses, Chervenak and McCullough acknowledge that the legal option of abortion constitutes an impediment to their being patients. They claim, however, that women who reach a "settled" decision to continue their pregnancies are obliged to present their previable fetuses to the physician, and once they do that, the physician is morally obliged to treat the fetus as a patient whose interests may be at odds with hers. In other words, a woman's decision to continue her pregnancy commits her to accept what others decide on behalf of her fetus. As with viable fetuses, however, Chervenak and McCullough still maintain that previable fetuses have dependent rather than independent moral status.

From the standpoint of those who impute full moral status to embryos or fetuses, Chervenak and McCullough are correct that fetuses are patients in their own right. Had these authors supported that starting position, however, they would have no need to argue for either viability or the woman's decision to continue her pregnancy as determinative of patienthood. Rather, all fetuses would then be considered patients precisely because they are persons. From that standpoint, viability suggests an analogy with patients who are indisputably persons, such as children and individuals dependent on life support, whose survival or viability is not simply a matter of developmental level or decisional capacity but also, and sometimes only, a function of whether others are willing and able to treat them. The woman's decision to continue her pregnancy is simply irrelevant to determination of whether human embryos or fetuses have rights and responsibilities that are objectively and independently attributable to them as persons—that is, as individuals with full moral status. Fetal personhood thus implies fetal patienthood, regardless of whether pregnant women themselves make that determination.

Full moral status is generally attributed to persons as such, and partial moral status is attributed to individuals who are not persons but who have some moral status or standing of their own, regardless of whether it is attributed to them by others. For those who impute partial moral status to fetuses, obligations to people already born are clearly more compelling than those that apply to persons who are born. But Chervenak and McCullough's distinction between dependent and independent moral status is unrelated to the important difference between partial and full moral status. Instead, their position is that fetuses either have it or don't have it. Once fetuses meet either of their criteria for patienthood, their interests may be as compelling as, or even override, those of the pregnant woman. The dependent moral status they attribute to some fetuses is thus equivalent to full moral status or personhood.

Because some practitioners believe that fetuses are patients with moral status of their own, but others do not, clinical practice varies with regard to ethical issues involving reproduction. Some physicians, for example, perform abortions only for compelling medical reasons; some never perform them, and others perform them routinely if the woman wishes to terminate her pregnancy. Some practitioners support coercive treatment for the sake of the fetus after viability (e.g., Chervenak), while others oppose coercive treatment of pregnant women for any reason. In light of these differences among their members, professional health care organizations usually provide guidance that respects their different moral standpoints as well as the different standpoints of researchers and study subjects. Similarly, federal regulations and state statutes attempt to articulate requirements applicable to all citizens, whose moral positions on key issues differ considerably. To be just in their provisions about women, laws and policies must take account of the distinguishing features of women's health care, as well as the variable standpoints of those who provide treatment or conduct research.

Notes

1. Albert R. Jonsen, Mark Siegler, and William J. Winslade, *Clinical Ethics*, 5th ed. (New York: McGraw-Hill, 2002).

2. Frank A. Chervenak and Laurence B. McCullough, "Perinatal Ethics: A Practical Method of Analysis of Obligations to Mother and Fetus," *Obstetrics and Gynecology* 66 (1985): 443. The authors elaborate on the meaning of "interests" and on "beneficence-based obligations" in obstetrics in Chervenak and McCullough, *Ethics in Obstetrics and Gynecology* (New York: Oxford University Press, 1994), 25–42, 113–22.

3. Thomas H. Strong, *Expecting Trouble: The Myth of Prenatal Care in America* (New York: New York University Press, 2000).

A Realistic Approach to Maternal-Fetal Conflict

DEBORAH HORNSTRA

Hastings Center Report 28, no. 5 (1998): 7–12.

It is the first of my three pregnancies. I am twenty years old and in my senior year of college at Syracuse. *Roe v. Wade* is seven years old, and my girlfriends and I are confident of our right to safe, accessible abortion. We are all sexually active, and though we use various forms of birth control, including the pill, the IUD, and the diaphragm, the availability of legal abortion as a backup is essential to our peace of mind. My college pregnancy, for instance, is the result of diaphragm failure (of either the device or the user, who knows).

Like most American women who have abortions, I want to have children some day. I am only trying to delay the first birth until I am domestically, educationally, and financially stable. This contrasts with the situation in developing countries, where the majority of women seeking abortion are mothers trying to bring an end to their constant childbearing. In many cultures, of course, twenty-year-olds are considered quite old enough for motherhood. But in our culture, education, employment, travel, romance, and leisure are considered more appropriate pursuits for this age group, and I certainly find them more appropriate for myself. As I see it, having a baby will bar my further participation in all of the above, at least until some time in the inconceivably distant future. And without having had these experiences, I fear I am not ready for motherhood and will not be able to do it well. Getting an abortion will give me the best of both worlds: I can continue to enjoy my youth unencumbered, while reserving the right to have a child when I am ready to care for it.

So I never consider having the baby. I am concerned only with when and where I can get an abortion, and how I will find the $300 to pay for it when I am clearing about $20 a week from my work-study job. Knowing the baby will never be born, I do not concern myself with his health (for some reason, I always think of it as a boy). I feel no compulsion to modify my diet or otherwise keep myself fit. I carry on as before, maintaining myself on pizza, cup-a-soup, beer, No-Doz, and pot, no one's welfare at stake but my own. Under the circumstances, I would consider miscarriage a lucky break, a $300 windfall.

This is not to say I do not feel any remorse about the abortion. I sincerely hope the baby understands that its time has not come. I hope it knows I love it, love the *idea* of it, but cannot and will not live with the timing, both for my sake and his. But these thoughts are rather ethereal and fleeting; I have other things on my mind, practical things, important arrangements to make. In this respect I am like a grieving spouse grateful for necessary distractions. I know I do not wish to think too hard about the baby that might have been. I quench my natural curiosity and do what I honestly feel I must.

There is an affecting poem posted on the Internet, written in the voice of an aborted child. The child is forgiving its mother for what she did, and promising her understanding and a reunion sometime. I think all women who have abortions hope this is how our couldn't-be babies feel. The pain we feel at the loss of the innocent child is compounded by some measure of guilty complicity on our part. There is, or at least there can be, an emotional bond between a woman who has conceived and the fetus she will abort, one that reflects the potential of the more complex mother-baby relationship that will not be realized this time around.

Fast forward six years. I've got my degree and some work experience under my belt. I'm living in Amsterdam with my Dutch husband, and I'm pregnant again, but this time I intend to carry to term. Now the fetus inside me is not merely a potential child, but as Bonnie Steinbock puts it, a "child-who-will-be-born." What a difference an attitude makes! The unborn child assumes personhood in my mind, and I graciously assume obligations toward him. Having decided to bring this new life into the world—that is, having decided not to abort—I am already feeling "maternal" in the most traditional sense: protective and responsible. I realize it is not in my power to ensure a healthy baby, but I resolve to give this tiny future person the best possible chance by following my midwife's orders. Some of these I find a trifle burdensome, especially the nasty iron tablets, but in general I am willing and able to subordinate my own needs to those of the baby-to-be for the finite period of time this is necessary.

Fortunately for me, I am living in a country where pregnant women are not held to undue standards of purity and perfection. My midwife, for example, allows her cigarette-smoking patients to light up four times a day. She has concluded that requiring pregnant women to quit tobacco cold turkey only exacerbates the anxiety that is a common feature of all pregnancies. When I go out, I am not confronted by oversized signs warning me of the dangers of drinking alcohol while pregnant. Even after I start to show, waiters continue to pour me wine, which I drink in moderation until it no longer tastes good.

So what changed in the six years between my first two pregnancies? Certainly not the definition of life. Not my own moral compass. In fact, the only significant change was in my circumstances, and as a consequence thereof, in my relationship to the baby I was carrying. It is my contention that this is the defining element in the mother-baby pas de deux: the mother's emotional connection to her unborn child. When this is intact and flourishing, as in most wanted pregnancies, women have little difficulty behaving during pregnancy. In fact, many take the opportunity to better their nutrition, start an exercise program,

and quit or curtail their bad habits. Pregnancy is widely recognized as a time when women decide to put their lives in order. But when the emotional connection is lacking, when the mother views the baby as an interloper, a disruption, even a threat, it becomes possible, perhaps necessary as a survival technique, to detach and put your own needs first. The ultimate example of detachment and self-interest is the decision to abort, but some degree of ambivalence, if not hostility, is manifested whenever a pregnant woman willfully undertakes activities known to be harmful to the baby she expects to bear.

An unborn child is in a very real sense at its mother's mercy, and thrives more or less at her pleasure. What is the baby's relationship to the mother, and what rights does it hold against her? It is dependent on another to a degree without parallel in human relations, and it is completely helpless to affect that other's behavior. The baby can in no way engender the emotional bond necessary to sustain its own existence. That bond may be present in the mother's psyche or it may be lacking. The mother may respond to the call, or she may ignore it. Her circumstances may encourage her to desire the baby or to fear it with an angst so palpable that it overrides her previous convictions.

Nonetheless, my view is that we cannot speak of a fetal "right" to be born healthy when this can never be guaranteed, and our attempts to do so intrude in the most intimate way on personal behavior. First, what do we mean by "healthy," anyway? Is healthy synonymous with "perfect"? Does it mean free of any defects that are known to be preventable or correctable? If we answer in the affirmative, we seem to imply that certain people should never have been born. I maintain that this is the logical conclusion of a philosophy that emphasizes fetal rights, or of the premise that a fetus has separate interests equal to or greater than those of a pregnant woman. While we may desire perfect babies, the desire does not justify doing whatever is necessary to achieve them. Such thinking leads directly to the horror of eugenics and its evil offspring, Nazism.

Interestingly, people with disabilities are among the leading opponents of fetal rights. They rightly perceive it as an attack on their right to exist as they are, and as an attack on their mothers, to whom they may feel nothing but gratitude. People with disabilities, especially those with disabilities targeted for extinction, such as Down syndrome and spina bifida, fear that an overemphasis on turning out perfect babies will result in the devaluation of their less-than-perfect selves. As Lisa Blumberg has argued, a concern for fetal rights misconstrues the nature of the mother-baby relationship:

> Fetal rights proponents believe that if a child is born with a disability, there must be someone to blame for it. Fetal rights is really fetal quality control. [The fetal rights proponents] do not stop and consider how the children will feel when they eventually learn about how their mothers were treated for producing them.[1]

Protecting Whom? From What?

The whole notion of regulating the behavior of pregnant women in order to ensure the "health" of their unborn children goes back to long-discredited theories of "improving" the species. But in spite of our abhorrence of such extremism, it may seem we should not accept any and all behavior from expectant mothers who opt to carry to term. Occasionally when mothers willfully refuse to do what is in their power to ensure the health of their babies, they engage in behavior they ought not to. Obvious examples of pregnant women whose behavior is dangerous to their babies are those who smoke cigarettes, abuse drugs or alcohol, engage in risky sexual practices, refuse to follow medical advice, or fail to eat properly and otherwise take care of themselves (and, by extension, the baby within). Less obvious examples might include pregnant women who work at hazardous or stressful occupations, those who participate in dangerous athletic activities, those who are obese, those who ride in cars without seatbelts, those over the age of thirty-four, those who expose themselves to secondhand smoke or environmental toxins, those who frequent saunas, and those who remain with men who abuse them. Even such seemingly benign activities as owning a cat and eating feta cheese have been linked to consequences as serious as fetal death. Indeed, since few activities in life are completely risk-free, virtually anything a pregnant woman does could be considered potentially harmful to her baby.

Plainly, then, one of the plethora of problems to which attempts to encourage "gestational responsibility" give rise is the delineation of the activities and conditions to be proscribed. And that problem leads to others: It is necessary to prove causality? How do we prove it, especially when multiple factors are so often involved, and what do we do when we cannot prove it? How much risk must be present before a duty to protect, and if necessary to intervene, emerges? Practically speaking, how can such intervention be implemented on the scale that may be necessary?

Thus a further problem is the practicability and moral acceptability of enforcement. The simple solution, of course, is to somehow compel responsibility in otherwise irresponsible expectant mothers. This would not be unprecedented, as the law already compels personal responsibility in many ways. We risk punishment if we drink and drive, if we beat our children, and if we let our dog run loose in Central Park. These activities are held to harm (or potentially harm) other living persons, and we can be forbidden from engaging in them at no great cost to our own personal freedom. They are cases of moral obligation made legal obligation. This is the approach favored by fetal rights activists, but otherwise condemned as unworkable and potentially contributory to the harm it would be instituted to prevent. A woman who gets drunk or high while pregnant may be harming her baby, but in any case, the baby must remain inside her body and completely dependent on her. He cannot be rescued from his maternal environment, however potentially damaging it may be. At least until late in the pregnancy (beyond the period during which most birth defects become detectable), the two living entities are irretrievably intertwined, a biologically unified dyad. Conceptually, pregnancy confounds our cherished notion of the autonomous self. Mother, perfect or not, is all baby's got, and indeed, all he needs. There is no way to usurp her position as baby's lifeline; their relationship is truly "for better or worse."

To protect an unborn child from the potentially harmful actions of its mother, therefore, requires controlling the mother's behavior to a degree incompatible with our notions of due process and individual freedom. It may also be detrimental to the baby's welfare, to the extent that normal bonding is hindered, the mother is dissuaded from seeking prenatal care, or the mother is herself harmed by the external control of her body and behavior.

Wholes—or Parts?

This last set of problems suggests another, deeper one. There is something unnatural about positing a fetus at odds with its own mother, since until recently pregnancy was viewed as a cooperative interaction. Wendy Chavkin of the Columbia University School of Public Health traces the genesis of this line of thinking to the 1973 *Roe v. Wade* decision. *Roe* gave the decisionmaking authority concerning reproductive choices to women and physicians, says Chavkin, and ever since, fathers and churches have been trying to regain some authority in this domain. Associated with this effort is the development of a maternal-fetal conflict, which Chavkin characterizes as a perception not dictated by the laws of nature but "socially constructed."[2] The courts participate in this social construction by forcing women to bear the costs of making fetal rights real. As Lisa Maher has written, it is part of an attempt to regain control over women by controlling their pregnancies.

This trend has been greatly aided by relentless technological advances, to which we mere mortals have not yet adjusted. Since the Second World War, increasingly routine use of ultrasonography has rendered the pregnant woman transparent, which is to say invisible, while revealing the previously hidden baby to a chorus of delight and confusion. One writer describes the evolution of the accompanying attitudinal change:

> [Traditionally] unable to interact with the fetus in clear distinction from its host, physicians conceptualized the maternal-fetal dyad as one complex patient, the gravid female, of which the fetus was an integral part. Now we have tools that penetrate the diagnostic environment. The biological maternal-fetal relationship has not changed, of course, but the medical model of that relationship has shifted emphasis from unity to duality.[3]

Organizations ranging from the Right to Life Committee to the National Institutes of Health acknowledge that the use of ultrasound and other prenatal tests has had a profound conceptual effect on medical practice:

> While [cesarean section] has been performed largely to protect the health of the mother, more recently the health of the fetus has played a larger role in decisions to go to surgery. Ultrasound … provided medical personnel with valuable information, but it also influenced attitudes toward the fetus. When the fetus could be visualized and its sex and chromosomal makeup determined … it became more of a person.[4]

For the perinatologist, then, there is now not one patient, but two. The fetus is no longer a sheltered recluse, and can even be treated surgically and phamaceutically in utero, which changes the emotional and financial investment of both medical practitioners and parents. One writer notes that our overdependence on the technological fix has created a "perfect-child mentality" that blames women for turning out children with any preventable defect.

In keeping with that mentality, current approaches typically incorporate no role for the larger society other than those of spy and enforcer, leaving individual mothers-to-be to respond to the new demands for vigilance on their own. This is the unfortunate result of our culture's obsession with personal responsibility and its flip side, our disdain for collective solutions. Society claims an interest in the developing fetus, but no responsibility.

Part of this focus upon personal responsibility is that an expectant mother who does not properly care for herself during pregnancy is viewed as evil. But this attitude fails to recognize that the mother may not truly be free to do what is right for her baby. Arguing in favor of fetal rights, one writer remarks that "these infants are not given a choice as to whether or not they want to be born addicted, yet their mothers have direct control over their status of addiction or non-addiction." If a woman is addicted to drugs, alcohol, or tobacco, however, all the evidence shows she will need a tremendous amount of expensive, time-consuming assistance, not to mention willpower and support, to kick her habit. If she is poor, she may not be able to afford to eat properly or obtain adequate prenatal care. If she is ignorant, she may not be capable of understanding what is required of her. If she is an undocumented alien, she may need to avoid any contact with authorities who can have her deported. If she is a victim of domestic violence, she may be trapped in a cycle of fear and dependence made worse by her pregnancy. In such cases, it cannot be said that the pregnant woman is in "direct control" of her addictive status.

Easy Targets

To be fair and effective, our approaches must address not only individual choices, but also the environments in which those choices are made. When these are far from optimum, holding pregnant women to a standard they cannot meet can only be seen as blame shifting, and blame shifting that doesn't even accomplish its putative goals. Pregnant women are easy targets for this. They are conspicuous, under stress, and by now, preconditioned to assume guilt for their behavior. The strange bedfellows of modern technology and traditional sexism have spawned a new paradigm, represented at its most extreme by the prolife slogan that declares the womb the most dangerous place for an unborn baby. (It must be the safest place as well, for it is the only place.)

Pregnant women who fall short of the prevailing standard for maternal self-sacrifice are scapegoated and held in contempt. Not only are they blamed for their own inappropriate actions, they are held liable for the failings of the larger society, including sexism, spousal abuse, environmental hazards, and poverty. This diverts our attention from those unfashionable root causes of deviance, while conveniently releasing us from the need to address our collective failures on the systemic level.

The push for fetal rights is the consummate product of our age. It could not have occurred without the present-day confluence of high technology, a serious backlash against women's rights, and widespread duplicity in the mass media. Perhaps the issue will be sorted out as part of a larger paradigm shift, the beginning of which we may be witnessing in the right-to-die movement, as well as in the recent resurgence of interest in alternative medicine. These trends portend a rediscovery of the power of individuals and of the limitations of medical technology and legal machination. We have been led to believe that doctors and judges can rescue us from ourselves and cleanse society of deviance. This is dangerously wishful thinking that distracts from the formidable tasks of striving toward justice and learning love.

Notes

1. Lisa Blumberg, "Why Fetal Rights Must Be Opposed," *Social Policy* 18 (1987): 40–41, at 40.
2. Wendy Chavkin, "Women and Fetus: The Social Construction of Conflict," in *The Criminalization of a Woman's Body*, edited by Clarice Feinman (New York: Harrington Park Press, 1992), pp. 193–201, at 196.
3. Susan S. Mattingly, "The Maternal-Fetal Dyad: Exploring the Two-Patient Obstetric Model," *Hastings Center Report* 22, no. 1 (1992): 13–18, at 13.
4. Department of Health and Human Services, National Institutes of Health, National Library of Medicine, *Cesarean Section—A Brief History* (Washington, DC: Government Printing Office, 1996), 1.

What Are Families For?

Getting to an Ethics of Reproductive Technology

THOMAS H. MURRAY

Hastings Center Report 32, no. 3 (2002): 41–45.

Procreative liberty, as the regnant contemporary framework for thinking about the ethics of reproductive technologies, has its defects. It begins with a pair of confusions and disregards a central, vital interest: it ignores the values at the heart of family life and relies on a thin and unsatisfying conception of human flourishing.

Intellectual frameworks matter: They direct our attention toward certain moral considerations over others, and they implicitly tell us what, like the cents column on income tax returns, can be ignored. Once the shortcomings of procreative liberty as the dominant framework in ethical discourse on assisted reproduction become obvious, so does the need for a more fulsome and nuanced framework, one that begins with the moral significance of the relationship between parents and children, the values at the heart of that relationship, and the ways in which people flourish, or shrivel—physically, emotionally, and morally,

I want to describe briefly the defects in procreative liberty as a framework for thinking about parents and children. I also want to propose a different starting point—a more challenging and complex one to be sure, that begins with what we value most highly and insists on keeping the broader picture in view, however difficult that may sometimes be. Finally. I want to explore what difference it would make to begin with one rather than the other framework.

An Impoverished Worldview

The confusions in the standard account of procreative liberty are twofold. First, procreative liberty seems confused as to its purpose. Does it mean to be an insightful ethical analysis that illuminates what is morally important about families, parents, and children? Or is it only a quasi-moral, quasi-legal algorithm for considering questions about law and policy in reproductive technologies? Its proponents often write as if procreative liberty was indeed a comprehensive moral account of the ethics of initiating parenthood, and implicitly of parenthood in general.

The second confusion abides in the claim that decisions about what sort of child to have and what means to employ to create a child are merely the flip side of decisions *whether* to have a child—that is, decisions about abortion and contraception. Advocates of procreative liberty fix on the free choices of presumably autonomous adults. But abortion and contraception are means *to not have* a child, at least not at this time, or not under these circumstances. The not-so-flip side is the decision *to have* a child, to create a new person who will have interests, hopes, and concerns of her or his own. It is also a decision to initiate a vital, life-long relationship.

The most egregious defect of procreative liberty is its nearly complete disregard of the interests of children created through reproductive technologies.

It permits adults to use virtually any reproductive means for virtually any end; it prohibits or condemns almost nothing. The test of an analytic moral framework cannot be limited to those cases for which it gives the answers one wants; if it provides morally dubious or outrageous answers in other cases, or feeble answers where moral judgments should be clear and ringing, then we have reason to doubt its insightfulness and completeness.

The third defect, procreative liberty's failure to acknowledge values at the heart of family life, is the most sweeping difficulty and at the same time the most difficult to remedy. Control and choice—the values at the heart of procreative liberty—are not entirely out of place in the relationship between parents and children. But they are hardly the entire story, or even the most important themes, and excesses of control and choice can distort and destroy what is most precious in families.

Families, Values, and Human Flourishing

The standard account of procreative liberty is truncated and impoverished. It limits its moral universe to a few values, primarily autonomous adult choice and control. Left out are the values served by parenthood and families, and the role that enduring relationships play in our flourishing as human beings.

Advocates of procreative liberty might argue that the decision about which particular values to pursue is left to the adults making the choice. They can point to the analogy with a woman's right to choose whether to become pregnant or to carry that pregnancy to term.

Here, I think, is where procreative liberty makes a fundamental mistake. Whatever one believes about women's moral rights concerning birth control or abortion, it is undeniable that becoming pregnant and giving birth to a child have an enormous impact on women's lives and on their possibilities for flourishing. Having, raising, and loving a child is a profoundly life-altering experience for both women and men. We must not lose sight of this. At the same time, unpredictable and uncontrolled fertility can restrict women's opportunities for education and work; it consigns some women to deep, enduring poverty.

Procreative liberty's problems began when it appropriated the abstract principle—the right to choose—and ripped it out of the rich context that provided its moral heft: women's prospects for flourishing are diminished when they have no control over their fertility. Procreative liberty then applied that abstracted idea to a very different context—parents, children, and families—with little or no reflection on how these affect our flourishing.

We need a richer ethical framework. We need a framework that acknowledges what should be obvious: decisions about *having* a child are not merely the other side of the moral/legal coin of decisions *not to have* a child. Many people—indeed, probably a robust majority of Americans—support women's access to abortion yet have qualms about the commercialization of reproduction, the growing powers of control over the traits of our children, and reproductive cloning. Our framework must acknowledge the moral significance and interests of the children created through reproductive technologies and do so in a full and robust manner, not as a side-constraint that proves meaningless in practice. And this framework must attend carefully to the values central to the relationship between parents and children, and not be satisfied with the valorization of choice and control in the hands of autonomous adults.

Having and raising children is not the only way to find the enduring, intimate relationships that typify families. But it is the path chosen by many, including those who use reproductive technologies. There are central human values that are either found only in the context of enduring, committed human relationships such as families, or that rely upon such relationships for their realization. Values such as love, loyalty, intimacy, steadfastness, acceptance, and forgiveness are crucial to well-functioning families, which are also the most robust settings in which to raise children to become confident, competent, loving, and emotionally resilient adults.

I do not mean to romanticize families: families can be riven by selfishness, betrayal, and mistrust, or shattered by injustice and oppression. Humans are fallible and all families are imperfect. Yet families are also astonishingly powerful communities of shared memory and experience. Those memories can be scorching and bitter—consider children who were victims of sexual abuse within their family. But they can also be sweet or, perhaps as powerful an emotional glue, a bittersweet mingling of disappointment and loss with love and enduring mutual constancy.

How We Got Here

The roots of our current way of framing the ethics of reproduction are old and deep, manifested in the nascent bioethics movement in the latter half of the twentieth century. As bioethics began to gather steam as a field of scholarly inquiry with an accompanying commentary on practical ethical issues, there arose parallel social and political currents concerning women's reproductive capabilities, the emergence of effective and reasonably safe means for controlling those capabilities, and with those new means of control, new possibilities for women's lives. Women could now think about what a good life for them would entail, a good life that had no need to deny a central role to having, raising, and loving children, yet one that also envisioned creative work and other activities outside the household, activities that uncontrolled fertility made difficult or impossible.

A sharp division of capacities between men and women has never struck me as convincing. Women can be more or less competitive; so can men. Men can be better or worse nurturers: the same for women.

Reflections such as these have convinced me that we must take seriously conceptions of human flourishing if we are to have any chance for meaningful moral dialogue or robust and sensible public policy on a variety of issues concerning conceiving, bearing, and raising children. Any wise inquiry into ideas about human flourishing must acknowledge diversity. It must also, I believe, pay great attention to the similarities and the disparities between the conceptions held about flourishing for women and for men.

It would be unforgivably foolish to presume that all people everywhere shared the same notions of human flourishing. The Taliban, for one, made very sharp distinctions in their perceptions of good lives for women and for men, differences that are likely to reflect and be reflected by assumptions about the nature of women and men. As this example suggests, diversity must be given its due—but not more than its due. If you ask your neighbors where they find meaning in their lives, they will tell you in overwhelming numbers that it is in their families. If you talk with someone who has recently had their first child, as my daughter Kate and her husband Matt did with Grace Emilia, our first grandchild, they are likely to tell you—through the haze of exhaustion—that the experience is life-transforming and wondrous.

Of course, there are families in which deep affection never takes hold, or loses out to selfishness or indifference. And there are times and places when grinding poverty and uncontrolled fertility led to the abandonment of many children who could not be cared for. But the fact that all parents are imperfect and some downright awful, and that some families are blighted by poverty or illness or oppression or any of a multitude of factors that can stunt the growth of love and mutual concern, should not blind us to what is morally and emotionally important about families, to the central role families play in many people's flourishing.

We will find better insight about what it means to be human, I believe, by reflecting on the central relationships in our lives and the significance of those relationships for our flourishing, than by focusing exclusively on the liberty of autonomous adults. We must take care to acknowledge and understand differences among conceptions of flourishing, but we should not reflexively set aside the best and most broadly shared understandings of human flourishing simply because no single one commands universal accord.

Those different conceptions lie barely beneath the surface of some of our most bitter public disputes, yet we regularly fail to acknowledge or probe for possible areas of agreement. The obvious example is the debate over abortion, where the disputants prefer to battle over intractable metaphysical questions about the moral status of fetuses and embryos or the limits of state control over women's bodies. These are important questions, to be sure, but they are not the only wedges into the broader disagreements. They are merely the ones that allow partisans on both sides to feel righteous.

It is neither likely nor desirable that only one rich, full-fledged conception of human flourishing prevail in our public policy debate. But I do believe that failing to engage each other about competing conceptions of human flourishing and the values central to family life results in a moral debate in which many of the most important elements remain hidden or scarcely noticed. It likewise results in public policies that are fiercely resisted—as in abortion—or virtually non-existent—regrettably true of reproductive technologies in the United States (a lack that makes us an object of curiosity in other countries). The divide between right-to-life and prochoice factions in the United States has resulted in an enormous hole in American public policy. Any political leader who takes on the world of infertility treatment, IVF, and the like does so at risk of his or her political life.

Where to Start Thinking

In practice, procreative liberty and what we could call a flourishing-centered approach diverge especially in what moral considerations they include. Take, for example, the case of the Nash family. Their daughter, Molly, would die without a life-saving infusion of healthy, immunologically compatible blood stem cells. One possible source: the stem cell-rich umbilical cord blood from a new brother or sister. The Nashes used preimplantation genetic diagnosis for two simultaneous purposes—to avoid having another child with Fanconi anemia, a life-threatening illness, and to choose an embryo that might become, upon birth, a compatible cord blood donor for its older sister. Procreative liberty dictates a two-step analysis: Was this choice an authentic, informed expression of the prospective parents' autonomy? Would the child have been better off never being born at all? If the answers are, respectively, yes and no, then procreative liberty gives its blessing.

An approach centered on human flourishing requires much more. It begins with reflections on parents and children, on the values served by and intrinsic to this relationship, and on the significance of the proposed act, practice, or policy for the flourishing of children and parents. This is not a simple or easy task. It's more like a complex life-long inquiry.

The process is not mysterious, however. We must reflect on the values that are most important and most widely shared for parents, children, and families; on what makes for good lives for children, women, and men. There will not be one and only one morally defensible account of human flourishing. But not all accounts will be equally convincing. Some seek fulfillment and pleasure through tyranny and oppression or by inflicting physical or emotional cruelty, by employing manipulation and deceit, resulting in emotional emptiness. If someone wishes to defend that as a morally desirable form of human flourishing, let them try.

Thinking about the Nash case by attending to values, flourishing, and context compels us to ask difficult questions. Does preimplantation testing and selection in this instance support or undermine the values central to parents and children? Will it strengthen that family's prospects for flourishing, or erode them? What effect will this case have on practices and policies in preimplantation genetic testing?

Each of these questions deserves extended reflection, more than I can provide here. My sense is that, in the end, we would conclude that the Nash family's choice was an ethically defensible action, born in compassion for the suffering of one child, and not an effort to exert excessive control over the traits of another. We could come to a very different conclusion about parents wanting to impose their preferences for less compelling ends. By contrast, procreative liberty has difficulty summoning the ethical will to curb the indulgence of almost any parental whim. That is a vitally important difference.

What are families for? This is the question we must ask when we think about the ethics of reproductive technologies. Choice and control are to be valued, but not limitlessly, and not as decisive moral panaceas. Choice is not the universal moral solvent, dissolving all moral dilemmas.

We should turn first to that which shapes our lives and gives them meaning, and especially to those enduring relationships of mutual caring that grow between parents and children. Those relationships occupy crucial places in the grand tapestries of images and narratives that depict our richest and fullest images of human flourishing, as well as human failure, cruelty, and misery. When we avert our gaze from those tapestries, we blind ourselves to what ought to be our starting point for thinking insightfully about ethical issues in creating children.

Whose Bodies? Which Selves?

Appeals to Embodiment in Assessments of Reproductive Technology

PAUL LAURITZEN

From *Embodiment, Morality, and Medicine,* edited by L. Sowle Cahill and M.A. Farley, (Dordrecht, the Netherlands: Kluwer Academic Publishers, 1995): 113–26.

Now men are far beyond the stage at which they expressed their envy of women's procreative power through couvade, transvestism, subincision. They are beyond merely giving spiritual birth in their baptismal-font wombs, beyond giving physical birth with their electronic fetal monitors, their forceps, their knives.

Now they have laboratories.

This passage from Gena Corea's book, *The Mother Machine,* typifies the reaction of one important strand of feminist thought to the new technologies of reproduction and birth. It is fairly representative, for example, of the grave suspicion with which feminists associated with FINRRAGE (Feminists International Network of Resistance to Reproductive and Genetic Engineering) have greeted such possibilities as *in vitro* fertilization, embryo flushing and transfer, and gene therapy. According to this general line of thinking, the new reproductive technologies should be resisted because they concentrate power in the hands of a predominantly male and patriarchal medical establishment by disembodying procreation. By separating procreation from women's bodies, reproductive technology simultaneously reduces women to bodies, or body parts, and strips women of one traditional source of power, namely, the power to procreate. Hence Corea's warning. Previously men were denied direct control over the process of procreation; they might give birth symbolically or intervene medically in this process, but these were only simulacra of control. The existence of *in vitro* fertilization, however, and the distinct possibility of *in vitro* gestation turn resemblance into reality. Laboratory conception and gestation are a threat to women.

At the same time that FINRRAGE has mobilized to resist the new reproductive technologies, opposition has come from other quarters as well. The most substantial opposition has come from groups at the opposite end of the political spectrum, most notably the Roman Catholic Church. For example, the Catholic Church has also condemned *in vitro* fertilization, embryo flushing and transfer, and genetic engineering. Indeed, the Vatican has rejected virtually every application of the new reproductive technology (NRT), and, like FINRRAGE, the Vatican is worried about disembodiment. Thus, in the Vatican *Instruction* on reproductive technology, we hear an echo of Corea's concern. We must take seriously the embodied nature of our existence, and failure to do so results in the reduction of a person to a product. So, for example, we find the Vatican insisting that "an intervention on the human body affects not only the tissues, the organs and their functions but also the person himself on different levels."

This apparent convergence of two such different traditions of thought is interesting in itself. It is doubly so when attention is focused on "how the realities of embodiment influence moral relationships in practical health care settings." Despite very serious differences between these traditions of thought – even on issues of embodiment – they agree in their rejection of reproductive technology, and they do so for reasons connected to worries about treating procreation as an out-of-the-body laboratory production. If we attend to the similarities and differences between feminist appeals to embodiment and those of the Catholic Church, we may come to appreciate how the meaning of embodiment may vary from context to context. We may see, for example, how a religious appeal to embodiment in the Christian tradition takes quite a different form from an appeal to embodiment rooted in feminist thought, even if there are also substantial similarities between the two appeals.

Feminist Opposition to Reproductive Technology

We can begin, then, with feminist opposition to reproductive technology. That one significant strand of feminist resistance is fueled by concerns about embodiment is clear. Yet, how precisely does the appeal to embodiment function in this particular feminist critique of reproductive technology? To answer that question, we can return to Gena Corea's work. According to Corea, reproductive technology is best understood in terms of two analogies that have implications for how we think about women's bodies and thus for how

we think about, and treat, women. On the one hand, techniques for assisting human reproduction bear a striking resemblance to techniques used to facilitate reproduction in livestock. On the other hand, the commercial transactions frequently associated with reproductive technology bear a striking resemblance to those associated with sexual prostitution. Let us consider each of these analogies in turn.

Corea makes the comparison between reproductive technology in humans and scientific breeding of animals repeatedly and forcefully in her writings. Consider, she says, the techniques commonly used for breeding animals. Artificial insemination, superovulation, estrus synchronization, ova recovery, embryo evaluation, embryo transfer, and caesarean section are all available to animal breeders, just as they are to physicians of reproductive medicine. Indeed, many applications of this technology used in infertility clinics have been adapted from their original use in the livestock breeding industry. This, says Corea, should give us pause because women have frequently been symbolically associated with animals in western thought, as "parts of nature to be controlled and subjugated."

The point of the comparison between reproductive medicine and animal breeding is to invite an inspection of the attitudes that stand behind the practice of animal breeding. Once we see the attitudes driving animal reproduction, we may come to ask whether similar attitudes do not also drive reproductive medicine. And, as Corea shows [in *The Mother Machine*], there is no mistaking the attitudes of animal breeders.

> When reproductive engineers manipulate the bodies of female animals today, they are clear, blunt and unapologetic about why they are doing it. They want to turn the females into machines for producing "superior" animals or into incubators for the embryos of more "valuable" females. They want, as one entrepreneur told me, to "manufacture embryos at a reduced cost." They aim to create beef cows yielding "quality carcasses of high cutability," and dairy cows producing more milk on the same amount of feed.

Corea's point is clear: When the bodies of animals are treated in this fashion, when the animal is essentially reduced to its reproductive parts, the animal ceases to have any individuality or spiritual worth. The upshot of reproductive technology is thus that the animal is reduced to a reproductive commodity and nothing more. The worry is that we may come to think of women and their bodies in precisely the same terms.

This worry informs Corea's second analogy as well. If comparing reproductive medicine to livestock production is meant to highlight the possibility that employing reproductive technology may lead us to think about women's bodies as commodities, comparing reproductive medicine to prostitution is meant to highlight the fact that our society already conceptualizes women's bodies in market terms. Drawing on Andrea Dworkin's work, Corea shows that the reduction of women to commodities has already taken place. As Corea notes, our society already markets parts of women's bodies. Pornography is a thriving industry and sexual prostitution is widely perceived to be harmless and is thus tolerated as largely benign. But if women can sell vagina, rectum, and mouth, Corea asks, why not wombs, embryos, or eggs? Given how women are conceptualized in our society, the answer, of course, is that there is no reason to object to the marketing of women as reproductive commodities, and indeed, Corea says, that is precisely what we see with the development of a commercial surrogate mother industry and egg "donor" programs.

In fact, says Corea, we do not need to attend merely to the obvious comparison case, namely, surrogate motherhood. Talk to women who have been through *in vitro* fertilization programs.

Corea notes [in "What the King Can Not See"], for example, that many women report undergoing a process of emotional distancing during IVF. They attempt to separate mind from body and in fact come to feel disconnected from their bodies in ways that interfere with bodily love making with their partners. Here, Corea says, the comparison to prostitution is direct and disturbing.

What kind of spiritual damage does it do to women when they emotionally separate their minds and bodies? … We have heard some prostitutes say that during intercourse with strangers who have rented the use of their bodies, they too separate their minds from their bodies as a means of self protection. We have heard some people with multiple personalities say that during extreme sexual abuse and torture in childhood, they split off into separate personalities in order to make what was happening to them endurable. In order to survive.

What does it do to women in IVF "treatment" programs when, to varying extents, they separate their minds and bodies in order to make all the poking and prodding and embarrassments endurable?

Corea is not the only feminist asking such questions, nor is she the only one to focus on the importance of embodiment to assessments of reproductive technology.

In fact, a careful reading of feminist responses to the technologies of reproductive medicine shows this to be a pervasive theme: reproductive technology encourages women to separate their selves from their bodies, and the resulting fragmentation leaves women vulnerable. Women become vulnerable because, with fragmentation comes a willingness to treat women's bodies as biological machines that can be manipulated and controlled. Reproductive technology thus alienates women from their bodies and thereby strips them of an important source of personal fulfillment and power.

Catholic Opposition to Reproductive Technology

If we turn now to the Vatican's response to reproductive technology, we see that the Catholic Church is also concerned about issues of embodiment. Consider, for example, the *Instruction* on reproductive technology issued by the Congregation for the Doctrine of the Faith in 1987, in which the position of the Church is set out at length. For our purposes, the introduction and the first two sections of this document are of particular interest, because the introduction sets out the basic moral considerations that are then applied in sections one and two to arrive at particular conclusions about reproductive technology. A careful reading of these three sections reveals that Vatican opposition to reproductive technology is supported by two lines of argument, both of which are rooted in concerns about embodiment. The first line of argument is set out in the introduction in terms of what the Vatican describes as "a proper idea of the nature of the human person in his bodily dimension." The Congregation asks: What moral criteria must be used to assess reproductive technology? The first answer it gives is that any adequate criteria must recognize the bodily and spiritual unity of the person. In the Vatican's view, a person is a "unified totality," and thus it is wrong to treat a person in a way that reduces that person either to mere body or mere spirit. It is particularly important to keep this principle in mind, the Vatican says, when addressing ethical issues in medicine because there is a tendency in medicine to treat the body as "a mere complex of tissues, organs, and functions." Indeed, this is one of the central difficulties with reproductive medicine: it approaches human reproduction as if it were nothing more than the union of bodily parts, namely, of gametes. So one of the most serious problems with reproductive technology, the Vatican concludes, is precisely that it fails to treat the person as a unified whole. Instead, it treats the body in just the way the Vatican says it must not be treated, as a mere complex of tissues and organs. In other words, this technology treats our bodies functionally, the consequence of which is that persons get objectified and treated merely as means to an end. When this happens, technology is not simply assisting, but dominating the process of reproduction.

The second line of argument used to oppose interventions in the reproductive process is less obviously rooted in a concern about embodiment, but, once again, a careful reading of the text highlights the relevance of considerations of embodiment. This second line of reasoning is related to what the Vatican calls "the special nature of the transmission of human life in marriage." In the Vatican's view, since human procreation is the fruit of a "personal and conscious act," it is irreconcilably different from the transmission of life in other animals. It is intentional and purposive and therefore governed by laws. What laws? Laws, says the Vatican, given by God and "inscribed in the very being of man and woman."

As the language here suggests, the appeal is to a natural law conception of human nature, according to which we must understand the telos of human sexual life, marriage, and the family in order to discern the range of acceptable reproductive interventions. Moreover, the appeal is to a particular understanding of this telos, one in which intercourse, love, procreation, marriage, and the family belong together. In the Vatican's view, procreation is properly undertaken in the context of a loving monogamous marriage through an act of sexual intercourse. Here, then, is a second standard by which to assess interventions in the reproductive process. Any type of assisted reproduction that conforms to the procreative norm just articulated, i.e., any procreative attempt that includes sexual intercourse between partners in a loving monogamous marriage, helps facilitate the natural process of procreation and is therefore acceptable. Any intervention that fails to conform to the norm is a departure from the natural law with respect to human sexuality and is therefore morally problematic.

Two points are worth noting at this juncture. First, in rejecting reproductive technology as a violation of natural law, the Vatican is invoking the "inseparability thesis," set out in *Humanae Vitae*, and which supports Catholic opposition to contraception. Just as the Catholic Church condemns contraception because it separates what is never permitted to be separated by allowing for sex without procreation, so it condemns reproductive technology because it provides for the possibility of procreation without sex.

This observation suggests a second one. To say that reproductive technology separates procreation from sex is not equivalent to saying that reproductive technology disembodies procreation. So opposition to reproductive technology is not just opposition to those techniques, like IVF, that actually disembody conception, but opposition to how the body is used and viewed by reproductive technology generally. To be sure, the Vatican objection is not merely reducible to the consequentialist concern that all forms of reproductive technology move us toward the objectionable endpoint of extracorporeal gestation. Nevertheless, whether emphasis is placed upon the bodily and spiritual unity of a person, or upon the importance of keeping sex and procreation together, the Vatican is concerned that reproductive technology leads us to treat our bodies merely as a source of gametes, and that so treating our bodies is the first step to disembodying procreation altogether.

At this point it is worth noting that Vatican opposition to reproductive technology appears strikingly similar to feminist opposition to this technology, and that both groups couch their opposition in terms of the unfortunate consequences of disembodying procreation. Indeed the language of complaint is almost identical. Technological intervention in the process of procreation reduces reproduction to a production process in which humans are themselves reduced to products. Given the similarity of complaint, may we conclude that Vatican appeals to embodiment are essentially identical to feminist appeals to embodiment?

Janice Raymond has argued [in "Fetalists and Feminists"] that the answer to this question should be an emphatic and unequivocal "no!" The similarities, she says, are apparent only. In fact, according to Raymond, feminists should resist this equation, not only because it will be used by their opponents to discredit them as latter day Luddites, but because it is offensive to women. Linking fetalists – the term she uses for conservative religious opponents of reproductive technology – and feminists, she writes, "is

an insult of the first order to women. It's tantamount to saying that behind every female idea or movement is male impetus, that women cannot stand on our own and create a woman-defined opposition to the NRTs for autonomous feminist reasons…." "Feminists and fetalists," she says flatly, "are not aligned in any way."

Raymond's total rejection of the similarities between Vatican opposition and feminist opposition is too extreme, but her argument is instructive nonetheless, for it demonstrates how an appeal to embodiment is inextricably tied to the context in which it is made. We therefore do well to take up her argument in some detail.

Raymond begins by noting that there are essentially two groups that have mounted substantial opposition to reproductive technology, feminists and the Roman Catholic Church, and that supporters of reproductive technology have an interest in trying to link feminist opposition to Catholic opposition as a way of discrediting both. Not only will advocates of reproductive technology adopt this "politics of guilt by association," but some conservative religious groups may attempt "to co-opt feminist language, ethics, and politics for their own cause." So there may be a variety of reasons why individuals or groups might seek to conflate feminist opposition and Catholic opposition. Nevertheless, there are philosophical and political differences that make these traditions irreconcilable.

Raymond acknowledges that both the Catholic Church and feminists appeal to the language of embodiment in their critique of reproductive technology, but she says they "are talking about different bodies." Feminists locate their appeal to embodiment within a context of opposition to violence against women. "Feminists," Raymond writes:

> are concerned about the ways in which the NRTs destroy a woman's bodily integrity and the totality of her personal and political existence. Many feminists criticize the way in which the 'technodocs' sever the biological processes of pregnancy and reproduction from the female body while at the same time

making ever more invasive incursions into the female body for eggs, for implantation, for embryo transfers, and the like. Through such incursions, women can only come to be distanced from their autonomous bodily processes. And the net result of this is that women's bodies are perceived by themselves and others as a reproductive resource, as a field to be seeded, ploughed and ultimately harvested for the fruit of the womb. The feminist value of 'embodiment' translates to bodily integrity and the control of one's body."

By contrast, Raymond argues, Catholic opposition to disembodiment is located within a context of opposition to violence against fetuses. Consequently, in the Vatican *Instruction*, a document that, as we saw, appeals repeatedly to the language of embodiment, an entire section is devoted to a discussion of the effects of disembodied procreation on the fetus, but scarcely a word to the effects on women. "Nowhere," writes Raymond about the Vatican *Instruction*:

> is there one mention of the 'disrespect' that is accorded to the woman's 'human life' by these technologies. One might expect that a document whose title purports to talk about the 'origin' of human life might at least mention women. But the so-called 'dignity of procreation' is applied in a general sense to the dignity of the human person and certainly not specifically to the dignity and integrity of the woman's body.

Moreover, Raymond argues, even when the Vatican is not focused exclusively on the bodies of fetuses, even when women's bodies come into view, the consequences of reproductive technology on women's bodies are seen against the backdrop of concern about sexuality, parenthood, or marriage, and not against a backdrop of concern about the bodily integrity of women, nor of concern that women have control of their bodies. So whereas feminist appeals to embodiment are rooted in a commitment to subverting "the entire fabric of sexual subordination and the ways in which that subordination has insured for men

both sexual and reproductive access to women," Vatican appeals to embodiment are rooted in a pro-natalist world view that embraces compulsory motherhood for women and thus subsumes "the autonomy and independence of the woman to the 'interests' of the family."

Given the striking similarities that we noted above between feminist opposition to reproductive technology and Vatican opposition, is Raymond right? The answer is that Raymond is both partly right and partly wrong. Although Raymond is right to point out the very real differences between some of the feminist objections and some raised by the Catholic Church, she is wrong to dismiss as quickly as she does the mutual concern about disembodiment. To be sure, there are good reasons for feminists to be skeptical about Catholic opposition to reproductive technology. As we saw, the rather glaring omission of any explicit discussion of how reproductive technology affects women is one. Nevertheless, a healthy skepticism here does not justify Raymond's hasty dismissal of Vatican concerns about disembodiment.

For example, Raymond claims that while the Vatican uses the language of embodiment in criticizing reproductive technology, it is only concerned about women's body derivatively. That is, the Catholic Church is only concerned about women's bodies to the extent that these bodies serve the reproductive interest of men or are necessary to safeguarding the bodies of fetuses. She says, "for feminists, women are our bodies," and the unstated implication is that for the Catholic Church this is not true. If we look closely at the Vatican *Instruction*, however, we see nearly identical language, language that, I believe, is meant to express the same worry. Quoting Pope John Paul II, the Congregation for the Doctrine of the Faith endorses a claim that might well be summarized as, "touch the body, touch the person." "Each human person," we read, "in his absolutely unique singularity, is constituted not only by his spirit, but by his body as well. Thus, in the body and through the body, one touches the person himself in his concrete reality." "Touch the body, touch the person" might well be substituted without loss of meaning for "women are our bodies."

Yet, if this comparison highlights the fact that Raymond states her case too strongly by claiming that the Vatican and feminists are not aligned in any way, it also reveals the truth of her observation that the context of appeals to embodiment is all important. Feminists apply the insight behind the aphorism "women are our bodies" from a context in which there is an explicit and unequivocal commitment to women's bodily integrity and to securing personal and political liberty for women. So feminists move directly from a concern about the disembodiment of procreation that appears to come with reproductive technology to an explicit discussion of how this technology affects women's bodies and thus women's hope for freedom and equality.

By contrast, the Catholic Church appeals to embodiment from within a context in which there has not traditionally been a significant commitment to women's equality. The upshot is that when the Vatican talks about embodiment, it is not typically speaking about women's bodies. So although "touch the person, touch the body" in fact articulates the same view of the human person as "women are our bodies," the former aphorism refers primarily to male bodies. Thus, when the Vatican turns to apply this insight in an assessment of reproductive technology, we should not be altogether surprised—though we may still be outraged — by the fact that it takes up the effects this technology has on the bodies of fetuses, but says nothing about its impact on the bodies of women.

Indeed, Raymond's emphatic repudiation of Vatican appeals to embodiment forces us to confront the fact that the Church's discussion of the effects of disembodiment takes place against the backdrop, not merely of an undistinguished record of commitment to the rights of women, but against a significant legacy of denigration of the body, women, and sexuality. Margaret Farley, for example, has pointed out [in "Feminist Theology and Bioethics"] that any appeal to embodiment within the Christian tradition must come

to grips with the fact that the Christian tradition has frequently embraced a dualism that pits spirit against body, man against woman, reason against emotion, a dualism that has served to oppress women.

Has the Church come to grips with this legacy in its appeal to embodiment in the *Instruction* on Reproductive Technology? Raymond has shown decisively that the answer to this question is 'no.' The lesson to be drawn here is that the Church's own best insights have been undermined by a continuing legacy of sexism and dualistic thinking. It is regrettable that the *Instruction* does not do justice to the Church's own vision of the human person as "a unified totality" of body and spirit, but we should not dismiss the vision itself as sexist or misogynist for that reason.

If Raymond's juxtaposition of feminist criticism with Vatican criticism of reproductive technology helps us to see that any appeal to embodiment must be taken in context, and, if attending to the context of Vatican appeals to embodiment helps us to discern the shortcomings of Catholic opposition to reproductive technology, it is worth asking whether this juxtaposition does not also highlight the shortcomings of some feminist appeals to embodiment. I want in closing to suggest that it does and, indeed, to show how the Vatican *Instruction* might offer an important corrective to one strand of the feminist critique precisely at the point where the context of feminist appeals to embodiment undermines feminist insights.

To see once again that the comparison of feminist and Catholic opposition to reproductive technology is instructive, we may return to the analogy Gena Corea draws between sexual prostitution and the commodification of reproduction. We saw above that this comparison is made to highlight the dangers of an activity that appears to commodify women's bodies in a cultural context where women's bodies are already for sale in the marketplace. To explain the full force of this analogy, however, we must ask why sexual prostitution is morally problematic. If feminism is committed to the bodily autonomy of women, why should women not be able to sell their bodies if they would so choose? This is a difficult question for feminism, and it is instructive to see how one strand of feminist thought has answered this question. One answer to the question has essentially been to suggest that prostitution is so degrading and so dehumanizing, that no woman would choose to be a prostitute unless she were coerced.

It is this line of reasoning, for example, that Catharine MacKinnon has in mind when she writes [in *Feminism Unmodified*] that the fact that "prostitution and modeling are structurally women's best economic options should give pause to those who would consider women's presence there a true act of free choice." As MacKinnon points out, in other contexts, we readily acknowledge that people do degrading work for lack of better economic options, and we neither deny that the work is degrading nor deceive ourselves by thinking that the work is freely chosen. Indeed, even where a woman "chooses" prostitution in a context where she is not doing so, say, to feed herself or her children, we have good reason to suspect that other forms of coercion are at work. Perhaps self esteem has been so undermined by a society that systematically devalues women that there is not a sufficient sense of self worth to recognize the degradation of prostitution.

Thus, whether we are talking about economic coercion or other, perhaps less obvious forms of coercion, the important point is that this approach to prostitution challenges the presumption that prostitution is freely chosen.

I have argued elsewhere that this is in fact a powerful argument and that the critique of "liberal" conceptions of autonomy implicit in it is also significant. For our purposes, it is important to see how the logic of this argument must be extended to reproductive technology if the comparison of assisted reproduction to sexual prostitution is to carry any weight. Take, for example, the argument that IVF turns a woman into a sort of reproductive prostitute. Part of the force of this argument comes from the suggestion that women are coerced into IVF, just as

they are coerced into becoming prostitutes. Yet, if we consider the claim that to offer IVF to a childless woman is coercive, we discover that for this claim to be plausible we require a conviction comparable to the belief that eliminating prostitution could not conflict with any legitimate interest a woman of self respect might have.

In one sense, of course, this is not true even of prostitution. If a woman sells her body in order to feed herself or her children, she is obviously pursuing a legitimate interest. Nevertheless, the point opponents of prostitution and of reproductive technology wish to make is that there is nothing in the activity of selling one's body or in the procedures of assisted reproduction that is itself rewarding for women, and, consequently, if women choose either activity, the only explanation is that they have been coerced. The problem with pressing this line of argument, however, is that there is a more direct connection between assisted reproduction and the good of bearing and begetting a child than between prostitution and the good of feeding children. The upshot is that opponents of reproductive technology can only utilize this analogy with prostitution effectively, if they are simultaneously prepared to reject or devalue the importance of begetting and bearing children.

Unfortunately, when we examine the work of some who have opposed IVF on the grounds that it may be coercive, we see precisely this sort of skepticism about the value of children. For example, in an article entitled '"Women Want It": *In-Vitro* Fertilization and Women's Motivations for Participation,' Christine Crowe argues that women participate in IVF programs largely because they accept the dominant ideology of motherhood in Western culture, an ideology that includes the belief that biological motherhood is valuable.

Here we see how the context of feminist appeals to embodiment may also subvert the full significance of embodiment. To appeal to embodiment from within a context that emphasizes the way in which pregnancy, childbirth, and the care of children have been oppressive to women, poses the danger of neglecting the value of the decidedly embodied experience of pregnancy and the embodied goodness of children.

This is not to say that all, or even most, feminists who have opposed reproductive technology out of concerns over embodiment devalue children. Nor do I wish to deny that pregnancy is sometimes oppressive for women and perceived by women as such. Nor would I deny that having and rearing children can be unfulfilling or even disastrously burdensome. Still, those feminists who have categorically discounted the value to women of pregnancy and parenthood have not taken embodiment seriously enough. Given a preoccupation with combatting an ideology that sacralizes pregnancy and motherhood, it is easy to conflate the socially sanctioned belief that having children is desirable (and pregnancy uniquely fulfilling) with the very different proposition that women cannot be fulfilled unless they have children. Thus, in their eagerness to reject the latter claim, some feminists have been blinded to the fact that women may legitimately value carrying and caring for children. To celebrate is not to sacralize, and any view that fully embraced the importance of embodiment, could not but celebrate the experiences of bearing and rearing children.

In the final analysis, careful attention to Vatican and to feminist appeals to embodiment reveals striking differences that in turn highlight the short-comings of both Vatican and some feminist opposition to reproductive technology. At the same time, however, we can see striking similarities. Both traditions of thought draw our attention to the potential dangers of disembodying procreation, and in doing so, both traditions properly highlight the importance of attention to issues of embodiment when reflecting morally on medicine. It is perhaps ironic, therefore, that, in assessing reproductive technology in light of the embodied character of human life, critics in both traditions go so wrong. For, surely, no adequate account of embodiment and reproductive technology would conclude that this technology always or necessarily violates the embodied quality of human procreation. On the contrary, for many infertile individuals, reproductive technology mediates embodiment, not the reverse. That both Catholic opposition and some feminist opposition to reproductive technology appear blind to this fact demonstrates how important the context of appeals to embodiment can be.

Bibliography

Bynum, C. W. *Fragmentation and Redemption*. New York: Zone Books, 1991.

Congregation for the Doctrine of Faith. *Instruction of Respect for Human Life in Its Origin and on the Dignity of Procreation*. Washington, DC: United States Catholic Conference, 1987.

Corea, G. *The Mother Machine*. New York: Harper & Row, 1985.

————. "The Reproductive Brothel." In *Man-Made Women*, edited by G. Corea, Reuate Duelli Klein, Jalrnax Hanmer, Helen B. Holmes, Betty Hoskins, Madhu Kishwar, Janice Raymond, Robyn Rowland, and Roberta Steinchader, Bloomington: Indiana University Press, 1987.

————. "What the King Can Not See." In *Embryos, Ethics, and Women's Rights*, edited by E. H. Baruch, A.F. Adomo Jr., and J. Seager, 77–93. New York: Harrington Park Press, 1988.

Crowe, C. "Women Want It: *In Vitro* Fertilization and Women's Motivations for Participation." *Women's Studies International Forum* 8, no. 6 (1985): 547–52.

Farley, M. "Feminist Theology and Bioethics." In *Women's Consciousness, Women's Conscience*," edited by B. H. Anderson, C. E. Gudorf, and M. D. Pellauer, 285–305. San Francisco: Harper and Row, 1985.

MacKinnon, C. *Feminism Unmodified*. Cambridge, MA: Harvard University Press, 1987.

Raymond, J. "Fetalists and Feminists: They Are Not the Same." In *Made to Order*, edited by P. Spallone and D. L. Steinberg, 55–66. Oxford: Pergamon, 1987.

Rothman, B. K. *Recreating Motherhood*. New York: W. W. Norton, 1989.

————. *The Tentative Pregnancy*. New York: Viking Press, 1985.

Reproductive Gifts and Gift Giving

The Altruistic Woman

JANICE G. RAYMOND

Hastings Center Report no. 6 (1990): 7–11.

Gifts and Gift Giving

In his well-known study, *The Gift Relationship: From Human Blood to Social Policy*, Richard Titmuss opposed commercial systems of blood supply to noncommercial and altruistic systems of blood giving. Titmuss's concern was to shore up the spirit of altruism and voluntarism which he saw declining in western societies. His analysis is, in the main, a positive assessment of the possibilities of altruistic blood donation. But Titmuss also understood that giving was influenced by "the relationships set up, social and economic, between the system and the donor," and that these relationships are "strongly determined by the values and cultural orientations permeating the donor system and the society in general." The dialectic between values and structural factors emerges strongly in his work. We must ask, he wrote, if there is truly "no contract of custom, no legal bond, no functional determinism, no situations of discriminatory power, domination, constraint or compulsion, no sense of shame or guilt, no gratitude imperative and no need for the penitence of a Chrysostom" (239). The role of cultural values and constraints in shaping gift-giving arrangements is vital.

In the case of many new reproductive practices, and surrogacy especially, "the donor system" mainly depends on women as the gift givers—women who donate the use of their bodies and the fruit of their wombs. Those who endorse altruistic surrogacy as an alternative to commercial surrogacy accept, without comment or criticism, that it is primarily women who constitute the altruistic population called upon to contribute gestating capacities. The questions that Titmuss raised about "contract of custom," "functional determinism," "situations of discriminatory power," "domination,

constraint or compulsion," as well as possible "shame or guilt" and a "gratitude imperative" form part of the unexamined hallowing of altruistic surrogacy.

This unexamined acceptance of women as reproductive gift givers is very much related to a longstanding patriarchal tradition of giving women away in other cultural contexts—for sex and in marriage, for example. Following Titmuss, we must continually in these discussions of altruism ask: who gives and why? But further, who has been given away historically and why? In this sense, women are not only the gift givers but the gift as well. The pervasiveness of women's personal and social obligation to give shapes the contexts of reproductive gifts and gift giving. We see this most clearly in the situation of so-called altruistic surrogacy.

Altruism Versus Commercialism

Those critical of commercial surrogacy often contrast it to noncommercial or altruistic surrogacy. The New Jersey Supreme Court, in its appellate judgment, *In the Matter of Baby M*, found surrogate contracts contrary to the law and public policy of the state. Nonetheless, it concluded that there were no legal impediments to arrangements "when the surrogate mother volunteers, without any payment, to act as a surrogate." Altruism and voluntarism emerge as moral virtues in opposition to commercialism. George Annas, who has opposed commercial surrogacy, is sympathetic to the view that "one can distinguish between doing something out of love and doing it for money. As long as existing adoption laws are followed, voluntary relinquishment of a child to a close relative (such as an infertile sister) seems acceptable." Such a scenario has in fact already been played out.

In this country, one publicized case of altruistic surrogacy occurred in 1985 when Sherry King offered to become pregnant for her sister, Carole, who had undergone a hysterectomy eighteen years before. Sherry King provided both egg and womb. "I know I couldn't be a surrogate mother for money.... I'm doing this for love and for my sister."

Such agreements have not been confined only to sisters. In 1987, a forty-eight-year-old woman, Pat Anthony, acted as a surrogate mother for her daughter and gave birth to triplets in South Africa. The attending obstetrician, Dr. Bernstein, commented: "We feel that what Pat Anthony has done for Karen is the acceptable face of surrogacy.... There was no payment, no commercialism. It was an act of pure love." Thus altruism becomes the ethical standard for an affirmative assessment of noncommercial surrogacy.

Altruism also is invoked to soften the pecuniary image of commercial surrogacy. Noel Keane, the well-known surrogate broker, has made an educational video called "A Special Lady," which is often shown to teenage girls in high schools and other contexts, encouraging them to consider "careers" as surrogates. The video promotes the idea that it takes a special kind of woman to bear babies for others, and that women who engage in surrogacy do so not mainly for the money but for the special joy it brings to the lives of those who can't have children themselves.

Altruism holds sway. Part of its dominance as an ethical norm derives from its accepted opposition to commercialism. Particularly in the current debate about legalizing surrogate contracts, opponents contend that these contracts make children into commodities to be bought and sold. They allege that this is tantamount to baby selling, and some have renamed the practice commercialized childbearing. Many have focused on the economic exploitation of the women who enter surrogate contracts, women who are in need of money or are financially dead-ended. In these perspectives, the ethical objection is restricted to the fact that a price tag is attached to that which should have no price. The corollary

is often that surrogacy "for free" is morally and legally appropriate.

The Moral Celebration of Women's Altruism

The cultural norm of the altruistic woman who is infinitely giving and eternally accessible derives from a social context in which women give and are given away, and from a moral tradition that celebrates women's duty to meet and satisfy the needs of others. The cultural expectation of altruism has fallen most heavily on pregnant women, so that one could say they are imaged as the archetypal altruists. As Beverly Harrison notes:

> Many philosophers and theologians, although decrying gender inequality, still unconsciously assume that women's lives should express a different moral norm than men's, that women should exemplify moral purity and self-sacrifice, whereas men may live by the more minimal rational standards of moral obligation ... perfection and self-sacrifice are never taken to be a day-to-day moral requirement for any moral agent except, it would seem, a pregnant woman.[1]

Harrison calls this a "supererogatory morality," acts that are expected to go beyond the accepted standards of obligation. Although traditionally women have been exhorted to be passive, simultaneously they are expected to be more responsible than men for meeting the needs of others. "We live in a world where many, perhaps most, of the voluntary sacrifices on behalf of human well-being are made by women, but the assumption of a special obligation to self-giving or sacrifice... is male-generated ideology" (62). The other side of this altruistic coin is male self-interest. A man is allowed to be more self-seeking, to go to great lengths to fulfill his self-interests, and this has been rationalized, in the case of surrogacy, as genetic continuity and "biological fulfillment."

This is not merely an ideological pronouncement about female self-giving and male self-seeking. It raises complex questions about moral double standards in a cultural context where men as a class set the standards and women live them out, where inequality is systemic, and where women have an investment in their own subordination. This does not mean that every man is self-interested and every woman is altruistic. Were that the case, surely the biological determinists would be right!

There is, moreover, a distinct moral language that is part of this tradition that celebrates women's altruism. It is the language of selflessness and responsibility toward others in which women's very possibilities are framed. It is the discourse of maternalism, which traditionally has been the discourse of devotion and dedication in which women turn away from their own needs. It is also the discourse of maternal destiny in which a real woman is a mother, or one who acts like a mother, or more specifically, like the self-sacrificing, nurturant, and care-taking mothers women are supposed to be. If a woman chooses a different destiny and directs her self elsewhere, she risks placing herself outside female nature and culture. This language also encases women's activities in mothering metaphors, framing many of the creative endeavors that women undertake. Motherhood becomes an inspirational metaphor or symbol for the caring, the nurturing, and the sensitivity that women bring to a world ravaged by conflict.

A body of recent feminist literature, exemplified in the work of Carol Gilligan, has valorized women's altruistic development as the morality of responsibility, emphasizing that this is morality "in a different voice" from men. Formerly a mainstay of separate but equal ideology—as in "vive la différence"—this same discourse is now being transformed by some feminists into an endorsement of women's difference in human and moral development. Yet as Catharine MacKinnon notes,

> For women to affirm difference, when difference means dominance, as it does with gender, means to affirm the qualities and characteristics of powerlessness... So I am critical of affirming what we have been, which nec-

essarily is what we have been permitted.... Women value care because men have valued us according to the care we give them[2]

Altruism has been one of the most effective blocks to women's self-awareness and demand for self-determination. It has been an instrument structuring social organization and patterns of relationship in women's lives. The social relations set up by altruism and the giving of self have been among the most powerful forces that bind women to cultural roles and expectations.

The issue is not whether altruism can have any positive content in the lives of women, but rather that we cannot abstract this question from the gender-specific and gender-unequal situation of cultural values and structures in which new reproductive practices are arranged. This is not to claim that voluntary and genuine magnanimity does not exist among women. It is to say that more is at stake than the womb, the egg, or the child as gift—and the woman as gift giver.

Creating Women in the Image of Victim

Altruism is not crudely obligatory. The more complex issue is what kind of choices women make within the context of a culture and tradition that orients them to give and give of themselves. To paraphrase Marx, women make their own choices, but they often do not make them just as they please. They often do not make them under conditions they create but under constraints they are powerless to change. The social construction of women's altruism should not reduce to creating women in the victim image.

Yet when feminists stress how women's choices are influenced by the social system and how women are channeled into giving, for example, they are reproached for portraying women as passive victims. Lori Andrews in her essay "Alternative Modes of Reproduction" for the Rutgers *Reproductive Laws for the 1990s* project faults feminist critics of the new reproductive technologies for embracing arguments based on "a presumed incapacity of women to make decisions." For such detractors, pressure seems to exist only at the barrel of a gun.

For women gifts play many roles. They generate identity, they protect status, and they often regulate guilt. Women who don't give—time, energy, care, sex—are often exposed to disapproval or penalty. But the more important element here is that on a cultural level women *are expected* to donate themselves in the form of time, energy, and body.

Family Ties, Gifts, and the Inducement of Altruism

The potential for women's exploitation is not necessarily less because no money is involved and reproductive arrangements may take place within a family setting. The family has not always been a safe place for women. And there are unique affective "inducements" in familial contexts that do not exist elsewhere. Although there is no "coercion of contract" or "inducement" of money, there could be the coercion of family ties in which having a baby for a sister or another family member may be rationalized as the "greatest gift" one woman can give to another.

Thus we must also examine the power and role of gifts in shaping social life. In *The Gift: Forms and Functions of Exchange in Archaic Society*, Marcel Mauss contends that gifts fulfill certain obligations. These obligations vary, but in all these instances—whether gifts are used to maintain social affection or to promote unity or loyalty within the group—they are experienced as prescriptive and exacting. This is true on a cultural level, as Mauss has pointed out, but it is even more true on a family level, the context most often cited as the desirable site of altruistic reproductive exchanges.

Family opinion may not force a woman, in the sense of being outrightly coercive, to become pregnant for another family member. However, where family integration is strong, the nature of family opinion may be so engulfing that, for all practical purposes, it exacts a reproductive donation from a female source. And representing the surrogate arrangement as a gift holds the woman in tutelage to the norms of family duty, represented as giving to a family member in need.

Within family situations, it may also be considered selfish, uncaring, even dishonorable for a woman to deprive a relative of eggs or her gestating abilities. The category of altruism itself is *broadened* in family contexts to include all sorts of nontraditional reproductive "duties" that would be frowned on if women undertook them for money. Within families, it may be considered selfish for a woman to deprive her husband of children by not allowing the reproductive use of another female family member, especially *because* the arrangements will be kept within the family.

We might ask further what is suitable matter for exchange. When we speak of reproductive gifts and donations, but more especially in the case of surrogacy, where the gift and donation is the woman's body and ultimately the child who may be born of such a practice, we put the donation of persons side by side with the exchange of objects and things.

Gender-Specific Ethics, Public Policy, and Legislation

While the altruistic woman may be at the center of noncommercial reproductive exchanges, so too is a portrait of science and technology as altruistic. The new reproductive technologies provide science with one part of this image: *in vitro* fertilization is represented as offering "new hope for the infertile"; surrogacy gives infertile couples the gift of a child; egg donation is helping others to have children. But it is not the technologies that are the sources of these reproductive gifts. It is women, and the historical medicalization of women's bodies in the reproductive context. Women are taken for granted in the name of reproductive research, the advancement of reproductive science, and, of course, the giving of life.

Altruism cannot be separated from the history, the values, and the political structures reinforcing women's reproductive inequality in our society. Questions such as, Who is my stranger? which Titmuss designates as the altruistic question with respect to blood donation, cannot be asked within the context of reproductive donations without asking the prior question of Who is my Samaritan?

Reproductive gift relationships must be seen in their totality, not just as helping someone to have a child. Noncommercial surrogacy cannot be treated as a mere act of altruism, for more is at issue than the ethics of altruism. Any valorizing of altruistic surrogacy and reproductive gift giving for women must be assessed within a context of political inequality, lest it help dignify inequality. Moral meaning and public policy should not be governed by the mere absence of market values. Moral meaning and public policy should be guided by the presence of gender specificity.

What does this mean? For one thing, it means that any assessment of reproductive exchanges, whether they involve commerce or not, takes as its ethical starting point the question of women's status and how the exchange enhances or diminishes gender inequality. Gender-specific ethics devotes primary attention to the consequences to women. It recognizes not only the harm but the devaluation that happens to all women when some are used for reproductive exchanges.

A gender-specific ethics and public policy confronts the degradation of women in the "private" sphere of reproduction and recognizes the gender inequality that exists as a result, for example, of women's expected altruism. Validating altruistic surrogacy on the level of public policy leaves intact the image and reality of a woman as a *reproductive conduit*—someone through whom someone passes. The woman used as a conduit for someone else's procreative purposes, most evident in the case of surrogacy, becomes a mere instrument in reproductive exchanges, an incidental incubator detached from the total fabric of social, affective, and moral meanings associated with procreation. Thus the terminology of "donor" is inaccurate; women are more appropriately "sources" of eggs, wombs, and babies in

the context of reproductive exchanges. Further, we are not really talking about "donations" here but about "procurement."

Surrogacy, situated within the larger context of gender inequality, is not simply the commercialization of women and children. On a political level, it reinforces the perception and use of women as a breeder class and reinforces the gender inequality of women as a group. This is not symbolic or intangible but strikes at the core of what a society allows women to be and become. Taking the commerce out of surrogacy but leaving the practice intact on a noncommercial and contractual basis glosses over that essential violation.

Proposals that the law keep clear of reproductive exchanges where no money changes hands are based on gender-neutral assumptions. If the harm of surrogacy, for example, is based only on the commercialization and commodification of reproduction, then the reality that *women* are always used in systems of surrogacy gets no fundamental legal notice. We must note that babies are not always born of surrogate contracts but women are always encumbered.

Gender-specific ethics and public policy raise serious doubt about the concept and reality of altruism and the ways it is used to dignify women's inequality. The focus on altruism sentimentalizes and thus obscures the ways women are medicalized and devalued by the new reproductive technologies and practices. An uncritical affirmation of reproductive gifts and gift givers—of egg donations, of "special ladies" who serve as so-called surrogate mothers for others who go to such lengths to have their own biological children, and of reproductive technology itself as a great gift to humanity—fails to examine the institutions of reproductive science, technology, and brokering that increasingly structure reproductive exchanges.

Altruistic reproductive exchanges leave intact the status of women as a breeder class. Women's bodies are still the raw material for other's needs, desires, and purposes. The normalization of altruistic exchanges may have, in fact, the effect of promoting the view that women *should* engage in reproductive exchanges free of charge. In the surrogacy context, altruism reinforces the role of women as *mothers for others* and creates a new version of *relinquishing motherhood.*

The new reproductive altruism is very old in that it depends almost entirely upon women as the givers of these reproductive gifts. This is not to say that women cannot give freely. It is to say that things are not all that simple. It is also to say that this emphasis on giving has become an integral part of the technological propaganda performance. And finally, it is to say that the altruistic pedestal on which women are placed by these reproductive practices is one more way of glorifying women's inequality.

Notes

1. Beverly Wildung Harrison, *Our Right to Choose: Toward a New Ethic of Abortion* (Boston: Beacon Press, 1983), 39–40.
2. Catharine A. MacKinnon. *Feminism Unmodified: Discourses on Life and Law* (Cambridge, MA: Harvard University Press, 1987), 39.

Two Questions About Surrogacy and Exploitation

ALAN WERTHEIMER

Philosophy and Public Affairs, 21, no. 3 (1992): 211–39.

I. Introduction

Commercial surrogacy has been criticized on many fronts. It has been argued that surrogacy is baby-selling, that it is harmful to the children born to surrogates, that it is harmful to all children, whose sense of security is undermined by the practice, and that it is harmful to women as a class. Another line of argument maintains that surrogacy involves the wrongful "commodification" of persons or relationships, or that it violates the Kantian maxim that persons should never be treated merely as means but always as ends-in-themselves.

In addition to these (and other) arguments, it is frequently alleged that surrogacy exploits the surrogate mothers and that such exploitation is grounds for prohibiting commercial surrogacy. I say "alleged" not to prejudge the coherence or validity of such claims, but because they have typically been advanced without much analysis or argument. Instead, it is simply said that surrogacy is exploitative, as if the meaning, validity, and moral force of these claims were self-evident. They are not.

In this article I will consider two related questions about surrogacy and exploitation: (1) Is surrogacy exploitative? (2) If surrogacy is exploitative, what is the moral force of this exploitation? Briefly stated, I shall argue that whether surrogacy is exploitative depends on whether exploitation must be *harmful* to the exploited party or whether (as I think) there can be mutually advantageous exploitation. It also depends on some facts about surrogacy about which we have little reliable evidence and on our philosophical view on what *counts* as a harm to the surrogate. Our answer to the second question will turn in part on the account of exploitation we invoke in answering the first question and in part on the way in which we resolve some other questions about the justification of state interference. I shall suggest, however, that if surrogacy is a form of voluntary and mutually advantageous exploitation, then there is a strong presumption that surrogacy contracts should be permitted and even enforceable, although that presumption may be overridden on other grounds.

II. Exploitation

Although there is no canonical (non-Marxist) account of exploitation, we typically say that A wrongfully exploits B when A takes unfair advantage of B. Now the notion of an "unfair advantage" seems to reflect two dimensions of an exploitative transaction, what I shall refer to as the dimension of *value* and the dimension of *choice*. With respect to the dimension of value, it seems that A must benefit from the transaction, for A would not *exploit* B if A were to *abuse* B without benefiting from the abuse. In addition, A exploits B only when the transaction is harmful or unfair to *B*. With respect to the dimension of choice, we typically say that A exploits B only when B's choice is somehow compromised, even if, as I believe, exploitation does not require that B's choice be strictly involuntary. It appears that exploitation requires at least *some* defect in choice, because A does not exploit B when B makes an entirely voluntary and altruistic transfer of disproportionate value to A.

Given these two dimensions of exploitation, to say that the surrogate is exploited seems to imply some defect in the values exchanged. On one view, surrogacy is exploitative because the intended parents gain from the transaction while the surrogate is—on balance—harmed. Call this *harmful exploitation*. On a second view, the surrogate gains from the transaction but in a way that is unfair to her, perhaps because the intended parents gain much more than the surrogate. Call this *mutually advantageous exploitation*. Third, it may be argued that surrogacy is exploitative because the intended parents gain from a transaction that is fundamentally immoral, perhaps because the relationship involves an exchange of radically incommensurate values, or because the transaction wrongly commodifies procreational labor. For want of a better term, call this *moralistic exploitation*. Now it is not clear, at this point, why incommensurability or commodification should be taken to involve exploitation. But since the link between commodification and exploitation has been made in the literature and because I think there is a way in which it might be sustained, I shall try to see what moralistic exploitation might involve.

With respect to the dimension of choice, it may be argued that some women are effectively coerced into serving as surrogates. It may also be argued that women do not and cannot have sufficient information to make a fully voluntary choice or that even with sufficient "external" information, they cannot anticipate the degree of their attachment to the baby. In the next two sections, I shall consider both dimensions—value and choice—in more detail.

III. Value

Is surrogacy a case of harmful exploitation, mutually advantageous exploitation, or moralistic exploitation? Because I believe that moralistic exploitation must involve some sort of harm to the surrogate, I shall consider harmful exploitation under the rubrics of "nonmoral harm" and "moral harm" before going on to consider mutually advantageous exploitation.

A. Harmful Exploitation

I. Nonmoral Harm

Rosemarie Tong says that surrogacy is harmful in straightforward nonmoral terms—"Since there is evidence that surrogacy arrangements … harm contracted mothers … a ban on commercial surrogacy needs to rely only on the harm principle [as opposed to legal moralism]."[1] As it stands, this is a non sequitur. After all, if surrogacy is harmful but consensual, a ban on commercial surrogacy cannot rely only on the harm (to others) principle; it would need to rely on a principle of paternalism. But the present question is not whether the surrogate is harmed with her consent, but whether she is harmed at all.

And here there are two reasons why we must be careful. First, in deciding whether surrogacy is harmful, we must adopt an "all things considered" conception of harm. There are, after all, negative *elements* in virtually all employment contracts, indeed, in virtually all uncontroversially beneficial transactions. We do not say that a worker is harmed by employment, although the worker may prefer leisure to work. We assume that the benefits received by employment are greater than the costs. So the question is not whether surrogacy has harmful elements, but whether it is a *net* harm, whether the costs to the surrogate outweigh the benefits. We know that some surrogates, such as Mary Beth Whitehead, have regarded surrogacy as a net harm. But this is largely irrelevant even if we assume that retrospective judgments are accurate indicators (and they may not be) in an individual case. For, and secondly, the question is not whether surrogacy is harmful *ex post* in a particular case, but whether it is typically or *ex ante* harmful. If a worker is severely injured on the job, such that employment is a net harm to that worker, we do not say that such employment is harmful as a practice. Similarly, the question is not whether an *individual* surrogate such as Ms. Whitehead is harmed, but whether (all things considered) the expected value of surrogacy is negative, where the expected value is a function of the probability distribution of the various outcomes.

Surrogacy presents a particularly difficult context for making an "all things considered" judgment because some of the crucial benefits and harms are explicitly psychological and subjective. They are hard to measure and will vary substantially from person to person. On the positive side of the ledger, we have to put the value of the monetary compensation, whatever psychological gratification the surrogate obtains from bringing a child into the world, and the surrogate's knowledge that she has made the intended parents very happy. These benefits may or may not be considerable. There is much that might appear on the debit side of the ledger: the risk of physical harm or death resulting from

the pregnancy or the delivery, restraints on the surrogate's choices during pregnancy, and the inconvenience and discomfort associated with a normal pregnancy. Perhaps most important, the surrender of the baby to the intended parents may be psychologically harmful to the surrogate. And, unlike the previous harms, some of which last no longer than the pregnancy, this harm may endure for an indefinite period thereafter.

At this point, the defender of surrogacy might reply that the *ex ante* value of the surrogacy arrangement simply could *not* be negative, for, if that were so, women would not agree to serve as surrogates. But that statement is false. That a woman agrees to serve as a surrogate does not show that an accurate judgment of her *ex ante* value is positive; it only shows that she *thought* it would be positive. She may have miscalculated, perhaps because surrogates are unable to make accurate predictions of their future psychological reactions. Thus surrogacy may be harmful even though most surrogates believe it will be beneficial.

In addition, it might be argued that a surrogate may be "objectively" harmed even if she does not feel harmed, *ex post*. It is a commonplace that B's interests—*as B defines them*—can be harmed even if B is unaware that the harm has occurred. For example, B's interest in her reputation or the fidelity of her spouse can be damaged by libel or infidelity even if she is unaware that either has occurred. More controversially, it may be argued that a person's objective interests can be harmed even if she does not now and never will regard these as her interests.

Given all this, is surrogacy *ex ante* harmful, all things considered? Given our limited factual knowledge and unresolved theoretical controversies over what counts as "objective" harm, I am inclined to think that we should now remain agnostic. For, depending on the answers to these questions, surrogacy could turn out to be a case of harmful exploitation, mutually advantageous exploitation, or neither.

Suppose that most surrogates are worse off for the experience, all things considered. Could surrogacy be advantageous to the surrogate if the monetary compensation were high enough? If surrogacy is typically harmful, all told, because "for what amounts to very little money for a nine-month, twenty-four-hour-a-day 'job,' the contracted mother risks and usually experiences a variety of physical but especially psychological harms," this can be rectified by imposing an adequate mandatory minimum wage. Moreover, if surrogacy is typically mutually advantageous but asymmetrically and unjustly so, this dimension of the exploitation can be remedied in the same way.

Now it is entirely possible, indeed inevitable, that an increase in compensation would convert a net harm into a net benefit for some women. Moreover, if surrogacy were mutually advantageous but unjust at $10,000, then the arrangement would be less unjust or not unjust for a higher fee. Yet, unlike other contexts in which it is uncontroversial that exploitation can be eliminated or decreased by increasing the compensation to the exploited party, it is rarely argued that surrogacy would be less exploitative if the surrogate were paid more. In fact, unpaid surrogacy is typically regarded as less exploitative than paid surrogacy. Among the critiques of surrogacy, higher pay is the dog that doesn't bark.

Why does the dog not bark? I suspect that higher pay is not offered as a solution to the problem of exploitation in part because the very receipt of monetary compensation may actually cause some of the psychological harm experienced by some surrogate mothers, who may feel they are doing something "sleazy." If so, increasing the compensation may add to both the negative and positive sides of the ledger, although it is not clear how much it would add to each. After all, even if increased compensation caused increased psychological harm, the value of the increased compensation may be *greater* than the increased psychological harm it causes.

2. Moral Harm

I suspect, however, that the main reason a wage increase is rarely advanced as a solution to exploi-

tation is not that it would be psychologically harmful to the surrogate, but that it is thought that procreative labor should not be exchanged for money—period. And if procreative labor should not be exchanged for money, it will not improve things to exchange procreational labor for *more* money. If, as I have argued, exploitation involves a defect in the values exchanged, the task is to see how this perspective can be related to exploitation. There are two ways in which the connection might be drawn: one focuses on the incommensurability of the values exchanged, and the other focuses on commodification.

Elizabeth Anderson says that "a kind of exploitation occurs when one party to a transaction is oriented toward the exchange of 'gift' values, while the other party operates in accordance with the norms of the market."[2] But *incommensurability*, as such, does not take us very far. First, to say that the values exchanged in a transaction are incommensurable does not establish that a market transaction is wrong, at least not without further argument. The permissibility of market transactions does not require that the goods exchanged be commensurable on a single metric. It requires that the parties transact voluntarily and, perhaps, with a (reasonable) belief that the value received is at least as great as the value given. One can and (arguably) should be able to buy or sell a "priceless" painting without claiming that its value is "commensurate" with the money that is paid. Second, even if incommensurability provides a reason for thinking that a transaction is *wrong*, it does not entail that a party's interests are negatively affected by the transaction. So more will have to be said if incommensurability is going to support the claim that surrogacy is exploitative.

Incommensurability aside, it is widely thought that some goods and services are appropriately exchanged for money whereas others are not. On the one hand, automobiles, houses, books, television sets, and at least *some* forms of labor can legitimately be exchanged for money. By contrast, there are some things that should *not* be exchanged for money—citizenship, human beings, criminal justice, marriage rights, exemption from military service, and perhaps other forms of human labor (e.g., sexual and procreational labor). On this view, surrogacy is exploitative not because it comes too cheap, but because it *commodifies* that which should not be commodified.

If procreational labor should not be commodified, does it follow that surrogacy is harmful to the surrogate? It is not clear. It may have been wrong to commodify exemptions from military service during the Civil War, when citizens were allowed to pay $300 to purchase the services of a substitute, but it was hardly harmful to those who *bought* exemptions. And while the commodification of exemptions may have *caused* harm—by injury or death—to the substitutes, it is much less clear that the commodification of exemptions, as such, *constituted* a harm to them. And so we must ask whether the commodification of the surrogate's labor is (1) harmful, (2) harmful *because* it is wrong, or (3) wrong but not harmful (to the surrogate).

It may be thought that the commodification of the surrogate's labor is *psychologically* harmful to her, but the extent to which that is so is an empirical question, and little evidence has been adduced. We might say that the commodification of procreational labor is *objectively* harmful to the surrogate's interests, even if she does not feel harmed. This could occur in two ways.

First, as with nonmoral forms of objective harm, we might say that a woman has an interest in not being commodified, degraded, or treated merely as a means. But to say that a woman may be objectively harmed is one thing; to identify the nature of that harm is another. And it is not quite clear in what ways a woman is thought to be harmed by commodification or degradation, in the absence of the psychological connection.

Second, it might be claimed that a person can lose the respect of others or be degraded in *their* eyes, even if she does not lose *self*-respect or become degraded in her own eyes. So to the extent that a person has an interest in the way she is regarded by others, surrogacy may injure

those interests. But that raises at least two points. First, it is not clear that surrogacy actually does have these effects. Second, to the extent that these effects stem solely from the way surrogacy is regarded by the society—as a matter of fact and without separate normative justification—it is not clear that it represents a basis for condemning the practice rather than a basis for condemning society's reaction. Although homosexuality was (or is) a basis for a loss of social respect, this provides no reason to condemn homosexuality.

In any case, even if commodification or degradation constituted objective harms to the surrogate, it cannot show that surrogacy is harmful to the surrogate, all things considered. Surrogacy would produce a *net* harm to the surrogate only if the degree of harm that resulted from commodification or degradation was *greater* than the benefits that she received *from* the compensation.

But there is a second way in which commodification or degradation might be regarded as harmful to the surrogate. It may constitute a *moral* harm, and this in one or both of two ways. First, we may harm someone by violating her *rights*, independent of any other physical, economic, or psychological harm. A trespasser harms the property owner by violating her rights to exclusive use of her property, even though there is no "ordinary" harm to her property. A man harms a woman by fondling her without her consent, even if the touching causes no physical pain or lasting psychological damage. If a woman has a right not to have her labor commodified, then surrogacy is harmful precisely because it is a violation of her rights. The problem here, of course, is that many acts that would constitute a violation of B's rights if done without B's consent are not rights violations if done with B's consent. It is no violation of a person's rights if her property is entered with her consent or if she is fondled with her consent. More generally, we do not treat a person *merely* as a means rather than an end-in-herself if we treat her in a certain way only if she consents to be treated in that way. Thus commodification is no obvious violation of this Kantian maxim if the commodification is consensual—absent some additional argument, for example, that the rights involved are inalienable or that consent given under objectionable background conditions is not sufficiently voluntary.

Surrogacy might involve a different and second form of moral harm. It may be thought that surrogacy is injurious to the surrogate precisely because she participates in something bad. The structure of the argument from moral harm might look something like this:

(1) Surrogacy is wrong, say, because it is wrong to commodify procreational labor.
(2) Because surrogacy is wrong, it is immoral for a woman to serve as a surrogate.
(3) Participating in an immoral activity is bad for the participant.
(4) Combining (1), (2), and (3), because it is immoral for a woman to serve as a surrogate, surrogacy "sets back" her interest in being a moral person, that is, it constitutes a harm to her.
(5) Because the surrogate is harmed by the transaction for the benefit of the intended parents, surrogacy is exploitative.

Two points about this line of argument. First, to the extent that commodification constitutes a serious moral harm, it also harms the intended parents, and thus it may entail that surrogacy is *mutually* exploitative, although the surrogate might be *more* exploited because this harm is added to other harms that the intended parents do not suffer. And this raises the second point. Even if we accept (3)—and that is the crucial question—the argument from moral harm only allows us to claim that surrogacy has additional harmful *elements*. Assuming, however, that surrogacy is otherwise advantageous to the surrogate, it is not clear that the harmful moral elements necessarily outweigh the beneficial nonmoral elements, unless it is assumed that moral harms always trump nonmoral benefits. And it is not clear whether an increase in compensation to the surrogate would yield an increase in the amount of moral harm or

whether the degree of moral harm is inelastic with respect to price.

I am well aware that there is something very odd about the attempt to understand commodification as a harm and to assess its place in overall harm and benefit to the surrogate. Nonetheless, I believe that commodification *must* be considered a harmful element in the transaction if it is to be related to the claim that surrogacy is *exploitative*. Of course, commodification may be better understood as a basis for thinking that surrogacy is wrong although not exploitative. After all, apart from its effects on the surrogate, the commodification of procreational labor may have undesirable effects on the offspring, women (as a class), or society as a whole. And even if commodification is not harmful to specific persons in any straightforward way, it may fail to reflect the best "conception of human flourishing."

B. Mutually Advantageous Exploitation

Suppose that the typical surrogate is *not* harmed by surrogacy, all things considered, or would not be harmed if the compensation were higher. All things considered, surrogacy is or would be a mutually advantageous transaction. Might we still regard the transaction as exploitative? I think so. I see no reason to assume that voluntary and mutually advantageous transactions cannot be unfair.

The problem, of course, is that if we are going to say that a transaction is exploitative because it is insufficiently beneficial to the exploited party, we may reasonably be asked to specify the criteria by which we are making this assessment. And that is a difficult matter. It is, for example, frequently said that a fair transaction is one in which both parties gain (roughly) equally. On that account, we can say that a surrogate is exploited if she receives *less* value from the transaction than the intended parents. Unfortunately, this definition of a fair transaction is clearly wrong. If a physician performs a procedure (for a normal price) that saves a patient's life, we do not say that the patient has exploited the physician's labor, although the patient has gained far more from the transaction than the physician. Indeed, I suspect that the exploit*ee* often gets much more utility from a transaction than the exploiter. It is precisely because the exploitee stands to gain so much from the transaction (relative to the exploiter) that his bargaining position is comparatively weak. This does not, of course, show that it is the intended parents who are exploited. It does suggest that the fact that the surrogate receives less value from the transaction than the intended parents is not sufficient to show that *she* is exploited.

In any case—notwithstanding the difficulties in formulating criteria for fair transactions, and notwithstanding that I do not have an alternative account to propose—I see no reason to think that a voluntary and mutually advantageous transaction cannot be unfair. At this point in the history of moral philosophy, it seems more reasonable to suppose that we have not yet developed an ade-quate theory of fair transactions than to conclude that these difficulties demonstrate that there cannot be independent criteria for fair transactions. So I prefer to suppose that the surrogate may be exploited if the compensation is insufficient or if the contractual terms are unacceptably harsh. On the other hand, if the compensation is adequate and if the contractual terms are not unacceptably harsh, then we will have to conclude that the surrogate has not been exploited, whatever else we may want to say about surrogacy.

Notes

1. Rosemarie Tong, "The Overdue Death of a Feminist Chameleon: Taking a Stand on Surrogacy Arrangements," *Journal of Social Philosophy* 21 (1990): 47.
2. Elizabeth S. Anderson, "Is Women's Labor a Commodity?" *Philosophy and Public Affairs* 19, no. 1 (1990): 71–92, at 84.

Preventing a *Brave New World*
Why We Should Ban Cloning Now

LEON R. KASS

The New Republic 21, May (2001): 30–39.

The urgency of the great political struggles of the twentieth century, successfully waged against totalitarianisms first right and then left, seems to have blinded many people to a deeper and ultimately darker truth about the present age: all contemporary societies are traveling briskly in the same utopian direction. All are wedded to the modern technological project; all march eagerly to the drums of progress and fly proudly the banner of modern science; all sing loudly the Baconian anthem, "Conquer nature, relieve man's estate." Leading the triumphal procession is modern medicine, which is daily becoming ever more powerful in its battle against disease, decay, and death, thanks especially to astonishing achievements in biomedical science and technology—achievements for which we must surely be grateful.

Yet contemplating present and projected advances in genetic and reproductive technologies, in neuroscience and psychopharmacology, and in the development of artificial organs and computer-chip implants for human brains, we now clearly recognize new uses for biotechnical power that soar beyond the traditional medical goals of healing disease and relieving suffering.

Human nature itself lies on the operating table, ready for alteration, for eugenic and psychic "enhancement," for wholesale re-design.

Years ago Aldous Huxley saw it coming. In his charming but disturbing novel, *Brave New World* (it appeared in 1932 and is more powerful on each re-reading), he made its meaning strikingly visible for all to see. Unlike other frightening futuristic novels of the past century, such as Orwell's already dated *Nineteen Eighty-Four*, Huxley shows us a dystopia that goes with, rather than against, the human grain. Indeed, it is animated by our own most humane and progressive aspirations. Following those aspirations to their ultimate realization, Huxley enables us to recognize those less obvious but often more pernicious evils that are inextricably linked to the successful attainment of partial goods.

Huxley depicts human life seven centuries hence, living under the gentle hand of humanitarianism rendered fully competent by genetic manipulation, psychoactive drugs, hypnopaedia, and high-tech amusements. At long last, mankind has succeeded in eliminating disease, aggression, war, anxiety, suffering, guilt, envy, and grief. But this victory comes at the heavy price of homogenization, mediocrity, trivial pursuits, shallow attachments, debased tastes, spurious contentment, and souls without loves or longings. The Brave New World has achieved prosperity, community, stability, and nigh-universal contentment, only to be peopled by creatures of human shape but stunted humanity. They consume, fornicate, take "soma," enjoy "centrifugal bumble-puppy," and operate the machinery that makes it all possible. They do not read, write, think, love, or govern themselves. Art and science, virtue and religion, family and friendship are all passé.

In Huxley's novel, everything proceeds under the direction of an omnipotent—albeit benevolent—world state. Yet the dehumanization that he portrays does not really require despotism or external control. To the contrary, precisely because the society of the future will deliver exactly what we most want—health, safety, comfort, plenty, pleasure, peace of mind and length of days—we can reach the same humanly debased condition solely on the basis of free human choice. No need for World Controllers. Just give us the technological imperative, liberal democratic society, compassionate humanitarianism, moral pluralism, and free markets, and we can take ourselves to a Brave New World all by ourselves—and without even deliberately deciding to go. In case you had not noticed, the train has already left the station and is gathering speed, but no one seems to be in charge.

Some among us are delighted, of course, by this state of affairs: some scientists and biotechnologists, their entrepreneurial backers, and a cheering claque of sci-fi enthusiasts, futurologists, and libertarians. There are dreams to be realized, powers to be exercised, honors to be won, and money—big money—to be made. But many of us are worried, and not, as the proponents of the revolution self-servingly claim, because we are either ignorant of science or afraid of the unknown. To the contrary, we can see all too clearly where the train is headed, and we do not like the destination. We can distinguish cleverness about means from wisdom about ends, and we are loath to entrust the future of the race to those who cannot tell the difference.

Yet for all our disquiet, we have until now done nothing to prevent it. We hide our heads in the sand because we enjoy the blessings that medicine keeps supplying, or we rationalize our inaction by declaring that human engineering is inevitable and we can do nothing about it. In either case, we are complicit in preparing for our own degradation, in some respects more to blame than the bio-zealots who, however misguided, are putting their money where their mouth is. Denial and despair, unattractive outlooks in any situation, become morally reprehensible when circumstances summon us to keep the world safe for human flourishing. Our immediate ancestors, taking up the challenge of their time, rose to the occasion and rescued the human future from the cruel dehumanizations of Nazi and Soviet tyranny. It is our more difficult task to find ways to preserve it from the soft dehumanizations of well-meaning but hubristic biotechnical "recreationism"—and to do it without undermining biomedical science or rejecting its genuine contributions to human welfare.

Truth be told, it will not be easy for us to do so, and we know it. But rising to the challenge requires recognizing the difficulties. For there are indeed many features of modern life that will conspire to frustrate efforts aimed at the human control of the biomedical project. First, we Americans believe in technological automatism: where we do not foolishly believe that all innovation is progress, we fatalistically believe that it is inevitable ("If it can be done, it will be done, like it or not"). Second, we believe in freedom: the freedom of scientists to inquire, the freedom of technologists to develop, the freedom of entrepreneurs to invest and to profit, the freedom of private citizens to make use of existing technologies to satisfy any and all personal desires, including the desire to reproduce by whatever means. Third, the biomedical enterprise occupies the moral high ground of compassionate humanitarianism, upholding the supreme values of modern life—cure disease, prolong life, relieve suffering—in competition with which other moral goods rarely stand a chance.

There are still other obstacles. Our cultural pluralism and easygoing relativism make it difficult to reach consensus on what we should embrace and what we should oppose; and moral objections to this or that biomedical practice are often facilely dismissed as religious or sectarian. Many people are unwilling to pronounce judgments about what is good or bad, right and wrong, even in matters of great importance, even for themselves—never mind for others or for society as a whole. It does not help that the biomedical project is now deeply entangled with commerce: there are increasingly powerful economic interests in favor of going full steam ahead, and no economic interests in favor of going slow. Since we live in a democracy, moreover, we face political difficulties in gaining a consensus to direct our future, and we have almost no political experience in trying to curtail the development

of any new biomedical technology. Finally, and perhaps most troubling, our views of the meaning of our humanity have been so transformed by the scientific-technological approach to the world that we are in danger of forgetting what we have to lose, humanly speaking.

But though the difficulties are real, our situation is far from hopeless. Regarding each of the aforementioned impediments, there is another side to the story. Though we love our gadgets and believe in progress, we have lost our innocence regarding technology. The environmental movement especially has alerted us to the unintended damage caused by unregulated technological advance, and has taught us how certain dangerous practices can be curbed. Though we favor freedom of inquiry, we recognize that experiments are deeds and not speeches, and we prohibit experimentation on human subjects without their consent, even when cures from disease might be had by unfettered research; and we limit so-called reproductive freedom by proscribing incest, polygamy, and the buying and selling of babies.

Although we esteem medical progress, biomedical institutions have ethics committees that judge research proposals on moral grounds, and, when necessary, uphold the primacy of human freedom and human dignity even over scientific discovery. Our moral pluralism notwithstanding, national commissions and review bodies have sometimes reached moral consensus to recommend limits on permissible scientific research and technological application. On the economic front, the patenting of genes and life forms and the rapid rise of genomic commerce have elicited strong concerns and criticisms, leading even former enthusiasts of the new biology to recoil from the impending commodification of human life. Though we lack political institutions experienced in setting limits on biomedical innovation, federal agencies years ago rejected the development of the plutonium-powered artificial heart, and we have nationally prohibited commercial traffic in organs for transplantation, even though a market would increase the needed supply. In recent years, several American states and many foreign countries have successfully taken political action, making certain practices illegal and placing others under moratoriums (the creation of human embryos solely for research; human germ-like genetic alteration). Most importantly, the majority of Americans are not yet so degraded or so cynical as to fail to be revolted by the society depicted in Huxley's novel. Though the obstacles to effective action are significant, they offer no excuse for resignation. Besides, it would be disgraceful to concede defeat even before we enter the fray.

Not the least of our difficulties in trying to exercise control over where biology is taking us is the fact that we do not get to decide, once and for all, for or against the destination of a post-human world. The scientific discoveries and the technical powers that will take us there come to us piecemeal, one at a time and seemingly independent from one another, each often attractively introduced as a measure that will "help [us] not to be sick:" But sometimes we come to a clear fork in the road where decision is possible, and where we know that our decision will make a world of difference—indeed, it will make a permanently different world. Fortunately, we stand now at the point of such a momentous decision. Events have conspired to provide us with a perfect opportunity to seize the initiative and to gain some control of the biotechnical project. I refer to the prospect of human cloning, a practice absolutely central to Huxley's fictional world. Indeed, creating and manipulating life in the laboratory is the gateway to a *Brave New World*, not only in fiction but also in fact.

"To clone or not to clone a human being" is no longer a fanciful question. Success in cloning sheep, and also cows, mice, pigs, and goats, makes it perfectly clear that a fateful decision is now at hand: whether we should welcome or even tolerate the cloning of human beings. If recent newspaper reports are to be believed, reputable scientists and physicians have announced their intention to produce the first human clone in the coming year. Their efforts may already be under way.

The media, gawking and titillating as is their wont, have been softening us up for this possibility by turning the bizarre into the familiar. In the four years since the birth of Dolly the cloned sheep, the tone of discussing the prospect of human cloning has gone from "Yuck" to "Oh?" to "Gee whiz" to "Why not?" The sentimentalizers, aided by leading bioethicists, have downplayed talk about eugenically cloning the beautiful and the brawny or the best and the brightest. They have taken instead to defending clonal reproduction for humanitarian or compassionate reasons: to treat infertility in people who are said to "have no other choice" to avoid the risk of severe genetic disease, to "replace" a child who has died. For the sake of these rare benefits, they would have us countenance the entire practice of human cloning, the consequences be damned.

But we dare not be complacent about what is at issue, for the stakes are very high. Human cloning, though partly continuous with previous reproductive technologies, is also something radically new in itself and in its easily foreseeable consequences—specially when coupled with powers for genetic "enhancement" and germline genetic modification that may soon become available, owing to the recently completed Human Genome Project. I exaggerate somewhat, but in the direction of the truth: we are compelled to decide nothing less than whether human procreation is going to remain human, whether children are going to be made to order rather than begotten, and whether we wish to say yes in principle to the road that leads to the dehumanized hell of Brave New World.

II

What is cloning? Cloning, or asexual reproduction, is the production of individuals who are genetically identical to an already existing individual. The procedure's name is fancy—"somatic cell nuclear transfer"—but its concept is simple. Take a mature but unfertilized egg; remove or deactivate its nucleus; introduce a nucleus obtained from a specialized (somatic) cell of an adult organism. Once the egg begins to divide, transfer the little embryo to a woman's uterus to initiate a pregnancy. Since almost all the hereditary material of a cell is contained within its nucleus, the re-nucleated egg and the individual into which it develops are genetically identical to the organism that was the source of the transferred nucleus.

An unlimited number of genetically identical individuals—the group, as well as each of its members, is called "a clone"—could be produced by nuclear transfer. In principle, any person, male or female, newborn or adult, could be cloned, and in any quantity; and because stored cells can outlive their sources, one may even clone the dead. Since cloning requires no personal involvement on the part of the person whose genetic material is used, it could easily be used to reproduce living or deceased persons without their consent—a threat to reproductive freedom that has received relatively little attention.

Some possible misconceptions need to be avoided. Cloning is not Xeroxing: the clone of Bill Clinton, though his genetic double, would enter the world hairless, toothless, and peeing in his diapers, like any other human infant. But neither is cloning just like natural twinning: the cloned twin will be identical to an older, existing adult; and it will arise not by chance but by deliberate design; and its entire genetic makeup will be pre-selected by its parents and/or scientists. Moreover, the success rate of cloning, at least at first, will probably not be very high: the Scots transferred two hundred seventy-seven adult nuclei into sheep eggs, implanted twenty-nine clonal embryos, and achieved the birth of only one live lamb clone.

For this reason, among others, it is unlikely that, at least for now, the practice would be very popular; and there is little immediate worry of mass-scale production of multicopies. Still, for the tens of thousands of people who sustain more than three hundred assisted-reproduction clinics in the United States and already avail themselves of in vitro fertilization and other techniques, cloning would be an option with virtually no added fuss. Panos Zavos, the Kentucky reproduction specialist who has announced his plans to clone a child, claims that he has already received thousands of e-mailed requests from people eager to clone, despite the known risks of failure and damaged offspring. Should commercial interests develop in "nucleus-banking" as they have in sperm-banking and egg-harvesting; should famous athletes or other celebrities decide to market their DNA the way they now market their autographs and nearly everything else; should techniques of embryo and germline genetic testing and manipulation arrive as anticipated, increasing the use of laboratory assistance in order to obtain "better" babies—should all this come to pass, cloning, if it is permitted, could become more than a marginal practice simply on the basis of free reproductive choice.

What are we to think about this prospect? Nothing good. Indeed, most people are repelled by nearly all aspects of human cloning: the possibility of mass production of human beings, with large clones of look-alikes, compromised in their individuality; the idea of father-son or mother-daughter "twins"; the bizarre prospect of a woman bearing and rearing a genetic copy of herself, her spouse, or even her deceased father or mother; the grotesqueness of conceiving a child as an exact "replacement" for another who has died; the utilitarian creation of embryonic duplicates of oneself, to be frozen away or created when needed to provide homologous tissues or organs for transplantation; the narcissism of those who would clone themselves, and the arrogance of others who think they know who deserves to be cloned; the Frankensteinian hubris to create a human life and increasingly to control its destiny; men playing at being God. Almost no one finds any of the suggested reasons for human cloning compelling, and almost everyone anticipates its possible misuses and abuses. And the popular belief that human cloning cannot be prevented makes the prospect all the more revolting.

Revulsion is not an argument; and some of yesterday's repugnances are today calmly accepted—not always for the better. In some crucial cases, however, repugnance is the emotional expression of deep wisdom, beyond reason's power completely to articulate it. Can anyone really give an argument fully adequate to the horror that is father-daughter incest (even with consent), or bestiality, or the mutilation of a corpse, or the eating of human flesh, or the rape or murder of another human being? Would anybody's failure to give full rational justification for his revulsion at those practices make that revulsion ethically suspect?

I suggest that our repugnance at human cloning belongs in this category. We are repelled by the prospect of cloning human beings not because of the strangeness or the novelty of the undertaking, but because we intuit and we feel, immediately and without argument, the violation of things that we rightfully hold dear. We sense that cloning represents a profound defilement of our given nature as pro-creative beings, and of the social relations built on this natural ground. We also sense that cloning is a radical form of child abuse. In this age in which everything is held to be permissible so long as it is freely done, and in which our bodies are regarded as mere instruments of our autonomous rational will, repugnance may be the only voice left that speaks up to defend the central core of our humanity. Shallow are the souls that have forgotten how to shudder.

III

Yet repugnance need not stand naked before the bar of reason. The wisdom of our horror at human cloning can be at least partially articulated, even if this is finally one of those instances about which the heart has its reasons that reason cannot entirely know. I offer four objections to human cloning: that it constitutes unethical experimentation; that it threatens identity and individuality; that it turns procreation into manufacture (especially when understood as the harbinger of manipulations to come); and that it means despotism over children and perversion of parenthood. Please note: I speak only about so-called reproductive cloning, not about the creation of cloned embryos for research. The objections that may be raised against creating (or using) embryos for research are entirely independent of whether the research embryos are produced by cloning. What is radically distinct and radically new is reproductive cloning.

Any attempt to clone a human being would constitute an unethical experiment upon the resulting child-to-be. In all the animal experiments, fewer than two to three percent of all cloning attempts succeeded. Not only are there fetal deaths and stillborn infants, but many of the so-called "successes" are in fact failures. As has only recently become clear, there is a very high incidence of major disabilities and deformities in cloned animals that attain live birth. Cloned cows often have heart and lung problems; cloned mice later develop pathological obesity; other live-born cloned animals fail to reach normal developmental milestones.

The problem, scientists suggest, may lie in the fact that an egg with a new somatic nucleus must re-program itself in a matter of minutes or hours (whereas the nucleus of an unaltered egg has been prepared over months and years). There is thus a greatly increased likelihood of error in translating the genetic instructions, leading to developmental defects some of which will show themselves only much later. Considered opinion is today nearly unanimous, even among scientists: attempts at human cloning are irresponsible and unethical. We cannot ethically even get to know whether or not human cloning is feasible.

If it were successful, cloning would create serious issues of identity and individuality. The clone may experience concerns about his distinctive identity not only because he will be, in genotype and in appearance, identical to another human being, but because he may also be twin to the person who is his "father" or his "mother"—if one can still call them that. Unaccountably, people treat as innocent the homey case of intra-familial cloning—the cloning of husband or wife (or single mother). They forget about the unique dangers of mixing the twin relation with the parent-child relation. (For this situation, the relation of contemporaneous twins is no precedent; yet even this less problematic situation teaches us how difficult it is to wrest independence from the being for whom one has the most powerful affinity.) Virtually no parent is going to be able to treat a clone of himself or herself as one treats a child generated by the lottery of sex. What will happen when the adolescent clone of Mommy becomes the spitting image of the woman with whom Daddy once fell in love? In case of divorce, will Mommy still love the clone of Daddy, even though she can no longer stand the sight of Daddy himself?

Most people think about cloning from the point of view of adults choosing to clone. Almost nobody thinks about what it would be like to be a cloned child. Surely his or her new life would constantly be scrutinized in relation to that of the older version. Even in the absence of unusual parental expectations for the clone—say, to live the same life, only without its errors—the child is likely to be ever a curiosity, ever a potential source of deja-vu. Unlike "normal" identical twins, a cloned individual—copied from whomever—will be saddled with a genotype that has already lived. He will not be fully a surprise to the world: people are likely always to compare his doings in life with those of his alter ego, especially if he is a clone of someone gifted or famous. True, his nurture and his circumstances will be different; genotype is not exactly destiny. But one must also expect parental efforts to shape this new life after the original—or at least to view the child with the original version always firmly in mind. For why else did they clone from the star basketball player, the mathematician, or the beauty queen—or even dear old Dad—in the first place?

Human cloning would also represent a giant step toward the transformation of begetting into making, of procreation into manufacture (literally, "handmade"), a process that has already begun with in vitro fertilization and genetic testing of embryos. With cloning, not only is the process in hand, but the total genetic blueprint of the cloned individual is selected and determined by the human artisans. To be sure, subsequent development is still according to natural processes; and the resulting children will be recognizably human. But we would be taking a major step into making man himself simply another one of the man-made things.

How does begetting differ from making? In natural procreation, human beings come together to give existence to another being that is formed exactly as we were, by what we are—living, hence perishable, hence aspiringly erotic, hence procreative human beings. But in clonal reproduction, and in the more advanced forms of manufacture to which it will lead, we give existence to a being not by what we are but by what we intend and design.

Let me be clear. The problem is not the mere intervention of technique, and the point is not that "nature knows best." The problem is that any child whose being, character, and capacities exist owing to human design does not stand on the same plane as its makers. As with any product of our making, no matter how excellent, the artificer stands above it, not as an equal but as a superior, transcending it by his will and creative prowess. In human cloning, scientists and prospective "parents" adopt a technocratic attitude toward human children: human children become their artifacts. Such an arrangement is profoundly dehumanizing, no matter how good the product.

Finally, the practice of human cloning by nuclear transfer—like other anticipated forms of genetically engineering the next generation—would enshrine and aggravate a profound misunderstanding of the meaning of having children and the parent-child relationship. When a couple normally chooses to procreate, the partners are saying yes to the emergence of new life in its novelty—are saying yes not only to having a child, but also to having whatever child this child turns out to be. In accepting our finitude, in opening ourselves to our replacement, we tacitly confess the limits of our control.

Embracing the future by procreating means precisely that we are relinquishing our grip in the very activity of taking up our own share in what we hope will be the immortality of human life and the human species. This means that our children are not our children: they are not our property, they are not our possessions. Neither are they supposed to live our lives for us, or to live anyone's life but their own. Their genetic distinctiveness and independence are the natural foreshadowing of the deep truth that they have their own, never-before-enacted life to live. Though sprung from a past, they take an uncharted course into the future.

Much mischief is already done by parents who try to live vicariously through their children. Children are sometimes compelled to fulfill the broken dreams of unhappy parents. But whereas most parents normally have hopes for their children, cloning parents will have expectations. In cloning, such overbearing parents will have taken at the start a decisive step that contradicts the entire meaning of the open and forward-looking nature of parent-child relations. The child is given a genotype that has already lived, with full expectation that this blueprint of a past life ought to be controlling the life that is to come. A wanted child now means a child who exists precisely to fulfill parental wants. Like all the more precise eugenic manipulations that will follow in its wake, cloning is thus inherently despotic, for it seeks to make one's children after one's own image (or an image of one's choosing) and their future according to one's will.

Is this hyperbolic? Consider concretely the new realities of responsibility and guilt in the households of the cloned. No longer only the sins of the parents, but also the genetic choices of the parents, will be visited on the children—and beyond the third and fourth generations; and everyone will know who is responsible. No parent will be able to blame nature or the lottery of sex for an unhappy adolescent's big nose, dull wit, musical ineptitude, nervous disposition, or anything else that he hates about himself. Fairly or not, children will hold their cloners responsible for everything,

for nature as well as for nurture. And parents, especially the better ones, will be limitlessly liable to guilt. Only the truly despotic souls will sleep the sleep of the innocent.

IV

The defenders of cloning are not wittingly friends of despotism. Quite the contrary. Deaf to most other considerations, they regard themselves mainly as friends of freedom: the freedom of individuals to reproduce, the freedom of scientists and inventors to discover and to devise and to foster "progress" in genetic knowledge and technique, the freedom of entrepreneurs to profit in the market. They want large-scale cloning only for animals, but they wish to preserve cloning as a human option for exercising our "right to reproduce"—our right to have children, and children with "desirable genes." As some point out, under our "right to reproduce" we already practice early forms of unnatural, artificial, and extra-marital reproduction, and we already practice early forms of eugenic choice. For that reason, they argue, cloning is no big deal.

We have here a perfect example of the logic of the slippery slope. The principle of reproductive freedom currently enunciated by the proponents of cloning logically embraces the ethical acceptability of sliding all the way down: to producing children wholly in the laboratory from sperm to term (should it become feasible), and to producing children whose entire genetic makeup will be the product of parental eugenic planning and choice. If reproductive freedom means the right to have a child of one's own choosing by whatever means, then reproductive freedom knows and accepts no limits.

Proponents want us to believe that there are legitimate uses of cloning that can be distinguished from illegitimate uses, but by their own principles no such limits can be found. (Nor could any such limits be enforced in practice: once cloning is permitted, no one ever need discover whom one is cloning and why). Reproductive freedom, as they understand it, is governed solely by the subjective wishes of the parents-to-be. The sentimentally appealing case of the childless married couple is, on these grounds, indistinguishable from the case of an individual (married or not) who would like to clone someone famous or talented, living or dead. And the principle here endorsed justifies not only cloning but also the future artificial attempts to create (manufacture) "better" or "perfect" babies.

Proponents of cloning urge us to forget about the science-fiction scenarios of laboratory manufacture or multiple-copy clones, and to focus only on the sympathetic cases of infertile couples exercising their reproductive rights. But why, if the single cases are so innocent, should multiplying their performance be so off-putting? (Similarly, why do others object to people's making money from that practice if the practice itself is perfectly acceptable?) The so—called science-fiction cases—say *Brave New World*—make vivid the meaning of what looks to us, mistakenly, to be benign. They reveal that what looks like compassionate humanitarianism is, in the end, crushing dehumanization.

V

Whether or not they share my reasons, most people, I think, share my conclusion: that human cloning is unethical in itself and dangerous in its likely consequences, which include the precedent that it will establish for designing our children. Some reach this conclusion for their own good reasons, different from my own: concerns about the distributive justice in access to eugenic cloning; worries about the genetic effects of asexual "inbreeding"; aversion to the implicit premise of genetic determinism; objections to the embryonic and fetal wastage that must necessarily accompany the efforts; religious opposition to "man playing God." But never mind why: the overwhelming majority of our fellow Americans remain firmly opposed to cloning human beings.

For us, then, the real questions are: What should we do about it? How can we best succeed? These questions should concern everyone eager to secure deliberate human control over the

powers that could re-design our humanity, even if cloning is not the issue over which they would choose to make their stand. And the answer to the first question seems pretty plain. What we should do is work to prevent human cloning by making it illegal.

We should aim for a global legal ban, if possible, and for a unilateral national ban at a minimum—and soon, before the fact is upon us. To be sure, legal bans can be violated; but we certainly curtail much mischief by outlawing incest, voluntary servitude, and the buying and selling of organs and babies. To be sure, renegade scientists may secretly undertake to violate such a law, but we can deter them by both criminal sanctions and monetary penalties, as well as by removing any incentive they have to proudly claim credit for their technological bravado.

Such a ban on clonal baby-making will not harm the progress of basic genetic science and technology. On the contrary, it will reassure the public that scientists are happy to proceed without violating the deep ethical norms and intuitions of the human community. It will also protect honorable scientists from a public backlash against the brazen misconduct of the rogues. As many scientists have publicly confessed, free and worthy science probably has much more to fear from a strong public reaction to a cloning fiasco than it does from a cloning ban, provided that the ban is judiciously crafted and vigorously enforced against those who would violate it.

Five states—Michigan, Louisiana, California, Rhode Island, and Virginia—have already enacted a ban on human cloning, Internationally, the movement to ban human cloning gains momentum. France and Germany have banned cloning (and germline genetic engineering), and the Council of Europe is working to have it banned in all of its forty-one member countries, and Canada is expected to follow suit. The United Nations, UNESCO, and the Group of Seven have called for a global ban on human cloning.

Given the decisive actions of the rest of the industrialized world, the United States looks to some observers to be a rogue nation. A few years ago, soon after the birth of Dolly, President Clinton called for legislation to outlaw human cloning, and attempts were made to produce a national ban. Yet none was enacted, despite general agreement in Congress that it would be desirable to have such a ban.

Two major anti-cloning bills were introduced into the Senate in 1998. The Democratic bill (Kennedy-Feinstein) would have banned so-called reproductive cloning by prohibiting transfer of cloned embryos into women to initiate pregnancy. The Republican bill (Frist-Bond) would have banned *all* cloning by prohibiting the creation even of embryonic human clones. Both sides opposed "reproductive cloning," the attempt to bring to birth a living human child who is the clone of someone now (or previously) alive. But the Democratic bill sanctioned creating cloned embryos for research purposes, and the Republican bill did not. The pro-life movement could not support the former, whereas the scientific community and the biotechnology industry opposed the latter; indeed, they successfully lobbied a dozen Republican senators to oppose taking a vote on the Republican bill (which even its supporters admit now was badly drafted). Owing to a deep and unbridgeable gulf over the question of embryo research, we did not get the congressional ban on reproductive cloning that nearly everyone wanted.

To find a way around this impasse, several people (myself included) advocated a legislative "third way," one that firmly banned only reproductive cloning but did not legitimate creating cloned embryos for research. This, it turns out, is hard to do. It is easy enough to state the necessary negative disclaimer that would set aside the embryo-research question: "Nothing in this act shall be taken to determine the legality of creating cloned embryos for research; this act neither permits nor prohibits such activity." It is much more difficult to state the positive prohibition in terms that are unambiguous and acceptable to all sides.

Given both these difficulties, and given the imminence of attempts at human cloning, I now believe that what we need is an all-out ban on human cloning, including the creation of embry-

onic clones. I am convinced that all halfway measures will prove to be morally, legally, and strategically flawed, and—most important—that they will not be effective in obtaining the desired result. Anyone truly serious about preventing human reproductive cloning must seek to stop the process from the beginning. Our changed circumstances, and the now evident defects of the less restrictive alternatives, make an all-out ban by far the most attractive and effective option.

A ban only on reproductive cloning would turn out to be unenforceable. Once cloned embryos were produced and available in laboratories and assisted-reproduction centers, it would be virtually impossible to control what was done with them. Biotechnical experiments take place in laboratories, hidden from public view, and, given the rise of high-stakes commerce in biotechnology, these experiments are concealed from the competition. Huge stockpiles of cloned human embryos could thus be produced and bought and sold without anyone knowing it. As we have seen with in vitro embryos created to treat infertility, embryos produced for one reason can be used for another reason: today "spare embryos" once created to begin a pregnancy are now used in research, and tomorrow clones created for research will be used to begin a pregnancy.

Assisted reproduction takes place within the privacy of the doctor-patient relationship, making outside scrutiny extremely difficult. Many infertility experts probably would obey the law, but others could and would defy it with impunity, their doings covered by the veil of secrecy that is the principle of medical confidentiality. Moreover, the transfer of embryos to begin a pregnancy is a simple procedure (especially compared with manufacturing the embryo in the first place), simple enough that its final steps could be self-administered by the woman, who would thus absolve the doctor of blame for having "caused" the illegal transfer.

Even should the deed become known, governmental attempts to enforce the reproductive ban would run into a swarm of moral and legal challenges, both to efforts aimed at preventing transfer to a woman and—even worse—to efforts seeking to prevent birth after transfer has occurred. A woman who wished to receive the embryo clone would no doubt seek a judicial restraining order, suing to have the law overturned in the name of a constitutionally protected interest in her own reproductive choice to clone. (The cloned child would be born before the legal proceedings were complete.) And should an "illicit clonal pregnancy" be discovered, no governmental agency would compel a woman to abort the clone, and there would be an understandable storm of protest should she be fined or jailed after she gives birth. Once the baby is born, there would even be sentimental opposition to punishing the doctor for violating the law—unless, of course, the clone turned out to be severely abnormal.

For all these reasons, the only practically effective and legally sound approach is to block human cloning at the start, at the production of the embryo clone. Such a ban can be rightly characterized not as interference with reproductive freedom, nor as even interference with scientific inquiry, but as an attempt to prevent the unhealthy, unsavory, and unwelcome manufacture of and traffic in human clones.

IV

I appreciate that a federal legislative ban on human cloning is without American precedent, at least in matters technological. Perhaps such a ban will prove ineffective; perhaps it will eventually be shown to have been a mistake. (If so, it could be reversed.) If enacted, however, it will have achieved one overwhelmingly important result, in addition to its contribution to thwarting cloning: it will place the burden of practical proof where it belongs. It will require the proponents to show very clearly what great social or medical good can be had only by the cloning of human beings. Surely it is only for such a compelling case, yet to be made or even imagined, that we should wish to risk this major departure—or any other major departure—in human procreation.

Americans have lived by and prospered under a rosy optimism about scientific and technological progress. The technological imperative has probably served us well, though we should admit that there is no accurate method for weighing benefits and harms. And even when we recognize the unwelcome outcomes of technological advance, we remain confident in our ability to fix all the "bad" consequences—by regulation or by means of still newer and better technologies. Yet there is very good reason for shifting the American paradigm, at least regarding those technological interventions into the human body and mind that would surely effect fundamental (and likely irreversible) changes in human nature, basic human relationships, and what it means to be a human being. Here we should not be willing to risk everything in the naive hope that, should things go wrong, we can later set them right again.

Some have argued that cloning is almost certainly going to remain a marginal practice, and that we should therefore permit people to practice it. Such a view is shortsighted. Even if cloning is rarely undertaken, a society in which it is tolerated is no longer the same society—any more than is a society that permits (even small-scale) incest or cannibalism or slavery. A society that allows cloning, whether it knows it or not, has tacitly assented to the conversion of procreation into manufacture and to the treatment of children as purely the projects of our will. Willy-nilly, it has acquiesced in the eugenic re-design of future generations. The humanitarian superhighway to a Brave New World lies open before this society.

But the present danger posed by human cloning is, paradoxically, also a golden opportunity. In a truly unprecedented way, we can strike a blow for the human control of the technological project, for wisdom, for prudence, for human dignity. The prospect of human cloning, so repulsive to contemplate, is the occasion for deciding whether we shall be slaves of unregulated innovation, and ultimately its artifacts, or whether we shall remain free human beings who guide our powers toward the enhancement of human dignity. The humanity of the human future is now in our hands.

Human Reproductive Cloning

A Look at the Arguments Against It and a Rejection of Most of Them

RAANAN GILLON

Journal of the Royal Society of Medicine 92 (1999): 3–12.

Human reproductive cloning—replication of genetically identical or near identical human beings—can hardly be said to have had a good press. Banned in one way or another by many countries including the UK, execrated by the General Assembly of the World Health Organization as 'ethically unacceptable and contrary to human integrity and morality', forbidden by the European Commission through its Biotechnology Patents Directive, by the Council of Europe through its Bioethics Convention and by UNESCO through its Declaration on the Human Genome and Human Rights, clearly human cloning arouses massive disapproval reactions . . . What are the reasons, and especially the moral reasons, offered as justifications for this wholesale disapproval? In brief summary these seem to be: 'yuk—the whole thing is revolting, repellent, unnatural and disgusting'; 'it's playing God, hubris'; 'it treats people as means and not as ends, undermines human dignity, human rights, personal autonomy, personality, individuality and individual uniqueness; it turns people into carbon copies, photocopies, stencils and fakes'; 'it would be dangerous and harmful to those to whom it was done, as well as to their families; it would particularly harm the women who would be bearing the babies, and especially so if they were doing so on behalf of others as would probably be the case; it would harm societies in which it happened, changing and demeaning their values, encouraging vanity, narcissism and avarice; and it would be harmful to future generations.' 'Altogether it would be the first massive step on a ghastly slippery slope towards'— here fill in the horror—'Hitler's Nazi Germany, Stalin's USSR, China's eugenic dictatorship; or, from the realms of literature, *Boys from Brazil*,

mad dictators and of course mad scientists in science fiction, Big Brother in *Nineteen Eighty-Four*, and the human hatcheries of *Brave New World*'. 'It would be unjust, contrary to human equality, and, as the European Parliament put it, it would lead to eugenics and racist selection of human beings, it would discriminate against women, it would undermine human rights, and it would be against distributive justice by diverting resources away from people who could derive proper and useful medical benefits from those resources'. So, clearly, where it has not already been legally prohibited it should be banned as soon as possible.

Note that I have grouped these objections into five categories. The first constitute a highly emotionally charged group that includes yuk, horror, offence, disgust, unnaturalness, the playing of God and hubris. Then come four clearly moral categories—those concerned with autonomy (in which for reasons given later I have included dignity); those concerned with harm; those concerned with benefit; and those concerned with justice of one sort or another, whether in the sense of simply treating people equally, of just allocation of inadequate resources, of just respect for people's rights, or in the sense of legal justice and the obeying of morally acceptable laws.

Two types of cloning have generated particular moral concern: the first involves taking a cell from a human embryo and growing it into a genetically identical embryo and beyond; the second, made famous by the creation of 'Dolly' the sheep, involves taking out the nucleus of one cell and putting into the resulting sac, or cell wall, the nucleus of another cell to be cloned. With either of these cloning techniques, the process can be carried to early stages of development for a variety of potentially useful purposes, without any intention or prospect of producing a developed human being (lumped together here as non-reproductive human cloning and referred to only in passing). The human cloning that produces the greatest concern, and is the main subject of this paper, is of course reproductive human cloning, which would aim to produce a human person with the same genes as some other human being.

HUBRIS, YUK, ETC.

First, then, the group of responses based on yuk, it's unnatural, it's against one's conscience, it's intuitively repellent, it's playing God, it's hubris—a group of responses that one hears very frequently. I have to admit that this sort of essentially emotional response tends to evoke a negative emotional response in me when it is used in moral argument, as it often is. The trouble is that these gut responses *may* be morally admirable, but they may also be morally wrong, even morally atrocious, and on their own such gut responses do not enable us to distinguish the admirable from the atrocious. Think of the moral gut responses of your favourite bigots—for example, the ones who feel so passionately that homosexuality is evil, that black people are inferior, that women should be subservient to men, that Jews and Gypsies and the mentally retarded or mentally ill ought to be exterminated. People have existed—some still exist—who have these strong 'gut beliefs' which they believe to be strong *moral* feelings, which indeed they believe to be their consciences at work; and my point here is that gut responses provide no way for us to distinguish those moral feelings that we know or strongly believe to be wrong, from the moral feelings that we ourselves have, which we know or strongly believe to be right. To discriminate between emotional or gut responses, or indeed between the promptings of deeply felt moral intuitions or of conscience, we must reflect, think, analyse, in order to decide whether particular moral feelings are good or bad, whether they should lead to action or whether they should be suppressed (and yes, I think moral reflection shows that it is important to suppress,

or even better re-educate so as to change, one's moral feelings when on analysis one finds they are wrong). Without such moral reflection the feeling itself, while it may be an important flag that warns us to look at the issues it concerns, is no more than that. With such reflection we may find that the flag is signalling an important moral perspective that we should follow; or we may find that the flag is signalling us to respond in a morally undesirable way.

An analogy which I like to use concerns medical practice. Doctors, especially surgeons, cut people up quite a lot; they (we) also stick their fingers in people's bottoms. Most of us, I imagine, would feel quite deeply that both of those activities are rather disgusting and not to be done; yet we know, through thought and reflection in our medical studies, that we had better overcome these deep feelings because in some circumstances it is right to cut people and in some circumstances it is right to put our fingers in people's bottoms. Both are extraordinary and counterintuitive things to do, but on analysis we find that they are sometimes the *right* thing to do. The same need for reflection, thought and analysis applies to our deeply felt moral feelings in general. We need those deep moral feelings, those deep moral gut responses. Moral feelings are—here we may agree with Hume—the main springs or drivers of our moral action. They lead us to action against social injustice and corruption, against the tyrant, the torturer, the sadist, the rapist, the sexual aggressor of children but—and now I part company with Hume—we need to reflect on and educate our moral feelings so as to select and develop the good ones, and deter and modify or preferably abolish the bad ones.

Brave New World

In the context of our deep feelings let's just remind ourselves about Huxley and his *Brave New World*. It has become a trigger title, only needing utterance to provoke strong negative feelings, especially about the use of science and technology to control and predetermine people's feelings, attitudes and behaviour. From a rereading of *Brave*

New World I was satisfied that Huxley's main target is not science and technology but rather their misapplication by the despotic state that systematically sets out to undermine the possibility of freedom—freedom in the sense of humanity's ability to make thought-out choices and live by them, autonomous freedom. Recall, as an example itself of conditioning (of Huxley's readers), the ghastly example early on in which babies are naturally attracted to books and to flowers, and then, to ensure that the particular class of worker that the babies are destined to become will detest flowers and books, are subjected to nasty noises, terrifying explosions, sirens, alarm bells and finally, to make sure, electric shocks. Two hundred repetitions of the pavlovian conditioning would cause them to grow up with what the psychologists used to call an 'instinctive' hatred of books and flowers. 'Reflexes unalterably conditioned. They'll be safe from books and botany all their lives', declared the Director of Hatcheries.

Later on infants are socially programmed while they sleep through 'hypnopaedia', in which they are conditioned to have predetermined attitudes. Thus children predestined to be in the beta class of citizen hear over and over again:

> "Alpha children wear grey. They work much harder than we do because they're so frightfully clever. I'm really awfully glad I'm a Beta, because I don't work so hard. And then we are much better than the Gammas and Deltas. Gammas are stupid. They all wear green, and Delta children wear khaki. Oh no, I *don't* want to play with Delta children. And Epsilons are still worse. They're too stupid."

So, the Director concludes,

> "At last the child's mind *is* these suggestions, and the sum of the suggestions *is* the child's mind ... The adult's mind too—all his life long ... But all these suggestions are *our* suggestions." The Director almost shouted in his triumph. "Suggestions from the State," he banged the nearest table ... "Oh, Ford! ... I've gone and woken the children."

We will return to *Brave New World*, but I do not think we need Huxley's warnings about childhood conditioning of our attitudes and beliefs and prejudices to know that, even in our ordinary lives, many of our strong attitudes and prejudices and beliefs have emerged as a result of childhood patterning. We have been programmed to some extent into our attitudes. The big difference, of course, is that as we grow up and are educated we are able to reflect on these attitudes and beliefs and to *decide* whether to own them or reject them. Nonetheless many of our deep moral attitudes and beliefs are firmly embedded from early childhood (as the book of *Proverbs* reminds us 'Train up a child in the way he should go: and when he is old he will not depart from it') and, even if we decide that some of them are wrong, we have to work very hard if we want to change them. Huxley in *Brave New World* warns against despotic *misuse* of science and technology that, by painfully embedding attitudes and feelings in early infancy, and by later social prohibition or discouragement of reflection about those attitudes, makes the development of moral agency impossible or at least extremely difficult.

However, we have not been the recipients of such state conditioning and control in our own societies and I find it difficult to understand the strength and depth and origins of the contemporary widespread hostility to the very idea of cloning human beings. Certainly the existence of contemporary nature's own human clones, identical twins, seems harmless enough *not* to account for such deep hostility to the idea of deliberate cloning.

We will return to the issue of identity, because the myth that genetic identity equals personal identity lies at the root of much misunderstanding about cloning. First, let us pursue in more detail the argument that cloning is *unnatural* and therefore wrong. What role does 'unnatural' play in moral argument? Our first requirement is to disambiguate the term—what do we *mean* by unnatural in this context? Anything that occurs in nature could be said to be natural, but that sense of natural is not going to do much moral work for us, for we and what we do are natural, not unnatural, in this sense. In any case, right and wrong, good and bad, in so far as they occur in nature, also are equally natural in this sense, so that to say that something is natural will hardly help us distinguish between the two. Another sense of natural means unaffected by human intervention. But unless we wish to argue that all human interventions are bad and or wrong and all states of nature are good and/or right, then this sense of natural too is not much help for moral judgment. Think of all the truly horrible and morally undesirable things that occur in nature uninfluenced by humans; think too of all the human interventions in nature that are clearly morally desirable, but 'unnatural' in this sense—including all medical interventions, and all the other activities by which we help each other, including the provision of food, housing, clothing and heating.

There is another sense of unnatural which I think is also of potential moral relevance. If we do something that weakens, undermines, destroys or harms our human moral nature, then this is immoral and unnatural in the sense of anti-natural or against nature; and that of course is of enormous moral significance not just in relation to cloning but for the whole of the new genetics enterprise. So, to show that any activity, such as cloning, is unnatural in a morally relevant sense we need to give *reasons* that demonstrate why it is contrary to our human moral nature, or why it will undermine that human moral nature. Until we can give such reasons let us be particularly careful to avoid pejorative claims about cloning being unnatural, not simply for the reasons I have just given, but also because it must be very hurtful for the world's identical twins to hear that they, by association, are considered to be 'unnatural' and therefore that their existence is morally undesirable.

To continue with this range of somewhat mysterious objections to cloning and sometimes to the new genetics as a whole, we need to look now at hubris and playing God. Hubris is a pejorative term meaning a contemptuous arrogance, especially against God or the gods. 'Playing at God' combines both an implicit accusation of hubris with an implicit accusation of immaturity and lack of skill—as when children play doctors, somewhat inefficiently. Suffice it to agree that contempt, arrogance, puerile immaturity and lack of skill are all morally undesirable in one fulfilling a responsible task. But are these accusations justifiably made against the whole enterprise of human cloning, or indeed against the whole enterprise of the new genetics? One would require specific cases and examples rather than sweeping generalizations, which otherwise boil down to mere abuse. There clearly is an important moral issue here, especially in relation to the question of whether at present we can safely and sufficiently skilfully carry out reproductive cloning, even if we wish to do so, and I shall return to this. But, without specific evidence, it seems straightforwardly tendentious to brand the whole enterprise of human cloning, let alone the whole of the new genetics, as 'hubris' and 'playing God'.

Autonomy and Personal Identity

The next set of objections against cloning concerns personal identity and dignity, the undermining of autonomy, of individuality, of personality, of uniqueness, the production of carbon copies, photocopies, stencils and fakes of human beings.

Even if reproductive cloning were to produce a person identical with the person from whom he or she were cloned, it is not clear to me why this should be immediately condemned as morally unacceptable, though the idea so greatly strains the imagination that one might argue that it would be irresponsible to try any such trick even if it were possible. But of course reproductive cloning would *not* produce two identical people—only two people with identical (or in the case of 'Dolly-type cloning' near identical) sets of genes. Genetic identity neither means nor entails personality identity.

Once again the proof of this exists all around us, for genetically identical twins are obviously different people, even though their genes are identical or near identical. But this genetic type–type identity of people who are clones does not make them identical as people, in either sense.

Some commentators make a different criticism. It is not only personal identity that must not be replicated; nor must genetic identity, for that itself is morally important, indeed even a right according to the European Parliament. They assert that every one of us has a right to his or her own genetic identity. If I have such a right, then no-one else is entitled to have the (type–type) identical genes that I have. It might be described as a claim right that one's genetic identity, in the sense of token identity, must be unique—in other words, a claim right *not* to have type–type genetic identity. But if that is the European Parliament's claim it is not merely bizarre; if taken seriously it is morally malignant, for it implies morally malignant consequences for identical twins, nature's existing examples of people who are clones. If we have this right to genetic uniqueness, then somebody must have the corresponding duty—the duty to destroy one of each pair of existing identical twins, both born and *in utero*. Fortunately such counter-examples, plus the general tendency of morally reflective people to be morally and legally unconcerned about the lack of genetic uniqueness of identical twins, indicate that genetic uniqueness is unlikely, *pace* the European Parliament, to be of moral importance, let alone a moral right, and still less a right that ought to be enshrined in law.

But maybe there is a difference between cloning that occurs naturally and cloning that occurs by intention? Perhaps it is deliberate cloning that is the problem, rather than the cloning that occurs naturally, in the sense of unmediated by human beings? And perhaps the problem is that such deliberate reproductive cloning somehow demeans human dignity? Certainly both the World Health Organization and the European Parliament have stated that such cloning would

offend against human dignity. Well, once again we need to know what we mean by human dignity. We all know that human dignity is good and ought to be promoted and respected, but most of us, I suspect, would find it very difficult to say what we actually mean by human dignity and to explain why its violation is wrong.

Those who wish to use infringement of human dignity as an argument against human reproductive cloning thus need to explain what they mean by the term. For me the most plausible account of human dignity is Immanuel Kant's. For him human dignity resides in our ability to be autonomous, to will or choose to act according to the moral law. I suspect that many uses of the term 'human dignity' are consistent with this Kantian notion that our human dignity is our ability to make autonomous choices for ourselves according to what we believe to be right. If so, when we commit ourselves to respecting human dignity, to treating others in ways that respect their human dignity, we mean roughly that we should treat them in ways that they themselves on reflection and deliberation would believe to be good or right ways; and that when we make decisions on behalf of people who cannot make their own decisions, we should try so far as we can to replicate the decisions they themselves would have autonomously chosen (or if they have not yet become autonomous, can be expected and desired to make were they autonomous).

If we accept some version of the Kantian meaning of human dignity and its basis in autonomous choice, then it is not at all clear to me why reproductive cloning should in any way undermine such dignity. Of course there might be ways of destroying or damaging that dignity by damaging the underlying genetic basis for such autonomous choice—and any such activity should be morally condemned precisely because of the damage to human dignity, a version of the reputable anti-human-nature argument above. But no reason has been offered for accusing reproductive human cloning of damaging human dignity in this way.

Another objection to cloning that may also reside in the notion of human dignity is that we must never treat other people merely as means to an end, but always as ends in themselves—one of the versions of Kant's categorical imperative. The issue is complicated with embryos because it is a matter of unresolved and passionate moral debate whether embryos and fetuses are within the scope of the Kantian requirement to treat each other as ends in themselves. Many of us believe that they are not, and thus would permit for example the cloning of human embryos for research purposes with disposal (i.e. destruction) of the experimented-on embryo at an early stage in its development. In the UK the law allows this sort of thing. On the other hand, many others would say that this is morally outrageous because the human embryo *does* fall within the scope of the Kantian categorical imperative, being itself a human person from the moment of its creation. I am not going to address that argument, but it is important to see how it complicates the issue of cloning, both sorts of cloning. For if in creating an embryo, by whatever method, we have created a person, then of course we must treat it as a person, and thus not use it merely as a means to an end. If, on the other hand, it is not yet a person then we may use it merely as a means to an end, as a research tool for example, and destroy it after such use. That is an unresolved philosophical and/or theological problem.

Suppose, however, we put aside that piece of the argument and revert to human reproductive cloning, then the requirement always to treat people as ends in themselves, even when we also treat them as means, is entirely compatible with reproductive cloning. The issue surely turns, not on the method of reproduction, cloning or otherwise, that one may choose, but rather on how one actually treats and regards the child that results.

Once there is another person created as a result of one's decision, then that person must be accorded the same moral respect as is due to all people and must not be treated merely as a means to an end, an object, a tool, an instrument. So while one may perfectly properly decide to have a child in order to provide a source of life-saving cord blood or marrow for one's existing child, one must of course then respect the new child as an end and never treat him or her merely as a means to an end. I can see no reason for the parents' instrumental motivation for having a child in any way necessitating their treatment of the new child merely as a means and not an end. If anything, I suspect that human psychological nature would tend to lead parents to treat such children even more lovingly and respectfully than usual.

I have given reasons for doubting that cloning would infringe the human dignity and autonomy of the cloned person. Let us now consider the dignity and autonomy of those who wish to engage in reproductive cloning. Such considerations favour non-interference on the grounds that in general people's autonomous choices for themselves should be respected, unless there are very strong moral reasons against doing so, and that this is particularly true in respect of those rather personal and private areas of choice, notably those concerning reproduction, sexuality, choice of partners, and decisions about babies. Intervention by the state, or anyone else, in these areas of private morality undermines the human dignity/autonomy of those people. Moreover, respect for people's dignity/autonomy in these areas is not only right in itself, but is also likely to lead to far greater overall good and far less harm than if we start erecting state apparatuses for intervention in these private areas.

I think this is Huxley's main message in *Brave New World*. Do not let government start to control our private decisions, our autonomy or our development. Do not let the apparatus for state control in these areas be developed. By leaving such choices decentralized not only will people's dignity/autonomy be respected—a good in itself—but human welfare generally will benefit. Similarly, beware state control of science and technology, for in the name of social order it will lead to the end of liberty. As Huxley later admits, this is an overstated case, and I am certainly not arguing for total libertarianism and absence of state controls either of citizens' behaviour or of science and technology. But I am arguing against excessive state control, and in favour of a substantial zone of respect by the state for private autonomous choices where such respect does not entail harm to others. And so I think was Huxley.

Harms and Benefits

Which brings us to the next group of arguments, based on the harms and benefits of cloning. Let us briefly examine these in relation to the people cloned, their families, their societies and future generations. It is in the context of the social and personal harms of human reproductive cloning that *Brave New World* (and also the Ira Levin book of 1976, *Boys from Brazil*, in which clones of Hitler are bred in an attempt to rekindle the Nazi enterprise) has done so much to turn us against cloning, even succeeding in rendering the term pejorative. What was common to both of those books, but was especially evident in Huxley's novel, was that the cloning they described involved either selection of already impaired humanity for cloning (e.g. Levin and the cloning of Hitlers) or the deliberate impairment of human embryos before they were cloned, as in Huxley's 'Bokanovsky's Process'.

Note that Huxley has here combined and conflated three quite separate ideas. One is reproductive cloning; the second is a crude and simplistic genetic determinism (ascribed to the rulers of course and rejected by Huxley himself) whereby genetic identity equals personal identity; and the third is intervention in the cloning process to impair the normal development of the human embryo. But we have seen that cloning does not entail personal identity, and so far as we know cloning need not harm or impair the embryo.

But of course we do not yet know. Cloning by nuclear substitution has only just begun in mammals.

Claims about the potential harms caused by human reproductive cloning are extensive. Animal experiments are reported to have produced many abnormal embryos and fetuses, many spontaneous abortions, and many abnormal births. Theoretical reasons are claimed to indicate that the offspring will be particularly prone to various diseases including those associated with premature ageing. Psychological harms are predicted for individual children thus born, including resentment at having their genetic structure predetermined by their parents, resentment at having been conceived merely as means to benefit others (for example as blood or bone marrow sources), a sense of overwhelming burden if they have been cloned from someone with great achievements that they are supposed to emulate; confusion about their personal identity and relationships (if, for example, they are clones of one of their parents). Physical and emotional harms are also predicted for women bearing cloned embryos, including the high rate of failure and abnormality of the pregnancies; and if the women are also surrogates even more emotional harms can be anticipated.

Once again we need to look at this range of harms rather more precisely. Let it be acknowledged immediately that *at present* the technique of human cloning is not well developed enough to be safely used in humans for reproduction, but this is not to acknowledge either that each of the preceding harm arguments is valid, or that the harm arguments that are currently valid are sufficiently strong to prevent further research into ways of reducing such harms—for example, by animal experimentation.

What then of the formidable lists of harms, mainly psychological harms, anticipated to affect children? In brief, I think we need to set against these purported and anticipated psychological harms of being a clone child the very important counter-consideration of what is the alternative for that particular child? This argument commonly irritates, sometimes enrages, but rarely convinces. Yet it seems valid and I have not encountered plausible counter-arguments. The alternative *for those children* is not to exist at all, so if we are genuinely looking at the interests of those children who are anticipated to have the various psychological problems of being clones, and the difficulties that undoubtedly we can anticipate those will raise, and if we are genuinely looking at those problems from the point of view of the child, then the proper question to ask is what is preferable for that child? To exist but to have those problems or not to exist at all? It is an argument that I learned from the so-called Pro Life movement, though I suspect this is not a use that they themselves would wish to make of it. I found that the argument radically changed the way I thought about anticipated harms. Of course, it in no way stops one from deciding, for example, not to have a baby, or to have an abortion, or not to pursue reproductive cloning. But it does force one, or should force one, to realize that one's reasons are unlikely to be the best interests of the child whom one is thinking of not having, but are instead one's own reasons and preferences, largely about the sort of world one wishes to participate in creating. And if that is the case, why should one's own reasons and preferences prevail over the reasons and preferences of those who do wish to carry out reproductive cloning? After all, they do not claim a right to prevent us from reproducing according to our preferences; why should we claim a right to prevent them from reproducing according to their preferences?

As for the arguments about the potential social harms of cloning, other than those based on safety of the techniques, it seems to me that they are either frankly implausible (the argument that cloning is a threat to further human evolution surely falls into this category, given the likely numbers of cloned versus more conventionally produced people); too weak to justify imposition on those who reject them (for instance the arguments that reproductive cloning encourages vanity, narcissism and avarice); or powerful but misdirected. Thus it is not cloning, nor the techniques of the new genetics more broadly considered, that might lead to the social harms of racism, eugenics, mass destruction, or the violation of the security of genetic material, but rather social structures that per-

mit dictatorships and other forms of immorally enforced control of people's behaviour by their rulers. Those are the harms that we need to be concerned about; and the most important way of avoiding them—of avoiding oppression of all those who are oppressed by the strong, including the widespread oppression of women by men—is not to ban cloning or to become obsessed with the new genetics, but rather to reform those social structures that result in such harms and to maintain in good order those social structures that do largely avoid these harms.

What about the germ-line argument of dangers to future generations? Well certainly the genome resulting from reproductive cloning is germ-line transmissible and any mistakes that occur can be passed on to future generations. But so too, of course, can any benefits. If, for example, a cloning technique results in the elimination of some genetic abnormality that would otherwise have been transmitted through the germ-line, then the cascade effect is geometrically beneficial, just as, if a 'mistake' results and is passed on through the germ-line, that too is geometrically inheritable. Clearly care is needed to minimize the chances of the latter and maximize the chances of the former. But in general, with ever increasing voluntary personal control over reproduction, it seems likely that even if genetic 'mistakes' do occur, if they are severe people will be reluctant to pass them on to their offspring, thus reducing the risks of a cascade of negative genetic effects down the generations.

In general, and in relation to possible harms of new techniques, we need I believe to beware excessive concern with the 'precautionary principle'. In so far as it tells us to avoid doing harm, it is an important moral concern to balance against our continuing search for new ways of doing good—of benefiting others. In other words, the principle of beneficence should always take into account the principle of non-maleficence, and the objective should be an acceptable probability of doing good with minimal and acceptable harm and risk of harm. But sometimes the precautionary principle is used as a sort of moral blunderbuss, like the use of *primum non nocere* when this is translated as 'above all do no harm'. That way lies a beneficence moratorium, with all applied medical research, indeed all new medical interventions, being banned, for whenever we seek to benefit we risk harming. The morally desirable use of the precautionary principle is to 'weigh' anticipated benefits and their probabilities against anticipated harms and their probabilities, always aiming at a likely outcome of net benefit with minimal and acceptable harm and risk of harm.

So what about the benefits? I have been able to find less in the published work about the potential benefits of reproductive human cloning than about its potential harms. The same is not true about non-reproductive human cloning, for which a wide variety of impressive potential benefits has been claimed. These include production of useful pharmaceuticals from cloned transgenic animals; basic research into DNA and aspects of genetics, human reproduction and infertility, ageing and oncogenesis; as well as the possible production of cloned human tissues and organs (for use, for example, in transplantation). But even human reproductive cloning can be anticipated to provide certain benefits. For example, in rare cases Dolly-type cloning techniques could prevent inheritance of rare and disabling mitochondrial genetic disorders. The genetic abnormality being in the mitochondria, these cloning techniques make it possible to replace the cell membrane containing the defective mitochondria with an unaffected cell membrane and then to insert into that the unaffected genetic material in the cell nucleus. For the affected people such reproductive cloning could be of major benefit. A second potential benefit could arise where parents wish to have a further child, as already suggested, in order to provide, for example, compatible bone marrow or cord blood for an existing child who needs it to survive. A third example of potential benefit might be where a car crash has led to the death of a husband and the fatal injury of the only child and where the surviving woman wishes to have a clone from the child as the only means of raising a child who is her husband's biological offspring. A further potential benefit of reproductive cloning might be to a couple who are carriers of a fatal recessive gene and prefer to clone a cell from one of them to avoid the genetic danger, rather than reproduce by means of other people's genetic material.

Given the limited potential benefits of reproductive human cloning, the benefit/harm analysis does not seem at present to create much moral pressure to undertake this activity (though in non-reproductive cloning there certainly seem to be a large number of potential benefits, with far fewer potential harms). Nonetheless, given that there are some benefits that may be anticipated from reproductive human cloning, given the counter-arguments offered above to many of the claims that this would create major harms, and given the arguments from respect for reproductive and scientific autonomy, then at the very least we should thoroughly question contemporary absolutist proposals to ban human reproductive cloning for ever and a day—even if prudence and precaution indicate a temporary ban until the safety of such techniques can be researched and developed.

Justice

But do the last set of moral arguments against human reproductive cloning—those based on justice—lead us to require a permanent ban on the technique? Justice arguments can usefully be considered from the point of view of rights-based justice; of straightforward egalitarian justice (according to the European Parliament, cloning is contrary to the principle of human equality because it leads to eugenics and racism), and finally, and perhaps in this context most importantly, of distributive justice—the fair or just distribution of scarce resources, including consideration of the opportunity costs of using such resources for one purpose rather than another.

The only rights-based arguments that I have found against reproductive human cloning are based on the right to have a genetic identity—a claim that I have examined above and found morally unacceptable in regard to identical twins. On the other hand, in favour of reproductive cloning are rights-based arguments claiming rights to reproductive autonomy and privacy and rights to carry out morally acceptable scientific research.

Egalitarian theories of justice are fine (everyone should be treated equally) provided they pass the Aristotelian test for theories of justice—notably, that it is equals who should be treated equally, while those who are not equal in a morally relevant sense ought *not* to be treated equally but treated unequally in proportion to the morally relevant inequality. Thus, cloning does not treat everyone as equal if it is not done for everyone, but that is not unjust; for not everyone *needs* cloning and not everyone *wants* cloning. However, the European Parliament has claimed that cloning is contrary to human equality because it leads to eugenics and racism. Suffice it to say that, while both racism and imposed eugenics are morally unacceptable (though not the sort of 'eugenics' that stems from uncoerced reproductive choice, against which there are I believe no convincing moral arguments), there seem to be no reasons for believing that cloning is or entails either of these morally unacceptable phenomena.

Distributive justice arguments seem to offer the most plausible case against development of human reproductive cloning, or at least against funding such development from community funds, simply because the anticipated benefit–harm ratio does not seem to justify the undoubted costs and especially the opportunity costs. But this argument does not rule out private funding of such research, nor does it result in a permanent ban on provision of state funding, should the anticipated benefits become substantially greater.

Conclusion

And so I conclude that all the arguments for a permanent ban on human reproductive cloning fail and that most of the arguments for even a temporary ban fail. However, four arguments in favour of a temporary ban do, I have indicated, currently succeed. The first is that at present the technique for human reproduction by cloning is simply not safe enough to be carried out in human beings. The second related argument is that, given these safety considerations, the benefits including respect for the autonomy of prospective parents and the scientists who would assist them, are at present insufficient to outweigh the harms. The third is the argument from distributive justice, but this is only sufficient to prescribe a low priority for state funding for human reproductive cloning. And finally, respect for autonomy within a democratic society requires adequate social debate before decisions are democratically made about socially highly contentious issues so a moratorium is also needed to provide time for this full social debate, and with luck for more informed, more deliberated and less frantic decisions.

The issues that underlie, and in my view are far more morally important than, the cloning debate and indeed much of the contemporary opposition to the new genetics are those that Huxley pointed to in *Brave New World*—notably that both science and government must be used as servants of the people and not as our masters. This is something that Huxley explicitly addresses in the foreword to his 1946 edition of *Brave New World*, where he points out that if he had written the book again he would not have had just two alternatives—essentially either the madness of state control or the madness of the savage's emotional and unreasoned lifestyle. He would also have included a middle way in which reason was used in pursuit of a reasonable life, in which science was applied for the benefit, for the *eudaemonia* or flourishing of human kind.

Like Huxley in his 1946 preface I think we should look more positively at our brave new world—the brave new world of genetics. We should learn Huxley's lessons, protect ourselves against the depredations of those who would unjustifiably control us, and realize that the potential problems lie less in cloning and genetics and more in politics and political philosophy—and of course in *their and our* underlying ethics.

CASES

Measure for Measure

In November 2008, South Dakota's ballot contained a proposal to place strict limitations on abortion. The law's supporters considered it a direct assault on *Roe v. Wade*. They thought that the ideal time had come to challenge *Roe*, because of President Bush's appointments of John Roberts and Samuel Alito to the Supreme Court.

In 2006, voters faced a similar proposition, which was defeated fifty-six percent to forty-four percent. The new proposition, Measure 11, contained something that the 2006 version did not: exceptions for rape, incest, and the health of the mother. The 2006 proposal allowed an exemption only to save the pregnant woman's life, which was also included in the new version. Even Measure 11, though, would have given South Dakota the strictest limits on abortion in the country.

Measure 11 declares that abortion "terminates the life of an entire, unique, living human being, a human being separate from his or her mother, as a matter of scientific and biological fact" and that this life begins from the point of fertilization. The exemptions are strictly defined and regulated; for example, rape and incest victims would be required to report those crimes to the police, and the abortions must be performed before the twentieth week of pregnancy. Physicians who violate the law are guilty of a Class 4 felony, and could receive up to ten years in prison.

Planned Parenthood criticized Measure 11, noting that South Dakota already has some of the most restrictive abortion laws and the lowest abortion rates in the nation. South Dakota requires a twenty-four-hour waiting period, mandatory education about the woman's options, parental notification for minors, and an offer to view the fetal sonogram. South Dakota only has one place that routinely performs abortions: Planned Parenthood's clinic in Sioux Falls. According to Sarah Stoesz, president and chief executive officer of Planned Parenthood of Minnesota, North Dakota, and South Dakota, "Women must overcome substantial geographic, legal and cultural obstacles to access abortion in South Dakota."

Some abortion opponents, such as South Dakota Right to Life, also criticized Measure 11, viewing it as being too lax. They saw the exemptions as failing to provide the direct attack on *Roe* that the 2006 proposal would have been. Leslie Unruh, who led the initiative efforts in both 2006 and 2008, dismissed the criticism, saying "I have to save as many children as I can."

Discussion Questions

1. Do you think that South Dakota's Measure 11 is too strict, too lenient, or about right?
2. Do you think that the penalty for doctors who violate Measure 11 is too strict, too lenient, or about right?
3. Should the women who hire doctors to perform illegal abortions also get punished?
4. Because Measure 11 defines human life as beginning at fertilization, what sense do you make out of the provision that any exempt abortions must be performed before the twentieth week of pregnancy?

Sources

Associated Press. "South Dakota Abortion Ban to Face Voters." *Sioux Falls Argus-Leader*, April 25, 2008. http://www.argusleader.com/apps/pbcs.dll/article?AID=/20080425/UPDATES/80425033 (accessed June 11, 2008).

Davey, Monica. "South Dakota to Revisit Restrictions on Abortion." *New York Times*, April 26, 2008. http://www.nytimes.com/2008/04/26/us/26abort.html (accessed June 7, 2008).

South Dakota Secretary of State. "Initiated Measure 11." http://www.sdsos.gov/electionsvoteregistration/electvoterpdfs/

2008/2008regulateperformanceofabortions.pdf (Accessed June 11, 2008).

Where the Boys Are

In April 2008, Indian Prime Minister Manmohan Singh called the widespread practice of aborting female fetuses a "national shame" and demanded stricter enforcement of laws designed to thwart the practice. "No nation, no society, no community can hold its head high and claim to be part of the civilized world if it condones the practice of discriminating against one half of humanity represented by women."

Over the past thirty years, the proliferation of ultrasound equipment has enabled Indians to act on a cultural and economic preference for sons. Although it is illegal for doctors to disclose the fetus's sex—the penalty is up to five years in prison—and parents must sign a form agreeing not to seek that knowledge, the law is frequently ignored and prosecution is rare.

The preference for sons stems from the patriarchal structure in which most social responsibilities are carried out by males, including sons' traditional role of caring for parents during old age, and the cultural practice of providing a dowry to the new son-in-law at a daughter's wedding. Girls thus are a social and financial liability. Surveys have confirmed the preference for sons, even among women. The desire is strongest among rural women (seventy percent) and women who have not yet had a male child (sixty-five percent). Armed with the knowledge that their fetus is female, twenty percent of women admitted that they would abort.

The overall female-male birth ratio has declined over the years. In 2001, there were 927 girls born for every 1,000 boys, down from 962 in 1981. A study published in The Lancet showed that the rate is lower if the first child was a girl (759 per 1,000 males) and even lower for a third child if the first two are female (719 per 1,000 males). The rate is about even if the first child is a male. Although rural women may more often express a desire for sons, in practice urban women apparently abort female fetuses more frequently if they already have one or more female children, because their female-male rate is lower. A higher education level also correlates with lower female-male ratio. Urban and more highly educated women can more readily act on their desires, likely because they have easier access to ultrasound testing. The Lancet study estimated that about ten million female fetuses were aborted over a twenty-year span.

Besides the prime minister's call for increased law enforcement, the government has developed a financial incentive program. It is offering to pay poor families nearly $3,000 to have and raise daughters. In regions with the worst female-male ratios, families will receive $385 when the girl is born and another $2,500 when she turns 18, provided that she has completed her education and remains unmarried.

Discussion Questions

1. Given the cultural context in India, do you think that abortion based on sex selection is ethical?
2. Given the very different cultural context of the United States, would abortion based on sex selection be ethical here? Would it make a difference if it were practiced only by Indian immigrants, rather than the general population?
3. In the earliest stages of pregnancy, does it matter what the woman's reasons are for having an abortion?

Sources

Gentleman, Amelia. "Indian Prime Minister Denounces Abortion of Females." New York Times, April 29, 2008. http://www.nytimes.com/2008/04/29/world/asia/29india.html (Accessed June 7, 2008).

Jha, Prabhat, Rajesh Kumar, Priya Vasa, Neeraj Dhingra, Deva Thiruchelvam, and Rahim Moineddin. "Low Male-To-Female Sex Ratio of Children Born in India: National Survey of 1.1 Million Households." Lancet 367 (2006): 211–18.

Reuters. "Cash Incentives for Raising Girls," New York Times, March 4, 2008.

Vadera, B.N., U.K. Joshi, S.V. Unadakat, B.S. Yadav, and Sudha Yadav. "Study on Knowledge, Attitude and Practices Regarding Gender Preference and Female Feticide Among Pregnant Women." *Indian Journal of Community Medicine* 32, no. 4 (2007): 300–301.

What's Plan C? Pharmacist Refusal to Distribute Plan B

In the aftermath of *Roe v. Wade*, most states passed legislation allowing doctors to refuse to perform abortions and hospitals to refuse to allow abortions in their facilities. Some conscience laws pertain to contraception, with eight states allowing physicians to refuse to provide contraception to patients. The legal right of refusal is now being extended to pharmacists. Several states now permit pharmacists to refuse to dispense contraceptives.

A few states, however, have moved in the opposite direction. In 2007, New Jersey enacted a law prohibiting pharmacists from refusing to dispense medication solely for philosophical, moral, or religious reasons, and three states require pharmacies (not individual pharmacists) to dispense or stock medication. The American Pharmacists Association (APhA) "recognizes the individual pharmacist's right to exercise conscientious refusal and supports the establishment of systems to ensure patient's access to legally prescribed therapy." According to the APhA, the pharmacist may "step away, not in the way" and "does not support lecturing a patient or taking any action to obstruct patient access to clinically appropriate, legally prescribed therapy."

Although some pharmacists refuse to fill prescriptions for long-term contraceptives such as birth control pills, most of the controversy surrounds the emergency contraceptive Plan B, which may be purchased by adults without a prescription. Because Plan B works better the sooner it is used after sexual intercourse, and must be used within seventy-two hours to be effective at all, delays in obtaining it could lead to more unwanted pregnancies.

Pharmacist refusal could be particularly problematic in sparsely populated areas that have few pharmacies.

Frank Soprano is a pharmacist in New Jersey. Soprano is a Catholic, and is quite distressed about New Jersey's law that prohibits him from refusing to dispense Plan B. He follows the Church's teaching about contraception and abortion, and so declines to fill prescriptions for contraception. What particularly bothers Frank about Plan B is that he believes it really to be an abortifacient, holding that most of the time it works *after* ovulation or fertilization by preventing implantation and thus destroys an embryo. Furthermore, Soprano refuses to be involved with Plan B or abortions in any way, and so is unwilling to provide referrals to other pharmacists or pharmacies. "If I'm not going to kill a human being, I'm not going to help the customer go do it somewhere else." As far as he is concerned, New Jersey is trying to force him to do something he knows is morally wrong.

Discussion Questions

1. Are pharmacists or pharmacies ethically obligated to dispense Plan B? Should they be legally required to do so?
2. What are the ethical obligations of pharmacists like Frank Soprano, who have conscientious objections to Plan B?

Sources

American Pharmacists Association. "Pharmacist Conscience Clause." *APhA2008 Government Affairs Issue Briefs.* 2008. http://www. pharmacist.com/AM/Template.cfm?Section =Search1&section=Federal_Government_ Affairs1&template=/CM/ContentDisplay. cfm&ContentFileID=3872 (accessed June 14, 2008).

National Conference of State Legislatures. "Pharmacist Conscience Clauses: Laws and Legislation." 2007. http://www.ncsl.org/ programs/health/ConscienceClauses.htm (accessed June 10, 2008).

Villa, Joan. "Right of Refusal." *Illinois Times*, June 16, 2005. http://www.illinoistimes.com/ gyrobase/Content?oid = oid%3A4635 (accessed March 20, 2006).

Safe in the Womb?

Sen. Sam Brownback won't take no for an answer. Annually since 2004, he has introduced legislation entitled the "Unborn Child Pain Awareness Act." Sen. Brownback contends that scientific evidence proves that fetuses can feel pain, and notes that they receive anesthesia during fetal surgery. The Act would require that women seeking abortions after twenty weeks of gestation receive information about the medical evidence for fetal pain. It also would require that women who still choose abortion have the option of choosing anesthesia for the fetus. Five states have similar laws, and three others mention fetal pain in their abortion-counseling materials.

Sen. Brownback's legislation was motivated by the testimony of Dr. Kanwaljeet Anand. In his work as a physician and researcher, Dr. Anand has noted that even the most premature infants (twenty-two to twenty-four weeks of gestation) show signs of experiencing pain. He is convinced that fetuses can feel pain by twenty weeks, and perhaps even earlier. Dr. Nicholas Fisk performs fetal surgery, and his research shows that fetuses as young as eighteen weeks react to invasive procedures much like infants and adults, with a large increase of stress hormones and increased blood flow to the brain.

Although fetuses do react physically, anesthesiologist Mark Rosen believes that they do not feel pain. Dr. Rosen agrees that fetuses should receive anesthetics during surgery for various reasons, such as inhibiting fetal movement and relaxing the uterus to prevent damage to the fetus, but he thinks that pain perception does not occur before the third trimester of pregnancy. Pain signals must travel from the receptors all the way to the cerebral cortex, which is the part of the brain necessary for consciousness. Until the cortex develops and nerve fibers connect it to the thalamus, there is no consciousness and therefore no experience of pain. Before that, all we have are reflexive responses. Other scientists disagree with Dr. Rosen, claiming that consciousness is possible without a cortex. Dr. Bjorn Merker contends that the brain stem, which develops before the cortex, is sufficient for at least some level of awareness.

But even if Dr. Merker is correct about brain function, Dr. David Mellor contends that the uterine environment plays a crucial role in negating conscious awareness of pain. Biochemicals suppress brain activity, relieve pain, and induce sleep. No matter the stage of brain development, the fetus is unconscious while in the womb.

Discussion Questions

1. Do you think that Congress should pass the Unborn Child Pain Awareness Act?
2. Although he supports anesthesia for fetal surgery, Dr. Rosen rejects it for abortion. He thinks that a fetus feels no pain, and with abortion there is no reason to worry about physical damage to the fetus. Do you agree with Rosen?
3. How far should the concern for fetal pain go? The birth process may well be painful for the fetus, not just the mother. Should fetuses receive anesthesia before birth?

Sources

Brownback, Sam. "Unborn Child Pain Awareness Act." http://brownback.senate.gov/english/ legissues/cultureoflife/unbornchildpainact.cfm (accessed June 10, 2008).

Paul, Annie Murphy. "The First Ache." *New York Times Magazine*, February 10, 2008, 45–49.

McKnight v. South Carolina

In May 2008, Regina McKnight finally won her case. She had been in jail for seven years following her conviction on a "homicide by child abuse" charge for killing her fetus by using cocaine. The South Carolina Supreme Court overturned her conviction, unanimously ruling that McKnight had inadequate legal representation; her public defender attorney made several errors. The Court rejected a previous appeal in 2003, which was based on other grounds.

Nine years before her conviction was overturned, McKnight gave birth to a stillborn, five-pound girl. Gestational age was estimated at thirty-four to thirty-seven weeks. The state supreme court had previously ruled that a viable fetus is a person under state child-abuse and child-neglect laws, and so McKnight became one of at least ninety South Carolina women prosecuted through the end of 2005 for using drugs while pregnant. The first woman convicted of killing her fetus by using cocaine was Talitha Garrick, who in 1995 pleaded guilty to involuntary manslaughter for the stillborn death of her thirty-eight-week-old fetus. Garrick received probation for the offense.

At McKnight's trial, the pathologist who performed the autopsy testified that McKnight's baby had a substance in her system that could only have been caused by the mother's use of cocaine. He believed the cocaine use to be the cause of death, and so it was a homicide. The jury convicted McKnight on the basis of his testimony. In her 2003 appeal, the South Carolina Supreme Court held that a pregnant woman who unintentionally heightens the risk of a stillbirth could be found guilty of homicide based on "extreme indifference to human life." It noted that "it is public knowledge that cocaine use is potentially fatal" and that "McKnight took cocaine knowing she was pregnant." In contrast, the state supreme court's 2008 opinion noted that expert defense witnesses could have testified that while cocaine can be harmful to fetuses, recent studies show that it is "no more harmful to a fetus than nicotine use, poor nutrition, lack of prenatal care, or other conditions commonly associated with the urban poor."

Discussion Questions

1. Did McKnight act unethically by using cocaine while pregnant?
2. Should McKnight have gone to jail for homicide?
3. Should pregnant women who smoke, drink alcohol, or do any legal activity that could endanger a fetus (e.g., skiing) also be punished?

Sources

Brundrett, Rick. "Reprieve in Homicide by Child Abuse Case: Court Overturns Ruling of Woman Whose Fetus Died." *Columbia State*, May 13, 2008.

South Carolina Supreme Court. *State v. McKnight*. Opinion No. 25585 (2003).

_____. *McKnight v. State*. Opinion No. 26484 (2008).

Amber Alert

In 2004, Amber Marlowe was pregnant for the seventh time. When she went into labor, doctors at Wilkes-Barre (Pennsylvania) General Hospital told her that the eleven-pound, nine-ounce baby could only be delivered by caesarian section. Marlowe explained that she had delivered her first six children—all weighing nearly twelve pounds at birth—vaginally, but the doctors insisted on the surgical procedure.

Marlowe left the hospital in search of a new doctor. Hospital lawyers quickly went to court to get legal guardianship of Marlowe's fetus. A judge ruled that if she returned, the hospital had the authority to perform the procedure, even against Marlowe's wishes, if they felt it was medically necessary. She did not return, but went to another hospital, where she gave birth to a healthy baby girl.

Unlike with Marlowe, Melissa Rowland's case does not have a happy ending. Rowland was pregnant with twins in 2004, and a doctor at LDS Hospital in Salt Lake City recommended an immediate caesarian section because the fetuses were in poor health. She left the hospital against the doctor's advice, and a nurse claimed that Rowland said she would rather "lose one of the babies than be cut like that." Ten days later, Rowland gave birth at another hospital; one child was born alive, but the other was stillborn. Rowland was charged with first-degree murder, demonstrating "depraved indifference to human life" by failing to pursue immediate medical treatment for the twins, including having the C-section. "It was her omissions that caused the death of the child," said Kent Morgan of the Salt Lake City District Attorney's Office. "She was given three or four opportunities to get a C-section to save that baby." Rowland eventually accepted a plea bargain to reduced charges of two counts of child endangerment, with a sentence of eighteen months of probation and completion of a drug treatment program. (Rowland had used drugs during her pregnancy, but prosecutors did not claim that the drugs caused the child's death.)

Discussion questions:

1. A caesarian section is an invasive procedure. Who should decide whether a pregnant woman should have the procedure?
2. When, if ever, may a woman's decision against a caesarian be overridden?

Sources

Associate Press. "What Are Mothers' Rights During Childbirth? Debate Revived Over Pregnant Woman's Choice of Delivery." MSNBC.com. May 19, 2008. http://www.msnbc.msn.com/id/5012918/ (accessed June 14, 2008).

Thomson, Linda. "Mother Is Charged in Stillbirth of a Twin." *Deseret News,* March 12, 2004. http://deseretnews.com/dn/view/0,1249,595048573,00.html (accessed June 15, 2008).

A Person, No Matter How Small?

In November 2008, Colorado's ballot contained Amendment 48, a measure to amend the state's constitution, defining person as "any human being from the moment of fertilization." The petition drive was organized by a group called Colorado for Equal Rights, founded by twenty-year-old Kristi Burton. "The main thing the Constitution is supposed to do is to protect us," she said. "But who is that 'us'? There is currently no definition of personhood in the constitution." According to Michael Norton, a lawyer representing the proposal's supporters, "Whatever rights and liberties and duties and responsibilities are guaranteed under the Constitution or other state laws would flow to that life." Those rights would include life, liberty, equality of justice, and due process of law.

If passed, Amendment 48 could have a sweeping impact on birth control, abortion, reproductive technology, and biomedical research. Criminal and civil laws would be extended to fertilized eggs, and lawsuits could be filed on their behalf. Oral contraceptives and intrauterine devices could be threatened, because they inhibit implantation of a fertilized egg. All abortion could become illegal. *In vitro* fertilization might end, because doctors would be reluctant to offer the procedure when any accident that harmed an embryo could bring a wrongful death lawsuit. Embryos in storage would have rights, which could mean that all of them would have to be implanted, and in small numbers, to avoid the risk of multiple pregnancy. It also could mean that they could not be destroyed or used in research. Fertility drugs also would be problematic, because of the risk of multiple pregnancy, which could be harmful to the developing embryos/fetuses.

Discussion Questions

1. Should fertilized human eggs be considered people?
2. If Amendment 48 appeared on your own state's ballot, would you vote for it?

Sources

Draper, Electa. "Personhood Push Headed for Ballot." *Denver Post,* May 13, 2008. http://www.denverpost.com/legislature/ci_9248327 (accessed June 15, 2008).

Johnson, Kirk. "Proposed Colorado Measure on Rights for Human Eggs." *New York Times,* November 18, 2007.

Veto Power

In contrast to Colorado's Amendment 48, courts in Massachusetts and New Jersey have ruled that dispositional authority regarding embryos lies with the parents. In fact, it lies with both parents. They must agree that the embryos should be implanted, or they cannot be. Each person has veto power; the wishes of the person wanting to avoid procreation have priority.

The Massachusetts case involved a forty-four-year-old woman, who wanted to make one last attempt at pregnancy using four frozen embryos left from her fertility treatments. Her ex-husband objected, in spite of the consent form he had signed years earlier when they were married. Massachusetts' Supreme Judicial Court stated that it "would not enforce an agreement that would compel one donor to become a parent against his or her will. As a matter of public policy, we conclude that forced procreation is not an area amenable to judicial enforcement." Rather, "respect for liberty and privacy requires that individuals be accorded the freedom to decide whether to enter into a family relationship."

The New Jersey case also involved a divorced couple with stored embryos left over from their marriage. This time, the ex-husband wanted to donate the seven frozen embryos, so that they could be implanted in other women seeking to have children. The ex-wife objected. As in Massachusetts, the New Jersey Supreme Court held that the embryos could not be used to produce a child without the consent of both parties. "Ordinarily, the party wishing to avoid procreation should prevail....Implantation, if successful, would result in the birth of her biological child and could have lifelong emotional and psychological repercussions."

Discussion Questions

1. The Massachusetts and New Jersey courts give priority to avoiding procreation. Has procreation already occurred in these cases?

2. Do you think that the courts made the right decision?

3. What do you think should happen to the embryos in cases where the two parties disagree?

Sources

"Court Says Woman Can Bar Embryos' Use." *New York Times*, August 15, 2001. http://www.nytimes.com/2001/08/15/nyregion/15EMBR.html (accessed August 15, 2001).

Goldberg, Carey. "Court Says a Partner Can Veto an Embryo Implantation." *New York Times*, April 4, 2000.

Surrogacy Specialists of America (SSA)

The following material is reproduced from the SSA.com website:

By statute, court-approved "gestational agreements" between intended parents and their gestational mothers (surrogates) are valid and enforceable in Texas. The gestational mother may be compensated for her efforts and the intended parents will be recognized as the legal parents of the child upon his or her birth without the need for an adoption. The names of the intended parents go directly onto the birth certificate. Out-of-state couples can also take advantage of the Texas surrogacy law if they work with a gestational mother residing in Texas.

Texas law authorizes a wide variety of gestational arrangements. The most common would be one in which the gestational mother carries a child that is biologically related to one or both of the intended parents. But it is also possible to have a court-approved enforceable arrangement in Texas where there is no biological connection whatsoever between either of the intended parents and the child. This would be the case where the intended parents choose to work with both an egg donor and sperm donor and transfer the resulting embryos to a gestational mother.

The parties have their rights determined by the court prior to any embryo transfer to the gestational mother. A contract must satisfy numerous requirements before the court will approve it as a "gestational agreement". The principal requirements are as follows:

- The intended parents must be married to each other
- The parties must sign the agreement more than fourteen days before the date of the transfer of embryos to the gestational mother
- There must be medical necessity for the arrangement (for example, the intended mother is unable to carry and deliver a child or the pregnancy would pose an unreasonable risk to her physical or mental health or to the health of the child)
- The gestational mother must have had at least one previous pregnancy and delivery and carrying another pregnancy to term and giving birth will not pose an unreasonable risk to her physical or mental health or the child's health
- The gestational mother's eggs cannot be used in the procedure and
- Unless waived by the court, the intended parents must complete a home study

The agreement must also provide various other safeguards for the health of the gestational mother and disclosures designed to ensure that all parties have full knowledge of the arrangement and its risks.

Although the Texas surrogacy statute is broad, it does not protect so-called "traditional" arrangements in which the gestational mother carries and relinquishes custody of her own biological child to the intended parents. It also does not apply to single persons. Even in these situations, however, Texas law is not unduly harsh. Although the statute makes a contract that does not qualify as a "gestational agreement" unenforceable, it does not make it illegal. In this event the parties must look to general Texas family law to determine their parental relationships.

Discussion Questions

1. Texas law enforces gestational surrogacy agreements, as long as the baby is not the biological child of the surrogate. In other words, the surrogate mother must surrender custody when she is not the source of the egg, but is not legally obligated to do so when she is. Do you think that this distinction in the Texas law is ethical?
2. Among the requirements for an enforceable agreement is that the intended parents be married. Should surrogacy also be available to unmarried couples or homosexual couples?
3. The requirements stipulate that the arrangement must be a "medical necessity." Is that ethically important?
4. The requirements also stipulate that the gestational mother must have had at least one previous pregnancy. Does this seem like a good idea?

Source

Surrogacy Specialists of America, LLC. "Legal Aspects of Assisted Reproduction in Texas." http://www.ssa-agency.com/index.cfm?menuitemid=106 (accessed June 15, 2008).

Free to Be Me (Again?)

Liz Catalan is forty-one and infertile. Her ovaries went into premature failure years ago. Catalan still dreams of having a child of her own. She does not want to use a donor egg or adopt. She wants a child that is genetically related to her. In order to get that child, Catalan wants to be cloned.

Catalan has considered the various ethical issues about cloning, and is convinced that she should be allowed to clone herself when the technology is available. Her child would feel unique, not like she was living her mother's life over again. Identical twins know that they are unique, so why wouldn't clones?

Safety concerns should not be a barrier. Catalan points to *in vitro* fertilization, and how that technique brings an increased risk of medical and developmental problems for the resulting children. Nevertheless, parents are free to take those risks. "I know it's not right for everyone. But I do personally believe that it should be up to each person. And if the only way a person can have a child of their own is to do this, and if they are willing to take a chance, then they should be able to."

Discussion Questions

1. Do you think Catalan should be able to have herself cloned?
2. How would Kass and Gillon evaluate Catalan's case? How does your view compare with theirs?

Source

Weiss, Rick. "Free to Be Me: Would-Be Cloners Pushing the Debate." *Washington Post*, May 12, 2002.

CHAPTER 5

Distributing and Procuring Health Care Resources

INTRODUCTION

Does everyone deserve good health and access to health care? Even if they do, medical resources are sometimes sufficiently scarce that it is impossible to treat every patient who might need them. How should we decide who receives treatment in such cases? And what factors should we consider when trying to determine whether and how to increase the supply of medical resources? This chapter explores such questions, which all in one way or another concern the principle of justice. The first section focuses on justice in relation to health and patient access to the health care system. The second section concerns the rationing of care when there are insufficient resources, and whether physicians should act as gatekeepers. The third section considers the institutional setting for health care, and how organizational structure can facilitate or inhibit patient access to health care. Finally, the fourth section focuses on the specific area of organ transplantation, and the issues associated with distributing scarce life-saving resources as well as procurement options to increase their supply.

Health and Access to Health Care

Even if good health has no price, we cannot deny that it has a cost.

—Jacques Barrot, *Le Concours Médical*

The conditions necessary for good health and access to health care present some of the most critical ethical and public policy issues in bioethics today. Many of these issues have not changed much over time, but the landscape has become more complex because of new developments in health care delivery and because of wider concerns about various factors that affect health. The natural environment significantly impacts human health (see chapter 8), as do the social and workplace environments. For example, social class strongly influences both quality of life and longevity. The more education and income people have, the less likely they are to suffer from heart disease, stroke, diabetes, and many types of cancer, based upon where and how they live and work. When they do suffer from one or more of these things, they are less likely to die from them than are people poorer or less well educated. Although the illness (e.g., heart attack) may be the same, social class shapes its circumstances, including the type of care the patient receives, the patient's relationship with doctors, familial support, and prospects of returning to his or her job.

The 1997 film *As Good as It Gets* illustrates the differences social class makes regarding the circumstances of illness and access to health care. Jack Nicholson plays Melvin Udall, a misanthropic character who is a successful author with obsessive-compulsive disorder. Melvin is quite wealthy and can afford to pay for the best health care available. Helen Hunt plays Melvin's love interest, Carol Connelly, a poor waitress and single mother whose own mother also lives with her. Carol's son, Spencer, is frequently ill because of asthma and allergies. Carol's employer does not provide benefits, so she has purchased insurance through a health maintenance organization (HMO). Unfortunately, Spencer's condition has failed to improve and he needs frequent trips to a hospital emergency room. Spencer's ill-health sometimes forces Carol to miss work, which reduces her income. Because Melvin strongly prefers Carol to be his waitress at the restaurant, he decides to address Spencer's health needs, and requests that his physician, Dr. Martin Bettes, make a house call. Dr. Bettes, who brings along a nurse, inquires about previous examinations of Spencer, and considers it "amazing" that basic skin allergy tests had not been done. Unlike previous physicians, Dr. Bettes also provides advice about altering Spencer's living environment. The difference in quality of care is so startling for Carol that she blurts out, "Fucking HMO bastard pieces of shit!" Dr. Bettes replies, "Actually, I think that's their technical name." (Audiences usually laugh approvingly at the exchange.) Dr. Bettes gives Carol his business card, which includes his home telephone number, so that she can call him regarding the lab results and if Spencer needs further attention. When inquiring about the costs, Carol learns that they are "considerable," but that Melvin will be paying them.

Although Carol's situation may look bad, other people are even worse off. Unlike Carol, they have no health insurance at all, and if they do not qualify for government assistance, they have no access to care, except for emergency services. According to a 2007 U.S. Census Report, forty-seven million people living in the United States (15.8 percent of the population) lacked health insurance in 2006, which is a 3.26 percent increase from 2005. When divided into various demographic characteristics, the report notes that coverage increases as age, income, and employment increase, yet 17.9 percent of people employed full-time still lack health coverage. Race, ethnicity, nativity, family status, and region also were statistically relevant in terms of identifying who is more and less likely to have health care coverage. For example, in 2006 10.8 percent of non-Hispanic whites, 15.5 percent of Asians, 20.5 percent of African Americans and 34.1 percent of Hispanics lacked health insurance. People without insurance coverage are less likely to receive preventive health services and adequate treatment, and are more likely to die from treatable illnesses.

The growing number of uninsured Americans, and the frustration that many patients and physicians experience with insurers, have led to calls for health care reform. This is the context for Michael Moore's controversial film *Sicko*, which was released in 2007. Moore profiles U.S. citizens who have been denied access to adequate health care and contrasts the United States with other nations, such as Canada, Cuba, France, and the United Kingdom, which have universal health care systems. Moore lauds those systems as superior, contending that they would provide adequate care to the patients featured in his film.

Justice and Access to Health Care

Although he does not say so directly, Moore implies that access to health care is a matter of justice, and that the U.S. health care system is unjust. Quite often people associate the term justice with criminal law, as in "the justice system." Philosophically, this is called retributive justice, and it concerns the appropriate punishment for criminal acts. The type of justice pertaining to access to health care is *distributive justice*, which concerns a fair allocation of the benefits and burdens of social and economic goods. That is, it addresses who should benefit from the goods, and who should bear the burdens associated with their production (e.g., paying for them).

To achieve this fair allocation, distributive justice involves using both formal and material criteria. The *formal* principle of distributive justice simply establishes that there should be consistency in how we distribute benefits and burdens. The *material* principles specify who, exactly, is entitled to receive the goods in question and under what circumstances. Philosophers, religious ethicists, and others have supported various material criteria of justice, such as merit, ability to pay, effort, social status, equality, and need. The challenge, of course, is to decide which of these criteria are appropriate in which contexts.

Material Criteria of Justice

1. To each person the same thing
2. To each person according to merit or achievement
3. To each person according to effort
4. To each person according to need
5. To each person according to social status
6. To each person according to social contribution
7. To each person according to contracts and free-market exchanges

Visions of justice, including the relevant material criteria and rules for how they should be applied, emerge from religious and secular frameworks. Moore's vision grows out of the Catholic tradition in which he was raised. His comment in the film that health care is about "the we, not the me," comes from his Catholic education. He was explicit about that in an interview, saying "Instead of calling it 'socialized medicine,' it should be called 'Christianized medicine.'" Moore's remarks correspond with the U.S. Catholic bishops' claim that a "just health care system will be concerned both with promoting equity of care—to assure that the right of each person to basic health care is respected—and with promoting the good health of all in the community." To this end, the bishops maintain that Catholic health care is distinguished by its particular concern for the poor and disadvantaged, and that health care should be allocated on the basis of need. Many other religious traditions (e.g., Buddhism, Islam, and Judaism) also support universal access to health care and a special concern for the poor.

Among secular visions of justice, philosopher John Rawls has provided the most influential modern articulation. Rawls's notion of "justice as fairness" focuses on procedures for ensuring the fair distribution of primary goods—the things that people would want, no matter their position or goals in life, like liberty and opportunity, wealth and income, and the bases for self-respect. He develops two principles of justice, which he thinks all people would endorse if they were able to set aside their own particular stations in life and focus on what they would want regardless of position. The first principle is egalitarian (i.e., "to each the same thing"), claiming that everyone should have a comprehensive set of liberties that is compatible with everyone having that same set (the liberty principle). The second principle governs social and economic inequalities, and contains two parts. The first part states that these inequalities should be attached to offices and positions "open to everyone under conditions of fair equality of opportunity" and the second part states that they must be to "the greatest benefit of the least-advantaged members of society" (the difference principle). This second principle assumes that everyone could be better off under some unequal distribution of social and economic goods than they would under a strictly egalitarian distribution, although the degree of benefit could vary considerably. It thus invokes multiple material criteria of justice, the first part arguably attending to several (e.g., the same thing regarding equal opportunity, but then merit and free-market exchanges would govern), and the second part attending to need.

Rawls did not originally include health or health care among the primary goods of life, but did so in subsequent revisions of his theory. This shift came in response to the work of other scholars, including **Norman Daniels**, who extends Rawls's theory into the health care setting. In the first reading selection of this chapter, Daniels addresses three central questions regarding justice for health and health care: (1) Is health care special? (2) When are health inequalities unjust? and (3) How can health care needs be met fairly when resources are inadequate? He views health as having special importance for the "fair equality of opportunity" in society; without health, people are less able to participate fully as citizens or to pursue various life plans. For this reason, Daniels holds that access to health care is a matter of justice. He recognizes that practical limitations prevent all health needs from being met, but contends that unequal outcomes can be either fair or unfair, as per Rawls's difference principle.

Whereas Daniels criticizes Rawls's inattention to health and health care, several other scholars find more fundamental problems with Rawls's theory of justice. Libertarians like Robert Nozick and **H. Tristram Engelhardt** find Rawls's vision to be coercive, undermining personal freedom. They accept his liberty principle, but reject the difference principle. Engelhardt claims that goods and services, including health care, should be assigned according to merit and/or contracts and free-market exchanges, not need. Health care should be provided only to those who can pay for it (directly or through insurance), or by others who agree to contribute voluntarily. Any redistribution of resources must be voluntary in order to be moral, otherwise it is an oppressive use of state power. A community or society may freely decide to devote commonly held resources to the provision of health care, but there is no moral requirement to do so. As Engelhardt puts it, it is unfortunate, but not necessarily unfair, if an unhealthy person does not receive needed care. (There are several other notable justice perspectives, such as communitarian, feminist, and "capabilities," that provide other important criticisms of Rawls, and alternative approaches to justice issues in health and health care. For examples, see the References and Further Reading section in this chapter.)

Implementing Access to Health Care

Financial barriers to receiving health care have largely arisen along with the development of modern medicine beginning in the late nineteenth century. By that time, various European nations had so-called "sickness funds," some voluntary, and some compulsory for particular occupations, such as mining. These funds were more like contemporary disability insurance than health insurance, because they provided for wages lost by ill or injured workers. Although the payments could be used for medical care expenses, that was a secondary concern. During the twentieth century, these European nations developed universal health care programs.

In the United States, companies, labor unions, and fraternal organizations also established sickness funds by the late 1800s, with workers contributing to the funds. Unlike in Europe, various efforts to establish public health insurance at the state and national level failed. One of the reasons was that alternatives to government-based programs had developed during the 1930s. Hospital groups had established the nonprofit organization Blue Cross, and physician groups established Blue Shield (these later merged into the giant Blue Cross/Blue Shield), which provided hospital service and health insurance to subscribers. The insurance industry, which had primarily provided different types of property insurance (such as fire insurance) and life insurance, entered the health market at this time, because the development of actuarial science in this area made it profitable for them to do so. (Actuarial science is a mathematical discipline that uses statistical methods to calculate risk.) In the public sphere, the federal government eventually enacted Medicare (an entitlement program primarily for citizens and legal residents over age sixty-five or who are disabled and meet other qualifications) and Medicaid (a health insurance program for low-income people managed by the individual states), which were established in 1965.

The present-day U.S. health care system is funded by a blend of private insurance (for-profit and nonprofit), personal expenditure, public finance, and charity. In spite of Medicare and Medicaid, not everyone has access to health care beyond emergency services, and not all forms of care are accessible even for people who

Table 5.1 Select Health Care Statistics for the United States and Other Countries, 2004

Country	Health Care Expenses (Percentage of GDP)	Health Expenditures Per Capita (U.S.$)	Percentage Funding from Public Sector	Life Expectancy at Birth	Infant Morality Rate Per 1,000 Live Births
Australia	9.5	3128	67.5	80.6	4.7
Canada	9.8	3161	70.2	80.2	5.3
France	11.0	3191	79.4	80.3	3.9
Germany	10.6	3169	76.9	78.6	4.1
Japan	8.0	2358	81.7	82.1	2.8
United Kingdom	8.1	2560	86.3	78.9	5.0
United States	15.2	6037	44.7	77.8	6.8

From the Organization for Economic Co-operation and Development (2007).

have insurance—health care thus is not universal in the United States. Although it is widely known that the United States has perhaps the best health care facilities in the world and spends more money per capita on health care than any other nation (15.3 percent of gross domestic product in 2006), it has a larger percentage of uninsured residents than any other developed nation, has among the fewest physicians relative to the population (2.4 per thousand), and has relatively poor health outcomes relative to other nations (life expectancy of 77.8 years and infant mortality rate of 6.8 per 1,000 live births).

What is keeping the United States from reforming its health care system so that it will provide universal access? One key barrier is the insurance industry, which fears a loss of profitability. Another has been the lack of physician support, and even outright opposition to change. Although many physicians supported state and national health insurance in the early part of the twentieth century, the American Medical Association (AMA) opposed any government-sponsored insurance programs, including Medicare and Medicaid.

Although the AMA still opposes a single-payer health system, it now advocates for universal health care. Individual physicians, however, are increasingly expressing their support for national health insurance. Aaron Carroll and Ronald Ackerman's 2007 survey of U.S. physicians shows that fifty-nine percent support legislation to establish national health insurance, while thirty-two percent oppose it. A slightly smaller majority of fifty-five percent support achieving universal coverage through incremental reform, with twenty-five percent opposing incremental reform. It is not clear how much of the opposition reflects disagreement with the need for reform or disagreement with the particular approach to reform. It is also unclear whether it matters to most physicians which type of reform is implemented, as long as it leads to universal coverage. One thing that the survey did make clear was that overall physician support for national health insurance has increased significantly in the new millennium. Support was at forty-nine percent in 2002, and within five years had increased by a twenty percent margin.

Universal health care is often seen as proceeding from a politically liberal perspective, and is frequently derided as "socialized medicine," without regard to the various forms it could take. But as **Paul Menzel and Donald Light** argue in their article, conservative values also support universal health care: "being able to take care of oneself and others, preventing irresponsible free-riding, and alleviating the inefficiency, waste, and other weaknesses that limit business and entrepreneurial activity. Access to medical services, regardless of income, is as necessary to individual freedom, opportunity, and self-responsibility as is access to the protective services of fire or police departments."

Even assuming that justice requires universal access to health, what is the scope of "universal"? If the patient is not a citizen or legal resident, but an illegal immigrant or perhaps just a person abroad on vacation, does justice demand equal access? In his 2007 proposal to address California's health care crisis, Governor Arnold Schwarzenegger set out a plan to "Cover All Californians." Who counts as a Californian? According to Schwarzenegger's plan, all children count, regardless of immigration status, but only adults who are legal residents count. Although excluding illegal residents could reflect an ethnic or nationalistic bias and so be unjust, it also could reflect a notion of fairness, using desert and/or social contribution as material criteria of justice. **James Dwyer** contrasts the view of two groups: "nationalists" claim that illegal immigrants have no right to health care in their new place of residence, while "humanists" claim that health is a human right that should be provided to everyone regardless of residential status. In rejecting both views, Dwyer contends that a better way to frame the problem is that of social justice and social responsibility. As part of that framework, Dwyer thinks that all workers and their families should receive health care, whether or not those workers are legal residents.

Rationing

Although it sounds comforting and secure, universal access to health care would still not guarantee that everyone would receive all of the health care that they need, simply because medical resources are limited in supply. The distribution of these resources can be a relatively easy or difficult process depending upon how much is available, and can be just or unjust depending on how the process is conducted. Allocation of health care resources occurs at the macro and micro levels. There are at least four types of *macroallocation* considerations. First, a society must determine how much of its resources to devote to health care relative to other important social goods, such as education, transportation, and the arts. Second, of this total health care budget, a society must determine how much to allocate among preventive medicine, primary care, critical or emergency care, and chronic care. Third, a society must determine which treatment technologies get priority. Finally, a society must determine which diseases get priority regarding treatment availability and research funding.

After these decisions are made, *microallocation* determines which patients actually receive the medical resources. Some microallocation problems can be eliminated by increasing the available resources. It would be impossible, however, to eliminate all microallocation decisions, even if funding were unlimited, such as with organ transplantation (see the discussion later in this chapter).

In any situation involving scarce resources, some type of rationing must occur, and health care is no exception. *Rationing* is the controlled distribution of some resource, usually one in scarce supply. What makes it particularly problematic in this setting is that although rationing paradigms exist, they come from outside the Hippocratic tradition and its focus on particular patients and the doctor-patient relationship. The military, for example, engages in a practice called *triage*. When a large number of wounded soldiers require medical attention, they are classified according to diagnosis and prognosis, and then prioritized. The "walking wounded" and the hopeless cases wait, while the severely wounded with a chance for recovery are treated first, followed by those whose injuries are less severe. Another example comes from Departments of Public Health, which have had to allocate vaccines in limited supply, and have utilized various methods, such as lotteries and targeting at-risk groups.

An ethical microallocation framework might use one or more of the material criteria of justice we listed. Besides relative need and survivability, as in the triage model, resources might be rationed using some type of objective criteria, such as age, gender, or body mass index (BMI). The decision to ration on this basis is not itself objective, but the criteria utilized are objective in that they are readily observed or measured. The United Kingdom uses an objective criterion when it limits joint replacement to people whose BMI is less than thirty. Another possible allocation standard would be social contribution or utility, weighing the social benefit of potential recipients against each other. This type of framework was utilized in Seattle in the 1960s to allocate kidney dialysis. Although it is generally rejected today, we still see limited versions of the "social utility" model. For example, Nicki Pesik, Mark Keim, and Kenneth Iserson reject the broad use of social utility, but accept a limited version that they call the "direct multiplier effect." They contend that emergency caregivers should receive priority treatment after a terrorist attack, because they can in turn provide medical care to others. Finally, allocation might be made through the impersonal mechanisms of queuing (first-come-first-served) or a lottery. Oregon now uses a lottery to determine which eligible citizens get to join the state's health plan.

Because health care resources are inadequate to fill all patient needs, rationing is unavoidable. But who should do the rationing? Physicians often reject the responsibility. Some claim that any rationing should be done by public servants and health plan administrators, while physicians focus on the needs of each patient. According to Norman Levinsky, former chief of medicine at Boston University: "Physicians are required to do everything that they believe may benefit each patient without regard to costs or other societal considerations. In caring for an individual patient, the doctor must act solely as that patient's advocate, against the apparent interests of society as a whole, if necessary." Along these lines, many physicians lie to insurance companies and "game" the system in order to provide the treatment that they think their patients need.

Some physicians, bioethicists, and public policy experts, however, are willing to admit that in certain instances, bedside rationing of care by physicians is necessary and can be done ethically. In his article, **Milton Weinstein** asks, "If there is general consensus that resources should be allocated in such a way as to maximise aggregate health benefit, who is responsible for allocating the resources?" He contends that physicians play a key role along with patients in providing the most efficient allocation of health care resources. Weinstein envisions a decentralized system in which physicians are empowered to be stewards, and consider how the costs of treating a particular patient impact the welfare of their entire patient population. In his vision, the physician as good steward remains an agent and advocate for patients.

Robert Truog and colleagues, writing for the Task Force on Values, Ethics, and Rationing in Critical Care, contend that in the intensive care unit (ICU), physicians must engage in rationing. Critical care services account for at least twenty percent of hospital costs and impinge on the resources available to other patients, so they argue that "rationing is not only unavoidable but essential to ensuring the ethical distribution of medical goods and services." Some rationing decisions are morally justifiable while others are not. In order to help guide physician decisions, Truog et al. develop a framework for ethical analysis, dividing rationing decisions into three categories: external constraints (e.g., resource availability), clinical guidelines (e.g., effectiveness and efficiency of potential diagnostic and therapeutic procedures), and individual clinical judgment (e.g., applying clinical guidelines and triage of ICU beds).

Organizational Ethics

Although Weinstein and Truog consider rationing at the level of the physician, the availability of resources and clinical guidelines is generally set at the organizational level. Today, the managed care organization (MCO) dominates health care provision in the United States, with the HMO as the most commonly recognized version. (Other MCOs include preferred provider organizations and diagnosis-related groups.) MCOs were envisioned as providing efficient health care delivery—quality service at lower costs. Their popular reputation, however, is that they deny beneficial care to patients in order to cut costs and attain a high profit margin. This reputation explains why the films *As Good as It Gets* and *Sicko* resonate with many viewers.

Many people assume that cost-consciousness, especially when it is tied to a for-profit organization, is incompatible with justice and medical practice. They consider business and medicine to operate under competing paradigms. For example, Arnold Relman, former editor of the *New England Journal of Medicine* and professor at Harvard Medical School, contends that while physicians have always had business concerns, those interests generally were superseded by the professional commitment to serve patient needs. He claims that the "entrepreneurial imperative" of for-profit health care now dominates medical practice, and forces nonprofit and academic centers to behave along the same lines. MCOs thus are necessarily unethical enterprises in this environment, because this profit imperative undermines the goals of medicine.

Is there a possible alternative, such that MCOs can support quality medical care and high ethical standards, rather than act in opposition to them? **Ezekiel Emanuel** contends that four principles exist for the just allocation of health resources within MCOs. He admits that the principles could be construed in different ways, but maintains that they nevertheless provide "significant implications for the structure, practices, and allocation policies" of MCOs. Unlike Relman, Emanuel contends that MCOs can be structured to allocate health care resources justly.

John Gallagher and Jerry Goodstein borrow concepts from business ethics and organizational ethics to assess health organizations based upon their mission and how well they attend to it. They view organizational ethics as being "fundamentally concerned with questions of integrity, responsibility, and choice," providing a framework that seeks to ensure that the organization adheres to its fundamental purpose and/or ethical aims. The organization's mission thus should provide its identity, and insofar as the mission is ethical, then the organization can be ethical. Gallagher and Goodstein draw upon a response ethic and adapt it to the organization, claiming that the organization must find the fitting action or response that takes into account its own identity and values in relation to external forces. They call this process "mission discernment." In contrast to Relman, they contend that organizations are not necessarily compelled to adopt the entrepreneurial imperative, and can in fact engage in ethical actions.

Organ Transplantation—Distribution and Procurement

Organ transplantation is the area where moral tension over the distribution and procurement of health care resources is perhaps most acute. Although transplantation is expensive and requires special expertise on the part of health care workers and hospital centers, the scarcity problem is not primarily related to costs or personnel. Organs themselves are scarce. Their shortage creates distribution problems, and an interest in increasing their supply creates procurement issues. On January 2, 2009, the waiting list for organs had 108,559 total registrations, including 83,058 for kidneys, 16,512 for livers, and 2,726 for hearts. Since 2001, over 7,000 patients have died annually while on the waiting list for organs, and between about 1,600 and 2,500 patients each year were removed from the list because they became too sick for transplant surgery.

The United Network for Organ Sharing (UNOS) operates the U.S. Organ Procurement and Transplantation Network, which maintains the transplant recipient waiting lists. Several allocation standards are combined into a method that utilizes a point system to prioritize patients, and organizes the lists by organ and by region (there are eleven regions). The regional system is one of the ways in which the allocation method attends to the criterion of medical utility, because the procedure is more likely to succeed by minimizing the time between organ harvest and transplantation. Unfortunately, the geographical waiting lists are imbalanced, with some much larger than others because of population density. There are also more potential donors in the regions with larger populations, and indeed more transplants are performed there, but median waiting time tends to be longer. This imbalance in waiting time causes concerns about fairness, especially when some wealthier candidates register in more than one region and so increase their chances of receiving an organ and getting it sooner. Organs are sometimes shared between regions on the basis of a complex algorithm and point system that varies according to organ (kidneys require more careful blood antigen matching than do livers, for example). This point system ranks patients within regions by organ, and considers such things as degree of urgency, blood type, organ size, and waiting time. Waiting time used to figure more prominently in prioritizing recipients than it does today, although it remains a factor among candidates whose conditions are similar. Relative need and medical utility are the primary considerations in the point system.

Ability to pay and social utility are seemingly absent from the calculation, but may play a role in who gets on the transplant list in the first place. Some organ transplants are covered by government programs in the United States, but in other cases there is a "green screen" that prevents potential patients from getting on the transplant list. A patient who does not qualify for Medicare may lack insurance coverage for transplantation and be unable to pay the large expense, or may lack insurance altogether and so not receive the care that could have prevented organ damage or else provided a timely diagnosis. Social utility may also screen people from this list when physicians consider whether a patient is a good candidate for transplantation. For example, one of the factors is whether a patient has a strong social network of support. Such support correlates well with survivability, and so is defensible on the grounds of medical utility, but does raise the possibility of making value judgments about patients.

A particular instance of social utility being a prominent consideration is in the case of liver transplantation for alcoholics. **Walter Glannon** claims fairness as his justification when making the argument that patients with liver cirrhosis caused by alcohol abuse deserve lower priority for receiving transplants because they bear some responsibility for their condition. He views the lower priority not as punishment that they deserve, but rather as affirming responsibility for their autonomous choices. He contends that "the strength of one's claim to scarce medical resources like livers is inversely proportional to the control one has over one's health." Alcoholics may be sufficiently autonomous to be "responsible both for the addiction and the end-stage liver disease."

Organ Procurement

There are many possible methods of procuring organs, and problems exist with each of them. The United States has used *express donation* as the primary method of procuring human organs for transplantation, both for the donation of one's own organs and for those of deceased family members who have not made a declaration of intent. Since 2004, over 14,000 people have donated organs annually. The main problem with express donation is that while it respects individual autonomy and promotes altruism, it has failed to generate a sufficient supply of organs to meet patient need. Various methods have been used to increase donations, such as promoting awareness through marketing campaigns, "mandated choice" when renewing drivers licenses (in some cases even offering a discount on license fees for agreeing to become an organ donor), and the "required request" made by hospital personnel when admitting a new patient to the hospital, or of families when patients die. Although the vast majority of donated organs are cadaveric, a smaller number come from "living donors"—people who are willing to donate a kidney or a portion of their liver. The U.S. now permits more living donations than it had previously. Organs from living donors tend to perform better, but the practice has not been promoted because there are some risks to the donor (e.g., infection) and because of a concern that the donor might have been paid for the organ. Living donations still occur primarily for family members, but donations are becoming more frequently accepted from friends and altruistic strangers.

Two articles provide arguments for how the supply of organs can be increased while maintaining the express donation method. **Joseph Verheijde, Mohamed Rady, and Joan McGregor** question the recent practice of permitting organ harvesting after cardiac or circulatory function has ceased. They argue that this practice violates the "dead donor rule" (donors must be legally dead before their organs can be removed), because the legal standard for death is brain death. Although James Bernat accepts "cardiac death" as a sufficient standard before organ donation (see his article in chapter 3), Verheijde, Rady, and McGregor are unwilling to follow suit. They argue that rather than modifying the determination of death depending upon whether the patient is an organ donor, the dead donor rule should be abandoned.

David Steinberg provides another way that supply can be increased by voluntary donation, moving the United States from being a nation of "organ-takers" to a nation of "organ-givers." His proposal is to provide incentives for posthumous donation based on reciprocal altruism. In exchange for "opting in" with a pledge to donate their organs after death, people would receive preferential treatment in the form of reduced waiting time should they need a transplant. Steinberg views this plan as satisfying the utilitarian concern for good consequences for more people, and also satisfying notions of fairness and respect for autonomy by preserving individual choice.

Unlike the United States, a few countries like Austria, Belgium, and Spain have a policy of *presumed consent* for cadaveric organs. Unless a person officially registers his or her refusal to donate, the person has presumably consented to be an organ donor. These countries have organ retrieval programs that require opting-out, rather than opting-in. **Michael Gill** argues that the United States should follow suit, and shift to a policy of presumed consent for the donation of cadaveric organs for transplantation. Gill recognizes that under presumed consent, personal autonomy will doubtlessly be violated because cases will arise when people who did not want to donate nevertheless have their organs harvested. Nonetheless, he finds that scenario morally equivalent to cases when willing donors' organs are not removed. He also thinks that there will be fewer mistakes violating unwilling donors wishes than we currently have with willing donors. Thus, he holds that the principle of respect for autonomy supports presumed consent, rather than rejects it.

Another proposed method of increasing the organ supply is to create a human organ market and permit people to sell their organs. Organ donation would still be permitted, but now so would organ "vending." People could sell one of their kidneys or a portion of their liver, or there could even be a "futures market" where people will commit to providing an organ posthumously in exchange for money today. Sales could occur in private transactions (directly to individuals or through brokerages), or could be part of a larger system like UNOS, where there is a single buyer for organs that are then distributed in a manner similar to the way they are today. Organ sales are illegal in the United States and in most nations, although in 1999 a kidney was put up for auction on eBay (the bidding reached over five million dollars before the auction was stopped), and various stories have emerged about organ markets in developing countries. A prominent attempt to purchase an organ occurred in the United Kingdom in 2000, when the winner of the national lottery was a twenty-six-year-old kidney dialysis patient named Mick Taylor, who stated at a news conference that he would swap his lottery winnings for a new kidney.

Barbro Björkman argues against the market approach to increasing organ supply. He contends that the arguments favoring organ sales—usually based on consequentialist or individual rights—are unpersuasive and run counter to our moral intuitions. Nevertheless, he finds a viable moral argument can proceed from the perspective of virtue ethics, and contends that virtuous people are more likely to donate their organs, and less likely to sell them.

REFERENCES AND FURTHER READING

AMA Health Policy Group. *Expanding Health Insurance Coverage and Choice: The AMA Proposal for Reform.* 2008. http://www.ama-assn.org/ama1/pub/upload/mm/478/2008brochure.pdf (accessed May 12, 2008).

Beauchamp, Tom L., and James F. Childress. *Principles of Biomedical Ethics.* 6th ed. New York: Oxford University Press, 2009.

Carroll, Aaron, E., and Ronald T. Ackerman. "Support for National Health Insurance Among U.S. Physicians: 5 Years Later." *Annals of Internal Medicine* 148, no. 7 (2008):566.

Daniels, Norman. *Just Health: Meeting Health Needs Fairly*. New York: Cambridge University Press, 2008.

DeNavas-Walt, Carmen, Bernadette D. Proctor, and Jessica Smith. *Income, Poverty, and Health Insurance Coverage in the United States: 2006*. U.S. Census Bureau, Current Population Reports, P60–233. Washington, DC: U.S. Government Printing Office, 2007.

Dutton, Paul V. *Differential Diagnoses: A Comparative History of Health Care Problems and Solutions in the United States and France*. Ithaca, NY: Cornell University Press, 2007.

Health Canada. *Canada Health Act—Annual Report 2006–2007*. HC Pub. Ottawa: 1257.

Levinsky, Norman. "The Doctor's Master." *New England Journal of Medicine* 311 no. 24 (1984):1573–75.

MacIntyre, Alasdair. *After Virtue*. 3rd ed. Notre Dame, IN: University of Notre Dame Press, 2007.

Murray, John E. *Origins of American Health Insurance: A History of Industrial Sickness Funds*. New Haven, CT: Yale University Press, 2007.

Novak, David. "A Jewish Argument for Socialized Medicine." *Kennedy Institute of Ethics Journal* 13, no. 4 (2003): 313–28.

Nozick, Robert. *Anarchy, State, and Utopia*. New York: Basic Books, 1974.

Numbers, Ronald L. *Almost Persuaded: American Physicians and Compulsory Health Insurance, 1912–1920*. Baltimore, MD: Johns Hopkins University Press, 1978.

Nussbaum, Martha. *Frontiers of Justice: Disability, Nationality, Species Membership*. Cambridge, MA: Harvard University Press, 2006.

Okin, Susan Moller. *Justice, Gender, and the Family*. New York: Basic Books, 1989.

Outka, Gene. "Social Justice and Equal Access to Health Care." *Journal of Religious Ethics* 2, no. 1 (1974): 11–32.

Pesik, Nicki, Mark E. Keim, and Kenneth V. Iserson. "Terrorism and the Ethics of Emergency Medical Care." *Annals of Emergency Medicine* 37, no. 6 (2001): 642–46.

President's Commission for the Study of Ethical Problems in Medicine and Biomedical and Behavior Research. *Securing Access to Health Care: A Report on the Ethical Implications of Differences in the Availability of Health Services*. Washington, DC: U.S. Government Printing Office, 1983.

Rawls, John. *A Theory of Justice*. Cambridge, MA: Harvard University Press, 1971.

Relman, Arnold. *A Second Opinion: Rescuing America's Health Care*. New York: Public Affairs, 2007.

Rosenberg, Charles E. *The Care of Strangers: The Rise of America's Hospital System*. New York: Basic Books, 1987.

United States Conference of Catholic Bishops (USCCB). *Ethical and Religious Directives for Catholic Health Care Services*. 4th ed. Washington, DC: USCCB Publishing. http://www.usccb.org/bishops/directives.shtml (accessed May 12, 2008).

Walzer, Michael. *Spheres of Justice: A Defense of Pluralism and Equality*. New York: Basic Books, 1984.

Whitall, Susan. "Moore Outrage: He Taps Anger Over 'Sicko' Health Care System." *Detroit News*, June 8, 2007. http://www.detnews.com/apps/pbcs.dll/article?AID=/20070608/ENT02/706080379 (accessed May 12, 2008).

Young, Iris Marion. *Justice and the Politics of Difference*. Princeton, NJ: Princeton University Press, 1990.

DISCUSSION QUESTIONS FOR THE READINGS

Justice, Health, and HealthCare

1. If health care is "special," what makes it so?
2. Should efforts to ensure justice in health outcomes focus on social conditions in addition to access to health care?
3. Will following Daniels's four conditions ensure justice in the allocating of health care resources?

Rights to Health Care, Social Justice, and Fairness in Health Care Allocations: Frustrations in the Face of Finitude

1. Is Engelhardt correct that humans do not share a common view of justice and beneficence?
2. Are the natural and social lotteries as readily distinguishable as Engelhardt claims?
3. Should the unfortunate also have a right to receive health care?
4. What are the advantages and disadvantages of Engelhardt's proposed "diverse health care packages"?
5. Engelhardt lauds "open democratic dialogue" as a way "to fashion a basic package of health care for all citizens." How does this notion compare with Daniels's four procedural justice conditions for distributing health care?

A Conservative Case for Universal Access to Health Care

1. Menzel and Light define conservativism as cautious pragmatism. Is it pragmatic to support universal access to health care?
2. Is access to health care like police and fire protection?
3. Is the free rider problem better addressed by universal access or refusing to provide care to the uninsured?
4. Assuming that conservative values support universal access to health care, what level of access would satisfy those values?

Illegal Immigrants, Health Care, and Social Responsibility

1. Is desert the appropriate material criterion of justice for access to health care?
2. Would California's Proposition 187 justly or unjustly deny health care to illegal immigrants?
3. Are the professional ethics of physicians sufficient for addressing Proposition 187?
4. Is social ethics easily distinguishable from bioethics?
5. What is the social responsibility of the United States regarding illegal immigrants?

Should Physicians Be Gatekeepers of Medical Resources?

1. How is health care like and unlike a commons?
2. Are QALYs a good way to determine the cost-effectiveness of health care?
3. Is it in your best interests for physicians to be constrained to act in the collective interest of society?
4. Are constrained physicians able to maintain fiduciary trust with patients?

Rationing in the Intensive Care Unit
1. Is bedside rationing ethical?
2. What role should values play in rationing decisions?
3. What should guide clinical judgment when making rationing decisions?

Justice and Managed Care: Four Principles for the Just Allocation of Health Care Resources
1. Are Emanuel's four principles adequate for the just allocation of health care resources? Are there additional principles necessary to ensure just allocation?
2. Should for-profit MCOs be eliminated?
3. What is the relationship between market choice and consent?
4. Why is consent important for justice in the allocation of health care resources?

Fulfilling Institutional Responsibilities in Health Care: Organizational Ethics and the Role of Mission Discernment
1. To whom do organizational ethics apply? Physicians? Administrators? Everyone connected to the organization?
2. Because organizational ethics is responsive to multiple stakeholders, not only patients, is it an appropriate framework for health care?
3. Does the Holy Cross Health System and its mission discernment process satisfy the four principles and six practical implications outlined by Emanuel in the previous article?
4. How does the ethic of response or responsiveness compare with the moral theories and methods discussed in chapter 1?

Responsibility, Alcoholism, and Liver Transplantation
1. Is the medical argument to give lower priority to alcoholics for liver transplants clearly distinct from moral argument?
2. How much control is necessary to impute responsibility for the consequences of one's actions?
3. Should alcoholics receive lower priority for liver transplantation?
4. Does Glannon provide a convincing argument that lower priority is not punishment?
5. If it is fair for alcoholics to receive lower priority for liver transplantation, what are the implications for other diseases and injuries caused by chosen activities (e.g., smoking, auto accidents, and sports injuries)?

Recovery of Transplantable Organs After Cardiac or Circulatory Death: Transforming the Paradigm for the Ethics of Organ Donation
1. Why does donation after cardiac or circulatory death (DCD) violate the dead donor rule?
2. Does DCD materially violate general consent to become an organ donor?
3. Of the three strategic options, which are ethically acceptable? Which one is ethically preferable to the others?

Why We Are Not Allowed to Sell That Which We Are Encouraged to Donate
1. Do the arguments supporting organ sales correlate with your moral intuitions?
2. Is it possible to be a virtuous person and *not* be an organ donor?

3. Are there any situations where a virtuous person might sell rather than donate organs?

4. What can be done to increase your society's sense of virtue? What is the probability that such projects will be successful?

Presumed Consent, Autonomy, and Organ Donation

1. What is the "fewer mistakes" claim? Does it provide a good basis for adopting a policy of presumed consent for organ donation?

2. Are mistaken removals morally worse than mistaken nonremovals?

3. Gill and some of his opponents (Veatch and Pitt) both appeal to nonconsensual emergency room treatment. Who makes the stronger case?

4. Do Gill's concluding remarks favoring a family veto strengthen or weaken his previous argument supporting presumed consent?

An "Opting In" Paradigm for Kidney Transplantation

1. On balance, is living kidney donation more praiseworthy or more problematic?

2. By giving priority to organ donors, is the "opting in" paradigm more fair than the current system, which permits people to be "organ takers?"

3. What are some potential problems that could occur if the "opting in" paradigm were put into practice?

READINGS

Justice, Health, and Health Care

NORMAN DANIELS

From *Medicine and Social Justice*, edited by Rosamond Rhodes, Margaret Pabst Battin, and Anita Silvers (New York: Oxford University Press, 2002), 6–23.

Three Questions of Justice

A theory of justice for health and health care should help us answer three central questions. First, is health care special? Is it morally important in ways that justify (and explain) the fact that many societies distribute health care more equally than many other social goods? Second, when are health inequalities unjust? After all, many socially controllable factors besides access to health care affect the levels of population health and the degree of health inequalities in a population. Third, how can we meet competing health-care needs fairly under reasonable resource constraints? General principles of justice that answer the first two questions do not, I argue, answer some important questions about rationing fairly. Is there instead a fair process for making rationing decisions?

My goal is to sketch the central ideas behind my approach to all three questions and to suggest how they all fit together. By pushing a theory of justice toward providing answers to all three questions, and not simply the first, I hope to give a fuller demonstration that justice is good for our health.

What Is the Special Moral Importance of Health Care?

For purposes of justice, the central moral importance of preventing and treating disease and disability with effective health-care services (construed broadly to include public health and environmental measures, as well as personal medical services) derives from the way in which protecting normal functioning contributes to protecting opportunity. Specifically, by keeping people close to normal functioning, health care preserves for people the ability to participate in the political, social, and economic life of their society. It sustains them as fully participating citizens—normal collaborators and competitors—in all spheres of social life.

By maintaining normal functioning, health care protects an individual's fair share of the normal range of opportunities (or plans of life) that reasonable people would choose in a given society. This normal opportunity range is societally relative, depending on various facts about its level of technological development and social organization. Individuals' fair shares of that societal normal opportunity range are the plans of life it would be reasonable for them to choose were they not ill or disabled and were their talents and skills suitably protected against misdevelopment or underdevelopment as a result of unfair social practices and the consequences of socioeconomic inequalities. Individuals generally choose to develop only some of their talents and skills, effectively narrowing their range of opportunities. Maintaining normal functioning preserves, however, their broader, fair share of the normal opportunity range, giving them the chance to revise their plans of life over time.

This relationship between health care and the protection of opportunity suggests that the appropriate principle of distributive justice for regulating the design of a health-care system is a principle protecting equality of opportunity. Any theory of justice that supports a principle assuring equal opportunity (or giving priority to improving the opportunities of those who have the least opportunity) could thus be extended to health care. At the time I proposed this approach, the best defense of such a general principle was to be found in John Rawls's theory of justice as fairness. One of the principles that Rawls's social contractors would choose is a principle assuring them *fair equality of opportunity* in access to jobs and offices. This principle not only prohibits discriminatory barriers to access, but requires positive social measures that correct for the negative effects on opportunity, including the underdevelopment of skills and talents, that derive from unfair social practices (e.g., a legacy of gender or race bias) or socioeconomic inequalities. Such positive measures would include among other things the provision of public education and other opportunity improving early childhood interventions.

Rawls, however, had deliberately simplified the formulation of his general theory of justice by assuming that people are fully functional over a normal life span. His social contractors thus represented people who suffered no disease or disability or premature death. By subsuming the protection of normal functioning under (a suitably adjusted version of) Rawls's principle assuring fair equality of opportunity, I showed how to drop that idealization and apply his theory to the real world.

The fair equality of opportunity account does not use the impact of disease or disability on welfare (desire satisfaction or happiness) or utility as a basis for thinking about distributive justice. One might have thought, for example, that what was special about health care was that good health was important for happiness. But illness and disability may not lead to unhappiness, even if they restrict the range of opportunities open to an individual. Intuitively, then, there is something attractive about locating the moral importance of meeting health-care needs in the more objective impact on opportunity than in the more subjective impact on happiness.

Health care is of special moral importance because it helps to preserve our status as fully functioning citizens. By itself, however, this does not distinguish health care from food, shelter, and rest, which also meet the basic needs of citizens by preserving normal functioning. Because medical needs are more unequally distributed than these other needs and can be catastrophically expensive, they are appropriately seen as the object of private or social insurance schemes. It might be argued that we can finesse the problem of talking about the medical needs we owe it to each other to meet if we assure people fair income shares from which they can purchase such insurance. We cannot, however, define a minimal but fair income share unless it is capable of meeting such needs.

The account sketched here has several implications for the design of our health-care institutions and for issues of resource allocation. Perhaps most important, the account supports the provision of universal access to appropriate health care—including traditional public health and preventive measures—through public or mixed public and private insurance schemes. Health care aimed at protecting fair equality of opportunity should not be distributed according to ability to pay, and the burden of payment should not fall disproportionately on those who are ill.

Properly designed universal coverage health systems will be constrained by reasonable budgets, for health care is not the only important good. Reasonable resource constraints will then require judgments about which medical needs are more important to meet than others. Both rationing and setting priorities are requirements of justice; this is because meeting health-care needs should not and need not be a bottomless pit.

One controversial implication of my approach provides a way to contrast the fair equality of opportunity view with some alternative egalitarian accounts. In aiming at normal functioning, my approach views the prevention and treatment of disease and disability as the primary rationale for what we owe each other by way of assistance in cooperative health-care schemes. Enhancing otherwise normal conditions—even when they put us at a disadvantage compared to others through no fault of our own—is then viewed as "not medically necessary." For example, there is support in my view for the common insurance practice of covering treatment for very short children who have growth-hormone deficiencies but not covering it for equally short children who are otherwise normal.

The objection to my view is that this coverage policy seems to place too much weight on the presence of disease and disability and too little on what really should matter to an account aiming at protecting opportunity—namely, reducing the disadvantage that extreme shortness brings. This objection might be pressed by those who defend "equal opportunity for welfare or advantage" (Arneson, 1988; G.A. Cohen, 1989). Their view rests on claiming that anyone who suffers bad "brute luck"—a deficit in welfare or advantage that is no fault of their own—has a claim on others for assistance or compensation. In contrast, bad "option luck," the result of the choices we make or are responsible for making, does not give rise to claims on others. A disadvantage in talents or skills or even height that is not our fault thus provides a basis for claims on others for compensation or possibly enhancement.

A similar objection might be raised from a perspective grounded in the importance of positive liberty or freedom, thought of as our capability to do or be what we choose (Sen 1980, 1992, 1999). The claim is that we should not necessarily be focused on a concept such as disease or disability but rather on whether individuals have the appropriate set of capabilities to do or be what they choose. Perhaps the very short child who is otherwise normal still lacks a key trait or capability that we should address.

If we consider more carefully, however, when differences in capabilities give rise to claims on others, support for treating the short but normal child may disappear. The short but normal child, for example, may have an excellent temperament or wonderful social or cognitive skills. The cases where there is likely to be agreement that someone is clearly worse off in capabilities are likely to be captured by the categories of (serious) disease and disability. In practice, then, this view converges much more with the view I defend than it appears at first.

Which Health Inequalities Are Unjust?

Universal access to appropriate health care—health care that is just—does not break the link between social status and health that I noted earlier, a point driven home in studies of the effects on health inequality of the British National Health Service and confirmed by work in other countries as well. Our health is affected not simply by the ease with which we can see a doctor—though that surely matters—but also by our social position and the underlying inequality of our society. We cannot, of course, infer causation from these correlations between social inequality and health inequality (though later I explore some ideas about how the one might lead the other). Suffice to say that, although the exact processes are not fully understood, the evidence suggests that social determinants of health exist (Marmot, 1999).

If social factors play a large role in determining our health, then efforts to ensure greater justice in health outcomes should not focus simply on the traditional health sector. Health is produced not merely by having access to medical prevention and treatment, but also, to a measurably greater extent, by the cumulative experience of social conditions over the course of one's life.

As I noted earlier, Rawls's theory of justice as fairness was not designed to address issues of health care. Rawls assumed a completely healthy population, and he argued that a just society must assure people equal basic liberties, guarantee that the right of political participation has roughly equal value for all, provide a robust form of equal opportunity, and limit inequalities to those that benefit the least advantaged.

The conjecture I explore is that by establishing equal liberties, robustly equal opportunity, a fair distribution of resources, and support for our self-respect—the basics of Rawlsian justice—we would go a long way in eliminating the most important injustices in health outcomes. To be sure, social justice is valuable for reasons other than its effects on health. And social reform in the direction of greater justice would not eliminate the need to think hard about fair allocation of resources within the health-care system. Still, acting to promote social justice is a crucial step toward improving our health because there is this surprising convergence between what is needed for our social and political well being and for our mental and physical health.

One especially important factor in explaining the health of a society is the distribution of income: The health of a population depends not just on the size of the economic pie, but on how the pie is shared. Differences in health outcomes among developed nations cannot be explained simply by the absolute deprivation associated with low economic development—lack of access to the basic material conditions necessary for health such as clean water, adequate nutrition and housing, and general sanitary living conditions. The degree of relative deprivation within a society also matters.

Numerous studies support this *relative-income hypothesis*, which states, more precisely, that inequality is strongly associated with population mortality and life expectancy across nations (Wilkinson 1992, 1994, 1996). Rich countries vary in life expectancy, and that variation dovetails with income distribution. In particular, wealthier countries with more equal income distributions, such as Sweden and Japan, have higher life expectancies than does the United States, despite their having lower per capita GDP. Likewise, countries with low GDPpc but remarkably high life expectancy, such as Costa Rica, tend to have a more equitable distribution of income.

At the individual level, we also find that inequality is important. Numerous studies have documented what has come to be known as the "socioeconomic gradient": At each step along the economic ladder we see improved health outcomes over the rung below (including in societies with universal health insurance). Differences in health outcomes are not confined to the extremes of rich and poor; they are observed across all levels of socioeconomic status.

The slope of the socioeconomic gradient varies substantially across societies. Some societies show a relatively shallow gradient in mortality rates: Being better off confers a health advantage, but not so large an advantage as elsewhere. Others, with comparable or even higher levels of economic development, show much steeper gradients. The slope of the gradient appears to be fixed by the level of income inequality in a society: The more unequal a society is in economic terms, the more unequal it is in health terms. Moreover, middle-income groups in a country with high income inequality typically do worse in terms of health than comparable or even poorer groups in a society with less income inequality. We find the same pattern within the United States when we examine state and metropolitan area variations in inequality and health outcomes.

Earlier, I cautioned that correlations between inequality and health do not necessarily imply causation. Still, there are plausible and identifiable pathways through which social inequalities appear to produce health inequalities to make a reasonable case for causation. In the United States, the states with the most unequal income distributions invest less in public education, have larger uninsured populations, and spend less on social safety nets. Studies of educational spending and educational outcomes are especially striking: Controlling for median income, income inequality explains about 40% of the variation between states in the percentage of children in the fourth grade who are below the basic reading level. Similarly strong associations are seen for high school dropout rates. It is evident from these data that educational opportunities for children in high income-inequality states are quite different from those in states with more egalitarian distributions. These effects on education have an immediate impact on health, increasing the likelihood of premature death during childhood and adolescence (as evidenced by the much higher death rates for infants and children in the high-inequality states). Later in life, they appear in the socioeconomic gradient in health.

These societal mechanisms—for example, income inequality leading to educational inequality leading to health inequality—are tightly linked to the political processes that influence government policy. For instance, income inequality appears to affect health by undermining civil society. Income inequality erodes social cohesion, as measured by higher levels of social mistrust and reduced participation in civic organizations. Lack of social cohesion leads to lower participation in political activity (such as voting, serving in local government, volunteering for political campaigns). And lower participation, in turn, undermines the responsiveness of government institutions in addressing the needs of the worst-off. States with the highest income inequality, and thus lowest levels of social capital and political participation, are less likely to invest in human capital and provide far less generous social safety nets.

Rawls's principles of justice thus turn out to regulate the key social determinants of health. One principle assures equal basic liberties, and specifically provides for guaranteeing *effective* rights of political participation. The fair equality of opportunity principle assures access to high-quality public education, early childhood interventions, including day care, aimed at eliminating class or race disadvantages, and universal coverage for appropriate health care. Rawls's "Difference Principle" permits inequalities in income only if the inequalities work (e.g., through incentives) to make those who are worst-off as well-off as possible. This is not a simple "trickle down" principle that tolerates any inequality as long as there is some benefit that flows down the socioeconomic ladder; it requires a maximal flow downward. It would therefore flatten socioeconomic inequalities in a robust way, assuring far more than a "decent minimum." In addition, the assurances of the value of political participation and fair equality of opportunity would further constrain allowable income inequalities.

The conjecture is that a society complying with these principles of justice would probably flatten the socioeconomic gradient even more than we see in the most egalitarian welfare states of northern Europe. The implication is that we should view health inequalities that derive from social determinants as unjust unless the determinants are distributed in conformity with these robust principles. Because of the detailed attention Rawls's theory pays to the interaction of these terms of fair cooperation, it provides us—through the findings of social science—with an account of the just distribution of health.

The inequalities in the social determinants that are still permitted by this theory may still produce a socioeconomic gradient, albeit a much flatter one than we see today. Should we view these residual health inequalities as unjust and demand further redistribution of the social determinants?

I believe the theory I have described does not give a clear answer. If the Rawlsian theory insists that protecting opportunity takes priority over other matters and cannot be traded for other gains (and Rawls generally adopts this view), then residual health inequalities may be unjust. If health can be traded for other goods—and all of us make such trades when we take chances with our health to pursue other goals—then the account may be more flexible. Still, Rawls's principles provide more specific guidance in thinking about the distribution of the social determinants than is provided by the fair equality of opportunity account of a just health-care system alone.

When Are Limits to Health Care Fair?

Justice requires that all societies meet health-care needs fairly under reasonable resource constraints. Even a wealthy, egalitarian country with a highly efficient health-care system will have to set limits to the health care it guarantees every-

one (whether or not it allows supplementary tiers for those who can afford them). Poorer countries have to make even harder choices about priorities and limits. However important, health care is not the only important social good. All societies must decide which needs should be given priority and when resources are better spent elsewhere.

How should fair decisions about such limits be made? Under what conditions should we view such decisions as a legitimate exercise of moral authority?

Answering these questions would be much simpler if people could agree on principles of distributive justice that would determine how to set fair limits to health care. If societies agreed on such principles, people could simply check social decisions and practices against the principles to determine whether they conform with them. Where decisions, practices, and institutions fail to conform, they would be unjust and people should then change them. Disagreements about the fairness of actual distributions would then be either disagreements about the interpretation of the principles or about the facts of the situation. Many societies have well-established and reliable, if imperfect, legal procedures for resolving such disputes about facts and interpretations.

Unfortunately, there is no consensus on such distributive principles for health care. Reasonable people, who have diverse moral and religious views about many matters, disagree morally about what constitutes a fair allocation of resources to meet competing health-care needs—even when they agree on other aspects of the justice of health care-systems, such as the importance of universal access to whatever services are provided. We should expect, and respect, such diversity in views about rationing health care. Nevertheless, we must arrive at acceptable social policies despite our disagreements. This moral controversy raises a distinctive problem of legitimacy: Under what conditions should we accept as legitimate the moral authority of those making rationing decisions?

I shall develop the following argument: (1) We have no consensus on principled solutions to a cluster of morally controversial rationing problems, and general principles of justice for health and health care fail to provide specific guidance about them. (2) In the absence of such a consensus, we should rely on a fair process for arriving at solutions to these problems and for establishing the legitimacy of such decisions. (3) A fair process that addresses issues of legitimacy will have to meet several constraints that I shall refer to as "accountability for reasonableness"; these constraints tie the process to deliberative democratic procedures. This issue of legitimacy and fair process arises in both public and mixed public–private health-care systems, and it must be addressed in countries at all levels of development.

To support the first step of the argument, consider a problem that has been labeled the "priorities problem": How much priority should we give to treating the sickest or most disabled patients? To start with, imagine two extreme positions. The Maximin position ("maximize the minimum") says that we should give complete priority to treating the worst-off patients. The Maximize position says that we should give priority to whatever treatment produces the greatest net health benefit (or greatest net health benefit per dollar spent) regardless of which patients we treat.

In practice, most people are likely to reject both extreme positions. A definite but very small minority are inclined to be *maximizers* and a definite but very small minority are inclined to be *maximiners*. Most people fall in between, and they vary considerably in how much benefit they are willing to sacrifice to give priority to worse off patients.

If we have persistent disagreement about principles for resolving rationing problems, then we must retreat to a process all can agree is a fair way to resolve disputes about them. The "retreat to procedural justice" as a way of determining what is fair when we lack prior agreement on principles is a central feature of Rawls's account (thus "justice as [procedural] fairness").

We would take a giant step toward solving the problems of legitimacy and fairness that face public agencies and private health plans making limit-setting decisions if the following four conditions were satisfied:

- *Publicity condition*: Decisions regarding coverage for new technologies (and other limit-setting decisions) and their rationales must be publicly accessible.
- *Relevance condition*: The rationales for coverage decisions should aim to provide a *reasonable* construal of how the organization (or society) should provide "value for money" in meeting the varied health needs of a defined population under reasonable resource constraints. Specifically, a construal will be "reasonable" if it appeals to reasons and principles that are accepted as relevant by people who are disposed to finding terms of cooperation that are mutually justifiable.
- *Appeals condition*: There is a mechanism for challenge and dispute resolution regarding limit-setting decisions, including the opportunity for revising decisions in light of further evidence or arguments.
- *Enforcement condition*: There is either voluntary or public regulation of the process to ensure that the first three conditions are met.

The guiding idea behind the four conditions is to convert private health plan or public agency decisions into part of a larger public deliberation about how to use limited resources to protect fairly the health of a population with varied needs. Meeting these conditions also serves an educative function: The public is made familiar with the need for limits and appropriate ways to reason about them.

The first condition (Publicity condition) requires that rationales for decisions be publicly accessible to everyone affected by them. One American health plan, for example, decided to cover growth-hormone treatment but only for children who are growth hormone deficient or who have Turner syndrome. It deliberated carefully and clearly about the reasons for its decision. These included the lack of evidence of efficacy or good risk benefit ratios for other groups of patients, and a commitment to restrict coverage to the treatment of disease and disability (as opposed to enhancements). It did not, however, state these reasons in its medical director's letter to clinicians or in support materials used in "shared decision making" with patients and families about the procedure. Its reasons were defensible ones aimed at a public good that all people can understand and see as relevant, the provision of effective and safe treatment to a defined population under resource constraints. The restriction to treatment rather than enhancement requires a moral argument, however, and remains a point about which reasonable people can disagree.

One important effect of making public the reasons for coverage decisions is that, over time, the pattern of such decisions will resemble a type of "case law." A body of case law establishes the presumption that if some individuals have been treated one way because they fall under a reasonable interpretation of the relevant principles, then similar individuals should be treated the same way in subsequent cases. In effect, the institution generating the case law is saying, "We deliberate carefully about hard cases and have good reasons for doing what we have done, and we continue to stand by our reasons in our commitment to act consistently with past practices." To rebut this presumption requires showing either that the new case differs in relevant and important ways from the earlier one, justifying different treatment, or that there are good grounds for rejecting the reasons or principles embodied in the earlier case. Case law does not imply past infallibility, but it does imply giving careful consideration to why earlier decision makers made the choices they did. It involves a form of institutional reflective equilibrium, a commitment to both transparency and coherence in the giving of reasons.

The benefits of publicity in the form of case law are both internal and external to the decision-making institution. The quality of decision making improves if reasons must be articulated. Fairness improves over time, both formally, because like cases are treated similarly, and substantively, because there is systematic evaluation of reasons. To the extent that we are then better able to discover flaws in our moral reasoning, we are more likely to arrive at fair decisions. Over time, people will understand better the moral commitments of the institutions making these decisions.

The Relevance condition imposes two important constraints on the rationales that are made publicly accessible. Specifically, the rationales for coverage decisions should aim to provide (a) a *reasonable* construal of (b) how the organization (or society) should provide "value for money" in meeting the varied health needs of a defined population under reasonable resource constraints. Both constraints need explanation.

We may think of the goal of meeting the varied needs of the population of patients under reasonable resource constraints as a characterization of the *common* or *public good* pursued by all engaged in the enterprise of delivering and receiving this care. Reasoning about that goal must also meet certain conditions. Specifically, a construal of the goal will be "reasonable" only if it appeals to reasons (evidence, values, and principles) that are accepted as relevant by "fair-minded" people. By "fair-minded" I mean people who seek mutually justifiable terms of cooperation. The notion is not mysterious; we encounter it all the time in sports. Fair-minded people are those who want to play by agreed-upon rules in a sport and prefer rules that are designed to bring out the best in that game. Here we are concerned with the game of delivering health care that meets population needs in a fair way.

The Appeals and Enforcement conditions involve mechanisms that go beyond the publicity requirements of the first two conditions.

When patients or clinicians use these procedures to challenge a decision, and the results of the challenge lead effectively to reconsideration of the decision on its merits, the decision-making process is made iterative in a way that broadens the input of information and argument. Parties that were excluded from the decision-making process, and whose views may not have been clearly heard or understood, find a voice, even if after the original fact. The dispute resolution mechanisms do not empower enrollees or clinicians to play a direct, participatory role in the actual decision-making bodies, but that does not happen in many public democratic processes as well. Still, it does empower them to play a more effective role in the larger social deliberation about the issues, including deliberation within those public institutions that can play a role in regulating private health plans or otherwise constraining their acts. The mechanisms we describe thus play a role in assuring broader accountability of private organizations to those who are affected by limit-setting decisions. The arrangements required by the four conditions provide connective tissue to, not a replacement for, broader democratic processes that ultimately have authority and responsibility for guaranteeing the fairness of limit-setting decisions.

Together these conditions hold institutions—public or private—and decision makers in them "accountable for the reasonableness" of the limits they set. All must engage in a process of establishing their credentials for fair decision making about such fundamental matters every time they make such a decision. Whether in public or mixed systems, establishing the accountability of decision makers to those affected by their decisions is the only way to show, over time, that arguably fair decisions are being made and that those making them have established a procedure we should view as legitimate. This is not to say that public participation is an essential ingredient of the process in either public or mixed systems, but the accountability to the public in both cases is necessary to facilitate broader democratic processes that regulate the system.

In many public systems the reasoning that lies behind decisions that affect the length of queues—a rationing device—are inscrutable to the public. They are made in a "black box" of budgetary decisions. Queues may then be adjusted if the public complains too much—there is this kind of accountability to the squeaky wheel. But there is in general too little accountability of the sort demanded by the four conditions I describe. Only through such accountability and the way in which it facilitates or enables a broader social deliberation will there be a wider perception that rationing decisions are fair and are made through an exercise of legitimate authority.

One issue facing this "process" approach to rationing seems to be more problematic in public systems than it does in mixed ones. In a mixed system, two different insurers or health plans might arrive at different judgments about what limits to set. I have suggested both might be "right" if their decisions are the results of fair procedures. The anomaly is that some patients will then have access to services that others will not have, and this might seem to violate a formal constraint on fairness—that society treat like cases similarly. In a mixed system, we might see this variation as a price we pay for whatever virtues (if any) the mixed system brings (the variation might ultimately lead us to better decisions over time). In a public system, however, such variation (e.g., between districts) might seem more objectionable if all are governed by the same public legislation and funding. Still, despite such anomalies, fair process may be the best we can do wherever we have no prior consensus on fair outcomes.

Concluding Remarks

A comprehensive approach to justice, health, and health care must address all three questions I have discussed. My extension of Rawls's theory of justice to health and health care provides a way to link answers to the first and second questions.

There are also three ways in which Rawls's theory also provides support for my approach to the third question. First, I propose that we use a fair process to arrive at what is fair in rationing; this is because we lack prior consensus on the relevant distributive principles. This "retreat to procedural justice" is at the heart of Rawls's own invocation of his version of a social contract. Second, Rawls places great emphasis on the importance of publicity as a constraint on theories of justice: Principles of justice and the grounds for them must be publicly acknowledged. This constrain is central to the conditions that establish accountability for reasonableness. Finally, Rawls develops the view that "public reason" must constrain the content of public deliberation and decision about fundamental matters of justice, avoiding special considerations that might be elements of the comprehensive moral views that people hold (Rawls 1993). Accountability for reasonableness pushes decision makers toward finding reasons all can agree are relevant to the goals of cooperative health-delivery schemes. In this way, accountability for reasonableness promotes the democratic deliberation that Rawls also advocates.

In pointing out these connections, I am not suggesting that this is the only approach to developing a theory of justice that applies to all aspects of health and health care. Indeed, I have pointed to other theories that converge in practice and to some extent in theory with the approach adopted here. I am proposing that concerns about justice and fairness in health policy should look to political philosophy for guidance and that some specific guidance is forthcoming. At the very same time, seeing how we have to modify and refine work in political philosophy if it is to apply to real issues in the world suggests that we should abandon the unidirectional implications of the term "applied ethics" or "applied political philosophy".

References

Arneson, R.J. Equality and equal opportunity for welfare. *Philosophical Studies* 54 (1988): 79–95.

Cohen, G.A. On the currency of egalitarian justice. *Ethics* 99 (1989): 906–44

Marmot, M.G. *Social Causes of Social Inequalities in Health*. Harvard Center for Population and Development Studies, Working Paper Series 99.01, January 1999.

Rawls, J. *A Theory of Justice*. Cambridge, MA: Harvard University Press, 1971.

Rawls, J. *Political Liberalism*. New York: Columbia University Press, 1993.

Sen, A.K. Equality of what? In *Tanner Lectures on Human Values: Vol. 1*, edited by S. McMurrin. Cambridge: Cambridge University Press, 1980.

Sen, A.K. *Inequality Reexamined*. Cambridge, MA: Harvard University Press, 1992.

Sen, A.K. *Development as Freedom*. New York: Alfred A. Knopf, 1999.

Wilkinson, R.G. Income distribution and life expectancy. *British Medical Journal* 304 (1992): 165–68.

Wilkinson, R.G. The epidemiological transition: From material scarcity to social disadvantage? *Daedalus* 123 (1994): 61–77.

Wilkinson, R.G. *Unhealthy Societies: The Afflictions of Inequality*. London: Routledge, 1996.

Rights to Health Care, Social Justice, and Fairness in Health Care Allocations

Frustrations in the Face of Finitude

H. TRISTRAM ENGELHARDT, JR.

From The *Foundations of Bioethics*, 2nd ed. (New York: Oxford University Press, 1996), 375–410.

The imposition of a single-tier, all-encompassing health care system is morally unjustifiable. It is a coercive act of totalitarian ideological zeal, which fails to recognize the diversity of moral visions that frame interests in health care, the secular moral limits of state authority, and the authority of individuals over themselves and their own property. It is an act of secular immorality.

A basic human secular moral right to health care does not exist—not even to a "decent minimum of health care." Such rights must be created.

The difficulty with supposed rights to health care, as well as with many claims regarding justice or fairness in access to health care, should be apparent. Since the secular moral authority for common action is derived from permission or consent, it is difficult (indeed, for a large–scale society, materially impossible) to gain moral legitimacy for the thoroughgoing imposition on health care of one among the many views of beneficence and justice. There are, after all, as many accounts of beneficence, justice, and fairness as there are major religions.

Most significantly, there is a tension between the foundations of general secular morality and the various particular positive claims founded in particular visions of beneficence and justice. It is materially impossible both to respect the freedom of all and to achieve their long-range best interests. Loose talk about justice and fairness in health care is therefore morally misleading, because it suggests that there is a particular canonical vision of justice or fairness that all have grounds to endorse.

Rights to health care, unless they are derived from special contractual agreements, depend on particular understandings of beneficence rather than on authorizing permission. They may therefore conflict with the decisions of individuals who may not wish to participate in, and may indeed be morally opposed to, realizing a particular system of health care. Individuals always have the secular moral authority to use their own resources in ways that collide with fashionable understandings of justice or the prevailing consensus regarding fairness.

Health Care Policy: The Ideology of Equal, Optimal Care

It is fashionable to affirm an impossible commitment in health care delivery, as, for example, in the following four widely embraced health care policy goals, which are at loggerheads:

1. The best possible care is to be provided for all.
2. Equal care should be guaranteed.
3. Freedom of choice on the part of health care provider and consumer should be maintained.
4. Health care costs are to be contained.

One cannot provide the best possible health care for all and contain health care costs. One cannot provide equal health care for all and respect the freedom of individuals peaceably to pursue with others their own visions of health care or to use their own resources and energies as they decide. For that matter, one cannot maintain freedom in the choice of health care services while containing the costs of health care. One may also not be able to provide all with equal health care that is at the same time the very best care because of limits on the resources themselves. That few openly address these foundational moral tensions at the roots of contemporary health care policy suggests that the problems are shrouded in a collective illusion, a false consciousness, an established ideology within which certain facts are politically unacceptable.

These difficulties spring not only from a conflict between freedom and beneficence, but from a tension among competing views of what it means to pursue and achieve the good in health care (e.g., is it more important to provide equal care to all or the best possible health care to the least-well-off class?). The pursuit of incompatible or incoherent health care is rooted in the failure to face the finitude of secular moral authority, the finitude of secular moral vision, the finitude of human powers in the face of death and suffering, the finitude of human life, and the finitude of human financial resources. A health care system that acknowledges the moral and financial limitations on the provision of health care would need to

1. endorse inequality in access to health care as morally unavoidable because of private resources and human freedom;
2. endorse setting a price on saving human life as a part of establishing a cost-effective health care system established through communal resources.

Even though all health care systems de facto enjoy inequalities and must to some extent ration the health care they provide through communal resources, this is not usually forthrightly acknowledged. There is an ideological bar to recognizing and coming to terms with the obvious.

Only a prevailing collective illusion can account for the assumption in U.S. policy that health care may be provided (1) while containing costs (2) without setting a price on saving lives and preventing suffering when using communal funds and at the same time (3) ignoring the morally unavoidable inequalities due to private resources and human freedom. There has been a failure to acknowledge the moral inevitability of inequalities in health care due to the limits of secular governmental authority, human freedom, and the existence of private property, however little that may be.

It is difficult to know why such a unique place should be given to health care versus other undertakings such as education, housing, and personal security, where individuals are allowed to secure better private basic education and housing, as well as private security services. The answers must lie in the ways in which personal health care appears to be central to the human struggle with finitude and death.

Reflections concerning the difficulties in limiting the use of health care resources have an ancient lineage and reveal a tight bond with the obsession to postpone death at all costs. Plato in Book 3 of the *Republic* recognizes the quandary of infinite expectations and finite resources that characterizes the challenge of health care choices. He concludes that the protracted treatment of chronic illnesses is boonless when medicine cannot restore citizens to their occupations and duties. Such individuals should instead accept death. The *Republic* endorses acute health care, if it promises to restore individuals to a useful life, but very little, if any, chronic health care. Preventive health care would be provided in the form of gymnastics. Plato's reflections suggest the following general points: (1) humans have a difficulty in accepting their own limits; (2) limits should be acknowledged regarding the proper amount of resources to be invested in health care; (3) resources invested in health care often do not secure a high quality of life for those treated; and (4) such investments frequently constitute a major drain on common resources. For Plato, concerns regarding health care were expressed in terms of the goal of maintaining the polis, not in terms of isolated individual rights to health services.

But individuals are the source of secular moral authority.

Justice, Freedom, and Inequality

Interests in justice as beneficence are motivated in part by inequalities and in part by needs. That some have so little while others have so much properly evokes moral concerns of beneficence. Still, the moral authority to use force to set such inequalities aside is limited. These limitations are in part due to the circumstance that the resources one could use to aid those in need are already owned by other people. One must establish whether and when inequalities and needs generate rights or claims against others.

The Natural and Social Lotteries

"Natural lottery" is used to identify changes in fortune that result from natural forces, not directly from the actions of persons. The natural lottery shapes the distribution of both naturally and socially conditioned assets. The natural lottery contrasts with the social lottery, which is used to identify changes in fortune that are not the result of natural forces but the actions of persons. The social lottery shapes the distribution of social and natural assets. The natural and social lotteries, along with one's own free decisions, determine the distribution of natural and social assets. The social lottery is termed a lottery, though it is the outcome of personal actions, because of the complex and unpredictable interplay of personal choices and because of the unpredictable character of the outcomes, which do not conform to an ideal pattern, and because the outcomes are the results of social forces, not the immediate choices of those subject to them.

All individuals are exposed to the vicissitudes of nature. Some are born healthy and by luck remain so for a long life, free of disease and major suffering. Others are born with serious congenital or genetic diseases, others contract serious crippling fatal illnesses early in life, and yet others are injured and maimed. Those who win the natural lottery will for most of their lives not be in need of medical care. They will live full lives and die painless and peaceful deaths. Those who lose the natural lottery will be in need of health care to blunt their sufferings and, where possible, to cure their diseases and to restore function. There will be a spectrum of losses, ranging from minor problems such as having teeth with cavities to major tragedies such as developing childhood leukemia,

inheriting Huntington's chorea, or developing amyelotrophic lateral sclerosis.

These tragic outcomes are the deliverances of nature, for which no one, without some special view of accountability or responsibility, is responsible (unless, that is, one recognizes them as the results of the Fall or as divine chastisements). The circumstance that individuals are injured by hurricanes, storms, and earthquakes is often simply no one's fault. When no one is to blame, no one may be charged with the responsibility of making whole those who lose the natural lottery on the ground of accountability for the harm. One will need an argument dependent on a particular sense of fairness to show that the readers of this volume should submit to the forcible redistribution of their resources to provide health care for those injured by nature. It may very well be unfeeling, unsympathetic, or uncharitable not to provide such help. One may face eternal hellfires for failing to provide aid. But it is another thing to show in general secular moral terms that individuals owe others such help in a way that would morally authorize state force to redistribute their private resources and energies or to constrain their free choices with others. To be in dire need does not by itself create a secular moral right to be rescued from that need. The natural lottery creates inequalities and places individuals at disadvantage without creating a straightforward secular moral obligation on the part of others to aid those in need.

Individuals differ in their resources not simply because of outcomes of the natural lottery, but also due to the actions of others. Some deny themselves immediate pleasures in order to accumulate wealth or to leave inheritances; through a complex web of love, affection, and mutual interest, individuals convey resources, one to another, so that those who are favored prosper, and those who are ignored languish. Some as a consequence grow wealthy and others grow poor, not through anyone's malevolent actions or omissions, but simply because they were not favored by the love, friendship, collegiality, and associations through which fortunes develop and individuals prosper. In such cases there will be neither fairness nor unfairness, but simply good and bad fortune.

In addition, some will be advantaged or disadvantaged, made rich, poor, ill, diseased, deformed, or disabled because of the malevolent and blameworthy actions and omissions of others. Such will be unfair circumstances, which just and beneficent states should try to prevent and to rectify through legitimate police protection, forced restitution, and charitable programs. Insofar as an injured party has a claim against an injurer to be made whole, not against society, the outcome is unfortunate from the perspective of society's obligations and the obligations of innocent citizens to make restitution. Restitution is owed by the injurer, not society or others. There will be outcomes of the social lottery that are on the one hand blameworthy in the sense of resulting from the culpable actions of others, though on the other hand a society has no obligation to rectify them. The social lottery includes the exposure to the immoral and unjust actions of others. Again, one will need an argument dependent on a particular sense of fairness to show that the readers of this volume should submit to the forcible redistribution of their resources to provide health care to those injured by others.

When individuals come to purchase health care, some who lose the natural lottery will be able at least in part to compensate for those losses through their winnings at the social lottery. They will be able to afford expensive health care needed to restore health and to regain function. On the other hand, those who lose in both the natural and the social lottery will be in need of health care, but without the resources to acquire it.

The Rich and the Poor: Differences in Entitlements

The existence of any amount of private resources can be the basis for inequalities that secular moral authority may not set aside. Insofar as people own things, they will have a right to them, even if others

need them. Because the presence of permission is cardinal, the test of whether one must transfer one's goods to others will not be whether such a redistribution will not prove onerous or excessive for the person subjected to the distribution, but whether the resources belong to that individual. Consider that you may be reading this book next to a person in great need. The test of whether a third person may take resources from you to help that individual in need will not be whether you will suffer from the transfer, but rather whether you have consented—at least this is the case if the principle of permission functions in general secular morality. The principle of permission is the source of authority when moral strangers collaborate, because they do not share a common understanding of fairness or of the good. As a consequence, goal-oriented approaches to the just distribution of resources must be restricted to commonly owned goods, where there is authority to create programs for their use.

Drawing the Line Between the Unfortunate and the Unfair

How one regards the moral significance of the natural and social lotteries and the moral force of private ownership will determine how one draws the line between circumstances that are simply unfortunate and those that are unfortunate and in addition unfair in the sense of constituting a claim on the resources of others.

Life in general, and health care in particular, reveal circumstances of enormous tragedy, suffering, and deprivation. The pains and sufferings of illness, disability, and disease, as well as the limitations of deformity, call on the sympathy of all to provide aid and give comfort. Injuries, disabilities, and diseases due to the forces of nature are unfortunate. Injuries, disabilities, and diseases due to the unconsented-to actions of others are unfair. Still, outcomes of the unfair actions of others are not necessarily society's fault and are in this sense unfortunate. The horrible injuries that come every night to the emergency rooms of major hospitals may be someone's fault, even if they are not the fault of society, much less that of uninvolved citizens. Such outcomes, though unfair with regard to the relationship of the injured with the injurer, may be simply unfortunate with respect to society and other citizens (and may licitly be financially exploited). One is thus faced with distinguishing the difficult line between acts of God, as well as immoral acts of individuals that do not constitute a basis for societal retribution on the one hand, and injuries that provide such a basis on the other.

A line must be created between those losses that will be made whole through public funds and those that will not. Such a line was drawn in 1980 by Patricia Harris, the then secretary of the Department of Health, Education, and Welfare, when she ruled that heart transplantations should be considered experimental and therefore not reimbursable through Medicare. To be in need of a heart transplant and not have the funds available would be an unfortunate circumstance but not unfair. One was not eligible for a heart transplant even if another person had intentionally damaged one's heart. From a moral point of view, things would have been different if the federal government had in some culpable fashion injured one's heart. So, too, if promises of treatment had been made. For example, to suffer from appendicitis or pneumonia and not as a qualifying patient receive treatment guaranteed through a particular governmental or private insurance system would be unfair, not simply unfortunate.

Drawing the line between the unfair and the unfortunate is unavoidable because it is impossible in general secular moral terms to translate all needs into rights, into claims against the resources of others. One must with care decide where the line is to be drawn. To distinguish needs from mere desires, one must endorse one among the many competing visions of morality and human flourishing. One is forced to draw a line between those needs (or desires) that constitute claims on the aid of others and those that do not. The line distinguishing unfortunate from unfair circumstances justifies by default certain social and economic inequalities in the sense of determining who, if any one, is obliged in general

secular morality to remedy such circumstances or achieve equality.

The Moral Inevitability of a Multitier Health Care System

Public health care systems are communal attempts to ensure against losses at the natural and social lotteries through planned human beneficence. They function to blunt the tragedies of nature as well as the uncaring and evil choices of persons, including those who will not respond with sympathy to those in need. They are social constructs established to relieve individuals of some of the anxieties associated with the fear of disability, suffering, disease, and death. They are one of many human attempts to render nature congenial to persons.

The principles of permission and beneficence and of entitlements to property support a multitier system of health care. On the one hand, not all property is privately owned. Nations and other social organizations may invest their common resources in ensuring their members against losses in the natural and social lotteries. On the other hand, not all property is communal. There are private entitlements, which individuals may freely exchange for the services of others. The existence of a multitier system (whether officially or unofficially) in nearly all nations and societies reflects the existence of both communal and private entitlements, of social choice and individual aspiration. A two-tiered system with inequality in health care distribution is both morally and materially inevitable.

In the face of unavoidable tragedies and contrary moral intuitions, a multitiered system of health care is in many respects a compromise. On the one hand, it provides some amount of health care for all, while on the other hand allowing those with resources to purchase additional or better services. It can endorse the use of communal resources for the provision of a decent minimal or basic amount of health care for all, while acknowledging the existence of private resources at the disposal of some individuals to purchase better basic as well as luxury care. While the propensity to seek more than equal treatment for oneself or loved ones is made into a vicious disposition in an egalitarian system, a multitier system allows for the expression of individual love and the pursuit of private advantage, though still supporting a general social sympathy for those in need. Whereas an egalitarian system must suppress the widespread human inclination to devote private resources to the purchase of the best care for those whom one loves, a multitier system can recognize a legitimate place for the expression of such inclinations. A multitier system (1) should support individual providers and consumers against attempts to interfere in their free association and their use of their own resources, though (2) it may allow positive rights to health care to be created for individuals who have not been advantaged by the social lottery.

The serious task is to decide how to define and provide a decent minimum or basic level of care as a floor of support for all members of a society, while allowing money and free choice to fashion special tiers of services for the affluent. In addressing this general issue of defining what is to be meant by a decent minimum basic level or a minimum adequate amount of health care, the American President's Commission in 1983 suggested that in great measure content is to be created rather than discovered by democratic processes, as well as by the forces of the market. "In a democracy, the appropriate values to be assigned to the consequences of policies must ultimately be determined by people expressing their values through social and political processes as well as in the market place." The Commission, however, also suggested that the concept of adequacy could in part be discovered by an appeal to that amount of care that would meet the standards of sound medical practice. "Adequacy does require that everyone receive care that meets standards of sound medical practice." But what one means by "sound medical practice" is itself dependent on particular understandings within particular cultures. Criteria for sound medical practice are as much created as discovered. The moral inevitability of multiple tiers of care brings with it multiple standards of proper or sound medical practice and undermines the moral plausibility

of various obiter dicta concerning the centralized allocation of medical resources.

Indeed, concepts of adequate care are not discoverable outside of particular views of the good life and of proper medical practice. In nations encompassing diverse moral communities, an understanding of what one will mean by an adequate level or a decent minimum of health care will need to be fashioned, if it can indeed be agreed to, through open discussion and by fair negotiation. In some small-scale communities such as the BaMbuti, there may be little commitment of common resources to the endeavors of modern health care. For such communities, a decent level of such care may be little or no care. In nations such as the United Kingdom, the decent minimum of care may not include hemodialysis for individuals over a particular age or coronary bypass surgery for any but the most promising candidates (or at least there will be informal ways of discouraging such treatment). For many elsewhere, such a minimal level of investment will not count as a decent level. For Roman Catholics and others in the United Kingdom, the provision of abortions through the National Health Service will be unacceptable, making the United Kingdom's basic package morally problematic.

One creates through negotiation an amount of health care that becomes de facto the decent minimal amount for a polity, though it always remains open to further critique, discussion, and alteration. In smaller social groups that share a common view of the good life, one may be able to appeal to a common vision to discover what should count as a decent minimum of health care. But across communities there will be different moral visions along with different understandings of what should count as a decent minimum of health care or a standard of services that comports with sound medical practice. This diversity will provide a motivation for particular groups to provide particular packages of health care that reflect moral concerns regarding the character of proper health care delivery, rather than concerns to have access to better basic or to luxury health care. For example, out of concerns to avoid supporting morally inappropriate care (e.g., abortion and euthanasia), and in order to establish a worldwide basic package for all its members, one might imagine the Roman Catholic church requiring all of its members to devote 40 percent of their tithe to the church for health care. In this way, all Roman Catholics could carry with them through the world a basic guaranteed package of services, which would be in accord with their moral commitments. Those who wish more could purchase it. One would receive care *secundum status*.

Or one could envisage various groups creating their own special health care packages integrated with the basic package for a polity. Just as in Germany, citizens who are Roman Catholic or members of the Evangelical Reformed church are visited with a tax surcharge for spiritual services, different groups could pay different amounts (or receive refunds) for their special moral commitments with respect to abortion, sterilization, third-party-assisted suicide, euthanasia, and the like, insofar as these are made part of health care agreements. There might be special discounts for signing agreements to limit treatment or be euthanatized. Among the moral advantages of this approach would be that one would not need to be involved in the provision of health care one knew to be immoral. In particular, one would not be taxed to support what one recognizes to be immoral endeavors. Moreover, one could clearly distance oneself from their provision.

These diverse health care packages could in some circumstances be provided in the same building, just as hospitals now have private and semiprivate rooms. In other cases, such moral diversity could be realized in separate facilities. In either case, there could be special criminal and civil law that would protect against health care being provided to patients or in areas where it had by agreement been held to be morally offensive. Thus, for example, those who opposed euthanasia and joined a noneuthanasia health insurance system or sickness fund could be assured against being euthanatized. Those who performed abortions in a

nonabortion hospital could be held criminally and civilly liable.

Outside of communities that share a moral vision, one will need to create policy for the use of common resources. Often this will proceed best through a dialogue among citizens, politicians, and health care experts. In this way, one may be able to fashion a basic package of health care for all citizens. But there will inevitably be different levels of care and different standards. Those who have the resources will demand first-class basic along with supplementary care.

The best example of an open democratic dialogue creating a basic package of health care is what was forwarded as the so-called Oregon Plan. The plan was developed in order to cover all Oregonians below the poverty line. The idea was to decrease the use of high-cost, low-yield interventions in order to provide all indigents with a level of care likely to secure morbidity and mortality relief on a par with that achieved by the basic health care guaranteed in many countries. The hope was to require all employers to provide this minimal package to all their employees. A poll was taken to determine how citizens ranked the various health care services that could be provided. Public meetings were held in forty-seven of the forty-nine counties of Oregon to explore the balancing of interest in different treatments. After all, one must decide whether a basic package of care will cover root-canal work as well as critical care for neonates with birth weights under 500 grams. The plan was clearly committed to multitier health care provision. Providers would not be held criminally or civilly liable for the nonprovision of treatment, if when the treatment was not covered under the basic Oregon Plan they indicated its merit and the need to purchase it privately. Nor would individuals or companies be coercively prevented by state force from buying or selling private basic or luxury health care or health care insurance.

Because federal law and limited effective states' rights constrained the Oregon Plan to address only issues of Medicaid and basic mandated

Principle of Health Care Allocation

People are free to purchase the health care they can buy and to provide the health care others wish to give or to sell.

A. The principle of permission allows persons with common resources to act beneficently by creating a package of health care that can be guaranteed to others, thus creating basic expectations for care and treatment. The principle recognizes the following secular moral constraints:

   1. A private tier of health care is morally unavoidable.
   2. A public or communal tier of health care may, but need not, be created out of communal funds.
   3. There is no canonical, secularly discoverable normative comparison or ranking of health care needs and desires with other needs and desires, or among health care needs and desires; all such orderings or rankings must be created. There is no secularly obligatory rule of rescue that is independent of particular agreement.
   4. Health care in almost all morally defensible circumstances will be multitier so that when a basic package is provided for the indigent, more ample or better quality basic as well as luxury care may be purchased by the affluent.
   5. An all-encompassing, single-payer plan, as has existed in Canada, is morally impermissible because it violates fundamental principles of secular morality. It is in this sense immoral.
   6. Inequalities in health care are morally inescapable because individuals are free and differ in the scope of their needs and resources.
   7. Whether or not they are geographically located, given the limited secular moral authority of large-scale governments spanning pluralist societies, communities (e.g., the Roman Catholic) may develop their autonomous health care systems so that they need not be involved in morally objectionable health care services (e.g., be involved in abortion and euthanasia) and so that such services may be forbidden in their own facilities.

B. Maxim: Give to those who need or desire health care that which they, you, or others are willing to pay for or provide gratis.

---

insurance for employees, and because of the intrusions of the Americans with Disabilities Act (the plan would not have provided neonatal intensive care for newborns with birth-weights under 500 grams, or liver transplants for alcoholics, which omissions were held to be invidiously discriminatory), the Oregon Plan was not allowed to proceed as first envisioned. Still, the plan showed that it was possible for citizens, politicians, and health care experts to enter into a dialogue aimed at creating a basic package of health care without interfering in the rights of individuals to purchase better basic or supplementary care. It laid the basis for an important cultural achievement: recognizing and working within the constraints set by the probabilistic character of health care reality and the limits of moral authority, human life, and human resources.

The Oregon Plan represented a first hesitant and difficult break with the American health care ideology and its regnant deceptions. Understood in this light, the original Oregon Plan had the special virtue of recognizing: (1) the moral inevitability of inequality in health care; (2) the moral necessity of creating the proper character of basic health care packages, rather than discovering their appropriate content; (3) the moral necessity of recognizing the finitude of life and resources and then setting a price on saving life and treating suffering, disability, and deformity; (4) the moral allowability of responding with sympathy and altruism as expressed in the fashioning of a basic health care package from communal resources; (5) the moral challenge of sustaining a secular culture able to gamble with human life and suffering in the face of limited moral authority and vision; and (6) the moral necessity of the limited character of all secular projects, including that of treating disease, disability, and deformity.

Understood most generally, these reflections can be seen as indicating the moral inevitability of the displayed principle in fashioning health care allocations:

The principle of health care allocation does not disclose what concretely is good, proper, praiseworthy, or morally appropriate for individuals to provide to others in need of health care. That can only be discovered within the right community of moral friends.

Conclusions: Creating Rights to Health Care in the Face of Moral Diversity

Particular health care systems with particular guaranteed basic minimums of health care services reflect explicit as well as implicit choices of particular goals and values, rather than others. They involve ranking some goals and values higher, and others lower. In general secular moral terms, the circumstance that patients in one system or tier will be guaranteed care not provided in another, that patients who are salvageable in one system or tier will die in another tier for lack of the same care, is not a testimony to secular moral malfeasance, but to the different powers, fortune, choices, and visions of free men and women. There are limits to our capacity secularly to discover what we ought to do together. There are limits to our secular moral authority to require others to conform to one moral vision or one content-full understanding of justice or fairness.

Our secular moral limitations argue against uniformity in health care packages and in favor of the affirmative acceptance of a diversity of approaches to providing health care. If one takes moral diversity seriously, whether expressed in religious understandings or in desires for augmented or superior care, one will need to tolerate the fashioning of parallel health care systems with diverse basic packages of care. When we meet as moral strangers, we must settle for deciding fairly what we will do together. When we cannot together discover what we ought to do, then we must often agree peaceably to go our own ways. Partially parallel health care systems can allow the segmentation of health care delivery in areas of significant moral disagreement. Our moral differences need not lead us to total separation, but only to parting company in certain areas of health care delivery.

A Conservative Case for Universal Access to Health Care

PAUL MENZEL AND DONALD W. LIGHT

Hastings Center Report 36, no.4 (2006): 36–45.

For decades, the advocates of implementing universal access to needed health care in the United States—the only remaining industrialized country not to provide it—have been talking largely to each other. To them, the arguments for universal access usually seem so obvious that they can hardly believe that tens of millions do not agree. Conservative opposition still prevails, however, especially among powerful leaders in business, health care, and government. To many in this opposition, universal health care would mean something akin to socialism, making people more dependent on hand-outs, expanding the clumsy hand of regulation, and hobbling individual choice.

One of the more striking aspects of this continued opposition to universal health care in the United States is that conservative parties in every other industrialized country, while they often criticize certain features of the particular form that universal access takes in their country, nonetheless support it. There is disagreement about what exactly conservatism means for this basic question in health policy. At a fundamental philosophical level it would seem that either American conservatives are wrong, or conservatives elsewhere are. And so we are drawn to ask: what really *are* the implications of conservative values for universal health care?

We will argue emphatically that a strong case exists for universal access to basic care that is politically and morally conservative. It is conservative because it is based on values that conservatives share and emphasize—the values of being able to take care of oneself and others, preventing irresponsible free-riding, and alleviating the inefficiency, waste, and other weaknesses that limit business and entrepreneurial activity. Access to medical services, regardless of income, is as necessary to individual freedom, opportunity, and self-responsibility as is access to the protective services of fire or police departments. In a voluntary system, employers who do not arrange insurance for their employees, as well as many individuals who do not insure themselves, irresponsibly free-ride on the unintended largesse of others. When roughly 40 percent of all employers do not participate in this "system," when only 61 percent of American workers receive insurance through their employers, and when over three thousand people a day lose their existing health insurance, the practical extent of this compromise of conservative values is hardly minor.

Do typical U.S. conservatives, however, really oppose universal access? Many of them, too, object to a situation in which forty-five million residents are uninsured and talk of universal "access" as something that they would like to achieve. Conservative spokespersons certainly laud voluntary efforts, often boosted by financial incentives from government, to expand coverage in the population. Numerous publications from conservative think tanks such as the Heritage Foundation and the Galen Institute, for example, urge converting the current regressive, employment-based, unlimited taxable income exclusion to a fixed, universal tax credit that can be applied to the purchase of insurance by anyone, even when their tax level is less than the tax credit. While such proposals may sound like "universal access," however, conservative politicians are seldom its advocates in a realistic sense. They usually oppose any sort of compulsory, government-mandated insurance, and even conservative institute publications typically do not mention the question of mandating insurance. Only a very few have supported a requirement that everyone be insured. If conservatives are generally unwilling to enact a requirement that everyone be insured, coverage will remain far less than universal. Opposition to the mandating of insurance is just opposition to effective universal access.

Conservatism, Here and Elsewhere

The contrast between the conservative support for real universal access elsewhere and opposition to it in the United States can perhaps be best seen initially in economic terms. Even if an argument focused on consumer choice and liberty could justify opposition to universal access, from an economic and business point of view the opposition is strange. Foreign competitors get medical benefits for all their workers at little more than half the cost, while American employers are weighed down by ever-growing costs for health care. In a global competitive environment, companies like Nokia, Toyota, and Siemens, for example, enjoy a significant competitive advantage over their American competitors, Motorola, Ford, and GE.

It is thus easy to see the practical basis of support from conservatives and business executives abroad for universal access to basic care. It minimizes costs and waste and increases economic growth by raising worker productivity, lowering labor costs, and allowing employers to focus on their business. Clinicians, too, are relieved from spending time and money coping with an ever-changing complex of coverages, forms, and unpaid bills. In the United States, by contrast, large secondary and questionably efficient industries have arisen around a voluntary, competitive health insurance and health care system in order to manage its administrative complexity. Health care plans design and market thousands of different policies, helping companies minimize coverage of high-risk people but resulting in an inequitable, costly, and fragmented system that compromises the choice and freedom of those with the greatest risk and need.

Do the reasons for conservative support for universal access to basic health care in other developed countries reflect mere pragmatism, or do they also reflect some central values espoused by political conservatism? We believe they reflect both. To see this one needs to understand three things: (1) something about the essential nature of political and moral conservatism, (2) the relationship of health care to self-care and individual responsibility for others, and (3) the objectionable nature of free-riding.

Consider the spirit of conservatism first. Unlike reactionary ideologies that more indiscriminately resist change, conservatism is usually defined not as a doctrine, but as a cautious, pragmatic predisposition toward change. While it typically opposes drastic change—and is cautious about any change—its caution is essentially pragmatic. Orthodoxy defends existing institutions as legitimate simply because they exist; conservativism "defends existing institutions because their very existence creates a presumption that they have served some useful function." That presumption can be overcome, however, especially when an existing institution begins to conflict with specific conservative values.

This essential pragmatism of the conservative outlook has eventually led most conservatives in every other industrialized country to support universal access to basic health care. As would be expected from an essentially pragmatic conservative approach, universal access gets provided in those countries in a variety of different ways. Arguably, in any of its forms, universal health care helps to contain costs.

The Ability to Take Care of Oneself and Immediate Others

Conservatives' wariness of government power is based in part on the belief that "individuals should make their own way in the world." A common conservative argument against "government health insurance" is thus that people should take care of themselves. Paradoxically, however, this belief also forms an argument *for* universal health insurance: people need universal access to basic health care in order to maximize their ability to care for themselves. When people are ill, individual liberty and personal responsibility are quickly compromised. Even small disorders like mild depression or a bad back can turn liberty and responsibility into dependency. For the chronically or seriously ill, medical care can become a great financial burden. Losses in wages and earned income make matters even worse, particularly when able-bodied citizens can no longer care for themselves and their dependents. Medical bankruptcy is virtually unknown in the rest of the developed world, but it is quite common in the United States. Forty percent of U.S. personal bankruptcies are attributed to medical bills people are unable to pay. Out-of-pocket costs that total 10 percent or more of household income are not uncommon, especially among the working class. This can hardly be an attractive picture of a workforce for American business.

Financial losses and threats to one's wellbeing that hobble or cripple individual freedom, opportunity, and responsibility are among the major reasons why most conservatives support public police and fire departments. These same arguments, however, also apply to health care. Many common illnesses and injuries are just as incapacitating or threatening to individual opportunities and responsibility as being robbed or having one's home catch fire. Basic protections are necessary to provide everyone opportunities to improve their lives. These typically include services for fire protection, police protection, and education. American conservatives seem unique among their peers in the West in not adding basic medical services to this short list.

Irresponsible Free-Riding

Another important value that conservatives ordinarily emphasize, the irresponsibility of free-riding, has rarely been raised in the debates about the 45 million Americans who do not have health insurance and the many more whose employers choose policies that leave large portions of bills for serious diseases uncovered. Inadequate or no coverage typically leaves uncovered bills to be paid by others, but letting *others* pay for the consequences is tacit endorsement of free-riding. Sometimes free-riders, in exercising their individual choice, claim to be "conservative," but they are abusing the label by doing that. Serious conservatives regard themselves as responsible for the effects of their behavior on others when they exercise choice.

Perhaps U.S. political conservatives simply do not recognize how much free-riding is built into and rewarded by a voluntary system of insurance. In 2001 the uninsured used $98.9 billion in health care, $34.5 billion of which was "uncompensated"—paid for neither out-of-pocket by the uninsured nor by any discrete source of private or public insurance. In a major 2005 report using a cautious estimation method, Families USA calculated that $43 billion of the care that the uninsured received was "uncompensated," with $29 billion of that cost-shifted to those who pay higher premiums for private health insurance. As a result, private insurance premiums are 8.5 percent higher than they would otherwise be, adding $922 to the annual cost of family health insurance provided by private employers. The thousands of employers who do not offer health insurance or offer only thin coverage, as well as the millions of individuals who choose not to buy coverage, cause this cost-shifting.

To make matters worse, a vicious cycle then unfolds. When people go without insurance, premiums rise for the less healthy who are more likely to stay insured, exacerbated by the fact that they end up paying many of the cost-shifted expenses of other sick patients who are uninsured and underinsured. In turn, these rising premiums lead even more people to drop out, causing premiums to rise still more for those who remain. Then still more people drop insurance, causing an even higher increment in insurance premiums to cover cost-shifted, uncompensated care. This cycle, combined with increases in health care costs that are already outstripping inflation and increases in real income, leads to "an actuarial disaster in the making" that increasingly renders health insurance unaffordable to the working classes.

Much of the cost of the rising volume of care for the uninsured will continue to be borne by others. This will inevitably happen in any moral culture where a rescue ethic trumps other values when health care providers encounter uninsured patients with serious medical needs. To be sure, such cost-shifting could be avoided if providers steeled themselves and simply did not provide care to the uninsured who land on their doorsteps. While such a response may be theoretically conceivable, it is hardly an option that political conservatives have chosen. They, too, have supported the "antidumping" legislation that requires hospitals to treat even the uninsured in emergency situations, and many politically conservative physicians are proud to be among those who provide considerable care to patients who cannot realistically be expected to pay their bills. Thus, most uninsured patients still get treated for many conditions (although often, of course, in nonideal situations such as emergency rooms). The costs get shifted to the individuals and employers who pay higher premiums, or to the hospitals and physicians who are forced to decide how hard they want to work without pay.

The anti-free-riding principle that holds cost-shifting objectionable is based on larger conservative values about individual responsibility. These apply to the cost-shifting and free-riding inherent in a voluntary health insurance system. The same phenomena have led to making auto liability insurance mandatory, a development apparently accepted by conservatives to correct an analogous instance of free-riding—drivers who go without liability insurance and shift costs for their negligence onto other drivers who then feel compelled to purchase "uninsured motorist" insurance. The situation that free-riding creates in health care should similarly lead U.S. conservatives to support mandatory health insurance.

Mandatory health insurance is part of an "ordered liberty" within the state that enhances people's ability to take care of themselves and immediate others and does not tolerate free-riding. Mandatory insurance corrects for the ruinous market failures of voluntary private health insurance and supports a conservative conception of liberty. Conservatives in other western nations apparently think so; U.S. conservatives should, too.

Other Conservative Problems with Voluntary Insurance

Beyond these flaws in voluntary health insurance—to allow free-riding and submit millions to the risk of losing their life savings—other problems may attract conservatives to mandatory insurance and thus universal access: barriers to self-employment; highly risk-segmented insurance markets that provide the least coverage to those who most need insurance and increase the wastefulness of the huge variety of market generated plans; and difficulties in cost control.

In political argument conservatives often claim that any needs-based, restoration-of-capacity argument cited for universal access confuses health *care* with health care *insurance*. They argue that illness, accident, and disease reduce people's ability to take care of themselves and others, but that insurance to protect against these hazards is an individual choice and should be left to free exchange in an open competitive market. Such a claim, however, needs to reckon with the inherent limitations of voluntary, competitive insurance in carrying out its principal function of helping seriously ill individuals regain their capacities to take care of themselves. Reports routinely describe forms of "disinsurance" through higher deductibles, larger copayments, and more limits on services covered.

In any case, the market for individual insurance policies is so affected by the risk aversion of insurance companies that individuals often cannot find coverage at a remotely affordable price. The resultant effect on people who want to be self-employed—a portion of the population often esteemed by conservatives—is one of the most sinister aspects of a voluntary insurance market. Self-employed entrepreneurs discover that "even affluence and good health may not matter when you shop for health insurance." Conservatives' strong support for entrepreneurship should leave them up in arms about this damaging aspect of a voluntary insurance market.

In a voluntary health insurance market, the most effective way for companies to compete is to minimize coverage for higher-risk persons or conditions—precisely those who most need coverage to restore their individual capacities. Competitive voluntary insurance follows the inverse coverage law: the more that people need coverage, the more they have to pay for it and the less likely they are to get it. Selective marketing, exclusion clauses, waiting periods, coverage caps, rapid policy switching ("churning"), claims harassment, and risk-based premiums are among the techniques that insurers in a voluntary competitive system have developed and refined. If even a few insurers use them, others must follow or lose market share. All these techniques increase the personal expense for people with disabilities and disease, who then suffer the double burden of limited ability to work, as well as uncovered medical bills and higher premiums. Employers are often partners in participating in these techniques and have shifted an increasing portion of their health cost increases to employees. The result is that those with greater need and modest income are forced to use up their savings and impoverish themselves. If we want to enhance the capacity of individuals to be self-sufficient and to exercise choice and responsibility, we need a health insurance system that does not discourage coverage of those who most need it.

The fact that the market rewards niche strategies and isolating segmentation also helps to explain why voluntary health insurance becomes wasteful. A study of the mature market in the

Seattle area, for example, found that a sample of 2,277 people were covered by 755 different policies linked to 189 different health care plans. The expense of designing, marketing, and servicing so many policies and of establishing and operating so many plans, all of which claim to be "better" than the others, only benefits those who profit from private health insurance with its seven times greater overhead than Medicare. The $420 billion (31 percent!) paid for managing, marketing, and profiting from the current fragmented system could be drastically cut and the difference used either to pay for medical costs of the underinsured or uninsured or to keep the profits of companies and the savings of individuals from being drained.

Voluntary health insurance increases costs in an even larger way when compared with more structured frameworks for universal health care. Universal health care helps control costs by providing a common structure of basic benefits and financing that can more easily be used to minimize duplication, unnecessary procedures, and price inflation. Even the largest corporations in the United States cannot manage the dynamics of supply-induced demand; excessive, unnecessary tests and procedures; pricing structure; and the introduction of new technology that is at best marginally better but much more expensive. Costs still need to be contained, but in a voluntary insurance arrangement, the levers of downward pressure on utilization, supply, use of capital, and prices are relatively weak. Many employers feel they are getting poor value and being blamed for problems not of their making. They are right. With properly structured universal health insurance, the charges for a CAT scan, a prescription, a day in the hospital, or a general check-up would drop closer to Western European levels.

Reasons for Continued Opposition

So why do most political conservatives in the United States, including many business leaders, continue to defend an unraveling system?

For one thing, there is probably more general repugnance in the United States toward government. Most conservatives outside the United States are wary of government, too, but they have more readily recognized that fair choice is possible only in a fair system. Thus they have come to regard their society's arrangements to assure universal access to health care as justified in order to foster fair opportunity, individual freedom, and a more productive society, while their U.S. counterparts focus more on the fear that universal access will lead to a uniform, government-run, one-size-fits-all health plan that restricts patient choices. Conservatives in other countries know what many American conservatives seem not to believe—that most universal health insurance makes considerable use of private care and provides a good deal of choice.

Related to the U.S. conservative fear of one-size-fits-all is a wider fear of rationing that is also shared by many liberals. But that fear, too, is misconceived if translated into continued opposition to universal access to basic care. Rationing is at least as extensive in our competitive voluntary system through the inverse coverage law and managed care. In nonuniversal systems, rationing is built into competition in myriad ways that are seldom acknowledged. The public framework provided by universal access enables individuals to voice their preferences and concerns so that limits to services can be set through a fair process. This helps to make limits on care reflect people's own values when faced with scarce resources. In a voluntary market, executive and corporate decisions to ration usually take place behind closed doors and often result in plans chosen specifically to keep members from knowing what their policies do not cover.

Political conservatives typically hold a different conception of what equity demands in regard to the distribution of income and wealth. They tend to tolerate and defend a wider spectrum of distribution than liberals do, and they are much more suspicious of redistribution. Insofar as taxation for the support of universal access to basic health care is seen as another "redistribution," conservatives are inclined to oppose it.

First, though, conservatives need to compare such a basis for opposition carefully with their endorsement of taxation for other needs such as police and fire departments and education. If the protection of responsibility for self and others, the prevention of free-riding, and the efficiency of collective provision is persuasive enough for conservatives to support universal provision of these other three goods without seeing them as "redistribution," why do the same considerations not lead conservatives to support universal access to health care?

Another objection often voiced by conservatives of a more academic stripe concerns the inefficiency of so-called "moral hazard." Any good provided to a user when the full expense is not paid by the user runs the danger of being used in excess, past the point where the real benefit of investing further resources in it is equal to the real gains in human welfare that can be achieved by alternative investments. In health care, this means overinsurance—insurance coverage for care beyond an efficient level. This kind of efficiency objection is certainly germane to decisions about the scope of care that universal access should encompass, but it is a weak reason for objecting to bringing the forty-five million people in the United States who are currently uninsured under some sort of basic coverage. Is moral hazard going to characterize the amount of insurance that would be mandated or provided *for them*? If conservatives think that it will, why do they not favor demolishing existing Medicare and Medicaid programs? And why have not moral hazard objections led conservatives to try to rescind the taxable income exclusion for employer-paid insurance? This last question is not hard to answer, though: without some sizable incentive such as this taxable income exclusion, the ranks of the uninsured would grow by leaps and bounds, utterly demolishing conservative hopes that voluntary insurance can do a reasonably good job of covering the population.

A crucial political factor is undoubtedly the power of U.S. insurance companies. U.S. conservatives, as supportive as they are of private business, are reticent to do what is seen by most insurance companies as severely bridling their activities in any fairly regulated framework for universal access, even one that would preserve a significant role for private insurance. Perhaps, on this score, the explanation of the differing views of U.S. and other conservatives is that in other countries, private health insurance plans have historically had a shorter tenure before a framework for universal access was enacted. Or perhaps it is that U.S. conservatives are less willing to look at the overall effects of a whole health care system on business activity in general and more willing to listen to the cries of particular well-heeled portions of the private sector, such as insurance.

What Could Make Conservative Support Feasible?

Regardless of its many actual varieties, no universal access to basic care can be accomplished except by a mixture of insurance mandate and insurance subsidy. To many in the United States, the prospect of enough conservative support to accomplish the actual adoption of some such mixture seems daunting.

To be sure, any such development will require ingenuity, savvy, persistence, political fence-mending and compromise, and no doubt simply the sheer luck of a rare combination of events and forces that congeal at a particular moment of history. The current decade of Republican and conservative ascendancy may hardly seem encouraging. But then again, in mid-2005, *Fortune* magazine (of all places) published an article headlined "Socialized Medicine? From Republicans?" The author, Matt Miller, surmised that business's woes about health insurance, driven in part by international competition, are getting so intense that it is Republicans who will start carrying the ball for universal coverage. Business executives are beginning to realize how untenable today's system is. For them, says Miller, the attractions of greater cost certainty and a level playing field (another way of saying "no free-riding") provided by universal access may be getting to the point where they tip the balance of opinion.

Perhaps, in fact, something like this vision has already come to some fruition in one U.S. state. On April 3, 2006, the Massachusetts legislature passed legislation predicted to extend coverage to 95 percent of the state's residents currently without health insurance. While not strictly mandating that everyone be insured, both individuals and businesses will pay financial penalties for failing to obtain insurance. In addition to providing pooling mechanisms and subsidies to make insurance to the uninsured more affordable, supporters of the plan invoke the responsibility of people who can afford insurance to get it. Republican Governor Mitt Romney pushed the idea of the "individual mandate" to require those who can afford insurance to buy it. While the legislation does not actually mandate insurance, after 2007 the penalties for those who do not insure are estimated to grow to half the cost of an affordable premium.

For a fertile political setting to emerge from such reconceived business interests, it will be important that political conservatives grasp the *moral* case that can be made for universal access on philosophical terms that *they share*. The chances of this occurring are diminished if liberals, who have thought and spoken to universal access out of deep moral conviction for so long, insult their conservative counterparts by implicitly assuming that the case for universal access to basic care cannot be based on conservative moral values. That moral case exists in a powerful form, ready to be made by conservatives themselves. If articulated, it would be an important component among many factors, including business self-interest, that could combine to create significantly greater political pressure for universal access.

One of the constructive developments that could emerge if political conservatives make their own constructive moral case for universal access is the opening of a serious dialogue that would help liberals break some of their preconceptions about what is involved in moving toward universal access. If hope for universal access in the United States is ever to bloom, political and moral imagination aplenty will be needed on all sides. Already, however, we can imagine that a fair plan for universal access embraceable by both liberals and conservatives would have the following features:[1]

1) Everyone is provided access to needed health care. The fact that one has insurance for basic, needed care should not depend on one's "insurance risk" or health condition.
2) Nonfinancial barriers by class, language, education, and geography are minimized.
3) Decisions about all matters are open and publicly debated. Accountability for costs, quality, and the value of providers, suppliers, and administrators is public.
4) Administrative overhead, markups, and overtreatment are minimized.
5) Self-responsibility, prevention, strong primary care, and public health are emphasized to maximize people's ability to exercise their freedom, choice, and responsibility.
6) Individuals will still have considerable discretion to buy up to more expensive coverage and intensive services than the services to which universal access is guaranteed.
7) Providers are paid fairly and equitably for treating any patient.

It is time for American conservatives to add health care to fire and police services as minimum government services needed to enable individuals to thrive at minimum financial cost. The question for conservative leaders who deplore wasted human potential, free-riding, financial waste, and inefficiency is not whether they can support universal access to needed health care. It is how they *cannot* support universal access without betraying their own values.

Note

1. N. Daniels, D.W. Light, and R. Carson, *Benchmarks of Fairness for Health Care Reform* (New York: Oxford University Press, 1996).

Illegal Immigrants, Health Care, and Social Responsibility

JAMES DWYER

Hastings Center Report 34, no. 5 (2004): 34–41.

Illegal immigrants form a large and disputed group in many countries. Indeed, even the name is in dispute. People in this group are referred to as illegal immigrants, illegal aliens, irregular migrants, undocumented workers, or, in French, as *sans papiers*. Whatever they are called, their existence raises an important ethical question: Do societies have an ethical responsibility to provide health care for them and to promote their health?

This question often elicits two different answers. Some people—call them nationalists—say that the answer is obviously no. They argue that people who have no right to be in a country should not have rights to benefits in that country. Other people—call them humanists—say that the answer is obviously yes. They argue that all people should have access to health care. It's a basic human right.

I think both these answers are off the mark. The first focuses too narrowly on what we owe people based on legal rules and formal citizenship. The other answer focuses too broadly, on what we owe people qua human beings. We need a perspective that is in between, that adequately responds to the phenomenon of illegal immigration and adequately reflects the complexity of moral thought. There may be important ethical distinctions, for example, among the following groups: U.S. citizens who lack health insurance, undocumented workers who lack health insurance in spite of working full time, medical visitors who fly to the United States as tourists in order to obtain care at public hospitals, foreign citizens who work abroad for subcontractors of American firms, and foreign citizens who live in impoverished countries. I believe that we—U.S. citizens—have ethical duties in all of these situations, but I see important differences in what

these duties demand and how they are to be explained.

In this paper, I want to focus on the situation of illegal immigrants. I will discuss several different answers to the question about what ethical responsibility we have to provide health care to illegal immigrants. (I shall simply assume that societies have an ethical obligation to provide their own citizens with a reasonably comprehensive package of health benefits.) The answers that I shall discuss tend to conceptualize the ethical issues in terms of individual desert, professional ethics, or human rights. I want to discuss the limitations of each of these approaches and to offer an alternative. I shall approach the issues in terms of social responsibility and discuss the moral relevance of work. In doing so, I tend to pull bioethics in the direction of social ethics and political philosophy. That's the direction I think it should be heading. But before I begin the ethical discussion, I need to say more about the phenomenon of illegal immigration.

Human Migration

People have always moved around. They have moved for political, environmental, economic, and familial reasons. They have tried to escape war, persecution, discrimination, famine, environmental degradation, poverty, and a variety of other problems. They have tried to find places to build better lives, earn more money, and provide better support for their families. A strong sense of family responsibility has always been an important factor behind migration.

But while human migration is not new, *illegal* immigration is, since only recently have nation-states tried to control and regulate the flow of immigration. Societies have always tried to exclude people they viewed as undesirable: criminals, people unable to support themselves, people with contagious diseases, and certain ethnic or racial groups. But only in the last hundred years or so have states tried in a systematic way to control the number and kinds of immigrants.

Modern attempts to control residency are not remarkably effective. There are illegal immigrants residing and working all over the globe. When people think about illegal immigrants, they tend to focus on Mexicans in the United States or North-Africans in France. But the phenomenon is really much more diverse and complex. Illegal immigrants come from hundreds of countries and go wherever they can get work. There are undocumented workers from Indonesia in Malaysia, undocumented workers from Haiti in the Dominican Republic, and undocumented workers from Myanmar in Thailand. Thailand is an interesting example because it is both a source of and a destination for undocumented workers: while many people from poorer countries have gone to work in Thailand, many Thais have gone to work in richer countries.

I believe that a sound ethical response to the question of illegal immigration requires some understanding of the work that illegal immigrants do. Most undocumented workers do the jobs that citizens often eschew. They do difficult and disagreeable work at low wages for small firms in the informal sector of the economy. In general, they have the worst jobs and work in the worst conditions in such sectors of the economy as agriculture, construction, manufacturing, and the food industry. They pick fruit, wash dishes, move dirt, sew clothes, clean toilets.

In the global economy, in which a company can shift its manufacturing base with relative ease to a country with cheaper labor, illegal immigrants often perform work that cannot be shifted overseas. Toilets have to be cleaned, dishes have to be washed, and children have to be watched *locally*. This local demand may help to explain a relatively new trend: the feminization of migration. Migrants used to be predominantly young men, seeking work in areas such as agriculture

and construction. But that pattern is changing. More and more women migrants are employed in the service sector as, for example, maids, nannies, and health care aides.

Women migrants are also employed as sex workers. The connection between commercial sex and illegal immigration is quite striking. As women in some societies have more money, choices, schooling, and power, they are unwilling to work as prostitutes. These societies seem to be supplying their demands for commercial sex by using undocumented workers from poorer countries.

Even when prostitution is voluntary, it is difficult and dangerous. And for some illegal immigrants, prostitution is not a voluntary choice. Some are deceived and delivered into prostitution. Others are coerced, their lives controlled by pimps, criminal gangs, and human traffickers.

Some of the worst moral offenses occur in the trafficking of human beings, but even here it is important to see a continuum of activities. Sometimes traffickers simply provide transportation in exchange for payment. Sometimes, they recruit people with deceptive promises and false accounts of jobs, then transport them under horrible and dangerous conditions. If and when the immigrants arrive in the destination country, they are controlled by debt, threat, and force. Some become indentured servants, working without pay for a period of time. Others are controlled by physical threats or threats to expose their illegal status. A few are enslaved and held as property.

Not all illegal immigrants are victims, however, and an accurate account of illegal immigration, even if only sketched, must capture some of its complexity. My task is to consider how well different ethical frameworks deal with that complexity.

A Matter of Desert

The abstract ethical question of whether societies have a responsibility to provide health care for illegal immigrants sometimes becomes a concrete political issue. Rising health care costs, budget reduction programs, and feelings of resentment sometimes transform the ethical question into a political debate. This has happened several times in the United States. In 1996, the Congress debated and passed the "Illegal Immigration Reform and Immigrant Responsibility Act." This law made all immigrants ineligible for Medicaid, although it did allow the federal government to reimburse states for emergency treatment of illegal immigrants.

In 1994, the citizens of California debated Proposition 187, an even more restrictive measure. This ballot initiative proposed to deny publicly funded health care, social services, and education to illegal immigrants. This law would have required publicly funded health care facilities to deny care, except in medical emergencies, to people who could not prove that they were U.S. citizens or legal residents.

This proposition was approved by 59 percent of the voters. It was never implemented because courts found that parts of it conflicted with other laws, but the deepest arguments for and against it remain very much alive. Because they will probably surface again, at a different time or in different place, it is worthwhile evaluating the ethical frameworks that they assume.

The first argument put forward is that illegal aliens should be denied public benefits because they are in the country illegally. Although it is true that illegal aliens have violated a law by entering or remaining in the country, it is not clear what the moral implication of this point is. Nothing about access to health care follows from the mere fact that illegal aliens have violated a law. Many people break many different laws. Whether a violation of a law should disqualify people from public services probably depends on the nature and purpose of the services, the nature and the gravity of the violation, and many other matters.

Consider one example of a violation of the law. People sometimes break tax laws by working off the books. They do certain jobs for cash in order to avoid paying taxes or losing benefits. Moreover, this practice is probably well quite

common. I recently asked students in two of my classes if they or anyone in their extended family had earned money that was not reported as taxable income. In one class, all but two students raised their hands. In the other class, every hand went up.

No one has suggested that health care facilities deny care to people suspected of working off the books. But undocumented work is also a violation of the law. Furthermore, it involves an issue of fairness because it shifts burdens onto others and diminishes funding for important purposes. Of course, working off the books and working without a visa are not alike in all respects. But without further argument, nothing much follows about whether it is right to deny benefits to people who have violated a law.

Proponents of restrictive measures also appeal to an argument that combines a particular conception of desert with the need to make trade-offs. Proponents of California's Proposition 187 stated that, "while our own citizens and legal residents go wanting, those who chose to enter our country ILLEGALLY get royal treatment at the expense of the California taxpayer." Proponents noted that the legislature maintained programs that included free prenatal care for illegal aliens but increased the amount that senior citizens must pay for prescription drugs. They then asked, "Why should we give more comfort and consideration to illegal aliens than to *our* own needy American citizens?"

The rhetorical question is part of the argument. I would restate the argument in the following way: Given the limited public budget for health care, U.S. citizens and legal residents are more deserving of benefits than are illegal aliens. This argument frames the issue as a choice between competing goods in a situation of limited resources.

There is something right and something wrong about this way of framing the issue. What is right is the idea that in all of life, individual and political, we have to choose between competing goods. A society cannot have everything: comprehensive and universal health care, good public schools, extensive public parks and beaches, public services, and very low taxes. What is false is the idea that we have to choose between basic health care for illegal aliens and basic health care for citizens. Many other trade-offs are possible, including an increase in public funding.

The narrow framework of the debate pits poor citizens against illegal aliens in a battle for health care resources. Within this framework, the issue is posed as one of desert. Avoiding the idea of desert is impossible. After all, justice is a matter of giving people their due—giving them what they deserve. But a narrow conception of desert seems most at home in allocating particular goods that go beyond basic needs, in situations where the criteria of achievement and effort are very clear. For example, if we are asked to give an award for the best student in chemistry, a narrow notion of desert is appropriate and useful. But publicly funded health care is different and requires a broader view of desert.

The discussion of restrictive measures often focuses on desert, taxation, and benefits. Proponents tend to picture illegal immigrants as free riders who are taking advantage of public services without contributing to public funding. Opponents are quick to note that illegal immigrants do pay taxes. They pay sales tax, gas tax, and value-added tax. They often pay income tax and property tax. But do they pay enough tax to cover the cost of the services they use? Or more generally, are illegal immigrants a net economic gain or a net economic loss for society?

Instead of trying to answer the economic question, I want to point out a problem with the question itself. The question about taxation and benefits tends to portray society as a private business venture. On the business model, investors should benefit in proportion to the funds they put into the venture. This may be an appropriate model for some business ventures, but it is not an adequate model for all social institutions and benefits. The business model is not an adequate model for thinking about voting, legal defense, library services, minimum wages, occupational safety, and many other social benefits.

Consider my favorite social institution: the public library. The important question here is not whether some people use more library services than they pay for through taxation, which is obviously true. Some people pay relatively high taxes but never use the library, while others pay relatively low taxes but use the library quite often. In thinking about the public library, we should consider questions such as the following. What purposes does the library serve? Does it promote education, provide opportunity, and foster public life? Does it tend to ameliorate or exacerbate social injustice? Given the library's purposes, who should count as its constituents or members? And what are the rights and responsibilities of the library users? In the following sections, I shall consider analogous questions about illegal immigrants and the social institutions that promote health.

A Matter of Professional Ethics

Some of the most vigorous responses to restrictive measures have come from those who consider the issue within the framework of professional ethics. Tal Ann Ziv and Bernard Lo, for example, argue that "cooperating with Proposition 187 would undermine professional ethics."[1] In particular, they argue that cooperating with this kind of restrictive measure is inconsistent with physicians' "ethical responsibilities to protect the public health, care for persons in medical need, and respect patient confidentiality."

Restrictive measures may indeed have adverse effects on the public health. For example, measures that deny care to illegal aliens, or make them afraid to seek care, could lead to an increase in tuberculosis. And physicians do have a professional obligation to oppose measures that would significantly harm the public health. But the public health argument has a serious failing, if taken by itself. It avoids the big issue of whether illegal immigrants should be considered part of the public and whether public institutions should serve their health needs. Instead of appealing to an inclusive notion of social justice, the argument suggests how the health of illegal immigrants may influence citizens' health, and then appeals to citizens' sense of prudence. The appeal to prudence is not wrong, but it avoids the larger ethical issues.

The second argument against Proposition 187 is that it restricts confidentiality in ways that are not justified. It requires health care facilities to report people suspected of being in the country illegally and to disclose additional information to authorities. Ziv and Lo argue that "Proposition 187 fails to provide the usual ethical justifications for overriding patient confidentiality." Thus this restriction on confidentiality is a serious violation of professional ethics.

But if restrictive measures work as designed, issues of confidentiality may not even arise. Illegal aliens will be deterred from seeking medical care or will be screened out before they see a doctor. Thus the issue of screening may be more important than the issue of confidentiality. First, if the screening is carried out, it should not be by physicians, because it is not their role to act as agents for the police or the immigration service. Professional ethics requires some separation of social roles, and terrible things have happened when physicians have become agents of political regimes. The bigger issue, though, is not who should do the screening, but whether it should be done at all.

Ziv and Lo argue that physicians bear some responsibility for arrangements that conflict with professional ethics. In their view, screening out illegal aliens conflicts with physicians' ethical responsibility to "care for persons in medical need."

This claim is important, but ambiguous. It could mean simply that physicians have an obligation to attend to anyone who presents to them in need of emergency care. That seems right. It would be wrong not to stabilize and save someone in a medical emergency. It would be inhumane, even morally absurd, to let someone die because her visa had expired. But a claim that physicians have an enduring obligation to provide emergency care is consistent with measures like Proposition 187 and the 1996 federal law.

The claim might also mean that the selection of patients should be based only on medical need, never on such factors as nationality, residency, immigration status, or ability to pay. This is a very strong claim. It means that all private practice is morally wrong. It means that most national health care systems are too restrictive. It means that transplant lists for organs donated in a particular country should be open to everyone in the world. It might even mean that physicians have an ethical responsibility to relocate to places where the medical need is the greatest. This claim goes well beyond professional ethics. It is an ethical claim that seems to be based on a belief about the nature of human needs and human rights.

Finally, Ziv and Lo's claim about physicians' responsibility to care for people in medical need might be stronger than the claim about emergency care but weaker than the universal claim. Perhaps we should interpret it to mean that it is wrong to turn patients away when society has no other provisions and institutions to provide them with basic care. The idea then is that society should provide all members with basic health care and that physicians have some responsibility to work to realize this idea.

There is something appealing and plausible about this interpretation, but it too goes beyond professional ethics. It has more to do with the nature of social justice and social institutions than with the nature of medical practice. It makes an ethical claim based on a belief about social responsibility and an assumption that illegal aliens are to be counted as members of society. I shall try to elaborate this belief and assumption later.

Let me sum up my main points so far. Political measures that restrict medical care for illegal immigrants often involve violations of professional ethics, and health care professionals should oppose such measures. But the framework of professional ethics is not adequate for thinking about the larger ethical issues. It fails to illuminate the obligation to provide medical care. Furthermore, it fails to consider factors such as work and housing that may have a profound impact on health. In the next two sections I shall consider broader frameworks and discourses.

A Matter of Human Rights

To deal with the issue of health care and illegal immigrants, some adopt a humanistic framework and employ a discourse of human rights. They tend to emphasize the right of all human beings to medical treatment, as well as the common humanity of aliens and citizens, pointing to the arbitrary nature of national borders.

National borders can seem arbitrary. Distinctions based on national borders seem even more arbitrary when one studies how borders were established and the disparities in wealth and health that exist between countries. Since it doesn't seem just that some people should be disadvantaged by arbitrary boundaries, it may also seem that people should have the right to emigrate from wherever they are and to immigrate to wherever they wish. But does this follow from the fact that national borders can be seen as arbitrary?

Even if boundaries depend on historical circumstances, a defined territory may allow a people to form a government that acts as their agent in a fair and effective way. A defined territory may allow a people to form a government that enables them to take responsibility for the natural environment, promote the well-being of the human population, deal with social problems, and cultivate just political institutions.

From functions like these, governments derive a qualified right to regulate immigration. This right is not an unlimited right of communal self-determination. Societies do not have a right to protect institutions and ways of life that are deeply unjust. Furthermore, even when a society has a right to regulate immigration, there are ethical questions about whether and how the society should exercise that right. And there are ethical questions about how immigrants should be treated in that society.

Of course, the humanist need not be committed to an abstract position about open borders.

The humanist might accept that states have a qualified right to regulate immigration, but insist that all states must respect the human rights of all immigrants—legal and illegal. That idea makes a lot of sense, although much depends on how we specify the content of human rights.

The idea that all human beings should have equal access to all beneficial health care is often used to critique both national and international arrangements. In an editorial in the *New England Journal of Medicine*, Paul Farmer reflects on the number of people who go untreated for diseases such as tuberculosis and HIV. He writes:

> Prevention is, of course, always preferable to treatment. But epidemics of treatable infectious diseases should remind us that although science has revolutionized medicine, we still need a plan for ensuring equal access to care. As study after study shows the power of effective therapies to alter the course of infectious disease, we should be increasingly reluctant to reserve these therapies for the affluent, low-incidence regions of the world where most medical resources are concentrated. Excellence without equity looms as the chief human-rights dilemma of health care in the 21st century.[2]

I too am critical of the gross inequalities in health within countries and between countries, but here I only want to make explicit the framework and discourse of Farmer's critique. His critique appeals to two ideas: that there is a lack of proportion between the medical resources and the burden of disease and that there is a human right to equal access.

What is wrong with the claim that equal access to health care is a human right? First, to claim something as a right is more of a conclusion than an argument. Such claims function more to summarize a position than to further moral discussion. A quick and simple appeal to a comprehensive right avoids all the hard questions about duties and priorities. When faced with grave injustices and huge inequalities, claiming that all human beings have a right to health care is easy. Specifying the kind of care to which people are entitled is harder. Specifying duties is harder yet. And getting those duties institutionalized is hardest of all.

In addition to the general problems with claims about rights, a problem more specific to the issue of illegal immigration exists. Since a claim based on a human right is a claim based on people's common humanity, it tends to collapse distinctions between people. Yet for certain purposes, it may be important to make distinctions and emphasize different responsibilities. We may owe different things to, for example, the poor undocumented worker in our country, the middle-class visitor who needs dialysis, the prince who wants a transplant, people enmeshed in the global economy, and the most marginalized people in poor countries.

Rather than claiming an essentially limitless right, it makes more sense to recognize a modest core of human rights and to supplement those rights with a robust account of social responsibility, social justice, and international justice. I do not know if there is a principled way to delineate exactly what should be included in the core of human rights. But even a short list of circumscribed rights would have important consequences if societies took responsibility for trying to protect everyone from violations of these rights.

A Matter of Social Responsibility

Framing the issue in terms of social responsibility helps to highlight one of the most striking features of illegal immigration: the employment pattern within society. As I noted before, illegal immigrants often perform the worst work for the lowest wages. Illegal immigrants are part of a pattern that is older and deeper than the recent globalization of the economy. Societies have often used the most powerless and marginalized people to do the most disagreeable and difficult work. Societies have used slaves, indentured servants, castes, minorities, orphans, poor children, internal migrants, and foreign migrants. Of course, the pattern is not exactly the same in every society, nor even in every industry within a society, but the similarities are striking.

I see the use of illegal immigrants as the contemporary form of the old pattern. But it is not a natural phenomenon beyond human control. It is the result of laws, norms, institutions, habits, and conditions in society, and of the conditions in the world at large. It is a social construction that we could try to reconstruct.

Some might object that no one forces illegal immigrants to take unsavory jobs and that they can return home if they wish. This objection is too simple. Although most undocumented workers made a voluntary choice to go to another country, they often had inadequate information and dismal alternatives, and voluntary return is not an attractive option when they have substantial debts and poor earning potential at home. More importantly, even a fully informed and voluntary choice does not settle the question of social justice and responsibility. We have gone through this debate before. As the industrial revolution developed, many people agreed to work under horrible conditions in shops, factories, and mines. Yet most societies eventually saw that freedom of contract was a limited part of a larger social ethic. They accepted a responsibility to address conditions of work and to empower workers, at least in basic ways. Decent societies now try to regulate child labor, workplace safety, minimum rates of pay, workers' rights to unionize, background conditions, and much more. But because of their illegal status, undocumented workers are often unable to challenge or report employers who violate even the basic standards of a decent society.

We need to take responsibility for preventing the old pattern from continuing, and the key idea is that of "taking responsibility." It is not the same as legal accountability, which leads one to think about determining causation, proving intention or negligence, examining excuses, apportioning blame, and assigning costs. Taking responsibility is more about seeing patterns and problems, examining background conditions, not passing the buck, and responding in appropriate ways. A society need not bear full causal responsibility in order to assume social responsibility.

Why should society take responsibility for people it tried to keep out of its territory, for people who are not social members? Because in many respects illegal immigrants are social members. Although they are not citizens or legal residents, they may be diligent workers, good neighbors, concerned parents, and active participants in community life. They are workers, involved in complex schemes of social cooperation. Many of the most exploited workers in the industrial revolution—children, women, men without property—were also not full citizens, but they were vulnerable people, doing often undesirable work, for whom society needed to take some responsibility. Undocumented workers' similar role in society is one reason that the social responsibility to care for them is different from the responsibility to care for medical visitors.

I can already hear the objection. "What you propose is a perfect recipe for increasing illegal immigration. All the practical measures that you suggest would encourage more illegal immigration." Whether improving the situation of the worst-off workers will increase illegal immigration is a complex empirical question. The answer probably depends on many factors. But even if transforming the worst work and empowering the worst-off workers leads to an increase in illegal immigration, countries should take those steps. Although we have a right to regulate immigration, considerations of justice constrain the ways we can pursue that aim. A society might also decrease illegal immigration by decriminalizing the killing of illegal immigrants, but no one thinks that would be a reasonable and ethical social policy.

I have left out of my account the very point with which I began, namely, health and health care, and I ended up talking about work and social responsibility. Surely work and social responsibility are at the heart of the matter. Where then does health care fit in?

Good health care can, among other things, prevent death and suffering, promote health and well-being, respond to basic needs and vulnerabilities, express care and solidarity, contribute to equality of opportunity, monitor social problems (such as child abuse or pesticide exposure), and accomplish other important aims. But health care is just one means, and not always the most effective means, to these ends. To focus on access to and payment of health care is to focus our ethical concern too narrowly.

I believe that societies that attract illegal immigrants should pursue policies and practices that (1) improve the pay for and conditions of the worst forms of work; (2) structure and organize work so as to give workers more voice, power, and opportunity to develop their capacities; and (3) connect labor to unions, associations, and communities in ways that increase social respect for all workers. I cannot justify these claims in this paper, but I want to note how they are connected to health care. Providing health care for all workers and their families is a very good way to improve the benefit that workers receive for the worst forms of work, to render workers less vulnerable, and to express social and communal respect for them. These are good reasons for providing health care for all workers, documented and undocumented alike. And they express ethical concerns that are not captured by talking about human rights, public health, or the rights of citizens.

Notes

1. T.A. Ziv and B. Lo, "Denial of Care to Illegal Immigrants," *New England Journal of Medicine* 332 (1995).
2. P. Farmer, "The Major Infectious Diseases in the World–To Treat or Not to Treat?" *New England Journal of Medicine* 345 (2001): 208–10.

Should Physicians Be Gatekeepers of Medical Resources?

MILTON C. WEINSTEIN

Journal of Medical Ethics 27 (2001): 268–74.

The Medical Commons

Resources available for health care are finite. This means that it is impossible for physicians collectively to offer all technologically feasible and clinically beneficial medical services to all patients. Individually, though, physicians practise medicine under a basic ethical tenet which compels them to do whatever is in their power to help their patients. Herein lies one of the fundamental ethical issues in modern medicine: how can physicians fulfil their moral obligations as fiduciary agents for individual patients while being responsible stewards of the finite pool of resources?

In a 1975 article in the *New England Journal of Medicine*, Howard Hiatt likened the situation in medical care to a parable described by Garrett Hardin in a classic article, entitled The tragedy of the commons. According to Hiatt's adaptation of Hardin's parable, physicians are like herdsmen who used to feed their cattle (patients) on a common pasture. Acting in their own interests, the herdsmen could allow their cattle to feed on the land without limit, as long as their numbers and appetites were small compared to the resources on the land. As the number and appetites of the cattle grew to the point where, collectively, their wants exceeded the capacity of the common resource, the desires of the herdsmen to extract the maximal nutrition for their cattle led to overgrazing. At first, the less aggressive cattle failed to get adequate nutrition and died. Later, herdsmen were forced out of business. And, in the end, the rich pasture turned into an overgrazed wasteland.

Although Hardin's essay was written in the context of population growth, Hiatt saw its relevance to health care. Physicians, each acting in the best interests of their own patients, collectively reach the limits of health care resources, with the result that access to care and quality of care are compromised. There is no obvious ethical solution to the problem of rationing the medical commons, because any solution involves comparisons between the value of health services provided to different patients with different conditions. None the less, the remedy must lie in some form of collective action: physicians, like the herdsmen in Hardin's parable, can save the commons only by adhering to a set of mutually acceptable covenants which govern and limit their use of the shared resource.

If health care were "free," there would be no need to limit its use. Health care is not "free," because the use of resources (physician time, hospital beds, health care budgets) by some precludes the use of those resources by others. The overall result of failing to adopt covenants that lead to restrained use of resources by well-meaning physicians is unacceptable. If a society mandates universal access to health care, and if all physicians provide their patients with the most beneficial treatments available, then the cost of health care will be unacceptably high to their patients, either as taxpayers, payers of insurance premiums, at the point of care, or in combination. The alternatives are compromises, either with the principle of universal access, or with the principle of unlimited care. Failure to acknowledge these trade-offs can lead to inefficiencies and inequities that compromise both principles: hidden barriers to access such as queues and administrative hassles, exclusion of entire segments of the population, or erecting rigid and arbitrary barriers to introducing new treatments while older treatments of questionable efficacy continue to be used.

The Cost-Effectiveness Paradigm

Suppose that a society wants to provide the maximum aggregate health improvement in its population, but it has limited resources to do so. Each potential health intervention delivered to a defined group of persons with a particular condition yields a health improvement and entails a cost. If health improvement is measured in units which reflect the values of the society, and if costs are measured in units which reflect the extent to which the resource budget is depleted by the intervention, then the maximum societal health improvement can be achieved by applying the following simple decision rule: rank order medical interventions in decreasing order of their expected health improvement per unit expected cost, and adopt them from the top of the rank list to the point on the list that resources are depleted. The ratio of benefit to cost from each intervention represents its "value for money." To make this decision rule operational even at the societal level, one needs measures of predicted health improvement or benefit, and predicted resource cost. (For present purposes, complexities arising from uncertainty regarding anticipated benefits and costs are set aside, and are summarised in terms of the average, or expected, values of each.)

The health benefit can be measured in units that reflect the preferences of the community, considering their desire for increased longevity but also the value they place on limitation of function, pain, and other dimensions of health related quality of life. One such measure is the quality adjusted life year (QALY). Quality adjusted life years measure the number of years of remaining life, each adjusted by a preference weight (generally between zero and one, or possibly even less than zero for health states judged worse than dead) that reflects the relative value of the health state on a scale between perfect health (one) and dead (zero). Since the amount of health benefit is uncertain before the intervention, the measure of benefit for a health care intervention can be expressed as an average across similar persons in the target population, in terms of quality adjusted life expectancy. The QALY gain for an intervention should include all health consequences, both positive

and negative, and is therefore a measure of net health benefit.

Monetary Terms

Costs are usually measured in monetary terms–dollars, pounds, euros–but it should always be remembered that money is only a proxy for the real resources–physicians, nurses, hospital facilities, pharmaceutical development and production–that are consumed in providing the service. From society's perspective, costs are also net of any savings in future health care resources that might have been consumed but for the intervention–such as the costs of treating strokes that are averted because of a blood pressure control programme. From a societal perspective, costs also include resources contributed by patients and family members and other caregivers, including their time, and not just resources financed through health insurance (public or private) or billed to the patient.

In common practice, the ratio reported from cost-effectiveness analyses is the reciprocal of "value for money," namely the cost per quality adjusted year of life gained. Thus, interventions having low values of this ratio go to the top of the rank list, and those with high values may fall below the line for a particular budget.

What is the ethical basis for seeking to allocate society's health care resources with the aim of maximising quality adjusted life expectancy? If each individual measured the value of his or her own health in terms of quality adjusted life expectancy, and if each of them paid for his or her own health care through individual savings accounts, then economic theory would lead them each to allocate their own assets according to the cost-per-QALY rule. Because of the uncertainties about the need for health care during one's life, however, and for reasons of equity, health care services are typically covered by pooled risk-sharing arrangements, in the form of insurance or national health care. Under these arrangements, the measure of aggregate QALYs at the societal level entails an interpersonal comparison: the implicit assumption is that a QALY is a QALY, no matter who gets it.

Whether a society wishes to count all QALYs equally, or to weight them inversely to the health status of the beneficiary, the result is a utilitarian measure of societal health benefit that could be used to guide resource allocations in health care through an appropriately constructed ratio.

The fundamental question in this essay is this: if there is general consensus that resources should be allocated in such a way as to maximise aggregate health benefit, who is responsible for allocating the resources? Should the patient voluntarily deny himself health services out of a sense of communal obligation to conserve the commons? Should physicians be expected to balance their responsibilities to do the best they can for their patients with a responsibility to be the gatekeeper of the commons at each and every encounter with patients? Or is some form of collective action required, whereby citizens empower their physicians to practise medicine within a system that imposes limits on the resources available to them? My conclusion is that a combination of all three is necessary in order to allocate medical resources efficiently.

The Role of Patients

Patients expect physicians, as fiduciary agents, to do everything in their power to provide them with the best possible health care. Americans in particular, perhaps in contrast with citizens of other industrialised countries, demand the maximal use of available technologies. They are none the less accustomed to the fact that their physicians are already forced to ration care because of constraints that are neither financial nor under their control. For example, physicians have limited time during the day, which results in barriers to scheduling office appointments or conducting the most thorough possible examinations. Access to facilities, such as hospital beds, and especially diagnostic technologies such as magnetic resonance imaging and computed tomography, may be limited, forcing physicians to delay, or even forgo, some diagnostic information. In sum,

physicians ration care to some extent, or at least set priorities, and patients know that other patients may take precedence for their physician's attention, depending on the urgency and severity of their problems. Unfortunately, the services that physicians are most likely to forgo under these pressures are those which patients do not actively seek, much less demand. Some of these services, such as periodic screening for colorectal and breast cancer, or blood pressure monitoring and treatment, may be far more cost-effective (by the cost-per-QALY criterion) than the services that physicians are compelled, by their sense of obligation to patients, to provide.

Patients themselves ration their own health care to some degree. In the United States, insured patients often face copayments or deductibles. Looming even larger as resource constraints upon patients are their own time, including travel to the doctor's office, and other out-of-pocket costs such as transportation and child care.

In general, these constraints on physicians and patients are relatively weak deterrents to the use of maximally beneficial medical care. They are not strong enough by themselves to allocate the commons, and to the extent that they limit care, they may not do so efficiently.

The Role of Consumers (Patients *Ex Ante*)

As patients, people have a different view of health care costs than they have as consumers. While people may expect that physicians do everything possible for them when they are sick, they complain bitterly when their insurance premiums rise, when the prices of goods and services go up because labour costs to employers reflect rising health care benefits, or when their taxes go up.

Consumers have to pay for their collective use of health care resources, but they don't want to bear responsibility for the collective costs at the point of their own care. Part of the motivation for individuals is explained by the economic theory of insurance–groups of people can become better off by pooling risks and avoiding major losses in the event they become sick. As a result, citizens demand that health insurance be provided by their employers (or made available at nominal cost) or by government. Moreover, subsidised health insurance enables citizens who would not otherwise be able to afford basic health care to obtain it; there is a redistributional aspect to the provision of health insurance.

When patients have medical insurance, they face different incentives in going to the doctor to seek care. Price becomes less of a factor because the patient does not bear the full cost of care at the time care is sought. In effect, the price facing the patient is lower than the full social cost of health care. The gap between perceived price and resource cost creates an incentive to utilise more health care than the patient would otherwise be willing to buy. This phenomenon is known as "moral hazard" in the economics literature. It tends to promote excessive use of the "medical commons," leading to increases in the cost of health insurance beyond what consumers believe is reasonable.

Ironically, the word "moral" in "moral hazard" suggests that patients are at risk of being "immoral" if they *over*utilise health care services relative to the value of the services they receive. This nomenclature stands in sharp contrast to the predominant ethical problem faced by physicians in the presence of limited resources: their ethical obligation to the patient at hand makes them immoral if they *under*utilise services relative to the maximum they could do. In reality, neither the physician placed in the fiduciary role as agent for the patient, nor the patient facing artificially low prices at the point of care, can be faulted for providing and expecting, respectively, the best health care technology can offer.

The Role of Physicians

Physicians and patients engage in what economists refer to as principal-agent relationships. This refers to the fiduciary trust that patients (the principals) place in physicians (the agents) to make decisions that maximise the wellbeing of their patients, and to act as advocates for their patients in the health care system.

As ideal agents for patients, physicians would consider not only the health consequences of their decisions, but also the economic and psychological consequences for their patients. Out-of-pocket costs, time and inconvenience, and reassurance from diagnostic tests are all part of what patients value. A perfect agent would consider all of these, and weigh them against one another if necessary, as would the patient.

Principal-agent relationships do not always achieve the goal of perfect proxy decision making and selfless advocacy, if the incentives facing the agent lead to deviations from the decision that is best for the principal. For example, physicians may obtain different levels of remuneration, professional stature, or satisfaction, from their actions, and these incentives compete with the incentives that are aligned with the interests of their patients, such as a sense of obligation and cognisance of external monitoring of their quality of care.

As noted before, physicians are often unable to be perfect agents for their patients because of constraints placed upon them. They have limited time during the day (and even if they work extra hours, their performance may suffer). They are limited by resource constraints in hospitals and laboratories, such as intensive care beds and magnetic resonance equipment.

Sometimes constraints force the physician to make explicit choices between the interests of different patients, as in the setting of emergency triage or in the selection of organ transplant recipients. In these situations, the choices concern patients with names and faces, all of whom are under the care of a single physician or provider organisation. The question at the societal level is whether physicians should be expected to allocate resources between their patients and other nameless, faceless patients who could, perhaps, obtain more benefit if the resources were conserved to benefit them. The question, in other words, is whether physicians should consider the cost-effectiveness of the decisions they make for their patients, recognising that resources are limited. Is it the physician's responsibility to protect the medical commons?

An entirely different view of the physician's ethical responsibility would be as an agent for society at large, rather than for individual patients. Under this view of agency, the physician would be compelled to allocate resources in the most cost-effective manner, in order to achieve maximal value for money on behalf of society. In such a world, physicians would make decisions that are in less than the best interests of their individual patients, because not all medically beneficial procedures would be provided. But, on aggregate, consumers would be better off because more health benefit would be achieved.

Or would they? Such an ethic would compromise the fiduciary relationship between patient and physician. It would place the physician in a position of making trade-offs with faceless patients, and then explaining to patients why it was not "cost-effective" to do extra computed tomography (CT) or to prescribe the more expensive drug with a slightly better side effect profile. Physicians trained to do the best for individual patients would balk at this social agency role.

Major Sea Change

The dilemma, then, is that consumers collectively, concerned about health care costs, have an interest in cost-consciousness in the clinic and at the bedside, while as patients they expect a perfect agency relationship. One possible class of solutions may entail collective action, to constrain (not necessarily regulate!) physicians to act in the collective interest while allowing them to strive to maximise the welfare of their individual patients. This is the type of solution that economists advocate, for example, to induce manufacturers to restrict pollution or to induce consumers to recycle. But in health care, it is not clear that consumers will accept such collective solutions until they first buy into the premise that resources are limited. I believe that a combination of incentives, constraints, and a major sea change in citizen attitudes toward the finitude of medical care will be required to save the medical commons.

The Role of Collective Action

The goal of a collective solution to protect the medical commons would be served by placing constraints on physicians' choices such that, even as they strive to do the best they can on behalf of their patients, the result of their doing so leads to cost-effective resource allocation. The constraints would, in effect, force physicians to consider the opportunity cost of their decisions, just as shopping consumers are bound by the cash in their wallet and their credit balance. The consumer seeks to maximise her wellbeing, subject to a budget constraint. The idea is to get the physician to take cognisance of the collective budget constraint.

If physicians consider both QALYs (or another socially desirable measure of health outcome) and cost when deciding how to allocate their budgets, the result would produce the societal allocation implied by cost-effectiveness analysis. Physicians in that setting would be led to consider the cost per QALY of alternative decisions, and the result would be the maximum possible production of QALYs by that physician. If physicians consider other values, for example if they give additional priority to the sickest patients as suggested by Nord, then the result would reproduce the cost-effective result based on those values.

While some economists might applaud the decentralised, provider-centred solution in theory, it does have a number of practical flaws. For one, physicians would have to fend off patients whose demands for health care services were not being met. There would be a tendency to give more attention to the loudest, most assertive patients, relative to the cost-effectiveness of their claims on the resource pool, and relatively less attention to more passive patients. Perhaps a major barrier to successful implementation of the provider-centred model is the need for buy-in on the part of both physicians and consumers. I will return to this essential ingredient later.

The Role of Physicians Under Resource Constraints

A responsible physician who cares for a panel of patients, but who is either faced with a resource budget or accountable for the resources he consumes, would be placed in a situation similar to the emergency room physician performing triage. The physician would be responsible for setting or implementing priorities for care and could invoke cost-effectiveness data to help guide these priorities. This would enable physicians to consider the incremental health benefit they could offer to each patient, with perhaps some added moral consideration given to applying resources to the most desperate cases. Whatever metric the physicians use, whether implicitly or explicitly, they would be striving to maximise the welfare of *their* patient population. Like parents taking care of their several children–decisions about what clothing to buy for each, which ones to send to sports camp, which to send to college–physicians could approach these interpersonal comparisons in a caring, compassionate way.

Given the complexity of medical decisions, and in light of the growing recognition of the role of evidence on effectiveness and cost in medical decisions, physicians must work together to develop and interpret the evidence to support a mutually acceptable framework for cost-effective decision making. This entails physician participation at two levels: helping to set the constraints within which they practise, and formulating flexible guidelines to help them allocate the resources under their stewardship. These, then, are the additional roles physicians must play in order to ensure resource allocations that are responsive to patients' needs and preferences. If physicians accept this role of stewardship for their portion of the medical commons, they can continue to exercise their roles as agents and advocates for patients.

Concluding Remarks: The Need for "Buy-In"

Should physicians do cost-effectiveness analysis at the bedside, even if they are not compelled to ration care by externally imposed constraints? To do so would place them in an untenable position as agents for two, sometimes adversarial, principals–the individual patient in the clinic and the larger community. Patients would lose the undivided advocacy to which they are accustomed, and the pressures on physicians to be responsive would be overwhelming.

Collective action is required to constrain individual providers of health care to practise within their collective means. These constraints could be implemented in and by organisations as diverse as managed care organisations and national health services. Or they could be agreed upon by consensus of provider organisations and citizens. Decision making within these constraints would invite cost-effectiveness analysis by individual providers, but now the choices would be among members of the physician's own "family" of patients, just as the parent decides how to tend to the needs and wants of her several children. The physician would be free to advocate for each patient, to do the best he can to "[preserve] life capacities for the realization of a reasonable, realistic life plan."

Such a means of protecting the "medical commons" could result in resentment on the part of physicians and patients alike, unless both accept the underlying rationale for the constraints. The system of utilisation review by managed care organisations in the United States has spawned a movement in support of a return to physician control of decision making. But a return to unconstrained use of technologies and resources will fail because of the limits at the societal level. The only way out of this dilemma is for citizens and physicians to accept the concept and consequences of resource limits, just as they accept speed limits, zoning laws, and other self-imposed constraints in the interest of the greater good.

Attitude of Consumers

How can this acceptance of resource constraints come about? There is some indication that physicians are already willing to accept the idea of limits, as long as they have some degree of control or participation of the process of setting them. Medical specialty societies have begun to incorporate cost-effectiveness into their formulation of clinical guidelines. A recent study showed good concordance between the rankings by a consensus panel of physicians of appropriateness of a medical technology in different indications–coronary angiography after myocardial infarction–and cost-effectiveness ratios for these indications.

The biggest obstacle to cost-effective resource allocation along these lines is the attitude of consumers. People who expect everyone to have access to all possible medical care regardless of cost are bound to be disappointed. In the United States, the sustenance of this myth has come at a high price. Even in times of economic prosperity, an increasing proportion of Americans is uninsured, and millions of them have limited or no access to medical care. Some of the most cost-effective but least glamorous medical interventions, such as screening for colorectal cancer and adult vaccinations against influenza and pneumonia, are underutilised in favour of the procedures consumers want and demand. An informed populace, aware of the finite benefits of health care services and of the rationale for constrained choice in the clinic and at the bedside, is an essential ingredient if physicians are to be burdened with the responsibility for cost-effective decision making. The evidence suggests that the medical profession will accept that responsibility if it is given the authority to set the rules by which its members are to play, and if their patients are at peace with the principle of living within their means.

Rationing in the Intensive Care Unit

ROBERT D. TRUOG, DAN W. BROCK, DEBORAH J. COOK, MARION DANIS, JOHN M. LUCE, GORDON D. RUBENFELD, AND MITCHELL M. LEVY

Critical Care Medicine 34, no. 4 (2006): 958–63.

Critical care physicians are at the front lines of the current economic crisis in health care. Critical care services account for >1% of the gross domestic product in the United States and represent an increasing proportion of hospital costs—up from 8% in 1980 to 20% today. Since physicians have control over many of the costs of caring for critically ill patients, they are under pressure, both implicit and explicit, to rein in these expenditures.

Decisions to limit the use of beneficial services in the intensive care unit (ICU) are particularly difficult, however, because they potentially have life or death consequences for patients. In addition, many patients and families believe they are entitled to the full range of critical care services.

Although many ICU clinicians acknowledge that they have rationed care, some physicians have asserted that it is unethical to withhold any therapy that may benefit a patient. Even so, no health care system can provide all patients with all treatments that may have the potential for benefit. Many people could benefit, even if only marginally, from greater utilization of health care resources. Even if it were possible to provide these benefits to all patients, it would not be desirable, since this approach would siphon resources from other worthwhile societal goals, such as improving education or the economic infrastructure.

Some insist that "rationing at the bedside" can never be ethical. In other words, they argue that even if critical care services must be limited to preserve resources for other societal purposes, intensivists should never be placed in the role of rationing these services but rather should be strong advocates for all of their patients' needs, regardless of scarcity or expense. According to this argument, if rationing is necessary, it must be done away from the bedside, through the development of clear and specific rules (such as restricting procedures to those who meet certain clinical criteria) or through public policy (such as by limiting the construction of ICU beds and thereby rationing their availability). Although agreeing that many types of rationing should be done through public policy and regulatory structures, we believe that no bright line can be drawn that will protect the bedside clinician from the need to make rationing decisions. Even very specific rules that define how services should be limited to certain patient populations must be interpreted by the intensivist within the context of each patient's clinical situation, and decisions to limit critical care services by restricting the availability of ICU beds necessarily force intensivists to use their judgment in deciding which patients to admit to those beds. Any systematic approach to rationing therefore requires intensivists to use their clinical judgment to link rationing principles to specific clinical situations.

Furthermore, beyond those decisions that are readily recognized as rationing are many commonplace and mundane decisions made by intensivists on a daily basis that effectively direct resources toward some patients and away from others and thereby also represent rationing. Consider, for example, deciding whether to cancel surgery for a patient undergoing elective hepatectomy to make room for a patient who might benefit from intensive monitoring in the ICU, or choosing whether to send the ICU house officer to accompany an unstable patient to the computed tomography scanner rather than remain at the bedside of a patient with impending respiratory failure. In each case, a physician must choose to make a health benefit available to one patient but not to another.

Some have resisted the view that rationing is necessary by invoking euphemisms that allow them to deny that rationing decisions are being made. One approach, for example, is to argue that an inferior therapy is ethically acceptable because it is sufficient to meet the "standard of care," even when an alternative therapy would be superior. Another is to justify withholding a treatment on grounds that it would be "medically inappropriate," based, for example, on a patient's age or comorbidities. Yet another approach is to distinguish between treatments that are necessary and those that are merely beneficial and to argue that denial of necessary treatment is rationing and unethical, whereas denial of merely beneficial treatment does not count as rationing and may be permissible. Appeals to the standard of care, to what is medically appropriate, or to what is necessary vs. merely beneficial are complex claims that seek to combine assessments about medical effectiveness, social utility, and economic feasibility into a judgment about whether an intervention should be provided. The advantage of these strategies is that they allow clinicians to believe they are not rationing; the disadvantage is that they justify denial of potentially beneficial treatments for reasons that may be implicit, unexamined, and unarticulated—even to physicians themselves—under the guise of presumably objective medical criteria.

The Task Force on Values, Ethics, and Rationing in Critical Care (VERICC) is an *ad hoc* working group, not affiliated with any institution or society, formed to address ethical issues raised by rationing in the ICU. The task force was funded by an unrestricted grant from Eli Lilly and Company, which played no role in either the deliberations of the task force or the content of this manuscript. The task force has defined rationing as "the allocation of healthcare resources in the face of limited availability, which necessarily means that beneficial interventions are withheld from some individuals." Although others have proposed alternative definitions, all recognize that rationing decisions have become part of the fabric of routine decision making for every practicing physician. Indeed, a system that failed to ration resources would likely be catastrophic, quickly undermining the ability of clinicians to effectively deliver health care. The ethical peril lies in holding the persistent view that rationing can be avoided rather than in developing strategies for allocating resources in ways that optimize medical care while treating all patients fairly.

Types of Rationing in the ICU

Many rationing decisions are morally justifiable and indeed essential to achieve a just allocation of health care resources. Others are unethical and deny patients potentially beneficial treatments that they are entitled to receive. How can those that are ethical be differentiated from those that are not?

Rationing occurs at many levels, from governmental budgetary decisions to clinical decisions by individual physicians. In this article, we do not address the ethics of rationing across all of these levels but examine rationing through a more focused lens, as it is experienced by the physician at the bedside in the ICU. We propose a stepwise process for determining whether a rationing decision is ethical, beginning with an examination of the reasons behind the physician's decision to withhold a potentially beneficial intervention.

To more clearly understand rationing decisions, we propose three general categories of reasons that physicians might use to justify a decision about the use of an intervention when they believe that the intervention may offer at least some net benefit to a patient (Table 5.2). We do not propose that reasons offered within any of

Table 5.2. Rationing Decisions

Categories of Reasons	Rationing Decision	Reason Given to Support the Decision
Reasons that refer to external constraints	Not ordering an MRI for a nonemergent indication	No MRI booking slots are available
	Not admitting a patient from the emergency department who needs intensive care	All available ICU beds are full and no patient can be safely discharged
	Not placing a patient on continuous hemofiltration	All machines for continuous hemofiltration are currently in use by patients with appropriate indications
Reasons that refer to clinical guidelines	Ordering a CT as a first-line imaging study, even though an MRI would have greater diagnostic yield	Local hospital policy to manage utilization of imaging resources and control costs
	Using narrow-spectrum prophylactic antibiotics and switching only for documented infections	Clinical guidelines developed to control emergence of multiply resistant organisms
	Reserving expensive nonionic contrast agents for those at high risk for contrast nephropathy	Clinical guidelines developed to avoid unnecessary expenditures
Reasons based on clinical judgment	Instructing a house officer to stay at the bedside of a patient with evolving sepsis rather than accompany an unstable patient to CT	Clinical judgment about which decision would optimize the clinical outcome overall
	Filling the last bed in the ICU with a trauma patient from the emergency department rather than an oncology patient from the ward	Clinical judgment about which decision would optimize the clinical outcome overall
	Not offering liver transplantation to a recovered alcoholic with liver failure	Personal belief that organs should not be allocated to those with self-induced disease

Note. MRI, magnetic resonance imaging; ICU, intensive care unit; CT, computed tomography.

these categories are necessarily superior to others in all circumstances but rather that the categories provide insight into the types of evidence that would be most appropriate for the rationing decision under consideration. Table 5.2 illustrates how a variety of rationing decisions may be evaluated differently depending on which of the three categories of reasons is used to justify the decision.

Rationing and External Constraints

The first category consists of reasons related to external constraints. An example would be accepting a long turnaround time for an important test result because the hospital has made the decision to outsource the test to an external laboratory rather than to do the test internally.

In many cases, reasons that refer to external constraints are compelling and sufficient, since these external constraints impose large barriers to any alternative decision. Appeals to external constraints do not always justify rationing decisions, however. If a patient needs an emergency craniotomy for an epidural hematoma but the hospital's only neurosurgeon is already occupied in a lengthy surgery, then clearly a physician would be ethically obligated to go beyond this external constraint and to do whatever was necessary to urgently transfer the patient to a facility where the procedure could be performed promptly. Similarly, even when the barriers to alternative choices are high, they may not be insurmountable. For example, medications that are not available on the hospital formulary can be obtained in compelling circumstances, although physicians who routinely make such requests might be rightly criticized for trying to circumvent a legitimate and important institutional mechanism for cost control. An argument could be made that patients who are willing to pay out-of-pocket for off-formulary medications should be allowed to do so, although in most practice settings, patients are neither informed that these rationing decisions are being made nor that they could choose to obtain the medications at their own expense.

Rationing and Clinical Guidelines

The second category of reasons that can be used to justify rationing decisions are those that refer to clinical guidelines. In the context of rationing decisions, clinical guidelines have the potential to inform clinical decisions relative to both clinical efficacy and cost. Historically, clinical guidelines have focused primarily on the relative clinical efficacy of alternative diagnostic and therapeutic strategies. Given the volume and complexity of clinical decision making in the ICU, clinical guidelines have become an essential tool for physicians in supporting decisions about clinical efficacy. The content, format, and strength of clinical guidelines vary, however. Some are developed by rigorous guideline methodology and are reflective of high-quality research evidence. Others are much less reliable, because the data to support them are inadequate or out of date, reflect only expert opinion, or have been developed using weak guideline methodology. Even in the best of circumstances, clinical judgment is necessarily a part of the development and use of clinical guidelines, since the data informing these guidelines must always be synthesized, interpreted, and integrated.

Most important, however, clinical guidelines only inconsistently address the economic side of clinical decision making. Many clinical guidelines, for example, make recommendations based exclusively on scientific evidence of whether the intervention's benefits exceed its risks, without regard to cost. Although this type of analysis can be helpful, it is incomplete. Physicians are commonly willing to recommend treatments that have limited evidence of benefit if they are inexpensive and safe yet cautious in recommending interventions that are expensive or risky when evidence of benefit is modest or ambiguous.

One method for bringing cost considerations explicitly into the development of guidelines is cost-effectiveness analysis (CEA). CEA provides a quantitative method for comparing the value of interventions across a broad spectrum, from public health initiatives affecting millions of individuals to high-technology interventions intended for only a very few. A comprehensive review of CEA is beyond the scope of this article, but it is worth noting that although the methodology has scientific appeal, it has led to some spectacularly counterintuitive conclusions. When this approach was used to develop the Oregon rationing plan for Medicaid, for example, it gave a higher priority for tooth capping than for appendectomies. This example illustrates how CEA fails to capture some of the values that must be included in rationing guidelines. Despite these limitations, CEA does have the potential to inform rationing decisions by formalizing and quantifying the clinical and economic consequences of alternative health care interventions.

However even if clinical guidelines were always based on the highest quality scientific evidence and always included the most sophisticated comparisons of costs vs. benefit, they could never provide a scientific answer to the question of whether any given test or treatment is "worth it." Ultimately, questions about how much to spend on health care overall, and questions about how to allocate those funds among different health priorities, are values questions that can never be answered by scientific or economic methodology alone. Furthermore, although development of a comprehensive health policy with explicit priorities would help to minimize uncertainty, both the pace at which health technologies are developing and the complexity of the choices mean that guidelines will never be able to provide rote solutions for all of the rationing decisions that clinicians face on a regular basis.

Rationing and Clinical Judgment

The third category of reasons that could be used to support a rationing decision is clinical judgment. Stated most generally, clinical judgment is required for rationing decisions in at least two circumstances: when it is unclear how guidelines should be applied, and when guidelines do not exist. The application of any clinical guideline requires clinical judgment, and deviation from the guideline in appropriate circumstances is both acceptable and necessary.

Clinical judgment is also necessary when guidelines are available but express views that lack widespread consensus. With regard to triaging ICU beds, for example, evidence indicates that clinicians rarely follow published guidelines and that most rationing decisions with respect to ICU admission are based on clinical judgment.

Many daily routine decisions made by intensivists can be characterized as rationing decisions made by clinical judgment. For example, all ICU physicians must decide how to allocate their time among all of the patients in the ICU each day. How much time to spend making rounds in the morning and how to divide one's time among all the patients are rationing decisions that can have important effects on clinical outcomes and patient safety.

Other examples of rationing by clinical judgment are more open to criticism. A rich debate is ongoing about the merits of age-based rationing, that is, whether medical care should be limited for individuals who are beyond a certain age. Evidence suggests that this occurs, particularly with regard to expensive treatments for the elderly. Physicians are therefore apparently making individualized judgments not to offer potentially beneficial interventions based on their own views about the appropriate way to allocate these resources, in the absence of a societal consensus. Although rationing by clinical judgment can be ethical, it is particularly susceptible to unethical subjectivity and bias. For example, one study showed that the likelihood of a patient being given a "do not attempt resuscitation" order in the ICU was negatively correlated with that patient's preillness employment status. Another study showed that surgical ICU beds were allocated with respect to the political power of the surgical services within the institution rather than based on patient-centered factors. Deep-seated prejudices can be particularly difficult to both recognize and rectify, as illustrated by the fact that fewer cardiovascular procedures are done on African Americans than Caucasians, even after risk adjustment. An ethnographic study suggested that, as a group, intensivists were more likely than surgeons to consider the scarcity of resources as a factor in end of life decision making.

These biases can influence rationing at even the most personal level, such as when physicians direct resources disproportionately toward patients and families who they know or like particularly well or who are more demanding about receiving the interventions they desire. Acknowledging that these are rationing decisions and revealing the reasons behind the decisions is a necessary first step toward eliminating those decisions that derive from unrecognized prejudice or bias.

Disclosure of Rationing Decisions

Do patients need to be informed of rationing decisions? When clinicians withhold interventions based on their interpretation of the standard of care, one could argue that the decisions are technical in nature and that the patient need neither consent to the limitation nor even be informed about it. When these decisions are framed as rationing, however, it becomes clear that a potentially beneficial intervention is being withheld for reasons other than the best interests of the patient. Under these circumstances, it is likely that many (even most) patients would want to be aware that their health care was being rationed and would perhaps want the opportunity to question these decisions or even appeal them.

Although the frequency of these decisions makes it highly impractical to discuss each one of them with every patient or family, honesty and transparency are required if physicians are to maintain the trust and confidence of their patients and the public. Future discussion should elucidate the place for patient notification and dialogue about rationing decisions and the conditions under which physicians should seek the patient's informed consent.

Which Rationing Decisions Are Ethical?

How can we determine which rationing decisions are ethical? Our taxonomy identifies three types of reasons that physicians may use to justify rationing decisions. This taxonomy does not by itself determine which decisions are ethical but rather clarifies the type of evidence that must be used to support the decision that is made. Some of this evidence is scientific in nature and can be judged in terms of the strength of the research that supports it. Some of the reasons, however, appeal to fundamental ethical principles. Although not "evidence-based," these principles are rooted in deeply held and widely respected values. Using race or ethnic origin as a criterion for allocating resources between patients would be prohibited under these precepts, for example. The algorithm of "first-come, first-served" is an ethical guideline that could be used to justify a choice between two patients who would otherwise have an equal claim to a resource, or the practice of triage could be used to justify rationing decisions when resources are diverted to those who have the greatest chance of benefiting from them.

Although rationing is necessary, it can clearly never be mechanical; all three types of rationing described here require the involvement of physicians who possess integrity of character and sound clinical judgment. Additional work is needed to elucidate how both empirical evidence and ethical analysis can illuminate and inform the rationing decisions that arise in the taxonomy described here.

Justice and Managed Care

Four Principles for the Just Allocation of Health Care Resources

EZEKIEL J. EMANUEL

Hastings Center Report 30, no. 3 (2000): 8–16.

The American health care system has long been criticized for its injustice. The absence of universal coverage and the reliance on employer-based health insurance and patient ability to pay create financial barriers that limit access and produce high levels of under- and uninsured. Further, the diffuseness of decisionmaking within the American health care system precludes a coherent process for allocating health care resources. The growing dominance of managed care organizations raises both expectation and apprehension about improving the justice of the American health care system. How can we evaluate the justice of a managed care organization's allocation of resources? What set of criteria can we use to determine when managed care's denial of benefits is just or unjust?

Two Dimensions of Justice in Health Care

Issues related to justice in health care can be divided along two dimensions: access and allocation. Access refers to whether people who are—or should be—entitled to health care services receive them. Allocation refers to determining what resources should be devoted to health care, at three distinct levels. At the social level, allocation refers to the proportion of Gross National Product, the government budget, or a company's revenues that should be devoted to health care. At the service level, allocation refers to what health services people should be guaranteed as part of a basic benefits package, or which services should receive the highest funding priority. At the patient care level, allocation refers to which specific patients should obtain naturally or socially scarce services, such as organ transplantation or in-patient psychiatric care for depression. Managed care organizations are involved in allocation at both the service and patient care level.

Access and allocation are related. One of the main allocating decisions is whether to use resources to increase the number of people entitled to specific services or to expand the range of services provided. For instance, the Oregon Medicaid reform plan opts "to assure everyone basic health care rather than to offer a larger but unevaluated collection of benefits to some of the poor while excluding others from anything but emergency services." Nevertheless, access and allocation are conceptually distinct: After we decide that people should have access to health services, it is always a further question to delineate precisely what services they will be guaranteed.

While some managed care organizations have accepted some responsibility to ensure access for the uninsured, whether managed care organizations—and those who fund them—have such an obligation and how far such an obligation extends are complex and unresolved issues. Conversely, the fair allocation of resources at the service level is an obligation all parties, including managed care organizations themselves, agree they have. The very nature of managed care financing and delivery makes defining benefits inescapable; receiving a fixed budget to provide services for a defined population necessitates judgments about what services should be guaranteed and what should be left to members' discretion. Indeed, an advantage of managed care is that there finally is a natural locus in the American health care system for service level allocation decisions. What constitutes a just allocation of health care resources at the service level for managed care organizations?

Principles for the Just Allocation of Health Care Resources

There have been many different substantive methods proposed for the just allocation of health care resources, including cost-effectiveness, age-based rationing, the prudent insurer method, and the fair opportunity method. Yet even their proponents acknowledge that these substantive methods have serious philosophical and practical problems that constrain their use for the just allocation of resources.

In the absence of defensible substantive methods for the just allocation of health care resources, how can a managed care organization determine what services should be guaranteed as a matter of justice? How can members determine whether a managed care organization's benefit package is just? I propose four principles for the just allocation of health care resources that articulate widely held truisms about the American health care system. The principles do not describe the allocation of health care resources per se, but they bear on how allocation decisions are made. They are about the allocation of power over key resource decisions and thus integrally related to justice.

Improving Health Should Be the Primary Goal

The allocation of health care resources should aim at and be justified by the improvement in people's health.

In some sense, this principle needs no justification; it seems self-evident, almost a tautology. After all, what else are a health care system, physicians, hospitals, and specific medical services for except to improve people's health? If formal justification is attempted, however, it should appeal to the idea that health care is dedicated to a special set of aims or purposes and that it is the obligation of health care professionals to pursue these aims. The special aim or purpose of health care is curing disease, relieving pain and suffering, promoting public health, pursuing research to improve health, and so on. What distinguishes the health care system from the educational or law enforcement or banking systems is pursuing

this aim rather than improving reading ability or reducing crime or enhancing return on capital. Similarly, pursuing this aim as a primary interest also distinguishes the professional obligations and norms of clinicians from teachers, policemen, and bankers as well as the obligations of health care institutions from schools, jails, and banks.

The principle of improving health restates this aim for the allocation of resources. While there may be disagreement about which allocation is better at improving people's health, this principle specifies and restricts the kinds of reasons that can be given to justify guaranteeing certain services rather than others.

Patients and Members Should Be Informed

Patients, members, and prospective members of managed care organizations should be informed about the allocation of health care resources and the underlying data and justification for the allocation.

The justification of this principle has many sources, but the strongest derives from the necessity of respecting individuals as rational and autonomous moral agents, a fundamental ideal of American society, as well as the related value of publicity. Individuals should be accorded the opportunity to devise, revise, and pursue their own life plans. For these choices to be autonomous and based not merely on whim, they must be informed and they need to be made by free and rational individuals acting from values they affirm.

To respect people as autonomous moral agents in the health care context requires (1) forging the conditions necessary for their making free and rational choices and (2) respecting their choices.[1] Providing patients information about their illness, options for diagnostic tests, and the risks and benefits of alternative treatments is necessary because such information permits "individuals to develop their own aims and interests and to make their values effective in the living of their lives" (p. 18). This reasoning has generated the standards of informed consent. The same rationale also justifies providing people with other information relevant to health care, including information about the range of services a managed care organization makes available. Indeed, the new institutionalization of health care delivery requires reconceiving the notion of informed consent to include the information on institutional policies that have a high likelihood of affecting people's health and opportunities.

The principle of information is also justified by the ideal of publicity. It has been argued that a necessary condition for an action to be moral is that it can be made public and justified to those who are affected by it. If we cannot offer reasons for an action or policy that others can accept—or if we deliberately keep the reasons secret because others will not accept them—then the action or policy cannot be deemed moral. Publicity is a fundamental requirement of the democratic process because it lets people participate in deliberation and approving decisions, but it does not apply only to political actions and governmental policies. Publicity is a necessary value generally for actions by private entities that affect critically important goods and that involve issues of justice. Thus for the allocation of health care resources to be fair, publicity requires that it be made public, whether the allocation is by a public or private entity. Importantly, the standard benefits language stating that "medically necessary and appropriate" services are covered fails to meet publicity; it has too many interpretations, obscuring rather than accurately informing patients about what services are covered and why.

Patients and Members Should Have the Opportunity to Consent

Patients, members, and prospective members of managed care organizations should be given the opportunity to consent to the allocation of health care resources that will affect them.

As with the principle of information, the justification for this principle of consent ultimately rests on respect for persons as autonomous moral agents; it also appeals to the closely related reason of democratic legitimacy.

As noted, respecting people as autonomous moral agents requires not only creating conditions necessary for them to make free and rational choices but also respecting their choices. With regard to allocating health care resources, treating people as autonomous agents requires not just disclosing the allocation enacted or listing covered services, but providing an opportunity for them to consent to the allocation. Therefore, justice requires that those who have to live with the consequences of the allocation be afforded the opportunity to affirm that the allocation reflects their values.

A related way of justifying the principle of consent is to appeal to democratic legitimacy. In a democracy, decisions by politicians about the distributions of social resources that affect the citizens' lives, and the quality of their lives, are legitimate only when they are based on consent, or only if they are justified by reasons citizens affirm. Importantly, citizens have a correlative obligation to obey decisions that are legitimate. Because the allocation of health care resources is a matter of justice and of fundamental importance to citizens, it must be viewed as legitimate even if it is most frequently handled by private organizations. And citizens will view such allocation decisions as legitimate only if they—or their representatives—can consent to them.

Conflicts of Interest Should Be Minimized

People entrusted to allocate health care resources should not make allocating decisions under conditions that could reasonably be expected to be influenced by direct, personal financial benefits or penalties.

Conflict of interest rules are meant to minimize the influence of secondary interests on decisions and judgments, to ensure that the primary motivation of those who make decisions that affect the well-being of others is, in fact, the well-being of others. Since in most cases it is impossible to eliminate the role of secondary interests, these rules use a sliding scale, tailoring limits to the magnitude of the conflict and the potential harm that can result.

How does this apply to the allocation of health care resources? As the principle of improving health indicates, the primary interest of those making judgments about the allocation of health care resources should be improving people's health. Personal financial gain or other secondary interests should not influence the allocation decisions. Conflict of interest rules should minimize—or, in the ideal, eliminate—the possibility that the financial interests of those making allocating decisions unduly influence the task of improving people's health.

Differing Interpretations and Implementations of the Four Principles

Like laws and constitutional amendments, these principles provide a shared framework expressed in general phrases. Inevitably, reasonable people will offer differing interpretations of the principles and disagree about how they should be implemented. For instance, with regard to the principle of improving health there are at least two sources of potential controversy. "Improvement in people's health" could be interpreted in a strictly utilitarian manner, such as maximizing longevity or QALYs. Alternatively, improvements might require not maximization of health but more evenly distributed improvements so each person's average life span is improved.

Different interpretations of each principle can lead to significantly different policies implementing them. Each managed care organization will have to offer its own coherent and defensible interpretations of these principles and develop policies that cohere with them. Fortunately, such interpretations are not immutable. Like constitutional interpretation, interpreting and applying these principles should be viewed as an iterative process of elaboration and refinement of the interpretations based on new policy challenges and revisions of policies based upon refined interpretations of the principles. However, some interpretations of the principles are likely to be better, more justifiable, than others. For instance, a strict maximizing interpretation of the principle of improving health, while consistent with utilitarian theory, seems ethically unpersuasive.

Yet even without elaborating and justifying a particular interpretation of these principles, relying solely on their general phrasing, there are significant implications for the structure, practices, and allocation policies of managed care organizations. I identify six implications, some of which are familiar and commonly advocated in the current debate, while others have received significantly less attention.

Practical Implications of the Four Principles of Justice in Managed Care

First, the goal dictated by the principle of improving health provides a performance-driven standard for evaluating the allocation of health care resources. While for-profit managed care organizations are not inherently unethical, this principle establishes an ethical presumption to prohibit such entities insofar as their allocation of resources to investor profits inevitably diverts funds that could improve people's health. Both nonprofit and for-profit managed care organizations must allocate resources for the provision of health services, administrative expenses, and investments in the future such as quality improvement programs, capital expenditures for new equipment and facilities, and training of personnel. The difference is that for-profit organizations must also allocate resources for profit. Consequently, the justification for the allocation is not only improving people's health but also providing investors a financial return.

This is not to argue that the allocation decisions of nonprofit managed care organizations will always sustain the principle of improving health simply because those decisions are made by nonprofit organizations. Nonprofit managed care organizations might divert resources to ends other than improving members' health— for example, into amenities or disproportionately generous salaries and/or benefits for executive staff. But nonprofit organizations do not have an obligation to return a profit on shareholders investment, and thus do not face the same constraint as for-profit organizations on how their resources may be allocated. Much of the antipathy toward for-profit managed care arises because profit seems inherently to divert resources away from the performance standard of improving people's health.

This means there is a prima facie presumption against for-profit managed care plans. According to their proponents, the claim that profits divert resources from health is deceptive, however. The amount of resources expended for a given improvement of health is not fixed. Through better coordination of care; redesign of information, laboratory, and other systems; lower supply costs; and providing care in more cost-effective settings, it is possible to improve people's health at lower cost. Profit, it is argued, is an essential incentive to achieve these efficiencies. Moreover, efficient for-profit managed care organizations force competing nonprofit organizations to re-examine and streamline their operations.

If allocating health care resources to profit truly creates a more efficient health care system that improves people's health, then it would overcome this prima facie presumption. Because it is a performance-driven standard, such a claim is not a matter of market or antimarket ideology; it can be assessed empirically. There are minimal data on this issue, and data comparing other for-profit and nonprofit health providers are contradictory and inconclusive. The experiences of some for-profits are not encouraging in ensuring that the focus is improving health care. A CEO of a for-profit managed care organization explained his experience:

> The difficulty is that market pressures are extremely short term. Stock analysts who follow companies want them to perform to the calculated profit estimates every quarter.... [W]hen [Wellpoint Health Networks] became publicly held, and listed on the stock exchange, for the first time ever there were incredible pressures for achieving our goals for quarterly earnings.[2]

If studies are needed to vindicate the allocation of health care resources to profit as justifiable and just, current for-profit managed care organizations are justified only if they are participating in these studies. Their future status depends on the results of the studies.

The principle of improving health also compels critical examination of the allocation of resources within managed care organizations according to whether they promote people's health. Some programs, such as persuasive advertising, high administrative costs, and plush hospital rooms, appear less justifiable than others. Billboards, newspaper ads, and commercials divert health resources from improving health to marketing and appear unjust. Again, this prohibition on allocating resources to advertisements is prima facie; advertising could be justified as an essential mechanism to the ultimate goal of improving people's health.

But the claim seems implausible. Advertisements do not seem to be an essential incentive to creating better information systems or to providing care in the most appropriate setting. Advertising that informed people about the allocation of resources and the reasons for including certain services and excluding others could be justified by the principle of information, which provides a useful standard for regulating appropriate advertising in health care. However, billboards that proclaim "We are your health plan, not your doctor" or "We hear you" do not seem justified either by the principle of improving health or the principle of information.

The principle of information offers a third implication: "gag rules" are unjust. "Gag rules" are intended to prevent physicians from informing patients about services that may be appropriate to their medical condition but are not offered or covered by their managed care organization. They prevent patients from knowing what services the managed care organization covers and, therefore, why it has not covered the specific service that may be appropriate to their disease. Clearly, hiding essential information about the allocation of resources both fails to treat patients as autonomous moral agents and violates publicity. Protecting the managed care organization against patients' negative reactions is certainly not a valid justification for withholding information.

Consenting to Allocation Decisions

The principle of consent leads to a fourth implication: the creation of forums for patients to consent to the allocation of resources within managed care organizations. The implications of the principles of improving health and information are negative, since they lead to prohibitions of unethical practices; the implication of the principle of consent is positive, requiring the creation of practices. Consequently, it can generate more disagreement. Not only do reasonable people disagree about what constitutes valid consent, judgments about what policies and practices are appropriate to the unique circumstances of different managed care organizations will vary.

At best, four core organizational elements must be considered to operationalize consent: who, what, when, and how. The first element, "who," concerns the locus of consent—what forums, committees, or boards will consent to the allocation and how will patients be represented? Some managed care organizations could—and do—have members and patients represented on their boards of directors that must ultimately approve all allocation decisions.

The second element is the domain of consent: what substantive allocation decisions are patients supposed to consent to? There is interpretive latitude here. Consent might be to the broad principles or values that guide the allocation of resources; or to the ranking of broad categories of coverage, such as preventive services or rehabilitative services; or to the coverage of paradigmatic or salient services, such as mammograms for women under fifty, or chiropractors. Alternatively, consent could be to the weighting of outcomes to be used in cost-effectiveness analyses, or even more comprehensively, the ranking of intervention-condition pairs such as were used in Oregon.

The third element broaches the matter of timing: when in the process of allocating resources is patients' consent solicited? Members and patients could be asked to consent early in the process, when broad principles or the general benefits language are designed. Alternatively, they could be consulted at the end to endorse allocation decisions or assess particularly controversial coverage decisions.

"How" refers to the pervasiveness of consent: how systematic is patient involvement in the process of allocating resources? Patient consent could be a one-time event in which members and patients comment on the organization's list of covered services, covering or disallowing controversial services, or endorsing broad allocation principles that affect specific coverage decisions made by others. At the other end of the spectrum, consent could be integrally woven into an organization's culture. Members and patients could participate in all phases of the allocation process, from the articulation of broad principles and decisions about paradigmatic services to surveys about the ranking of services, to the establishment of research priorities and the specification of a comprehensive list of intervention-condition pairs.

Consent and the Market

There are many different ways of combining these four elements, creating a spectrum of consent processes that range from the minimal to the comprehensive. One appealing way to implement consent is through the market: people could consent to the allocation of resources by choosing in the market among competing managed care organizations that offer different benefits packages, embodying different schemes of allocating resources. Market consent provides people, as individual consumers, with a choice over a benefits package that they can "take or leave" but not modify. And this may be part of its great appeal. It is simple—it requires no changes in the internal structure of most managed care organizations; familiar—it uses the existing mechanism of annual enrollment; and not demanding—it permits members and patients to determine how much effort they will invest in consenting to the allocation of resources.

Market consent in health care has two weaknesses. Philosophically, annual choice among competing alternatives is, at best, a very minimal version of consent. It emphasizes individualistic choices and precludes—or does not encourage—collective deliberation and weighing of options. Further, it does not permit changing or modifying the options offered. In addition, for complex issues, such as allocating health care resources, consent is rarely thought of as a single event. In politics, for example, periodic elections for office do not alone constitute consent. Choice among alternative candidates for office occurs within an elaborate system that permits citizens multiple other opportunities to voice their opinions and advocate and lobby on particular issues.

Even more problematic are the practical problems of implementing market consent in the American health care system. Choice in the market can qualify as consent only (1) if consumers actually have choices and (2) if the range of options from which people can choose is reasonably diverse. Neither of these criteria currently is—or is likely to be—fulfilled in the American health care market. The majority of workers have no choice of health plan; their employers decide from whom they will receive health care. With no choice of managed care organization, consent to allocation is not even a theoretical possibility. Furthermore, through mergers and consolidation, the system is evolving toward a few large managed care organizations offering fairly similar benefit options competing in each market. Even if people were offered the opportunity, choosing among two or three similar alternatives would hardly qualify as consent to the allocation decisions represented by the individual plans.

Importantly, overcoming these limitations of the market model of consent requires systematic reform of how employers offer health insurance and the diversity of options in the market; managed care organizations cannot resolve the problems if each is acting alone. Such systematic reform seems improbable, and in its absence managed care organizations aspiring to make their allocation of resources just cannot sincerely claim that choice in the market is effective consent; they must incorporate into their internal procedures these four elements of consent. The problems and difficulties of doing so are significant, ranging from skepticism, lack of knowledge, and lack of participation on the part of members to inefficiency and capture by extremists. Further, while some managed care organizations and other health care institutions have experience with eliciting member participation and consent, what we know frequently comes from cases that may not be generalizable. Consequently, establishing and institutionalizing consent is likely to be an iterative process requiring a sustained commitment by managed care organizations.

However, such efforts at consent should not be immediately dismissed as inherently impractical. First, there may be practical benefits from establishing consent procedures: greater acceptance of and adherence to restrictions of services, less litigation, and an improvement in the sense of community essential to the most cost-effective delivery of health services. Second, procedures for consent to the allocation of health care resources are necessary for the allocation to be ethically defensible and broadly endorsed. Third, in their drive for efficiency, managed care organizations have demonstrated the ability to undertake long-term commitments in areas fraught with problems and barriers that defied prior efforts, such as developing, implementing, and reporting outcomes and quality measures. Redirecting such experience could be quite useful in developing procedures for consent.

Consent and Appeals

The principle of consent further suggests a fifth practical implication: establishing appeals processes to review patient grievances about the denial of services. On this view, grievance procedures should be viewed less as giving patients what they want and more as a supplementary consent process. Even in a well-designed consent process integrated into the culture of a managed care organization, both that process and substantive allocation decisions may be imperfect. An appeals process is a safety check on both procedural and substantive errors. It allows those excluded from the consent process to express their views and a reassessment of actual allocations in light of their implications in particular cases. If the original allocation is sustained, the legitimacy of the allocation decision and its justification are strengthened; if the original allocation is overturned, the allocation principles and decisions are revised to reflect more accurately the values of the managed care organization's members.

Conflicts of Interest

Finally, the principle of minimizing conflicts of interest provides the sixth practical implication: financial incentives for physicians and managers linked to the reduced use of resources or profitability should be minimized or, ideally, eliminated. Many managed care organizations use financial incentives that are linked to withholding tests, interventions, and specialist referrals. Those with authority for a managed care organization's allocation of resources may have financial incentives that are linked to profits, low medical-loss ratios, or reduced use of services. These incentives attempt—or appear—to make the physicians' and managers' personal financial interests rather than improvements in people's health guide allocating decisions.

It may be impossible completely to disconnect financial incentives from the allocation of resources and profitability. Even salaried physicians who receive no bonus recognize that the level of their salary next year, the number of patients they must see, and even the existence of their managed care organizations may be linked to financial performance and, therefore, the allocation of resources. Nevertheless, it is possible to prohibit the financial incentives that create the most flagrant conflicts of interest, namely those directly linking—or appearing to link—payment with the withholding of services. These links create conditions that increase the likelihood of personal gain. By developing rules that attenuate the link between financial reward and allocation decisions, it may be possible to minimize the likelihood that other financial arrangements threaten patients' health.

Beyond Managed Care

Managed care organizations have pursued cost reductions with tremendous zeal. They have developed strategic plans that require the complete restructuring of delivery systems, invested millions of dollars in information systems, purchased practices, and engaged in various other activities. Often, however, they have done these things without substantial data assuring the production of high quality health care at lower prices. While efficiency is a legitimate and important goal in the provision of health care, it is not the only goal. We also demand that the health care system be just. With the pursuit of efficiency well established, it is now appropriate for managed care organizations to give justice a high priority. No one can trivialize the difficulties that will accompany the implementation of these four principles for the just allocation of resources. As with all worthy endeavors, being just requires sustained effort and resources over time. If the market rewards cost-reductions but not justice, then—if we believe in the importance of ethics—maybe we need to create incentives and forces that also reward the sustained effort needed to realize justice.

Notes

1. G. Dworkin, *The Theory and Practice of Autonomy* (New York: Cambridge University Press, 1988); see T.L. Beauchamp and J.F. Childress, *Principles of Biomedical Ethics,* 4th ed. (New York: Oxford University Press, 1994), ch. 6.
2. J. K. Ingelhart, "Inside California's HMO Market: A Conversation with Leonard D. Schaeffer," *Health Affairs* 14, no. 4 (1995); 131–42.

Fulfilling Institutional Responsibilities in Health Care

Organizational Ethics and the Role of Mission Discernment

JOHN A. GALLAGHER AND JERRY GOODSTEIN

Business Ethics Quarterly 12, no. 4 (2002): 433–50.

Introduction

Change has been an endemic feature of American health care throughout the twentieth century. Hospitals have grown from community institutions caring for the homeless and dying into modern technological corporations. Where once only meager forms of palliative care could be offered, the contemporary hospital offers the residents of a community an armamentarium of diagnostic and therapeutic interventions undreamed of a century ago. In order to sustain this transition, American hospitals have acquired a corporate structure that is similar to that of commercial enterprises.

The role of the physician has undergone a similar transformation. In the living memory of many Americans, physicians were either general practice physicians or surgeons. Today the scope of medical practice ranges from family practice physicians and general internists to a vast array of specialists and sub-specialists. As new therapies emerge for specific diseases and more is learned about specific organ systems, as new technologies make possible the viewing and treatment of discrete aspects of the human body, new specializations arise. These new technologies have not only changed the practice of medicine, they have also altered the role of the physician within the health care delivery system. Increasingly, physicians are becoming investors or owners of ambulatory surgery centers, radiology clinics, heart and birthing hospitals. In many instances physicians financially benefit not only from providing a service, but also benefit from the profits of the facility in which the services are rendered.

For health care organizations, a significant ethical challenge is to determine how to fulfill institutional responsibilities to patients, physicians and other health care professionals, payers, and the community. An interest in the ethical responsibility and integrity of institutions has already begun to capture the interest of writers in the domains of business ethics and health care ethics.

Below we explore in greater detail the forces prompting the emergence of organizational ethics issues within health care institutions. We highlight the significance of mission discernment as a core organizational process that allows health care institutions to actively reflect on their mission and core values and confront the ethical challenges posed by the contemporary health care context.

Organizational Ethics

Organizational ethics is fundamentally concerned with questions of integrity, responsibility, and choice. It involves a comprehensive framework that involves the creation and implementation of processes, procedures, and policies that seek to ensure that the performance of an organization or institution is consistent with its fundamental purpose(s) or ethical aims and values. There is a core concern with fulfilling key responsibilities to appropriate stakeholders and ensuring that the choices made on behalf of the institution are responsive to market, financial, and legal realities.

Integrity

The preservation of institutional integrity is a central focus for organizational ethics. At issue is how to ensure that organizational decisions and actions are carefully considered and implemented in a manner that is consistent with the mission statement and core values of the organization. The mission and core values should be an important driving force for an organization.

> Ethical values shape the search for opportunities, the design of organizational systems, and the decision-making process used by individuals and groups. They provide a common frame of reference and serve as a unifying force across different functions, lines of business, and employee groups. Organizational ethics helps define what a company is and what a company stands for. (Paine, 1994)

Such a commitment to core values and institutional integrity, institutionalized through formal and informal structures and processes, is an important foundation for long-run organizational success in health care and in other sectors. Collins and Porras (1994) undertook an extensive six-year study to identify the determinants of enduring success within large corporations. They found that the most significant factors differentiating companies that thrived over the long-term from those that merely survived were (1) the compelling presence of a core ideology (mission and values) that transcends purely economic considerations and mechanisms, and (2) processes to translate the core ideology into actions that preserve the core, while motivating progress and change.

Complementing this work, Paine studied a variety of organizations (e.g., Martin Marietta, NovaCare, and Wetherill Associates) that had successfully implemented integrity-oriented strategies. While the way in which the mission and values were integrated into each organization varied, what was key was the fact that the mission and values were integrated into the "driving systems" of each organization. Summarizing this research Paine noted, "In each case, management has found that the initiative has made important and often unexpected contributions to competitiveness, work environment, and key relationships on which the company depends."

Such a focus on organizational integrity is not easily achieved. As Selznick (1992) suggests,

institutional values are precarious in nature and must be protected:

> Institutions embody values, but they can do so only as operative systems or going concerns. The trouble is that what is good for the operative system does not necessarily serve the standards or ideals the institution is supposed to uphold. Therefore institutional values are always at risk. Insofar as organizational, technological, and short-run imperatives dominate decision-making, goals and standards are vulnerable. They are subject to displacement, attenuation, and corruption.

The challenge of sustaining organizational integrity is complicated by the context within which health care organizations operate. Health care organizations must take account of multiple internal (e.g., medical staff, employees) and other (e.g., patients, communities, insurers, government) stakeholders. The current health care delivery system is constituted by a variety of stakeholders, each with its own self-interests. Physicians, employees, patients, vendors, the civic community, and payers each have their expectations of what the system will "do for them." In this environment, tensions among stakeholder values can be high and institutional integrity may become more difficult to preserve.

Responsibility

It is therefore crucial that the challenge of sustaining organizational integrity in health care be framed in a manner that acknowledges multiple stakeholder relationships, the responsibilities owed to these stakeholders, and the influence of stakeholders on the values, decisions, and actions of health care organizations. Within the past few years, there has been an important call within the health care ethics literature to develop a stronger organizational focus on ethical issues in health care.

Organizational ethics departs from the individual patient focus of bioethics or the broad systemic orientation of many business ethics writers and looks to how the health care institutions can respond to multiple stakeholder responsibilities in a manner that upholds critical institutional purposes and values. It is fundamentally grounded in a response ethic. Health care organizations are conceived of as moral agents that respond, answer, and are in dialogue with the multiple organizations, persons, political, social, and economic forces acting upon them. A response ethic draws on a particular conception of moral agency, one that involves intentionality of purpose and embodiment of values.

While such a view of moral agency among formal organizations has been disputed, others have emphasized that corporations do have organizational processes and decision-making structures that require a collective sense of responsibility, accountability, and moral agency. Collier (1998) points out that while individual agents may make decisions and carry out actions, these individuals do so "in the name of and by the authority of the organization, frequently in contexts where it is not possible to identify and attribute responsibility to any single individual or group."

Choice

Operating from a response ethic, an organization is not focused primarily on an abstract notion of the good or the right. A response ethic prompts an organization to find the fitting action or response that embodies its mission, values, and corporate identity in a manner that takes account of the forces acting upon it. Organizational ethics is therefore concerned primarily with concrete notions of the good or the right as these are defined in a particular context and enacted through the choices made within organizations.

Selznick (1992) notes that a strategy of responsiveness that fulfills core responsibilities in a specific context entails a "burden of choice." There are likely to be tensions and conflicts associated with multiple stakeholder responsibilities and commitments. It is through the specific choices a health care organization makes (e.g., affiliations

with other health care providers, establishing budget priorities) and how the institution makes these choices that the character of the institution is defined and institutional integrity either reinforced or undermined.

Organizational ethics attempts to identify the structures, processes, and policies that support choices that are made in a reflective and responsive manner. Responsiveness is morally bounded and constrained through taking into account organizational and community values that are grounded in the organization's implicit contract with society. The goal is to foster a certain kind of value-attuned responsiveness or reflexive responsibility that can rule out morally illegitimate missions, e.g., the Mafia.

How can this capacity for institutional responsiveness and responsibility be achieved and built into the social structure of health care organizations? Below we discuss one process. Mission Discernment, created by Holy Cross Health System in South Bend, Indiana. Mission Discernment represents a morally grounded and practical process integrated health care systems can implement to make the mission and core values a central determinant of institutional choice and responsiveness in a changing and uncertain health care context.

Mission Discernment

Developing Mission Discernment at Holy Cross Health System

The Mission Discernment Process (Mission Discernment) discussed in this paper was developed within the Holy Cross Health System. The Holy Cross Health System (which merged into Trinity Health in 2000) consists of seven hospitals/ organized delivery systems and one long-term care company. The subsidiary organizations are spread across the United States. Prior to the development of Mission Discernment, the health care systems had relied upon a process, "An Ethical Framework," grounded in the work of Charles McCoy (1985), to assess major decisions. "An Ethical Framework" was generally regarded as not "user friendly." Executives expressed confusion about when the "Framework" was to be used. Further, they were uncertain about how the process was to be conducted, who was to be involved, and how outcomes were to be reported and to whom.

Mission Discernment was created during the early 1990s with these concerns in mind. The leadership of Holy Cross Health System was committed to developing this process in order to ensure that as Holy Cross Health System responded to an increasingly turbulent health care environment, the mission of the member organizations was as much a driver of corporate strategic decisions as financial, marketing, and operational considerations.

The mission statement identified the fundamental purpose for the corporation's existence. Decisions inconsistent with its mission could only alter the character of the corporation in a manner that would be alienating from its own self-identity and the legitimate interests of a variety of stakeholders. Thus, Mission Discernment was designed to ensure the integrity of the organization in its strategic decisions while at the same time identifying choices responsive to the concerns of a variety of stakeholders.

Holy Cross Health System's mission statement reads:

> *Faithful* to the spirit of the Congregation of the Sisters of the Holy Cross, the Holy Cross Health System exists to witness to Christ's love through *excellence* in the delivery of health services motivated by respect for those we serve. We foster a climate that *empowers* those who serve with us while *stewarding* our human and financial resources.

The words in italics were identified by Holy Cross Health System leadership as key operational values within the mission statement. These values are used to frame major documents and initiatives within the company, including Mission Discernment.

The Mission Discernment Process begins with a review of the proposal or initiative under consideration. Any major initiative that would affect the self-identity of the organization, any merger, acquisition or partnership, the addition or deletion of a service line, anything that might have a significant impact on the local community, care of the poor or vulnerable populations was generally recognized as requiring Mission Discernment. These issues defined the scope or range of issues subject to Mission Discernment.

Those individuals with the relevant capabilities to address the key issues associated with a particular proposal, and who represent key stakeholders, are brought together to deliberate the ethical implications latent within the proposal. Mission-driven values guide the discussion. For example, under Fidelity, participants are asked to analyze issues pertaining to the self-identity of the organization as well as potential ethical concerns. Issues of integrity, self-identity, and institutional character come to the fore within this aspect of the process.

The next phase of Mission Discernment prompts participants to inquire about the manner in which the proposal under discussion is responsive to the interests of the multiple stakeholders who might be affected by a pending decision. The key values in this phase are Empowerment and Stewardship of human resources. In this phase of the process, participants are explicitly charged to assess the impact of a potential decision on patients, employees, other providers, payers, vendors, and the community.

The final component of Mission Discernment directs attention to the health needs of the community. Does a pending decision have a potential positive or negative impact on the organization's commitment to care of the poor (uncompensated care), vulnerable populations, community health and community benefit programs? Two core values of the Holy Cross Health System drive this discussion: social justice and human dignity. As this point in the process, the organization is consciously addressing its duties as a not-for-profit, religious institution.

Mission Discernment in Practice

The value of Mission Discernment has been demonstrated in a variety of situations facing Holy Cross Health System. In one region, a member organization saw an opportunity to enhance its market presence by creating a new for-profit joint enterprise with a group of physicians. The leadership of Holy Cross Health System was committed to the goal of becoming an "indispensable" provider in the markets in which it operated, but not at the risk of undermining its other core values.

Participants in the Mission Discernment Process, including the Board of Trustees at the final review stage, were able to directly confront this issue by actively posing and engaging questions around whether this initiative was consistent with crucial core values at Holy Cross Health System. Financial, marketing, and legal considerations were clearly brought into these discussions as key elements of indispensability and financial stewardship. However, the Mission Discernment Process also gave stakeholders an opportunity to ask whether this initiative upheld the core values of fidelity and social justice. Through deliberation and dialogue around the meaning of these values in relation to this proposed physician partnership, the participants were able to address Holy Cross Health System's core service commitment to the poor and vulnerable and to draw attention to the importance of the new joint partnership assuming responsibility for community service and care of the poor and other vulnerable populations. Mission Discernment played a central role in this instance by elevating the importance of institutional integrity in the discussions.

The on-going practice of Mission Discernment within Holy Cross Health System has also been vital in clarifying choices among potentially competing goods and fostering a greater awareness of the multiple stakeholders potentially affected by a particular proposal—early in the decision-making process. One of the most complex mission discernment discussions involved a proposal to replace an older hospital in a community and to rebuild at a new site. In order to account for the diverse stakeholders and their interests implicated in this proposal, a series of questions were formulated to guide discussion: What would be the impact on the community surrounding the current facility and the wider civic community? Would a move to a new location be readily accessible to the elderly, Medicaid beneficiaries, and the underinsured that were dependent upon the current facility? What effect would this move have on physicians, nurses, and other employees?

These questions surfaced important conflicts and prompted Holy Cross Health System to undertake a series of studies to determine accessibility at the new site, whether the move would overburden the emergency department of the other local hospital, and an internal impact study of the move on health care professionals and other employees within the hospital. Ultimately the studies provided critical information that the Board of Trustees of Holy Cross Health System was able to draw on in making this difficult decision in an ethical and reflective manner.

Confronting the Limits of Mission Discernment

In each of these situations and in others faced by Holy Cross Health System, the Mission Discernment Process helped the institution confront major strategic decisions while attending to the issues of power and conflict. The danger for Holy Cross Health System, like any other large corporate entity, is to fail to recognize and control its power and self-interest. Through establishing new ventures, developing physician-partnerships, or at times closing down facilities and rebuilding elsewhere, Holy Cross Health System and other health care organizations seek to enhance market share, attract insurers to negotiate contracts, and to enrich the range and quality of services they provide within a community. Such plans necessarily entail the self-interest and power of the organization. In the name of responsiveness, an organization can use a process such as Mission Discernment to create and reinforce its own moral universe—one that defines meaning and value in self-serving terms, as a bastion of corporate power and purpose unfettered by moral restraints.

The Mission Discernment Process also directs attention to issues of power and self-interest by eliciting joint reflection concerning the impact of a potential decision on the multiple stakeholders who might be negatively affected by the decision. At Holy Cross Health System the framing of questions around the values of social justice and human dignity, and the discussion of how initiatives will affect patients, employees, other providers, payors, and the community, makes the interests of these stakeholders and the broader society an explicit and important element in the deliberations.

Strategic decisions often raise important conflicts among stakeholder interests. A virtue of the Mission Discernment Process is that it provides a formal forum for identifying and discussing conflicts between the interests of the corporation, its multiple stakeholders, and, at times, the wider community. The weight and legitimacy of competing interests or commitments must be discerned. Such conflicts are rarely resolved in perfect accordance with the desires and goals of each stakeholder. What Mission Discernment does in this regard is twofold. First, by having a formalized means for taking into account mission and values, it better ensures that economic and bottom line considerations do not overwhelm or crowd out other institutional values and stakeholder commitments in making strategic decisions.

Second, within the context of these forums for discussion, Mission Discernment encourages its practitioners to address conflicting commitments by encouraging participants to pursue options that are "fitting," concrete responses to the problem at hand. The fitting response is one that takes into account corporate integrity and institutional responsibilities and is sensitive to the interests and goals of others. It is not an ideal or perfect solution, but rather it is likely to be discovered in the convergence of possibilities and natural limitations that Mission Discernment prompts participants to think about.

The on-going success of Mission Discernment at Holy Cross Health System represents an explicit strategy within this institution to weave organizational ethics and the core mission and values into the fabric of the organization. The success of these efforts has been sustained by a deep commitment on the part of senior leadership within the organization and the broad participation of administrative and clinical staff.

Ethical Theory and Mission Discernment

A series of convictions drawn from ethical theory and closely connected to the core themes of organizational ethics (i.e., integrity, responsibility, and choice) underlie the development and institutionalization of Mission Discernment.

Integrity needs to be the basic virtue of health care institutions. Such institutions need to develop a clearly articulated sense of purpose and ask, what is this organization most fundamentally about? Such a sense of purpose is customarily expressed in an organization's mission statement. It is the mission statement and associated core values that drive the Mission Discernment Process at Holy Cross Health System.

Mission statements are the hubs, which enable an organization to become "a system of consciously coordinated activities" (Selznick, 1992). Purpose or mission statements also serve as articulations of the ethical aims of the organization, as indicators of the kind of organization it intends to be, and the scope of goods and services it provides. In addition, such statements provide boards of directors, management teams, physicians, nurses, patients, and the community a sense of the kind of health care organization it is and what it is willing to commit itself to.

With a well thought out and explicit statement of mission and core values, an organization can measure its fidelity to its self-defining principles. Selznick (1992) sees this moral accountability as central to the notion of institutional responsibility. "In short," he argues, "to be responsive is a way of being responsible. Responsibility runs to an institutional self identity; to those upon whom the institution depends; and to the community whose well-being it affects." Indeed, external factors such as the expectations of payers and patients, the dynamics of the local market along with a host of other issues will all contribute to the concrete manner in which the organization implements its mission and responds to environmental forces. But such issues ought not to be the sole determinants of the activities of an organization that strives to maintain its corporate identity. Integrity requires that health care organizations not act in an opportunistic manner, but rather align decisions and actions to be consistent with their fundamental missions and social values.

The second conviction is that institutions such as hospitals, integrated health care systems, insurers, and other health care organizations are moral agents. Mission Discernment supports a view of institutions as responsible "participants in the moral order, as potential objects of moral concern" (Selznick, 1992). An institution's actions and failure to act have moral consequences for the institution and its stakeholders. The Mission Discernment Process is grounded in a recognition that contemporary medical practice occurs within institutionalized structures, within specific policies and procedures; individual practitioners in the context of the ad hoc physician/patient relationship do not determine the rules of the game.

Mission Discernment is premised upon the conviction that institutions are moral agents that through their reflective processes plan and thus incur responsibility for their actions. The nature and attributes of the institution as a moral agent are grounded in its reflective, deliberative processes by which it charts its path within an environment.

The third conviction is that a response ethic, an understanding of health care institutions as responsive moral agents, most adequately depicts the decision-making functions of such institutions. Niebuhr (1963) enunciated his theory of moral responsiveness as an alternative to teleological and deontological ethical models.

The ethic of response depicts the moral agent as "man-the-answerer" or man engaged in "dialogue" or "man acting in response to actions upon him" (Niebuhr, 1963). This theory of moral responsiveness seems to be most aligned with the decision-making activities of corporations and is inherent in Mission Discernment. Rarely do corporations initiate a service or program simply to foster human benefit. Corporations do, however, respond to forces in their environment such as clinical pathways, outcomes studies, technological advances, as well as financial and market indicators To revert to Niebuhr again, to understand an institution as responsive is to understand it as a moral agent, "which in all its actions answers to action upon it in accordance with its interpretation of such action" (Niebuhr, 1963).

The goal of moral reasoning associated with the responsive model is to choose the fitting response. Health care organizations struggle to respond to needs of patients, the expectations of various stakeholders, and advances in clinical medicine. The fitting response is a concrete response found within the interpretation of these competing demands upon a corporation; it is found in the identification of what an organization can do and cannot do; it is found in the recognition of a decision that is honestly responsive to such demands and congruent with the self-identity of the organization. The mission and values of an institution provide vital guideposts for the construction of the fitting response.

Conclusion

We have argued throughout this paper for adopting a definition of organizational ethics in health care that embraces three core themes: (1) the creation of structures and processes that promote integrity with respect to the mission and core organizational values; (2) identification and the fulfillment of critical institutional responsibilities to stakeholders; and (3) institutional reflection on critical choices with potentially broad organizational implications. We have connected these themes of integrity, responsibility, and choice to the manner in which the mission and values directly enter in organizational strategic and policy decision making.

Corporations and health care institutions, as moral agents, will increasingly be challenged to take responsibility not only for outcomes, but also for the processes by which these outcomes are achieved. In the midst of great uncertainty and change, Mission Discernment offers these institutions a theoretically grounded and practical process for making the core mission and values the foundation for institutional integrity and responsible choice.

Bibliography

Collier, J. "Theorising the Ethical Organization." *Business Ethics Quarterly* 8, no. 4 (1998): 621–54.

Collins, J. C., and Porras, J. I. *Built to Last*. New York: HarperCollins, 1994.

McCoy, Charles. *The Management of Values*. New York: Harper and Row, 1985.

Niebuhr, H. R. *The Responsible Self*. New York: Harper and Row, 1963.

Paine L. S. "Managing for Organizational Integrity." *Harvard Business Review* 72, no. 2 (1994): 106–17.

Selznick, P. *The Moral Commonwealth*. Berkeley: University of California Press, 1992.

Responsibility, Alcoholism, and Liver Transplantation

WALTER GLANNON

Journal of Medicine and Philosophy 23, no. 1 (1998): 31–49.

I. Introduction

Medical and moral arguments have been advanced in response to the question of whether patients with alcohol-related end-stage liver disease should be given lower priority for a liver transplant than those whose disease is not alcohol-related. According to the medical argument, alcoholics should have lower priority than nonalcoholics because the survival rate of the former after transplantation is lower than that of the latter, owing to a fairly high probability of relapse into alcohol abuse. According to the moral argument, alcoholics should be given lower priority for a new liver because their moral vice of heavy drinking makes them responsible for their condition and effectively forfeit their claim to medical treatment.

Two challenges have been issued to the moral argument. First, Carl Cohen and Martin Benjamin maintain that the argument is defective because there is no agreement about what constitutes moral virtue and vice. Moreover, E. Haavi Morreim argues that "it is generally wrong to deny medical care because of patients' lifestyles" on similar grounds. And a task force on individual responsibility for health at the University of Minnesota Center for Biomedical Ethics concluded that "the state of knowledge about what causes behavior and disease is inadequate to support the imposition of punitive measures" (Caplan *et al.*,), which includes giving alcoholics lower priority for liver transplants. Thus, it seems that moral evaluation of patients of *any* sort should be excluded from consideration of who should be treated for liver disease. Second, Alvin Moss and Mark Siegler hold that alcoholism is a disease and, as such, legitimizes medical intervention to treat it, including receiving a new liver. However, they claim that while *retrospective* considerations involving causal factors leading to the disease of alcoholism should be excluded from consideration, *prospective* considerations with respect to whether they seek treatment once they already have the disease may serve to justify giving higher priority to non-alcoholics for liver transplantation. This would be the case if a person failed to enter or comply with a recovery program such as Alcoholics Anonymous to try to keep his alcoholism in remission. These considerations are not prospective in the usual sense concerning how a patient will do with a transplant, but in the sense concerning the period after alcoholism has developed but before a decision about treatment for it is made.

I shall focus on the moral rather than medical aspects of a patient's candidacy for liver transplantation and argue that neither of these two challenges refutes the claim that some patients may be given lower priority than others on the grounds that they have retrospective responsibility for their disease. My argument will proceed in two steps.

I will argue that even if disease often befalls people due to some factors beyond their control, it does not follow that it is entirely beyond their control to prevent. We have to examine the history of the disease and determine whether or to what extent one has control over the events that lead to it. Furthermore, I take issue with the claims that it is unfair or indeed punitive to exclude alcoholics from consideration for liver transplantation because of moral vice or an irresponsible lifestyle. Whether alcoholics are vicious or non-alcoholics virtuous is not what matters, but rather whether patients who need a new liver have the capacity to exercise causal control over the events that lead to end-stage liver disease.

II. Control and Responsibility

The idea that some people may have higher or lower priority than others concerning claims to organs or other medical resources is motivated by the fact that these resources are scarce and by the belief that some people have more control over their bodily and mental functionings than others. Generally, the more control one has over one's health, the more responsible one is for a diseased condition, defined as a physical or mental state of impaired functioning. Conversely, the less control one has, the more one's diseased condition befalls him through no fault of his own and the less responsible he is for it. Responsibility for health is a matter of degree, as is the strength of claims to be treated for a disease.

To the extent that a person has causal control over the events that determine his healthy or diseased condition, he is causally responsible for these events as well as for this condition. Furthermore, he is morally responsible for his condition just in case he is able but fails to exercise the control he has in accord with how he reasonably can be expected to behave. It is important to emphasize that it is not whether a person actually exercises causal control, but whether he has the capacity for this control, which grounds attributions of causal and moral responsibility for his good or bad health.

Causal control over one's health consists of four components. First, a person's choices and actions must not be coerced by external factors or compelled by internal factors such as literally irresistible impulses. Broadly construed, a person's choices and actions may be externally coerced if social and economic conditions such as an abusive upbringing or extreme poverty rule out genuine alternative possibilities of choice over time concerning such things as lifestyle and diet. In this regard, social and political institutions have to be in place to ensure adequate conditions for the choices necessary to have control over one's health. That a person's choices and actions are neither coerced nor compelled is not sufficient for them to be autonomous, however. Autonomy, the second component of causal control, also requires the capacity for reflective self-control regarding the desires, beliefs, and intentions that issue in choices and actions. One must be able critically to evaluate these springs of action and eliminate, modify, or reinforce them and come to identify with them as one's own. Third, a person must have the cognitive capacity to foresee his diseased condition at a later time as the likely consequence of his autonomous preferences, choices, and actions at earlier times. Fourth, the consequence that is a diseased condition must be sensitive to the choices and actions (or omissions) that a person makes over time, where sensitivity is formulated in counterfactual terms. That is, holding fixed all other events external to the individual, if the patient in question had made different choices and performed different actions, then the consequence of his diseased condition would not have obtained. Causal sensitivity is a necessary, not a sufficient, condition for having causal control over one's health.

Fairness in giving an ex-alcoholic lower priority to receive a liver transplant requires a fifth condition beyond the four conditions of causal control and responsibility which I have just articulated. When the person begins to drink at an earlier time, he must know, not only that his behavior may cause the disease and the need for treatment at a later time, but also that his behavior may result in his having lower priority to receive treatment for his disease. It seems quite reasonable to assume that most people are capable of knowing that medical resources like livers are scarce, and that they are capable of inferring from this knowledge that such scarcity might require some system of priority based on control and responsibility. Assuming that an alcoholic has causal control over his condition, and that when he begins to drink he is capable of knowing that he may be given lower priority concerning treatment for his disease, it may be fair to give him lower priority.

One might object that when persons currently in need of liver transplants began to drink, say fifteen to twenty years ago, the idea that drinking could cause liver failure would not have occurred to them. Nor did medicine have a priority system in place which might have been based on people's responsibility for their health care needs. But both the link between drinking and cirrhosis and the scarcity of livers for transplantation have been common knowledge for some time, and even twenty years ago most people had the capacity to know the likely consequences of heavy drinking. If one is not persuaded by these points, then at the

very least we can respond by saying that henceforth basing claims to health care on responsibility should become public policy, especially given the limited supply of medical resources.

Intuitively, entitlements to health care for a diseased condition are inversely proportional to control and responsibility. The more control one has over one's health, and thus the more responsible one is for it, the weaker is one's claim to receive treatment for one's condition from the health care system. Conversely, the less control one has over one's health and thus the less responsible one is for it, the stronger is one's claim to treatment.

Applied to the case at hand, if alcoholics have control over the events that lead to cirrhosis but fail to exercise it, and if non-alcoholics with cirrhosis or some other form of end-stage liver disease do exercise this control and yet it befalls them through no fault of their own, then it seems both reasonable and fair to conclude that alcoholics should be given lower priority than non-alcoholics in receiving a liver transplant. To uphold this claim, however, I will have to examine the idea that alcoholism as a disease involves causal factors beyond our control. Moreover, I will have to address the claim that giving lower priority to alcoholics for liver transplantation unfairly singles out and even punishes them for displaying the moral vice of heavy drinking, when in fact we all display other moral vices that lead to other diseases for which we are equally responsible.

III. Alcoholism as a Disease

Some believe that we are influenced to such a degree by our genetic inheritance, upbringing, and social and economic factors that we lack the control necessary to be responsible for most diseases and alcoholism would be included among them. But from the fact that one has a disease with a genetic component, it does not follow that one cannot be responsible for contracting the disease. A gene that makes one susceptible to alcoholism only indicates the likelihood of developing the disease, not that the gene itself causally determines the disease. In most diseases with a genetic component, a faulty gene is a necessary but not sufficient cause. Sometimes an environmental insult may also be needed, as for example in schizophrenia. In the case of alcoholism, even if the A1 allele makes it more likely that a person will become addicted to alcohol over time, it seems implausible to claim that it compels a person to take the first drinks that eventually lead to the addiction and liver failure.

In order to ascertain whether a person who has a disease is responsible for it, we need to examine the etiology or history of that disease. To what extent did environmental factors external to the person (e.g., an abusive upbringing) play a causal role? To what extent did a mutant gene affect one's brain biochemistry to make one more likely to become addicted to alcohol? To what extent did the patient's own autonomous choices and actions causally contribute to the disease? Retrospective as well as prospective aspects of responsibility for one's state of health need to be considered.

One could take the tack of Moss and Siegler and claim that what one is responsible for is failure to get treatment that would successfully eliminate one's alcoholism. This seems plausible, given that alcohol-related end-stage liver disease typically results from something on the order of ten to twenty years of heavy drinking. And one could insist that what is at issue here is not prospective but retrospective responsibility, where we evaluate a person's candidacy for a liver transplant depending on whether they made an effort to get treatment. Yet a recent study sponsored by the National Institute on Alcohol Abuse and Alcoholism concluded that of all the alcoholics who get treatment, at least half will relapse in two to four years. Among other things, this conclusion shows the importance of prevention and thus the need to trace responsibility for alcoholism back further to the events that brought it about in the first place. Aristotle points out in Book III of the *Nicomachean Ethics*, a person may be responsible for an event or condition beyond his control at a later time if, at an earlier time, he freely performs an action or series of actions

which he is capable of foreseeing will lead to an impaired condition.

The following transfer principle of responsibility can be invoked to support my claim: if a person is causally and morally responsible for freely and knowingly performing an action or series of actions at an earlier time which he ought not to have performed, and if he is responsible for the fact that these actions entail certain harmful health consequences at a later time, then he is also causally and morally responsible for these consequences. In the case at hand, the responsibility transfers from the earlier presumed free acts of drinking to the later consequences, which include both the disease and the liver disease that results from it. The history of how his alcoholism developed may include enough autonomy and control for him to be at least partly responsible for both the alcoholism and the end-stage liver disease. And if, when he drinks at the earlier time, he is capable of knowing that he may be given lower priority for a liver transplant at a later time on the basis of his responsibility, then it would be fair to give him lower priority.

Except for diseases caused solely by a mutation of a single gene, like Huntington's or Tay-Sachs, or where a mutation implies an extremely high risk of disease, as in the five to ten percent of breast cancer cases caused by the BRCA1 or BRCA2 gene, most diseases result from the combination of genetic and environmental factors, as well as from people's autonomous choices and actions. So most diseases are not entirely beyond one's control, and one can be at least partly responsible for them. For example, while people with Type-II (adult-onset) diabetes mellitus may be genetically susceptible to the disease, usually they develop it by combining a high-fat diet with lack of exercise. Unless they live in extreme poverty and have little or no choice concerning diet and mobility, they seem to have some control over whether or not they develop diabetes and therefore may be at least partly responsible for it. Similarly, those who are more susceptible than others to become alcoholics because they have the A1 allele of the dopamine D_2 receptor gene, but are not effectively coerced into drinking by adverse environmental factors, may have enough control over their desires, choices, and actions to refrain from drinking and thus avoid the type of behavior that leads to the disease. If so, then they may be responsible for acquiring the disease.

It may seem unfair to give lower priority for a liver transplant to a person whose alcoholism has a genetic component, when another person who also took the risk of beginning to drink did not become an alcoholic and did not later need treatment *only* because he lacked the gene which would have led to alcoholism. Are we not punishing the first individual for having the gene? Punishment is not really the issue here. Rather, the issue is whether having the gene merely disposes one to drink or compels one to drink. If the latter is true, then the person should not be given lower priority for needed health care because his condition is caused by factors completely beyond his control and thus he is not causally or morally responsible for it. If the former is true, however, then he may be given lower priority because whether he drinks or not arguably is at least partly within his control. Crucially, the D$_2$ gene by itself is not sufficient to cause alcoholism, but is one causal factor among others. Responsibility for alcoholism and cirrhosis is a matter of degree, depending on the degree of control one has over the events leading to these conditions. Consequently, the strength of one's claim to treatment or a transplant may also be a matter of degree, depending on the degree of one's control and responsibility.

As Ferdinand Schoeman has pointed out, determining when these factors do or do not undermine control is a notoriously difficult task. In some cases, a person does seem to have enough control over his drinking to be held responsible for his alcoholism. In others, internal or external causes may undermine his control over his drinking and thereby excuse him from responsibility for his condition.

My aim is not to take sides, but only to emphasize the difficulty in determining whether, or to what extent, one can have control over

and be responsible for alcoholism. Ultimately, it depends on the desires, choices, and actions that cause the disease, specifically whether they are autonomous or else made in ignorance or under compulsion or coercion. And because some of these conditions may hold but not others, responsibility for the disease may be a matter of degree, falling somewhere between complete excuse and complete accountability.

The idea that one may be compelled to drink by certain desires raises the important issue of addiction. Many claims have been made recently about the addictive nature of alcohol, given certain features of a person's genes and brain biochemistry. If alcohol is addictive, the argument goes, then alcoholics really are compelled to have certain desires and act on them. Accordingly, they cannot appropriately be held responsible for cirrhosis because they do not have sufficient control over the events leading to this disease. There are two responses to this argument.

First, it is important to distinguish willing from unwilling addicts, only the latter of which may be excused from responsibility from behavior presumably caused by the addiction. A person is an unwilling addict and thus does not act freely only if the desire associated with the addiction compels him to act in a way that defeats a contrary desire to refrain from drinking. Insofar as the addiction makes him act on a desire that he does not want to have or act on, it undermines his autonomy and, correspondingly, his responsibility for his actions and their consequences. However, if the desire to drink associated with the addiction is unopposed by a competing desire to refrain from drinking, then the addict acts freely and can be held responsible for his behavior. The upshot is that addictions *per se* do not necessarily undermine one's autonomy or one's responsibility for alcoholism.

Second, we must examine the *history* of the addiction and how it affects brain biochemistry. An addiction usually develops only after a person repeatedly takes in a particular substance over time. Addictive drugs like cocaine, nicotine, and alcohol affect the neurotransmitter dopamine by causing heightened metabolic activity in the mesolimbic dopamine system. Taking these drugs repeatedly over time perturbs the dopamine system, which adapts by making dopamine less effective. Once the relevant cells adopt this defensive maneuver and become less responsive, the cells are left without normal levels of the neurotransmitter if a person stops taking a substance that floods the mesolimbic system with dopamine. These changes in turn cause a person to crave more of the drug, and the shift to addiction occurs as dopamine dependence produces chronic unpleasant feelings, depression, and the loss of motivation, which causes the need to take the drug in order to feel better.

Significantly, the dopamine system becomes altered only when nicotine, cocaine, or alcohol is taken repeatedly over time. The addiction does not explain or causally determine why the person first takes the drug which subsequently leads to the addiction. If a person is not compelled or coerced into drinking by social factors beyond his control, and is not so young or cognitively disabled as not to be capable of knowing the likely addictive consequences of drinking repeatedly over time, then he can be responsible for acquiring the addiction, as well as for its deleterious effects on his health. Even if a person becomes addicted to alcohol, the history of how this condition came about may include enough autonomy and control for him to be deemed responsible both for the addiction and the end-stage liver disease.

It is worth emphasizing that the strength of one's claim to scarce medical resources like livers is inversely proportional to the control one has over one's health. Someone who fits the description I gave above will have a weaker claim to receive a liver than someone whose end-stage liver failure is beyond his control and thus contracted through no fault of his own. Precisely because livers are scarce, it seems both reasonable and fair to employ the notions of control and responsibility in setting this order of priority.

It may well be the case that an alcoholic with end-stage liver disease *does* have as strong a claim to receive a liver as a non-alcoholic with the same disease. Yet this would be so only if the combination of genetic and environmental causes beyond his control actually coerced or compelled him to drink as he gradually acquired the disease, or if he was incapable of knowing the likely consequences of his drinking.

IV. Moral Vice and Punitive Measures

The second objection to using control and responsibility as moral grounds for giving some with end-stage liver disease lower priority than others is that alcoholics are unfairly and punitively singled out for the moral vice of heavy drinking. It is unfair because *all* of us display different vices to varying degrees (overeating, failure to exercise, etc.) which have deleterious effects on our health. It is punitive in the sense that by giving the alcoholic lower priority for, or categorically denying him from, liver transplantation, we are in effect punishing him for a morally vicious form of behavior which is more repugnant and blameworthy than others.

Cohen and Benjamin maintain that "we could rightly preclude alcoholics from transplants only if we assume that qualification for a new organ requires some level of moral virtue, or is canceled by some level of moral vice. But there is absolutely no agreement – and there is likely to be none – about what constitutes moral virtue and vice and what rewards and penalties they deserve." This view is supported by Caplan *et al.*, who, as I noted earlier, claim that we lack sufficient knowledge of the causes of disease to justify the imposition of punitive measures. On this basis, they conclude that moral evaluation should be excluded altogether from consideration of people's need for medical treatment.

This argument is flawed because it wrongly assumes that moral evaluation of a person's candidacy for a scarce organ is understood solely in terms of virtue and vice. Surely we can discuss causal control over and moral responsibility for the actions that lead to a disease without invoking virtue and vice. To say that a person is virtuous or vicious is to make a judgment of that person's character, which consists in a general disposition to act in a certain way. But not every type of action which a person autonomously performs repeatedly over time is reflective of his character, and therefore our actions are underdetermined by our characters.

Generally vicious people with bad characters may at times perform a praiseworthy action or series of actions. A noteworthy example of this is Oskar Schindler, the self-serving German industrialist who saved more than a thousand Jews from the Holocaust. By contrast, generally virtuous people with good characters sometimes freely perform a blameworthy action or series of actions out of weakness of will or negligence. For instance, someone who is otherwise concerned about his health may continue to smoke, even though he knows that it is bad for him. But this irrational behavior does not mean that the person who engages in it is himself vicious. Autonomous choices and actions that display a failure to exercise control and which adversely affect one's health when performed over time need not and indeed should not be construed as vicious or reflective of a vicious character. Reframing the issue in terms of control and responsibility instead of virtue and vice more adequately reflects the rationale behind the shift in emphasis in health care from treatment of disease by health care professionals to prevention by people whose own choices and actions can determine whether they are diseased or healthy.

Earlier, I noted the problem of social cost, which says that it is unreasonable to expect some people to bear the social costs of others' conditions that are at least partly within their control to prevent. In risky activities like alpine skiing or mountain climbing, we can distribute these costs more equally and fairly by taxing people for engaging in that behavior. Or with respect to people who ride motorcycles without helmets, the costs of head injuries can be dealt with by increasing the insurance premiums of motorcycle riders. In the case of a scarce, nonrenewable organ like a liver, though, the measures that I have just mentioned are ineffectual because liver transplantation involves not *economic* but rather *physical* scarcity of a resource. Assigning priority to receive the organ on the basis of the control the person reasonably can be expected to exercise over the preferences, choices, and actions that lead to his diseased condition is perhaps the only fair way of resolving the problem of balancing physical scarcity of medical resources with entitlements to these resources.

The policy I have proposed should not be understood as implying that the alcoholic did something wrong and is denied a liver transplantation as punishment for this wrong. Instead, it should be understood in the following way. If a person acts on autonomously formed preferences and choices, and if he is capable of knowing what the probable consequences of his behavior will be, then he weakens his entitlement to receive treatment for a diseased condition he has brought upon himself. The weakening of the entitlement is not a form of punishment imposed on him externally, but something that he brings upon himself as the consequence of his *own* preferences, choices, and actions over time.

If we do not employ the criteria of control and responsibility in assessing whether some people should be given higher priority over others in their claims to a scarce medical resource, then we risk undermining what may very well be the fairest policy available. Perhaps more importantly, we would debase rather than affirm the value of autonomy. Autonomy and responsibility are mutually entailing notions. Freedom to make choices and act on these choices entails the capacity to take responsibility for them and their consequences. By the same token, responsibility for choices, actions, and consequences presupposes that a person makes, performs, and brings them about autonomously. To say that alcoholics cannot be responsible for end-stage liver failure because alcoholism is a disease, or that it unfairly singles them out for a moral vice when non-alcoholics display other vices, threatens to divorce autonomy from responsibility. It is as if we were saying that, even if the choices that lead to the disease are not compelled or coerced, it is unfair to hold the person making those choices responsible for their consequences because we are all "sinners" capable of making bad choices that can adversely affect our health (as Caplan *et al.* claim). Yet autonomy and responsibility are essential features of our personhood. And the responsibility we are capable of taking for our autonomous choices and actions as well as their consequences is what makes each of us unique as a person.

So to dismiss moral responsibility from assessment of our claims to scarce medical resources in general, and to liver transplantation in particular, is to debase our autonomy and personhood. Provided that they are capable of being responsible for their choices and actions as well as for the healthy or diseased consequences of these choices and actions, giving lower priority to alcoholics than non-alcoholics is not punitive but an affirmation of people's ability to take responsibility for their own health.

V. Conclusion

In an era of scarce medical resources, there has been a necessary shift in emphasis from treatment to prevention of disease. This shift presupposes that people are able to make autonomous choices and actions and to take responsibility for their health. If we are to make good on this claim, and to affirm the value of autonomy and responsibility so essential to our personhood,

then we have to hold people responsible for diseases they contract when they are able but fail to exercise control over the events that cause these diseases. This may mean giving lower priority to some versus others concerning claims to medical treatment. But provided that these decisions are based on control and responsibility, it may be fair to discriminate on these grounds.

References

Caplan, A. *et al. Sinners, Saints and Health Care: Individual Responsibility for Health-Ethical, Legal and Economic Questions*, University of Minnesota Center for Biomedical Ethics, Minneapolis, 1994.

Cohen, C., and Benjamin, M. "Alcoholics and liver transplantation," *Journal of the American Medical Association* 265 (March 13, 1991): 1299–1301.

Morreim, E.H. "Lifestyles of the risky and infamous," *Hastings Center Report* 25 (November–December 1995), pp. 5–13.

Moss, A., and Siegler, M. "Should alcoholics compete equally for liver transplantation?" *Journal of the American Medical Association* 265 (March 13, 1991): 1295–1298.

Schoeman, F. "Alcohol addiction and responsibility attributions," in *Philosophical Psychopathology*, ed. G. Graham and G.L. Stephens, (183–204), Cambridge, MA: MIT Press, 1994.

Recovery of Transplantable Organs After Cardiac or Circulatory Death

Transforming the Paradigm for the Ethics of Organ Donation

JOSEPH L. VERHEIJDE, MOHAMED Y. RADY, AND JOAN MCGREGOR

Philosophy, Ethics, and Humanities in Medicine 2 (2007): 8.

Background

Medical and pharmacologic advancements have made it possible to transplant organs successfully and thereby to save the lives of many persons who otherwise would die from irreversible end-stage organ disease. The greatly enhanced technical ability to transplant organs has also led to an ever-increasing need for transplantable organs. The explosive growth in the demand for and the marginal increase in the supply of transplantable organs have together been characterized as an 'evolving national health care crisis'. In fact, organ donation rates nationally have changed little in the past 15 years, whereas the need for donated organs has grown 5 times faster than the number of available cadaveric organs. It is therefore no surprise that the transplantation community and society as a whole now consider balancing the demand for and the supply of transplantable organs as one of their biggest challenges.

The continually increasing need for organs led to the reintroduction of the principle of donation after cardiac or circulatory death (DCD) in the early 1990s with the Pittsburgh protocol to complement already available organ procurement from brain-dead persons. A new federal mandate requires hospitals as of January 2007 to design policies and procedures for organ procurement in DCD to increase the rate of organ donation and recovery from decedents to 75% or greater.

However, DCD is controversial because of medical, ethical, and legal uncertainties about the premise that donors are indeed dead before their organs are procured. In this article, we contend that the recovery of viable organs useful for transplantation in DCD is not compat-ible with the dead donor rule and we explain the ethical and legal ramifications of DCD. We also examine the current process of consent for organ donation and whether it includes the necessary elements for voluntary informed consent (i.e., the full disclosure of information relevant to decision making and respect for the person's autonomy). Finally, we will conclude by positing that in order for the current principle of DCD to proceed with recovery of transplantable organs from decedents, a paradigm change in the ethics of organ donation is necessary. The paradigm change to ensure the legitimacy of DCD practice must include (1) societal agreement on abandonment of the dead donor rule, (2) legislative revisions reflecting abandonment of the dead donor rule, and (3) the requirement of mandated choice to facilitate individual participation in organ donation and to ensure that DCD is in compliance with the societal values of respect for autonomy and self-determination.

DCD and the Dead Donor Rule

The criteria for determining death play a prominent role in the acceptability of DCD. The recovery of viable organs for successful transplantation must be achieved with the donor already dead at the time of procurement in order to comply with the dead donor rule. Whereas some have considered a person dead after 2 minutes of apnea, unresponsiveness, and absent arterial pulse, the Institute of Medicine recommended waiting for 5 minutes of absent consciousness, respiration, and mechanical pump function of the heart (zero pulse pressure through arterial catheter monitoring), irrespective of the presence of electric activity of the heart (evident on electrocardiographic monitoring). In 2001, the American College as well as the Society of Critical Care Medicine concluded in a position statement that a waiting period of either 2 minutes or 5 minutes was physiologically and ethically equivalent and therefore either was an acceptable timeline for beginning the process of organ retrieval. Waiting for longer than 5 minutes can cause warm ischemia and detrimentally affect the quality of procured organs and impair their suitability for transplantation. However, critics have argued more than a decade ago that the waiting time to determine death by respiratory and circulatory criteria is based on insufficient scientific evidence. The spontaneous return of circulation and respiration (i.e., the Lazarus phenomenon or autoresuscitation) has been reported to occur in humans as long as 10 minutes after cessation of circulation and respiration. Autoresuscitation appears to validate previous concerns that viable organs may be procured from persons who are in the process of dying yet are not truly dead.

According to the Uniform Determination of Death Act (UDDA) of 1981, a person is determined dead after having sustained either irreversible cessation of circulatory and respiratory functions or irreversible cessation of all brain function, including that of the brain stem, and the determination of death must be made in accordance with accepted medical standards. The President's Commission for the Study of Ethical Problems in Medicine and Biomedical and Behavioral Research defined the statute for the determination of death so that "Death is a Single Phenomenon." The statute is intended to address the question "how, given medical advances in cardiopulmonary support, can the evidence that death has occurred be obtained and recognized." The President's Commission defined the cessation of circulation to be irreversible for death determination "[i]f deprived of blood flow for at least 10–15 minutes, the brain, including the brainstem, will completely cease functioning … A 4–6 minute loss of blood flow – caused by, for example, cardiac arrest – typically damages the cerebral cortex permanently, while the relatively more resistant brainstem may continue to function."[1]

The challenge in determining death for organ procurement is twofold: (1) the use of an arbitrary set of criteria and time frames to define irreversible cessation of circulatory and respiratory functions without evidence of the uniformity for death determination and (2) the variability of the criteria used by different institutions for organ procurement protocols.

The notion of irreversibility of cessation of circulatory and respiratory functions has been a contentious medical and ethical issue. Tomlinson proposed a definition of irreversibility as "a requirement that arises only at the level of the *criteria for the determination* of death, rather than at the level of the concept of death, just as 'beyond reasonable doubt' is not a part of the *concept* of 'guilty', but instead is a requirement for the legitimate determination of guilt within a judicial system."[2] The requirement for irreversibility therefore depends on the context in which, and the purposes for which, the concept of death is being used. The notion of irreversibility is commonly understood as meaning either that the heart cannot be restarted spontaneously (a weaker construal) or that the heart cannot be restarted despite standard cardiopulmonary resuscitation (a stronger construal). The stronger construal of irreversibility as meaning "can never be reversed" implies in its extreme that *at no time* can organ procurement ever be permissible because future possibilities of resuscitation can never be fully ruled out. In practical terms, the weaker definition of "not reversible now" implies that a person is considered irreversibly dead based on that person's moral choice to forego resuscitative interventions; thus, as long as the probability of autoresuscitation is negligible, the dead donor rule is not violated. On the basis of that argument, the notion of irreversibility depends on the person's choice to forego resuscitative interventions after spontaneous cessation of circulatory and respiratory functions. However, the argument that irreversibility can be understood as a moral choice is flawed. First, the issue is not whether there are good reasons not to resuscitate a person but whether the person is truly dead. Second, resuscitative interventions are performed during the procurement process to keep organs viable for transplantation after the cessation of vital functions. The use of artificial cardiopulmonary bypass machines, external mechanical cardiac compression devices, and reinflation of the lungs to preserve organs for procurement also results in the resuscitation of the heart and the brain after the formal declaration of death. Resuscitation of the brain with a return of consciousness is particularly problematic because the Institute of Medicine announced in its 2006 report that expansion of the organ donor pool by procuring organs from living persons with normal brain function who sustain sudden cardiac death is morally acceptable.

Longer than 10 minutes of absent circulation is required for irreversible cessation of the entire human brain, including brain stem function. The administration of medications to suppress heart and brain functions is therefore required when the procurement process begins within 5 minutes of cessation of circulation.

The use of resuscitative methods and medications to suppress heart and brain functions during organ procurement raises a host of additional ethical and legal questions. Organ donors consent to the withholding of all resuscitative interventions after cessation of circulatory and respiratory functions through a do-not-resuscitate (DNR) directive. Under such conditions, the use of resuscitative methods for organ procurement violates not only the dead donor rule but also the person's health directives. The strong probability of a return of heart and brain functions during procurement also means that the act of organ removal is the immediate and proximate cause of death for that person.

The need for criteria to sharpen "the indeterminate boundary between life and death" for death determination has been widely recognized. The dependence on both circulatory and respiratory criteria only for the determination of death

in DCD is problematic and conceptually inconsistent because of (1) there is a likelihood of spontaneous reversibility of circulatory and respiratory functions when organ procurement begins, and (2) the possibility for the brain to recover function long after circulatory arrest, particularly when artificial circulation is used for organ procurement. Therefore, the practice of DCD conflates a prognosis of death with a diagnosis of death. The application of criteria for irreversible cessation of neurologic, circulatory and respiratory functions requires a waiting time well in excess of 10 minutes to sharpen the determination of death for organ procurement. However, that waiting time can also make it more difficult to recover viable organs for transplantation. The simultaneous determination of total cessation of the activity of the entire brain, including the brain stem, is required for the determination of death when respiration and circulation are artificially supported during organ procurement.

The Dead Donor Rule and the Law

DCD has been recommended on the basis of the utilitarian rationale of maximizing the number of organ transplants in order to save more lives. This utilitarian approach has also provided implicit justification for manipulation of some aspects of the death process. Intervention has been justified not only in the dying process but also in defining the word *dead*. The uncertainty of the uniformity of determination of death in DCD has legal implications. The act of procurement or the removal of organs from persons who may still be in the process of dying but who are labeled as being dead, becomes the direct and proximate cause of death or of "killing" rather than the natural illness itself. Medically redefining death arbitrarily to permit DCD for organ procurement has been a necessary prerequisite for the circumvention of homicide law. Declaration of death or calling someone dead takes the burden off procurement personnel and provides the appearance that it is acceptable to remove organs under such conditions without being found guilty of murder. The purposeful manipulation of the criteria for the determination of death serves the desired goal of increasing the opportunities for procurement of transplantable organs, but it also represents a knowing gerrymandering of the existing legal definition. The President's Commission indicated in the 1981 report on defining death that the UDDA is intended to aid in the process of recognition and providing a legal standard to distinguish the dead from the dying and, ought not to reinforce the misimpression that there are different "kinds" of death, defined for different purposes, and hence that some people are more "dead" than others.

Problems with Consent for Organ Donation

Obtaining consent is considered one of the guiding principles that provide moral validation of organ transplant programs. Consent for organ donation is obtained in two different situations. The first situation is to acquire consent from healthy persons for future organ donation. It is generally achieved by inviting members of the public to complete donor cards (e.g., as part of a driver's license application) providing general consent for organ donation or to consent to organ donation by signing up on a state registry when they visit an OPO Web site. The second situation occurs when consent is obtained from a surrogate decision maker for a brain-dead person or a person for whom death is imminent and who has not expressed intent for organ donation through a driver's license, a donor card or donor registry.

Studies show that half of the families who are asked to consider donation after a relative's death refuse consent. It should therefore come as no surprise that in addition to educating the public, the Institute of Medicine Committee on Increasing Rates of Organ Donation has identified among its primary objectives an increase in the number of opportunities for people to record the decision to donate and the enhancement of donor registries to ensure full access to and sharing of donor registration data.

Requiring consent is consistent with one of the corner stones of medicine and bioethics: respect for individual autonomy. Among other things, the process of obtaining consent must include the provision of an appropriate quantity and quality of information so that the person can make an informed decision. Currently, the consent for DCD is requested with disclosure of similar information as with brain-death donation. Given the medical and ethical uncertainties surrounding DCD, its consent process should be expected to be different from that used in brain-death donation. The differences between the two types of organ donation with regard to timing and the nature of the procurement procedure, nonbeneficial interventions, and trade-offs in end-of-life care are not often clarified to potential donors or surrogate decision makers at the time of consent. DCD also exposes donors to the risk of failing to die within the allotted time frame for successful organ procurement after the performance of predonation procedures.

Considering that actual donation or procurement processes differ according to the death criteria, one might expect the consent process to include details about the various death scenarios. In 2006, Woien et al examined the quality and quantity of information about consent that is disclosed to the public and to potential organ donors on OPO Web sites. The information content about relevant aspects of medical interventions, procedures, protocols and changes to the quality of end-of-life care was found to be deficient because it was focused primarily on the encouragement and reinforcement of consent to donation.[3] This lack of disclosure on OPO Web sites and in online consent documentation raises doubts about whether organ donors actually receive and understand the pertinent information necessary to making an informed decision about whether to participate in deceased organ donation. The lack of detailed and accurate disclosure violates the tenet of informed consent and abuses the public's trust in the deceased organ donation system.

Paradigm Transformation of Organ Donation Ethics

There is growing doubt among scholars and medical practitioners that DCD can comply with the principles on which it was introduced into society as an ethically acceptable practice. We have highlighted several concerns indicating that the current DCD practice not only violates the dead donor rule but also puts the moral legitimacy of consent for donation in question. Unless the current DCD practice is reevaluated, the erosion of public trust and damage to the integrity of the medical profession are likely to develop over time. To avoid these negative consequences, we are faced with implementing any or all of three strategic options. The first strategy would be to discontinue DCD and instead focus on reducing the demand for transplantable organs by promoting healthy lifestyles (i.e., primary and secondary prevention programs for chronic diseases such as diabetes and hypertension). This strategy might decrease the future incidence of end-stage organ disease and the resulting need for transplantation; however, it would not resolve the current imbalance between the supply of and the demand for organs. The second strategy would be to revise the uniform definition of death to allow the definition of "dead" to be applied to dying persons so that the recovery of transplantable organs from DCD can be continued in an ethical and legal manner. Bernat, for instance, has argued for a change in the standard determination of death that would substitute "permanence" for "irreversibility" and thereby permit the classification of dying persons as truly dead.[4] Bernat's proposal to change the death determination implicitly acknowledges that the current DCD practice is inconsistent with the dead donor rule. Bernat justifies violation of the dead donor rule and there is no need to distinguish between the "dying" and the "dead" for the purpose of organ procurement for transplantation. The justification put forward by Bernat conflicts with the President's Commission views on when and how the death statute is applied "to distinguish the dead from the dying" and to prevent "the mistaken impression that a special 'definition' of death needs to be applied to organ transplantation, which is not the case" and that it "ought not to reinforce the misimpression that there are different 'kinds' of death, defined

for different purposes, and hence that some people are [more dead] than others."

The word "permanence" conveys the absolute accuracy of the "prognosis" rather than a determination or diagnosis of death. However, opponents of the criterion of absolute certainty of prognosis of death may consider as homicide its application to persons for whom the consent to withdraw artificial life support is made. Revising the UDDA in this manner would have far-reaching ethical implications not only for society but also for criminal and homicide laws. Criminal prosecution, inheritance, taxation, treatment of cadaver, and mourning are all affected by the way society draws the dividing line between life and death. More importantly, it can violate the principle of nonmaleficence by allowing the introduction of errors in prognostication that may have a detrimental effect on end-of-life care and palliation. The third strategy would be to abandon the dead donor rule for organ procurement so that procuring organs becomes permissible during the terminally ill person's dying phase after voluntary informed consent has been obtained. The abandonment of the dead donor rule would constitute a paradigm switch in the ethics of deceased organ procurement for transplantation from donor beneficence to autonomy and nonmaleficence. Donors would be solely responsible for their decisions, and the medical community would have to comply with the do-no-harm principle at the end of life. As is the case with revising the determination of death, this paradigm switch would require changes in criminal and homicide laws to legitimize DCD legally, ethically, and medically. In addition, changing the paradigm would require public discourse about permitting autonomy-based end-of-life decisions. The preservation of a person's autonomy and the voluntary nature of the decision are fundamental for such a profound paradigm shift and, as such, they require comprehensive public education and disclosure of all relevant information. The mandated personal choice in conjunction with the paradigm shift would protect an individual's right to agree or refuse and thereby would eliminate coercion in the organ donation consent process with minimal infringement on privacy. Within this context, mandated choice restores the public trust and eliminates the individual's fear of manipulation of the dying and death process for the intent of organ procurement. Mandated choice is compatible with the principle of respect for individual autonomy and decision making, and it does not require additional consent from a person's family to procure organs after death.

Conclusion

The long-term solution for overcoming the shortage of transplantable organs is to focus on, and to broadly implement, universally accessible preventive health-care programs. For the short term, increasing the number of potential donors while also maintaining the public trust and the integrity of medicine requires public education, a consent process characterized by full disclosure of relevant information about organ donation and procurement procedures critical to the decision making about organ donation, and a switch of the ethics paradigm from beneficence to nonmaleficence and respect for individual autonomy to allow for DCD to comply with legal and ethical standards. The implementation of mandated

choice for obtaining consent would appear reasonable and morally justifiable to assist with the objective of increasing the number of people who consent to organ donation after death. Ultimately, the outcome of public debate must be the decisive factor in determining the conditions under which DCD should be considered legitimate.

Notes

1. President's Commission for the Study of Ethical Problems in Medicine and Biomedical and Behavioral Research, *Defining Death: A Report on the Medical, Legal and Ethical Issues in the Determination of Death.* Washington, DC: Government Printing Office, 1981.
2. T. Tomlinson, "The Irreversiblity of Death: Reply to Cole," *Kennedy Institute of Ethics Journal* 3 (1993): 157–65.
3. S. Woien, M.Y. Rady, J.L. Verheijde, and J. McGregor, "Organ Procurement Organizations Internet Enrollment for Organ Donation: Abandoning Informed Consent," *BMC Medical Ethics.* 7, no. 1 (2006): 14.
4. J.L. Bernat, "Are Organ Donors After Cardiac Death Really Dead?" *Journal of Clinical Ethics* 17, no. 2 (2006): 122–32.

Why We Are Not Allowed to Sell That Which We Are Encouraged to Donate

BARBRO BJÖRKMAN

Cambridge Quarterly of Healthcare Ethics 15 (2006): 60–70.

Introduction

It is a reality today that people die waiting in line for transplant organs. Something needs to be done to remedy this dire situation and alleviate the suffering. Broadly speaking, barring scientific progress that might make artificial organs and stem cell therapy viable alternatives, three options are available to us: increase voluntary donation,

compel access to organs via government policy, or open up for a commercial market in organs.

It has proven hard to explain why so many of us are convinced that donation is the only morally permissible form of transaction when it comes to organs from the living. This is particularly surprising in light of the fact that we live in a liberal, capitalist society that has seen fit to not only commodify, but, indeed, also commercialize just about everything else. Naturally it would be a different matter altogether if organs were non-transferable, that come what may no human being could be allowed to part with his/her organs. But this is not so—quite the contrary, the citizens of the Western world are exposed to campaigns encouraging donations. It is quite difficult to come up with other examples of objects that we are encouraged to donate and at the same time morally forbidden to sell. Bearing in mind the current organ shortage, ethical questions relating to organ procurement are becoming increasingly pressing—what can we allow ourselves, and others, to do with our bodies?

In this paper I attempt to show that virtue ethics could provide an explanation of why it is morally permissible to donate but not to sell organs, which seems to correlate with our moral intuitions on this matter. The position defended here is that it is morally wrong to sell organs because this is something a virtuous person would not do. Given the choice between selling and donating an organ the virtuous agent would choose the latter, and this is why it is not permissible to sell one's organs. I, first, however take a closer look at some standard arguments for and against the selling of organs. Then I move on to a discussion about whether virtue ethics can give us the necessary tools for explaining why we are not allowed to sell that which we are encouraged to donate. The purpose is to show that a strong case can be made that, given the choice, a virtuous person would donate rather than sell his or her organs.

Some Common Arguments in Favor of Organ Commodification

A number of arguments in favor of allowing for a market, especially in kidneys, have surfaced in the increasingly heated debate surrounding transplant organs. Broadly speaking, such arguments can be split into two groups: consequence- and rights-based ones. It should be noted that very few people, however, go all the way and propose an unregulated global market for organ transplantation. Arguments are commonly put forward in defense of a limited market, one that is rigged such that the active participants can be protected against the most blatant forms of harmful exploitation.

Consequentialist arguments are often structured along the following lines: It is a fact that most people do not donate their organs, at least not to the extent that is required to make up for the organ shortage. It is said to follow that we ought to create a market for selling and buying organs because that would have the best consequences in the sense that fewer people would suffer, and die, in line for a transplant. The underlying assumption is that payment would result in more available organs. It is suggested that many people who are not prepared to part with their organs given the current legislation might well rethink their decision if they were paid. Evidently this is an empirical assumption, but it does not seem to be too far-fetched.

A standard critique is to draw a parallel with the case made for blood donation by Titmuss in his book *The Gift Relationship*.[1] In that text, he argued that paying for blood would not increase the supply significantly, as those who had previously donated would be repulsed by the introduction of money in this transaction. The available empirical data do not suffice to determine whether this is true in the case of organ transplantation. However, it should be noted that donations are in this case—contrary to blood donation—essentially restricted to close relatives. It is a plausible hypothesis that the choice of giving one's kidney to a close relative is less influenced by a parallel market than the act of donating one's blood to an unknown recipient. Moreover Titmuss argued that such a financial compensation would attract the wrong kind of people, for example, drug addicts, and thus threaten the quality of the blood. The scientific progress made since the 1970s has made it possible to test for a much larger range of diseases, a development that disqualifies Titmuss's concerns that commercialization would increase the spreading of infectious diseases.

The second broad category of arguments consists of *rights-based* ones. The underlying assumption is that we have a right to our own bodies such that we are also entitled to sell parts thereof that we can make do without. It is suggested that the ruling out of a market in organs is, in fact, a grave violation of people's most fundamental rights. Briefly, the gist of the argument is the following: We do not live in a fair world, resources and opportunities are not evenly distributed, and, as a result, the vast majority of the world's population lives in poverty. We should all do our best to lessen poverty and suffering and make the world a more equal place. This is not done, however, by denying them what might be their best option to improve their lives, which well could be to sell an organ. To do so, it is said, is to violate their rights, rob them of their autonomy, and, to make matters even worse, will do nothing to alleviate the real problem. Julian Savulescu takes the argument one step further and calls a ban on organ selling "paternalism in its worst form". He advocates that people should be allowed to make this choice (on the condition that it is informed consent) if it provides them with the means to realize what they value in life.[2]

Although the arguments outlined above might seem reasonable on one level (i.e., that people should not have to die queuing for an organ if there are alternatives), they fail to correlate with most people's moral intuitions on this matter. It appears that we have strong intuitions, in the sense that they are stable and withstand the test of time, that the selling of organs is plain wrong and no reasonable consequence- or rights-based argument can make it more palatable. Few of us sincerely feel that creating a market for transplant organs would make the world a better place from a moral point of view, even if the consequences were favorable and important rights would be protected.

Virtue Ethics

Most mainstream moral theories, such as utilitarianism, Kantian ethics, and contract theories, occupy themselves with the issues of rightness and obligation. Virtue theory, on the other hand, approaches ethics by asking "what traits of character make one a good person?" Note, however, that this does not imply a total disregard for the actual action as such, nor for its consequences. We can well imagine cases where the virtuous agent would, in fact, be highly concerned with the consequences and then, naturally, so should we be. A key claim made by virtue ethicists is that we *ought* to do what a (fully informed) virtuous person would have done. So how can we meet this requirement and how do we determine whether virtuous persons would donate rather than sell their organs? Broadly speaking, there are two answers to this question, the classic Aristotelian approach and a more modern one. Aristotle claimed that the virtuous character traits are those we need to live humanly flourishing/fulfilled lives. He argued that it is only when we live virtuously that our rational capacity can guide our lives. Character traits have to be stable—that is, the disposition has to be firm and unchanging—and should, in this context, be understood as something that is manifested in habitual action. However, habitual should not be interpreted as "automatic." Describing an action as habitual does not necessarily mean that it is also effortless or spontaneous, although it could well be; in fact, most decisions would be reached through deliberation. In short, moral virtues are those virtues that are good for everyone to have. The more modern approach, partly seeking to avoid references to human nature, claims that the virtues come from the commonsense views about which character traits we typically find admirable, traits manifested by people we look up to. These are the kind of people we ought to model ourselves on when seeking to act virtuously. It seems plausible to argue that it is more admirable to donate than to sell one's organs—we look up to those who take personal risks not for the sake of economic compensation but simply because they "see" that helping their fellow man is a fine and worthwhile thing to do. Presumably this could be the practical expression of a number of virtues such as unselfishness, generosity, kindness, beneficence, and so forth.

The Transplant Issue

So how does one tell if it is more virtuous to donate than to sell one's organs? From a virtue ethics perspective, there are two answers to that question: It is either that which will help us flourish as human beings *or* what is admirable to do.

Let us first briefly recapitulate what Aristotle had to say about human flourishing and what is required of us to lead a flourishing/fulfilled life. We recall that a virtue is here to be understood as the golden mean, an intermediate, between two vices. Acting virtuously does not require us to maximize the good; we can do this without bringing about the best consequences. What should be aimed for is instead excellence; rather than seeking to have the best friendship we can have we should strive to have *excellent* friendships. This could be understood in relation to the golden mean—that we are under no obligation to maximize but, rather, to strike a balance in life. According to Aristotle, to flourish is a desirable state for any human being because it is only then we can lead fully human lives realizing our full capacities.

Let us construct an example to examine whether a case can be made that organ donation is more likely to promote human flourishing. We imagine two men each wanting to make a kidney available for transplantation. A wants to donate and B wants to sell. Let us now investigate whether A, by wanting to donate, is successful in fulfilling several of the virtues as listed by Aristotle.

By being *courageous*, we bravely sacrifice ourselves and jeopardize our own well-being and health; we choose to perform an act that we know involves some risk. "The courageous person is the one who stands firm and keeps his head in the midst of danger." She/he is neither a coward nor does she/he take foolish risks, that is, such a person has the right attitude to personal safety. This appears to hold true for both A and B—regardless of why they are contemplating giving up their organs, the two of them run the same medical risks. However, one of the strengths of virtue ethics is that it provides an account of moral motivation. The theory recognizes that we can only get a satisfactory account of moral life when we look to the motives of an action. It seems reasonable to suggest that a contributing motive for selling a kidney, in a situation where one could have chosen to donate, would be personal gain (monetary or otherwise). It can then be argued that the fact that B will be compensated monetarily for the risk

he is about to take partially detracts the element of self-sacrifice, which is central to the virtue of courage. It follows that A, by donating, is more courageous than B on this account.

Being *open-handed* involves attempting to share your good fortune with those in need. Now, perhaps having two working kidneys might not be considered affluence under normal circumstances, but when contrasted with a dialysis patient, it just might. Irrespectively, it is clear that giving something away out of the goodness of your heart, not seeking any reward, would objectively qualify as (more) generous than selling that same thing. When applying this to the example above, it is clear that A displays an open-handed behavior whereas B, by requiring compensation, does not.

The second possible reply to the question "How do we know if it is more virtuous to donate than to sell?" is whether or not donating rather than selling will make us more admirable human beings.

To make the problem clearer we can imagine the following, somewhat Singeresque, situation. On my way home from the office, I walk by a pond where a man is drowning. Standing on the shore, I can hear his shrill, panic-stricken cries for help. As he disappears under the water for the second time, I suddenly remember that I have a lifebuoy in my backpack and, as luck has it, I will not have any personal use for it on this particular evening. As I unpack the lifebuoy I have two options. I can either (A) take advantage of the man's desperate situation and tell him that I will throw him the buoy if he promises to pay me the equivalent of his monthly salary or (B) I can save his life for free. Presumably there is not much doubt as to what a virtuous person would do in this situation. To help others unselfishly without expecting a reward is surely the virtuous thing to do, and, as outlined above, indeed, what an admirable person would have done.

Virtue ethics claims that the virtuousness of the act is not decided by the consequences, yet option A above might seem more morally appealing if I were to use the money for charity rather than splurging on a new handbag. Let us revisit the example. The setting is the same, only this time the man in the water is a very wealthy but extremely stingy person and I am the local Red Cross representative who has spent the past decade trying to persuade him to part with if only a small fraction of his wealth, but to no avail. As I unpack my lifebuoy, I have two options. I can either (A) throw him the buoy on the condition that he donate a substantial part of his wealth to the Red Cross or some other aid foundation or (B) save his life for free. It appears relatively uncontroversial to say that engaging in charity, the giving of a part of one's wealth to those who are less fortunate, is a virtuous thing to do. But in the example above this admirable act is preceded by blackmail. It hardly seems admirable to take advantage of people's predicaments, to force them to agree to terms that they would not otherwise have accepted because they fear for their lives. We might be sympathetic to the person on the shore, but it seems odd to suggest that we would admire her when she exploits the circumstances. The fact that option A in the second example might have good consequences does not justify the blackmail. The good, the virtuous in this sense, ought to be chosen for its own sake, not for what it might lead to. Again, the virtues are not to be understood as instrumental. Virtuous actions do not cause fulfillment in the sense that an appropriate medicine might cause health. Living the fulfilled life is the carrying out of fine and noble acts. The focus is on the virtuous character, not the right action, and it is hardly conceivable that a person of virtuous character would engage in blackmail with someone who fears for his/her life. This does not seem to be what one ought to do.

In conclusion, a case can be made that donating rather than selling can bring us closer to a state of flourishing and that we act in accordance with several, and do not seem to violate any, of the central virtues when we refrain from monetary compensation in these instances.

Conclusion

One way of answering the question of why we are encouraged to donate that which we are not allowed to sell is to adopt a virtue ethics approach. In this paper I have attempted to show that virtue ethics can provide a strong support for keeping organ commodification at the gates. I propose that virtue ethics can be action guiding in the sense that it is clear what decision virtuous persons, admirable persons, would reach when facing the choice between donating their organs for free or giving them up conditioned on a price. Further to that point, I have also concluded that donating organs will bring us closer to a state of Aristotelian flourishing because it means that we act in accordance with several of the central virtues when we refrain from monetary compensation in these instances.

It is worth pointing out that this argument does not collapse virtue ethics into some form of duty- or rule-based ethic. Admittedly, such ethical theories might well yield the same result (in most realistic situations) but not on the same grounds. Virtue ethics rejects commodification of organs because it fails to make us flourish, not because it has bad consequences or breaks some rule. The theory is able to help us in these situations partly because it does not focus on the consequences but rather on the character of the decisionmaker. The root of the problem today, according to the virtue ethics approach, is that people are not virtuous enough. The current, dire situation would not improve (ethically speaking; whether it would, in fact, free up more organs is a purely empirical matter) in the least if we were to create a market for organs because a virtuous person would not sell her/his organs anyway. Virtuous persons would not sell their organs but rather donate them because they wish to help their less fortunate fellow man, they "see" that this is fine, noble, and worthwhile. The fact that this is not the current practice in society today only shows that people in general are not virtuous. The way to redeem the problems of organ shortage in a given society is not to create a market but rather to increase the sense of virtue.

Notes

1. Titmuss R.M. *The Gift Relationship: From Human Blood to Social Policy.* London: George Allen and Unwin, 1970.
2. J. Savluescu. Is the sale of body parts wrong? *Journal of Medical Ethics* 29 (2003): 138–39.

Presumed Consent, Autonomy, and Organ Donation

MICHAEL B. GILL

Journal of Medicine and Philosophy 29, no. 1 (2004): 37–59.

I. Introduction

The current American system of cadaveric organ procurement includes the default assumption that individuals prefer *not* to donate their organs for transplantation after their death. Thus, if there is no evidence that an individual either wanted or did not want to donate her organs after her death, she is currently treated as though she did not want to donate.

"Presumed consent" is the name that has been given to a proposal to change the current system. A policy of presumed consent would include the default assumption that individuals *do* prefer to donate their organs for transplantation after their death. Under such a policy, every individual would be given the opportunity to register her desire not to have her organs removed for transplantation, and that registered desire would be respected in every case. But if a person died without leaving any indication of her desires – and if family members provided no reason to believe the individual did not want to donate – we would proceed on the assumption that she would have preferred that her organs be removed for transplantation.

I believe that a policy of presumed consent would be a moral improvement over the current American system of organ procurement. In what follows, I will try to make the case for presumed consent by addressing what I take to be the most important objection to it. The objection is that if we implement presumed consent we will end up removing organs from the bodies of people who did not want their organs removed, and that this situation is morally unacceptable because it violates the principle of respect for autonomy that underlies our concept of informed consent. I will argue that while removing organs from the bodies of people who did not want them removed

is unfortunate, it is morally no worse than not removing organs from the bodies of people who did want them removed, and that presumed consent will produce fewer of these unfortunate results than the current system. The principle of respect for autonomy, I will argue, does not conflict with presumed consent but speaks in its favor.

II. The Two Sides: Cohen vs. Veatch and Pitt

There is some dispute about whether a policy of presumed consent would increase the number of organs available for transplantation. I believe that it is probable that a policy of presumed consent would produce more organs, but I will not argue that point here. What I want to focus on instead is the dispute over whether or not a policy of presumed consent would do a better job than the current system at respecting people's wishes about what should happen to their bodies after death.

Cohen has given the following argument for the claim that presumed consent would do a better job than the current system at respecting people's wishes. About 70% of Americans would prefer to donate their organs for transplantation after their death. But fewer than 70% of the organs suitable for transplantation are donated. This is because many people who want to donate their organs do not leave indications of their desires that are clear enough to overcome the current system's initial presumption against removing organs for transplantation. As a result, many who wanted to donate their organs after death are buried with all their organs intact inside their bodies. This violates their wishes about what should happen to their bodies after death. A policy of presumed consent, however, would result in people's wishes being respected at least 70% of the time, and probably much more than that, so long as the policy includes a well-publicized opt-out opportunity. This would almost certainly constitute an increase over the current system in the number of decedents whose wishes are respected.

Veatch and Pitt have given the following argument for the claim that presumed consent is morally unacceptable because it violates persons' wishes about what should happen to their bodies after death. About 30% of Americans prefer not to donate their organs for transplantation after their death. But if presumed consent was implemented, some portion of that 30% would fail to indicate their desire not to donate. As a result, some people who wanted to buried with all their organs intact would have their organs removed. This would violate their wishes about what should happen to their bodies after death. Under the current system, in contrast, it is very unlikely that organs will be removed from the body of someone who did not wish to donate. The current system thus does a better job than presumed consent at respecting the wishes of those who do not want to donate their organs after death.

It's striking that the argument for presumed consent and the argument against it both start from the same datum: that about 70% of Americans want to donate their organs after death; or, if you like, that about 30% of Americans do not want to donate their organs after death. Where does this 70%–30% figure come from? It comes from a 1993 Gallup Poll, to which most recent commentators on both sides of the issue have referred. Now there are a number of problems with using these poll numbers. But the fact is that the 1993 Gallup Poll still constitutes the best estimate we have of Americans' attitudes towards organ donation. It is important to keep in mind, however, that the arguments that follow do depend on this imperfect estimate of Americans' desires to donate their organs after death. As such, the conclusions I draw should be taken to be conditional, based as they are on an empirical assumption that may have to be revised in light of future evidence.

III. The Fewer Mistakes Claim

I believe both sides have to admit that mistakes will occur under either system. No matter how

well the current system is instituted, there will still be cases in which people who would have preferred to donate their organs will be buried with all their organs intact; call these mistaken non-removals. And no matter how well presumed consent is instituted, there will still be some cases in which people who would have preferred to be buried with all their organs intact will have some of their organs removed; call these mistaken removals.

Proponents of presumed consent can plausibly claim that under their proposal there will be fewer mistakes than under the current system. They can claim this not only because a majority of Americans prefer to donate their organs, but also because it is plausible to believe that a person who does not want to donate is more likely to opt out under a system of presumed consent than a person who does want to donate is to opt in under the current system. This belief is based on the idea that most of those opposed to organ transplantation have conspicuous religious or moral objections of which they themselves are very aware, and that as a result these people are unlikely to neglect to opt out of a system of presumed consent, unlikely in the same way a Quaker is unlikely to forget to register as a conscientious objector to the draft, or as a Jehovah's Witness is to forget to inform her physician of his opposition to blood transfusion. The wish to donate one's organs, in contrast, is usually tied to religious and moral values that are relatively unremarkable, and so people who wish to donate are less likely to register their preference.

Proponents of presumed consent maintain, then, that their policy will lead us to follow the wishes of more decedents than the current system does, that the current system produces more mistakes than a policy of presumed consent will. Those who argue for presumed consent in this way believe that from the standpoint of trying to respect the wishes of decedents, mistaken removals and mistaken non-removals are morally equivalent or symmetrical. Both kinds of mistakes violate the wishes of decedents, and so they are both morally unfortunate in the same way. We should, therefore, implement the policy that produces the fewest mistakes, without regard to the ratio of mistaken removals to mistaken non-removals. That means that even if presumed consent will lead to more mistaken removals than the current system, it will still be the right policy to implement if, as a result of greatly decreasing the number of mistaken non-removals, it leads to fewer mistakes overall. Call this the "fewer mistakes claim" for presumed consent.

The opposition to presumed consent that is insulated from the fewer mistakes claim is based on the idea that mistaken removals are morally much worse than mistaken non-removals. Those who subscribe to this idea hold that it would be wrong to implement a policy of presumed consent because even if it does lead to fewer mistakes overall, it will also inevitably lead to more mistaken removals. And the moral harm of increasing the number of mistaken removals is greater than – or trumps – the moral benefit of decreasing the number of mistakes overall.

We can sharpen this picture of one kind of mistake's being worse than another by comparing it to our differing attitudes toward punishing the innocent and not punishing the guilty. We all want the guilty to be punished and the innocent to go free. But we also have to acknowledge that our legal system cannot be perfect, that some mistakes will be made. We do not, however, believe that all legal mistakes are morally equivalent and that therefore we should simply try to reduce the number of legal mistakes overall. Mistaken convictions and mistaken acquittals are both bad, but mistaken convictions are worse. It's worse to punish an innocent person than not to punish a guilty one. Because of this belief that one kind of mistake is worse than (or trumps) the other kind, we have constructed a system based on the presumption of innocence. We have tried to ensure that we err on the side of not punishing the guilty so as never to punish the innocent. The core opposition to presumed consent holds that mistaken removals are worse than mistaken non-removals in much the same way that punishing the innocent is worse than not punishing the guilty.

Why do opponents of presumed consent believe that mistaken removals are morally worse than mistaken non-removals? Why do they believe that we are morally required to place higher priority on preventing mistaken removals than on preventing mistaken non-removals? They believe it, I think, because they take it to be a necessary consequence of the principle of respect for autonomy underlying our commitment to informed consent.

The origin of the requirement that physicians gain informed consent from their patients is the belief that it is wrong to invade a person's body unless that person has given permission. This belief is an essential aspect of the moral principle of respect for autonomy, as a person cannot engage in autonomous decision-making if she cannot control what happens to her own body. And this is why medical ethics generally takes informed consent to be a sacrosanct requirement: it is the guardian of patients' control over what happens to their own bodies.

Opponents of presumed consent seem to believe that mistaken removals violate the right of bodily control while mistaken non-removals do not. They seem to believe that when we remove organs from the body of someone who did not want them removed, we invade her body against her wishes, which constitutes a blatant violation of her autonomy. Mistaken non-removals, in contrast, merely fail to help bring about a state of affairs the individual desired. And while it is unfortunate if we fail to help a person achieve one of her goals, this failure pales in comparison to the violation of a person's right to decide whether an invasive procedure is performed on her body.

Proponents of presumed consent believe, in contrast, that mistaken removals and mistaken non-removals are morally equivalent, that each kind of mistake is morally unfortunate in the same way. Because proponents of presumed consent believe that mistaken removals and mistaken non-removals are morally equivalent, they believe that we should implement the organ procurement policy that results in the fewest mistakes overall – i.e., that we should base organ procurement policy on the fewer mistakes claim. And the fewer mistake claim (along with the empirical assumption discussed in section II) implies that presumed consent is superior to the current system of organ procurement.

IV. Why the Fewer Mistakes Claim Should Guide Organ Procurement Policy

Does the fact that a person is legally dead mean that she will not be wronged if we remove her organs even though she did not want them removed? No, it does not mean that. A person *is* wronged if after her death we treat her body in a way that she did not want it to be treated. Treating a person's body after her death in a way she did not want it to be treated is a wrong done to her in the same way disposing of a person's estate in a way she did not want it to be disposed of is a wrong done to her. We have a powerful moral duty to respect a person's wishes about what should happen after her death to the things that belonged to her. But mistaken non-removals violate that duty in the same way that mistaken removals do.

The key to seeing the moral equivalence between mistaken removals and mistaken non-removals is to distinguish between two models of respect for autonomy. These two models are closely related and usually overlap when the treatment of competent persons is concerned, but they will almost always come apart when the treatment of the bodies of brain-dead individuals is concerned. The first is what we can call the non-interference model of autonomy: it tells us that it is wrong to interfere with a person's body unless that person has given us explicit permission to do so. The second is what we can call the respect-for-wishes model of autonomy: it tells us that we ought to treat a person's body in the way that he wishes it to be treated.

It is reasonable to hold that the non-interference model of autonomy ought to govern our treatment of competent individuals. If someone is awake and aware, then we ought to assume that he would tell us if he wanted us to do anything to his body. So we ought not to do anything to the body of someone who is awake and aware unless he gives us explicit permission to do so.

But it is not reasonable to hold that the non-interference model ought to govern our treatment of brain-dead individuals. For the non-interference model implies that we would have to refrain from doing anything at all to the bodies of brain-dead individuals who had left no explicit instructions about how they wanted their bodies to be treated. But we have to do *something* to the bodies of such people. We have to treat them in one way or another. Literal non-interference – letting their bodies lay untouched where they fall – is not an option. So how do we go about trying to respect the autonomy of the brain-dead? We do so by acting under the respect-for-wishes model of autonomy, which tells us to do our best to treat persons' bodies in the ways they wanted them to be treated. On this model, each type of mistake is on a moral par, for each type of mistake involves treating a person's body in a way the person did not want.

If, then, our goal is to respect the autonomy of brain-dead individuals, we have no choice but to operate under the respect-for-wishes model of autonomy. And according to the respect-for-wishes model, we ought to implement the organ procurement policy that results in the fewest mistakes. If, therefore, presumed consent will result in fewer mistakes than the current system, presumed consent will be more respectful of autonomy than the current system.

This point will become clearer when we compare the decision of whether or not to remove organs for transplantation to the closely related decision of what to do, ultimately, with the body of someone recently deceased. Some people wish to have their bodies embalmed and displayed in an open casket before burial, while other people are religiously opposed to embalming and wish to have their bodies buried within 48 hours of death. Some people wish to be buried in family plots, while others wish their ashes to be scattered in a place of spiritual significance. We have a moral duty to try to respect these various wishes. But is failing to respect one kind of wish morally worse than failing to respect another kind of wish? I don't think so. It would be unfortunate if we cremated someone who wanted to be buried in a family plot, but it would be just as unfortunate if we buried in a potter's field someone who had a fervent desire to have her ashes scattered in the Ganges. The wrong done to a person cremated against her wishes and the wrong done to a person buried against her wishes are symmetrical or morally equivalent. If, therefore, we do not know what a particular person wanted done to her body after death, we should do what it is most likely she would have wanted done. The duty to respect persons' wishes about what should happen to their bodies after death implies that we should follow the policy that can reasonably be expected to lead to the fewest mistakes.

The decision of whether or not to remove organs for transplantation parallels these other decisions of how to treat the things that belonged to a person after the person has died. There is not nearly as much of a parallel between the decision of whether or not to remove organs for transplantation and the decision of how to treat a competent, living person.

It is, consequently, illegitimate to equate a mistaken removal of organs to an operation on a competent, living person against her will. For operating on a competent person against her will is a violation of the non-interference model of autonomy. But the non-interference model of autonomy does not apply to our treatment of the bodies of individuals who are brain-dead. The illegitimate equation of a mistaken removal of organs to an unwanted operation on a competent, living person is, however, just what opponents of presumed consent rely upon when they dismiss the fewer mistake claim. Veatch and Pitt, for instance, maintain that mistaken removals violate "the right of the individual not to have his or her body invaded".

But this comparison ignores the crucially important disanalogy between the person we might physically interfere with and the person whose organs we might remove. The person we might physically interfere with is competent and living; she can be left alone to determine her own fate. But the person whose organs we might remove is no longer capable of determining the fate of her body; other people are going to have to treat her body in one way or another. And this disanalogy vitiates Veatch and Pitt's comparison between mistaken removals and unwanted physical interference with a competent, living person.

Let me emphasize again that I do believe that our commitment to respect for autonomy implies that we have a moral duty to treat the body of a person who is brain-dead in the way she wanted it to be treated. My point is that the noninterference model of respect for autonomy does not apply to the treatment of the body of such a person. The model of respect autonomy that does apply is that of trying to fulfill a person's wishes when she is no longer capable of fulfilling them herself. And that second model coheres perfectly with the fewer mistakes claim that is at the heart of the case for presumed consent.

Moreover, even if we disregard the fact that potential organ donors meet the legal criteria of death, the moral principles underlying the requirement of informed consent still do not imply the asymmetry between mistaken removals and mistaken non-removals upon which the core opposition to presumed consent is based. To see this, consider the decision of whether to perform an invasive procedure on an unconscious person who has arrived at the emergency room. Of course we would do everything we could to ensure that we made the decision that accorded with that person's own values and beliefs. But if the decision had to be made immediately and we had no way of determining the patient's proclivities, we would not necessarily refrain from operating. And we would not necessarily refrain because we do not think a mistaken operation is of a morally more significant kind than a mistaken non-operation. Current emergency room procedure seems to suggest, rather, that the principles underlying informed consent do not imply that the mistake of invading the body of an incompetent patient who would not have wanted to be invaded is morally worse than the mistake of not invading the body of an incompetent patient who did want to be invaded. The goal of preventing mistaken operations does not morally trump the goal of preventing mistaken non-operations in a manner that requires us to presume that all unconscious people do not want to be operated on. But if the principles of informed consent do not imply that mistaken bodily invasions are always worse than mistaken bodily non-invasions, then it's hard to see why the principles of informed consent should commit us to the idea that mistaken organ removals are significantly worse than mistaken organ non-removals.

Now I should mention that Veatch and Pitt explicitly address emergency room procedure and draw from it the opposite conclusion. They write,

> In the case of the emergency room treatment of the patient incapable of giving explicit consent, the presumption of consent is surely valid. Were we to conduct a survey of the population asking its members whether they would want such a presumption made, agreement would be close to unanimous. To be sure, some small group would object. A patient who is a Jehovah's Witness may refuse blood products; a Christian Scientist may refuse treatment altogether. This reveals that on occasions the presumption of consent in the emergency room may be an erroneous presumptions (it will, on occasion, yield *false positives*). But it will be accurate an overwhelming percentage of the time, and the presumption is therefore justified. By contrast if we presume consent in the case of organ procurement, we will be wrong at least 30% of the time.

In this clear dismissal of the fewer mistakes claim, Veatch and Pitt argue that we are justified in treating a person without her explicit permission only if the chance that we are making a mistake is virtually non-existent. But this idea does not accord with either our current medical procedure or our moral intuitions.

To see that it does not accord with current medical procedure, consider that a non-negligible portion of elderly and terminal patients would prefer not to be resuscitated if they go into cardiac arrest. Unfortunately, many of these patients have not completed advance directives, and some of those who have completed advance directives do not have the documents on their person at the moment emergency medical teams arrive. So what do EMTs do when they encounter an unconscious patient but have no way of determining in time whether she would prefer to be treated or not to be treated? The fact is, in such a situation, EMTs treat the unconscious patient,

even if they know full well that there is a non-negligible chance that the person would prefer not to have been treated, and even if the treatment involves an invasive procedure. Indeed, our current practice, which involves treating even elderly and terminal patients unless there is a clear indication that they did not want to be treated, seems to embody the idea that it is morally worse not to perform an invasive procedure on someone who wanted the procedure done than it is to perform the invasive procedure on someone who did not want it done.

To see that Veatch and Pitt's idea does not necessarily accord with our moral intuitions, consider the following scenario. You are a doctor in a community in which there is an unusually high percentage of Christian Scientists, who oppose all medical treatment. Indeed, as much as 30% of the local population are Christian Scientists. But the other 70% have no religious objections to conventional medical care. One day, a 30-year-old adult male is brought into your emergency room. He is unconscious and will die without immediate surgery. A quick search of his wallet gives no indication of whether or not he is a Christian Scientist, and you do not have time to try to contact any of his family or friends. So what do you do? Veatch and Pitt are committed to saying that the 30% chance that the person does not want to be operated on makes operating on him the wrong course of action to take. But I doubt that this conclusion tracks our moral intuitions, and that is because I doubt that most of us would judge it wrong to operate on the unknown person. It's true that, if we operate, there's a 30% chance that we will invade the body of someone who would not have wanted us to do so. But there's also a 70% chance that we will treat the person's body in the way that he would have wanted. And I think that in this situation most of us would think it morally acceptable (if not morally required) to make the choice that would have the greatest chance of success.

I conclude, therefore, that the principles underlying informed consent do not imply that mistakenly removing organs for transplantation is morally much worse than mistakenly neglecting to remove organs for transplantation. Both mistakes fail to fulfill a person's wishes about what should happen to her body when she is no longer competent. Both mistakes, consequently, fail to live up to goal of respect for autonomy in the same way. The fewer mistake claim (combined with the empirical assumption that most people want to donate their organs) thus constitutes a powerful reason for thinking that a policy of presumed consent is morally superior to our current system of organ procurement.

VI.   Presumed Consent and a Family Veto

It might be worth noting that there is strong evidence that people who prefer not to donate their organs are more likely to be influenced by false beliefs about donation and transplantation; there is good reason to believe, that is, that the better informed a person is about donation and transplantation, the more likely she is to prefer to donate her organs. We should not, however, place too much weight on the fact that those who prefer not to donate are more likely to be misinformed. And that is because the more we base the case for presumed consent on this point, the closer we come to the morally problematic strategy of trying to justify treating a person contrary to her actual wishes by claiming that we are treating her as she would wish to be treated were she fully rational.

The more salient response the proponent of presumed choice can make is to acknowledge that some of the people who answered the polls may be misinformed, and thus to concede that we should not place all the weight of our organ procurement policy on the poll numbers. The poll numbers and the existence of a well-publicized opportunity for opting out of organ donation would give us reason to presume that removing a person's organs for transplantation does not run contrary to her wishes. But they are no guarantee. A person may have forgotten to opt out, even though she meant to. Or she may have been willing to donate her organs

only because she was misinformed. Because these two scenarios are possible, a policy of presumed consent must include a mechanism that can override the presumption that a person who did not opt out would not have objected to having her organs removed for transplantation.

The mechanism for overriding the presumption should be discussion with the family of the potential donor. If a person has not opted out, we should presume that removing her organs for transplantation does not run contrary to her wishes. But we should also ask her family whether they have any reason for thinking that that presumption is false in this person's case. One point that it is important to keep in mind, however, is that when we are asking this question, we should inform the family as best we can about the circumstances of donation and transplantation. For the principles underlying informed consent tell us that we fully respect autonomy not merely by acting in accord with persons' statements about how they want to be treated but only by acting in accord with persons' *informed* decisions.

I conclude, then, that, at the present time, the organ procurement policy that best lives up to the principle of autonomy underlying informed consent is a system of presumed consent with a provision for family veto. Such a system may not procure as many organs as a system of presumed consent without a provision for family veto. But living up to the principle of autonomy underlying informed consent must be our first priority. We should procure as many organs as possible only after that priority has been met.

References

Cohen, C. The case for presumed consent to transplant human organs after death. *Transplantation Proceedings* 24 (1992): 2168–72.

Veatch, R.M., & Pitt, J.B. "The Myth of Presumed Consent: Ethical Problems in Organ Procurement Strategies." *Transplantation Proceedings* 27 (1995): 1888–92.

An "Opting In" Paradigm for Kidney Transplantation

DAVID STEINBERG

The American Journal of Bioethics 4, no. 4 (2004): 4–14.

The Motivating Force of Scarcity

Transplants using organs from live donors are now common, especially in kidney transplantation where the use of live donors has become a critical source of organs. In 2001, for the first time in recent decades, the number of live kidney donors exceeded the number of deceased donors. Although live donors have also provided a lobe of liver, a lobe of lung, and pancreatic and small intestinal tissue, live kidney donation was more than ten times as common as the live donation of all other organs combined. Long- and short-term outcomes using living kidney donors are superior to those with deceased organs.

The vast majority of live organ transplants have been between genetically or emotionally bonded individuals such as brothers and sisters and husbands and wives. Paired exchanges permit a couple with incompatible blood types to exchange kidneys with another suitable couple. Tissue incompatibility is surmounted because the donor in couple A gives a kidney to a compatible recipient in couple B and the donor in couple B simultaneously gives a kidney to a compatible recipient in couple A. A similar exchange program rewards the intended recipient of a willing but incompatible donor with the next available matched kidney after that donor gives a kidney to a compatible stranger on the transplant waiting list. In these exchanges organs are donated to strangers, but the quid pro quo aspect of the arrangements makes them different than organ donation by altruistic strangers.

The Altruistic Stranger

Organ donation by altruistic strangers has become accepted practice in the United States. It is approved in the live organ donor consensus statement; case reports have been published and major transplant centers have retrieved organs from strangers. Although donation by altruistic strangers can be expected to increase as this type of organ donation is publicized, it is currently uncommon and constitutes less than 1 percent of all live kidney donations.

Donation by altruistic strangers exists in two forms. Donors and recipients may locate each other, often using the Internet. When they approach a transplant center they have established a relationship and may be classified by the transplant center as emotionally bonded. However, because they would have remained strangers were it not for the sole stimulus of organ transplantation, it is more accurate to consider these donors altruistic strangers. The second form of donation by altruistic strangers exists when the donor permits the transplant center to select any recipient on their waiting list ("non-directed donation").

A variant of the second form of donation allows the selection of any donor, but with restrictions; in one case a Buddhist donor did not want her kidney given to anyone in a killing profession such as a fisherman, a hunter, or a soldier. Restrictions placed by altruistic strangers on who can receive their organ have been controversial. Genetically and emotionally bonded individuals are permitted to precisely specify their recipient; with the exception of offensive religious or racial groupings it is reasonable to accept donor restrictions. No one is hurt by the stranger's donation, and everyone below the designated recipient moves up the list.

Two aspects of organ donation by altruistic strangers should be influential. By not selecting a genetically or emotionally bonded specific individual as their recipient, the altruistic stranger expresses a solidarity with all humankind. The altruistic stranger is willing to help anybody, even someone they don't know, because they are sensitive to all suffering without distinction to specific persons. Altruistic strangers consider themselves part of a common humanity and probably have a broader sense of relationship than the rest of us.

Our embrace of altruistic strangers as kidney donors creates a moral dilemma because most people, if they required dialysis, would accept a donated kidney if that would improve the quality of their life or, as is occasionally the case, save their life; yet most people have made no provision to donate a kidney after they die. That some people give a live kidney with no expectation of a return in kind whereas others would take a kidney without ever having committed to giving when they are deceased should disturb our sense of fairness. By taking organs from altruistic strangers we place in sharp relief a distinction that pervades the field of organ transplantation: the existence of two classes of persons, "organ takers" and "organ givers."

A person who would accept a deceased donor kidney if they needed one for relief from the burdens of dialysis, or perhaps to save their life, is an "organ taker." An organ taker should acknowledge that a donated kidney, in view of its benefits, is a valuable gift. Because the deceased donor will have given the kidney free to relieve another person's suffering, the donation can be considered a morally valuable act.

An "organ taker" should recognize that other persons are also entitled to moral respect and might have a valid need for a donated kidney. Nagel (1970) claims that "the principle underlying altruism requires all reasons to be construable as expressing objective rather than subjective values." Reasons, according to Nagel, should express values that apply to all persons. If it is morally valuable for me to receive a kidney, objectivity requires that the donation of a kidney to someone else also be considered morally valuable. The "organ taker" must decide whether they would be willing to perform the same morally valuable act they would want and accept from others and become an "organ giver" by agreeing to donate their kidneys when they die. An ethical position is contaminated by subjectivity if it applies only to oneself and not to other similarly situated people.

There is also a practical contradiction in adopting the position that people can choose to be "organ takers" with no obligation to also be "organ givers." An ethical position that cannot be generalized should be suspect. If everyone could decide they wanted a kidney should they develop end stage renal disease and everyone could also decide they would not donate a kidney themselves, this would contradict the interests of "organ takers" because no one would receive a kidney.

Reciprocal Altruism

In contrast to pure altruism, the behavior characterized by a willingness to accept the benefits of altruism that is balanced by a willingness to similarly be altruistic when the circumstances are reversed has been called *reciprocal altruism*.

Sociobiologists have noted "the evolutionary value of mutual assistance" and that cooperation between animals is advantageous and "maximizes genetic proliferation." Wright (1994) describes vampire bats who feed regurgitated blood to hungry bats because they know the recipient bats will eventually return the favor in a "tit for tat" exchange that benefits them both. Wright notes that reciprocal altruism to promote itself has generated feelings such as affection, guilt, compassion, sympathy, obligation and gratitude that serve as "logic executers" of the "proper strategy" out of "genetic self-interest." Gratitude is a measure of the benefit received that helps determine the repayment owed.

Reciprocal altruism in deceased donor kidney transplantation is beneficial for humankind in a manner similar to bats feeding each other. A tolerable sacrifice is made for a significantly greater good to the group. If everyone donated a deceased kidney they no longer needed, more people would be relieved of the burdens of dialysis, some of them would live longer, and the cost to humankind considered as a group would be minimal and far outweighed by the benefits.

Any new paradigm for kidney transplantation not only should take into account the problems inherent in a system with organ givers and organ takers; it should also aim to decrease dependence on live kidney donors. I will review the flawed nature of the reasons commonly used to justify live kidney donation to explain why we should, to the extent possible, decrease our dependence on live organ donation. I will then discuss an "opting in" paradigm, which mimics reciprocal altruism and has the potential to advance this goal.

The Paradigm for Live Kidney Donation

The paradigm most commonly used to justify live kidney donation rests on several premises: the low risk to the donor, the favorable risk/benefit ratio, the psychological benefits to the donor, altruism, and autonomy coupled with informed consent. Although these premises are partly valid, each requires significant qualification and that weakens the entire paradigm.

Low Risk to the Donor

In a three-year period from 1999 to 2001 of 15,782 kidney retrievals from live donors seven deaths were reported for a rate of one death for every 2255 donors (0.04%). Although some donors have subsequently required a renal transplant themselves, no large series has demonstrated progressive deterioration of renal function. Donors also suffer pain, time lost from work, and, for altruistic strangers, forfeiture of the ability to donate a kidney should a genetic relative or emotionally bonded individual need one in the future.

Transplant centers can accurately note that individual donors face a statistically low risk of death; however, until the mortality of donor nephrectomy becomes zero, the global enterprise of live kidney transplantation will continue to be a form of human sacrifice because, although it cannot be known which donors will die, it can be known with statistical inevitability that some healthy donors will die. For perspective, the likelihood of death in living kidney donation is about 400 times higher than the risk of death from smallpox vaccination.

A Favorable Risk/Benefit Ratio

Calculating the risk/benefit ratio in live organ transplantation is problematic because the risks and benefits can be qualitatively different and the entity that accepts the risk is not the entity that reaps the benefit.

The use of live kidney donors makes utilitarian sense if we simply count and compare those who benefit and those who suffer. The retrieval of a kidney from 2500 live donors, assuming a one-year graft survival of 95 percent, would eliminate the need for dialysis for 2375 patients. The approximate cost of this benefit would be the death of one healthy donor. (I am ignoring the lesser risks previously noted.) Live kidney donation makes utilitarian sense because many more people benefit than are harmed. However, this analysis ignores a crucial issue. Most patients do not die without a kidney transplant because they can be sustained on dialysis.

Unlike most medical and public health interventions, in live kidney donation the person who accepts the risk has no probability of a medical benefit. Unless risk and benefit are apportioned among the same entity, risk/benefit calculations are problematic. This difficulty should become more troubling when the risk is higher, as it is in live liver transplantation.

The Psychological Benefit to the Donor

Live kidney donation may benefit the donor because, except in the case of most altruistic strangers, they will have the companionship of a healthier recipient. They will also avoid feelings of guilt that might accompany a refusal to donate. However, more sweeping claims of psychological benefit, such as improved self-esteem and a heightened sense of well-being, warrant scrutiny for several reasons. Not all donors will benefit psychologically; donors who die will not benefit psychologically. In a quality-of-life follow-up study, kidney donation was associated with an increase in self-esteem and sense of well-being; but not everyone benefited. Four percent of respondents said they wished they had not donated, and 3% were unsure whether they should have donated. Donor suicide following transplant failure and the death of the recipient has been described in a few cases.

If a donor wants psychological enhancement, it has not been shown that other less dangerous means, such as earning an advanced degree or doing charity work, would not be just as effective. Claims of a psychological benefit to the donor can be used to justify exposing a donor to risk because they allow us to believe the donor is getting something in return for their donation; but that return entails risk, and alternative and safer means for achieving psychological enhancement exist.

Altruism

The basic dictionary definition of altruism is the unselfish concern for the welfare of others. An altruistic act benefits another person without any quid pro quo commensurate compensation; the donation of a kidney for free is an altruistic act. The paradigm of altruism conveys positive connotations because it is endorsed by many religions and most people would preferentially applaud actions that help others over those that are either indifferent or hurtful. Altruistic acts merit scrutiny because their altruistic nature does not guarantee that they are morally appropriate. The fact that live kidney donation is an altruistic act does not automatically entail its endorsement. A man who gives his assets to a poor elderly aunt has performed an altruistic act; however, if he were left destitute and unable to care for his young children, the moral appropriateness of his altruism would be doubtful. A healthy person would not be permitted to donate their heart because altruistic acts remain subject to other moral principles.

Live organ donation differs from other accepted acts of medical altruism such as blood, sperm, and bone marrow donation because those acts are associated with low risk. By calling it "the gift of life" and honoring live kidney donors as praiseworthy and noble heroes, altruism is employed to justify an intervention that may cause death. This extension of the permissible risk boundaries of altruism should make us wary of automatically equating altruism with justification.

An "Opting in" Paradigm for Kidney Transplantation

We rely on live kidney donors because there are insufficient deceased donations. I have outlined both practical and conceptual problems in using live kidney donors. Is there a defensible paradigm that might bring the supply of cadaveric kidneys closer to demand and lessen the need for live donations? I will suggest one that responds to the unfairness inherent in the existence of "organ takers" and "organ givers" and also takes into account reciprocity and concern for the welfare of the group. This paradigm, which I will refer to as "opting in," is based on utility and fairness.

Utility

Although conceptual difficulties exist in calculating the net benefit of kidney transplantation, organs are transplanted because we believe that organ transplantation increases the total medical good. The dominant reason for kidney transplantation is utilitarian. Although some people may suffer because of transplantation, overall it is considered beneficial for the group. The starting premise in any justification of organ transplantation should be unabashedly utilitarian because that is the dominant motivating force.

"Opting In" and Fairness

The current system of kidney allocation based on need combined with organ procurement based on voluntary donation has failed to satisfy the demand for kidneys. This failure has spawned discussion of plans to provide a financial incentive for kidney donation, an approach that would unfairly separate "organ givers" and "organ takers" by economic status.

An alternate approach would preferentially distribute organs to people who have previously agreed to donate an organ. Currently, organ allocation considerations are essentially restricted to the time frame that begins after it is known who needs a kidney and who is an available and eligible donor. The process could begin earlier, at a time when potential recipients and potential donors are healthy and it is unknown who will need a kidney and who will be able to donate one.

Planning at this point could avoid the unfair separation of persons into "organ givers" and "organ takers." Jarvis (1995) has used the judgmental but colorful phrase "free riders," for people who would accept an organ if they needed one but would not donate one themselves and advocates that only those who have previously identified themselves as potential organ donors be allowed to receive organs. Eaton (1998) favors a similar but less draconian social contract. She would not exclude "free riders" as organ recipients but would penalize them for their "uncharitable views." If there were equally needy recipients, the "free rider" would lose out; no one would be forced to donate their organs, but those who refuse would have to accept the practical consequences of being discriminated against in the allocation of organs.

Gubenats and Kliemt (2000) suggested a "solidarity rule" that would provide a nonmonetary incentive to donate. People who, prior to developing a disease, declare a willingness to donate their organs would be given priority in organ allocation. Kleinman and Lowy (1992) called for an advance directive organ registry. All persons over age 18 would voluntarily provide their advance directive to a central registry, agreeing to donate their organs at death. Those who registered would get priority in organ allocation.

A system that offered preference in organ allocation to those who chose to "opt in" would be a very attractive form of organ insurance. You would not be presumed to be a kidney donor until you voluntarily "opted in" and agreed to donate a kidney. If you became ill, you would more quickly receive an organ that would substantially improve the quality of your life or save your life, and at the minimal cost of promising to donate your organs after you die, have no use for them, and can no longer suffer. It is an opportunity a rational person should willingly accept as very attractive.

An "opting in" kidney transplantation system comes with a significant moral cost. Medical care based on factors other than need is problematic, especially if failure to "opt in" is considered morally blameworthy. Criminals and our enemies in mortal combat are entitled to medical care. Patients who brought on their illness because they smoked or drank too much are entitled to medical care. The unavailability of medical care, including transplants, for those in need simply because they lack money or cannot afford health insurance is deplorable. Gillon (1995) notes the important moral tradition in medicine that treatment should be given on the basis of medical need and "scarce resources should not be prioritized on the basis of a patient's blameworthiness." I am sympathetic to Gillon's concern that if we discriminate against the sick who are considered blameworthy because they did not choose to "opt in," then what other fault might next be used to deny health care.

Organ allocation based on factors other than need currently exists. UNOS lists waiting patients only for transplant centers that are part of UNOS. Geography is a determining factor because organs are first distributed within a specific geographic region. Patients are denied transplants because they lack insurance or adequate funds. UNOS gives preference to prior organ donors by assigning four points to a person who has previously donated a vital organ or a segment of a vital organ within the United States. The distribution of healthcare based on factors other than need requires justification. In the case of an "opting in" organ transplantation system, justification would be based on the promise of making more organs available for transplantation, with an increase in overall health and a diminished requirement for living donors; nonetheless, we should acknowledge this moral transgression with regret and be reluctant to repeat it in other situations. Unfortunately, whatever mechanism is chosen to reduce the scarcity of kidneys will entail compromise.

An "opting in" system avoids many of the moral problems associated with living organ donation. One inequity would be resolved because the entity assuming risk—the members of the "opting in" pool—would also be the entity that incurred the benefit. Because everyone in the pool is potentially both an "organ giver" and an "organ taker," that unfair distinction would disappear, and within the pool there would be no "free riders." The conundrum of when altruism is appropriate would become irrelevant because those who donate a kidney would get something in return: the promise of a lesser wait for a kidney were they fated to need one. Autonomy would be respected because entrance to the transplantation pool would be voluntary. Each member could make risk/benefit calculations according to individual values before they joined the pool. Members of the pool would be expressing solidarity with each other, though with a greater degree of self-interest than the altruistic stranger.

Conclusion

Ideally, everyone should agree to donate their salvageable organs at death. Since that has not happened, an "opting in" program becomes a reasonable option. Although an "opting in" program mimics altruism, it is based on enlightened self-interest. The emotions that foster reciprocal altruism have been conserved in nature because they confer an evolutionary survival advantage. Cultural evolution works faster than genetic evolution and can be used to take advantage of the lessons of nature. An "opting in" policy, despite being rooted in enlightened self-interest, would be a cultural meme that simulates reciprocal altruism. If an "opting in" program is successful it might ironically, by demonstrating the utilitarian value of reciprocal altruism, promote the attitude that self-interest sometimes requires the perception that we are all part of a common humanity.

References

Eaton, S. "The Subtle Politics of Organ Donation: A Proposal." *Journal of Medical Ethics* 24 (1998): 166–70.

Gillon, R. "On Giving Preference to Prior Volunteers When Allocating Organs for Transplantation." *Journal of Medical Ethics* 21 (1995): 195–96.

Gubenats, G., and H. Kliemt. "A Superior Approach to Organ Allocation and Donation." *Transplantation* 70 (2000): 699–707.

Jarvis, R. "Join the Club: A Modest Proposal to Increase Availability of Donor Organs." *Journal of Medical Ethics* 21 (1995): 199–204.

Kleinman, I., and F. H. Lowy. "Ethical Considerations in Living Organ Donation and a New Approach: An Advance Directive Organ Registry." *Archives of Internal Medicine* 152 (1992): 1484–88.

Nagel, T. 1970. *The possibility of altruism.* Princeton, NJ: Princeton University Press.

Wright, R. *The Moral Animal: Why We Are the Way We Are; the New Science of Evolutionary Psychology.* New York: Pantheon Books, 1994.

CASES

The Health of Nations

It is widely known that the United States has perhaps the best health care facilities in the world and spends more money per capita on health care than any other nation (15.3 percent of gross domestic product in 2006), but it fails to achieve outcomes that would match these advantages. The United States has a larger percentage of uninsured people than any other developed nation, has among the fewest physicians relative to the population (2.4 per 1,000), and fails to achieve better overall results than many other nations (life expectancy of 77.8 years and infant mortality rate of 6.8 per 1,000 live births). Furthermore, wide disparities in access to health care exist, based on socioeconomic, race, gender, and immigrant status.

The United States spends more than double what England spends per person and about twice what Canada spends, yet the citizens of those nations are much healthier. A comparison study published in the *Journal of the American Medical*

Association shows that middle-aged, non-Hispanic white Americans are more likely to suffer from diabetes, hypertension, heart disease, myocardial infarction, stroke, lung disease, and cancer than are their counterparts in England. Health disparities are the largest for those with the lowest incomes and levels of education, with the health of wealthy Americans being similar to that of the poorest in England.

A comparison study published in the *American Journal of Public Health* showed that U.S. residents were less able to access health care than were Canadians, and so were less likely to have a regular doctor, more likely to have unmet health needs, and more likely to forgo needed medicines. Health disparities based on race, income, and immigrant status exist in both countries, but are more pronounced in the United States. Insured Americans and Canadians have about the same disease rates, but uninsured Americans made the overall U.S. figures worse.

About 13 percent of non-Hispanic white Americans lack health insurance, compared with 19 percent of Asian and Pacific Islanders, 21 percent of African Americans and 34 percent of Hispanics. People without insurance coverage are less likely to receive preventive health services and adequate treatment, and are more likely to die from treatable illnesses. For all cancers combined, uninsured patients are 60 percent more likely to die than are patients with private insurance.

Discussion Questions

1. Based upon these comparisons, does the U.S. health care system seem unjust?
2. Because our health care system is outperformed by those of Canada and England, should the United States switch to a system like one of these two nations with universal health care?
3. Can you think of some possible reasons why large expenditures on health care in the United States do not translate into better health?
4. Why is a lower rate of nonwhite than white Americans insured? What could be done to improve the access of nonwhite Americans to health care?

Sources

Banks, James, Michael Marmot, Zoe Oldfield, and James P. Smith. "Disease and Disadvantage in the United States and in England." *JAMA* 295, no. 17 (2006): 2037–45.

Lasser, Karen E., David U. Himmelstein, and Steffie Woolhandler. "Access to Care, Health Status, and Health Disparities in the United States and Canada: Results of a Cross-National Population-Based Survey." *American Journal of Public Health* 96, no. 7 (2006): 1300–1307.

Organization for Economic Co-operation and Development. "OECD Health Data 2007— Frequently Requested Data." http://www.oecd.org/document/16/0,3343,en_2825_495642_2085200_1_1_1_1,00.html (accessed May 12, 2008).

Ward, Elizabeth, Michael Halpern, Nicole Schrag, Vilma Cokkinides, Carol Desantis, Priti Bandi, Rebecca Siegel, Andrew Stewart, and Ahmedin Jemal. "Association of Insurance with Cancer Care Utilization and Outcomes." *CA: A Cancer Journal for Clinicians* 58, no. 1 (2008), 9–31.

The "Commonhealth" of Massachusetts

The Massachusetts Health Care Reform Plan was enacted in April 2006, utilizing what Fuchs and Emanuel call the "individual mandates with subsidies" model. Other states are watching, as they consider whether to adopt a similar approach. Massachusetts requires all adults to purchase health insurance, and imposes financial penalties for failure to comply. It also requires employers of eleven or more people to provide them with health coverage or pay a "Fair Share" contribution of up to $295 annually per employee. Many adults thus will be able to purchase their health insurance through employer-sponsored group plans. For people unable to obtain health care through their employers, Massachusetts established the Commonwealth Health Insurance Connector Authority to provide subsidized plans for people earning less than three hundred percent of the federal poverty level, and another program pooling together people earning more than that to reduce the cost of non-group insurance premiums. The state has also expanded Medicaid coverage for the poor.

While the Massachusetts plan is laudable, several problems have already emerged. Notably, there is a shortage of primary care physicians, which is exacerbated by the larger pool of patients, who may experience increasing delays in receiving care. A year after the plan was enacted, about 340,000 of the 600,000 uninsured gained coverage and began searching for doctors to schedule appointments. Because of the influx of new patients, Dr. Katherine Atkinson's patients are now having to schedule physical exams over a year in advance. According to Dr. Patricia A. Sereno, state president of the American Academy of Family Physicians, "It's a recipe for disaster. It's great that people have access to health care, but now we've got to find a way to give them access to preventive services. The point of this legislation was not to get people episodic care."

Affordability of insurance remains an issue as costs increase, and could prove difficult for the Connector Authority to manage. Insurance costs increased ten to twelve percent in 2008. Furthermore, a large number of residents, perhaps sixty thousand, could be exempt from the insurance mandate because they cannot afford to pay even the discounted premiums that the Connector Authority arranges.

Finally, some citizens—primarily young adults, who consider it unlikely that they will experience major health problems—object to the mandate and may choose to opt out of coverage. Ann McEachern, a thirty-three-year-old waitress and student, did not buy insurance in 2007. "The penalty in 2007 wasn't enough to kick it up to the top of my priority list. It's always nice to be insured, but I think I'm at pretty low risk for anything happening to me that would be financially devastating." Samuel Hagan is a courier who remains uninsured. "At 27, it's not like I'm thinking, 'Oh, man, what if I need an operation down the line?' Furthest thing from my head.'"

Discussion Questions

1. Do you think that the new Massachusetts health care plan is just?

2. Should people like Ann McEachern and Samuel Hagan be required to purchase health insurance?

3. Do you think that Massachusetts could make this kind of health care system work, or should they try a different model?

Sources

Fuchs, Victor R. and Ezekiel J. Emanuel. "Health Care Reform: Why? What? When?" *Health Affairs* 24, no. 6 (2005): 1399–1414.

Sack, Kevin. "Massachusetts Faces a Test on Health Care." *New York Times*, November 25, 2007. http://www.nytimes.com/2007/11/25/us/politics/25mass.html (accessed April 14, 2008).

——. "In Massachusetts, Universal Coverage Strains Care." *New York Times*, April 5, 2008. http://www.nytimes.com/2008/04/05/us/05doctors.html (accessed April 14, 2008).

Wilson, Jennifer Fisher. "Massachusetts Health Care Reform Is a Pioneer Effort, but Complications Remain." *Annals of Internal Medicine* 148, no. 6 (2008): 489–93.

Should Illegal Immigrants Have Access to Health Care?

The United States faces a health care crisis, with millions of residents lacking health care coverage. The problem is exacerbated by the presence of illegal immigrants who also lack access to health care. Two states that are especially impacted by this problem are Texas and California.

Hospitals face the dilemma of whether to demand immigration documents from patients and deny nonemergency care to anyone without it, or provide care to anyone who needs it. Two of the largest public hospitals in Texas take opposite approaches. Parkland Health and Hospital System in Dallas provides low-cost care to low-income people, without inquiring about immigration status. JPS Health Network in Fort Worth requires documentation to receive non-emergency treatment. Although uncomfortable with that decision, JPS views its first responsibility as attending to legal residents.

In attempting to address the health care needs of California's 6.5 million uninsured residents, Governor Arnold Schwarzenegger proposed a plan to "Cover All Californians." The plan does not, however, cover all California residents. It includes all children regardless of immigration status, but only adults who are legal residents. Among the criticisms of Gov. Schwarzenegger's plan are complaints that it covers too many people and that it covers too few. There is strong public sentiment that illegal immigrants, whatever their age, should receive no access to health care, especially when so many U.S. citizens lack adequate health care. On the other hand, the Catholic health care directives support health care for everyone, with an emphasis on the social responsibility of caring for the poor and uninsured.

Another justice-related argument in favor of providing health care for illegal immigrants concerns the lack of health care opportunities in their home countries. This problem is exacerbated by the migration of health professionals from developing nations to the United States, leaving many positions in those countries vacant. It may also be in the self-interest of the United States to provide health care access to illegal immigrants, because it could reduce the spread of disease among citizens.

Like the United States, Thailand has a problem with illegal immigration. Migrants and their families from Myanmar (formerly Burma), which has one of the world's worst health care systems, frequently cross the border seeking a better quality of life. The Thai government has established health clinics near the border that will provide care, even to undocumented migrants, and other nonprofit clinics also provide such care. They do so for "humanitarian reasons."

Discussion Questions

1. Do illegal immigrants have a right to health care? Do health care facilities have a duty to provide it? Or is providing such care praiseworthy, but not required?
2. Should doctors and hospitals be prevented from treating illegal immigrants?
3. Do you think that Governor Schwarzenegger's plan to cover all children, regardless of immigration status, but not adults, is ethically acceptable?

Sources

Isarabhakdi, Pimonpan. "Meeting at the Crossroads: Myanmar Migrants and Their Use of Thai Health Care Services." *Asian and Pacific Migration Journal* 13, no. 1 (2004): 107–26.

Preston, Julia. 2006. "Texas Hospitals Reflect Debate on Immigration." *New York Times*, July 18, 2006. http://www.nytimes.com/2006/07/18/us/18immig.html (accessed July 22, 2006).

State of California. "Governor's Health Care Proposal." http://gov.ca.gov/pdf/press/Governors_HC_Proposal.pdf (accessed April 10, 2007).

United States Conference of Catholic Bishops (USCCB). *Ethical and Religious Directives for Catholic Health Care Services*. 4th ed. Washington, DC: USCCB, 2001.

Blue Cross Seeks Physician Informants

Blue Cross, California's largest for-profit health insurer, decided to ask physicians to identify patients whose medical conditions would justify cancelling their coverage. Along with a copy of a new patient's health insurance application, Blue Cross included a letter stating that the company has "the right to cancel the member's policy back to its effective date for failure to disclose material medical history." The letter listed seven sources for identifying undisclosed preexisting health issues.

"We're outraged that they are asking doctors to violate the sacred trust of patients to rat them out for medical information that patients would expect their doctors to handle with the utmost secrecy and confidentiality," said Dr. Richard Frankenstein, president of the California Medical Association. Patients "will stop telling their doctors anything they think might be a problem for their insurance and they don't think matters for their current health situation. But they didn't go to medical school, and there are all kinds of obscure things that could be very helpful to a doctor."

Blue Cross initially defended its actions, stating that enrolling members who fail to disclose their health problems will utilize more resources and drive up costs for everyone. After much criticism, Blue Cross reversed its position the very next day. It released a statement, saying: "Today we reached out to our provider partners and California regulators and determined this letter is no longer necessary and, in fact, was creating a misimpression and causing some members and providers undue concern. As a result, we are discontinuing the dissemination of this letter going forward."

Governor Arnold Schwarzenegger was among those criticizing the practice. "That is outrageous," he said, and "one more reason why it is so important to have comprehensive healthcare reform."

Discussion Questions

1. Blue Cross was asking physicians to be gatekeepers of medical resources. Is it appropriate for doctors to take on that role?
2. How well does Blue Cross fare regarding Emanuel's four principles for the just allocation of health care resources?
3. Do Blue Cross's actions validate Emanuel's claim that ethical MCOs must be nonprofit?
4. Governor Schwarzenegger said that Blue Cross's actions demonstrated why we need "comprehensive healthcare reform." Do you agree with him?

Sources

Girion, Lisa. "Doctors Balk at Request for Data." *Los Angeles Times*, February 12, 2008. http://www.latimes.com/business/la-fi-bluecross12feb12,0,4319662.story (accessed February 19, 2008).

Girion, Lisa, and Jordan Rau. Blue Cross Halts Letters Amid Furor." *Los Angeles Times*, February 13, 2008. http://www.latimes.com/business/la-fi-bluecross13feb13,1,3811525.story (accessed February 19, 2008).

Age-Based Rationing

For years, Daniel Callahan has advocated limiting medical care for the elderly, so that more resources can be devoted to people who have not yet had the opportunity for a full life. More recently, he has claimed that the highest priority should go to children's health care. This should be an easy case to make, says Callahan, but we often fail to provide good health care for children. We fail them for four main reasons: (1) We are complacent after reducing infant and child mortality rates; (2) The health care system is biased toward cure over care, such that adult heart disease gets priority over chronic childhood conditions; (3) The rescue principle favors the dramatic problems over preventive care; and (4) Our cultural individualism favors personal welfare over that of groups, maximizing choice over outcomes. Callahan does not claim that we intentionally value adults over children, only that our priorities turn out to favor adults at the expense of children and their needs.

It is not only standard health care that favors adults, but also triage proposals. In the event of a global flu pandemic, two federal advisory panels recommended that vaccine first go to health care workers, who then will be able to help others, followed by the oldest, sickest patients. The policy is aimed at saving the most lives. Besides the elderly, the two highest-risk groups are those with heart disease and those with a history of pneumonia. Some panel members argued that children should be the top priority after health care workers, because more quality life-years are saved.

The panels' recommendations were challenged by Ezekiel Emanuel, head of bioethics at the National Institutes of Health, and Alan Wertheimer, but not in order to give children priority. After health care workers, they would give priority to young adults, then people ages forty-one to fifty, and finally those fifty-one and older. "Children under 13 could be confined to home instead of receiving a vaccine. Within this framework, 20-year-olds are valued more than 1-year-olds because the older individuals have more developed interests, hopes and plans but have not had an opportunity to realize them."

Discussion Questions

1. Do you think it is just to ration health care on the basis of age rather than relative need?

2. Should children's health care needs be addressed before adult health care needs?

3. Are Emanuel and Wertheimer right to value twenty-year-olds over thirteen-year-olds and one-year-olds?

Sources

Callahan, Daniel. "Health Care for Children: A Community Perspective." *Journal of Medicine and Philosophy* 26, no. 2 (2001): 137–46.

Connolly, Ceci. "Flu Vaccine Priorities Test Pandemic Planning." *Washington Post*, May 12, 2006.

Living the Mission

An institution's identity and integrity is linked to its mission and core values. Individual Catholic health care institutions in the United States have their own mission statements, but they are governed by the United States Conference of Catholic Bishops and its *Ethical and Religious Directives for Catholic Health Care Services*. A clash of mission and values often occurs when Catholic hospitals or health systems merge with non-Catholic facilities. Social justice, spirituality, and reproductive services are three key areas of the Catholic mission that merger agreements must address. Reproductive services frequently become the focal point.

In 2001, the U.S. bishops declared that sterilization is "intrinsically evil" and will no longer be tolerated at Catholic-affiliated hospitals, including non-Catholic hospitals now owned by Catholic health care groups. "I don't care what they impose on Catholics. I do care what they impose on the rest of society," said Stanley Korenman, professor of medicine at UCLA. "They are showing a striking disregard for the ethics of the rest of society. In lots of places, the Catholic hospital is the hospital. [They] are denying people who are not Catholics in that community the opportunity to have surgical sterilization, which is legal and accepted."

For many years, non-Catholic hospitals within a Catholic health network were able to provide reproductive services by creating a legally separate sphere within the hospital. For example, a hospital might designate a few beds

and operating room as belonging to the separate hospital. The 2001 directive made it clear that such practices could no longer continue.

In 2008, controversy continued regarding a Catholic hospital group acquiring non-Catholic hospitals in the Denver area. The Sisters of Charity of Leavenworth Health System (SCLHS) was set to take over three Exempla Healthcare facilities, one of which is Catholic (St. Joseph's Hospital in Denver), and two of which are not (Lutheran Medical Center in Wheat Ridge and Good Samaritan Medical Center in Lafayette). Exempla's board sued to block acquisition, because reproductive services could no longer be performed under the new arrangement. SCLHS stated that women had "more than adequate" access to these services elsewhere in the area.

On May 30, 2008, David Wollard, founding chairman emeritus of Exempla, published a commentary in the *Denver Post* explaining why Exempla maintained the individual identities of its three hospitals, and why he thinks that is still the right thing to do.

> When we established Exempla we took great pains to make certain that the role and mission of Catholic health care carried out by Saint Joseph Hospital would be fully protected and honored.
>
> To suggest that this debate is about either Catholic or non-Catholic is simply wrong.
>
> Exempla today opposes the SCLHS takeover because, as part of the founding agreements, it has an equally strong obligation to maintain the community hospital mission of Lutheran Medical Center, and now Good Samaritan Medical Center.
>
> By "community mission" we very clearly meant, and still mean, non-sectarian mission. If someone says that SCLHS will preserve the community mission of Lutheran and Good Samaritan while at the same time making them subject to the Catholic Ethical and Religious Directives, they are asking you to accept a logical contradiction.
>
> The ERDs should be rigorously applied at Saint Joseph Hospital. They should not be

imposed on Lutheran and Good Samaritan at all. We knew we were combining an apple and an orange when we created Exempla. And we intended that one should remain an orange and the other remain an apple.

Discussion Questions

1. Is it possible to adhere to the organization's mission by allowing individual units to play by different rules?
2. Would allowing the distinct identities of the Denver hospitals to continue be what Gallagher and Goodstein would call a "fitting concrete response" to the situation?
3. What if the acquisition of the Lutheran Medical Center and Good Samaritan Hospitals meant that all hospitals in the Denver area were now Catholic-owned. How does that impact the "fitting concrete response" to the situation?
4. Do women have a right to access reproductive health services?

Sources

Catholic News Agency. "Catholic Healthcare Group's Expansion in Colorado Triggers Dispute Over Abortion, Contraceptive Coverage." October 30, 2007. http://www.catholicnewsagency.com/new.php?n=10830. (accessed June 19, 2008).

Shannon, Thomas. "Living the Vision: Health Care, Social Justice and Institutional Identity." *Christian Bioethics* 7, no. 1 (2001): 49–65.

Stammer, Larry B. "Bishops Ban Sterilization Services at All Catholic-Affiliated Hospitals." *Los Angeles Times*, June 16, 2007.

Wollard, David. "Exempla's Priority is to Protect Catholic Health Care Values." *Denver Post*, May 30, 2008. http://www.denverpost.com/opinionheadlines/ci_9427973 (accessed June 19, 2008).

Early Harvest—Removing Organs After Cardiac Death

After the whole-brain standard for determining death was accepted in the 1970s, most organs were removed after the donor was declared brain-dead. This standard was implemented, in part, so that there would be no doubt that donors were dead, in spite of their bodies being artificially maintained to better preserve organs for harvesting by transplant teams. Now, in order to increase the supply of available organs, surgeons are using a new approach—donation after cardiac death (DCD). It is used primarily with dying patients who have suffered brain damage. There were 793 DCD donations during 2007, which was ten percent of the total number of deceased donors, and by far the largest number ever.

In DCD donations, life-sustaining treatment is discontinued, and shortly after the heart stops the transplant team enters the room and removes the organs. Because the heart can spontaneously start again, transplant doctors usually wait about five minutes before harvesting, but others remove the organs more quickly. Surgeons at Children's Hospital in Denver wait only 75 seconds to remove infant hearts, in order to maximize their usability. Doctors inject DCD donors with various drugs like morphine to ensure they do not suffer when life support is withdrawn. They also often inject the blood thinner heparin to help preserve the organs. It is possible that those measures hasten death.

Although many relatives of DCD donors support the procedure, questions surround the 2006 case of twenty-five-year-old Ruben Navarro, who was hospitalized at the Sierra Vista Regional Medical Center in San Luis Obispo, CA. Navarro had adrenoleukodystrophy, a severe neurological disorder, and lived in an assisted-care facility. On January 29, 2006, he was discovered unconscious in cardiac and respiratory arrest, revived, and then sent to Sierra Vista. Navarro's brain had been damaged from lack of oxygen. Within a few days, Navarro's mother was told that he would not recover. She agreed to donate Ruben's organs, and said that she did not want him "to suffer too long." On February 3, transplant surgeon Dr. Hootan Roozrokh arrived at the hospital, and according to a Sierra Vista nurse, was present in the room when Navarro's ventilator was removed. The nurse reported that Dr. Roozrokh gave orders for medication—excessive doses of morphine and Ativan (an anti-anxiety medication), which are typically given to comfort dying patients, as well as Betadine, which may cause death if ingested. Dr. Roozrokh is also accused of requesting that additional drugs be administered when Navarro did not die immediately after the removal of the ventilator. Navarro died eight hours later, but by that point his organs had deteriorated to the point that they were unsuitable for transplantation.

The United Network for Organ Sharing reprimanded the California Transplant Donor Network for breaking protocol in the case, and the California state medical board issued a complaint against Dr. Roozrokh, charging that he engaged in unprofessional conduct by "being present in the operating room prior to the patient's death, by actively monitoring the patient's vital signs for determination of death and by attending to the patient regarding the administration of pain medication." Dr. Roozrokh also faced criminal prosecution on three felony charges. In December 2008, he was acquitted of dependent adult abuse; the other two charges (administering a harmful substance and controlled substances without a medical purpose) had already been dropped. He still faces the state medical board complaint and a civil law suit filed by Navarro's mother.

Discussion Questions

1. Do you think that DCD is an ethical practice?
2. DCD accounted for ten percent of the deceased donors in 2007. Should the United States abandon the dead donor rule in order to further increase the organ supply?
3. Does learning about Dr. Roozrokh's actions impact your decision to be an organ donor?
4. Would it impact your decision to donate a family member's organs?

Sources

Arnquist, Sarah. "Surgeon Faces Trial for Felony." *San Luis Obispo Tribune*, March 20, 2008. http://www.sanluisobispo.com/183/story/309486.html (accessed June 20, 2008).

McKinley, Jessie. "Surgeon Accused of Speeding a Death to Get Organs." *New York Times*, February 27, 2008. http://www.nytimes.com/2008/02/27/us/27transplant.html (accessed February 27, 2008).

Parrilla, Leslie. "Medical Board Files Complaint Against Transplant Surgeon." *San Luis Obispo Tribune*, June 7, 2008. http://www.sanluisobispo.com/537/story/381047.html (accessed June 20, 2008).

——. "Transplant Surgeon Hootan Roozrokh Acquitted in Sierra Vista Organ Harvest Case." *San Luis Obispo Tribune*, December 18, 2008. http://www.sanluisobispo.com/183/story/564066.html (accessed January 27, 2009).

Stein, Rob. "New Trend in Organ Donation Raises Questions." *Washington Post*, March 18, 2007. http://www.washingtonpost.com/wp-dyn/content/article/2007/03/17/AR2007031700963.html (accessed March 19, 2007).

United Network for Organ Sharing. "Regional Meetings Data Update." http://www.unos.org/SharedContentDocuments/Spring_2008_Regional_Meeting_Data_Slides_Final.pdf (accessed June 20, 2008).

Presumed Consent and Organ Donation

Like the United States, the United Kingdom's organ procurement policy is to use express donation. Unfortunately, the United Kingdom's donation rate is very low. If it could increase the pool of donated organs, the United Kingdom could save more lives, decrease patient suffering, and even save money. Although it costs more up front, kidney transplants pay for themselves in just over two years when compared to kidney dialysis.

Prime Minister Gordon Brown has proposed that the United Kingdom move to a system like Spain's, where citizens must choose to opt out of donation rather than choose to opt in. Brown thinks that this policy of presumed consent for organ donation would dramatically increase the supply of donated organs as it has in other European nations, and still respect the wishes of patients and families who would prefer not to donate.

Dr. Evan Harris, a member of Parliament and also of the British Medical Association's Ethics Committee, supports the proposal. "Under an opt-out scheme donor's real wishes will be more often respected, more lives would be saved and grieving relatives will be spared the experience of making the wrong decision at the worst time," he said.

Several patient groups, however, are against the proposal, arguing that the state should not decide what happens to people's bodies when they die. Joyce Robins from Patient Concern said that presumed consent turned volunteers into conscripts, and was skeptical that the proposal would solve the problem of donor shortages. "Presumed consent is no consent at all," she said. Katherine Murphy, of the Patients Association, agreed: "We don't think a private decision, which is a matter of individual conscience, should be taken by the State. If people want to give the gift of life, that is their right, but it must be something that is a voluntary matter."

Discussion Questions

1. Do you think that presumed consent is an ethical organ procurement policy?
2. Do you think that presumed consent would increase the supply of organs for transplantation?
3. Would you support a policy of presumed consent in the United States?

Sources

British Broadcasting Corporation (BBC). "PM Backs Automatic Organ Donation." *BBC News*, January 13, 2008. http://news.bbc.co.uk/2/hi/health/7186007.stm (accessed June 19, 2008).

Webster, Philip. "Gordon Brown Seeks to Make Everyone an Organ Donor—with Opt-Out." *London Times*, January 14, 2008. http://www.timesonline.co.uk/tol/news/politics/article3182388.ece (accessed June 19, 2008).

Pat Summerall's New Liver

In August 2006, seventy-six-year-old Pat Summerall was feeling great. The former television sportscaster and NFL player had just published a book about his life, which just two years earlier almost ended. In 2004, Summerall nearly died from liver cirrhosis, but a transplant saved his life.

The life-saving arguably began twelve years before the transplant. Summerall was an alcoholic, and had spent much of his life drinking and carousing. "Nobody abused life as much as I did or had as good a time as I did," he said. In 1992, his performance as a sportscaster was suffering, and his friends and family persuaded him to enter the Betty Ford Clinic. He stayed for thirty-three days, got sober, and a month later had a religious conversion to Christianity. "I guess I knew I'd done this to myself, a realization I got at the Betty Ford Center," he said. "I knew that nobody was responsible but me, that I had done the damage."

Discussion Questions

1. If Summerall was responsible for his liver damage, what bearing, if any, does that have on him as a potential liver transplant recipient?
2. How do you think Glannon would evaluate Summerall's case?
3. Do you agree with Glannon?

Sources

Sandomir, Richard. "Summerall Gets New Liver, and Life, With a Transplant." *New York Times*, May 1, 2008. http://www.nytimes.com/2004/05/01/sports/football/01SUMM.html (accessed May 1, 2004).

——. "Summerall, Shocking and Sober." *New York Times*, August 19, 2006. http://www.nytimes.com/2006/08/18/sports/football/18sandomir.html (accessed June 18, 2008).

Matchmakers

Potential transplant recipients sometimes must wait years before receiving an organ, and some unfortunate patients never get one at all. In order to speed up the process, and to improve the supply of organs available, people have used the Internet to help themselves, or to set up a program to help others. Noteworthy among the programs are LifeSharers, which focuses on quicker access to cadaver organs for registered organ donors, and MatchingDonors, which focuses on encouraging living donation and matching donors with patients.

People who join LifeSharers pledge to donate their organs after they die, and to designate other LifeSharers members who need transplants as preferred recipients. The organization justifies this arrangement with an argument based on fairness. It is unfair to give organs to people who are unwilling to donate their own; it is fair to give priority to willing donors. LifeSharers claims that only about half of the transplanted organs in the United States go to other organ donors. The organization has grown tremendously since it was founded in 2003. As of May 31, 2008, it had nearly 11,500 members, but is still too young and too small to have resulted in a transplant from one member to another (although it may have increased the total number of organ donors). There were seventy-two LifeSharers members on waiting lists in May 2008, but so far no member has died in circumstances that would permit organ harvesting.

MatchingDonors had over five thousand registered donors and nearly 350 patient profiles in June 2008. It facilitated over sixty transplants between 2004 and 2007. Patients pay a membership fee to post a personal profile advertisement soliciting organ donations. The cost ranges from $49 for a one-time, seven-day trial membership, to $295 for thirty days, $441 for ninety days, and a lifetime membership for $25 monthly and $595 per profile listing. Patients have an opportunity to tell their stories and post pictures. Potential donors review the profiles and contact the patients; they work out the details themselves.

Perhaps the most prominent display of altruism associated with MatchingDonors comes from the Uribe family. Juan Uribe donated a kidney to Gail Fink in 2005, and then his wife Leigh Anne agreed to be a surrogate mother for Gail, giving birth to twins in October 2007. Because the patients are strangers and work out their own arrangements, there is some concern about patients paying donors. It is illegal to buy and sell organs in the United States.

Discussion Questions

1. Do you agree with LifeSharers that their network is more fair than the UNOS system, in that they give priority to willing donors, and that it is unfair to give organs to people who are unwilling to be donors?
2. Do you think that it would be fair to give preference to organ donors, but then give organs to nondonors if no donor can use them?
3. Do you think that it is ethical for patients to solicit other people to donate their organs to them? Does it discriminate against people who lack computer skills or persuasive story-telling ability, or who cannot afford the membership fee?
4. Would it be ethical if some patients using MatchingDonors were paying donors, or if donors were requesting payment?

Sources

LifeSharers. www.lifesharers.com (accessed June 20, 2008).

MatchingDonors. www.matchingdonors.com (accessed June 20, 2008).

Newbart, Dave. "The Greatest Gifts." *Chicago Sun-Times*, December 25, 2007.

CHAPTER 6

Biomedical Research

INTRODUCTION

Biomedical research (sometimes called experimental medicine) consists of basic and applied research aimed at increasing medical knowledge and understanding. Medical research has two main arms. *Preclinical research* tries to generate a better understanding of disease and new strategies for treatment. Almost all preclinical research is carried out on animals. A broad range of research can contribute to preclinical medical knowledge, including research in genetics, evolutionary biology, neuroscience, and biochemistry. *Clinical research* evaluates new treatments for safety and efficacy. Clinical research often takes the form of a *clinical trial*, which is a carefully designed experiment to test the safety and effectiveness of a drug, device, or preventive measure in a group of human patients.

Biomedical research is a huge and costly enterprise. In the United States about forty-five billion dollars are spent on biomedical research each year, with most of this funding coming from pharmaceutical companies, biotechnology companies, medical device companies, and the government—the National Institutes of Health (NIH) oversees the federal funding of medical research. A small percentage of research funding, around three percent, comes from philanthropic organizations such as the Bill and Melinda Gates Foundation. The Food and Drug Administration (FDA) is responsible for regulating the development of new drugs and devices.

Biomedical research has been a core issue in bioethics from its very beginnings as a discipline. Indeed, you will find in the second reading—*The Belmont Report*, published in 1979—one of the earliest articulations of the key moral principles in bioethics. This is no coincidence. Some of the early pioneers in bioethics sat on the National Commission for the Protection of Human Subjects of Biomedical Research, which wrote and then published *The Belmont Report*.

In this chapter, we focus on three areas of moral unrest in biomedical research: the ethics of using humans as research subjects, the ethics of using human embryonic stem cells for research, and the ethics of using nonhuman animals in medical experimentation. In each of these areas, certain key questions need to be answered: Who can ethically be used to test the safety and effectiveness of new drugs or therapies? What is an appropriate ratio of benefit to risk for a research subject? What is the potential value of a particular research project to society? How does this potential value weigh against the project's moral risks? Keep in mind, as you read this chapter, the four core principles of bioethics (beneficence, nonmaleficence, respect for autonomy, and justice). These are clearly at play in the readings on human research. But how well do these principles guide the discussion of research on animals and stem cells?

Research on Human Subjects

Dr. Lawrence Myrick: People die everyday. And for what? For nothing. What do we do? What do *you* do? You take care of the ones you think you can save. Good doctors do the correct thing. Great doctors have the guts to do the right thing. Your father had those guts.... If you could cure cancer by killing one person, wouldn't you have to do that? One person and cancer's gone tomorrow. When you thought you were paralyzed...what would you have done to be able to walk again? "Anything." You said it yourself. Anything.

Dr. Guy Luthan: Those men upstairs, maybe there isn't much point to their lives. Maybe they are doing a great thing for the world. Maybe they are heroes. But they didn't choose to be. You chose for them. You didn't choose your wife . . . or your granddaughter. You didn't ask for volunteers. You chose for them. And you can't do that, because you're a doctor, and you took an oath. And you're not God. . . . So, I don't care if you find a cure for every disease on the planet. You tortured and murdered those men upstairs, and that makes you a disgrace to your profession. And I hope you go to jail for the rest of your life.

—*Extreme Measures* (1996)

The practice of medicine has always been intertwined with the endeavor of scientists to understand more clearly biology, health, disease, and mortality. Medicine, in other words, has always been experimental, and humans have always been subjects of research. Doctors and scientists have used themselves, their families, their patients, and countless others to test their potions, hypotheses, scalpels, and pills.

Yet although the research enterprise has long been alive and well, prior to the mid-twentieth century there was little sustained discussion about the ethics of medical research. This began to change in the shadow of World War II, with revelations about doctors in Nazi Germany conducting extensive research on Jewish prisoners. Many of the experiments were gruesome and painful; all were conducted on unwilling victims, many of whom were "euthanized" afterwards. In 1946, twenty-three people—most of them doctors—were tried in front of a military tribunal in Nuremberg, Germany, in what is famously referred to as the Nuremberg Trials. In addition to convicting most of the twenty-three of war crimes and crimes against humanity, the trials provided the skeleton of a new code of ethics for medical research. **The Nuremberg Code** (the first reading selection) established ten principles for research with human subjects, including informed consent, absence of coercion, scientific rigor, and beneficence toward research participants. Although the Nuremberg Code had no legal status, it was profoundly influential in shaping how people thought about the ethics of research on humans, and is reflected in the content and language of the 1964 Declaration of Helsinki, *The Belmont Report*, and the United States regulations governing federally funded human research (Code of Federal Regulations, Title 45, Volume 46).

Unfortunately, the Nazi trials and the Nuremberg Code did not signal an end to unethical medical research, nor did they clarify exactly what constitutes the ethical use of humans as research subjects. Over the next several decades, numerous other problems surfaced, including the infamous Willowbrook State School experiments and the Tuskegee syphilis experiments. During the late 1950s, severely retarded children living at the Willowbrook State School in New York were injected with live hepatitis virus so that researchers could undertake a long-range study of the disease. Researchers justified their actions by arguing that fecally transmitted hepatitis was so prevalent in the institution that most of the children would have contracted the disease anyway.

In Tuskegee, Alabama, four hundred mostly poor and illiterate African American men with syphilis were monitored over a forty-year-period, so that researchers could study the progression of the disease. Soon after the study began, other research showed that penicillin would effectively treat syphilis, but the men in the study were not treated nor were they told that a treatment had been developed. Researchers were undoubtedly motivated by the belief that studying the full progression of syphilis would greatly enhance medical understanding of the disease. But in retrospect, the Tuskegee and Willowbrook studies appear to have had serious ethical shortcomings—notably a lack of informed consent, and the exploitation of vulnerable groups. But, like Dr. Myrick (Gene Hackman's character in *Extreme Measures*), the scientists involved likely were good people, and likely believed that they were doing good work and had, within their cultural milieu, reasonable justification for their actions. Tuskegee, Willowbrook, and other early studies prompted the publication, in 1979, of *The Belmont Report*, which gets it name from the conference center near Baltimore where the document was drafted. This government report, though written as a guide for human research, was profoundly influential in the development of the larger field of bioethics.

It is often much easier to identify problematic research, especially in retrospect, than to define exactly what constitutes *ethical* research. This is perhaps why research ethics remains such a hot topic within bioethics: there is profound disagreement about what makes a research project slide over that very thin and unstable line between ethical and unethical. The general principles codified at Nuremberg and Helsinki enjoy broad consensus. Yet how exactly to understand when, for example, consent is really informed, or research is really free from coercion, turns out to be exceedingly difficult. This is one reason that the regulations surrounding research are so long and so complex, and why the bioethics literature on research ethics is so extensive. Even today, there are many research protocols that raise questions and concerns. This is not a reflection of the poor character of biomedical researchers, but reflects rather the moral ambiguity of the research enterprise itself. This chapter explores some of these ambiguities.

First, though, a preliminary question must be asked: is research on humans ever morally justified? The central moral problem of research is this: the goal of research is to increase general knowledge, with the aim to improve health or treat disease and disability. But this knowledge cannot be pursued without placing some people at risk of harm. But placing some people at risk for the benefit of other people and for the common good is a form of exploitation. It goes against one of the most treasured moral principles: never use people merely as a means to an end, but only as ends in themselves—the essence of respect for human dignity. What moral justification might we give for using people as a means to acquire new knowledge? How do we avoid treating them *merely* as a means?

Research offers great benefit to society. Medicine relies on evidence; the more and better evidence we have, the better our medicine becomes. It is obvious that the entire history of medicine has been one of expanding knowledge: for example, learning that germs cause disease (leading to sterilization of hands and instruments) and that the body's own defense mechanisms can be put to use through vaccination. There is still much to learn. Each person is the recipient of the benefits of knowledge from past research, and for that reason each person owes a debt of gratitude to those who have sacrificed themselves in various ways to advance medicine (analogous in certain ways to the argument from chapter 2 that doctors don't "own" their medical knowledge, but use it in trust for the community). Individuals might, then, be said to have a duty to serve as research subjects.

Yet this is perhaps too strongly stated for most people. We might say that research on humans is justified only when the subjects have volunteered to be involved. If a person willingly accepts some risk in order to benefit others, then perhaps there is no exploitation—when, as Dr. Luthan (Hugh Grant's character in *Extreme Measures*) might say, they choose for themselves, rather than the doctor choosing for them. This presumption may be problematic, but let us set any problems aside for now. Let us assume that we agree that research is socially important, that medicine cannot really move forward without research, and that as long as people willingly volunteer to be involved we are not exploiting them. So the research enterprise, in itself, is justified. What, then, distinguishes ethical from unethical research? How can research be conducted without exploiting people? What are the problems that have so perplexed the ethicists?

Research and Therapy

Everyone who gets treated by a doctor is, in a most basic way, an experimental subject, since there is art and hypothesis in all diagnosis and treatment. Still, it is worth making a distinction between the enterprise of research and enterprise of medicine, even though we may want to keep in the back of our mind a question about how fine a line can be drawn between the two endeavors. In chapter 2, we talked about the profession of medicine, and the obligation of the physician to remain committed to the benefit of his or her patient. But research blurs the professional role.

The Belmont Report, your second reading selection, distinguishes between practice and research in this way: practice refers to "interventions that are designed solely to enhance the well-being of an individual patient and have a reasonable chance of success." Practice provides diagnosis and treatment to a particular individual. Research, on the other hand, is aimed at testing a hypothesis and then drawing conclusions that will contribute in some way to generalizable knowledge. Thus, research and practice are two distinct realms. Early ethicists also drew a distinction between therapeutic and nontherapeutic research. In *therapeutic research*, the subject is also the patient, and is expected to benefit medically from the research; the treatment is part of the research protocol. *Nontherapeutic research* offers no direct benefit to the subject. Because the subject does not benefit, nontherapeutic research is assumed to be more difficult to justify than therapeutic research.

Over the last decade, both distinctions have come under fire. The therapeutic/nontherapeutic distinction has been challenged because it obscures the relationship between researcher and subject. After all, no research has as its primary aim to benefit the individual subject; the goal is always to increase knowledge and understanding. Also, even therapeutic research often has nontherapeutic elements, such as extra blood draws.

Informed Consent and Other Ethical Rules for Research

If the ethics of research needs to be considered on its own terms, distinct from the ethics of medical practice, what moral principles should guide the research enterprise? There is broad agreement that the decision to participate in research should fall to the patient, and to the patient alone. No one should be coerced into being a research subject, or should be part of an experiment without his or her knowledge and agreement.

People have to agree to be subjects of research, and this agreement must be "informed," that is, subjects must understand fully what it is they are agreeing to. It is not considered ethical for a researcher to lie about or downplay risks, or to misrepresent the kind of research being proposed. The components of ethically valid informed consent include disclosure, understanding, voluntariness, competence and consent. According to the Health and Human Services provisions, legal requirements for informed consent involve the following:

> a statement that the study involves research, an explanation of the purposes of the research and the expected duration of the subject's participation, a description of the procedures to be followed, and identification of any procedures which are experimental; a description of any reasonably foreseeable risks or discomforts to the subject; a description of any benefits to the subject or to others which may reasonably be expected from the research.

Subjects must also be told how confidentiality of information will be protected, and whether there will be compensation for any harm or injury from the study.

Although the requirement of informed consent has been the cornerstone of research ethics, it has always been mired in controversy. Ethicists have long recognized that what exactly constitutes informed consent is ambiguous. There are certain groups of people for whom consent is not straightforward: patients who are in severe pain, patients with mental illness, older children, and elderly patients with some loss of intellectual capacity. In addition, there are groups of people who cannot give consent at all: young children, the unconscious, or the mentally incapacitated, such as people with Down syndrome and patients in a vegetative state. It is, on the one hand, desirable to do research that may benefit these very groups of people, but it is difficult to see past the exploitation, however mild, that accompanies their participation in research. This discussion overlaps with issues discussed in chapters 2 and 3: proxy consent and best interests versus community standards. Bioethicists disagree about whether research on those unable to give informed consent is ever ethical, though there is consensus that if research is conducted on these groups, the research must offer some promise *for those involved* and must pose only minimal risks.

Somewhere in the gray area between consenting adults and those who cannot give consent are certain classes of people who can ostensibly give informed consent, but who may be subject to subtle forms of coercion—so that consent, though perhaps informed, is not truly voluntary. These populations have been termed "vulnerable." For example, prisoners make wonderful research populations: they are captive; they will not walk out on the study; and their lives (when and what they eat, when they sleep, etc.) are regulated by others. Many variables that might confound a research study can be controlled. But some ethicists have raised concerns about whether captive populations can really give voluntary consent—might they be subject to subtle forms of coercion, for example, that participation in a study might be linked with "being a good citizen" and thus with earlier parole or other benefits.

Some ethicists have even begun to challenge the central dogma of informed consent itself, arguing that perhaps there are situations where people should be compelled to participate in research. For example, **David Orentlicher**, in his article "Making Research a Requirement of Treatment," argues that there is a need to relax the precautions taken to gain voluntary consent. In studies involving the comparison of two or more established therapies to see whether one is superior to the others, it is acceptable and perhaps even preferable to make treatment conditional on consent to participate.

Conditioning treatment on a patient's willingness to enroll in a trial is thought to be unduly coercive, but Orentlicher argues that it is ethically sound and could increase patient participation, which is important. He also argues that it could eliminate unnecessary impediments to progress, encourage more social sentiment in favor of participation in medical research (if people want to share in the benefits of research, they should also be willing to participate) and bolster patient trust. (On the move to expand beyond informed consent, see the box "Research Ethics, State of the Art circa 2000," and see the case "Medicare Requires Heart Patients to Enlist in Research" (for a real-life test of Orentlicher's argument).

Bioethicist **Carl Elliott's** essay "Guinea-pigging" moves beyond the abstractions of philosophers, and opens a window into the inner world of medical research, exploring the experiences of people who actually work as professional guinea pigs, hiring themselves out for one Phase I clinical trial after another. Elliott's piece raises troubling questions about exploitation, the rigor of regulatory and ethical oversight for research, the procurement of research volunteers, and the rigor of the science itself. Also woven through his narrative are nagging questions about fairness.

Justice and Research

There has long been concern that the people who serve as research subjects are not the same people who benefit from the drugs or devices being tested. Using prisoners in research, for example, raises concerns not only about voluntary consent but also a broader kind of social exploitation of certain groups. The prison population in the United States is predominantly black males, and some worry that this racial group is being exploited by pharmaceutical companies. Indeed, Tuskegee casts a long shadow across human subject research. A recent study by Giselle Corbie-Smith and colleagues found that minorities are two hundred percent more likely than whites to perceive harm coming from research and to distrust researchers. They are more likely to think that researchers would use them as guinea pigs and experiment on them without their knowledge or consent.

There have also been gender disparities in research, though the problems cut in a different direction. Men have more frequently been used as research subjects than women. In 1977, the U.S. Food and Drug Administration (FDA) issued guidelines that excluded women of child-bearing potential from Phase I and early Phase II testing. Caution about safety and liability of testing women, and concerns about protecting fetuses, led to some overprotection of women and reluctance to test drugs and devices in female populations. As a result, more research was done on male populations, and the consequent safety and dosing data was extrapolated to women. However, women's physiology differs from men's, so extrapolation of data to women is not always safe or effective. Research in pharmacokinetics (which studies how drugs are absorbed, distributed, metabolized, and excreted within the body) suggests a great deal of gender and individual variation in response to drugs. Furthermore, male bias in research shapes how medicine views certain diseases. For example, heart disease was long considered a man's problem, but this was largely because research on heart disease was conducted on male populations—which in turn reinforced the idea that it was a man's disease. But heart disease is a huge issue for women too, and is, in fact, the number one killer of women in the United States. Finally, research attention to women-specific problems such as vulvodynia and even premenstrual syndrome has lagged far behind research into male problems such as erectile dysfunction and premature hair loss.

The gender disparity began to subside in 1993 for two reasons: (1) the FDA rescinded its regulation excluding women, and (2) the National Institutes of Health Revitalization Act mandated that the directors of NIH ensure the inclusion of women in relevant clinical research. The NIH Act also stated that trials must be designed for a valid analysis of whether women as a subgroup differ from the rest of the study population. In 2001, the National Academy of Sciences issued a report urging the study of the sex differences in diseases and treatments. It recommended not only that women should be included in clinical trials, but that researchers should note whether the women have reached menopause and should try to identify the stages of female subject, menstrual cycles, which may affect hormone levels and body chemistry.

Using pregnant women in clinical trials presents additional issues, but the American College of Obstetricians and Gynecologists has said that "pregnant women should be presumed to be eligible for participation in clinical studies," with full disclosure of the risks so women can give informed consent if they wish. Obviously, pregnancy also has an impact on illnesses and the effect of treatments, so pregnant women must be tested in order to practice better medicine for this group of patients. Furthermore, there are some medical problems that only impact pregnant women, such as miscarriage and gestational diabetes. The only way to conduct research regarding these problems is to utilize pregnant women as subjects.

One of the most vigorous debates about justice in research ethics over the past decade has centered on research in third world countries. Pharmaceutical companies have increasingly been "outsourcing" research: they design and carry out clinical trials in developing countries, where the populations suffer from many health problems, and suffer from them in large numbers. There are many incentives for this global expansion. Often researchers can avoid ethics-related regulations that govern trials conducted in the United States. They can reduce the cost of the trial, because the populations are poor, and desperately need care or whatever other small incentives pharmaceutical companies might offer. They also arguably provide some benefits, because enrolling in a research study may be participants' only hope of receiving a medication or treatment.

Trials of drugs for HIV and AIDS carried out in Africa have been quite controversial, particularly several trials that were carried out on HIV-infected pregnant women. The experiments, which involved large numbers of women, were controversial because only half of the women were receiving treatment with the drug AZT, which is known to reduce the transmission of HIV from mother to infant by two thirds. Half of the women were given placebo pills. Many have spoken out against the experiments, arguing that it is unethical to give any women the placebo, knowing that the drug treatment is so effective. Furthermore, they argue, the drug therapy is expensive and these populations of women, on whom the drugs are tested, will never afford the medication. Defenders of the research note that without the study, no one would have received the drug, so at least some are better off. Furthermore, using placebos is the only way to get clear data on what kind of treatment regimen will work in the Third World, which is of ultimate benefit to the people there Fernando Meirelles's 2005 film *The Constant Gardener* revolves around the exploitation of Africa's poor by a large pharmaceutical company.

Philosopher **Alex John London**, in the essay "Justice and the Human Development Approach to International Research," wants to further broaden the debate about the ethics of research in developing countries. He seeks to make clear the links between medical research, social determinants of health, and global justice.

London argues that most discussion of international research has been framed by the "minimalist" view, which takes into account the needs and vulnerabilities of the host population, and the capacity of research to benefit and burden. Justice on this view is a matter of mutual advantage. But this framework, London asserts, is inadequate. There are two main problems with the minimalist view: first, it abstracts the health needs of the developing world from their broader social, political, and economic context. Second, it evaluates proposed collaborative research in isolation from the web of existing social, political, and economic relationships in which the partners are already engaged. The minimalist view assumes that questions of justice arise only within the terms of a cooperative relationship, which encourages a piecemeal and ad hoc approach to the needs of those in the developing world.

He suggests, instead, what he calls a human development view of justice in international research. This perspective treats clinical research as one important element within a larger division of labor of health-related institutions within a country. Research initiatives are permissible only if they contribute to a fair social division of labor in the host community and expand the capacity of the host community to meet the distinctive health needs of the population.

Research Ethics, State of the Art circa 2000

An important contribution to the research ethics literature is an essay published in 2000 by bioethicists Ezekiel Emanuel, David Wendler, and Christine Grady. They argue that informed consent is not enough to make research ethical. Consent has been an obsessive focus of most examination of ethics in research, reflecting a more general obsession in medical ethics with respect for autonomy. Informed consent is necessary in most, but not all, research situations, but it is never sufficient. The core documents written to guide research (Helsinki, Council for International Organizations of Medical Sciences, Nuremberg) were written in response to specific events, and thus the moral guidance is directed at specific issues and tends to ignore other concerns. Emanuel, Wendler, and Grady provide a set of guidelines for research that incorporate a much broader set of moral concerns. The values underlying these requirements go beyond beneficence, respect for autonomy, and justice to include the responsible use of finite resources and avoiding exploitation of potential subjects.

They propose seven ethical requirements for research:

1. Value. Research must be socially valuable; it must lead to improvements in treatment or diagnosis that will benefit humans.

2. Scientific validity. In addition to being socially valuable, research must be scientifically sound. Research must be well designed and rigorous, and use accepted methodologies and data analysis.

3. Fair subject selection. Criteria for inclusion and exclusion related to the recruitment of subjects must be consistent with principles of justice.

4. Favorable risk-benefit ratio. The potential benefits to individual research subjects and to society must outweigh risks.

5. Independent review. This will help maintain scientific rigor, allow for public accountability and transparency, and reduce the potential for conflicts of interest.

6. Informed consent. This requirement is based on the principle of respect for autonomy. Individual subjects must freely consent to participate in research, and must be fully apprised of the purpose, methods, risks, and benefits of the study.

7. Respect for potential and enrolled subjects. Obtaining informed consent is only the beginning; once subjects are enrolled in a study, they must continue to be treated with respect. Privacy of their information must be protected; they must be allowed to withdraw from a study; and they should be told about the results of the research.

The IRB

Institutional Review Boards for the Protection of Human Subjects (IRBs) are committees made up of clinicians, scientists, ethicists, and administrators. Their mandate is to review federally funded research according to the guidelines established by the Department of Health and Human Services in the Federal Code of Regulations (45 CFR 46). IRBs review the scientific value of proposed research, evaluate the methods to ensure scientific soundness, and make sure that subject selection is fair and non-coercive and that participants give informed consent. They give a kind of moral "green light" to research on human subjects.

IRBs have long been housed within academic medical centers, but as Carl Elliott notes, increasingly IRB approval is being "out-sourced."

How Are Experimental Drugs Tested?

A new drug or compound may take years to work its way to market. Before testing on human subjects begins, a drug will typically have been through years of preclinical and laboratory study, and will have been tested in human and animal cells, and then in live animals. At this point, the FDA will issue an Investigational New Drug application. Now testing in human subjects can begin.

Testing a new drug with human subjects usually occurs in three phases.

Phase I

These studies investigate a drug's safety. Testing involves a small number of healthy human subjects— maybe twenty to thirty—who are often paid for their service. (These are Carl Elliott's professional "guinea pigs.") Phase I trials are designed to study how a drug is metabolized, absorbed, and excreted by the body, what its side effects might be, and what might be an appropriate dosage.

Phase II

About three fourths of new drugs move on to Phase II testing. Here investigators want to discover whether a drug actually works: does it do what it promised?

Several hundred subjects may be tested, and most Phase II studies are randomized trials, comparing the new drug to existing drugs and/or a placebo. Phase II trials will typically test a drug on a group of patients who are suffering from an ailment that the drug is designed to treat. Roughly thirty percent of new drugs successfully pass Phase II.

Phase III

This is a large-scale investigation of the new drug, involving hundreds of patients and sometimes lasting several years. Phase III trials typically test a new drug against the best currently available treatment, with the hope that the new drug will prove even more efficacious. Once a Phase III trial is successfully complete (and most drugs successfully pass this stage of testing), the FDA will approve the drug and marketing will begin.

Phase IV

Sometimes pharmaceutical companies will run additional trials. Phase IV trials are done once a drug has proven effective and been approved by the FDA. These trials are designed to compare a drug's effectiveness against others on the market, or to determine cost-effectiveness of a new drug therapy.

Stem Cell Research

One area of biomedical research has been uniquely controversial: research into what are called "stem cells." This research explores the therapeutic potential of human embryonic stem cells derived from blastocysts (the stage of development between zygote and embryo, about four to five days of age). Stem cells are primitive and undifferentiated cells found in all animals. These special cells have the potential to develop into a vast array of functional and differentiated cells within the body. Human embryonic stem cells (hESC), which appear in the human blastocyst during the first few days of development, have two unique properties that make them of profound interest to medical research: hESCs are "pluripotent," which means that the cells can develop into any of the different and specialized cells or tissues in the body—into brain cells, or liver cells, or skin cells—and hESCs are also endlessly self-renewing in the undifferentiated state.

Medical researchers believe that stem cells have enormous scientific and therapeutic potential. Yet stem cell research has been mired in controversy. The reason: the only known successful method for harvesting and growing hESCs has involved harvesting the cells from the human blastocyst. The outer cellular layer of the blastocyst (which would develop as the placenta) is dissolved, revealing the inner cell mass, which is used for research. The inner cell mass, of course, would develop into the fetus. Here lies the heart of the moral controversy.

Many people are opposed to killing embryos, which they equate with killing people. The discussion of stem cell research ethics thus gets drawn into the highly politicized debate over the moral status of human embryos and into the vortex of the abortion controversy. Some believe that no medical benefit is worth the moral cost of researching on human embryos, while others believe that the promise of embryonic stem cell research has been exaggerated in order to justify the moral costs. Opponents also often note that *adult* stem cells may have as much potential to offer treatments, without the ethical costs, and that research should be focused here. On the other hand, supporters of the research point to its therapeutic potential: hESCs may offer treatments for spinal cord injuries and for neurodegenerative diseases such as Parkinson's and Alzheimer's, and may improve methods of organ transplantation. Basic research on hESCs is also helping scientists understand human developmental biology and the role of genes in causing disease. Proponents of stem cell research note that thousands of embryos are stored in fertility clinics, and will eventually be destroyed. These could be used for the benefit of humanity. Moreover, many women are eager to donate unused embryos, since they see some potential for benefiting others.

Some of the themes from human subject research carry into the stem cell debate: the scientific value of the research is a central point of discussion, since its scientific potential is offered in compensation for the morally problematic elements. Yet the stem cell debate also brings its own unique set of questions into focus: What is the status of the human blastocyst? Is it ethical to use embryos (and destroy them) for research purposes?

Stem cell research has also connected with the ongoing debate about the ethics of cloning. Scientists have found that embryonic stem cells can be created through somatic cell nuclear transfer, or cloning. Some researchers believe that cloning offers the best avenue for further research, since the quality of cloned embryos is superior to embryos that have been stored for long periods in IVF clinics. Furthermore, cloning could help overcome graft-host responses in organ transplantation, if organs or tissues could be developed using the recipient's own DNA. Ethical concern has focused on whether *therapeutic cloning* (cloning for the purposes of extracting stem cells) can be prevented from evolving into *reproductive cloning* (cloning to create a person).

The first reading selection is an excerpt from the **President's Council on Bioethics**, and serves as an introduction to the scientific and moral issues surrounding stem cell research. The report describes what stem cells are and why there is moral contention about using them in research—mainly because they are derived from early-stage human embryos. This reading also includes a discussion of the terms "embryo," "spare embryo," and "moral status." The report of the President's Council also offers a brief review of the central points of moral controversy.

The excerpts from the **National Bioethics Advisory Commission** (NBAC; the predecessor to the President's Council on Bioethics) provide a spectrum of religious perspectives on the use of stem cells in research, drawn from the testimony of a number of religious scholars who were asked to advise the NBAC in its deliberations about stem cell research. More than most areas of research ethics, the debate about embryonic stem cells touches on issues in which different perspectives are shaped by nuances of religious belief, particularly about when life begins and how we should understand the sanctity of human life.

The final reading in this section is by a group of scholars who served as an **Ethics Advisory Board** (EAB) for Geron Corporation, a large multinational biotechnology company involved in pioneering hESC research. Geron's website boasts that the company is the world leader in human embryonic stem cell–based therapeutics, and that its spinal cord injury treatment will likely be the first hESC-based product to enter clinical development. During the 1990s, Geron was at the forefront of early stem cell research, and announced in 1998 that it had successfully generated a handful of cell culture lines from human embryonic stem cells. Likely anticipating a moral storm, Geron hired a team of scholars to advise them on the ethics of their hESC research. The EAB unanimously agreed that embryonic stem cell research can be conducted ethically, and offered several conditions that must pertain for such research to be ethically justified.

Federal policy on stem cell research has evolved significantly during the first decade of this century. Stem cell research was legal during the George W. Bush administration (2001–2009), but reflected the president's belief that the human embryo is "human life" and should not be destroyed, even for the promise of potential life-saving benefits. In 2001, President Bush signed an executive order allowing federal funding *only* for research on embryonic stem cell lines already in existence—in other words, scientists could only research on cell lines created before 2001. No new embryos could be "sacrificed" to research. This restriction frustrated researchers, who felt that it jeopardized their work. In 2005, a team of scientists from the Salk Institute found that the available lines of human embryonic stem cells were contaminated with a non-human molecule—a cell-surface sialic acid called N-glycolylneuraminic acid (Neu5Gc)—which compromises their therapeutic usefulness. The contamination comes from the culture mediums in which the stem cells were grown; these culture mediums include so-called "feeder layers" which are derived from connective tissues of mice and fetal calves. Cells containing the Neu5Gc molecule will likely be attacked by the human immune system. Therapeutically useful stem cell lines thus need to be newly derived, which would require a change in the law.

The election of Barack Obama ushered in a new era for stem cell scientists. One of President Obama's first actions in office was to sign an executive order lifting the moratorium on federal funding for stem cell research. Hundreds of newer stem cell lines became eligible for research funding. During a campaign speech, Obama had made his position clear: "I believe that it is ethical to use these extra embryos for research that could save lives when they are freely donated for that express purpose."

Policy continues to move in a more pro-research and pro-science direction. During the 2008 elections, Michigan voters approved a proposal allowing surplus embryos from fertility treatments to be used by researchers to derive new stem cell lines. And voters in Colorado overwhelmingly rejected a so-called "Personhood Amendment," which sought to define a fertilized egg as a human being, with attendant constitutional protections.

Science is progressing rapidly as well. Among other things, researchers are exploring ways to develop pluripotent cells from adult cells. Work with adult skin cells has looked particularly promising. In 2008, two teams of researchers announced that they had successfully "reprogrammed" adult skin cells into stem cells with the same properties as human embryonic stem cells.

Stem Cell Research: President George Bush Addresses the Nation

August 9, 2001. 8:01 CDT.

Good evening. I appreciate you giving me a few minutes of your time tonight so I can discuss with you a complex and difficult issue, an issue that is one of the most profound of our time.

The issue of research involving stem cells derived from human embryos is increasingly the subject of a national debate and dinner table discussions. The issue is confronted every day in laboratories as scientists ponder the ethical ramifications of their work. It is agonized over by parents and many couples as they try to have children, or to save children already born. . . .

The United States has a long and proud record of leading the world toward advances in science and medicine that improve human life. And the United States has a long and proud record of upholding the highest standards of ethics as we expand the limits of science and knowledge. Research on embryonic stem cells raises profound ethical questions, because extracting the stem cell destroys the embryo, and thus destroys its potential for life. Like a snowflake, each of these embryos is unique, with the unique genetic potential of an individual human being.

As I thought through this issue, I kept returning to two fundamental questions: First, are these frozen embryos human life, and therefore, something precious to be protected? And second, if they're going to be destroyed anyway, shouldn't they be used for a greater good, for research that has the potential to save and improve other lives? . . .

I strongly oppose human cloning, as do most Americans. We recoil at the idea of growing human beings for spare body parts, or creating life for our convenience. And while we must devote enormous energy to conquering disease, it is equally important that we pay attention to the moral concerns raised by the new frontier of human embryo stem cell research. Even the most noble ends do not justify any means. . . .

I also believe human life is a sacred gift from our Creator. I worry about a culture that devalues life, and believe as your President I have an important obligation to foster and encourage respect for life in America and throughout the world. And while we're all hopeful about the potential of this research, no one can be certain that the science will live up to the hope it has generated.

As a result of private research, more than 60 genetically diverse stem cell lines already exist. They were created from embryos that have already been destroyed, and they have the ability to regenerate themselves indefinitely, creating ongoing opportunities for research. I have concluded that we should allow federal funds to be used for research on these existing stem cell lines, where the life and death decision has already been made.

Leading scientists tell me research on these 60 lines has great promise that could lead to breakthrough therapies and cures. This allows us to explore the promise and potential of stem cell research without crossing a fundamental moral line, by providing taxpayer funding that would sanction or encourage further destruction of human embryos that have at least the potential for life. . . .

I have made this decision with great care, and I pray it is the right one. Thank you for listening. Good night, and God bless America.

Research on Animal Subjects (or Objects)

Although aspects of human experimentation are controversial, the enterprise as such is generally considered a morally justified and good thing. Not so for animal research, which is controversial to its very core. As with the stem cell debate, the central moral questions have nothing to do with autonomy and consent—animals obviously cannot and do not consent to being the objects of research. Rather, there is deep moral disagreement about whether animal research should be conducted at all. Philosophical disagreements revolve around the moral status of animals, and whether it is morally acceptable to use them as a means to our own ends. Furthermore, there is considerable scientific controversy as well: people are divided over whether animal research is good science—or *goodenough* science—to justify the moral cost of so many animal lives.

Indeed, a great many animal lives are at stake. Animal research is an enormous enterprise. The British Nuffield Council on Bioethics estimates that fifty to one hundred million animals are used each year around the world in experimentation; precise numbers are hard to gauge. Within the United States, the Office of Technology Assessment (OTA) estimates that between seventeen and twenty-three million animals are used annually. Rats and mice make up about ninety percent of animals in biomedical research. The OTA estimates that about seventy thousand dogs are used each year. The OTA numbers refer only to vertebrates; invertebrates, such as nematodes and fruit flies, are not included in statistics, and research on them is essentially unregulated. Many more invertebrates are used than vertebrates.

Research on vertebrates is regulated in the United States by the Department of Agriculture, according to the Animal Welfare Act of 1966 (AWA). The AWA regulates things like housing (cage size, feeding requirements, and provision of light or dark), appropriate application of anesthesia, and which methods of euthanizing are appropriate for which kinds of animals. Federally funded research on animals must be reviewed by an Institutional Animal Care and Use Committee (IACUC), which functions rather like an IRB, although the ethical protections for animals vary dramatically from those for humans. The IACUC is charged with ensuring that each research protocol using animals is scientifically sound and takes appropriate measures to care for animals and minimize the potential for pain and suffering.

Bioethicist **David DeGrazia** outlines the central issues in the debate over animal research, taking as his points of reference the pro-research perspective of biomedicine and the anti-research perspective of animal advocates. As DeGrazia notes, the discussion of animal research often degenerates into political posturing and bumper-sticker ethics, and he offers some insights into why the debate has become so polarized and why people seem so afraid of real dialogue about the issue. He argues that when the various parties actually sit down and talk to each other, there is a broad area of consensus, and more points of agreement than disagreement. The points of divergence remain, of course, of ultimate significance.

The second reading is the code of ethics for animal research offered by the **Council for International Organizations of Medical Sciences** (CIOMS). The CIOMS document begins from the presumption that animal research is, on the whole, morally justified and seeks to provide guidance for those engaging in this researches. This document sets no particular boundaries on what kinds of research are acceptable on what species of animal, but does offer guidelines for balancing animal suffering with other considerations.

Studies published within the last few years have challenged the scientific validity of animal models and will likely shape the contours of the unfolding discussion. The onus of proof falls a bit more strongly on animal researchers than it has in the past, as scientists themselves have begun questioning the value of animal experiments, particularly in clinical trials of new drugs. One recent study, for example, found that a large number of animal studies were poorly designed, used less-than-ideal methodologies, and chose inappropriate animal models. These failings led to results that were inconclusive, inaccurate, or unusable (see, for example, the two articles by Knight, and one by Perel and colleagues listed in the References).

Many who believe that animal research is at its core unethical recognize that this kind of research will undoubtedly continue. The research industry is too large and too influential, and public opinion weighs too heavily in favor of research. Given this reality, we should give attention to developing careful ethical guidelines for using animals, and strengthening regulatory protections. One of the central concerns then becomes animal pain and suffering.

The long-standing presumption, often attributed to philosopher René Descartes, that animals are like machines and do not experience pain has begun to crumble over the past few decades. Scientists now widely agree that animals experience pain, though there are still differences in how such pain is understood, which leads to varying accounts of how disturbed we should be by it. The Humane Society has argued that although pain is taken into consideration in the animal protection rules, the more nebulous category of "distress" is not, and has urged the United States Department of Agriculture to revise its guidelines for the case and use of animals.

The **National Research Council** (NRC) in its *Guidelines for the Care and Use of Mammals in Neuroscience and Behavioral Research* defines distress as "an aversive state in which an animal is unable to adapt completely to stressors and the resulting stress, and shows maladaptive behaviors." Social animals such as chimpanzees, dogs, and rats suffer from isolation; and highly intelligent animals suffer from boredom and impoverished environments. These kinds of "distress," argue animal advocates, must be addressed alongside the more obvious category of pain. Scientists, too, see the need to address animal distress because recent research has shown that distress alters an animal's physiology, and may thus also alter or confound experimental data. For example, research on so-called "witnessing effects" in rats has found that levels of the hormone cortisol go up when rats witness another rat being decapitated or when a paper towel with blood from a decapitated rat is placed on top of their cage.

The excerpts in this chapter from the NRC suggest two things: first, there is an effort to improve attention to pain and distress and be conscientious about it. Second, researchers must be very well trained to appropriately understand distress, and often lack this training. The NRC readings show that understanding the signs of pain and distress in animals requires a fairly advanced and nuanced knowledge of animal behavior—which neither the average medical research scientist nor the average laboratory technicians who do most of the animal handling are likely to have.

Additional Codes of Ethics for Research on Humans

45 CFR 46 Protection of Human Subjects.
http://www.hhs.gov/ohrp/humansubjects/
guidance/45cfr46.htm.

Council for International Organizations of Medical
Sciences. "International ethical guidelines for biomedical research involving human subjects."
http://www.cioms.ch/frame_guidelines_
nov_2002.htm

Nuffield Council on Bioethics, "The ethics of
research related to healthcare in developing
countries."
http://www.nuffieldbioethics.org/go/ourwork/
developingcountries/introduction

National Bioethics Advisory Commission. 1998.
"Research Involving Persons with Mental Disorders
That May Affect Decisionmaking Capacity"
http://www.georgetown.edu/research/nrcbl/nbac/
capacity/Overview.htm#Promise

Documents on Ethics of Research with Stem Cells

National Institutes of Health, "Research ethics and
stem cells."
http://stemcells.nih.gov/info/ethics.asp

President's Council on Bioethics. 2004. "Report on
the Ethics of Stem Cell Research.
http://bioethicsprint.bioethics.gov/reports/stem-
cell/index.html [accessed 9/11/2006].

Additional Codes of Ethics for Research on Animals

Nuffield Council on Bioethics, "The ethics of research
using animals."
http://www.nuffieldbioethics.org/fileLibrary/pdf/
RIA_Report_FINAL-opt.pdf

Animal Welfare Regulations (U.S.).
http://www.access.gpo.gov/nara/cfr/waisidx_06/
9cfrv1_06.html

United States Department of Agriculture, Animal
Welfare Information Center.
http://riley.nal.usda.gov/nal_display/index.
php?tax_level = 1&info_center = 3&tax_
subject=169

REFERENCES AND FURTHER READING

"Protection of Human Subjects and Scientific Progress: Can the Two Be Reconciled?"
A series of replies to David Orentlicher. *Hastings Center Report* 36, no. 1 (2006): 4–9.

Benatar, Solomon R. "Justice and Medical Research: A Global Perspective." *Bioethics* 15,
no. 4 (2001):333–40.

Benatar, Solomon R., and Peter A. Singer. "A New Look at International Research Ethics."
British Medical Journal 321 (2000): 824–26.

Corbie-Smith, Giselle, Stephen Thomas, and Diane St. George. "Distrust, Race, and Research." *Archives of Internal Medicine* 162 (2002):2458–63.

Emanuel, Ezekiel J., and Christine Grady. "Four paradigms of clinical research and research oversight." *Cambridge Quarterly of Healthcare Ethics* 16 (2006):82–96.

——, David Wendler, and Christine Grady. "What makes clinical research ethical?" *JAMA* 283 (2000):2701–11.

Holland, Suzanne, Karen Lebacqz, and Laurie Zoloth. Eds. *The Human Embryonic Stem Cell Debate*. Cambridge, MA: MIT Press, 2001.

Jonsen, Albert R. "The Ethics of Research with Human Subjects: A Short History." *Sourcebook in Bioethics: A Documentary History*. Eds. Albert R. Jonsen, Robert M. Veatch, and LeRoy Walters. Washington, DC: Georgetown University Press, 1998, 5–10.

Knight, Andrew. "The poor contribution of chimpanzee experiments to biomedical progress." *Journal of Applied Animal Welfare Science* 10, no. 4 (2007):281–308.

——. "Systematic Review of Animal Experiments Demonstrate Poor Contributions Toward Human Healthcare." *Reviews on Recent Clinical Trials* 3 (2008):89–96.

Landes, Megan. "Can Context Justify an Ethical Double Standard for Clinical Research in Developing Countries?" *Globalization and Health* 1, no. 11 (2005). http://www.globalizationandhealth.com/content/1/1/11 (accessed September 18, 2006).

Leavitt, Frank J. "Is Any Medical Research Population Not Vulnerable?" *Cambridge Quarterly of Healthcare Ethics* 15 (2006): 81–88.

Miller, Franklin G., Donald Rosenstein, and Evan G. DeRenzo. "Professional Integrity in Clinical Research." *JAMA* 280, no. 16 (1998): 1449–54.

National Institutes of Health. *Stem Cells: Scientific Progress and Future Research Directions*. Honolulu, Hawaii: University Press of the Pacific, 2004.

Nussbaum, Martha. "The Moral Status of Animals." *The Chronicle of Higher Education* 52, no. 22 (February 3, 2006): B6-8.

Orlans, Barbara F., Tom Beauchamp, Rebecca Dresser, David B. Morton, and James P. Gluck. *The Human Use of Animals: Case Studies in Ethical Choice*. New York: Oxford University Press, 1998.

Perel, Pablo, Ian Roberts, Emily Sena, Philipa Wheble, Catherine Briscoe, Peter Sandercock, Malcolm Macleod, Luciano E Mignini, Pradeep Jayaram, and Khalid S Khan. "Comparison of treatment effects between animal experiments and clinical trial: Systematic review." *British Medical Journal* 334 (2007): 197.

Peters, Ted. *The Stem Cell Debate*. Minneapolis, MN: Fortress Press, 2007.

Rhodes, Rosamond. "Rethinking research ethics." *American Journal of Bioethics* 5, no. 1 (2005): 7–28.

Rollin, Bernard E. "The Regulation of Animal Research and the Emergence of Animal Ethics: A Conceptual History." *Theoretical Medicine and Bioethics* 27 no. 4 (2006): 285–304.

Ross, Lainie Friedman. "Children in Medical Research: Balancing Protection and Access: Has the Pendulum Swung Too Far?" *Perspectives in Biology and Medicine* 47, no. 4 (2004): 519–38.

Rudacille, Deborah. *The Scalpel and the Butterfly*. New York: Farrar, Straus and Giroux, 2000.

Ruse, Michael. *The Stem Cell Controversy: Debating the Issues*. Amherst, NY: Prometheus Books, 2006.

Sharav, Vera H. "Children in Clinical Research: A Conflict of Moral Values." *American Journal of Bioethics* 3, no. 1 (2003): W12-W59.

Slater, Lauren. *Opening Skinner's Box: Great Psychological Experiments of the Twentieth Century.* New York: W. W. Norton, 2004.

Snow, Nancy E., ed. *Stem Cell Research: New Frontiers in Science and Ethics.* Notre Dame, IN: University of Notre Dame Press, 2004.

Spriggs, M. "Canaries in the Mines: Children, Risk, Non-therapeutic Research, and Justice." *Journal of Medical Ethics* 30 (2004):176–81.

Washington, Harriet A. *Medical Apartheid: A Dark History of Medical Experimentation on Black Americans from Colonial Times to the Present.* New York: Doubleday, 2008.

Wendler, David. "Protecting Subjects Who Cannot Give Consent: Toward A Better Standard for 'Minimal' Risks." *Hastings Center Report* 35, no. 5 (2005): 37–43.

DISCUSSION QUESTIONS FOR THE READINGS

Nuremburg Code

1. Describe the historical context of the Nuremburg Code (look in the chapter introduction or in an encyclopedia).
2. To what does the *informed* in informed consent refer?
3. Which of the four core bioethics principles is *not* articulated in the Nuremburg Code?

The Belmont Report

1. How does the report distinguish between practice and research?
2. Why is the first principle formulated as "respect for persons" and not "respect for autonomy"?
3. What two moral rules are embedded in the principle of beneficence?
4. How would you describe the methodological framework of the Report (refer to chapter 1 in this text for help).

Declaration of Helsinki

1. What special obligations do *physician* researchers have when research is combined with patient care? Are the ethical rules different when the research subject is also a patient?
2. Under what conditions may research be conducted without informed consent of the research subject?
3. What are the practical implications of paragraph 33?

Making Research a Requirement of Treatment: Why We Should Sometimes Let Doctors Pressure Patients to Participate in Research

1. Exactly what kind of research trial does Orentlicher discuss in the essay? Does his argument extend to other kinds of research trials?
2. What are Orentlicher's central arguments for relaxing the rules on voluntary participation?
3. How does he answer the objection that requiring participation is coercive?
4. How might Orentlicher respond to the case "Medicare Requires Heart Patients to Enlist in Research"?

Guinea-Pigging

1. What is "guinea-pigging"?
2. What are some of the reasons that drug testing receives, in practice, relatively little ethical oversight?
3. After reading this piece, would you say that the people who volunteer for drug trials are being exploited? How might you propose to fix the system?

Justice and the Human Development Approach to International Research

1. What is his "human development" approach to research? How is it different from simply following the ethical requirements of the Declaration of Helsinki?
2. What would constitute ethical clinical research in a developing country, according to London?
3. Should the human development approach also be applied to research within the United States or other developed nations?

Monitoring Stem Cell Research: Introduction

1. What are embryonic stem cells, and what is their potential scientific and medical value?
2. What broader moral issues underlie the debate about stem cell research?
3. Why is the term "embryo" problematic? Why is "moral status" problematic?
4. What are the core moral issues in embryonic stem cell research?

Ethical Issues in Human Stem Cell Research: Religious Perspectives

1. In Rabbi Dorff's testimony, how does the Jewish position on abortion shape his moral argument about stem cell research? Is he supportive of stem cell research?
2. Why does Dorff say that the question of stem cell research can be reduced to a risk-benefit analysis? What risks and benefits does he think should be considered?
3. What does Farley mean when she says that natural law theory tells us where to "look" for answers to the stem cell controversy?
4. How can Catholicism provide a case both against and for stem cell research?
5. Why, according to Meilaender, is the stem cell issue distinct from the abortion issue?
6. Why, according to Meilaender, should we resist the promise of stem cells as a "saving solution"?
7. According to Sachedina, does Islamic law forbid or endorse embryonic stem cell research? On what grounds?
8. Which of these testimonies would you characterize as most strongly supportive of stem cell research? Which most prohibitive?

Research with Human Embryonic Stem Cells: Ethical Considerations

1. What does EAB mean by the "developmental" view of moral status? Do you agree with this view?
2. Bioethicists George J. Annas, Arthur Caplan, and Sherman Elias complained that the EAB's report is "more like 'ethical cover' . . . than ethics that can be taken seriously." What about the EAB statement might suggest "ethical cover"?

3. Annas, Caplan, and Elias go on to say:

> The ethics board seems to recognize what few, if any, Geron stockholders would concede: If only the rich are likely to benefit from stem cell research, it should not be pursued at all as a matter of social justice. This principle follows from ideas of respect for embryonic and fetal tissue that permit its instrumental use only to "alleviate human suffering and to promote the health and well-being of human populations," but obviously begs the question of whether for-profit corporations can ever have this as a realistic goal or how the company could be forced to adhere to this principle. As stated in the context of a policy that seems to have been created to provide an ethical rationalization rather than as an ethical guidance for research, it is not likely that it can or will be taken seriously.
>
> ("Stem cell politics, ethics, and medical progress" *Nature Medicine* 5(12), December 1999).

Would you agree with Annas, Caplan and Elias that principle 5 (on global justice) is "ethical rationalization" rather than "ethical guidance for research"? Do you think that therapeutic treatments developed from hESC research must be available to all people around the globe, in order for the research to be ethically justified?

The Ethics of Animal Research: What Are the Prospects for Agreement?

1. What is your view of the moral status of animals? How would you characterize DeGrazia's own view? How does your view compare with DeGrazia's?
2. How is the debate about animal research similar to and different from the debate about stem cell research?

International Guiding Principles for Biomedical Research Involving Animals (1985)

1. What are the moral parallels between human subjects research and animal subjects research? Where do the two issues diverge?
2. What would you say are the major weaknesses of the CIOMS principles?
3. The guidelines cover only vertebrate animals. Does recent research confirming that invertebrates experience pain suggest their inclusion under future revisions of these guidelines? What about research showing high levels of social intelligence in some species of invertebrate?

Guidelines for the Care and Use of Mammals in Neuroscience and Behavioral Research

1. What physiological or psychological experiences should count as harmful to animals? Is physical pain an adequate measure of suffering? How would you define animal suffering?
2. Why is pain research using animal models ethically troublesome?

READINGS

Nuremberg Code

From *Trials of War Criminals before the Nuremberg Military Tribunals under Control Council Law No. 10, vol. 2* (Washington, DC: U.S. Government Printing Office, 1949), 181–82.

1. The voluntary consent of the human subject is absolutely essential. This means that the person involved should have legal capacity to give consent; should be so situated as to be able to exercise free power of choice, without the intervention of any element of force, fraud, deceit, duress, overreaching, or other ulterior form of constraint or coercion; and should have sufficient knowledge and comprehension of the elements of the subject matter involved as to enable him to make an understanding and enlightened decision. This latter element requires that before the acceptance of an affirmative decision by the experimental subject there should be made known to him the nature, duration, and purpose of the experiment; the method and means by which it is to be conducted; all inconveniences and hazards reasonable to be expected; and the effects upon his health or person which may possibly come from his participation in the experiment. The duty and responsibility for ascertaining the quality of the consent rests upon each individual who initiates, directs or engages in the experiment. It is a personal duty and responsibility which may not be delegated to another with impunity.

2. The experiment should be such as to yield fruitful results for the good of society, unprocurable by other methods or means of study, and not random and unnecessary in nature.

3. The experiment should be so designed and based on the results of animal experimentation and a knowledge of the natural history of the disease or other problem under study

that the anticipated results will justify the performance of the experiment.

4. The experiment should be so conducted as to avoid all unnecessary physical and mental suffering and injury.

5. No experiment should be conducted where there is an a priori reason to believe that death or disabling injury will occur; except, perhaps, in those experiments where the experimental physicians also serve as subjects.

6. The degree of risk to be taken should never exceed that determined by the humanitarian importance of the problem to be solved by the experiment.

7. Proper preparations should be made and adequate facilities provided to protect the experimental subject against even remote possibilities of injury, disability, or death.

8. The experiment should be conducted only by scientifically qualified persons. The highest degree of skill and care should be required through all stages of the experiment of those who conduct or engage in the experiment.

9. During the course of the experiment the human subject should be at liberty to bring the experiment to an end if he has reached the physical or mental state where continuation of the experiment seems to him to be impossible.

10. During the course of the experiment the scientist in charge must be prepared to terminate the experiment at any stage, if he has probable cause to believe, in the exercise of the good faith, superior skill and careful judgment required of him that a continuation of the experiment is likely to result in injury, disability, or death to the experimental subject.

The Belmont Report

Ethical Principles and Guidelines for the Protection of Human Subjects of Research

THE NATIONAL COMMISSION FOR THE PROTECTION OF HUMAN SUBJECTS OF BIOMEDICAL AND

BEHAVIORAL RESEARCH

Summary

On July 12, 1974, the National Research Act (Pub. L. 93–348) was signed into law, there-by creating the National Commission for the Protection of Human Subjects of Biomedical and Behavioral Research. One of the charges to the Commission was to identify the basic ethical principles that should underlie the conduct of biomedical and behavioral research involving human subjects and to develop guidelines which should be followed to assure that such research is conducted in accordance with those principles.

Ethical Principles and Guidelines for Research Involving Human Subjects

Scientific research has produced substantial social benefits. It has also posed some troubling ethical questions. Public attention was drawn to these questions by reported abuses of human subjects in biomedical experiments, especially during the Second World War. During the Nuremberg War Crime Trials, the Nuremberg code was drafted as a set of standards for judging physicians and scientists who had conducted biomedical experiments on concentration camp prisoners. This code became the prototype of many later codes intended to assure that research involving human subjects would be carried out in an ethical manner.

The codes consist of rules, some general, others specific, that guide the investigators or the reviewers of research in their work. Such rules often are inadequate to cover complex situations; at times they come into conflict, and they are frequently difficult to interpret or apply. Broader ethical principles will provide a basis on which specific rules may be formulated, criticized and interpreted.

Three principles, or general prescriptive judgments, that are relevant to research involving human subjects are identified in this statement. Other principles may also be relevant. These three are comprehensive, however, and are stated at a level of generalization that should assist scientists, subjects, reviewers and interested citizens to understand the ethical issues inherent in research involving human subjects. These principles cannot always be applied so as to resolve beyond dispute particular ethical problems. The objective is to provide an analytical framework that will guide the resolution of ethical problems arising from research involving human subjects.

This statement consists of a distinction between research and practice, a discussion of the three basic ethical principles, and remarks about the application of these principles.

Part A: Boundaries Between Practice and Research

A. Boundaries Between Practice and Research

It is important to distinguish between biomedical and behavioral research, on the one hand, and the practice of accepted therapy on the other, in order to know what activities ought to undergo review for the protection of human subjects of research. The distinction between research and practice is blurred partly because both often occur together (as in research designed to evaluate a therapy) and partly because notable departures from standard practice are often called "experimental" when the terms "experimental" and "research" arc not carefully defined.

For the most part, the term 'practice' refers to interventions that are designed solely to enhance the well-being of an individual patient or client and that have a reasonable expectation of success. The purpose of medical or behavioral practice is to provide diagnosis, preventive treatment or therapy to particular individuals. By contrast, the term 'research' designates an activity designed to test an hypothesis, permit conclusions to be drawn, and thereby to develop or contribute to generalizable knowledge (expressed, for example, in theories, principles, and statements of relationships). Research is usually described in a formal protocol that sets forth an objective and a set of procedures designed to reach that objective.

When a clinician departs in a significant way from standard or accepted practice, the innovation does not, in and of itself, constitute research. The fact that a procedure is 'experimental,' in the sense of new, untested or different, does not automatically place it in the category of research. Radically new procedures of this description should, however, be made the object of formal research at an early stage in order to determine whether they are safe and effective. Thus, it is the responsibility of medical practice committees, for example, to insist that a major innovation be incorporated into a formal research project.

Research and practice may be carried on together when research is designed to evaluate the safety and efficacy of a therapy. This need not cause any confusion regarding whether or not the activity requires review; the general rule is that if there is any element of research in an activity, that activity should undergo review for the protection of human subjects.

Part B: Basic Ethical Principles

B. Basic Ethical Principles

The expression "basic ethical principles" refers to those general judgments that serve as a basic justification for the many particular ethical prescriptions and evaluations of human actions. Three basic principles, among those generally accepted in our cultural tradition, are particularly relevant to the ethics of research involving human subjects: the principles of respect of persons, beneficence and justice.

1. Respect for Persons

Respect for persons incorporates at least two ethical convictions: first, that individuals should be treated as autonomous agents, and second, that persons with diminished autonomy are entitled to protection. The principle of respect for persons thus divides into two separate moral requirements: the requirement to acknowledge autonomy and the requirement to protect those with diminished autonomy.

An autonomous person is an individual capable of deliberation about personal goals and of acting under the direction of such deliberation. To respect autonomy is to give weight to autonomous persons' considered opinions and choices while refraining from obstructing their actions unless they are clearly detrimental to others. To show lack of respect for an autonomous agent is to repudiate that person's considered judgments, to deny an individual the freedom to act on those considered judgments, or to withhold information necessary to make a considered judgment, when there are no compelling reasons to do so.

However, not every human being is capable of self-determination. The capacity for self-determination matures during an individual's life, and some individuals lose this capacity wholly or in part because of illness, mental disability, or circumstances that severely restrict liberty. Respect for the immature and the incapacitated may require protecting them as they mature or while they are incapacitated.

Some persons are in need of extensive protection, even to the point of excluding them from activities which may harm them; other persons require little protection beyond making sure they undertake activities freely and with awareness of possible adverse consequence. The extent of protection afforded should depend upon the risk of harm and the likelihood of benefit. The judgment that any individual lacks autonomy should be periodically reevaluated and will vary in different situations.

In most cases of research involving human subjects, respect for persons demands that subjects enter into the research voluntarily and with adequate information. In some situations, however, application of the principle is not obvious. The involvement of prisoners as subjects of research provides an instructive example. On the one hand, it would seem that the principle of respect for persons requires that prisoners not be deprived of the opportunity to volunteer for research. On the other hand, under prison conditions they may be subtly coerced or unduly influenced to engage in research activities for which they would not otherwise volunteer. Respect for persons would then dictate that prisoners be protected. Whether to allow prisoners to "volunteer" or to "protect" them presents a dilemma. Respecting persons, in most hard cases, is often a matter of balancing competing claims urged by the principle of respect itself.

2. Beneficence

Persons are treated in an ethical manner not only by respecting their decisions and protecting them from harm, but also by making efforts to secure their well-being. Such treatment falls under the principle of beneficence. The term "beneficence" is often understood to cover acts of kindness or charity that go beyond strict obligation. In this document, beneficence is understood in a stronger sense, as an obligation. Two general rules have been formulated as complementary expressions of beneficent actions in this sense: (1) do not harm and (2) maximize possible benefits and minimize possible harms.

The Hippocratic maxim "do no harm" has long been a fundamental principle of medical

ethics. Claude Bernard extended it to the realm of research, saying that one should not injure one person regardless of the benefits that might come to others. However, even avoiding harm requires learning what is harmful; and, in the process of obtaining this information, persons may be exposed to risk of harm. Further, the Hippocratic Oath requires physicians to benefit their patients "according to their best judgment." Learning what will in fact benefit may require exposing persons to risk. The problem posed by these imperatives is to decide when it is justifiable to seek certain benefits despite the risks involved, and when the benefits should be foregone because of the risks.

The obligations of beneficence affect both individual investigators and society at large, because they extend both to particular research projects and to the entire enterprise of research. In the case of particular projects, investigators and members of their institutions are obliged to give forethought to the maximization of benefits and the reduction of risk that might occur from the research investigation. In the case of scientific research in general, members of the larger society are obliged to recognize the longer term benefits and risks that may result from the improvement of knowledge and from the development of novel medical, psychotherapeutic, and social procedures.

The principle of beneficence often occupies a well-defined justifying role in many areas of research involving human subjects. An example is found in research involving children. Effective ways of treating childhood diseases and fostering healthy development are benefits that serve to justify research involving children – even when individual research subjects are not direct beneficiaries. Research also makes it possible to avoid the harm that may result from the application of previously accepted routine practices that on closer investigation turn out to be dangerous. But the role of the principle of beneficence is not always so unambiguous. A difficult ethical problem remains, for example, about research that presents more than minimal risk without immediate prospect of direct benefit to the children involved. Some have argued that such research is inadmissible, while others have pointed out that this limit would rule out much research promising great benefit to children in the future. Here again, as with all hard cases, the different claims covered by the principle of beneficence may come into conflict and force difficult choices.

3. Justice

Who ought to receive the benefits of research and bear its burdens? This is a question of justice, in the sense of "fairness in distribution" or "what is deserved." An injustice occurs when some benefit to which a person is entitled is denied without good reason or when some burden is imposed unduly. Another way of conceiving the principle of justice is that equals ought to be treated equally. However, this statement requires explication. Who is equal and who is unequal? What considerations justify departure from equal distribution? Almost all commentators allow that distinctions based on experience, age, deprivation, competence, merit and position do sometimes constitute criteria justifying differential treatment for certain purposes. It is necessary, then, to explain in what respects people should be treated equally. There are several widely accepted formulations of just ways to distribute burdens and benefits. Each formulation mentions some relevant property on the basis of which burdens and benefits should be distributed. These formulations are (1) to each person an equal share, (2) to each person according to individual need, (3) to each person according to individual effort, (4) to each person according to societal contribution, and (5) to each person according to merit.

Questions of justice have long been associated with social practices such as punishment, taxation and political representation. Until recently these questions have not generally been associated with scientific research. However, they are foreshadowed even in the earliest reflections on the ethics of research involving human subjects. For example, during the 19th and early 20th centuries the burdens of serving as research subjects fell largely upon poor ward patients, while the benefits of improved medical care flowed primarily to private patients. Subsequently, the exploitation of unwilling prisoners as research subjects in Nazi concentration camps was condemned as a particularly flagrant injustice. In this country, in the 1940's, the Tuskegee syphilis study used disadvantaged, rural black men to study the untreated course of a disease that is by no means confined to that population. These subjects were deprived of demonstrably effective treatment in order not to interrupt the project, long after such treatment became generally available.

Against this historical background, it can be seen how conceptions of justice are relevant to research involving human subjects. For example, the selection of research subjects needs to be scrutinized in order to determine whether some classes (e.g., welfare patients, particular racial and ethnic minorities, or persons confined to institutions) are being systematically selected simply because of their easy availability, their compromised position, or their manipulability, rather than for reasons directly related to the problem being studied. Finally, whenever research supported by public funds leads to the development of therapeutic devices and procedures, justice demands both that these not provide advantages only to those who can afford them and that such research should not unduly involve persons from groups unlikely to be among the beneficiaries of subsequent applications of the research.

Part C: Applications

C. Applications

Applications of the general principles to the conduct of research leads to consideration of the following requirements: informed consent, risk/benefit assessment, and the selection of subjects of research.

1. Informed Consent

Respect for persons requires that subjects, to the degree that they are capable, be given the opportunity to choose what shall or shall not happen to them. This opportunity is provided when adequate standards for informed consent are satisfied.

While the importance of informed consent is unquestioned, controversy prevails over the nature and possibility of an informed consent. Nonetheless, there is widespread agreement that the consent process can be analyzed as containing three elements: information, comprehension and voluntariness.

Information. Most codes of research establish specific items for disclosure intended to assure that subjects are given sufficient information. These items generally include: the research procedure, their purposes, risks and anticipated benefits, alternative procedures (where therapy is involved), and a statement offering the subject the opportunity to ask questions and to withdraw at any time from the research. Additional items have been proposed, including how subjects are selected, the person responsible for the research, etc.

However, a simple listing of items does not answer the question of what the standard should be for judging how much and what sort of information should be provided. One standard frequently invoked in medical practice, namely the information commonly provided by practitioners in the field or in the locale, is inadequate since research takes place precisely when a common understanding does not exist. Another standard, currently popular in malpractice law, requires the practitioner to reveal the information that reasonable persons would wish to know in order to make a decision regarding their care. This, too, seems insufficient since the research subject, being in essence a volunteer, may wish to know considerably more about risks gratuitously undertaken than do patients who deliver themselves into the hand of a clinician for needed care. It may be that a standard of "the reasonable volunteer" should

be proposed: the extent and nature of information should be such that persons, knowing that the procedure is neither necessary for their care nor perhaps fully understood, can decide whether they wish to participate in the furthering of knowledge. Even when some direct benefit to them is anticipated, the subjects should understand clearly the range of risk and the voluntary nature of participation.

Comprehension. The manner and context in which information is conveyed is as important as the information itself. For example, presenting information in a disorganized and rapid fashion, allowing too little time for consideration or curtailing opportunities for questioning, all may adversely affect a subject's ability to make an informed choice.

Because the subject's ability to understand is a function of intelligence, rationality, maturity and language, it is necessary to adapt the presentation of the information to the subject's capacities. Investigators are responsible for ascertaining that the subject has comprehended the information. While there is always an obligation to ascertain that the information about risk to subjects is complete and adequately comprehended, when the risks are more serious, that obligation increases. On occasion, it may be suitable to give some oral or written tests of comprehension.

Special provision may need to be made when comprehension is severely limited – for example, by conditions of immaturity or mental disability. Each class of subjects that one might consider as incompetent (e.g., infants and young children, mentally disabled patients, the terminally ill and the comatose) should be considered on its own terms. Even for these persons, however, respect requires giving them the opportunity to choose to the extent they are able, whether or not to participate in research. The objections of these subjects to involvement should be honored, unless the research entails providing them a therapy unavailable elsewhere. Respect for persons also requires seeking the permission of other parties in order to protect the subjects from harm. Such persons are thus respected both by acknowledging their own wishes and by the use of third parties to protect them from harm.

The third parties chosen should be those who are most likely to understand the incompetent subject's situation and to act in that person's best interest. The person authorized to act on behalf of the subject should be given an opportunity to observe the research as it proceeds in order to be able to withdraw the subject from the research, if such action appears in the subject's best interest.

Voluntariness. An agreement to participate in research constitutes a valid consent only if voluntarily given. This element of informed consent requires conditions free of coercion and undue influence. Coercion occurs when an overt threat of harm is intentionally presented by one person to another in order to obtain compliance. Undue influence, by contrast, occurs through an offer of an excessive, unwarranted, inappropriate or improper reward or other overture in order to obtain compliance. Also, inducements that would ordinarily be acceptable may become undue influences if the subject is especially vulnerable.

Unjustifiable pressures usually occur when persons in positions of authority or commanding influence – especially where possible sanctions are involved – urge a course of action for a subject. A continuum of such influencing factors exists, however, and it is impossible to state precisely where justifiable persuasion ends and undue influence begins. But undue influence would include actions such as manipulating a person's choice through the controlling influence of a close relative and threatening to withdraw health services to which an individual would otherwise be entitled.

2. Assessment of Risks and Benefits

The Nature and Scope of Risks and Benefits. The requirement that research be justified on the basis of a favorable risk/benefit assessment bears a close relation to the principle of beneficence, just as the moral requirement that informed consent be obtained is derived primarily from the principle of respect for persons. The term "risk" refers to a possibility that harm may occur. However, when expressions such as "small risk" or "high risk" are used, they usually refer (often ambiguously) both to the chance (probability) of experiencing a harm and the severity (magnitude) of the envisioned harm.

The term "benefit" is used in the research context to refer to something of positive value related to health or welfare. Unlike "risk," "benefit" is not a term that expresses probabilities. Risk is properly contrasted to probability of benefits, and benefits are properly contrasted with harms rather than risks of harm. Accordingly, so-called risk/benefit assessments are concerned with the probabilities and magnitudes of possible harm and anticipated benefits. Many kinds of possible harms and benefits need to be taken into account. There are, for example, risks of psychological harm, physical harm, legal harm, social harm and economic harm and the corresponding benefits. While the most likely types of harms to research subjects are those of psychological or physical pain or injury, other possible kinds should not be overlooked.

Risks and benefits of research may affect the individual subjects, the families of the individual subjects, and society at large (or special groups of subjects in society). Previous codes and Federal regulations have required that risks to subjects be outweighed by the sum of both the anticipated benefit to the subject, if any, and the anticipated benefit to society in the form of knowledge to be gained from the research. In balancing these different elements, the risks and benefits affecting the immediate research subject will normally carry special weight. On the other hand, interests other than those of the subject may on some occasions be sufficient by themselves to justify the risks involved in the research, so long as the subjects' rights have been protected. Beneficence thus requires that we protect against risk of harm to subjects and also that we be concerned about the loss of the substantial benefits that might be gained from research.

3. Selection of Subjects

Just as the principle of respect for persons finds expression in the requirements for consent, and the principle of beneficence in risk/benefit assessment, the principle of justice gives rise to moral requirements that there be fair procedures and outcomes in the selection of research subjects.

Justice is relevant to the selection of subjects of research at two levels: the social and the individual. Individual justice in the selection of subjects would require that researchers exhibit fairness: thus, they should not offer potentially beneficial research only to some patients who are in their favor or select only "undesirable" persons for risky research. Social justice requires that distinctions be drawn between classes of subjects that ought, and ought not, to participate in any particular kind of research, based on the ability of members of that class to bear burdens and on the appropriateness of placing further burdens on already burdened persons. Thus, it can be considered a matter of social justice that there is an order of preference in the selection of classes of subjects (e.g., adults before children) and that some classes of potential subjects (e.g., the institutionalized mentally infirm or prisoners) may be involved as research subjects, if at all, only on certain conditions.

Injustice may appear in the selection of subjects, even if individual subjects are selected fairly by investigators and treated fairly in the course of research. Thus injustice arises from social, racial, sexual and cultural biases institutionalized in society. Thus, even if individual researchers are treating their research subjects fairly, and even if IRBs are taking care to assure that subjects are selected fairly within a particular institution, unjust social patterns may nevertheless appear in the overall distribution of the burdens and benefits of research. Although individual institutions or investigators may not be able to resolve a problem that is pervasive in their social setting, they can consider distributive justice in selecting research subjects.

Some populations, especially institutionalized ones, are already burdened in many ways by their infirmities and environments. When research is proposed that involves risks and does not include a therapeutic component, other less burdened classes of persons should be called upon first to accept these risks of research, except where the research is directly related to the specific conditions of the class involved. Also, even though public funds for research may often flow in the same directions as public funds for health care, it seems unfair that populations dependent on public health care constitute a pool of preferred research subjects if more advantaged populations are likely to be the recipients of the benefits.

One special instance of injustice results from the involvement of vulnerable subjects. Certain groups, such as racial minorities, the economically disadvantaged, the very sick, and the institutionalized may continually be sought as research subjects, owing to their ready availability in settings where research is conducted. Given their dependent status and their frequently compromised capacity for free consent, they should be protected against the danger of being involved in research solely for administrative convenience, or because they are easy to manipulate as a result of their illness or socioeconomic condition.

Declaration of Helsinki
Ethical Principles for Medical Research Involving Human Subjects
WORLD MEDICAL ASSOCIATION

A. Introduction

1. The World Medical Association (WMA) has developed the Declaration of Helsinki as a statement of ethical principles for medical research involving human subjects, including research on identifiable human material and data.

   The Declaration is intended to be read as a whole and each of its constituent paragraphs should not be applied without consideration of all other relevant paragraphs.

2. Although the Declaration is addressed primarily to physicians, the WMA encourages other participants in medical research involving human subjects to adopt these principles.

3. It is the duty of the physician to promote and safeguard the health of patients, including those who are involved in medical research. The physician's knowledge and conscience are dedicated to the fulfilment of this duty.

4. The Declaration of Geneva of the WMA binds the physician with the words, "The health of my patient will be my first consideration," and the International Code of Medical Ethics declares that, "A physician shall act in the patient's best interest when providing medical care."

5. Medical progress is based on research that ultimately must include studies involving human subjects. Populations that are underrepresented in medical research should be provided appropriate access to participation in research.

6. In medical research involving human subjects, the well-being of the individual research subject must take precedence over all other interests.

7. The primary purpose of medical research involving human subjects is to understand the causes, development and effects of diseases and improve preventive, diagnostic and therapeutic interventions (methods, procedures and treatments). Even the best current interventions must be evaluated continually through research for their safety, effectiveness, efficiency, accessibility and quality.

8. In medical practice and in medical research, most interventions involve risks and burdens.

9. Medical research is subject to ethical standards that promote respect for all human subjects and protect their health and rights. Some research populations are particularly vulnerable and need special protection. These include those who cannot give or refuse consent for themselves and those who may be vulnerable to coercion or undue influence.

10. Physicians should consider the ethical, legal and regulatory norms and standards for research involving human subjects in their own countries as well as applicable international norms and standards. No national or international ethical, legal or regulatory requirement should reduce or eliminate any of the protections for research subjects set forth in this Declaration.

B. Principles for All Medical Research

11. It is the duty of physicians who participate in medical research to protect the life, health, dignity, integrity, right to self-determination, privacy, and confiden-

tiality of personal information of research subjects.

12. Medical research involving human subjects must conform to generally accepted scientific principles, be based on a thorough knowledge of the scientific literature, other relevant sources of information, and adequate laboratory and, as appropriate, animal experimentation. The welfare of animals used for research must be respected.

13. Appropriate caution must be exercised in the conduct of medical research that may harm the environment.

14. The design and performance of each research study involving human subjects must be clearly described in a research protocol. The protocol should contain a statement of the ethical considerations involved and should indicate how the principles in this Declaration have been addressed. The protocol should include information regarding funding, sponsors, institutional affiliations, other potential conflicts of interest, incentives for subjects and provisions for treating and/or compensating subjects who are harmed as a consequence of participation in the research study. The protocol should describe arrangements for post-study access by study subjects to interventions identified as beneficial in the study or access to other appropriate care or benefits.

15. The research protocol must be submitted for consideration, comment, guidance and approval to a research ethics committee before the study begins. This committee must be independent of the researcher, the sponsor and any other undue influence. It must take into consideration the laws and regulations of the country or countries in which the research is to be performed as well as applicable international norms and standards but these must not be allowed to reduce or eliminate any of the protections for research subjects set forth in this Declaration. The committee must have the right to monitor ongoing studies. The researcher must provide monitoring information to the committee, especially information about any serious adverse events. No change to the protocol may be made without consideration and approval by the committee.

16. Medical research involving human subjects must be conducted only by individuals with the appropriate scientific training and qualifications. Research on patients or healthy volunteers requires the supervision of a competent and appropriately qualified physician or other health care professional. The responsibility for the protection of research subjects must always rest with the physician or other health care professional and never the research subjects, even though they have given consent.

17. Medical research involving a disadvantaged or vulnerable population or community is only justified if the research is responsive to the health needs and priorities of this population or community and if there is a reasonable likelihood that this population or community stands to benefit from the results of the research.

18. Every medical research study involving human subjects must be preceded by careful assessment of predictable risks and burdens to the individuals and communities involved in the research in comparison with foreseeable benefits to them and to other individuals or communities affected by the condition under investigation.

19. Every clinical trial must be registered in a publicly accessible database before recruitment of the first subject.

20. Physicians may not participate in a research study involving human subjects unless they are confident that the risks

involved have been adequately assessed and can be satisfactorily managed. Physicians must immediately stop a study when the risks are found to outweigh the potential benefits or when there is conclusive proof of positive and beneficial results.

21. Medical research involving human subjects may only be conducted if the importance of the objective outweighs the inherent risks and burdens to the research subjects.

22. Participation by competent individuals as subjects in medical research must be voluntary. Although it may be appropriate to consult family members or community leaders, no competent individual may be enrolled in a research study unless he or she freely agrees.

23. Every precaution must be taken to protect the privacy of research subjects and the confidentiality of their personal information and to minimize the impact of the study on their physical, mental and social integrity.

24. In medical research involving competent human subjects, each potential subject must be adequately informed of the aims, methods, sources of funding, any possible conflicts of interest, institutional affiliations of the researcher, the anticipated benefits and potential risks of the study and the discomfort it may entail, and any other relevant aspects of the study. The potential subject must be informed of the right to refuse to participate in the study or to withdraw consent to participate at any time without reprisal. Special attention should be given to the specific information needs of individual potential subjects as well as to the methods used to deliver the information. After ensuring that the potential subject has understood the information, the physician or another appropriately qualified individual must then seek the potential subject's

freely-given informed consent, preferably in writing. If the consent cannot be expressed in writing, the non-written consent must be formally documented and witnessed.

25. For medical research using identifiable human material or data, physicians must normally seek consent for the collection, analysis, storage and/or reuse. There may be situations where consent would be impossible or impractical to obtain for such research or would pose a threat to the validity of the research. In such situations the research may be done only after consideration and approval of a research ethics committee.

26. When seeking informed consent for participation in a research study the physician should be particularly cautious if the potential subject is in a dependent relationship with the physician or may consent under duress. In such situations the informed consent should be sought by an appropriately qualified individual who is completely independent of this relationship.

27. For a potential research subject who is incompetent, the physician must seek informed consent from the legally authorized representative. These individuals must not be included in a research study that has no likelihood of benefit for them unless it is intended to promote the health of the population represented by the potential subject, the research cannot instead be performed with competent persons, and the research entails only minimal risk and minimal burden.

28. When a potential research subject who is deemed incompetent is able to give assent to decisions about participation in research, the physician must seek that assent in addition to the consent of the legally authorized representative. The potential subject's dissent should be respected.

29. Research involving subjects who are physically or mentally incapable of giving

consent, for example, unconscious patients, may be done only if the physical or mental condition that prevents giving informed consent is a necessary characteristic of the research population. In such circumstances the physician should seek informed consent from the legally authorized representative. If no such representative is available and if the research cannot be delayed, the study may proceed without informed consent provided that the specific reasons for involving subjects with a condition that renders them unable to give informed consent have been stated in the research protocol and the study has been approved by a research ethics committee. Consent to remain in the research should be obtained as soon as possible from the subject or a legally authorized representative.

30. Authors, editors and publishers all have ethical obligations with regard to the publication of the results of research. Authors have a duty to make publicly available the results of their research on human subjects and are accountable for the completeness and accuracy of their reports. They should adhere to accepted guidelines for ethical reporting. Negative and inconclusive as well as positive results should be published or otherwise made publicly available. Sources of funding, institutional affiliations and conflicts of interest should be declared in the publication. Reports of research not in accordance with the principles of this Declaration should not be accepted for publication.

C. Additional Principles for Medical Research Combined with Medical Care

31. The physician may combine medical research with medical care only to the extent that the research is justified by its potential preventive, diagnostic or therapeutic value and if the physician has good reason to believe that participation in the research study will not adversely affect the health of the patients who serve as research subjects.

32. The benefits, risks, burdens and effectiveness of a new intervention must be tested against those of the best current proven intervention, except in the following circumstances:

- The use of placebo, or no treatment, is acceptable in studies where no current proven intervention exists; or
- Where for compelling and scientifically sound methodological reasons the use of placebo is necessary to determine the efficacy or safety of an intervention and the patients who receive placebo or no treatment will not be subject to any risk of serious or irreversible harm. Extreme care must be taken to avoid abuse of this option.

33. At the conclusion of the study, patients entered into the study are entitled to be informed about the outcome of the study and to share any benefits that result from it, for example, access to interventions identified as beneficial in the study or to other appropriate care or benefits.

34. The physician must fully inform the patient which aspects of the care are related to the research. The refusal of a patient to participate in a study or the patient's decision to withdraw from the study must never interfere with the patient-physician relationship.

35. In the treatment of a patient, where proven interventions do not exist or have been ineffective, the physician, after seeking expert advice, with informed consent from the patient or a legally authorized representative, may use an unproven intervention if in the physician's judgement it offers hope of saving life, re-establishing health or alleviating suffering. Where possible, this intervention should be made the object of research, designed

to evaluate its safety and efficacy. In all cases, new information should be recorded and, where appropriate, made publicly available.

Making Research a Requirement of Treatment
Why We Should Sometimes Let Doctors Pressure Patients to Participate in Research

DAVID ORENTLICHER

Hastings Center Report 35, no.5 (2005): 20–28.

In recent years, a number of events have raised concerns about the adequacy of safeguards to protect people who volunteer for medical research. Individuals without a serious illness, like Jesse Gelsinger and Ellen Roche, have died unexpectedly while participating in clinical trials. The federal Office for Human Research Protections temporarily halted studies at several major academic centers for their failure to observe research guidelines. Overseas trials of HIV-therapy during pregnancy have been criticized for including a placebo control arm. For some studies, we must worry whether research subjects are placed at too great a risk by physicians seeking to advance medical knowledge.

At the same time, we must also question whether research safeguards are sometimes overly protective of people who might enter clinical trials. Progress in treating trauma patients, for example, was hampered for many years by the requirements of informed consent—seriously injured patients often lack the decision-making capacity necessary to agree to enrollment in a research trial, and family members may not be available to consent to the trial on their behalf. These difficulties in enrolling patients slowed the development of promising therapies—including more effective methods for cardiac resuscitation and substitutes for blood to transfuse patients who have suffered major blood loss. To address this problem, federal guidelines for informed consent were modified in 1996 to permit valuable research in the emergency setting.

This article argues that just as there was a need to relax the requirements of informed consent for trauma research, there is a need to relax the precautions taken to ensure voluntary participation of subjects in another kind of research trial—studies involving the comparison of two or more established therapies to see whether one is superior to the alternative(s). For many medical problems, physicians can choose among multiple therapeutic options, and the choice is typically based more on hunch than on data. Patients would benefit greatly from studies that clarify the relative benefits and risks of different options for their illnesses.

However, these studies can be delayed—and medical progress impeded—by difficulties in securing the participation of enough individuals.

Concerns about ensuring that patients participate in research truly voluntarily discourage or prevent physicians from employing such a measure. Conditioning treatment on a patient's willingness to enroll in a trial is thought to constitute unacceptable coercion. But in fact, linking treatment to participation in research could be a valuable and ethically sound way to increase patient participation, as long as the clinical trial involves a comparison of alternative, established therapies.

Hypothetical Case Study

As an illustration of the concern with current standards for informed consent in research, consider the following hypothetical case study, which is based on an important, federally funded clinical trial.

The clinical trial was the Atrial Fibrillation Follow-up Investigation of Rhythm Management (AFFIRM) trial. Sponsored by the National Heart, Lung, and Blood Institute, AFFIRM compared two established treatment strategies for persistent or recurrent atrial fibrillation to see if one offered either better outcomes or less adverse effects. In one strategy, physicians try to restore and maintain the atrium's normal sinus rhythm with cardioversion (the application of an electrical shock to jolt an abnormal heartbeat into a normal one) and antiarrhythmic drugs. This method is known as "rhythm control." Alternatively, physicians can try to control the response of the heart's ventricles to the atrial fibrillation by maintaining a good ventricular heart rate—a method known as "rate control." With this second strategy, physicians employ both drug and nonpharmacologic therapies. In the AFFIRM study, patients were randomized to receive one of the two treatment strategies, and the patients received their care from their current physician according to the study protocol's guidelines. Thus, while the patients were participating in a research trial, there was nothing experimental about their treatment. The only experimental part of the trial was the fact that a patient's own treatment strategy was chosen randomly. (Results from AFFIRM were published in December 2002, and they suggested that rate control has important advantages over rhythm control as a therapeutic option.)

Now assume one change in the trial. In the actual study, cardiologists invited patients with atrial fibrillation to enter the AFFIRM trial. Patients who chose to enroll were assigned to one of the treatment strategies randomly. If a patient declined enrollment, then the cardiologist provided one of the two treatment strategies according to the cardiologist's usual practice. But suppose instead that some cardiologists told their patients that they would treat the atrial fibrillation only if the patients enrolled in the study. If a patient did not want to participate in AFFIRM, the cardiologist would decline to accept the patient for care or would end the patient-physician relationship and instruct the patient to obtain care from another cardiologist. Participation in AFFIRM would have been a condition of receiving care from these cardiologists.

Today's Research Guidelines

Under current practice, it is highly unlikely that approval would be given to a study in which physicians made participation in the study a condition for receiving treatment. Studies that involve testing or observation of people must be authorized by an institutional review board (IRB), a committee that reviews the proposed study and considers whether it meets ethical standards for medical research. For example, an IRB would analyze the proposal to ensure that participation in the study is voluntary and that the health of the volunteers is not placed at too great a risk. For a study conditioning treatment on participation in research, IRBs would be concerned that potential subjects would be coerced into enrolling in the trial—that a decision to enroll would not be truly voluntary.

Making a Change

Although current practices discourage conditioning treatment on participation in research, physicians could make a strong case for having the freedom to treat patients only in the setting of a clinical trial, when a study is comparing well-established therapies.

Eliminating Unnecessary Impediments to Medical Progress

When a physician chooses between multiple therapies without knowing which therapy offers the greatest benefit, the physician may be subjecting many patients to inferior treatment. The physician could use the different alternatives equally to ensure that at least some patients receive the best treatment, or the physician could make a best guess as to the most appropriate treatment, knowing that either all or none of the patients will receive the optimal therapy.

The only way to ensure that all patients receive optimal therapy is to run a clinical trial comparing the alternatives. Moreover, the number who receive inferior treatment can be minimized by completing the trial rapidly. Physicians might therefore want to enroll all of their patients in a definitive study. If patients have the option of declining participation, the study could take much longer, as in the study of treatment for chronic lung disease for which recruitment took twice as long as expected.

Encouraging More of a Social Sentiment in Favor of Participation in Medical Research

Today's patients benefit greatly from the medical discoveries of yesterday, and those discoveries would not have occurred without the willingness of previous generations of patients to volunteer for clinical trials. In return for the benefits of earlier research, we might want to say that patients should be willing to participate in new trials. To put it another way, if people want to share in the benefits of their society, they arguably should share in its burdens, too. Moreover, we might say, no one is *required* to accept the benefits of medical treatment. Indeed, patients enjoy a constitutional right to refuse medical treatment, even life-sustaining treatment. Whether to receive medical treatment remains an option. As an option, its receipt could be made conditional on the willingness of the patient to participate in medical research.

Answering the Objections

Not only are there strong grounds for conditioning treatment on the willingness of patients to participate in some clinical trials, but the usual justifications for strictly voluntary participation

are not present in the kinds of studies suggested by this article.

Risk to Patient Welfare Is Not a Concern

Most importantly, we do not have to worry about patients being forced to assume a risk to their health. In many clinical trials, a patient may be randomized to either standard therapy or experimental therapy. In such cases, the experimental therapy may not fulfill its promise and may have serious side effects. Patients in the experimental therapy arm of the study would be harmed by their participation. Similarly, if an experimental therapy is compared to placebo when established treatments already exist for the medical condition being studied, patients in the placebo arm and possibly in the experimental arm of the study will suffer by virtue of their participation in the clinical trial. In studies comparing well-accepted treatments, on the other hand, the patient would be receiving the same care that would be provided in a visit to a physician's office. In fact, the patient might receive better care by virtue of enrollment in the study; patients participating in research studies receive greater attention to—and more rigorous observation of—their medical conditions than do patients receiving care in their physicians' offices.

The Possibility of Coercion Is Not Serious

Voluntary participation in medical research is important because patients may be reluctant to reject their physicians' invitation to enter a research study. A patient might unduly defer to the physician's judgment because of the physician's greater expertise or because of fear that a refusal to participate might jeopardize the patient's relationship with the physician. Patients might easily feel that they have no real choice when asked to enroll in a study. As a result, ethical guidelines for medical research include provisions to assure patients that they are free to choose not to participate.

But with studies comparing different, well-accepted treatments, it would not be troublesome if patients felt some pressure to enroll. If they agreed to participate, they would not be placed at any greater risk of harm than if they did not. Moreover, the purpose of the pressure is to encourage them to help society understand and treat disease. There is nothing wrong with reasonable efforts at persuasion when the persuasion is designed to foster socially desirable behavior.

Threat to Patient Trust

We might be concerned that conditioning treatment on participating in research would undermine patient trust in the medical profession. If patients felt coerced by their physicians' research requirements, they would be inclined to wonder whether their physicians were compromising their interests for the benefit of other interests.

We should be wary of measures that might undermine patient trust. Because patients lack medical expertise and because the patient's health and even life may hang in the balance, patients are highly dependent on their physicians. With so much at stake for the patient and so much power in the hands of the physician, patients will not be willing to rely on their physicians' judgment unless they can trust that physicians use their skills and power on their patients' behalf.

Concerns about patient trust are especially important in medical research. Medical research generally involves patients accepting some risks to their own health for the benefit of future patients. Because medical research is predicated on a sacrifice of patient welfare, it is important to assure patients that the risk will be minimized. Moreover, past abuses of patient welfare in research give patients grounds for skepticism about the trustworthiness of today's researcher. The Tuskegee syphilis study and the radiation studies of cancer patients are two of the more notable examples of abuse.

While these concerns about trust are important, they should not lead us to reject entirely the possibility of conditioning treatment on participation in research. Past abuses in medical research involved two problematic elements, neither of which is present in the kind of trial suggested by this article. First, many abusive studies involved the deception of the research subjects. They were not given accurate information about the trials in which they were participating. As previously indicated, the ability to condition treatment on research participation would not entail any other changes in the requirements of informed consent. Second, many of the abusive trials placed patients at an unacceptable risk to their health. In contrast, the kinds of studies that satisfy this article's proposal are those in which patients would receive one of two or more well-accepted therapies—therapies that they would receive from any number of doctors whom they might see for care.

Moreover, conducting research that compares established therapies in order to discover whether one is better may well bolster patient trust. Patients ought to be reassured by knowing that their physicians are trying to find out which treatments are optimal.

Too Lax or Too Strict

Many people have been unnecessarily harmed by research that did not adhere to sufficiently strict ethical safeguards. Steps should be taken to protect against future harm. At the same time, ethical safeguards can become too strict. Sometimes, important advances in medical understanding are slowed or stymied by unnecessary limits on the ability of physicians to encourage their patients to participate in clinical trials. When a clinical trial compares two or more well-established therapies to determine which is better, physicians ought to be able to condition treatment on a patient's willingness to enroll in the trial.

Guinea-Pigging

CARL ELLIOTT

The New Yorker (January 7, 2008): 36–41.

On September 11, 2001, James Rockwell was camped out in a clinical-research unit on the eleventh floor of a Philadelphia hospital, where he had enrolled as a subject in a high-paying drug study. As a rule, studies that involve invasive medical procedures are more lucrative—the more uncomfortable, the better the pay—and in this study subjects had a fibre-optic tube inserted in their mouths and down their esophaguses so that researchers could examine their gastrointestinal tracts.

Rockwell had enrolled in many previous studies at corporate sites at places like Wyeth and GlaxoSmithKline. But the atmosphere there felt professional, bureaucratic, and cold. This unit was in a university hospital, not a corporate lab, and the staff had a casual attitude toward regulations and procedures. "The Animal House of research units" is what Rockwell calls it. "I'm standing in the hallway juggling," he says. "I'm up at five in the morning watching movies." Although study guidelines called for stringent dietary restrictions, the subjects got so hungry that one of them picked the lock on the food closet. "We got giant boxes of cookies and ran into the lounge and put them in the couch," Rockwell says. "This one guy was putting them in the ceiling tiles." Rockwell has little confidence in the data that the study produced. "The most integral part of the study was the diet restriction," he says, "and we were just gorging ourselves at 2 A.M. on Cheez Doodles."

On the morning of September 11th, nearly a month into the five-week study, the subjects gathered around a television and watched the news of the terrorist attacks through a drug-induced haze. "We were all high on Versed after getting endoscopies," Rockwell says. He and the other subjects began to wonder if they should go home. But a mass departure would have ruined the study. "The doctors were, like, 'No, no!'" Rockwell recalls. "'No one's going home, everything's fine!'" Rockwell stayed until the end of the study and was paid seventy-five hundred dollars. He used the money to make a down payment on a house.

Rockwell is a wiry thirty-year-old massage-therapy student with a pierced nose; he seems to bounce in his seat as he speaks, radiating enthusiasm. Over the years, he estimates, he has enrolled in more than twenty studies for money. The Philadelphia area offers plenty of opportunities for aspiring human subjects. It is home to four medical schools and is part of a drug-industry corridor that stretches into New Jersey. Bristol-Myers Squibb regularly sends a van to pick up volunteers at the Trenton train station.

Today, fees as high as the one that Rockwell received aren't unusual. The best-paying studies are longer, in-patient trials, where subjects are often required to check into a research facility for days or even weeks at a time, so that their diet can be controlled, their blood and urine checked regularly, and their medical status carefully monitored. Occasionally, they also undergo invasive procedures, like a bronchoscopy or a biopsy, or something else unpleasant, such as being deprived of sleep, wearing a rectal probe, or having allergens sprayed in their faces. Because such studies require a fair amount of time in a research unit, the subjects are usually people who need money and have a lot of time to spare: the unemployed, college students, contract workers, ex-cons, or young people living on the margins who have decided that testing drugs is better than punching a clock with the wage slaves. In some cities, like Philadelphia and Austin, the drug-testing economy has produced a community of semi-professional research subjects, who enroll in one study after another. Some of them do nothing else. For them, "guinea-pigging," as they call it, has become a job. Many of them say that they know people who have been travelling around the country doing studies for fifteen years or longer. "It's crazy and it's sad," one drug-trial veteran told me. "For me, this is not a life. But it is a life for a lot of these people."

Most drug studies used to take place in medical schools and teaching hospitals. Pharmaceutical companies developed the drugs, but they contracted with academic physicians to carry out the clinical testing. According to *The New England Journal of Medicine*, as recently as 1991 eighty per cent of industry-sponsored trials were conducted in academic health centers. Academic health centers had a lot to offer pharmaceutical companies: academic researchers who could design the trials, publications in academic journals that could help market the products, and a pool of potential subjects on whom the drugs could be tested. But, in the past decade, the pharmaceutical industry has been testing more drugs, the trials have grown more complex, and the financial pressure to bring drugs to market swiftly has intensified. Impatient with the slow pace of academic bureaucracies, pharmaceutical companies have moved trials to the private sector, where more than seventy per cent of them are now conducted.

This has spurred the growth of businesses that specialize in various parts of the commercial-research enterprise. The largest of the new businesses are called "contract research organizations," and include Quintiles, Covance, Parexel, and P.P.D. (Pharmaceutical Product Development), a company that has operations in thirty countries, including India, Israel, and South Africa. (About fifty per cent of clinical trials are now conducted outside the United States and Western Europe.) These firms are hired to shepherd a product through every aspect of its

development, from subject recruitment and testing through F.D.A. approval. Speed is critical: a patent lasts twenty years, and a drug company's aim is to get the drug on the shelves as early in the life of the patent as possible. When, in 2000, the Office of the Inspector General of the Department of Health and Human Services asked one researcher what sponsors were looking for, he replied, "No. 1—rapid enrollment. No. 2—rapid enrollment. No. 3—rapid enrollment." The result has been to broaden the range of subjects who are used and to increase the rates of pay they receive.

Most professional guinea pigs are involved in Phase I clinical trials, in which the safety of a potential drug is tested, typically by giving it to healthy subjects and studying any side effects that it produces. (Phase II trials aim at determining dosing requirements and demonstrating therapeutic efficacy; Phase III trials are on a larger scale and usually compare a drug's results with standard treatments.) The better trial sites offer such amenities as video games, pool tables, and wireless Internet access. If all goes well, a guinea pig can get paid to spend a week watching "The Lord of the Rings" and playing Halo with his friends, in exchange for wearing a hep-lock catheter on one arm and eating institutional food. Nathaniel Miller, a Philadelphia trial veteran who started doing studies to fund his political activism, was once paid fifteen hundred dollars in exchange for three days and two G.I. endoscopies at Temple University, where he was given a private room with a television. "It was like a hotel," he says, "except that twice they came in and stuck a tube down my nose."

The shift to the market has created a new dynamic. The relationship between testers and test subjects has become, more nakedly than ever, a business transaction. Guinea pigs are the first to admit this. "Nobody's doing this out of the goodness of their heart," Miller says. Unlike subjects in later-stage clinical trials, who are usually sick and might enroll in a study to gain access to a new drug, people in healthy-volunteer studies cannot expect any therapeutic benefit to balance the risks they take. As guinea pigs see it, their reason for taking the drugs is no different from that of the clinical investigators who administer them, and who are compensated handsomely for their efforts. This raises an ethical question: what happens when both parties involved in a trial see the enterprise primarily as a way of making money?

In May of 2006, Miami-Dade County ordered the demolition of a former Holiday Inn, citing various fire and safety violations. It had been the largest drug-testing site in North America, with six hundred and seventy-five beds. The operation closed down that year, shortly after the financial magazine *Bloomberg Markets* reported that the building's owner, SFBC International, was paying undocumented immigrants to participate in drug trials under ethically dubious conditions. The medical director of the clinic got her degree from a school in the Caribbean and was not licensed to practice. Some of the studies had been approved by a commercial ethical-review board owned by the wife of an SFBC vice-president. (The company, which has since changed its name to PharmaNet Development Group, says that it required subjects to provide proof of their legal status, and that the practice of medicine wasn't part of the medical director's duties. Last August, the company paid $28.5 million to settle a class-action lawsuit.)

"It was a human-subjects bazaar," says Kenneth Goodman, a bioethicist at the University of Miami who visited the site. The motel was in a downtrodden neighborhood; according to later reports, paint was peeling from the walls, and there were seven or eight subjects in a room. Goodman says that the waiting area was filled with potential subjects, mainly African-American and Hispanic; administrative staff members worked behind a window, like gas-station attendants, passing documents through a hole in the glass.

The SFBC scandal was not the first of its kind. In 1996, the *Wall Street Journal* reported that the Eli Lilly company was using homeless alcoholics from a local shelter to test experimental drugs at budget rates at its testing site in Indianapolis. (Lilly's executive director of clinical pharmacology told the *Journal* that the homeless people were driven by "altruism," and that they enrolled in trials because they "want to help society." The company says that it now requires subjects to provide proof of residence.) The Lilly clinic, the *Journal* reported, had developed such a reputation for admitting the down-and-out that subjects travelled to Indianapolis from all over the country to participate in studies.

How did the largest clinical-trial unit on the continent recruit undocumented immigrants to a dilapidated motel for ten years without anyone noticing? Part of the answer has to do with our system of oversight. Before the nineteen-seventies, medical research was poorly regulated; many Phase I subjects were prisoners. Reforms were instituted after congressional investigations into abuses like the four-decade Tuskegee syphilis studies, in which researchers studied, instead of treating, syphilis infections in African-American men. For the past three decades, institutional review boards, or I.R.B.s, have been the primary mechanism for protecting subjects in drug trials. F.D.A. regulations require that any study in support of a new drug be approved by an I.R.B. Until recently, I.R.B.s were based in universities and teaching hospitals, and were made up primarily of faculty members who volunteered to review the research studies being conducted in their own institutions. Now that most drug studies take place outside academic settings, research sponsors can submit their proposed studies to for-profit I.R.B.s, which will review the ethics of a study in exchange for a fee. These boards are subject to the same financial pressures faced by virtually everyone in the business. They compete for clients by promising a fast review. And if one for-profit I.R.B. concludes that a study is unethical the sponsor can simply take it to another.

Moreover, because I.R.B.s scrutinize studies only on paper, they are seldom in a position to comment on conditions at a study site. Most of the standards that SFBC violated in Miami, for example, would not be covered in an ordinary off-site ethics review. I.R.B.s ask questions like "Have the subjects been adequately informed of what the study involves?" They do not generally ask if the sponsors are recruiting undocumented immigrants or if the study site poses a fire hazard. At some trial sites, guinea pigs are housed in circumstances that would drive away anyone with better options. Guinea pigs told me about sites that skimp on meals and hot water, or that require subjects to bring their own towels and blankets. A few sites have a reputation for recruiting subjects who are threatening or dangerous but work cheaply.

Few people realize how little oversight the federal government provides for the protection of subjects in privately sponsored studies. The Office for Human Research Protections, in the Department of Health and Human Services, has jurisdiction only over research funded by the department. The F.D.A. oversees drug safety, but, according to a 2007 H.H.S. report, it conducts "more inspections that verify clinical trial data than inspections that focus on human-subject protections." In 2005, F.D.A. inspectors were finally given a code number for reporting "failure to protect the rights, safety, and welfare of subjects," and an agency spokesman says that they plan to make more human-subject-safety inspections in the future, but so far they have cited only one investigator for a violation. (He had held a subject in his research unit against her will.) In any case, the F.D.A. inspects only about one per cent of clinical trials.

Most guinea pigs rely on their wits—or on word of mouth from other subjects—to determine which studies are safe. Some avoid particular kinds of studies, such as trials for heart drugs or psychiatric drugs. Others have developed relationships with certain recruiters, whom they trust to tell them which studies to avoid. In general, guinea pigs figure that sponsors have a financial incentive to keep them healthy. "The

companies don't give two shits about me or my personal well-being," Nathaniel Miller says. "But it's not in their interest for anything to go wrong." That's true, but companies also have an interest in things going well as cheaply as possible, and this can lead to hazardous tradeoffs.

The most notorious recent disaster for healthy volunteers took place in March, 2006, at a testing site run by Parexel at Northwick Park Hospital, outside London; subjects were offered two thousand pounds to enroll in a Phase I trial of a monoclonal antibody, a prospective treatment for rheumatoid arthritis and multiple sclerosis. Six of the volunteers had to be rushed to a nearby intensive-care unit after suffering life-threatening reactions—severe inflammation, organ failure. They were hospitalized for weeks, and one subject's fingers and toes were amputated. All the subjects have reportedly been left with long-term disabilities.

The Northwick Park episode was not an isolated incident. Traci Johnson, a previously healthy nineteen-year-old student, committed suicide in a safety study of Eli Lilly's antidepressant Cymbalta in January of 2004. (Lilly denies that its product was to blame.) I spoke to an Iraqi living in Canada who began doing trials when he immigrated. He was living in a hostel and needed money to buy a car. A friend told him, "This thing is like fast cash." When he enrolled in an immunosuppressant trial at a Montreal-based subsidiary of SFBC, he found himself in a bed next to a subject who was coughing up blood. Despite his complaints, he was not moved to a different bed for nine days. He and eight other subjects later tested positive for tuberculosis.

A decade ago, shortly after I began teaching bioethics and philosophy at the University of Minnesota, I got a phone call from a psychiatrist named Faruk Abuzzahab. He wanted to know if he could sit in on an ethics class that I was teaching. There had been some trouble in a research study that he had conducted, it seemed, and the state licensing board had ordered him to take a class in medical ethics.

Despite some misgivings about my class being used as an instrument of punishment, I agreed. He seemed affable enough on the phone, explaining that he had been a faculty member at the university before going into private practice, and had once chaired the Minnesota Psychiatric Society's ethics committee.

I did not give much more thought to Abuzzahab until about three years ago, when a for-profit testing site called Prism Research opened in St. Paul. Prism was advertising for healthy subjects in a local alternative weekly. I discovered, on the company's Web site, that Abuzzahab was one of its researchers. A few more clicks revealed that he was also conducting studies at his private practice, Clinical Psychopharmacology Consultants. I began to wonder what, exactly, the incident was that had brought him to my class.

As it turned out, the disciplinary action was a response to the injuries or deaths of forty-six patients under Abuzzahab's supervision. Seventeen of them had been research subjects in studies that he was conducting. These were not healthy-volunteer studies. According to the board, Abuzzahab had "enrolled psychiatrically disturbed and vulnerable patients into investigational drug studies without ensuring that they met eligibility criteria to be in the study and then kept them in the study after their conditions deteriorated." The board had judged Abuzzahab a danger to the public and suspended his license, citing "a reckless, if not willful, disregard of the patients' welfare."

One case, which was reported in the Boston *Globe*, concerned a forty-one-year-old woman named Susan Endersbe, who had struggled for years with schizophrenia and suicidal thoughts. She had been doing well on her medication, however, until Abuzzahab enrolled her in a trial of an experimental anti-psychotic drug. In the trial, she was taken off her regular medication and became suicidal. When Abuzzahab gave her a day pass to leave the hospital unsupervised, she threw herself into the Mississippi River and drowned. In another case cited by the board,

Abuzzahab had prescribed a "large supply of potentially lethal medications" to a woman with a history of substance abuse, "shortly after a serious suicide attempt." She committed suicide by taking an overdose.

The public portion of Abuzzahab's disciplinary file is freely available from the Minnesota licensing board, and has been posted on the Web site of Circare, a watchdog group that documents research abuse. When I ran a Google search on "Faruk Abuzzahab," the first hit I got was a 1998 article in the *Globe* on his trial disasters. Yet none of this seems to have derailed Abuzzahab's research career. Even after his suspension, the *Times* has reported, he continued to supervise drug trials, and to receive payments from at least a dozen drug companies. In 2003, the American Psychiatric Association awarded him a Distinguished Life Fellowship.

The U.S. regulatory system is built on the tacit assumption that the main threat to research subjects comes from overly ambitious academic researchers, who might be tempted to gamble with subjects' health in the pursuit of medical knowledge or academic fame. The system was intended to check this sort of intellectual ambition, mainly by insuring that studies are reviewed in advance by boards made up of the researcher's academic peers. But, like most physicians supervising clinical trials today, Abuzzahab does not work in an academic setting. The studies conducted at for-profit sites such as Prism are not the natural domain of academically ambitious researchers. They are rarely published and, even if they were, would bring little intellectual credit to the physicians carrying them out, because they are designed by the industry sponsor. A researcher like Abuzzahab would not become famous by supervising subjects in studies like these. But he might become rich.

Abuzzahab represents a new, entrepreneurial breed of physician-researcher; in fact, many of his colleagues have moved even farther from the academic realm. In 1994, according to the Tufts Center for Drug Development, seventy per cent of clinical researchers were affiliated with academic medical centers. By 2006, that figure had dropped to thirty-six per cent. The work can be lucrative, and some sponsors offer researchers additional financial incentives to recruit subjects. One doctor told the Department of Health and Human Services that he was offered twelve thousand dollars for each subject that he could enroll in a trial, plus a thirty-thousand-dollar bonus and an additional six thousand dollars per subject after the first six.

Some of the people conducting clinical trials have little training in how to conduct research. And, as the Abuzzahab case suggests, not all drug companies are especially selective about the researchers they hire. In 2001, the F.D.A. asked the pharmaceutical company Sanofi-Aventis to perform new studies of the antibiotic Ketek, which was suspected of causing liver failure. Reports later revealed that the top-recruiting investigator hired by P.P.D., the firm contracted to conduct the studies, was a graduate of an offshore medical school who tested the antibiotic on clients in an obesity clinic she ran in Alabama. She was sentenced to five years in federal prison for fraud. Another top-recruiting investigator was arrested when the police found him carrying a loaded semi-automatic handgun, and hiding cocaine in his underwear.

In early December of 2002, a man named Bob Helms took part in an industry-sponsored "drug delivery" study. Helms and his fellow guinea pigs were required to take a new anti-anxiety drug and, later, to defecate into a small basket. The unfortunate clinic staff members then searched for the remains of the tablet to determine how much had been absorbed by the body.

The guinea pigs were paid thirty-three hundred dollars and were required to live in the unit for five periods of four days each. But before the end of the first period, Helms says, the guinea pigs decided that they were getting a raw deal. The process of fecal collection was smelly and unpleasant; the amount of time allowed outside the unit had been shortened from three days to thirty-six hours; and the subjects were required to abstain from alcohol, even though the study—because of unexpected delays—was taking place over the Christmas and New Year's holidays. The guinea pigs wanted a raise.

Since the staff was collecting their feces, Helms suggested that the guinea pigs all swallow notes that said "More money." This idea was rejected. Instead, they presented a one-page memo to the staff, detailing their concerns and requesting a pay increase of eleven hundred dollars. When the memo was ignored, they began hinting that they might decamp for a better-paying study at another site. Eventually, the clinic agreed to pay each subject an additional eight hundred dollars.

Helms is a pioneer in the world of guinea-pig activism. A fifty-year-old housepainter and former union organizer, he has a calm, measured demeanor that masks a deep dissident streak. Before he started guinea-pigging, in the nineteen-nineties, he worked as a caregiver for mentally retarded adults living in group homes. There Helms began to understand the difficulties in organizing health-care workers who were employed by the same company but in far-flung locations—in this case, group homes that were spread over two hundred miles of suburbs. "The other organizers told me right off the bat that I could not organize workers who might meet each other once a year at best," Helms says. "How could we ask them to take risks together? They were strangers."

Helms saw that guinea pigs faced a similar problem, and, in 1996, he started a jobzine for research subjects called *Guinea Pig Zero*. With a mixture of reporting, advocacy, and dark humor (a cartoon in an early issue shows a young man surrounded by I.V. bags and syringes, exclaiming, "No more fast food work for me—I've got a career in science!"), *Guinea Pig Zero* published the sort of information that guinea pigs really wanted to know—how well a study paid, the competence of the venipuncturist, the quality of the food. It even published report cards, grading research units from A to F. "Overcrowding, no hot showers, sleeping in an easy chair, incredibly cheap shit for dinner, creepy guys from New York jails—all these are a poor man's worries," Helms says. "Where are these things in the regulators' paperwork?" *Guinea Pig Zero* was not aimed at sick people who sign up for studies in order to get new treatment. It was aimed at poor people who sign up for studies in order to get money.

And here is where its perspective diverged most radically from the traditional ethical perspective. *Guinea Pig Zero* assumed that subjects should get more money, while many ethicists and regulators argued that they should get none at all. The standard worry expressed by ethicists is that money tempts subjects to take part in dangerous, painful, or degrading studies against their better judgment. F.D.A. guidelines instruct review boards to make sure that payment is not "coercive" and does not exert an "undue influence" on subjects. It's a reasonable worry. "If there were a study where they cut off your leg and sewed it back on and you got twenty thousand dollars, people would be fighting to get into that study," a Philadelphia activist and clinical-trial veteran who writes under the name Dave Onion says.

Of course, ethicists generally prefer that subjects take part in studies for altruistic reasons. Yet, if sponsors relied solely on altruism, studies on healthy subjects would probably come to a halt. The result is an uneasy compromise: guinea pigs are paid to test drugs, but everyone pretends that guinea-pigging is not really a job. I.R.B.s allow sponsors to pay guinea pigs, but, consistent with F.D.A. guidelines, insist on their keeping the amount low. Sponsors refer to the money as "compensation" rather than as "wages," but guinea pigs must pay taxes, and they are given no retirement benefits, disability insurance, workmen's compensation, or overtime pay. And, because so many guinea pigs are uninsured, they are testing the safety of drugs that they will probably not be able to afford once the drugs have been approved. "I'm not going to get the benefit of the health care that is developed by this research," Helms says, "because I am not in the economic class to get health insurance."

Guinea pigs can't even count on having their medical care paid for if they are injured in a study. According to a recent survey in *The New England Journal of Medicine*, only sixteen per cent of academic medical centers in the United States provided free care to subjects injured in trials. None of them compensated injured subjects for pain or lost wages. No systematic data are available for private testing sites, but the provisions typically found in consent forms are not encouraging. A consent form for a recent study of Genentech's immunosuppressant drug Raptiva told participants that they would be treated for any injuries the drug caused, but stipulated that "the cost of such treatment will not be reimbursed."

Some sponsors withhold most of the payment until the studies are over. Guinea pigs who drop out after deciding that a surgical procedure is too disagreeable, or that a drug seems unpleasant or dangerous, must forfeit the bulk of their paycheck. Two years ago, when SFBC conducted a two-month study of the pain medication Palladone, it offered subjects twenty-four hundred dollars. But most of that was paid only after the last of the study's four confinement periods. A guinea pig could spend nearly two months in the study, including twelve days and nights in the SFBC unit, and get only six hundred dollars. SFBC even reserved the right to withhold payments from subjects whom it dropped from the study because of a drug's side effects.

Guinea-pig activists recognize that they are indispensable to the pharmaceutical industry; a guinea-pig walkout in the middle of a trial could wreak financial havoc on the sponsor. Yet the conditions of guinea-pigging make any exercise of power difficult. Not only are those in a particular trial likely to be strangers; if they complain to the sponsor about conditions, they risk being excluded from future studies. And, according to *Bloomberg*, when illegal-immigrant guinea pigs at SFBC talked to the press, managers threatened to have them deported.

Lawsuits on behalf of injured subjects are growing, though, and they have begun to target not just research sponsors but also institutional review boards and bioethicists. Alan Milstein, an attorney in Philadelphia, has pioneered this area of law, most notably with successful litigation against the University of Pennsylvania on behalf of the family of Jesse Gelsinger, who died in a gene-therapy trial in 1999. Milstein has represented volunteers injured at commercial sites, but most guinea pigs are in no position to hire a lawyer. "This is not something you or I do," Milstein says. "This is something the poor do so that the rich can get better drugs."

During our early years of medical school, my classmates and I were given a course in physical diagnosis. Usually, we practiced on one another. Each of us would percuss a classmate's chest, or listen to his heart with a stethoscope. But some procedures were considered too personal to practice on a classmate. For some of these, we were assigned a "model patient"—someone from the community who was "compensated" in exchange for undergoing an examination.

This was how I performed my first rectal exam. A large group of us were led into a room, where our model patient was bent over an examining table with his pants around his ankles. One by one, we approached him nervously from behind, inserted a gloved, lubricated finger into his rectum, and felt around for the prostate. "Thank you," we all said politely to the model patient as we removed our index fingers from his anus. The model patient stared straight ahead, saying nothing.

What made the experience oddly disturbing was not just the forced, pseudo normality of the instruction, or the fact that the exam could have been done more privately, but the instrumentality of the encounter: a pretend "patient" bending over naked for anonymous strangers in exchange for money. The fact that the model patient had been paid did not make his work seem any less degrading. (Tipping him would have made it even worse.)

Perhaps there is something inherently disconcerting about the idea of turning drug testing into a job. Guinea pigs do not do things in exchange for money so much as they allow things to be done to them. There are not many other jobs where that is the case. Meanwhile, our patchwork regulatory system insures that no one institution is keeping track of how many deaths and injuries befall healthy subjects in clinical trials. Nobody appears to be tracking how many clinical investigators are incompetent, or have lost their licenses, or have questionable disciplinary records. Nobody is monitoring the effect that so many trials have on the health of professional guinea pigs. In fact, nobody is even entirely certain whether the trials generate reliable data. A professional guinea pig who does a dozen drug-safety trials a year is not exactly representative of the population that will be taking the drugs once they have been approved.

The safety of new drugs has always depended on the willingness of someone to test them, and it seems inevitable that the job will fall to people who have no better options. Guinea-pigging requires no training or skill, and in a thoroughly commercial environment, where there can be no pretense of humanitarian motivation, it is hard to think of it as meaningful work. As Dave Onion puts it, "You don't go home and say to yourself, 'Now, that was a good day.'"

Justice and the Human Development Approach to International Research

ALEX JOHN LONDON

Hastings Center Report 35, no.1 (2005): 24–37.

The intimate relationship between disease and conditions of social and economic deprivation has been at the center of an intense debate about the ethics of international medical research for more than a decade. But while this debate has at times been high-pitched and divisive, behind it lies a broad area of agreement. On the one hand, most commentators accept that medical research can and should play an important role in efforts to address the profound health needs of developing world populations. It is often noted, for example, that 90 percent of the world's research dollars are spent on diseases that affect only 10 percent of the world's population—the so-called 10/90 research gap—and that this imbalance in research priorities contributes to the pervasive lack of access to effective medical care in the developing world. On the other hand, there is also widespread recognition that the sheer extent of health needs in the developing world, combined with poverty and social deprivation, make populations there highly susceptible to abuse and exploitation. While medical research is capable of generating important benefits, it can also impose significant burdens. Too often in the past, the burdens of research participation have been borne in the developing world while the fruits of those endeavors are enjoyed principally in developed nations.

Unfortunately, the debate about the ethics of international research has not adequately considered the relationship between research and basic issues of social justice that are raised by these background considerations. For instance, although it is recognized that clinical trials in the developing world must respond to the health needs and priorities of the host country, there has been little discussion of the fundamental relationship between a community's health needs and the broader conditions of social justice that help to shape those needs. And while an intense debate has raged over the standard of care that should be provided to research participants, most of it has centered on the interpretation of the international guidelines for research. Broader issues of social justice are centrally relevant to this topic as well, but they have been addressed only at the margins. In fact, the debate about justice has become synonymous with the question of who gets access to the fruits of successful research. An intense focus on the guidelines for international research has effectively confined this debate to the question of whether, and to what degree, research sponsors must ensure that any interventions shown effective in a clinical trial are made *reasonably available* to the host population.

In part, no doubt, the reluctance to address the relationship between international research and broader questions of social justice stems from a desire to stick to what are perceived as more tractable practical issues and to avoid thorny philosophical disagreements over different theories of justice. In the discussion that follows, however, I argue that the desire to avoid important background issues and social justice has structured debate so as to filter out and exclude information that connects relatively local topics in international research to broader issues of global justice, the social determinants of health, and human development. This results in a way of framing central issues in international research that is essentially biased in favor of what Brian Barry calls "justice as mutual advantage." As a result, someone who approaches this topic wanting to remain agnostic about controversial issues in global justice may find herself formulating the basic problem in a way that tacitly presupposes a particularly anemic theory of justice.

Any frank and straightforward account of the health needs in the developing world reveals that they are staggeringly pervasive, profound, and urgent. People in the developing world who live in poverty and toil under some of the world's poorest social conditions also bear some of the heaviest burdens of sickness and disease. Of the 3.5 million deaths from pneumonia each year, 99 percent take place in developing countries, where pneumonia claims the lives of more children than any other infectious disease. To some degree, people in the developing world are more likely to die from pneumonia because they cannot afford the low-cost antibiotics widely available in developed nations. Twenty-seven cents (U.S.) for a five-day regimen of antibiotics is more than a day's income for roughly 1 billion people. Also, in rural communities and other places where the health care infrastructure is not well entrenched, hospitals and clinics may be too far away to get to.

Poverty and poor social conditions also make those in the developing world more susceptible to a wider array of illnesses. Pneumonia is more common in the developing world, for example, because children are more likely to be malnourished and to suffer from medical conditions that weaken their immune systems. Where sanitation is poor and the drinking water is unsafe, diarrhea-related diseases such as cholera, dysentery, typhoid fever, and rotavirus claim the lives of nearly two million children under the age of five. In developed nations, in contrast, such infections are much less common and are more easily treated when they occur. Similarly, of the roughly 1,600 children infected with HIV every day, approximately 90 percent live in the developing world. Africa alone is home to some 70 percent of the world's HIV-positive individuals, even though the continent contains only about 10 percent of the world's population. In developed countries, the use of costly anti-retroviral medications has dramatically reduced the rate of mother-to-child transmission of HIV and greatly extended the lives of HIV-positive adults, but precisely where the burden of HIV/AIDS is the greatest, these interventions remain largely unavailable.

One of the goals of collaborative international medical research is to address the profound health-related needs of the developing world. At the same time, medical research is also capable of imposing additional burdens on participants and the communities in which they live. The problem, then, is how to ensure that research actually benefits people in the developing world without further exacerbating their already profound deprivation.

The Moral Relevance of Social and Political Determinants of Health

Consider some parallels between Amartya Sen's groundbreaking work on famine and the broader health needs of developing world populations. Famines are commonly viewed as natural disasters caused principally by a combination of poverty and poor food production. Sen showed, however, that these factors alone do not account for the occurrence of famines. For example, in 1979–1981 and 1983–1984, Sudan and Ethiopia experienced declines in food production of 11 or 12 percent and, like a number of other countries in sub-Saharan Africa, suffered massive famines. During the same period, however, food production declined by 17 percent in Botswana and by a precipitous 38 percent in Zimbabwe, yet these countries did not suffer the ravages of famine. According to Sen, the reason for this difference in outcomes can be traced to differences in the social and political structures of these countries. Botswana and Zimbabwe had rudimentary democratic social institutions that enabled them to stave off famine. They implemented a series of social support programs targeted at enhancing the economic purchasing power of affected groups, while also supplementing food supplies. Mass starvation occurred in Sudan and Ethiopia because the dictatorial regimes in those nations failed to take such relatively simple social and economic steps to safeguard their citizens' interests.

These lessons should broadly inform our view of sickness and disease in the developing world. For example, HIV-AIDS is devastating many populations in sub-Saharan Africa. In some nations, as much as 30 percent of the population is HIV-positive and infection rates continue to climb. In sharp contrast, Senegal has been able to limit both the prevalence of HIV-AIDS and the rate of new infections to about 1 percent of the population. The principal cause of Senegal's success lies not in advanced technology or great wealth, but in the government's longstanding, grassroots investment in its human resources. In Senegal, information about HIV-AIDS and many other sexually transmitted diseases has been disseminated through an assortment of educational programs. Such programs represent a particularly prominent instance of the government's willingness to forge ties with community and religious leaders in order to encourage social activism. Empowering individuals with information and opportunities for activism enhances the public's capacities for communal interaction, free expression, and political participation, and so creates a social context in which people can more effectively safeguard and secure their welfare.

This focus on education and activism has been further enhanced by the judicious use of scarce resources. Senegal closely monitors its blood supply and distributes millions of condoms free of charge. It invests in monitoring and treating many sexually transmitted diseases, especially in target populations such as commercial sex workers, young people, truck drivers, and the spouses of migrant workers. Additionally, as part of a program of perinatal care, it has begun to offer antiretroviral drugs to pregnant women, although on a very limited basis. There remains room for improvement in Senegal. Still, the country's multisectoral approach to HIV-AIDS, and to public health in general, illustrates the positive health effects of policies that strive to protect citizens' basic capacities for agency and welfare.

As these examples show, the basic political, legal, social, and economic institutions of a community have a profound impact on the health status of community members. Because they determine the distribution of basic rights and liberties within a society, these structures set the terms on which individuals may access basic goods and resources such as food, shelter, education, and productive employment, as well as more specialized health care resources. They therefore determine the opportunities available to individuals to develop and exercise their basic human capacities.

Whether members of a community have a justified claim to something beyond the status quo depends crucially on whether the terms of social cooperation set by the community's social structures can be endorsed by community members as basically fair. As a minimal condition of fairness, it must be possible to see the fundamental structures of a community as organized around, and functioning in the service of, the common good of the community's members. In other words, a morally permissible division of labor must strive to secure for individuals what Rawls called the "fair value" of their basic capacities for welfare and human agency—meaning that the division of social labor should be designed so as to give each person an effective opportunity to cultivate and use their basic intellectual, affective, and social capacities to pursue a meaningful life plan. Social structures that do not meet this minimal requirement create conditions in which some are denied effective opportunities to develop their basic capacities while others enjoy a rich array of opportunities and benefits. In the most extreme cases, these are the social conditions in which starvation, sickness, and disease flourish. The harms that result in such cases cannot be dismissed as accidents of nature or justified by reference to the common good. They represent a failure to use the state's monopoly on force and control over basic social structures to advance the interests of community members. Those who suffer in these cases can legitimately claim, as a strict obligation of justice, an entitlement to relief from such hardships.

Duties of Rectification

Now it remains to show how these and similar considerations might alter or affect the rights and obligations of researchers and their sponsoring entities. To do so, I shall distinguish three classes of issues that might affect the obligations of researchers and their sponsoring entities.

At the most general level, duties of rectification may attach to all citizens of democratic nations whose policies and international activities have contributed to the plight of those in the developing world. In a series of recent articles, Thomas Pogge has argued that Western democratic nations have contributed greatly to the poverty and poor health of the global poor simply by recognizing and supporting what he calls the "international resource privilege." Any group that succeeds in wresting control of the national government in a developing country is recognized as having the legitimate authority "to borrow in the name of its people and to confer legal ownership rights for the country's resources." Not only does the existence of this privilege provide a powerful incentive for the unscrupulous to seize power in a developing nation, but it provides a convenient mechanism for consolidating power and then wielding it for the enrichment of a privileged few. Employing power in this way, of course, can saddle a developing nation with disastrous long-term debt and prevent most of the population from sharing in the benefits generated by their country's natural resources. Instead, the benefits are enjoyed primarily by a ruling elite in the developing world and by governments and corporations in the developed world.

A duty to aid grounded in this kind of pre-existing relationship would apply to medical researchers insofar as they are citizens of the basically democratic nations that have contributed to and benefited from such policies. The obligations may be strengthened if researchers are employed or funded by governments or private entities that have actively supported such policies. Alternatively, duties of rectification may attach to researchers who work for or are funded by entities that have contributed more directly to the plight of developing world populations. For example, one reason drugs are so scarce in the developing world is their cost. Many individual pharmaceutical companies played an active role in the negotiation of the TRIPS agreement at the World Trade Organization, and the pharmaceutical lobby has used its considerable influence on U.S. and E.U. trade representatives to enforce the companies' patent rights. The TRIPS agreement allows countries to produce or import generic versions of beneficial medications in cases of national emergency, but the Western pharmaceutical industry has aggressively pressed for trade sanctions or taken active legal action against countries that have tried to implement this emergency clause. In doing so, it has blocked legitimate efforts to provide medicines to some of the populations that need them most.

Unmet Obligations within Host Communities

As I noted, one of the defining problems of social structures that violate the minimal condition of basic fairness is that those structures fail to allocate scarce social resources around the goal of serving the common good. By failing to invest scarce social resources in the basic capacities of community members and denying the population access to social resources to which they have a legislative claim, they help to create conditions of deprivation in which sickness and disease flourish.

In such cases, resources that domestic authorities may be willing to make available for research purposes may not be "available" in a more fundamental moral sense: those who control them may have a prior moral obligation to deploy them in the service of other ends. Moreover, although the use of monetary and material resources may be particularly important in this regard, there are other social resources that matter as well. For example, regimes can fail to serve the common good by neglecting basic social institutions altogether, by misappropriating or misdirecting the time and energies of their personnel, or by inappropriately restricting or occupying important institutional spaces. These failures can generate prior moral claims that the community members have against their own authorities, and such claims may constrain the range of cooperative or collaborative relationships in which researchers may permissibly engage.

The Human Development View

"Human development" is understood in this view as the project of establishing and fostering basic social structures that guarantee to community members the fair value of their most basic human capacities. This project is grounded in the recognition that perhaps the most important determinant of health within a community is the extent to which its basic social structures guarantee members of the community opportunities for education, access to productive employment, control over their person and their personal environment, access to the political process, and the protection of their basic human rights. More important than the sheer economic wealth of a community, in fact, is whether the community directs the available resources to creating and sustaining the right social conditions.

Because the health status of individuals is affected by a matrix of political, social, and economic factors, the project of creating and sustaining the conditions that foster health requires a coordinated, multisectoral approach that is sensitive to these interrelationships. The health-related institutions of a community, including its public health and health care institutions, can contribute to this process in

two fundamental ways. First, they can facilitate development by targeting rudimentary health problems that can impede the ability of community members to function in ways essential to the development process. Literacy and education are powerful determinants of a person's ability to safeguard her own health and take advantage of economic opportunities; providing basic nutrition and rudimentary health care are therefore important because the sick and undernourished are less likely to attend school and less able to concentrate and to learn if they do.

Second, health-related institutions address health needs of community members that persist as the process of development proceeds. In other words, although other elements of the basic social structures of the community provide individuals with some important social determinants of health—education, nutrition, and respect for basic human rights—the health-related institutions target the health needs of individuals that these other measures do not alleviate.

The human development approach treats clinical research as one important element within this larger division of labor. The research enterprise represents a permissible use of a community's scarce public resources and is a permissible target of social support when it functions to expand the capacity of the basic social structures of that community to better serve the fundamental interests of that community's members. Therefore, if clinical research is to be permissible, it must function as a part of a division of labor in which the distinctive scientific and statistical methods of the research enterprise target and investigate the means of filling the gaps between the most important health needs in a community and the capacity of its social structures to meet them.

When the human development approach is applied to the research carried out within liberal democratic nations of the developed world, it captures important ideals that are often explicitly embraced by developed communities. In different ways and with varying degrees of success, these communities recognize the need to invest in a robust array of social institutions that protect community members' basic social, political, and economic opportunities, thereby safeguarding the social determinants of health. These ideals help to attract public support for health care and public health institutions. Significant public support is also provided to domestic clinical research as an engine of discovery that can push back the boundaries of knowledge in order to enhance the community's health-related institutions. *As a result, these communities often assess research that receives public support by asking how it is contributing to equity in the capacity of the community's health care institutions to address the needs of the diverse populations that those institutions serve.*

In the international context, the human development approach holds that collaborative research initiatives are permissible only if they are a part of, or contribute to, a fair social division of labor in the host community. In particular, they must directly and indirectly expand the capacity of the host community's basic social structures either to meet the distinctive health priorities of that community's members or to meet their basic health needs under distinctive social or environmental circumstances. Health needs are distinctive and are prioritized according to whether they cannot be ameliorated through the application of existing knowledge and resources.

Once this necessary condition has been satisfied, the human development approach also provides a framework for assessing the extent to which researchers and their sponsoring entities must secure additional resources to make the fruits of successful research available to members of the host population, or to provide ancillary benefits. The imperative to try to make the results of successful research available within the host community increases in inverse proportion to the capacity of that community's basic social structures to translate those results into sustainable benefits for community members. To the extent that the host community

cannot translate the results into sustainable benefits for its population on its own, an imperative exists either to build partnerships with groups that would be willing to augment the community's capacity to do so, or to locate the research within a community with similar health priorities and a more appropriate health infrastructure. Similarly, the imperative to provide an array of ancillary benefits to community members increases in inverse proportion to the community's capacity to treat or ameliorate the ancillary health problems that researchers are likely to encounter. This imperative is best understood as a duty to partner with governmental and nongovernmental agencies to use the research enterprise as a kind of anchor point around which aid can be coordinated. Such obligations are most pressing in exactly those cases in which community members have the strongest claims to assistance.

Microbicides

Let me close with an illustration. Consider the justification for international research aimed at finding a safe and effective vaginal microbicide, an agent delivered in gel form that would reduce the odds of HIV transmission, and perhaps secondary STI transmission, during heterosexual, vaginal intercourse.

Enhancing the basic capabilities and social opportunities of women is an important development goal. Roughly half of the global burden of HIV/AIDS is borne by women, and in southern Africa more than one in five pregnant women are HIV-positive. The complications of HIV/AIDS are increasing maternal death rates during labor, and vertical or maternal-fetal transmission of HIV still accounts for approximately 90 percent of new pediatric HIV infections—600,000 annually—the vast majority of which occur in the developing world. When used properly, condoms are good at preventing horizontal or partner-to-partner transmission of the HIV virus. But condoms are often not used consistently because men often dislike them and men tend to have more control than women over what happens in their relationships. As a result, the range of options available to women—who are already a disadvantaged social group and have a higher susceptibility to contracting HIV from heterosexual intercourse than men—may be further restricted by men's preferences and behavior.

Developing a safe, effective, and affordable microbicide would thus contribute to several important development goals. It would provide an intervention that expands the range of options available to women to safeguard their own health. Given the influence of gender inequalities on condom use, this positive effect would not necessarily be achieved just by emphasizing condom usage more strongly. Also, because it could help to reduce the frequency of HIV transmission to women, it could contribute to a reduction in transmission to children. Finally, by targeting the needs of an often disadvantaged subpopulation within the larger host population, such research would contribute to social equity.

Monitoring Stem Cell Research

Introduction

PRESIDENT'S COUNCIL ON BIOETHICS

From http://bioethicsprint.boethics.gov/reports/stemcell/chapter1.html

This monitoring report has its origins in President George W. Bush's remarks to the nation on August 9, 2001. It was his first major national policy address, and the topic was unusual: federal funding of research on human stem cells. In the speech, the President announced that after several months of deliberation he had decided to make federal funding available, for the first time, for research involving certain lines of embryo-derived stem cells. At the end of the speech the President declared his intention to

> name a President's Council to monitor stem cell research, to recommend appropriate guidelines and regulations, and to consider all of the medical and ethical ramifications of biomedical innovation....This council will keep us apprised of new developments and give our nation a forum to continue to discuss and evaluate these important issues.

In keeping with the President's intention, the Council has been monitoring developments in stem cell research, as it proceeds under the implementation of the administration's policy. Our desire has been both to understand what is going on in the laboratory and to consider for ourselves the various arguments made in the ongoing debates about the ethics of stem cell research and the wisdom of the current policy. Although both the policy and the research are still in their infancy, the Council is now ready to give the President and the public an update on this important and dynamic area of research.

I. What Are Stem Cells, and Why Is There Contention About Them?

The term "stem cells" refers to a diverse group of remarkable multipotent cells. Themselves relatively undifferentiated and unspecialized, they can and do give rise to the differentiated and specialized cells of the body (for example, liver cells, kidney cells, brain cells). All specialized cells arise originally from stem cells, and ultimately from a small number of embryonic cells that appear during the first few days of development. As befits their being and functioning as progenitor cells, all stem cells share two characteristic properties: (1) the capacity for unlimited or prolonged *self-renewal* (that is, the capability to maintain a pool of similarly undifferentiated stem cells), and (2) the potential to produce *differentiated* descendant cell types. As stem cells within a developing human embryo differentiate in vivo, their capacity to diversify generally becomes more limited and their ability to generate many differentiated cell types generally becomes more restricted.

Stem cells first arise during embryonic development and exist at all developmental stages and in many systems of the body throughout life. The best described to date are the blood-forming (hematopoietic) stem cells of the bone marrow, the progeny of which differentiate (throughout life) into the various types of red, white, and other cells of the blood. It appears that some stem cells travel through the circulatory system, from their tissue of origin, to take up residence in other locations within the body, from which they may be isolated. Other stem cells may be obtained at birth, from blood contained in the newborn's umbilical cord. Once isolated and cultured outside the body, stem cells are available for scientific investigation. Unlike more differentiated cells, stem cells can be propagated in vitro for many generations—perhaps an unlimited number—of cell-doublings.

Stem cells are of interest for two major reasons, the one scientific, the other medical. First, stem cells provide a wonderful tool for the study of cellular and developmental processes, both normal and abnormal. With them, scientists hope to be able to figure out the molecular mechanisms of differentiation through which cells become specialized and organized into tissues and organs. They hope to understand how these mechanisms work when they work well, and what goes wrong when they work badly. Second, stem cells and their derivatives may prove a valuable source of transplantable cells and tissues for repair and regeneration. If these healing powers could be harnessed, the medical benefits for humankind would be immense, perhaps ushering in an era of truly regenerative medicine. No wonder that scientists around the world are actively pursuing research with stem cells.

Why, then, is there public contention about stem cell research? Not because anyone questions the goals of such research, but primarily because there are, for many people, ethical issues connected to the means of obtaining some of the cells. The main source of contention arises because some especially useful stem cells can be derived from early-stage human embryos, which must be destroyed in the process of obtaining the cells. Arguments about the ethics of using human embryos in research are not new. They date back to the mid-1970s, beginning not long after in vitro fertilization (IVF) was first successfully accomplished with human egg and sperm in 1969. A decade later, after IVF had entered clinical practice for the treatment of infertility, arguments continued regarding the fate and possible uses of the so-called "spare embryos," embryos produced in excess of reproductive needs and subsequently frozen and stored in the assisted-reproduction clinics. Although research using these embryos has never been illegal in the United States (except in a few states), the federal government has never funded it, and since 1995 Congress has enacted annual legislation prohibiting the federal government from using taxpayer dollars to support any research in which human embryos are harmed or destroyed.

Although the arguments about embryo research had been going on for twenty-five years, they took on new urgency in 1998, when the current stem cell controversy began. It was precipitated by the separate publication, by two teams of American researchers, of methods for culturing cell lines derived, respectively, from: (1) cells taken from the inner cell mass of very early embryos, and (2) the gonadal ridges of aborted fetuses. (In this report, we shall generally refer to the cell lines derived from these sources as, respectively, *embryonic stem cells* [or "ES cells"] and *embryonic germ cells* [or "EG cells"].) This work, conducted in university laboratories in collaboration with and with financial support from Geron Corporation, prompted great excitement and has already led to much interesting research, here and abroad. It has also sparked a moral and political debate about federal support for such research: Is it morally permissible to withhold support from research that holds such human promise? Is it morally permissible to pursue or publicly support (even beneficial) research that depends on the exploitation and destruction of nascent human life?

Persons interested in the debate should note at the outset that ES and EG cells are not themselves embryos; they are not whole organisms, nor can they be made (directly) to become whole organisms. Moreover, once a given line of ES or EG cells has been derived and grown in laboratory culture, no further embryos (or fetuses) need be used or destroyed in order to work with cells from that line. But it is not clear whether these lines can persist indefinitely, and only very few lines, representing only a few genetic backgrounds, have been made. Thus there is continuing scientific interest in developing new embryonic stem cell lines, and the existence of large numbers of stored cryopreserved embryos in assisted-reproduction clinics provides a potential source for such additional derivations. Complicating the debate has been the study of another group of stem cells, commonly called "adult stem cells," derived not from embryos but from the many different tissues in the bodies of adults or children—sources exempt from the moral debate about obtaining ES and EG cells. For this reason, we often hear arguments about the relative scientific merits and therapeutic potential of embryonic and adult stem cells, arguments in which the moral positions of the competing advocates might sometimes influence their assessments of the scientific facts. Further complicating the situation are the large commercial interests already invested in stem cell research and the competition this creates in research and development not only in the United States but throughout the world. The seemingly small decision about

the funding of stem cell research may have very large implications.

II. Broader Ethical Issues

While most of the public controversy has focused on the issue of embryo use and destruction, other ethical and policy issues have also attracted attention. Although entangled with the issue of embryos, the question of the significance and use of federal funds is itself a contested issue: Should moral considerations be used to decide what sort of research may or may not be funded? What is the symbolic and moral-political significance of providing national approval, in the form of active support, for practices that many Americans regard as abhorrent or objectionable? Conversely, what is the symbolic and moral-political significance of refusing to support potentially life-saving scientific investigations that many Americans regard as morally obligatory?

Even for those who favor embryo research, there are questions about its proper limits and the means of establishing and enforcing those limits through meaningful regulation. Under the present arrangement, with the federal government only recently in the picture, what is done with human embryos, especially in the private sector, is entirely unregulated (save in those states that have enacted special statutes dealing with embryo or stem cell research). Is this a desirable arrangement? Can some other system be devised, one that protects the human goods we care about but that does not do more harm than good? What are those human goods? What boundaries can and should we try to establish, and how?

Although well-established therapies based on transplantation of stem cell-derived tissues are still largely in the future, concern has already been expressed (as it has been about other aspects of health care in the United States) about access to any realized benefits and about research priorities: Will these benefits be equitably available, regardless of ability to pay? How should the emergence of the new field of stem cell research alter the allocation of our limited resources for biomedical research? How, in a morally and politically controverted area of research, should the balance be struck between public and private sources of support? As with any emerging discovery, how can we distinguish between genuine promise and "hype," and between the more urgent and the less urgent medical needs calling out for assistance?

There are also sensitive issues regarding premature claims of cures for diseases that are not scientifically substantiated and the potential exploitation of sick people and their families. Some advocates of stem cell research have made bold claims about the number of people who will be helped should the research go forward, hoping to generate sympathy for increased research funding among legislators and the public. A few advocates have gone so far as to blame (in advance) opponents of embryonic stem cell research for those who will die unless the research goes forward today. At the same time, other scientists have cautioned that the pace of progress will be very slow, and that no cures can be guaranteed in advance. Which of these claims and counterclaims is closer to the truth cannot be known ahead of time. Only once the proper scientific studies are conducted will we discover the potential therapeutic value of stem cells from any source. How, then, in the meantime should we discuss these matters, offering encouragement but without misleading or exploiting the fears and hopes of the desperately ill?

Finally, questions are raised by some about the social significance of accepting the use of nascent human life as a resource for scientific investigation and the search for cures. Such questions have been raised even by people who do not regard an early human embryo as fully "one of us," and who are concerned not so much about the fate of individual embryos as they are about the character and sensibilities of a society that comes to normalize such practices. What would our society be like if it came to treat as acceptable or normal the exploitation of what hitherto were regarded as the seeds of the next generation? Conversely,

exactly analogous questions are raised by some about the social significance of *refusing* to use these 150-to-200-cell early human embryos as a resource for responsible scientific investigation and the search for cures. What would a society be like if it refused, for moral scruples about (merely) nascent life, to encourage every thoughtful and scientifically sound effort to heal disease and relieve the suffering of fully developed human beings among us?

It is against the background of such moral-political discussion and argument that the Council has taken up its work of monitoring recent developments in stem cell research. We are duly impressed with the difficulty of the subject and the high stakes involved. All the more reason to enable the debate to proceed on the basis of the best knowledge available, both about science and medicine and about ethics, law, and policy.

III. Types of Stem Cells: An Introduction

A. Embryonic Stem (ES) Cells

As noted above, ES cells are derived from the inner cell mass of embryos at the blastocyst stage, roughly five to nine days after fertilization—after the zygote has divided enough times to result in about 200 cells, but before it has undergone gastrulation and differentiation into the three primary germ layers. The inner cell mass is the part of the blastocyst-stage embryo whose cells normally go on to become the body of the new individual. The outer cells of the blastocyst-stage embryo (the trophoblast cells) normally (that is, in vivo) go on to become the fetal contribution to the placenta and other structures that connect the developing individual to the mother's bloodstream and that otherwise support the embryo's further development. Collecting the cells of the inner cell mass results in the destruction of the developing organism. The embryos from which human stem cells can be derived are available (so far) only from in vitro fertilization (IVF): they have been conceived by a combination of egg and sperm, occurring outside the body.

B. Embryonic Germ (EG) Cells

EG cells are stem cells that are isolated from the gonadal ridge of a developing fetus. These are the cells that ultimately give rise to sperm cells or egg cells, depending on the sex of the fetus. The EG cells are collected from the bodies of five-to-nine-week-old fetuses that have been donated after induced abortions. In federally funded research, collection of the EG cells is governed by existing federal regulations for fetal-tissue donation, designed (among other things) to ensure the separation of the decision to terminate pregnancy from the decision to donate the fetal tissue for research.

Cell lines established from either of these two sources (ES and EG cells, from embryos and fetal gonads, respectively) have demonstrated two important properties: great ability to multiply and form stable lines that can be characterized, and great flexibility and plasticity. Their progeny can differentiate in vitro into cells with characteristics of those normally derived from all three embryonic germ layers (ectoderm, endoderm, and mesoderm), which layers (in vivo) give rise in turn to all the different types of cells in the body. Because they are so flexible, it also seems likely that they could be used to produce cell preparations that could then be transplanted (assuming that the recipient's immune response could be managed) to repopulate a part of the body such as the pancreas or spinal cord that has lost function due to disease or injury. As with stem cells derived from the various tissues of the adult body, ES cells and EG cells seem to hold out hope for an era of regenerative medicine.

C. Adult (or Non-embryonic) Stem Cells

Adult stem cells are more differentiated than ES or EG cells, but not yet fully differentiated. Like stem cells of embryonic origin, they can give rise to lineages of cells that are more specialized than themselves. The term "adult" is a bit of a misnomer ("non-embryonic" would be more accurate): these cells are found in various tissues in children as well as adults (and in fetuses as well), and they have been isolated from umbilical cord blood at the time of delivery. Despite its inaccuracy regarding the *origin* of the cells, the term "adult" helpfully emphasizes that the cells have been partially differentiated. Although they can give rise to various cell types, these non-embryonic stem cells are generally all within the same broad type of tissue (for example, muscle stem cells, adipose stem cells, neural stem cells). For this reason, it had long been thought that they are less flexible than those derived from embryos or fetal gonads. Yet this presumption has been disputed in recent years by those who think that certain forms of adult stem cells may be equally or nearly as plastic as non-adult stem cells. Indeed, possible exceptions to the generalization that adult stem cells give rise only to cell types found within their own broad type of tissue have recently been reported (though most of these cells may well be shorter-lived than ES cells, and, if so, potentially less useful in therapy). This finding has ignited a debate about the relative merits of embryonic stem cells and adult stem cells: which is more valuable, both for research and (especially) for clinical treatment?

Research involving adult stem cells raises few difficult ethical concerns, beyond the usual need to secure free and fully informed consent from donors and recipients, a favorable benefit-to-risk ratio for all participants in attempts at therapy and protection of privacy. Adult stem cells are less controversial than embryonic ones, as we have noted, because the former can be collected without lasting harm to the donor.

D. Cord Blood Stem Cells

Though clearly a type of non-embryonic stem cell, cord blood stem cells deserve some special mention. Blood found in the umbilical cord can be collected at birth and hematopoietic stem cells (and other progenitor cells) isolated from it. It has been proposed that individually banked cord blood cells may, at some later time, offer a good match for a patient needing stem cell-based treatments, whether the individual cord-blood-donor himself or a close relative, and in unrelated recipients may require a less exact genetic match than adult bone marrow.

IV. Terminology

In considering complicated or contested public questions, language matters—even more than it ordinarily does. Clear thinking depends on clear ideas, and clear ideas can be conveyed only through clear and precise speech. And fairness in ethical evaluation and judgment depends on fair framing of the ethical questions, which in turn requires fair and accurate description of the relevant facts of the case at hand. Such considerations are highly pertinent to our topic and to the arguments it generates.

Confounding the discussions of stem cell research, there are, to begin with, difficult technical concepts, referring to complicated biological entities and phenomena, that can cause confusion among all but the experts. But the more important terminological issues are those used to formulate the ethical and policy issues about which people so vigorously disagree. We pause to comment on three of them: "the embryo" (or "the human embryo"), "spare embryos," and "the moral status of the embryo."

Strictly speaking, there is no such *thing* as "*the* embryo," if by this is meant a distinctive being (or *kind* of being) that deserves a common, reified name—like "dog" or "elephant." Rather, the term properly intends a certain *stage of development* of an organism of a distinctive kind. Indeed, the very term comes from a Greek root meaning "to grow": an embryo is, by its name and mode of being, an immature and growing organism in an early phase of its development. The advent of in vitro fertilization, in which living human embryos from their first

moments are encountered as independent entities outside the body of a mother, before human eyes and in human hands, may also have contributed to this tendency to reify "*the* embryo" in its early stages (though such reification has likely always played a role in embryology). The ex vivo existence of nascent human life is genuinely puzzling and may invite terminology that can be distorting.

If the term "*the* embryo" risks conveying the false notion that embryos are distinct kinds of beings or things, the term "spare embryo" risks making a difficult moral question seem easier than it is. The term is frequently used to describe those embryos, produced (each with reproductive intent, but in excess of what is needed) in assisted-reproduction clinics, that are not transferred to a woman in attempts to initiate a pregnancy. No longer needed to produce a child, they are usually frozen and stored for possible later use, should the first efforts fail. But the "spareness" of a "spare embryo" is not a property of a particular embryo itself; it bespeaks rather our attitude toward it, now that it may no longer be needed to serve the purpose for which it was initially brought into being. Calling something "spare," or only "extra," invites the thought that nothing much is lost should it disappear, because one already has more than enough: one has "embryos to spare." It also abstracts from the distinct genetic individuality of each embryo and invites the view that embryos are, like commercial products, simply interchangeable—an outlook that may affect the further judgment of any embryo's moral standing. To be sure, most of these unused embryos will die or be destroyed. To be sure, if these unused embryos are otherwise destined for destruction, a case can be made—and debated—that their unavoidable loss should be redeemed by putting them to use beforehand. But the moral question regarding their possible use and destruction should not be decided—here, as elsewhere—on terminological grounds, in this case, by the naming of the embryo "*spare.*" Rather it should be decided on the basis of a direct moral appraisal of the rights and goods involved: on the basis of what we owe to suffering humanity and the obligations we have to seek the means of its relief; and on the basis of the nature of human embryos, what we owe them as proper respect and regard, and whether and why such respect or regard may be overridden. For many people, the moral question depends, in other words, on what some bioethicists call—and we ourselves will sometimes call—"the *moral status* of *the* embryo." If embryos lacked all "moral status," there would be little moral argument about their use and destruction.

Yet the notion "moral status" is problematic, even though it is easy to understand why it has come into fashion. For many people, the central ethical question regarding embryonic stem cell research is whether an embryonic organism from which cells may be removed to develop ES cells is fully "one of us," deserving the same kind of respect and protection as a newborn baby, child, or adult. What they want to know is the *moral* standing of these organisms—entities that owe their existence, their extra-uterine situation, and their "spare-ness" to deliberate human agency—at such early stages of development. As we shall see, some people try to find structural or functional markers—for example, the familiar human form or the presence or absence of sensation—to decide the moral worth of a human embryo. Others use an argument from continuity of development to rebut any attempt to find a morally significant boundary anywhere along the continuum of growth and change. But, to judge from countless efforts to provide a biologically based criterion for ascribing full human worth, it seems certain that we shall never find an answer to our moral question in biology *alone*, even as the answers we give must take into account the truths of embryology. At least until now, philosophical attempts to draw moral inferences from the biological facts have not yielded conclusions that all find necessary or sound.

Under these circumstances, some people believe that we have no choice but to stipulate or ascribe some degree of moral "status" to the entity, based either on how it strikes us and the limited range of what we are able to know about it, or on what we wish to do with it: we confer upon it some moral status *in regard to us*, much as we confer one or another class of immigration status upon people. For this very reason, others object to the term, fearing that it enables us to beg the question of the intrinsic moral worth or dignity of the entity *itself*, seen in its own terms and without regard to us. Different members of this Council hold different views of this terminological and ontological matter, but we all recognize the moral freight carried by attempts to speak about and ascribe "moral *status*" to human embryos in their earliest stage of development. We encourage readers to be self-conscious about this and similar terms, even as we proceed ourselves to make use of them.

Ethical Issues in Human Stem Cell Research

Vol. 3, Religious Perspectives

NATIONAL BIOETHICS ADVISORY COMMISSION 2000

From http://bioethics.georgetown.edu/nbac/stemcell3.pdf

Testimony of Rabbi Elliot N. Dorff, Ph.D., University of Judaism

Stem Cell Research

Jewish Views of Genetic Materials

1. Because doing research on human embryonic stem cells involves procuring them from aborted fetuses, the status of abortion within Judaism is a subject that immediately arises. Within Judaism, by and large, abortion is forbidden. The fetus, during most of its gestational development, is seen as "the thigh of its mother," and neither men nor women may amputate their thigh at will, because that would be injuring their bodies, which belong to God. On the other hand, if the thigh turns gangrenous, both men and women have the positive duty to have their thigh amputated in order to save their lives. Similarly, if a pregnancy endangers a woman's life or health, an abortion *must* be performed to save her life or protect her physical or mental health, for she is without question a full-fledged human being with all the protections of Jewish law, while the fetus is still only part of the woman's body. When there is an elevated risk to the woman beyond that of normal pregnancy, but insufficient risk to constitute a clear threat to her life or health, abortion is permitted, but it is not required. That is an assessment that the woman should make in consultation with her physician. Some recent authorities also would permit abortions in cases where genetic testing indicates that the fetus will suffer from a terminal disease such as Tay-Sachs or from serious malformations.

The Jewish stance on abortion, then, is that *if* a fetus was aborted for legitimate reasons under Jewish law, it may be used to advance our efforts to preserve the life and health of others. In general, when a person dies, we must show honor to God's body by burying it as soon as possible after death. To benefit the lives of others, however, autopsies may be performed when the cause of death is not fully understood, and organ transplants are allowed to enable other people to live. The fetus, as I have said, does not have the status of a full-fledged human being. Therefore, if we can use the body of a human being to enable others to live, how much the more so may we use a part of a body—in this case, the fetus—for that purpose. This all presumes that the fetus was aborted for good and sufficient reason within the parameters of Jewish law.

2. Stem cells for research purposes also can be procured from donated sperm and eggs mixed together and cultured in a petri dish. Genetic materials outside the uterus have no legal status in Jewish law, for they are not even a part of a human being until implanted in a woman's womb, and even then, during the first 40 days of gestation, their status is "as if they were simply water." Abortion is still prohibited during that time, except for therapeutic purposes, for in the uterus such gametes have the potential of growing into a human being. Outside the womb, however, at least at this time, they have no such potential. As a result, frozen embryos

may be discarded or used for reasonable purposes and so may the stem cells that are procured from them.

Other Factors in This Decision

1. Given that the materials for stem cell research can be procured in permissible ways, the technology itself is morally neutral. It gains its moral valence on the basis of what we do with it.

2. The question, then, is reduced to a risk-benefit analysis of stem cell research. I want to note only two things about [this] from a Jewish perspective:

   a. The Jewish tradition views the provision of health care as a communal responsibility, and so justice arguments have a special resonance for me as a Jew. Especially because much of the basic science in this area was funded by the government, the government has the right to require private companies to provide their applications of that science at reduced rates, or if necessary, at no cost, to those who cannot afford them. At the same time, the Jewish tradition does not demand socialism, and for many good reasons we in the United States have adopted a modified, capitalistic system of economics. The trick, then, will be to balance access to applications of the new technology with the legitimate right of a private company to make a profit on its efforts to develop and market those applications.

   b. The potential of stem cell research for creating organs for transplant and cures for diseases is, at least in theory, both awesome and hopeful. Indeed, in light of our divine mandate to seek to maintain life and health, one might even argue that from a Jewish perspective we have a *duty* to proceed with that research. As difficult as it may be, we must draw a clear line between uses of this or any other technology for cure, which are to be applauded, as opposed to uses of this technology for enhancement, which must be approached with extreme caution. Jews have been the brunt of campaigns of positive eugenics both here, in the United States, and in Nazi Germany, and so we are especially sensitive to creating a model human being that is to be replicated through the kind of genetic engineering that stem cell applications will involve. Moreover, when Jews see a disabled human being, we are not to recoil from the disability or count our blessings for not being disabled in that way; rather, we are commanded to recite a blessing thanking God for making people different. Thus, in light of the Jewish view that all human beings are created in the image of God, regardless of their levels of ability or disability, it is imperative from a Jewish perspective that the applications of stem cell research be used for cure and not for enhancement.

Recommendation

My recommendation is that we take the steps necessary to advance stem cell research and its applications in an effort to take advantage of its great potential for good. We should do so, however, in such a way that we provide access to its applications to all Americans who need them and at the same time prohibit the development of applications intended to make all human beings fit any particular model of human excellence. Through this technology, we should seek to cure diseases and to appreciate the variety of God's creatures.

Testimony of Margaret A. Farley, Ph.D., Yale University

Roman Catholic Views on Research Involving Human Embryonic Stem Cells

At the heart of the Catholic tradition, there is a conviction that creation is itself revelatory and knowledge of the requirements of respect for created beings is accessible at least in part to human reason. This is what is at stake in the Catholic tradition's understanding of natural law. For most of its history, a Catholic natural law theory has not assumed that morality can simply be "read off" of nature, not even with the important help of Scripture. Nonetheless, what natural law theory does is tell us where to look—that is, to the concrete reality of the world around us, to the basic needs and possibilities of human persons in relation to one another, and to the world as a whole. "Looking" (to concrete reality) means a complex process of discernment and deliberation, and a structuring of insights and determination of meaning, from the fullest vantage point available, given a particular history—one that includes the illumination of Scripture and the accumulated wisdom of the tradition. The limits, yet necessity, of this process account for many of the disagreements about specific matters, even within the faith community.

This brings us, then, to disagreements regarding human embryonic stem cell research. Those who stand within the Catholic tradition tend to "look" to the reality of stem cells and, what is more relevant in this instance, to the realities of the sources of stem cells for current research—that is, human embryos and fetuses. Within the Catholic tradition, a case can be made both against and for such research—each dependent upon different interpretations of the moral status of the human embryo and the aborted human fetus. There are, first, a significant number of Catholics, who make the case *against*. They argue that human embryos must be protected on a par with human persons—at least to the extent that they should not be either created or destroyed merely for research purposes. Moreover, the use of aborted fetuses as a source for stem cells, while not in one sense different from the harvesting of tissue from any human cadavers, nonetheless should be prohibited because it is complicit with and offers a possible incentive for elective abortion. (If the fetuses in question have been spontaneously aborted, however, some opening is allowed for their use in this research.) Part of the case against embryo stem cell research also rests on the identification of alternatives (the use of adult cells, dedifferentiated and redifferentiated into specific lineages). One can also presume that the case against embryo stem cell research includes a case against cloning, if and insofar as this research incorporates steps involved in procedures for cloning.

But on the other hand, a case *for* human embryo stem cell research can also be made on the basis of positions developed within the Catholic tradition. A growing number of Catholic moral theologians, for example, do not consider the human embryo in its earliest stages (prior to the development of the primitive streak or to implantation) to constitute an individualized human entity with the settled inherent potential to become a human person. The moral status of the embryo is, therefore (in this view), not that of a person, and its use for certain kinds of research can be justified. (Because it is, however, a form of human life, it is due some respect—for example, it should not be bought or sold.) Those who would make this case argue for a return to the centuries-old Catholic position that a certain amount of development is necessary in order for a conceptus to warrant personal status. Embryological studies now show that fertilization ("conception") is itself a process (not a "moment"), and such studies provide support for the opinion that in its earliest stages (including the blastocyst stage, when stem cells would be extracted for purposes of research) the embryo is not sufficiently individualized to bear the moral weight of personhood. Moreover, some of the concerns regarding the use of aborted fetuses as a source for stem cells can be alleviated if safeguards (such as ruling out "direct" donation for this purpose) are put in place—not unlike the restrictions articulated for the general use of fetal tissue for therapeutic transplantation. And finally, concerns about cloning may be at least partially addressed by insisting on an absolute barrier between cloning for research and therapeutic purposes on the one hand and cloning for reproductive purposes on the other (the latter, of course, raising many more serious ethical questions than the former).

We have, then, two opposing cases articulated within the Roman Catholic tradition. It would be a mistake to conclude that what this tradition has to offer, however, is only a kind of "draw." It offers, rather, an ongoing process of discernment that remains faithful to a larger set of theological and ethical convictions, that takes account of the best that science can tell us about some aspects of reality, and that aims to make one or the other case persuasive on the basis of reasons whose intelligibility is open to the scrutiny of all. I myself stand with the case *for* embryonic stem cell research, and I believe this case can be made persuasively both within the Catholic tradition and in the public forum. The newest information we have from embryological studies supports this case, and I would argue that it can be made without sacrificing the tradition's commitments to respect human life, promote human well-being, and honor the sacred in created realities. Further, to move forward with human embryonic stem cell research need not soften the tradition's concerns to oppose the commercialization of human life and to promote distributive justice in the provision of medical care.

Testimony of Gilbert C. Meilaender, Jr., Ph.D., Valparaiso University

As I understand it, I have been invited to speak specifically in my capacity as a Protestant theologian, and I will try to do so. At the same time, I cannot claim to speak for Protestants generally—alas, no one can. I will, however, try to draw on several theologians who speak from within different strands of Protestantism. I think you can and should assume that a significant number of my co-religionists more or less agree with the points I will make. You can, of course, also assume that other Protestants would disagree, even though I like to think that, were they to ponder these matters long enough, they would not.

I will make two points. For each of the points, I will take as my starting point a sentence from a well-known Protestant thinker—not in order to claim that theologian's authority for or agreement with what I have to say, but simply to provide some "texts" with which to begin my reflections.

First, a passage from Karl Barth, perhaps the greatest of twentieth-century theologians, who writes from the Reformed (Calvinist) tradition: "No community, whether family, village or state, is really strong if it will not carry its weak and even its very weakest members."

This sentence invites us to ponder the status of the human embryo—the source of many, though not all, of the stem cells that would be used in research. One of the complexities that I do not fully understand involves the question of whether stem cells are not themselves and cannot develop into embryos. I will assume that they are not and cannot, although perhaps I need to be instructed further on this matter. Even in making this assumption, however, we face the fact that procuring embryonic stem cells for research requires the destruction of the embryo. Hence, we cannot avoid thinking about its moral status.

No doubt in our society it is impossible to contemplate this question without feeling sucked back into the abortion debate, and we may sometimes have the feeling that we cannot consider any other related question without always ending up arguing about abortion. Perhaps there is something to that, and I will not entirely avoid it myself before I am done, but the question of using (and destroying) embryos in research is a separate question. The issue of abortion, as it has been framed in our society's debate and in Supreme Court decisions, has turned chiefly on a conflict between the claims of the fetus and the claims of the pregnant woman. It is precisely that conflict, and our seeming inability to serve the woman's claim without turning directly against the life of the fetus, that has been thought to justify abortion. But there is no such direct conflict of lives involved in the instance of embryo research.

Here, as in so many other areas of life, we must struggle to think inclusively rather than exclusively about the human species, about who is one of us, and about whose good should count in the common good we seek to fashion. The embryo is, I believe, the weakest and least advantaged of our fellow human beings, and no community is really strong if it will not carry its weakest members.

This is not an understanding shaped chiefly in the fires of recent political debate; rather, it has very deep roots in Christian tradition, and, invited as I have been to address you from within that tradition, I need to explore briefly those roots. We have become accustomed in recent years to distinguishing between persons and human beings, to thinking about personhood as something added to the existence of a living human being—and then to debating where to locate the time when such personhood is added. There is, however, a much older concept of the person—for which no threshold of capacities is required—that was deeply influential in Western history and that had its roots in some of the most central Christian affirmations.

Christians believed that in Jesus of Nazareth, divine and human natures were joined in one person, and, of course, they understood that it was not easy to make sense of such a claim. For if Jesus had both divine and human natures, he would seem to be two persons, two individuals, identified in terms of two sets of personal capacities or characteristics—a sort of chimera, we might say, in terms appropriate to this gathering.

So Christian thinkers turned in a different direction that was very influential in our culture's understanding of what it means to be an individual. In their view, a person is not someone who has a certain set of capacities; a person is simply, as Oliver O'Donovan puts it, a "someone who"—a someone who has a history. That story, for each of us, begins before we are conscious of it, and, for many of us, may continue after we have lost consciousness of it. It is nonetheless our personal history even when we lack awareness of it, even when we lack or have lost certain capacities characteristic of the species.

This is, as I noted, an insight that grew originally out of intricate Christological debates carried on by thinkers every bit as profound as any we today are likely to encounter. But starting from that very definite point, they opened up for us a vision of the person that carries deep human wisdom, that refuses to think of personhood as requiring certain capacities, and that therefore honors the time and place of each someone who has a history. In honoring the dignity of even the weakest of living human beings—the embryo—we come to appreciate the mystery of the human person and the mystery of our own individuality.

Second, a sentence from the late John Howard Yoder, a well-known Mennonite theologian: "I am less likely to look for a saving solution if I have told myself beforehand that there can be none, or have made advance provision for an easy brutal one."

Stem cell research is offered to us as a kind of saving solution, and it is not surprising therefore that we should grasp at it. Although I suspect that promises and possibilities could easily be oversold, none of us should pretend to be indifferent to attempts to relieve or cure heart disease, Parkinson's and Alzheimer's diseases, or diabetes. Suffering, and even death, are not the greatest evils of human life, but they are surely bad enough—and all honor goes to those who set their face against such ills and seek to relieve them.

The sentence from Yoder reminds us, however, that we may sometimes need to deny ourselves the handiest means to an undeniably good end. In this case the desired means will surely involve the creation of embryos for research—and then their destruction. The human will, seeing a desired end, takes control, subjecting to its desire even the living human organism. We need to ask ourselves whether this is a road we really want to travel to the very end. Learning to think of human beings as will and freedom alone has been the long and steady project of modernity. At least since Kant, ethics has often turned to the human will as the only source of value. But C. S. Lewis, an Anglican and surely one of the most widely read of twentieth-century Christian thinkers, depicted what happens when we ourselves become the object of this mastering will:

> We reduce things to mere Nature in order that we may 'conquer' them. We are always conquering Nature, because 'nature' is the name for what we have to some extent conquered. The price of conquest is to treat a thing as mere Nature. . . . The stars do not become Nature till we can weigh and measure them: the soul does not become Nature till we can psycho-analyse her. The wresting of powers from Nature is also the surrendering of things to Nature. As long as this process stops short of the final stage we may well hold that the gain outweighs the loss.

> But as soon as we take the final step of reducing our own species to the level of mere Nature, the whole process is stultified, for this time the being who stood to gain and the being who has been sacrificed are one and the same. This is one of the many instances where to carry a principle to what seems its logical conclusion produces absurdity. It is like the famous Irishman who found that a certain kind of stove reduced his fuel bill by half and thence concluded that two stoves of the same kind would enable him to warm his house with no fuel at all. . . . [I]f man chooses to treat himself as raw material, raw material he will be.

What Yoder reminds us is that only by stopping, only by declining to exercise our will in this way, do we force ourselves to look for other possible ways to achieve admittedly desirable ends. Only by declining to use embryos for this research do we awaken our imaginations and force ourselves to seek other sources for stem cells—as may be possible, for example, if recent reports are to be believed, by deriving stem cells from bone marrow or from the placenta or umbilical cord in live births. The discipline of saying no to certain proposed means stimulates us to think creatively about other, and better, possibilities.

Testimony of Abdulaziz Sachedina, Ph.D., University of Virginia

Islamic Perspectives on Research with Human Embryonic Stem Cells

The ethical-religious assessment of research uses of pluripotent stem cells derived from human embryos in Islam can be inferentially deduced from the rulings of the Shari`a, Islamic law, that deal with fetal viability and the sanctity of the embryo in the classical and modern juristic decisions. The Shari`a treats a second source of cells, those derived from fetal tissue following abortion, as analogically similar to cadaver donation for organ transplantation in order to save other lives, and hence, the use of cells from that source is permissible.

Based on theological and ethical considerations derived from the Koranic passages that describe the embryonic journey to personhood developmentally and the rulings that treat ensoulment and personhood as occurring over time almost synonymously, it is correct to suggest that a majority of the Sunni and Shi`ite jurists will have little problem in endorsing ethically regulated research on the stem cells that promises potential therapeutic value, provided that the expected therapeutic benefits are not simply speculative.

The inception of embryonic life is an important moral and social question in the Muslim community. Anyone who has followed Muslim debate over this question notices that its answer has differed at different times and in proportion to the scientific information available to the jurists. Accordingly, each period of Islamic jurisprudence has come up with its ruling (*fatwa*), consistent with the findings of science and technology available at that time. The search for a satisfactory answer regarding when an embryo attains legal rights has continued to this day.

The life of a fetus inside the womb, according to the Koran, goes through several stages, which are described in a detailed and precise manner.

In the chapter entitled "The Believers" (24), we read the following verses:

> We created (*khalaqna*) man of an extraction of clay, then We set him, a drop in a safe lodging, then We created of the drop a clot, then We created of the clot a tissue, then We created of the tissue bones, then we covered the bones in flesh; thereafter We produced it as another creature. So blessed be God, the Best of creators (*khaliqin*) (K. 24:12–14)!

In another place, the Koran specifically speaks about "breathing His own spirit" after God forms human beings:

> Human progeny He creates from a drop of sperm; He fashions his limbs and organs in perfect proportion and breathes into him from His own Spirit (*ruh*). And He gives you ears, eyes, and a heart. These bounties warrant your sincere gratitude, but little do you give thanks (K. 41:9–10).

> And your Lord said to the angels: 'I am going to create human from clay. And when I have given him form and breathed into him of My life force (*ruh*), you must all show respect by bowing down before him' (K. 38:72–73).

The commentators of the Koran, who were in most cases legal scholars, drew some important conclusions from this and other passages that describe the development of an embryo to a full human person. First, human creation is part of the divine will that determines the embryonic journey developmentally to a human creature. Second, it suggests that moral personhood is a process and achievement at the later stage in biological development of the embryo when God says: "*thereafter* We produced him as another creature." The adverb "thereafter" clarifies the stage at which a fetus attains personhood. Third, it raises questions in Islamic law of inheritance as well as punitive justice, where the rights and indemnity of the fetus are recognized as a person, whether the fetus should be accorded the status of a legal-moral person once it lodges in the uterus in the earlier stage. Fourth, as the subsequent juridical extrapolations bear out, the Koranic embryonic development allows for a possible distinction between a biological and moral person because of its silence over a particular point when the ensoulment occurs.

Earlier rulings on indemnity for homicide in the Shari`a were deduced on the premise that the life of a fetus began with the appreciation of its palpable movements inside the mother's womb, which occurs around the fourth month of pregnancy. In addition to the Koran, the following tradition on creation of human progeny provided the evidence for the concrete divide in pre- and post-ensoulment periods of pregnancy:

Each one of you possesses his own formation within his mother's womb, first as a drop of matter for forty days, then as a blood clot for forty days, then as a blob for forty days, and then the angel is sent to breath life into him (*Sahih al-Bukhari* [d. 870] and *Sahih al-Muslim* [d. 875], The Book of Destiny [*qadar*]).

Ibn Hajar al-`Asqalani (d. 1449) commenting on the above tradition says:

The first organ that develops in a fetus is the stomach because it needs to feed itself by means of it. Alimentation has precedence over all other functions for in the order of nature growth depends on nutrition. It does not need sensory perception or voluntary movement at this stage because it is like a plant. However, it is given sensation and volition when the soul (nafs) attaches itself to it (*Fath al-bari fi sharh al-Sahih al-bukhari, kitab al-qadar*, 11:482).

A majority of the Sunni and some Shi`ite scholars make a distinction between two stages in pregnancy divided by the end of the fourth month (120 days) when the ensoulment takes place. On the other hand, a majority of the Shi`ite and some Sunni jurists have exercised caution in making such a distinction because they regard the embryo in the pre-ensoulment stages as alive and its eradication as a sin. That is why Sunni jurists in general allow justifiable abortion within that period, while all schools agree that the sanctity of fetal life must be acknowledged after the fourth month.

The classical formulations based on the Koran and the Tradition provide no universally accepted definition of the term "embryo." Nor do these two foundational sources define the exact moment when a fetus becomes a moral-legal being. With the progress in the study of anatomy and in embryology, it is confirmed beyond any doubt that life begins inside the womb at the very moment of conception, right after fertilization and the production of a zygote. Consequently, from the earliest stage of its conception, an embryo is said to be a living creature with sanctity whose life must be protected against aggression. This opinion is held by Dr. Hassan Hathout, a physician by training, who was unable to be here today. This scientific information has turned into a legal-ethical dispute among Muslim jurists over the permissibility of abortion during the first trimester and the destruction of unused embryos, which would, according to this information, be regarded as living beings in the *in vitro* fertilization clinics. Some scholars have called for ignoring the sanctity of fetal life and permitting its termination at that early stage.

A tenable conclusion held by a number of prominent Sunni and Shi`ite scholars suggests that aggression against the human fetus is unlawful. Once it is established that the fetus is alive, the crime against it is regarded as a crime against a fully formed human being. According to these scholars, science and experience have unfolded new horizons that have left no room for doubt in determining signs of life from the moment of conception. Yet, as participants in the act of creating and curing with God, human beings can actively engage in furthering the overall good of humanity by intervening in the works of nature, including the early stages of embryonic development, to improve human health.

The question that still remains to be answered by Muslim jurists in the context of embryonic stem cell research is, When does the union of a sperm and an ovum entail sanctity and rights in the Shari`a? Most of modern Muslim opinions speak of a moment beyond the blastocyst stage when a fetus turns into a human being. Not every living organism in a uterus is entitled to the same degree of sanctity and honor as is a fetus at the turn of the first trimester.

The anatomical description of the fetus as it follows its course from conception to a full human person has been closely compared to the tradition about three periods of 40-day gestation to conclude that the growth of a well-defined form and evidence of voluntary movement mark the ensoulment. This opinion is based on a classical ruling given by a prominent Sunni jurist, Ibn al-Qayyim (d. 1350):

> Does an embryo move voluntarily or have sensation before the ensoulment? It is said that it grows and feeds like a plant. It does not have voluntary movement or alimentation. When ensoulment takes place voluntary movement and alimentation is added to it (*Ibn al-Qayyim, al-Tibyan fi aqsam al-qur'an*, 255).

Since there is no unified juridical-religious body representing the entire Muslim community globally, different countries have followed different classical interpretations of fetal viability. Thus, for instance, Saudi Arabia, might choose to follow Ibn Qayyim; while Egypt might follow Ibn Hajar al-`Asqalani. We need to keep in mind that the same plurality of the tradition is operative in North America when it comes to making ethical decisions on any of the controversial matters in medical ethics. Nevertheless, on the basis of all the evidence examined for this testimony, it is possible to propose the following as acceptable to all schools of thought in Islam:

1. The Koran and the Tradition regard perceivable human life as possible at the *later* stages of the biological development of the embryo.
2. The fetus is accorded the status of a legal person only at the later stages of its development, when perceptible form and voluntary movement are demonstrated. Hence, in earlier stages, such as when it lodges itself in the uterus and begins its journey to personhood, the embryo cannot be considered as possessing moral status.
3. The silence of the Koran over a criterion for moral status (i.e., when the ensoulment occurs) of the fetus allows the jurists to make a distinction between a biological and a moral person, placing the latter stage after, at least, the first trimester of pregnancy.

Finally, the Koran takes into account the problem of human arrogance, which takes the form of rejection of God's frequent reminders to humanity that God's immutable laws are dominant in nature and that human beings cannot willfully interfere to cause damage to others. "The will of God" in the Koran has often been interpreted as the processes of nature uninterfered with by human action. Hence, in Islam, research on stem cells made possible by biotechnical intervention in the early stages of life is regarded as an act of faith in the ultimate will of God as the Giver of all life, as long as such an intervention is undertaken with the purpose of improving human health.

Research with Human Embryonic Stem Cells

Ethical Considerations

GERON ETHICS ADVISORY BOARD: KAREN LEBACQZ, MICHAEL M. MENDIOLA, TED PETERS, ERNLÉ W. D. YOUNG, AND LAURIE ZOLOTH-DORFMAN

Hastings Center Report 29, no. 2 (1999): 31–36.

On 5 November 1998 Geron Corporation announced that scientists working in collaboration with Geron had succeeded in establishing cell culture lines of human embryonic stem (hES) cells. Because these cells are considered pluripotent (capable of being the precursors to a variety of human cell types) and immortal (sustainable in culture and reproducing themselves indefinitely), they represent a major breakthrough in scientific research, with potential for significant advances in tissue transplantation, pharmaceutical testing, and embryology.

Prior to the November announcement, the Geron Ethics Advisory Board developed "A Statement on Human Embryonic Stem Cells" as a set of guidelines for hES research.* This essay provides an expansion and elaboration of the particular warrants and moral reasoning for that statement.

Research with Embryonic Stem Cells

1. "The blastocyst must be treated with the respect appropriate to early human embryonic tissue."

The creation of hES cells involves isolation of cells from the blastocyst. The blastocyst consists of an outer cellular layer, which would develop as the placenta, and an inner cell mass, which would develop as the body of the fetus. The outer layer is dissolved and the resulting mass of cells is used for research. Thus a central ethical issue is the moral status of the blastocyst.

To raise the matter of "moral status" is to ask, Does a given entity possess the requisite qualities or characteristics that entitle it to moral consideration and concern? "Moral status" thus functions as a threshold idea: entities with moral status should be treated in a manner differently from entities without that status. The EAB affirms that the blastocyst has moral status and hence should be treated with respect.

What sort of moral status does the blastocyst have? Some have argued for conception as the relevant consideration, others for the development of the "primitive streak" (the precursor to the spinal cord of an individual fetus) as a defining moment, and some for utilizing implantation as the crucial threshold for moral status.

Reviewing the complex literature on this topic, Ted Peters, following Daniel Callahan, distinguishes three basic schools of thought. The *genetic school* locates the beginning of human personhood, and thus claims of moral status and dignity, at the genetic beginning—that is, at conception, at the point where one's individual genome is set. Here, a criterion for moral status (human genetic heritage) is linked to a particular point in human life (conception). The *developmental school*, while granting that human life begins at conception, holds equally that human *personhood*—and hence *full* moral status—is a later development. Here, moral status is understood developmentally: as the conceptus develops from blastocyst to fetus and beyond so too does moral status grow

---

* An Ethics Advisory Board, whose members represent a variety of philosophical and theological traditions with a breadth of experience in health care ethics, was created by Geron Corporation in 1998. The Board functions as an independent entity, consulting and giving advice to the corporation on ethical aspects of the work Geron sponsors. Members of the board have no financial interest in Geron Corporation.

(although proponents differ on when exactly the threshold of moral status is reached). The *social consequences school* shares with the developmental school the belief that human personhood is a process and an achievement over time. Advocates deny, however, that personhood is achieved at any particular moment. Rather, "personhood" is a matter of definition rather than biological fact, based on socially constructed norms.

In its work, the National Institutes of Health Human Embryo Research Panel focused less on the time when moral status might be acquired and more on the *criteria* for its determination. The panel noted two broad approaches in the debates: one proposes a single criterion as constitutive of moral personhood, while a second, "pluralistic," approach emphasizes a number of different, interacting criteria. As the panel noted

> Among the qualities considered under a pluralistic approach are those mentioned in single-criterion views: genetic uniqueness, potentiality for development, sentience, brain activity, and degree of cognitive development. Other qualities often mentioned are human form, capacity for survival outside the mother's womb, and degree of relational presence (whether to the mother herself or to others). Although none of these qualities is by itself sufficient to establish personhood, their developing presence in an entity increases its moral status until, at some point, full and equal protectability is required.

The panel proposed the pluralistic approach as the more adequate of the two, with moral status (and hence protectability) understood developmentally, culminating at birth in full and equal personhood.

Drawing upon this wealth of philosophical and theological reflection and situating ourselves relative to it, the EAB affirmed our understanding of moral status as developmental and consonant with the pluralistic approach. This developmental view is in accord with Jewish tradition, with the views of many Roman Catholics (although not the Vatican), and with the

majority of Protestant traditions as well as with legal traditions that provide different protections at different stages of fetal development.

We hold that a fundamental principle of respect for human life applies at all stages of human development. The developmental view that we affirm does not mean that the principle of respect can be ignored; it means that the principle requires different considerations and entails different obligations at different developmental stages. Once there is evidence of capacity for sensation, for example, respect requires minimization of pain. In this very early embryonic tissue there is no capacity for sensation; thus minimization of pain does not apply. Rather, early embryonic tissue is respected by ensuring that it is used with care only in research that incorporates substantive values such as reduction of human suffering. We believe that the purposes of the hES research—its potential to contribute to fundamental knowledge of human development and to medical and pharmaceutical interventions to alleviate suffering—provide such substantive values.

A second source of cells is human embryonic germ (hEG) cells derived from gamete ridge tissue removed from early fetal tissue following elective abortion. These cells have been cultured using similar but not identical methods as are used for the hES cells, and may have both properties of pluripotency and immortality. However, this research raises ethical questions distinct from those in the use of the early blastocyst. The tissue is taken (much as cadaver organs might be taken) from an aborted fetus within the first eight weeks after conception. At stake in this debate is whether licit use can be made of tissue collected after abortion in a society in which the act of abortion is seen by some as murderous and by others (and by law) as acceptable.

The EAB cannot resolve the contentious abortion debate. We are developing guidelines for hEG research. Preliminary reflections suggest at least the following concerns: First, all agree that the demise of the fetus is not caused by the research procedures. Second, the moral obligation to save life may be a sufficiently strong warrant to justify certain uses of the tissue of the dead and hence to support such research. Third, the tissue of the dead must be used with respect. Respect for tissue taken from a dead fetus would take into account the need for closure, grief, and ritual that families might have in these cases. Respect would include the confidential and dignified handling of the tissue when collected and used. Finally, issues of informed consent would apply with the same stringency required in the case of hES research (see below).

2. "Women/couples donating blastocysts produced in the process of in vitro fertilization must give full and informed consent for the use of the blastocysts in research and in the development of cell lines from that tissue."

Human embryonic stem cells are derived from embryos produced for clinical purposes and then donated for research purposes. Hence of crucial ethical significance is the character and quality of the consent given by women and couples to such donation. What is needed for valid consent to donate embryonic tissue for research purposes?

Consent to utilize embryos for *clinical* purposes of IVF does not suffice as consent for their use in research and cell-line development. Explicit consent must be elicited for such use. We concur with Arthur Caplan that "when research is the goal, whether for profit or not, those whose materials are to be used have a right to know and consent to such use." Couples donating embryos for this research should understand clearly the nature of the research and also should understand whether there are commercial implications and if so, whether they hold any proprietary rights in the tissue lines developed from embryonic cells.

Moreover, we believe that the context of embryo donation within the process of IVF renders the need for careful consent even more important. The IVF process is often physically painful, emotionally burdensome, and financially costly. These factors may make IVF patients particularly vulnerable.

In the course of our deliberations, we reviewed an exemplary form used in soliciting consent for embryo donation for research. This form states explicitly: "cells that may be derived from embryos donated for this research could have clinical and commercial value in the event that the study is successful." It further specifies:

> This research will not benefit your clinical care, and you will not benefit financially from it. The physicians/clinicians involved in your care will not benefit financially from this study. The investigators conducting this study could benefit financially from clinical or commercial values that may result from it. The cells derived in this study may be shared with Geron Corporation, located in Menlo Park, CA, as part of the study. Geron Corporation may benefit financially from the development and clinical use of the cells derived in this study.

Such explicit statements embody well the kinds of financial disclosure that a consent form should contain.

3. "The hES research will not involve any cloning for purposes of human reproduction, any transfer to a uterus, or any creation of human chimeras or human-animal hybrids."

Corporate representatives have stated clearly to the EAB that human reproduction was not a goal, purpose, or intent of Geron's research on hES (and hEG) cells. Any effort to produce a living being out of this research would raise a host of ethical issues, in particular the risk of harms to potential offspring, to parenting women and couples, and to the human community itself through genetic manipulation and transmission.

4. "Acquisition and development of the feeder layer necessary for the growth of hES cells in vitro must not violate accepted norms for human or animal research."

To keep hES cells in an undifferentiated state, they are cultured and maintained on layers of nutrients called "feeder layers." Currently, irradiated mouse embryonic fibroblast feeder layers are utilized, but it is possible that other tissues would be used in the future. The acquisition and development of the feeder layers must be in accord with norms for research appropriate to the source from which the feeder layers are drawn.

Geron's use of mouse embryonic cells would seem to fall well within a judgment of ethical use of animal tissue. The research holds great potential therapeutic value. In addition, mouse embryos fall below the threshold of sentience (the ability to experience pain) or of other capacities of organic animal being and activity. Nevertheless, we mandate continued attention to animal welfare.

5. "All such research must be done in a context of concern for global justice."

One of the primary justifications of hES research is beneficence based: its therapeutic potential to alleviate human suffering and to promote the health and well-being of human populations. However, to justify a practice on the basis of its benefits makes moral sense only if people in need actually have access to those benefits. Hence the justification gains credibility only when it is wedded to a commitment to justice, rooted in "a recognition of our sociality and mutual vulnerability to disease and death." *The EAB considers concerns about social justice in public health to be of overriding importance.* Thus in the EAB's judgment, it is morally paramount that research development include attention to the global distribution of and access to these therapeutic interventions.

Two features of Geron's research render this commitment to just access particularly challenging. First, the research is undertaken in the private sector—in the context of market forces, patenting of products, interests of shareholders and investors, and a consideration of profit. These varied interests may compete with—but should not override—a concern for equitable access. Second, the research is highly technological and expensive, as well as under the proprietary rights of a U.S. company. How to ensure adequate access for insured, underinsured, and noninsured patients in the United States, let alone on a global basis, will be an ethically and financially challenging task. The EAB will continue to work with Geron on these matters.

The Ethics of Animal Research
What Are the Prospects for Agreement?

DAVID DEGRAZIA

Cambridge Quarterly of Healthcare Ethics 8 (1999): 23–24.

Few human uses of nonhuman animals (hereafter simply "animals") have incited as much controversy as the use of animals in biomedical research. The political exchanges over this issue tend to produce much more heat than light, as representatives of both biomedicine and the animal protection community accuse opponents of being "Nazis," "terrorists," and the like. However, a healthy number of individuals within these two communities offer the possibility of a more illuminating discussion of the ethics of animal research.

One such individual is Henry Spira. Spira almost single-handedly convinced Avon, Revlon, and other major cosmetics companies to invest in the search for alternatives to animal testing. Largely due to his tactful but persistent engagement with these companies—and to their willingness to change—many consumers today look for such labels as "not tested on animals" and "cruelty free" on cosmetics they would like to buy.

Inspired by Spira, this paper seeks common ground between the positions of biomedicine and animal advocates. (The term "biomedicine" here refers to everyone who works in medicine or the life sciences, not just those conducting animal research. "Animal advocates" and "animal protection community" refer to those individuals who take a major interest in protecting the interests of animals and who believe that much current usage of animals is morally unjustified. The terms are not restricted to animal activists, because some individuals meet this definition without being politically active in seeking changes.)

This paper begins with some background on the political and ethical debate over animal research. It then identifies important points of potential agreement between biomedicine and animal advocates; much of this common ground can be missed due to distraction by the fireworks of the current political exchange. Next, the paper enumerates issues on which continuing disagreement is likely. Finally, it concludes with concrete suggestions for building positively on the common ground.

Background on the Debate over Animal Research

What is the current state of the debate over the ethics of animal research? Let us begin with the viewpoint of biomedicine. It seems fair to say that biomedicine has a "party line" on the ethics of animal research, conformity to which may feel like a political litmus test for full acceptability within the professional community. According to this party line, animal research is clearly justified because it is necessary for medical progress and therefore human health—and those who disagree are irrational, antiscience, misanthropic "extremists" whose views do not deserve serious attention. (Needless to say, despite considerable conformity, not everyone in biomedicine accepts this position.)

In at least some countries, biomedicine's leadership apparently values conformity to this party line more than freedom of thought and expression on the animal research issue. (In this paragraph, I will refer to the American situation to illustrate the point.) Hence the unwillingness of major

medical journals, such as *JAMA* and *The New England Journal of Medicine*, to publish articles that are highly critical of animal research. Hence also the extraordinary similarity I have noticed in pro-research lectures by representatives of biomedicine. I used to be puzzled about why these lectures sounded so similar and why, for example, they consistently made some of the same philosophical and conceptual errors (such as dichotomizing animal welfare and animal rights, and taking the latter concept to imply identical rights for humans and animals). But that was before I learned of the "AMA [American Medical Association] Animal Research Action Plan" and the AMA's "White Paper." Promoting an aggressive pro-research campaign, these documents encourage AMA members to say and do certain things for public relations purposes, including the following: "Identify animal rights activists as anti-science and against medical progress"; "Combat emotion with emotion (eg [sic], 'fuzzy' animals contrasted with 'healing' children)"; and "Position the biomedical community as moderate—centrist—in the controversy, not as a polar opposite."

It is a reasonable conjecture that biomedicine's party line was developed largely in reaction to fear—both of the most intimidating actions of some especially zealous animal advocates, such as telephoned threats and destruction of property, and of growing societal concern about animals. Unfortunately, biomedicine's reaction has created a political culture in which many or most animal researchers and their supporters do not engage in sustained, critical thinking about the moral status of animals and the basic justification (or lack thereof) for animal research. Few seem to recognize that there is significant merit to the opposing position, fewer have had any rigorous training in ethical reasoning, and hardly any have read much of the leading literature on animal ethics. The stultifying effect of this cultural phenomenon hit home with me at a small meeting of representatives of biomedicine, in which I had been invited to explain "the animal rights philosophy" (the invitation itself being exceptional and encouraging). After the talk, in which

I presented ideas familiar to all who really know the literature and issues of animal ethics, several attendees pumped my hand and said something to this effect: "This is the first time I have heard such rational and lucid arguments for the other side. I didn't know there were any."

As for the animal protection community, there does not seem to be a shared viewpoint except at a very general level: significant interest in animal welfare and the belief that much current animal usage is unjustified. Beyond that, differences abound. For example, the Humane Society of the United States opposes factory farming but not humane forms of animal husbandry, rejects current levels of animal use in research but not animal research itself, and condemns most zoo exhibits but not those that adequately meet animals' needs and approximate their natural habitats. Meanwhile, the Animal Liberation Front, a clandestine British organization, apparently opposes all animal husbandry, animal research, and the keeping of zoo animals. Although there are extensive differences within the animal protection community, as far as our paper topic goes, it seems fair to say that almost everyone in this group opposes current levels of animal research.

Points on Which the Biomedical and Animal Protection Communities Can Agree

The optimistic thesis of this paper is that the biomedical and animal protection communities can agree on a fair number of important points, and that much can be done to build upon this common ground. I will number and highlight (in bold) each potential point of agreement and then justify its inclusion by explaining how both sides can agree to it, without abandoning their basic positions, and why they should.

1. The use of animals in biomedical research raises ethical issues. Today very few people would disagree with this modest claim, and any who would are clearly in the wrong. Most animal research involves harming animal subjects, provoking ethical concerns, and the leading goal of animal research, promotion of human health, is itself ethically important; even the expenditure of taxpayers' money on government-funded animal research raises ethical issues about the best use of such money. Although a very modest assertion, this point of agreement is important because it legitimates a process that is sometimes resisted: *discussing* the ethics of animal research.

It is worth noting a less obvious claim that probably enjoys strong majority support but not consensus: that animals (at least sentient ones, as defined below) have moral status. To say animals have moral status is to say that their interests have moral importance independently of effects on human interests. ('Interests' may be thought of as components of well-being. For example, sentient animals have an interest in avoiding pain, distress, and suffering.) If animals have moral status, then to brutalize a horse is wrong because of the harm inflicted on the horse, not simply because the horse is someone's property (if that is so) or because animal lovers' feelings may be hurt (if any animal lovers find out about the abuse). The idea is that gratuitously harming the horse *wrongs the horse*.

2. Sentient animals, a class that probably includes at least the vertebrates, deserve moral protection. Whether because they have moral status or because needlessly harming them strongly offends many people's sensibilities, sentient animals deserve some measure of moral protection. By way of definition, sentient animals are animals endowed with any sorts of feelings: (conscious) sensations such as pain or emotional states such as fear or suffering. But which animals are sentient? Addressing this complex issue implicates both the natural sciences and the philosophy of mind. Lately, strong support has emerged for the proposition that at least vertebrate animals are very likely sentient. This proposition is implicitly endorsed by major statements of principles regarding the humane use of research animals, which often mention that they apply to vertebrates. (Hereafter, the unqualified term "animals" will refer to sentient animals in particular.)

3. **Many animals (at the very least, mammals) are capable of having a wide variety of aversive mental states, including pain, distress (whose forms include discomfort, boredom, and fear), and suffering.** In biomedical circles, there has been some resistance to attributing suffering to animals, so goverment documents concerned with humane use of animals have often mentioned only pain, distress, and discomfort. Because "suffering" refers to a *highly* unpleasant mental state (whereas pain, distress, and discomfort can be mild and transient), the attribution of suffering to animals is morally significant. An indication that resistance may be weakening is the attribution of suffering to sentient animals in the National Aeronautics and Space Administration's "Principles for the Ethical Care and Use of Animals." Whatever government documents may say, the combined empirical and philosophical case for attributing suffering to a wide range of animals is very strong.

4. **Animals' experiential well-being (quality of life) deserves protection.** If the use of animals raises ethical issues, meaning that their interests matter morally, we confront the question of what interests animals have. This question raises controversial issues. For example, do animals have an interest in remaining alive (life interests)? That is, does death itself—as opposed to any unpleasantness experienced in dying— harm an animal? A test case would be a scenario in which a contented dog in good health is painlessly and unwittingly killed in her sleep: Is she harmed?

Another difficult issue is whether animal well-being can be understood *entirely* in terms of experiential well-being–quality of life in the familiar sense in which (other things equal) pleasure is better than pain, enjoyment better than suffering, satisfaction better than frustration. Or does the exercise of an animal's natural capacities count positively toward well-being, even if quality of life is not enhanced? A test case would be a scenario in which conditioning, a drug, or brain surgery removes a bird's instinct and desire to fly without lowering quality of life: Does the

bird's transformation to a new, nonflying existence represent a harm?

Whatever the answers to these and other issues connected with animal well-being, what is not controversial is that animals have an interest in experiential well-being, a good quality of life. That is why animal researchers are normally expected to use anesthesia or analgesia where these agents can reduce or eliminate animal subjects' pain, distress, or suffering.

5. **Humane care of highly social animals requires extensive access to conspecifics.** It is increasingly appreciated that animals have different needs based on what sorts of creatures they are. Highly social animals, such as apes, monkeys, and wolves, need social interactions with conspecifics (members of their own species). Under normal circumstances, they will develop social structures, such as hierarchies and alliances, and maintain long-term relationships with conspecifics. Because they have a strong instinct to seek such interactions and relationships, depriving them of the opportunity to gratify this instinct harms these animals. For example, in some species, lack of appropriate social interactions impedes normal development. Moreover, social companions can buffer the effects of stressful situations, reduce behavioral abnormalities, provide opportunities for exercise, and increase cognitive stimulation. Thus in the case of any highly social animals used in research, providing them extensive access to conspecifics is an extremely high moral priority.

6. **Some animals deserve very strong protections (as, for example, chimpanzees deserve not to be killed for the purpose of population control).** Biomedicine and animal advocates are likely to disagree on many details of ethically justified uses of animals in research, as we will see in the next section. Still, discussants can agree that there is an obligation to protect not just the experiential well-being, but also the lives, of at least some animals. This claim might be supported by the (controversial) thesis that such animals have life interests. On the other hand, it might be supported by the goal of species preservation (in the

case of an endangered species), or by the recognition that routine killing of such animals when they are no longer useful for research would seriously disturb many people.

Without agreeing on all the specific justifications, members of the National Research Council's Committee on Long-Term Care of Chimpanzees were able to agree (with one dissent) that chimps should not be killed for the purpose of population control, although they could be killed if suffering greatly with no alternative means of relief. This recommended protection of chimps' lives is exceptional, because animal research policies generally state no presumption against killing animal subjects, requiring only that killings be as painless as possible. Since this committee represents expert opinion in biomedicine, it seems correct to infer that biomedicine and the animal protection community can agree that at least chimpanzees should receive some very strong protections—of their lives and of certain other components of their well-being, such as their needs for social interaction, reasonable freedom of movement, and stimulating environments.

7. **Alternatives should now be used whenever possible and research on alternatives should expand.** Those who are most strongly opposed to animal research hold that alternatives such as mathematical models, computer simulations, and in vitro biological systems should replace nearly all use of animals in research. (I say "nearly all" because, as discussed below, few would condemn animal research that does not harm its subjects.) Even for those who see the animal research enterprise more favorably, there are good reasons to take an active interest in alternatives. Sometimes an alternative method is the most valid way to approach a particular scientific question; often alternatives are cheaper. Their potential for reducing animal pain, distress, and suffering is, of course, another good reason. Finally, biomedicine may enjoy stronger public support if it responds to growing social concern about animal welfare with a very serious investment in nonanimal methods. This means not just using alternatives wherever they are

currently feasible, but also aggressively researching the possibilities for expanding the use of such methods.

8. **Promoting human health is an extremely important biomedical goal.** No morally serious person would deny the great importance of human health, so its status as a worthy goal seems beyond question. What is sometimes forgotten, however, is that a worthy goal does not automatically justify all the means thereto. Surely it would be unethical to force large numbers of humans to serve as subjects in highly painful, eventually lethal research, even if its goal were to promote human health. The controversy over animal research focuses not on the worthiness of its principal goal–promoting human health—but rather on the means, involving animal subjects, taken in pursuit of that goal.

9. **There are some morally significant differences between humans and other animals.** Many people in biomedicine are not aware that the views of animal advocates are consistent with this judgment. Indeed, some animal advocates might not realize that their views are consistent with this judgment! So let me identify a couple of ideas, to which all should agree, that support it.

First, the principle of respect for autonomy applies to competent adult human beings, but to very few if any animals. This principle respects the self-regarding decisions of individuals who are capable of autonomous decisionmaking and action. Conversely, it opposes paternalism toward such individuals, who have the capacity to decide for themselves what is in their interests. Now, many sentient beings, including human children and at least most nonhuman animals, are not autonomous in the relevant sense and so are not covered by this principle. Thus it is often appropriate to limit their liberty in ways that promote their best interests, say, preventing the human child from drinking alcohol, or forcing a pet dog to undergo a vaccination. We might say that where there is no autonomy to respect, the principles of beneficence (promoting best interests) and respect for autonomy cannot conflict; where there is autonomy to respect, paternalism becomes morally problematic.

Second, even if sentient animals have an interest, others things equal, in staying alive (as I believe), the moral presumption against taking human life is stronger than the presumption against killing at least some animals. Consider fish, who are apparently sentient yet cognitively extremely primitive in comparison with humans. I have a hard time imagining even very committed animal advocates maintaining that killing a fish is as serious a matter as killing a human being. Leaders in animal ethics consistently support—though in interestingly different ways— the idea that, ordinarily, killing humans is worse than killing at least some animals who have moral status. (It is almost too obvious to mention that it's worse to kill humans than to kill animals, such as amoebas, that *lack* moral status.)

10. Some animal research is justified. Many animal advocates would say that they disagree with this statement. But I'm not sure they do. Or, if they really do, they shouldn't. Let me explain by responding to the three likeliest reasons some animal advocates might take exception to the claim.

First, one might oppose all uses of animals that involve *harming them for the benefit of others* (even other animals)–as a matter of absolute principle— and overlook the fact that some animal research does not harm animal subjects at all. Although such nonharmful research represents a tiny sliver of the animal research enterprise, it exists. Examples are certain observational studies of animals in their natural habitats, some ape language studies, and possibly certain behavioral studies of other species that take place in laboratories but do not cause pain, distress, or suffering to the subjects. And if nonsentient animals cannot be harmed (in any morally relevant sense), as I would argue, then any research involving such animals falls under the penumbra of nonharming research.

Moreover, there is arguably no good reason to oppose research that imposes only *minimal* risk or harm on its animal subjects. After all, minimal risk research on certain human subjects who, like animals, cannot consent (namely, children)

is permitted in many countries; in my view, this policy is justified. Such research might involve a minuscule likelihood of significant harm or the certainty of a slight, transient harm, such as the discomfort of having a blood sample taken.

Second, one might oppose all animal research because one believes that none of it actually benefits human beings. Due to physical differences between species, the argument goes, what happens to animal subjects when they undergo some biomedical intervention does not justify inferences about what will happen to humans who undergo that intervention. Furthermore, new drugs, therapies, and techniques must always be tried on human subjects before they can be accepted for clinical practice. Rather than tormenting animals in research, the argument continues, we should drop the useless animal models and proceed straight to human trials (with appropriate protections for human subjects, including requirements for informed or proxy consent).

Although I believe a considerable amount of current animal research has almost no chance of benefitting humans, I find it very hard to believe that no animal research does. While it is true that human subjects must eventually be experimented on, evidence suggests that animal models sometimes furnish data relevant to human health. If so, then the use of animal subjects can often decrease the risk to human subjects who are eventually involved in experiments that advance biomedicine, by helping to weed out harmful interventions. This by itself does not justify animal research, only the claim that it sometimes benefits humans (at the very least human subjects themselves and arguably the beneficiaries of biomedical advances as well).

Note that even if animal research never benefited humans, it would presumably sometimes benefit conspecifics of the animals tested, in sound veterinary research. It can't be seriously argued that animal models provide no useful information about animals! Moreover, in successful *therapeutic* research (which aims to benefit the subjects themselves), certain animals benefit directly from research and are not simply used to benefit other animals. For that reason, blanket opposition to animal research, including the most promising therapeutic research in veterinary medicine, strikes me as almost unintelligible.

Almost unintelligible, but not quite, bringing us to the third possible reason for opposing all animal research. It might be argued that, whether or not it harms its subjects, all animal research involves *using animals (without their consent) for others' benefit*, since—qua research—it seeks *generalizable knowledge*. But to use animals in this way reduces them to *tools* (objects to be used), thereby *disrespecting* the animals.

Now the idea that we may never use nonconsenting individuals, even in benign ways, solely for the benefit of others strikes me as an implausibly strict ethical principle. But never mind. The fact that some veterinary research is intended to benefit the subjects themselves (as well as other animals or humans down the road) where no other way to help them is known shows that such research, on any reasonable view, is *not* disrespectful toward its subjects. Indeed, in such cases, the animals *would* consent to taking part, if they could, because taking part is in their interests. I fully grant that therapeutic veterinary research represents a minuscule portion of the animal research conducted today. But my arguments are put forward in the service of a goal that I think I have now achieved: demonstrating, beyond a shadow of a doubt, that some animal research is justified.

If animal advocates and representatives of biomedicine were aware of these ten points of potential agreement, they might perceive their opponents' views as less alien than they had previously taken them to be. This change in perception might, in turn, convince all parties that honest, open discussion of outstanding issues has a decent chance of repaying the effort.

Points on Which Agreement Between the Two Sides Is Unlikely

Even if biomedicine and the animal protection community approach the animal research issue in good faith, become properly informed about animal ethics and the facts of research, and so

forth, they are still likely to disagree on certain important issues. After all, their basic views differ. It may be worthwhile to enumerate several likely points of difference.

First, disagreement is likely on the issue of *the moral status of animals in comparison with humans*. While representatives of biomedicine may attribute moral status to animals, they hold that animals may justifiably be used in many experiments (most of which are nontherapeutic and harm the subjects) whose primary goal is to promote human health. But for animal advocates, it is not at all obvious that much animal research is justified. This suggests that animal advocates ascribe higher moral status to animals than biomedicine does.

Second, disagreement is likely to continue on the issue of *the specific circumstances in which the worthy goal of promoting human health justifies harming animals*. Biomedicine generally tries to protect the status quo of animal research. Animal advocates generally treat not using animals in research as a presumption, any departures from which would require careful justification. Clearly, animal advocates will have many disagreements with biomedicine over when it is appropriate to conduct animal research.

Third, in a similar vein, continuing disagreement is likely on the issue of *whether current protections for research animals are more or less adequate*. Biomedicine would probably answer affirmatively, with relatively minor internal disagreements over specific issues (e.g., whether apes should ever be exposed to diseases in order to test vaccines). Animal advocates will tend to be much more critical of current protections for research animals. They will argue, for example, that animals are far too often made to suffer in pursuit of less than compelling objectives, such as learning about behavioral responses to stress or trauma.

In the United States, critics will argue that the basic principles that are supposed to guide the care and use of animals in federally funded research ultimately provide very weak protection for research animals. That is because the tenth and final principle begins with implicit permission to make exceptions to the previous nine: "Where exceptions are required in relation to the provisions of these Principles,...." Since no limits are placed on permissible exceptions, this final principle precludes any absolute restraints on the harm that may be inflicted on research animals—an indefensible lack of safeguards from the perspective of animal advocates. (Although similar in several ways to these American principles, including some ways animal advocates would criticize, the *International Guiding Principles for Biomedical Research Involving Animals* avoids this pitfall of a global loophole. One of its relatively strong protections is Principle V: "Investigators and other personnel should never fail to treat animals as sentient, and should regard their proper care and use and the avoidance or minimization of discomfort, distress, or pain as ethical imperatives.")

Although protections of research animals are commonly thought of in terms of preventing unnecessary pain, distress, and suffering, they may also be thought of in terms of protecting animal life. A fourth likely area of disagreement concerns *whether animal life is morally protectable*. Return to a question raised earlier: whether a contented animal in good health is harmed by being painlessly killed in her sleep. Since government documents for the care and use of research animals generally require justification for causing pain or distress to animal subjects, but no justification for painless killing, it seems fair to infer that biomedicine generally does not attribute life interests to animals. Although I lack concrete evidence, I would guess that most animal advocates would see the matter quite differently, and would regard the killing of animals as a serious moral matter even if it is justified in some circumstances.

The four issues identified here as probable continuing points of difference are not intended to comprise an exhaustive list. But they show that despite the fact that the biomedical and animal protection communities can agree on an impressive range of major points, given their basic orientations they cannot be expected to agree on every fundamental question. Few will find this assertion surprising. But I also suggest, less obviously, that even if both sides cannot be entirely right in their positions, differences that remain after positions are refined through honest, open-minded, fully educated inquiry can be reasonable differences.

What Can Be Done Now to Build upon the Points of Agreement

Let me close with a series of suggestions offered in the constructive yet critical-minded spirit of Henry Spira's work for how to build on the points of agreement identified above. For reasons of space, these suggestions will be stated somewhat tersely and without elaboration.

First, biomedical organizations and leaders in the profession can do the following: openly acknowledge that ethical issues involving animals are complex and important; educate themselves or acquire education about the ethical issues; tolerate views departing from the current party line; open up journals to more than one basic viewpoint; and stop disseminating one-sided propaganda.

Second, the more "militant" animal advocates can acknowledge that there can be reasonable disagreement on some of the relevant issues and stop intimidating people with whom they disagree.

Third, biomedicine can openly acknowledge, as NASA recently did in its principles, that animals can suffer and invite more serious consideration of animal suffering.

Fourth, the animal protection community can give credit to biomedicine where credit is due—for example, for efforts to minimize pain and distress, to improve housing conditions, and to refrain from killing old chimpanzees who are no longer useful for research but are expensive to maintain.

Fifth, animal researchers and members of animal protection organizations can be required by their organizations to take courses in ethical theory or animal ethics to promote knowledgeable, skilled, broad-minded discussion and reflection.

Sixth, the animal protection community can openly acknowledge that some animal research is justified (perhaps giving examples to reduce the potential for misunderstanding).

Seventh, more animal research ethics committees can bring aboard at least one dedicated animal advocate who (unlike mainstream American veterinarians) seriously questions the value of most animal research.

Eighth, conditions of housing for research animals can be improved—for example, with greater enrichment and, for social animals, more access to conspecifics.

Ninth, all parties can endorse and support the goal of finding ways to *eliminate* animal subjects' pain, distress, and suffering.

Tenth, and finally, governments can invest much more than they have to date in the development and use of alternatives to animal research, and all parties can give strong public support to the pursuit of alternatives.

International Guiding Principles for Biomedical Research Involving Animals (1985)

COUNCIL FOR INTERNATIONAL ORGANIZATION OF MEDICAL SCIENCES

From http://www.cioms.ch/1985_texts_of_guidelines.htm

Introduction

The International Guiding Principles for Biomedical Research Involving Animals were developed by the Council for International Organizations of Medical Sciences (CIOMS) as a result of extensive international and interdisciplinary consultations spanning the three-year period 1982–1984.

Animal experimentation is fundamental to the biomedical sciences, not only for the advancement of man's understanding of the nature of life and the mechanisms of specific vital processes, but also for the improvement of methods of prevention, diagnosis, and treatment of disease both in man and in animals. The use of animals is also indispensable for testing the potency and safety of biological substances used in human and veterinary medicine, and for determining the toxicity of the rapidly growing number of synthetic substances that never existed before in nature and which may represent a hazard to health. This extensive exploitation by man of animals implies philosophical and moral problems that are not peculiar to their use for scientific purposes, and there are no objective ethical criteria by which

to judge claims and counterclaims in such matters. However, there is a consensus that deliberate cruelty is repugnant.

Suggestions had been received from several quarters that CIOMS, as an international nongovernmental organization representative of the biomedical community, would be ideally placed to propose a broadly based statement, acceptable worldwide in different cultural and legal backgrounds, and designed to create a greater understanding on the subject of biomedical research involving animals. Moreover, in several countries political action was being taken to stop or severely limit animal experimentation, and the Council of Europe had for some time been engaged in the elaboration of a convention to regulate the use of vertebrate animals for experiments or toxicity tests.

While many countries have general laws or regulations imposing penalties for ill-treatment of animals, relatively few make specific provision for their use for scientific purposes. In the few that have done so, the measures adopted vary widely, the extremes being: on the one hand, legally enforceable detailed regulations with licensing of experimenters and their premises together with an official inspectorate; on the other, entirely voluntary self-regulation by the biomedical community, with lay participation. Many variations are possible between these extremes, one intermediate situation being a legal requirement that experiments or other procedures involving the use of animals should be subject to the approval of ethical committees of specified composition.

In elaborating and publishing the International Guiding Principles the objective of CIOMS is not to duplicate such national regulations or voluntary codes as already exist but to provide a conceptual and ethical framework, acceptable both to the international biomedical community and to moderate animal welfare groups, for whatever regulatory measure each country or scientific body chooses to adopt in respect of the used animals for scientific purposes. The Principles strongly emphasize that there should not be such restrictions as would unduly hamper the advance of biomedical science or the performance of necessary biological tests, but that, at the same time, biomedical scientists should not lose sight of their moral obligation to have a humane regard for their animal subjects, to prevent as far as possible pain and discomfort, and to be constantly alert to any possibility of achieving the same result without resort to living animals.

International Guiding Principles for Biomedical Research Involving Animals

Preamble

Experimentation with animals has made possible major contributions to biological knowledge and to the welfare of man and animals, particularly in the treatment and prevention of diseases. Many important advances in medical science have had their origins in basic biological research not primarily directed to practical ends as well as from applied research designed to investigate specific medical problems. There is still an urgent need for basic and applied research that will lead to the discovery of methods for the prevention and treatment of diseases for which adequate control methods are not yet available – notably the noncommunicable diseases and the endemic communicable diseases of warm climates.

Past progress has depended, and further progress in the foreseeable future will depend, largely on animal experimentation which, in the broad field of human medicine, is the prelude to experimental trials on human beings of, for example, new therapeutic, prophylactic, or diagnostic substances, devices, or procedures.

There are two international ethical codes intended principally for the guidance of countries or institutions that have not yet formulated their own ethical requirements for human experimentation: The Tokyo revision of *the Declaration of Helsinki* of the World Medical Association (1975); and *the Proposed International Guidelines for Biomedical Research Involving Human Subjects* of the Council for International Organizations of Medical Sciences and the World Health Organization (1982). These codes recognize that while experiments involving human subjects are a *sine qua non of* medical progress, they must be subject to strict ethical requirements. In order to ensure that such ethical requirements are observed, national and institutional ethical codes have also been elaborated with a view to the protection of human subjects involved in biomedical (including behavioural) research.

A major requirement both of national and international ethical codes for human experimentation, and of national legislation in many cases, is that new substances or devices should not be used for the first time on human beings unless previous tests on animals have provided a reasonable presumption of their safety.

The use of animals for predicting the probable effects of procedures on human beings entails responsibility for their welfare. In both human and veterinary medicine animals are used for behavioural, physiological, pathological, toxicological, and therapeutic research and for experimental surgery or surgical training and for testing drugs and biological preparations. The same responsibility toward the experimental animals prevails in all of these cases.

Because of differing legal systems and cultural backgrounds there are varying approaches to the use of animals for research, testing, or training in different countries. Nonetheless, their use should be always in accord with humane practices. The varying approaches in different countries to the use of animals for biomedical purposes, and the lack of relevant legislation or of formal self-regulatory mechanisms in some, point to the need for international guiding principles elaborated as a result of international and interdisciplinary consultations.

The guiding principles proposed here provide a framework for more specific national or institutional provisions. They apply, not only to biomedical research but also to all uses of vertebrate animals for other biomedical purposes, including the production and testing of therapeutic, prophylactic, and diagnostic substances, the diagnosis of infections and intoxications in man and animals, and to any other procedures involving the use of intact live vertebrates.

Basic Principles

I. The advancement of biological knowledge and the development of improved means for the protection of the health and well-being both of man and of animals require recourse to experimentation on intact live animals of a wide variety of species.

II. Methods such as mathematical models, computer simulation and *in vitro* biological systems should be used wherever appropriate.

III. Animal experiments should be undertaken only after due consideration of their relevance for human or animal health and the advancement of biological knowledge.

IV. The animals selected for an experiment should be of an appropriate species and quality, and the minimum number required to obtain scientifically valid results.

V. Investigators and other personnel should never fail to treat animals as sentient, and should regard their proper care and use and the avoidance or minimization of discomfort, distress, or pain as ethical imperatives.

VI. Investigators should assume that procedures that would cause pain in human beings cause pain in other vertebrate species, although more needs to be known about the perception of pain in animals.

VII. Procedures with animals that may cause more than momentary or minimal pain or distress should be performed with appropriate sedation, analgesia, or anesthesia in accordance with accepted veterinary practice. Surgical or other painful procedures should not be performed on unanesthetized animals paralysed by chemical agents.

VIII. Where waivers are required in relation to the provisions of article VII, the decisions should not rest solely with the investigators directly concerned but should be made, with due regard to the provisions of articles IV, V, and VI, by a suitably constituted review body. Such waivers should not be made solely for the purposes of teaching or demonstration.

IX. At the end of, or, when appropriate, during an experiment, animals that would otherwise suffer severe or chronic pain, distress, discomfort, or disablement that cannot be relieved should be painlessly killed.

X. The best possible living conditions should be maintained for animals kept for biomedical purposes. Normally the care of animals should be under the supervision of veterinarians having experience in laboratory animal science. In any case, veterinary care should be available as required.

XI. It is the responsibility of the director of an institute or department using animals to ensure that investigators and personnel have appropriate qualifications or experience for conducting procedures on animals. Adequate opportunities shall be provided for in-service training, including the proper and humane concern for the animals under their care.

Methods Not Involving Animals: "Alternatives"

There remain many areas in biomedical research which, at least for the foreseeable future, will require animal experimentation. An intact live animal is more than the sum of the responses of isolated cells, tissues or organs; there are complex interactions in the whole animal that cannot be reproduced by biological or nonbiological "alternative" methods. The term "alternative" has come to be used by some to refer to a replacement of the use of living animals by other procedures, as well as methods which lead to a reduction in the numbers of animals required or to the refinement of experimental procedures.

The experimental procedures that are considered to be "alternatives" include nonbiological and biological methods. The nonbiological methods include mathematical modelling of structure-activity relationships based on the physico-chemical properties of drugs and other chemicals, and computer modelling of other biological processes. The biological methods include the use of micro-organisms, *in vitro* preparations (subcellular fractions, short-term cellular systems, whole organ perfusion, and cell and organ culture) and under some circumstances, invertebrates and vertebrate embryos. In addition to experimental procedures, retrospective and prospective epidemiological investigations on human and animal populations represent other approaches of major importance.

The adoption of "alternative" approaches is viewed as being complementary to the use of intact animals and their development and use should be actively encouraged for both scientific and humane reasons.

Guidelines for the Care and Use of Mammals in Neuroscience and Behavioral Research

NATIONAL RESEARCH COUNCIL

From *Guidelines for the Care and Use of Mammals in Neuroscience and Behavioral Research* (Washington, DC: National Academies Press), 15–20, 97–98, 99–101.

Pain and Distress

Pain may be inherent in the study of pain and/or distress, but it can also be an unintended aspect of the research (for example, in animal models of disease, as a byproduct of a survival surgical procedure, or in transgenic animals with a clinical phenotype). It is critical to recognize and manage animal pain and distress.

The International Association for the Study of Pain has defined pain in humans as an "unpleasant sensory and emotional experience associated with actual or potential tissue damage, or described in terms of such damage." Although animals cannot communicate verbally, they exhibit motor behaviors and physiologic responses similar to those of humans in response to pain. Those behaviors may include simple withdrawal reflexes; complex, unlearned behaviors such as vocalization and escape; and learned behaviors such as pressing a bar to avoid further exposure to noxious stimulation. However, there are species-specific behaviors that animals may express in response to pain, see Table 6.1 for review.

Stress (or the stress response) has been defined as "the biological response an animal exhibits in an attempt to cope with threats to its homeostasis." Threats to homeostasis are called "stressors." Stressors can be physical, environmental, or psychologic in origin, and adaptation can involve

TABLE 6.1 Indicators of Pain in Several Common Laboratory Animals[a]

Species	General Behavior	Appearance	Other
Rodents	Decreased activity; excessive licking and scratching; self-mutilation; may be unusually aggressive; abnormal locomotion (stumbling, falling); writhing; does not make nest; hiding	Piloerection; rough/stained haircoat; abnormal stance or arched back; porphyrin staining (rats)	Rapid, shallow respiration; decreased food/water consumption; tremors
Rabbit	Head pressing; teeth grinding; may become more aggressive; increased vocalizations; excessive licking and scratching; reluctant to locomote	Excessive salivation; hunched posture	Rapid, shallow respiration; decreased food/water consumption
Dog	Excessive licking; increased aggression; increased vocalizations, inclusive of whimpering, howling, and growling; excessive licking and scratching; self-mutilation	Stiff body movements; reluctant to move; trembling; guarding	Decreased food/water consumption; increased respiration rate/panting
Cat	Hiding; increased vocalizations, inclusive of growling and hissing; excessive licking; increased aggression	Stiff body movements; reluctant to move; haircoat appears rough, ungroomed; hunched posture; irritable tail twitching; flattened ears	Decreased food/water consumption
Nonhuman Primate	Increased aggression or depression; self-mutilation; often a dramatic change in routine behavior (e.g., locomotion is decreased); rubbing or picking at painful location	Stiff body movements; reluctant to move; huddled body posture	Decreased food/water consumption

[a]No single observation is sufficiently reliable to indicate pain; rather several signs, taken in the context of the animal's situation, should be evaluated. The signs of pain may vary with the type of procedure (e.g., orthopedic versus abdominal pain).

immunologic, metabolic, autonomic, neuroendocrine, and behavioral changes, but the type, pattern, and extent of the changes depend on the stressor involved. When the animal responds to a stressor in an adaptive way, the animal returns to a state of comfort. It is also possible for stressors to induce responses that have beneficial effects. Animals (and people) are normally exposed regularly to stressors to which they need to respond and adapt, and some stress is probably necessary for well-being.

When an animal is unable to completely adapt to a stressor and the resulting stress, an aversive state has developed defined as distress. The term distress encompasses the negative psychologic states that are sometimes associated with exposure to stressors, including fear, pain, malaise, anxiety, frustration, depression, and boredom. These can manifest as maladaptive behaviors, such as abnormal feeding or aggression, or pathologic conditions that are not evident in behavior, such as hypertension and immunosuppression.

Assessment of Pain

According to the National Research Council's *Guide for the Care of Laboratory Animals*, "fundamental to the relief of pain in animals is the ability to recognize its clinical signs in specific species" (p. 64). Pain can be assessed by evaluating behavioral measures such as eating, socializing, and withdrawal reflexes, and physiologic measures such as heart rate and respiration rate (see Table 6.1). However, species, and even strains and individuals of the same species, may vary widely in their perception of and response to pain. Even for an individual animal, pain sensitivity varies among different tissues and organs, and pain sensitivities can be altered by pathologic processes or experimental procedures. For example, during the initial phase of lipopolysaccharide-induced fever, rats exhibit hyperalgesia, whereas they exhibit hypoalgesia during the later stages of the illness. The existence of these differences underscores the point that pain and distress exist as a continuum of experience. In addition, some animals may hide signs of pain; for example, it has been suggested that rats may mask pain during the dark-cycle hours to avoid displaying abnormal activity and increasing their risk of predation.

The American Association for Laboratory Animal Science (AALAS) suggests that the magnitude of the pain that the animal is expected to experience be categorized in the protocol and monitored and that there be an opportunity to adjust the pain category once the study is under way. It is important that researchers and animal-care staff have a solid knowledge of the normal and abnormal physiology, behavior, and appearance of the animals in their care.

Acceptable levels of noxious stimulation are those that are well tolerated and do not result in maladaptive behaviors. Acceptable levels range from an animal's pain threshold to its pain tolerance level. Pain threshold is the stimulus level at which pain is first perceived, while pain tolerance is the highest intensity of painful stimulation that an animal will voluntarily accept. As the intensity of a stimulus approaches the pain tolerance level, an animal's behavior will become dominated by attempts to avoid or escape the stimulus, and this degree of pain must be alleviated.

It is important to note that it is usually incorrect to infer that an animal's pain tolerance level is signaled by the onset of avoidance or escape behavior, as some avoidance-escape behavior is an appropriate adaptive response. It is only when the animal's behavior is dominated by avoidance-escape attempts that the behavior becomes maladaptive, signaling unacceptable levels of pain.

In pain studies, giving animals control over the source of pain by allowing them to withdraw from a painful stimulus is an effective way to minimize pain and the distress associated with it. If an animal is denied control of the stimulus and it approaches the tolerance limit, maladaptive behaviors will appear, and the animal should be presumed to be in distress. Maladaptive behaviors include persistent attacks on the perceived source of the pain, self-mutilation at the injured or stimulated site, and a state of learned helplessness in which the animal gives up and no longer attempts to escape, avoid, or control the stimulus. To avoid the development of maladaptive behaviors and to minimize pain during experimental manipulations where the animal is denied control of the stimulus, it is critical that the neuroscientist attempt to define the level of pain produced by the stimulus, and ensure that the level imposed by the stimulus is below that which causes the development of maladaptive behaviors. In most cases, previous experimental or published data will indicate the level of pain produced by the stimulus; lacking this information, a pilot study to identify the level of stimulus that produces maladaptive behavior could be useful.

Pain assessment will vary with the pain scale or scoring system used. Scoring systems involve assigning a numeric score to constellations of behavioral, physical, and physiologic observations, and this process can be subjective. There are no generally accepted objective criteria for assessing the degree of pain that an animal is experiencing, and different species or strains can vary in their response to pain. Physiologic measures include heart rate, blood pressure, and respiration rate, but obtaining most of the measures requires some degree of intervention, which may not be feasible or desirable.

Recent studies on pain in animals include methods for quantifying specific motor behaviors as indirect measures of responses to mechanical, thermal, or chemical injury. Animals will withdraw an injured body part from a stimulus, where different levels of stimulation affect the latency or force of withdrawal. This withdrawal response is considered a measure of pain, which correlates highly with more integrative nocifensive behaviors (behaviors in response to pain), such as licking of the injured body part and guarding behavior.

Some behavioral signs are usually associated with pain. Animals often communicate through posture. They may exhibit guarding behavior in an attempt to protect the injured part. Vocalizations are important indicators of pain in several species. Animals in pain may lick, bite, scratch, shake, or rub the site of injury. Restlessness may also be observed, including pacing, lying down and getting up, and shifting weight. Animals in pain may stay in one place for abnormal lengths of time and be reluctant to move or rise. They may withdraw from contact with other animals. They may become listless and refuse to eat or reduce their eating and drinking. They may avoid being handled. These are all possible signs of pain, but none alone is sufficient to determine the presence or level of pain. For example, many animals vocalize intensely when they are handled even if they are not in pain. Multiple criteria should therefore be assessed.

Recent evidence indicates that some signs of pain may not be perceived by personnel, such as the ultrasonic vocalizations of infant mice, but are detectable with appropriate equipment.

Assessment of pain should not be influenced by the biases of the observer, and the observer should be well trained in both normal and abnormal behaviors of the species in question. Variability among observers can have a substantial effect on the interpretation of assessment data.

Chronic or persistent pain differs from acute pain because it may not be associated with any obvious pathologic condition and does not serve any protective function. Signs of chronic pain can be subtle and difficult to detect in that an animal's behavior may change slowly and incrementally. Chronic or persistent pain is also more likely to lead to distress and maladaptive behavior. Signs of chronic or persistent pain include decrease in appetite, weight loss, reduction in activity, sleep loss, irritability, and decrease in mating behavior and reproductive performance. Alterations in urinary and bowel activities and lack of grooming are often associated with persistent pain. Severe chronic pain can reduce body temperature, cause a weak and shallow pulse, and depress respiration. As noted above, animals cannot control chronic or persistent pain, and it is important to assess the intensity of the pain by using behavioral measures.

Animal Models Involving Pain

Experiments with animals have mostly used stimuli that produce acute pain of short duration and moderate intensity; these models have become standards in the screening of putative analgesics. More recently, investigators have begun to develop nonhuman animal models that mimic persistent pain conditions seen in humans. Tissue injury and inflammation are commonly associated with clinical conditions that lead to persistent pain. Accordingly, new animal models to study these conditions differ in important ways from earlier, acute pain models.

Animal models of pain and hyperalgesia (excessive sensitivity to pain) have been developed to study the functional changes produced by the injection of inflammatory agents into the rat or mouse hindpaw. The animals withdraw their limbs reflexively but also exhibit more complex organized behaviors, such as paw-licking and guarding. A paw-withdrawal latency measure and withdrawal duration can be used to infer pain and hyperalgesia in response to thermal or mechanical stimuli. Methods of measuring nocifensive behavior have also been applied to the orofacial region. In the above studies, most of the nocifensive behaviors provide an animal with control of the intensity or duration of the stimulus in that the behaviors result in removal of the aversive stimulus.

Animals in persistent-pain models do not have control of stimulus intensity or duration. For example, the writhing response is produced in rodents by injecting pain-producing chemical substances intraperitoneally. The acute peritonitis resulting from the injection produces a response characterized by internal rotation of one foot, arching of the back, rolling on one side, and accompanying abdominal contractions. The writhing response is considered a model of visceral pain. Not only does the animal lack stimulus control with this method, but the experimenter cannot control the duration of the stimulus. In another test, formalin is injected beneath the footpad of a rat or cat. The chemical produces complex response patterns that last for about an hour. Many response measures are used for assessing pain after formalin injection. They include single measures such as flinching, shaking, and jerking—or complex scores that are derived from several nocifensive behaviors, such as licking or guarding. However, the animals do not have complete control over the aversiveness of the persistent stimulus. Vocalization is another common, unlearned reaction to painful stimuli, and the stimulus intensity necessary to elicit a vocal response from the animal can be determined. The stimulus can be applied to any part of the body; again, the animals cannot control the intensity or duration of the stimulus.

Nerve-injury models that mimic neuropathic pain in humans have been developed recently. Partial nerve injury in the rat results in signs of hyperalgesia and spontaneous pain. In one model, loose ligatures are placed around the sciatic nerve; demyelination of the large fibers and destruction of some unmyelinated axons result. In another model, ligation and severing of the dorsal one-third to one-half of the sciatic nerve produce similar behavioral changes. Kim and Chung have developed a third model, in which the L5 and L6 spinal nerves are tightly ligated on one of the rat's sides. All three models mimic clinical conditions of painful neuropathy and yield evidence of persistent spontaneous pain, allodynia (pain resulting from a nonnoxious stimuli), and hyperalgesia. These nerve-injury models of neuropathic pain have been adapted for use in mice, in which they can be used to study pain mechanisms in transgenic models.

Ethical Considerations Associated with Pain Research

Anesthetic and pain-relieving methods and drugs generally act on the system under study—the nervous system—and neuroscientists and IACUCs must make difficult choices in selecting the means by which pain and distress are controlled and how much pain and/or distress is acceptable.

Several ethical issues have been proposed for IACUC consideration when reviewing protocols involving pain and/or distress in animals

- Of the animal-use protocols reviewed by the IACUC, those which include pain and/or distress should be subject to a full committee review rather than review by a designated member or with an expedited review process. If necessary, the committee should involve an outside consultant to understand better the ramifications of the study.
- The protocol should provide a compelling justification for the work, a description of the qualifications of the personnel who will perform the work and provide care for the animals, and a rationale for withholding analgesics or other pain-relieving or distress-relieving methods.
- The protocol should contain a complete and accurate description of the severity of pain and/or distress that will potentially be experienced by the animals.
- When it is not in conflict with the scientific goals of a well-designed study, pain relief should be provided by anesthetizing the animals; giving them analgesics; allowing them to escape or avoid the pain; or control the experimental trials.
- A humane endpoint for the use of an animal should be determined as an element of the protocol, before work begins.

Ethically, models of persistent pain present a particular challenge because they produce pain that most guidelines for the use of animals in research state should be avoided. Scientists should demonstrate a continuing responsibility for the proper treatment of the animals involved in these experiments. Because some models produce persistent pain that the animals cannot control, it is important that investigators assess the level of pain in these animals and provide analgesic agents when they do not interfere with the purpose of the experiment. A reduction in body weight or a significant deviation from normal behavior—such as a change in normal activity patterns, social adjustment, feeding behavior, and sleep-wake patterns—suggests that an animal is in severe and possibly intolerable pain.

In animal models of inflammation and nerve injury, the IACUC should ensure that steps are taken to safeguard animal welfare. The steps may include use of fail-safe devices to avoid excessive exposure to painful stimuli (for example, monitoring stimulus intensity and duration), having in place well-established humane endpoints to deal appropriately with intractable conditions (such as self-mutilation), and postprocedure monitoring of animal well-being.

CASES

Medicare Requires Heart Patients to Enlist in Research

Congestive heart failure (CHF) is a chronic disease in which a person's heart cannot pump sufficient blood to the body's other organs. A number of medical problems can lead to CHF, including coronary artery disease, high blood pressure, cardiomyopathy, and past heart attack. For someone with CHF, an arrhythmia (an irregular electrical impulse to the heart) can be fatal. An implantable cardioverter-defibrillator (ICD) is a battery-powered, pacemaker-like device that can be implanted into the chest of a patient with CHF. The ICD will detect an arrhythmia and deliver electrical impulses to the heart to correct the irregularity. Although ICDs have been approved for the treatment of heart patients for a number of years, new research by Bardy and colleagues has shown that increased use of the devices could reduce the risk of death from congestive heart failure by twenty-three percent. A much broader group of heart patients could potentially benefit from the devices.

In light of the new research on ICDs, Medicare, the publicly financed U.S. insurance program for the elderly, announced that it would supply ICDs to thousands of additional patients at risk of heart attack. The program will cost Medicare about three billion dollars a year, and will double or triple the number of patients eligible for treatment with an ICS. But there is a catch: patients who accept the pacemaker must agree to participate in A large-scale observational research study on the safety and efficacy of the device. This new initiative is called "Coverage with Evidence Development" and would create a registry of ICD patients and track their health outcomes.

Medicare's ICD registry has created a good deal of controversy. Medicare officials and other supporters of the data registry requirement argue that collection of data on the effectiveness of ICD treatments is essential. Data registries of the sort Medicare is using are a key to developing evidence-based medical care. Also, given the enormous costs of treatments and the growing population of elderly who need medical care, large-scale studies of cost, safety, and effectiveness are crucial in deciding how best to allocate Medicare dollars. ICD therapy averages about thirty thousand dollars per patient, so a large sum of money is at stake. Medicare has a fiduciary duty to taxpayers to spend their money in the most cost-effective manner, so that the greatest number of people can benefit from the program.

Supporters also note that patient data is strictly confidential, in keeping with federal HIPPA (Health Insurance Portability and Accountability Act) requirements. Furthermore, this is really no different from other clinical research: it is often the case that patients do not receive cutting-edge treatments unless they enroll in clinical trials, and many patients enroll in research to receive treatments they otherwise could not afford. Bioethicist Ezekiel Emanuel was enthusiastic about Medicare's program. "I do think it raises a question of when research and clinical care merge. But my own sense is that every patient ought to be a data point, because we would learn so much more about what does and what doesn't work in a clinical setting" (Wadman 2005).

Opponents, including one group that calls itself a human rights organization, argue that the program is coercive and goes against the ethical and legal requirements that patients give informed consent before being enrolled in a research project. It is true, they say, that patients sign up for research in order to receive otherwise unavailable treatments, but ICDs have already been extensively studied and are already approved by the FDA. In response to Medicare's plan, bioethicist Arthur Caplan argued that making the patients participate in the follow-up amounted to coercion and rendered the program unethical. Although receiving the device will certainly benefit the patient, participating in the follow-up study will not directly benefit the patient and thus falls into the category of "research." He argues that people must be free to participate in research, without any form of coercion.

Discussion Questions

1. Which ethicist do you agree with more—Caplan or Emanuel—and why?
2. Do you consider Medicare's proposal coercive? Unduly coercive? Does all clinical research have an element of coercion?
3. What do you think of Emanuel's comment, "Every patient ought to be a data point"?

Sources

Bardy, Gust H., et al. "Amiodarone or an implantable cardioverter-defibrillator for congestive heart failure." *New England Journal of Medicine* 352, no. 3 (205): 225–37.

Centers for Medicare and Medicaid Services. "ICD registry." http://www.cms.hhs.gov/MedicareApprovedFacilitie/04_ICDregistry.asp#TopOfPage. (accessed March 14, 2008).

Graham-Rowe, Duncan. "Hotwire my heart." *Nature* 435 (May 5, 2005): 14–15.

Wadman, Meredith. "Medicare compels heart patients to enlist in follow-up research." *Nature* 433 (January 27, 2005): 341.

Empathic Mice

In June 2006, researchers reported in the journal *Science* the first unequivocal evidence for empathy in mice. Dale Langford, of McGill University, and her colleagues demonstrated that mice suffer distress when they watch a cagemate experience pain. Langford and her team injected either single mice or pairs of mice with acetic acid, which causes the stomach muscles to contract and the mice to "writhe." The researchers then placed mice either singly or in pairs in a Plexiglas tube and observed. A mouse injected with acid writhed more violently if his or her partner had also been injected and was writhing in pain. Not only did the

mice who watched cagemates in distress become more sensitive to the same painful stimuli, they became generally more sensitive to pain, showing a heightened reaction, for example, to heat under their paws. The researchers speculated that mice probably used visual cues to generate the empathic response, which is interesting since mice normally rely most heavily on olfactory communication.

Jaak Panksepp, an expert on animal emotion, said of Langford's research, "If it turns out that the 'empathetic' effect in mice is mediated by the same brain mechanisms as human empathy, then the evidence would be truly compelling that their model actually reflects evolutionary continuity in a pro-social mechanism among many different mammalian species" (Ganguli 2006). Frans de Waal, a world renowned primatologist, commented, "This is a highly significant finding and should open the eyes of people who think empathy is limited to our species" (Carey 2006).

Discussion Questions

1. What implications—both scientific and moral—might the capacity for empathy in mice have for how we use them in scientific research?
2. What is the significance of Panksepp's comment? If it turned out that other social mammals had the same basic behavioral repertoire that in humans we call morality (being altruistic, fair, empathic, compassionate), would this alter our moral responsibilities to them?

Sources

Carey, Benedict. "Message from Mouse to Mouse: I feel your pain." *New York Times*, July 4, 2006.

Ganguli, Ishani. "Mice show evidence of empathy." *The Scientist*, June 30, 2006. http://www.the-scientist.com/news/display/23764/ (accessed May 4, 2007).

Langford, Dale J., Sara E. Crager, Zarrar Shehzad, Shad B. Smith, Susana G. Sotocinal, Jeremy S. Levenstadt, Mona Lisa Chanda, Daniel J. Levitin, and Jeffrey S. Mogil. "Social

Modulation of Pain as Evidence for Empathy in Mice." *Science* 312, no. 5782 (2006): 1967.

Orphan Diseases

An orphan disease is one that has not been "adopted" by the research and development arm of the drug industry. There are two classes of orphan disease.

1. A rare disease, which is defined as one that affects fewer than 200,000 people a year. Some examples of this type of orphan disease are glioma, multiple myeloma, and cystic fibrosis.
2. A disease that is uncommon in developed countries (where there is little market for drugs to treat it) but prevalent in the developing world. The five most important orphaned diseases, in terms of mortality and burden of disease, are generally considered to be Chagas disease, malaria, tuberculosis, sleeping sickness, and leishmaniasis.

Orphan Diseases, Type 1

Because research and development of new drugs is market-driven, pharmaceutical companies tend to invest most heavily in those drugs for which there is a large potential market: drugs to treat asthma, heart disease, diabetes, and high blood pressure. The U.S. Orphan Drug Act of 1983 tried to stimulate increased attention to rare diseases by offering tax incentives on clinical trials and ensuring pharmaceutical companies of seven years' marketing exclusivity—they are given a monopoly on the drug for this seven-year time period. Although big diseases still get the most attention from drug makers, the Orphan Drug Act has stimulated the development of a number of drugs for less common ailments. Similar legislation has been passed in other developed countries.

Orphan Diseases, Type 2

Many people in the international health community have chastised the pharmaceutical industry for neglecting, in their research efforts, diseases that profoundly affect the world's poor. Medicins Sans Frontieres (also known as Doctors Without Borders), for example, published a scathing attack on eleven of the world's largest pharmaceutical companies. According to the report, eight of the eleven companies spent nothing on research into the five orphan diseases listed earlier. Medicins sans Frontieres points to the so-called "ninety/ten" disequilibrium: about ninety percent of global health research is concentrated on just ten percent of the global health burden (the diseases of affluence such as heart disease, stroke, obesity), a striking example of social injustice. The neglect of orphan diseases is a result, they argue, "of market failure and public policy failure."

A disease can be considered neglected when "treatment options are inadequate or don't exist, and when their drug-market potential is insufficient to readily attract a private sector response." Tropical diseases, notes the report, are good examples of neglected diseases. "Of the 1,393 total new drugs approved between 1975 and 1999, only 1% (13 drugs) were specifically indicated for a tropical disease." They further note surveys taken by a U.S. drug industry group, PhRMA:

> Of the 137 medications for infectious diseases in the pipeline during 2000, only one mentioned sleeping sickness as an indication, and only one mentioned malaria. There were no new medicines in the pipeline for tuberculosis or leishmaniasis. PhRMA's current 'New Medicines in Development' list shows eight drugs in development for impotence and erectile dysfunction, seven for obesity, and four for sleep disorders.

Discussion Questions

1. Do pharmaceutical companies have a moral responsibility to engage in research to help the world's poor? Assuming there is such a responsibility, on what grounds might it rest?
2. What ethical tensions or problems might be raised in relation to type 1 orphan diseases?

Source

Medicins Sans Frontieres. *Fatal Imbalance: The Crisis in Research and Development for Drugs for Neglected Diseases*. Published by Medicins Sans Frontieres Access to Essential Medicines Campaign and the Drugs for Neglected Diseases Working Group, 2001.

In Defense of Animals (IDA) Urges NIH to Halt Animal Nicotine Experiments

From an e-mail sent by In Defense of Animals, April 23, 2008:

> Many people find this hard to believe, but the U.S. government continues to sink millions of dollars each year into funding cruel and outdated experiments on animals to test the effects of nicotine and tobacco.
>
> Please join IDA during this week's observance of World Week for Animals in Laboratories (WWAIL) to call attention to this outrage and speak out in opposition. IDA's Up in Smoke campaign (www.UpInSmokeCampaign.org) highlights the futility and inhumanity of nicotine experiments on newborn and pregnant animals.

These are some examples:

- Since 1992, Elliot Spindel at Oregon Health and Science University delivers steady doses of nicotine to pregnant monkeys through pumps implanted into their backs. The babies are cut out of their mothers' wombs in order to dissect their lungs.
- At Texas A&M University, Ursula Winzer-Serhan forces baby rats to consume nicotine mixed with baby formula at the equivalent of three packs of cigarettes a day. After about a week of being fed nicotine, the babies' heads are cut off and their brains are dissected for analysis.
- Researcher Kent Pinkerton at University of California, Davis, subjects pregnant rhesus monkeys to smoking chambers where they are forced to inhale cigarette smoke for six hours each day, five days a week. When the infants are ten weeks old, they are killed by lethal injection and their lungs are dissected for analysis.

Over the past five years, the National Institutes of Health (NIH) has given at least $16.5 million to this category of research. This appalling figure does not reflect the total cost of all nicotine research on animals, but only that which focuses on nicotine's effect on fetal and newborn development.

Animal researchers staunchly defend these experiments as necessary for improving maternal and newborn health. But answers don't come from animal studies. After decades of animal studies, we still have not addressed the problem of smoking during pregnancy. Only education, public health outreach, and prevention programs can address the human behaviors that lead to smoking.

What You Can Do:

Please contact the following individuals at the National Institutes of Health. Ask that the agency end the decades-long policy of funding nicotine experiments on animals and instead redirect funds towards prevention, education and smoking cessation programs. Please keep all correspondence polite. We are aware that NIH is deterring calls, saying that you should instead e-mail to scientificaffairs@od.nih.gov.

Sample letter to NIH: (Please customize for maximum effect)

Dear Decision maker:

I am writing to request that the National Institutes of Health (NIH) cease funding of all futile and inhumane animal experiments to purportedly test the effects of nicotine on human physiology and development.

These experiments, which have spanned decades, have failed to help us address the problem of smoking during pregnancy and its outcome on the developing newborn.

A review of the published literature on this topic shows that animal experiments have failed to consistently and reliably demonstrate nicotine's effect on learning and memory, behavioral abnormalities (such as attention-deficit/hyperactivity disorder or anxiety), and even birth weight. If we cannot reproduce results between animal experiments, and if we cannot even reliably reproduce in animals what we have observed in humans, there is no reasonable hope that continued animal experiments will elucidate the complex molecular pathways that scientists are currently using to justify this type of research.

Rather than continuing to pursue this dead-end type of research on animals, the NIH needs to redirect funding into effective social outreach programs that focus on prevention, education and assistance for smoking cessation.

In Oregon, for example, the Tobacco Prevention and Education Program launched in 1996, led to a 41 percent decline in tobacco use, outstripping the national trend. NIH has spent approximately $16.5 million on fetal nicotine studies alone. If those monies had been utilized for a national tobacco prevention effort, far more lives of women and children would have been improved.

The time has come to end reliance on outdated and cruel animal experiments. The landmark National Academy of Sciences report in June 2008 highlighted recent advances in non-animal technology that led three key government agencies, including NIH, to propose a shift away from animal data. Though that decision applied to animal toxicity testing, the same scientific principles apply to studying the physiological effects of nicotine. If we cannot assess the safety of chemicals in the human body by studying animals, likewise, we cannot learn about the molecular effect of nicotine on humans by cutting up rats' brains.

These costly and esoteric experiments fail to address the root causes that lead to human behaviors such as smoking, and they should be ended.

Sincerely,

———

Discussion Questions

1. Can you identify any examples of "loaded language" in the e-mail?
2. What do you think is IDA's most compelling argument in the letter to the NIH? What is their least compelling argument?

3. Are nicotine experiments on animals morally different from other kinds of medical research on animals?

Source

In Defense of Animals. http://www.idausa.org/ and https://secure.ga0.org/02/idadonations_spindel_march08.

Pharmacological Research on Pregnant Women

Although research on pregnant women is legal, there has been long-standing trepidation about experimenting on this "vulnerable" population. As a result, data about the safety of medical treatments for pregnant women and their fetuses is woefully incomplete. For example, a review of research on the safety of antipsychotic drugs for pregnant and postpartum women suggests a serious lack of objective clinical evidence; physicians instead must rely on their own personal experiences and clinical judgment in treating psychosis during pregnancy. Without hard data, it is very hard for physicians to counsel patients about the potential benefits and risks of treatment, including possible risks to the developing fetus.

Federal guidelines on the protection of human subjects (Department of Health and Human Services, 45 FCFR 46) specify protections that must be extended to pregnant women, fetuses, and neonates. These protections require that the following conditions be met before research involving pregnant women can proceed:

- the risk to the fetus is caused solely by interventions and procedures that hold out the prospect of direct benefit both to the pregnant woman and the fetus; or if there is no such prospect of benefit, the risk to the fetus is not greater than minimal, and the purpose of the research is the development of important biomedical knowledge that cannot be obtained by other means;
- any risk is the least possible risk for the achievement of the objectives of the research;

- individuals who are engaged in the research will have no part in any decisions as to the timing, method, or procedures that are used to terminate a pregnancy.

In the journal *American Journal of Obstetrics and Gynecology*, Laurence McCullough, John Coverdale, and Frank Chervenak argue that increased research on pregnant women is essential to providing them good medical care, and offer an ethical framework for "responsibly defining and conducting pharmacologic research that involves pregnant women." The federal guidelines, while allowing research on pregnant women, do not offer any framework for balancing maternal and fetal health-related interests. McCullough and colleagues try to provide a framework for this balancing. They base their framework on "the ethical concept of the fetus as a patient." They explain:

> The ethical concept of the fetus as a patient involves dependent moral status. Dependent moral status is conferred freely on an entity by others, not out of an obligation to do so. This contrasts with independent moral status, which others must confer as a matter of obligation, usually to respect the rights of an entity.

The previable fetus is a patient when the pregnant woman confers this dependent moral status on it, which she is free to do or not to do as she decides. Once she does confer this status, she and her physicians have beneficence-based obligations to protect the fetus' health-related interests. The previable fetus is a patient solely as a function of the pregnant woman's autonomy.

Discussion Questions

1. McCullough and colleagues suggest that a fetus has moral value only if and when the mother confers this value. Do you agree? Why or why not?
2. If not, who else should be making the determination about moral status of the fetus?
3. Are pregnant women a "vulnerable" population? Should there be special rules governing their participation?

Source

McCullough, Laurence B., John H. Coverdale, Frank A. Chervenak. "A comprehensive ethical framework for responsibly designing and conducting pharmacologic research that involves pregnant women." *American Journal of Obstetrics and Gynecology* 193 (2005) 901–7.

Stem Cell Research—"Dead" Embryos?

Another attempt to sidestep the moral impasse over stem cell research is to create stem cell lines from "dead" embryos. There is broad consensus that using dead embryos (ones that have died naturally) is less morally fraught than using live ones, and would remove some of the obstacles to stem cell research.

British researcher Miodrag Stojković recently developed a method for deriving stem cells from "arrested" embryos. During *in vitro* fertilization (IVF), many of the fertilized embryos arrest, or stop dividing, several days after fertilization. An arrested embryo is one that has stopped dividing for more than twenty-four hours after reaching various stages of development. The researchers labeled these arrested embryos "dead." These dead embryos, of course, are not suitable for transfer to a woman's womb and would normally be discarded. Stojković's team found that some of the cells within these arrested embryos remain healthy and can be induced to grow. These cell lines could then be used to generate other tissue types.

Scientist Donald Landry, who originally proposed the idea of obtaining stem cells from arrested embryos, remarked on the research: "Regardless of how you feel about personhood for embryos, if the embryo is dead, then the issue of personhood is resolved. This then reduces the ethics of human embryonic stem cell generation to the ethics of, say, organ donation. So now you're really saying, 'Can we take live cells from dead embryos the way we take live organs from dead patients?'" Landry believes that an embryo is dead "if the cells irreversibly stop working together to function as a single organism" (Ritter 2006).

Not everyone is convinced that the ethical problems have been resolved. Some critics have argued that Stojković's (and Landry's) determination that arrested embryos are dead is both arbitrary and ambiguous. Just as the question of when "life" begins is morally contentious, so too will be the question of when such "life" ends. If, indeed, cells within the embryo were induced to grow, this indicates some potential for life. Others note that the arrested embryos may have stopped growing because of lab conditions; they might very well have developed normally had they been implanted into a womb instead of placed in a petri dish. Still others worry that cells from arrested embryos may have defects—they obviously arrest for some reason—and these defects could cause problems if and when the stem cells are used for therapeutic purposes (Ritter 2006).

Discussion Questions

1. Do you think that arrested embryos should be labeled "dead"?
2. What do you make of Landry's "organ donation" analogy? Does it clarify or confuse the moral issues?
3. Does this method of obtaining stem cells seem ethically defensible?

Sources

Ritter, Malcolm. "Stem cells made from 'dead' embryo." Discovery News Online, 2006. http://dsc.discovery.com/news/2006/09/25/stems_hea.html (accessed April 14, 2008).

Zhang, Xin, Petra Stojkovic, Stefan Przyborski, Michael Cooke, Lyle Armstrong, Majlinda Lako, Miodrag Stojkovic. "Derivation of human embryonic stem cells from developing and arrested embryos." *Stem Cells* 24 (2006): 2669–76.

Dying Patients and the Right to Try Experimental Drugs

Do terminally ill patients have a right—moral or constitutional—to obtain experimental drugs that have not yet been approved by the FDA? This question has been brought to attention through the work of a group called the Abigail Alliance for Better Access to Developmental Drugs. The Abigail Alliance was formed in 2001 by Frank Burroughs, whose twenty-one-year-old daughter, Abigail, died of throat and head cancer. After her diagnosis with cancer, Abigail's family tried in vain to enroll her in a number of clinical trials for new cancer drugs. They were refused, since none of the drugs had yet been approved by the U.S. Food and Drug Administration (FDA).

The Abigail Alliance sued the FDA in 2003, claiming that terminally ill patients have the right to use experimental drugs that have passed through Phase I testing. The Abigail Alliance won its first victory against the FDA in 2006. The U.S. Court of Appeals for the D.C. Circuit upheld the Alliance's argument that access to experimental drugs is a constitutional right. The court ruled that dying patients have a basic "right of self-preservation" and "barring a terminally ill patient from the use of a potentially life-saving treatment impinges on this right of self-preservation." The court referred back to the landmark case of Nancy Cruzan, which established a "right to die." Judge Judith W. Rogers wrote: "If there is a protected liberty interest in self-determination that includes a right to refuse life-sustaining treatment, even though this will hasten death, then the same liberty interest must include the complementary right of access to potentially life-sustaining medication, in light of the explicit protection accorded 'life'" (Kaufman 2006).

Critics of the ruling argued that the FDA already has programs in place that make promising drugs available to patients, even before final approval has been given, through the so-called "compassionate use" provision. This FDA regulation allows drug companies to release a promising experimental drug to a particular patient who is not (for whatever reason) enrolled in a clinical trial. Furthermore, the drug-approval process exists—and is as lengthy and rigorous as it is—expressly for the protection of patients. Allowing large numbers of patients access to drugs about which little is known will place many people at risk.

It typically takes about 6 1/2 years for a drug company to gather enough data on a promising new substance or molecule to apply to the FDA for approval to test the drug. Clinical trials take, on average, another seven years. About ninety percent of new drugs that enter Phase I testing are eventually abandoned, either because of safety concerns or because they prove ineffective.

Discussion Questions

1. Assess the argument made by Judge Rogers that a person's freedom to refuse life-sustaining treatment includes the right of access to life-saving experimental drugs.
2. Should dying patients have a right to access experimental drugs? Why should the restriction be limited to dying patients?
3. If it were legally established that dying patients have a "right of self-preservation," what broader implications might this have for health care?

Sources

Kaufman, Marc. "Court backs experimental drugs for dying patients." *Washington Post*, May 3, 2006.

Groopman, Jerome. "Medical Dispatch: The Right to a Trial." *The New Yorker*, December 18, 2006. http://www.newyorker.com/archive/2006/12/18/061218fa_fact (accessed May 20, 2008).

Surgeon as Animal Rights Warrior

Dr. Jerry Vlasak is trauma surgeon by day, animal rights warrior by night. About ten years after finishing medical school, Vlasak was inspired by his wife to take up the cause of animals. Since then, he has been an active and vocal member of several animal rights groups, including Animal Liberation Press Office, for whom Vlasak works as a liaison between the underground activists and the press (those working underground remain anonymous because many of their activities are illegal).

In a hearing before a U.S. Senate committee in 2005, Vlasak said:

> Here in the U.S., there are thousands of physicians like myself who realize there is no need to kill animals in order to help humans, the vast majority of whom get sick and die because of preventable lifestyle variables such as diet, smoking, drugs and environmental toxins. In a country where 45 million people do without reliable access to ANY medical care, there is no reason to waste hundreds of millions of dollars testing drugs and procedures on non-human animals. In a world where 20,000 children are dying from lack of access to clean water each week world wide, there is no reason to waste hundreds of millions of dollars testing drugs and procedures on non-human animals.

Vlasak is controversial because he has also made statements that seem to justify the use of violence in the fight to stop animal research. For example, he said in an interview, "the animal rights movement has been the most peaceful and restrained movement the world has ever known considering the amount of terror, abuse and murder done to innocent animals for greed and profit. If by chance violence is used by those who fight for non-human sentient beings, or even if there are casualties, it must be looked at in perspective and in a historical context." He went on to say, "I am personally not advocating, condoning or recommending that anybody be killed. I am a physician who saves lives. I spend my entire day saving people's lives."

But according to an essay about Vlasak on the Animal Liberation Press Office's website, he defends the use of violence in the campaign for animal rights on both moral and pragmatic grounds. Violence against animal researchers, in the form of break-ins, sabotage, and even assault, is morally justified "given the suffering exploiters inflict on animals, the impossibility of ending their misery through legal systems that cater to exploitation industries and define animals as property, and the moral imperative to save animals from the violent clutches of exploiters" (Best 2008). On pragmatic grounds, Vlasak believes that violence and intimidation serve as a deterrent to researchers and potential researchers. In a newspaper interview, he defended the extreme tactics of animal liberationists. "I don't think you'd have to kill too many [researchers who experiment on animals]. I think for five lives, 10 lives, 15 human lives, we could save a million, 2 million, 10 million nonhuman lives." He went on: "No strictly peaceful movement has succeeded in liberation. John Brown dragged slave owners out of their beds and shot them in the street" (Mozingo 2006).

Discussion Questions

1. In his remarks to the Senate, Vlasak makes at least five different arguments against using animals in research. Identify these arguments and determine which ones are based on empirical claims and which on moral claims. In your view, which is the strongest and which is the weakest?
2. Does the fact that Vlasak is a doctor add to his moral authority on the ethics of using nonhuman animals?
3. Is his moral stance coherent? Can he condone violence in the fight against animal research, and at the same time be committed to his professional vocation?
4. What are the implications, positive and negative, of using the language of "liberation" to frame the moral agenda of animal advocates?

Sources

Best, Stephen. "Who's afraid of Jerry Vlasak?" Animal Liberation Press Office. 2008. http://www.animalliberationpressoffice.org/Writings_Speeches/whos_afraid_of_jerry_vlasak.html (accessed March 12, 2008).

"Statement of Jerry Vlasak." U.S. Senate, Wednesday, October 26, 2005. Committee on Environment and Public Works, Washington, DC. [A second hearing on ecoterrorism specifically examining Stop Huntingdon Animal Cruelty ("SHAC")]. http://www.naiaonline.org/pdfs/Oct.%2026,%202005%20eco-terrorism%20transcript.pdf (accessed March 12, 2008).

Mozingo, Joe. "Surgeon walks thin line on animal rights." *Los Angeles Times*, September 5, 2006.

Great Ape Protection Act

The Great Ape Protection Act (H.R. 5852) was introduced into Congress in April 2008. The bill seeks to phase out all invasive biomedical research and testing on great apes (chimpanzees, bonobos, gorillas, and orangutans) in U.S. laboratories.

The bill would prohibit the funding of research on great apes, in addition to the use, transport, or breeding of great apes. It also proposes that all federally owned great apes be released into permanent sanctuary. Of the estimated 1,200 great apes in U.S. laboratories, about 600 are federally owned and would be protected under the bill. A number of European countries have already enacted a ban on great ape research.

Spain has gone a step further. It has become the first country to grant formal legal standing to a nonhuman animal. Spain's parliament voted in June of 2008 to approve a resolution that would extend to great apes the legal rights to life and freedom. The resolution requires the Spanish government to protect apes from torture and abuse. It prohibits the imprisonment of apes without due process of law, prohibits killing apes except in strictly defined circumstances such as self-defense, and forbids the deliberate infliction of severe pain.

Discussion Questions

1. Would you support a ban on great ape research? Why or why not?
2. Why would research on great apes be different, morally speaking, from research on other animals?
3. How does our genetic relatedness to great apes factor into the moral equation?

Sources

H.R. 5852. http://www.govtrack.us/congress/bill.xpd?bill=h110–5852 (accessed March 12, 2008).

Humane Society of the United States, Fact Sheet on Chimpanzees in Research. http://www.hsus.org/web-files/PDF/legislation/chimps_research_factsheet.pdf (accessed March 12, 2008).

Abend, Lisa. 2008. "In Spain, Human Rights for Apes," http://www.time.com/time/world/article/0,8599,1824206,00.html (accessed March 12, 2008).

CHAPTER 7

Genetics, Biotechnology, and Posthuman Possibilities

INTRODUCTION

As we noted at the outset of chapter 6, the purpose of biomedical research is to increase scientific knowledge and to improve medical treatments. Not all areas of inquiry are equal, however, nor are all possible applications of knowledge. One of the most promising—yet also most controversial—areas of biomedical research has been in the field of genetics. Genetics is the study of patterns of inheritance, heredity, and variation among organisms. Developments in this area have fundamentally changed biological science and have profound implications for medical practice. We not only have discovered the basic structure of life, but now are acquiring the ability to alter that structure. Advances in our understanding of genetics have also fueled a revolution in biotechnology, an area of research that involves the use and modification of living organisms to create new products.

This chapter explores just a few examples of how genetics and biotechnology are raising new and pressing moral questions about manipulating human form and function and about applying and sharing genetic information. The first section of readings will broadly consider the ethical ramifications of emerging genetic and biotechnological knowledge. Each of the readings asks when and for what reasons it is appropriate to manipulate human form and functioning. As you will see, some people believe that manipulations should be limited to those with clear medical purpose, while others believe that at least some nonmedical applications of biotechnologies are justified. Still others embrace the potential of these developments to transform humanity into an entirely new "posthuman" species. The second section of readings focuses particularly on technologies and drugs that manipulate the human mind. Neuroscience is rapidly following genetics as "the next big thing," with profound implications for medicine and ethics, as well as many other fields. The third section of readings focuses on the application of genetics within medicine, particularly the use of genetic information to choose future children.

Genetic and Biotechnological Manipulations

In reality, of course, if any one age really attains, by eugenics and scientific education, the power to make its descendants what it pleases, all men who live after it are patients of that power. They are weaker, not stronger: for though we have put wonderful machines in their hands we have preordained how they are to use them.

—C.S. Lewis, *The Abolition of Man*

God and Nature first made us what we are, and then out of our own created genius we make ourselves what we want to be . . . Let the sky and God be our limit and Eternity our measurement.

—Marcus Garvey, *African Fundamentalism*

Science fiction is fast becoming science fact. In 1932, Aldous Huxley published his famous novel *Brave New World*, which depicted a negative utopia (sometimes called a dystopia) that was dominated by technology and a rigid social structure. Although the discovery of DNA, the ability to insert and delete genes to create new genetic combinations, *in vitro* fertilization, and cloning were still many years away, Huxley anticipated a world in which humans could deliberately create the types of people it wanted, and do so in bulk. As he made clear in his follow-up essay *Brave New World Revisited*, Huxley considered his book a warning about a potential future that we should try to avoid—our manipulation by commercial and political forces and consequent loss of freedom—but not as a call to reject the developing biotechnology itself. As you could see in the chapter 4 essays by Leon Kass and Raanan Gillon, *Brave New World* has been extremely influential in shaping bioethics perspectives regarding the potential dangers of genetics and reproductive technology. Powerful stories tend to have a strong impact, even among people who do not typically employ narrative ethics.

The biological and psychological manipulations of humans in *Brave New World* stand in sharp contrast to the historical standards and goals of medical practice, which have focused on healing the sick and injured, and restoring them to normal functioning insofar as that is possible. The immediate impact of medical intervention has always been limited to individual patients, whether that intervention ultimately succeeded or failed. Thus far, medical advances have not moved beyond healing or restoration, and their impact remains solely with the patient. Mechanical devices like pacemakers, cochlear ear implants, and LASIK eye surgery all are attempts to restore normal functioning.

The ability to manipulate the human genome, advancements in biotechnology, and developments in neuroscience all have the potential to reach beyond healing and restoring function to augmenting current capabilities and even adding new ones. Consequently, many people want to draw a clear line between *therapy*—the traditional role of medicine to attend to the sick, injured, and impaired—and *enhancement*—improving the capabilities of normally healthy people. Bioethics pioneer Paul Ramsey was influential in defending genetic therapy while condemning genetic enhancement. Whether such a clear line exists, however, has come into question. In chapter 2, Franklin Miller, Howard Brody, and Kevin Chung claim that while there are clear cases of ethically permissible and impermissible uses of reconstructive surgery, there is no sharp boundary between therapeutic and merely cosmetic applications. Instead, there is a continuum between the two. Many commentators now make similar claims regarding the blurred boundary between therapy and enhancement in genetics, biotechnology, and neuroscience.

Consider these two recent developments in biotechnology that have created cyborgs (humans that have computerized and/or mechanized parts). First, myoelectric arms now make it possible for amputees to regain some normal function, as well as perform specialized tasks that are impossible for people with standard appendages. Sgt. David Sterling, who lost his right hand and forearm to a grenade explosion in Iraq, "now wears an $85,000 myoelectric forearm, powered by a lithium battery, that approximates hand movements through electrical impulses when he flexes the remaining muscles in his arm." Besides a standard-looking artificial hand for "routine tasks like shaking hands and holding a glass," he can exchange the hand for a "hook or the pliers-like grip. . . . At home, he has snap-on kitchen devices, work tools and separate hands that help him write, play golf, shoot pool, even cast a fishing rod" (Janofsky 2004). Is Sgt. Sterling's myoelectric arm with multiple attachments therapy, or enhancement? Would you change your view if Sterling were adding attachments to a normally functioning arm, rather than a damaged one?

Second, neuromotor brain prosthetics—sensors implanted into the brain's motor cortex—allow patients with severe neurological injuries to interact with their environment. Andrew Nagle, who was paralyzed below his shoulders after being stabbed in the neck, was the first person to receive the 4mm-x-4mm implant in 2004. The sensor has one hundred electrodes, each connected to a single neuron. Like a character in the novel *Neuromancer* or the *Matrix* movies, Nagle can be plugged into a computer, where he can move a cursor, open e-mail, play a simple video game, change a television channel, and partially manipulate a mechanical arm (Hochberg et al. 2006; Pollack 2006). Does Nagle's regained ability to do things like control a TV and read e-mail make his brain implant strictly therapy, or, because he can do these things by thinking rather than acting, is it an enhancement? Would you change your view if Nagle had not been injured?

As Nagle's limited ability to move a mechanical arm indicates, these two examples are in the process of being combined. In a recent research project, two monkeys with brain prostheses were able to control a mechanical arm to grab food and feed themselves. They apparently discovered their own uses for the arm, such as bringing it to their mouths to lick marshmallow residue off the fingers. Researchers hope that eventually people like Nagle will be able to interact physically with their environment through the use of this technology (Carey 2008; Velliste et al. 2008).

But even when the distinction between therapy and enhancement is fairly clear, moral judgments may be more nuanced than simply supporting therapy and opposing enhancement. For example, in the context of genetics, David Resnick claims "that the distinction does not mark a firm boundary between moral and immoral genetic interventions, and that genetic enhancement is not inherently immoral. To evaluate the acceptability of any particular genetic intervention, one needs to examine the relevant facts in light of moral principles." Some therapies would be moral, others immoral; some enhancements would be moral, others immoral. Do they cause harm? Do they provide benefits? Do they respect or disrespect (or promote or diminish) autonomy? Are they fairly distributed? Mary Mahowald contends that the key moral considerations regarding enhancements are justice and equality. She finds enhancements to be more easily justified if they are given to the disadvantaged, thus improving their condition relative to the societal norm. Enhancements are more difficult to justify for people who are already "above average." Carl Elliot notes some additional concerns. He asks, who directs enhancement? Is it really us, exercising our autonomy and authentic choice, or is it the pharmaceutical industry and other corporate interests that drive our desires, making us feel inadequate about ourselves? Like Mahowald, he is concerned about distributive justice, but considers enhancements in relation to the larger problem of access to health care, not strictly in themselves. Elliot laments "that we will ignore important human needs at the expense of frivolous human desires.... We live in a country where 46 million uninsured people cannot get basic medical care, while the rest of us spend a billion dollars a year on baldness remedies."

A key distinction in the early bioethics debate over genetic manipulations was between *somatic cell* and *germ line* genetic interventions. A somatic cell is any cell in the body that is not a sperm or egg cell; the reproductive cells (cells of sperm or eggs) are called germ cells. ("Germ" is from L. *germen* [gen. *germinis*], "sprout, bud"; "somatic" is from Gk. *somatikos* "of the body," from *soma* [gen. *somatos*], "body.") Somatic cell genetic interventions modify only somatic cells in a person's body, and any changes impact only that person. A repaired genetic abnormality could still be passed along to the person's offspring. Germ line modifications, on the other hand, involve genetic alterations to egg or sperm cells (the germ cells). These changes will appear in the person who developed from that embryo, and are also passed along to any future offspring. This traditional terminology is beginning to change, and "germ line" interventions are now often referred to as "inheritable genetic modifications" because it is no longer clear that modification of germ cells is the only way to create inheritable changes. Just like the therapy/enhancement distinction, the somatic cell/inheritable genetic modification distinction has been a focal point of moral debate. Many ethicists have argued that somatic cell therapy is morally acceptable, while alteration of the gene pool is not. Some of these commentators object to human interference per se, while others focus on potentially negative consequences.

The 1982 President's Commission report discusses two metaphors that suggest caution toward, or even outright rejection, of germ-line manipulations and any genetic enhancements—Frankenstein and "playing God." Like *Brave New World*, these two metaphors continue to be influential in shaping ethical attitudes and judgments. Among the various, overlapping implications of the Frankenstein and playing-God metaphors are issues of power, control, fear, rebellion, isolation, and hubris.

Dr. Frankenstein sought the power to create new life; likewise, the ability to manipulate genes could result in the creation of new life forms. Dr. Frankenstein was unable to control his creation; genetic manipulations could prove harmful and beyond scientists' ability to control. Dr. Frankenstein worked in physical and moral isolation from others on his secret project, holding power over other people; a relatively small number of scientists work on genetic projects that are not necessarily well known among the general public, who (if they knew) might not support those projects. The Frankenstein metaphor is important for suggesting caution and areas of concern, but unless you think that it is absolutely wrong to engage in genetic manipulation or develop other biotechnology, then the alternative would be to adhere to another vision that avoids the problems that the metaphor evokes. Courtney Campbell contends that while the monster gets our attention, "the mythological meaning of Frankenstein lies not primarily in the objectively catastrophic outcome but in much more subtle and nuanced attitudes and dispositions of carelessness that give rise to such a project in the first place." The solution to avoiding such horror is "a caring and careful science and biotechnology."

As for playing God, there are several possible meanings for this metaphor. Although it could be construed as a prohibition against usurping powers that do not belong to humanity, the President's Commission instead views it as a call to accountability (unlike God, we have to answer to others for our actions) and responsibility (be careful to avoid bad consequences). The ability to manipulate the genome, even to the point of enhancement and creating new life forms, is a God-like power. The concern is that we lack the God-like knowledge and wisdom for using this power, and the ability to control the outcomes of its use. The metaphor "not only reminds human beings that they are only human and will some day have to pay if they underestimate their own ignorance and fallibility; it also points to the weighty and unusual nature of this activity, which stirs elusive fears that are not easily calmed."

Some religious bioethicists view the metaphor very differently, and as a call to responsible action. They view humanity's creation in the image of God as meaning that we have at least some of the same qualities as God. Because humans are called to imitate God, we are actually invited to play God, rather than prohibited from it. Nevertheless, Paul Ramsey claims that we must recognize that there is a right way to play God, which is how God plays God. Along these lines, Allen Verhey contends that the metaphor of playing God invokes a particular perspective or vision—we can be creators in the realm of genetics if our purpose is to heal, and if we take the side of the poor. God's justice demands that everyone should benefit from developments in genetics. Qaiser Shahzad finds an analogous paradigm in Islam.

Rather than interfering with God's creation, genetic and biological manipulations might also be understood as interfering with the natural processes of Mother Nature, that is, evolution. What will be the evolutionary impact on human beings as we tamper with the evolutionary process? We could in fact be harming ourselves as a species by utilizing gene therapy and other biotechnology, because it would keep weaker genes in the gene pool that otherwise could die out. We may be stopping the evolutionary process, making ourselves a stagnant species, unable to adapt to its changing environment. Germ-line therapy could also prove problematic if we delete certain genes that protect us from other diseases. It is well known that one version of the hemoglobin gene causes sickle-cell anemia if a person inherits two copies of it, but the same gene protects against malaria if paired with another variant, without causing sickle-cell disease. Similarly, people who carry two identical copies of the gene for prion protein are more susceptible to mad cow disease than if they were heterozygote, which most people are. Quite provocatively, Simon Mead et al. conjecture that resistance to mad cow disease exists because of widespread cannibalistic practices in prehistoric human populations. On the other hand, the capacity to manipulate genes arguably is itself a product of the evolutionary development of intelligence. Simon Young charges that failure to develop and utilize biotechnology would halt the evolutionary process, rather than the other way around. Evolution is about increasing complexity, and we humans have a "Will to Evolve" that provides a moral imperative to become posthuman.

Technological Manipulations and Posthuman Futures

Arthur Caplan contends that the arguments of people opposing efforts toward human improvement "cluster around three key worries: that the pursuit of perfection by biomedical means is vain, selfish, and unrewarding, that improving ourselves is unfair, and that enhancement or improvement violates human nature and may actually destroy it." He sees this last argument as their primary concern. "They fear that in applying new biomedical knowledge to improve human beings, something essential about humanity will be lost. If biomedical tinkering is allowed, we will destroy the very thing that makes us human—our nature." Caplan, however, is skeptical that there is such a thing as human nature, and would like people who express this concern first to specify what human nature is. What exactly will be altered for the worse by biotechnology?

You might consider whether Caplan's characterization applies to the readings in this chapter's first section, and whether these readings specify what important human quality biotechnology alters. The **President's Council on Bioethics** notes the great enthusiasm and concern regarding new developments in biotechnology, and acknowledges the potential for both great benefits and problems, emphasizing the importance of public discussion on these issues. The Council follows the recent trend of rejecting the strict distinction between therapy and enhancement, including nontherapeutic enhancement, viewing it only as a useful starting point for discussion. Focusing on the distinction can distract from the key moral questions. Of particular concern for the Council are dreams of human perfection and the "terrible consequences of pursuing it at all costs," which are important themes in Greek tragedy and in Nathaniel Hawthorne's short story "The Birthmark."

In his article, **Michael Sandel**, a member of the President's Council, seeks a moral language to frame the discussion about genetic engineering and other forms of biotechnology. He finds the language of individual autonomy insufficient for addressing the issues that arise with these technologies. An exclusive emphasis on autonomy is in fact the problem that he sees—the imperative to remake ourselves to suit whatever purposes and desires that we may have. Sandel proposes a secular version of the religious language of "giftedness." Rather than believe that everything is up to us, Sandel would like us to have sufficient humility to recognize our limitations. In spite of our best efforts, "our talents and powers are not wholly our own doing" and "not everything in the world is open to whatever use we may desire or devise." Such humility is crucial for human solidarity and concern for the least advantaged members of society. If everything truly were up to us and we were wholly responsible for our lot in life, then everyone would get what they deserved; there would be no reason to have sympathy for anyone who is disadvantaged. This is the dark side that he sees to the quest for human mastery and perfection.

Sara Goering explores the therapy/enhancement distinction by focusing specifically on genetic enhancements that have the purported goal of bettering our children. She asks, what exactly should count as "bettering" them? In exploring this question, Goering focuses on how we define "disease" and "disorder," and whether cultural assumptions about what it means to be normal may influence judgments about what needs "treatment." She considers, for example, the labeling of homosexuality, deafness, and short stature as abnormal, and thus (presumably) in need of treatment. Goering suggests using a kind of thought experiment to distinguish between legitimate genetic interventions aimed at alleviating physical ailments and discriminatory or arbitrary interventions.

The next reading focuses on genetic manipulations from the perspective of a religious tradition. **Jeffrey Burack** is a physician and bioethicist, and writes a Jewish reflection on genetic enhancement. Burack notes the importance of humility in Judaism, and how it is central to Jewish apprehension about genetic enhancement. Nevertheless, in contrast to the Promethean concerns raised by Sandel, Burack notes that Judaism envisions an exalted role for humanity. Similar to the views of the religious ethicists cited earlier, Burack thinks that we are called to be "co-creators" with God, and charged to improve the world. In doing so, we are not usurping God's power or "playing God," but rather acting in the role God has given us. Instead of a definitive answer regarding the legitimacy of genetic enhancement, he proposes a set of questions to consider. The key point for Burack is being clear regarding the purposes of enhancements. They must truly improve the world, and be in line with notions of humility, giftedness, and duty.

In contrast to the cautious warnings of Goering and the President's Council, philosopher **Nick Bostrom** offers an unabashed defense of using enhancement technologies—whether from neuroscience or any other area of research—to improve the human condition. Bostrom is founder of the World Transhumanist Association, and an ardent proponent of using technology to move beyond the human condition, to become first a "transhuman" and finally, if all goes well, a "posthuman." (A transhuman is a transitional being, moderately enhanced.) Transhumanism is an approach to understanding and evaluating the opportunities for enhancing the human condition and the human organism through technology. Transhumanists view human nature as a work in progress, a "half-baked beginning." They encourage the direct application of medicine and technology to overcome some of our technological limits, and are hopeful that we will soon become posthumans, or beings with vastly greater capacities than present human beings have. Bostrom considers some of the most basic limitations of the human mode of being: (1) life span, (2) intellectual capacity, (3) bodily functionality, (4) sensory modalities, special faculties, and sensibilities, and (5) mood, energy, and self-control. The core transhumanist value, Bostrom argues, is exploring the posthuman realm, and the basic conditions for realizing this project are global security, technological progress, and wide access to the fruits of technology.

Manipulating the Mind

Genetics and biotechnology raise important questions about manipulating the human person, and about whether manipulations that go beyond therapy are morally acceptable and, if so, under what conditions. Developments in the field of neuroscience raise, in particularly pointed ways, moral issues about therapy and enhancement—because the organ being manipulated in this case is the human brain. "Neuroethics" is a newly emerging subfield of bioethics that focuses on questions raised by technological advances in neuroscience. Many of the ethical issues raised by neuroscience are continuous with issues in other areas of bioethics, such as concerns about whether certain treatments benefit or harm patients, or whether new technology can be distributed fairly. However, the issues are also uniquely challenging because the brain is the seat of consciousness and of the "mind," and is thus critical to our sense of self.

Neuroscience is the study of the nervous system, which includes the brain, the spinal column, and the network of about one hundred billion neurons (sensory nerve cells) spread throughout the body. Chemicals called neurotransmitters help neurons communicate with each other by carrying electrical signals across synapses, which are small gaps between neurons. A great deal of neuroscience is *basic* research, which is theoretical or experimental work aimed at increasing our general understanding of thought, emotion, and behavior, without attention to specific medical or other applications. But the clinical applications of neuroscience are also important, and are where many of the moral concerns arise.

Neuroscience may offer effective treatments for degenerative brain disorders such as Alzheimer's disease, mental illness, and stroke phenomenon, and may improve diagnosis and treatment of behavioral disorders such as autism and Asperger's syndrome. Research in neuroscience is also relevant to the treatment and status of people in coma or persistent vegetative state, and also consequently to ethics discussions about removing life support from patients with impaired consciousness. For example, a research team claimed in 2006 to have discovered that a patient in a vegetative state had conscious awareness and could communicate through her thoughts (see the chapter 3 case, "Is There Anybody in There?"). This highly controversial research threw a wrench into the ongoing discussion of whether and when to remove life support from vegetative patients.

The therapeutic application of neuroscience poses its share of ethical challenges. But the real moral excitement tends to center around nontherapeutic applications—the use of neuroscience tools, techniques, and knowledge to enhance the human person. In the first reading in the "Enhancing the Mind" section of this chapter, bioethicist **Paul Root Wolpe** explores the role of emerging neurotechnologies in enhancement of mental traits or skills in people with no pathology. Enhancement, as he notes, raises questions about how we define "normal" and "diseased," and poses questions about whether we should encourage people to improve their mood and memory. Wolpe looks particularly carefully at "neuropharmaceuticals" or drugs that alter specific brain functions such as mood and memory. Various drugs are being designed for "brain enhancement," promising to lift our mood, improve our mental acuity and concentration, and sharpen our memory.

The next reading narrows in on one particular area of neurological enhancement: memory. The excerpt "Memory and Happiness" from the **President's Council on Bioethics'** *Beyond Therapy* explores in detail the ethics of developing and using drugs both to improve "good" memory and to wash away traumatic memories. Although these may sound like futuristic scenarios, there is already research that offers the potential to alter memory in both of these ways. "Memory and Happiness" is really a meditation on what memory is, and how memories—both good and bad—create in us a sense of who we are. Good memories contribute to our happiness, but bad memories can be essential to our growth as human beings. Perfect memory is not a desirable goal; rather, remembering well is "remembering at the right pitch." The Council discusses some of the biotechnologies that do or perhaps will alter memory, either by improving the memory of those who are losing it, or by removing or blunting the effects of bad memory. They give particular attention to the potential for treatment of people suffering from post-traumatic stress disorder, and argue that even for these people, treatment with memory-erasing drugs would not be a good idea. People have an obligation to remember truthfully, especially if they carry with them memories that the community needs to retain (of genocide, racism, etc.). Memory is intimately tied to moral responsibility.

Genetics and Future Children

Although gene therapy has enjoyed success in a few cases, we have not yet entered the era of genetic medicine where we can correct genetic problems and enhance characteristics. Even identifying the genes associated with particular diseases and traits is problematic, because often there is no direct correspondence between a single gene and a disease or trait. Nevertheless, there are some clearly identifiable genetic "signatures" for certain traits and maladies, some of which indicate a predisposition toward an outcome. Genetic tests can discern whether a person possesses that signature. Genetic tests also have important nonmedical uses, such as in criminal investigations and in determining paternity. This latter use was part of an investigation into the historical mystery of whether one of the American Founding Fathers, Thomas Jefferson, had fathered children with one of his slaves, Sallie Hemings. Although it is not absolutely certain that he did so, we now know that there is a genetic link between the Jefferson and Hemings descendants based upon Y-chromosome DNA samples. (It is possible, although less likely, that one of Jefferson's relatives fathered Hemings's youngest child on a visit to Jefferson's home, Monticello.)

Dena Davis considers a dilemma confronted by genetic counselors: should they help parents who desire a child that shares their disability? Davis frames the discussion as a conflict between parental autonomy and the child's right to autonomy, or its right to "an open future" (i.e., its options for the future should be as broad as possible, and not diminished by decisions made by others). In such a conflict, Davis views the child's right as having greater moral weight than parental autonomy. She considers the particular case of deaf parents choosing to have a deaf child, and explores whether that choice would violate the child's right to an open future.

In order to ensure that they would have a deaf child, the parents in Davis's case might choose to utilize *in vitro* fertilization, because they could then use preimplantation genetic diagnosis (PGD)—also called embryo screening—to select the appropriate embryo. **John Robertson** discusses potential new uses of PGD, which include detection for late-onset disorders like Huntington's and Alzheimer's, ensuring a compatible tissue donor for an existing child, gender selection, and selecting for various "nonmedical" traits like intelligence, athleticism, and perfect pitch. Robertson finds the new medical uses to be ethically acceptable. Regarding nonmedical uses, Robertson proposes five key questions for ethical evaluation of those uses, and then applies those questions to analyze two particular cases: gender selection and perfect pitch.

The Genetic Information Nondiscrimination Act

Genetic information is power. It not only can be used to make medical diagnoses and prognoses, but it can also be used as a barrier to employment and insurance coverage. On April 24, 2008—just one day before National DNA Day, which commemorates the discovery of the double helix and the completion of the Human Genome project—the U.S. Congress passed the Genetic Information Nondiscrimination Act (GINA). GINA prohibits insurance companies or employers from using genetic information about an individual to deny benefits or increase premiums. In other words, an individual's genetic predisposition to developing some disease in the future cannot be used against him or her in the present.

The law responds to the rapid progress medical science has made in the past decade in understanding the genetic variants at play in various diseases, from breast cancer to diabetes. The number of people who might benefit from genetic testing is growing quickly.

Francis Collins, director of the National Human Genome Research Institute, testified before Congress in 2007 to support GINA:

> Since the completion of the Human Genome Project (HGP) in 2003, major advances in our understandings of the causes of disease have been appearing at an accelerated pace. As one example, the HGP enabled the development of the "HapMap," a detailed map of variations in the spelling of our DNA instruction books.... It is the vision of NHGRI [National Human Genome Research Institute] that within the next ten years, the cost of sequencing the complete genome of an individual will be $1,000 or less. Should an individual so choose, this information could then be used as part of routine medical care, providing health care professionals with a more accurate means to predict disease, personalize treatment, and preempt the occurrence of illness.
>
> Even before the $1000 genome becomes a reality, advances from genome research are already leading to important new understanding of the role of genetic factors in a number of common diseases.

Unless Americans are convinced that their genetic information will not be used against them, the era of personalized medicine may never come to pass. The result would be a continuation of the current one-size-fits-all medicine, ignoring the abundant scientific evidence that the genetic differences among people help explain why some of us benefit from a therapy while others do not, and why some of us suffer severe adverse effects from a medication, while others do not.

In its findings related to the legislation, Congress also noted some of the dangers of increased genetic knowledge.

> The early science of genetics became the basis of State laws that provided for the sterilization of persons having presumed genetic "defects" such as mental retardation, mental disease, epilepsy, blindness, and hearing loss, among other conditions. The first sterilization law was enacted in the State of Indiana in 1907. By 1981, a majority of States adopted sterilization laws to "correct" apparent genetic traits.... The current explosion in the science of genetics, and the history of sterilization laws by the States based on early genetic science, compels Congressional action in this area.
>
> Although genes are facially neutral markers, many genetic conditions and disorders are associated with particular racial and ethnic groups and gender. Because some genetic traits are most prevalent in particular groups, members of a particular group may be stigmatized or discriminated against as a result of that genetic information.
>
> Congress has been informed of examples of genetic discrimination in the workplace. These include the use of pre-employment genetic screening at Lawrence Berkeley Laboratory. . ... Congress clearly has a compelling public interest in relieving the fear of discrimination and in prohibiting its actual practice in employment and health insurance (H.R. 493).

Proponents of the bill say that fear of genetic discrimination has prevented thousands of people from taking genetic tests that might provide valuable information, and which might shape the kinds of health care choices they make. Genetic Alliance, an umbrella coalition that brings together disease-specific advocacy groups, lobbied hard to get GINA through Congress. When the bill passed, the Genetic Alliance proclaimed that GINA "will be the first civil rights act passed by the Congress in almost twenty years."

Some lobbying groups for manufacturers and insurance companies opposed GINA. They claimed that the legislation may force employers to offer insurance coverage for all genetically related conditions, and may lead to frivolous and expensive lawsuits. Health policymakers acknowledged that expanding genetic information may alter the landscape of health insurance. Karen Pollitz, director of the Health Policy Institute at Georgetown University, responded to the law: "Ultimately unlocking all these genetic secrets will make the whole idea of private health insurance obsolete."

GINA is a federal law, but not the first of its kind in the United States. Oregon led the way with its 1995 genetic privacy act. The point of the act was to protect personal privacy by preventing disclosure of genetic information. It defined genetic information as the property of the individual from whom it was derived. In 1997, pharmaceutical corporation Smith Kline Beecham lobbied the Oregon legislature to repeal the property provision, claiming that it was having a negative impact on research. Under the law, research subjects might claim to own the fruits of research projects, because their genetic information is their property. In 2001, Oregon repealed the property provision, replacing it with a confidentiality clause and other protections.

REFERENCES AND FURTHER READING

Buchanan, Allen. *From Chance to Choice: Genetics and Justice*. Cambridge: Cambridge University Press, 2001.

Cahill, Lisa. *Genetics, Theology, and Ethics*. Crossroad Publishing New York, NY, 2005.

Campbell, Courtney S. "Biotechnology and the Fear of Frankenstein." *Cambridge Quarterly of Healthcare Ethics* 12 (2003): 342–52.

Caplan, Arthur, and Carl Elliot. "Is It Ethical to Use Enhancement Technologies to Make Us Better Than Well?" *PLoS Medicine* 1, no. 3 (2004): 172–75.

Carey, Benedict. "Monkeys Think, Moving Artificial Arm as Own." *New York Times*, May 29, 2008. http://www.nytimes.com/2008/05/29/science/29brain.html (accessed May 29, 2008).

Collins, Francis. "The Threat of Genetic Discrimination to the Promise of Personalized Medicine." (Hearing before the House of Representatives). http://waysandmeans.house.gov/Media/pdf/110/3–14–07/CollinsTestimony.pdf (accessed May 7, 2008).

Fischbach R.L. and Fischbach G.D. "Neuroethicists needed now more than ever." *American Journal of Bioethics* 8, no. 1 (2008): 47–48.

Fukuyama, Francis. *Our Posthuman Future: Consequences of the Biotechnology Revolution*. New York: Farrar, Straus, and Giroux, 2002.

Gazzaniga, Michael S. "Better Brains Through Genes." From *The Ethical Brain*, 37–54. New York: Dana Press, 2005.

——. and Franco Furger. *Beyond Bioethics. A Proposal for Modernizing the Regulation of Human Biotechnologies*. Washington, DC: The Paul H. Nitze School of Advanced International Studies, 2008.

Glover, Jonathan. *Choosing Children: Genes, Disability, and Design*. New York: Oxford University Press, 2008.

Hochberg, Leigh R., Mijail D. Serruya, Gerhard M. Friehs, Jan A. Mukand, Maryam Saleh, Abraham H. Caplan, Almut Branner, David Chen, Richard D. Penn, and John P. Donoghue. "Neuronal Ensemble Control of Prosthetic Devices by a Human with Tetraplegia." *Nature* 442 (July 13, 2006): 164–71.

Huxley, Aldous. *Brave New World*. New York: Harper & Bros, 1932.

____. *Brave New World Revisited*. New York: Harper & Bros., 1958.

Janofsky, Michael. "Redefining the Front Lines in Reversing War's Toll." *New York Times*, June 21, 2004. http://query.nytimes.com/gst/fullpage.html?res=9B07E2DA1239F932 A15755C0A9629C8B63(accessed May 28, 2008).

Kamm, Frances M. "Is There a Problem With Enhancement?" *American Journal of Bioethics* 5, no. 3 (2005): 5–14.

Mahowald, Mary. "Drawing Lines Between Extremes: Medical Enhancement and Eugenics." *The Pluralist* 1 no. 2 (2006): 19–34.

Mead, Simon, Michael P. H. Stumpf, Jerome Whitfield, Jonathan A. Beck, Mark Poulter, Tracy Campbell, James B. Uphill, David Goldstein, Michael Alpers, Elizabeth M. C. Fisher, John Collinge. "Balancing Selection at the Prion Protein Gene Consistent with Prehistoric Kurulike Epidemics." *Science* 300 (April 25, 2003): 640–43.

Pang, Tikki. "The Impact of Genomics on Global Health." *American Journal of Public Health* 92, no. 7 (2003): 1077–179.

Peters, Ted. *Playing God: Genetic Determinism and Human Freedom*. New York: Routledge, 1996.

Pollack, Andrew. "Paralyzed Man Uses Thoughts to Move a Cursor." *New York Times*, July 13, 2006. http://www.nytimes.com/2006/07/13/science/brain.html (accessed May 28, 2008).

President's Commission for the Study of Ethical Problems in Medicine and Biomedical and Behavioral Research. *Splicing Life: A Report on the Social and Ethical Issues of Genetic Engineering with Human Beings*. Washington, DC: U.S. Government Printing Office, 1982.

Ramsey, Paul. *Fabricated Man: The Ethics of Genetic Control*. New Haven, CT: Yale University Press, 1970.

____. *The Patient as Person: Explorations in Medical Ethics*. New Haven, CT: Yale University Press, 1970.

Resnick, David. "The Moral Significance of the Therapy-Enhancement Distinction in Human Genetics." *Cambridge Quarterly of Healthcare Ethics* 9 (2000): 365–77.

Shahzad, Qaiser. "Playing God and the Ethics of Divine Names: An Islamic Paradigm for Biomedical Ethics." *Bioethics* 21, no. 8 (2007): 413–18.

Smart, Andrew, Paul Martin, and Michael Parker. "Tailored Medicine: Whom Will It Fit? The Ethics of Patient and Disease Stratification." *Bioethics* 18, no. 4(2004): 322–43.

Society for Neuroscience. Homepage http://www.sfn.org/ (accessed April 1, 2008).

Velliste, Meel, Sagi Perel, M. Chance Spalding, Andrew S. Whitford & Andrew B. Schwartz. "Cortical Control of a Prosthetic Arm for Self-Feeding." *Nature*, May 28, 2008. http://www.nature.com/nature/journal/vaop/ncurrent/full/nature06996.html (accessed May 20, 2008).

Verhey, Allen. "Playing God and Invoking a Perspective." *Journal of Medicine and Philosophy* 20, no. 4 (1995): 347–64.

Young, Simon. *Designer Evolution: A Transhumanist Manifesto*. Amherst, MA: Prometheus Books, 2006.

DISCUSSION QUESTIONS ON THE READINGS

Biotechnology and the Pursuit of Happiness: An Introduction

1. How do the authors define "biotechnology"?
2. How do they define "therapy" and "enhancement"? Why is this distinction useful? What is problematic about the distinction?
3. Give several examples of biotechnology applications that might be morally problematic because of implicit assumptions about health and normality.

The Case Against Perfection

1. Sandel canvasses and ultimately rejects various arguments against genetic enhancements. Characterize three of these arguments, and say why Sandel considers each one insufficient to make a case against enhancement.
2. What does Sandel mean by an "ethics of giftedness"?
3. How does an ethic of giftedness foster a sense of social solidarity?

Jewish Reflections on Genetic Enhancement

1. What concept is at the core of Jewish apprehensions about enhancement?
2. What does Burack mean when he says that Judaism's moral framework is aspirational?
3. How does a Jewish perspective transform the therapy/enhancement question?
4. Compare Burack's account of giftedness with Sandel's.

Gene Therapies and the Pursuit of a Better Human

1. What are some problems with using a medical model for deciding which genetic therapies will "better" our children?
2. What thought experiment does Goering employ to help think through what might count as a justifiable genetic improvement?
3. What sorts of improvements might Goering endorse? Reject?

Transhumanist Values

1. What is a posthuman? A transhuman?
2. How does Bostrom characterize the posthuman project?
3. What might a transhumanist say about the distinction between theory and enhancement?
4. Compare Bostrom's view of a "better" human with Goering's. Whose vision do you find most compelling?
5. Is Bostrom interested in perfection, in Sandel's sense of the word?

Treatment, Enhancement, and the Ethics of Neurotherapeutics

1. Why are neurological enhancements unique, according to Wolpe? Why do they raise unique ethical questions?
2. What do you think about the use of neurological enhancements such as modafinil in soldiers, to improve combat readiness?
3. Does Wolpe generally embrace neurological enhancement, or reject it? On what moral grounds?

Memory and Happiness

1. Why is memory so essential to our sense of self?
2. How are emotions and memory linked?
3. Why does the President's Council consider the use of memory-blunters problematic? (Note both practical and philosophical problems.)
4. Why (and what) might we have a responsibility to remember?

Genetic Dilemmas and the Child's Right to an Open Future

1. How does Davis want to reconceive the moral conflict faced by genetic counselors working with parents who want to have a child with a disability?
2. What does a child's right to an open future encompass?
3. How does Davis's argument compare with Sara Goering's arguments about gene therapies? Do you think Goering would agree with Davis about deafness as a disability?

Extending Preimplantation Genetic Diagnosis: Medical and Non-Medical Uses

1. Does Robertson support the use of PGD in selecting for perfect pitch? For gender?
2. How does Robertson's medical/nonmedical distinction compare with the therapy/enhancement distinction discussed by the President's Council, Sandel, and Wolpe?
3. Would screening an embryo for deafness count as a medical use? Would Robertson likely support the use of PGD in this scenario? (What would Davis likely think?)

READINGS

Biotechnology and the Pursuit of Happiness

An Introduction

PRESIDENT'S COUNCIL ON BIOETHICS

From *Beyond Therapy: Biotechnology and the Pursuit of Happiness*. http://www.bioethics.gov/reports/beyond-therapy/beyond_therapy_final_webcorrected.pdf (accessed March 30, 2008) 1–20.

What is biotechnology for? Why is it developed, used, and esteemed? Toward what ends is it taking us? To raise such questions will very likely strike the reader as strange, for the answers seem so obvious: to feed the hungry, to cure the sick, to relieve the suffering—in a word, to improve the lot of humankind, or, in the memorable words of Francis Bacon, "to relieve man's estate." Stated in such general terms, the obvious answers are of course correct. But they do not tell the whole story, and, when carefully considered, they give rise to some challenging questions, questions that compel us to ask in earnest not only, "What is biotechnology for?" but also, "What should it be for?"

Before reaching these questions, we had better specify what we mean by "biotechnology," for it is a new word for our new age. Though others have given it both narrow and broad definitions, our purpose—for reasons that will become clear—recommends that we work with a very broad meaning: the processes and products (usually of industrial scale) offering the potential to alter and, to a degree, to control the phenomena of life—in plants, in (non-human) animals, and, increasingly, in human beings (the last, our exclusive focus here). Overarching the processes and products it brings forth, biotechnology is also a *conceptual and ethical outlook*, informed by progressive aspirations. In this sense, it appears as a most recent and vibrant expression of the technological spirit, a desire and disposition rationally to understand, order, predict, and (ultimately) control the events and workings of nature, all pursued for the sake of human benefit.

Thus understood, biotechnology is bigger than its processes and products; it is a form of human empowerment. By means of its techniques (for example, recombining genes), instruments (for example, DNA sequencers), and products (for example, new drugs or vaccines), biotechnology empowers us human beings to assume greater control over our lives, diminishing our subjection to disease and misfortune, chance and necessity. The techniques, instruments, and products of biotechnology—like similar technological fruit produced in other technological areas—augment our capacities to act or perform effectively, for many different purposes. Just as the automobile is an instrument that confers enhanced powers of "auto-mobility" (of moving *oneself*), which powers can then be used for innumerable purposes not defined by the machine itself, so DNA sequencing is a technique that confers powers for genetic screening that can be used for various purposes not determined by the technique; and synthetic growth hormone is a product that confers powers to try to increase height in the short or to augment muscle strength in the old. If we are to understand what biotechnology is for, we shall need to keep our eye more on the new abilities it provides than on the technical instruments and products that make the abilities available to us.

Defining the Topic

The "beyond therapy" uses of biotechnology on human beings are manifold. We shall not here consider biotechnologies as instruments of bioterrorism or of mass population control. The former topic is highly specialized and tied up with matters of national security, an area beyond our charge and competence. Also, although the practical and political difficulties they raise are enormous, the ethical and social issues are relatively uncomplicated. The main question about bioterrorism is not what to think about it but how to prevent it. And the use of tranquilizing aerosols for crowd control or contraceptive additions to the drinking water, unlikely prospects in liberal democratic societies like our own, raise few issues beyond the familiar one of freedom and coercion.

Much more ethically challenging are those "beyond therapy" uses of biotechnology that would appeal to free and enterprising people, that would require no coercion, and, most crucially, that would satisfy widespread human desires. Sorting out and dealing with the ethical and social issues of such practices will prove vastly more difficult since they will be intimately connected with goals that go with, rather than against, the human grain. For these reasons, we confine our attention to those well-meaning and strictly voluntary uses of biomedical technology through which the user is seeking some improvement or augmentation of his or her own capacities, or, from similar benevolent motives, of those of his or her children. Such use of biotechnical powers to pursue "improvements" or "perfections," whether of body, mind, performance, or sense of well-being, is at once both the most seductive and the most disquieting temptation. It reflects humankind's deep dissatisfaction with natural limits and its ardent desire to overcome them. It also embodies what is genuinely novel and worrisome in the biotechnical revolution, beyond the so-called "life issues" of abortion and embryo destruction, important though these are. What's at issue is not the crude old power to kill the creature made in God's image but the attractive science-based power to remake ourselves after images of our own devising. As a result, it gives unexpected practical urgency to ancient philosophical questions: What is a good life? What is a good community?

The Limitations of the "Therapy Versus Enhancement" Distinction

Although, as we have indicated, the topic of the biotechnological pursuit of human improvement has not yet made it onto the agenda of public bioethics, it has received a certain amount of attention in academic bioethical circles under the rubric of "enhancement," understood in contradistinction to "therapy." Though we shall ourselves go beyond this distinction, it provides a useful starting place from which to enter the discussion of activities that aim "beyond therapy." "Therapy," on this view as in common understanding, is the use of biotechnical power to treat individuals with known diseases, disabilities, or impairments, in an attempt to restore them to a normal state of health and fitness. "Enhancement," by contrast, is the directed use of biotechnical power to alter, by direct intervention, not disease processes but the "normal" workings of the human body and psyche, to augment or improve their native capacities and performances. Those who introduced this distinction hoped by this means to distinguish between the acceptable and the dubious or unacceptable uses of biomedical technology: therapy is always ethically fine, enhancement is, at least prima facie, ethically suspect. Gene therapy for cystic fibrosis or Prozac for major depression is fine; insertion of genes to enhance intelligence or steroids for Olympic athletes is, to say the least, questionable.

At first glance, the distinction between therapy and enhancement makes good sense. Ordinary experience recognizes the difference between "restoring to normal" and "going beyond the normal." Also, as a practical matter, this distinction seems a useful way to distinguish between the central and obligatory task of medicine (healing the sick) and its marginal and extracurricular practices (for example, Botox injections and other merely cosmetic surgical procedures). Because medicine has, at least traditionally,

pursued therapy rather than enhancement, the distinction helps to delimit the proper activities of physicians, understood as healers. And because physicians have been given a more-or-less complete monopoly over the prescription and administration of biotechnology to human beings, the distinction, by seeking to circumscribe the proper goals of medicine, indirectly tries to circumscribe also the legitimate uses of biomedical technology. Accordingly, it also helps us decide about health care costs: health providers and insurance companies have for now bought into the distinction, paying for treatment of disease, but not for enhancements. More fundamentally, the idea of enhancement understood as seeking something "better than well" points to the perfectionist, not to say utopian, aspiration of those who would set out to improve upon human nature in general or their own particular share of it.

But although the distinction between therapy and enhancement is a fitting beginning and useful shorthand for calling attention to the problem (and although we shall from time to time make use of it ourselves), it is finally inadequate to the moral analysis. "Enhancement" is, even as a term, highly problematic. In its most ordinary meaning, it is abstract and imprecise. Moreover, "therapy" and "enhancement" are overlapping categories: all successful therapies are enhancing, even if not all enhancements enhance by being therapeutic. Even if we take "enhancement" to mean "nontherapeutic enhancement," the term is still ambiguous. When referring to a human function, does enhancing mean making more of it, or making it better? Does it refer to bringing something out more fully, or to altering it qualitatively? In what meaning of the term are both improved memory and selective erasure of memory "enhancements"?

Beyond these largely verbal and conceptual ambiguities, there are difficulties owing to the fact that both "enhancement" and "therapy" are bound up with, and absolutely dependent on, the inherently complicated idea of health and the always-controversial idea of normality. The differences between healthy and sick, fit and unfit, are experientially evident to most people, at least regarding themselves, and so are the differences between sickness and other troubles. When we are bothered by cough and high fever, we suspect that we are sick, and we think of consulting a physician, not a clergy-man. By contrast, we think neither of sickness nor of doctors when we are bothered by money problems or worried about the threat of terror-ist attacks. But there are notorious difficulties in trying to define "healthy" and "impaired," "normal" and "abnormal" (and hence, "super-normal"), especially in the area of "behavioral" or "psychic" functions and activities. Some psychiatric diagnoses—for example, "dysthy-mia," "oppositional disorder," or "social anxiety disorder"—are rather vague: what is the differ-ence between extreme shyness and social anxi-ety? And, on the positive side, mental health shades over into peace of mind, which shades over into contentment, which shades over into happiness. If one follows the famous World Health Organization definition of health as "a state of complete physical, mental and social well-being," almost any intervention aimed at enhancement may be seen as health-promoting, and hence "therapeutic," if it serves to promote the enhanced individual's mental well-being by making him happier.

Yet even for those using a narrower defini-tion of health, the distinction between therapy and enhancement will prove problematic. While in some cases—for instance, a chronic disease or a serious injury—it is fairly easy to point to a departure from the standard of health, other cases defy simple classification. Most human capacities fall along a continuum, or a "normal distribution" curve, and individuals who find themselves near the lower end of the normal dis-tribution may be considered disadvantaged and therefore unhealthy in comparison with others. But the average may equally regard themselves as disadvantaged with regard to the above average. If one is responding in both cases to perceived dis-advantage, on what principle can we call helping someone at the lower end "therapy" and helping someone who is merely average "enhancement"? In which cases of traits distributed "normally" (for example, height or IQ or cheerfulness) does the average also function as a norm, or is the norm itself appropriately subject to alteration?

Further complications arise when we consider causes of conditions that clamor for modifica-tion. Is it therapy to give growth hormone to a genetic dwarf, but not to a short fellow who is just unhappy to be short? And if the short are brought up to the average, the average, now having become short, will have precedent for a claim to growth hormone injections. Since more and more scientists believe that all traits of personality have at least a partial biologi-cal basis, how will we distinguish the biological "defect" that yields "disease" from the biological condition that yields shyness or melancholy or irascibility?

For these reasons, among others, relying on the distinction between therapy and enhance-ment to do the work of moral judgment will not succeed. In addition, protracted arguments about whether or not something is or is not an "enhancement" can often get in the way of the proper ethical questions: What are the good and bad uses of biotechnical power? What makes a use "good," or even just "acceptable"? It does not follow from the fact that a drug is being taken solely to satisfy one's desires—for example, to increase concentration or sexual performance—that its use is objectionable. Conversely, certain interventions to restore functioning whole-ness—for example, to enable postmenopausal women to bear children or sixty-year-old men to keep playing professional ice hockey—might well be dubious uses of biotechnical power. The human meaning and moral assessment must be tackled directly; they are unlikely to be settled by the term "enhancement," any more than they are by the nature of the technological intervention itself.

The Case Against Perfection

What's Wrong with Designer Children, Bionic Athletes, and Genetic Engineering

MICHAEL J. SANDEL

The Atlantic Monthly (April 2004): 51–62.

Breakthroughs in genetics present us with a promise and a predicament. The promise is that we may soon be able to treat and prevent a host of debilitating diseases. The predicament is that our newfound genetic knowledge may also enable us to manipulate our own nature—to enhance our muscles, memories, and moods; to choose the sex, height, and other genetic traits of our children; to make ourselves "better than well." When science moves faster than moral understanding, as it does today, men and women struggle to articulate their unease. In liberal societies they reach first for the language of autonomy, fairness, and individual rights. But this part of our moral vocabulary is ill equipped to address the hardest questions posed by genetic engineering. The genomic revolution has induced a kind of moral vertigo.

Consider cloning. The birth of Dolly the cloned sheep, in 1997, brought a torrent of concern about the prospect of cloned human beings. There are good medical reasons to worry. Most scientists agree that cloning is unsafe, likely to produce offspring with serious abnormalities. (Dolly recently died a premature death.) But suppose technology improved to the point where clones were at no greater risk than naturally conceived offspring. Would human cloning still be objectionable? Should our hesitation be moral as well as medical? What, exactly, is wrong with creating a child who is a genetic twin of one parent, or of an older sibling who has tragically died—or, for that matter, of an admired scientist, sports star, or celebrity?

Some say cloning is wrong because it violates the right to autonomy: by choosing a child's genetic makeup in advance, parents deny the child's right to an open future. A similar objection can be raised against any form of bioengineering that allows parents to select or reject genetic characteristics. According to this argument, genetic enhancements for musical talent, say, or athletic prowess, would point children toward particular choices, and so designer children would never be fully free.

At first glance the autonomy argument seems to capture what is troubling about human cloning and other forms of genetic engineering. It is not persuasive, for two reasons. First, it wrongly implies that absent a designing parent, children are free to choose their characteristics for themselves. But none of us chooses his genetic inheritance. The alternative to a cloned or genetically enhanced child is not one whose future is unbound by particular talents but one at the mercy of the genetic lottery.

Second, even if a concern for autonomy explains some of our worries about made-to-order children, it cannot explain our moral hesitation about people who seek genetic remedies or enhancements for themselves. Gene therapy on somatic (that is, nonreproductive) cells, such as muscle cells and brain cells, repairs or replaces defective genes. The moral quandary arises when people use such therapy not to cure a disease but to reach beyond health, to enhance their physical or cognitive capacities, to lift themselves above the norm.

Like cosmetic surgery, genetic enhancement employs medical means for nonmedical ends—ends unrelated to curing or preventing disease or repairing injury. But unlike cosmetic surgery, genetic enhancement is more than skin-deep. If we are ambivalent about surgery or Botox injections for sagging chins and furrowed brows, we are all the more troubled by genetic engineering for stronger bodies, sharper memories, greater intelligence, and happier moods. The question is whether we are right to be troubled, and if so, on what grounds.

In order to grapple with the ethics of enhancement, we need to confront questions largely lost from view—questions about the moral status of nature, and about the proper stance of human beings toward the given world. Since these questions verge on theology, modern philosophers and political theorists tend to shrink from them. But our new powers of biotechnology make them unavoidable. To see why this is so, consider four examples already on the horizon: muscle enhancement, memory enhancement, growth-hormone treatment, and reproductive technologies that enable parents to choose the sex and some genetic traits of their children. In each case what began as an attempt to treat a disease or prevent a genetic disorder now beckons as an instrument of improvement and consumer choice.

Muscles

Everyone would welcome a gene therapy to alleviate muscular dystrophy and to reverse the debilitating muscle loss that comes with old age. But what if the same therapy were used to improve athletic performance? Researchers have developed a synthetic gene that, when injected into the muscle cells of mice, prevents and even reverses natural muscle deterioration. The gene not only repairs wasted or injured muscles but also strengthens healthy ones. This success bodes well for human applications. H. Lee Sweeney, of the University of Pennsylvania, who leads the research, hopes his discovery will cure the immobility that afflicts the elderly. But Sweeney's bulked-up mice have already attracted the attention of athletes seeking a competitive edge. Although the therapy is not yet approved for human use, the prospect of genetically enhanced weight lifters, home-run sluggers, linebackers, and sprinters is easy to imagine. The widespread use of steroids and other performance-improving drugs in professional sports suggests that many athletes will be eager to avail themselves of genetic enhancement.

Suppose for the sake of argument that muscle-enhancing gene therapy, unlike steroids, turned out to be safe—or at least no riskier than a rigorous weight-training regimen. Would there be a reason to ban its use in sports? There is something unsettling about the image of genetically altered athletes lifting SUVs or hitting 650-foot home runs or running a three-minute mile. But what, exactly, is troubling about it? Is it simply that we find such superhuman spectacles too bizarre to contemplate? Or does our unease point to something of ethical significance?

It might be argued that a genetically enhanced athlete, like a drug-enhanced athlete, would have an unfair advantage over his unenhanced competitors. But the fairness argument against enhancement has a fatal flaw: it has always been the case that some athletes are better endowed genetically than others, and yet we do not consider this to undermine the fairness of competitive sports. From the standpoint of fairness, enhanced genetic differences would be no worse than natural ones, assuming they were safe and made available to all. If genetic enhancement in sports is morally objectionable, it must be for reasons other than fairness.

Memory

Genetic enhancement is possible for brains as well as brawn. In the mid-1990s scientists managed to manipulate a memory-linked gene in fruit flies, creating flies with photographic memories. More recently researchers have produced smart mice by inserting extra copies of a memory-related gene into mouse embryos. The altered mice learn more quickly and remember things longer than normal mice. The extra copies were programmed to remain active even in old age, and the improvement was passed on to offspring.

Human memory is more complicated, but biotech companies, including Memory Pharmaceuticals, are in hot pursuit of memory-enhancing drugs, or "cognition enhancers," for human beings. The obvious market for such drugs consists of those who suffer from Alzheimer's and other serious memory disorders. The companies also have their sights on a bigger market: the 81 million Americans over fifty, who are beginning to encounter the memory loss that comes naturally with age. A drug that reversed age-related memory loss would be a bonanza for the pharmaceutical industry: a Viagra for the brain. Such use would straddle the line between remedy and enhancement. Unlike a treatment for Alzheimer's, it would cure no disease; but insofar as it restored capacities a person once possessed, it would have a remedial aspect. It could also have purely nonmedical uses: for example, by a lawyer cramming to memorize facts for an upcoming trial, or by a business executive eager to learn Mandarin on the eve of his departure for Shanghai.

Some who worry about the ethics of cognitive enhancement point to the danger of creating two classes of human beings: those with access to enhancement technologies, and those who must make do with their natural capacities. And if the enhancements could be passed down the generations, the two classes might eventually become subspecies—the enhanced and the merely natural. But worry about access ignores the moral status of enhancement itself. Is the scenario troubling because the unenhanced poor would be denied the benefits of bioengineering, or because the enhanced affluent would somehow be dehumanized? As with muscles, so with memory: the fundamental question is not how to ensure equal access to enhancement but whether we should aspire to it in the first place.

Height

Pediatricians already struggle with the ethics of enhancement when confronted by parents who want to make their children taller. Since the 1980s human growth hormone has been approved for children with a hormone deficiency that makes them much shorter than average. But the treatment also increases the height of healthy children. Some parents of healthy children who are unhappy with their stature (typically boys) ask why it should make a difference whether a child is short because of a hormone deficiency or

because his parents happen to be short. Whatever the cause, the social consequences are the same.

In the face of this argument some doctors began prescribing hormone treatments for children whose short stature was unrelated to any medical problem. By 1996 such "off-label" use accounted for 40 percent of human-growth-hormone prescriptions. Although it is legal to prescribe drugs for purposes not approved by the Food and Drug Administration, pharmaceutical companies cannot promote such use. Seeking to expand its market, Eli Lilly & Co. recently persuaded the FDA to approve its human growth hormone for healthy children whose projected adult height is in the bottom one percentile—under five feet three inches for boys and four feet eleven inches for girls. This concession raises a large question about the ethics of enhancement: If hormone treatments need not be limited to those with hormone deficiencies, why should they be available only to very short children? Why shouldn't all shorter-than-average children be able to seek treatment? And what about a child of average height who wants to be taller so that he can make the basketball team?

Some oppose height enhancement on the grounds that it is collectively self-defeating; as some become taller, others become shorter relative to the norm. Except in Lake Wobegon, not every child can be above average. As the unenhanced began to feel shorter, they, too, might seek treatment, leading to a hormonal arms race that left everyone worse off, especially those who couldn't afford to buy their way up from shortness.

But the arms-race objection is not decisive on its own. Like the fairness objection to bioengineered muscles and memory, it leaves unexamined the attitudes and dispositions that prompt the drive for enhancement. If we were bothered only by the injustice of adding shortness to the problems of the poor, we could remedy that unfairness by publicly subsidizing height enhancements. As for the relative height deprivation suffered by innocent bystanders, we could compensate them by taxing those who buy their way to greater height. The real question is whether we want to live in a society where parents feel compelled to spend a fortune to make perfectly healthy kids a few inches taller.

Sex Selection

Perhaps the most inevitable nonmedical use of bioengineering is sex selection. For centuries parents have been trying to choose the sex of their children. Today biotech succeeds where folk remedies failed.

One technique for sex selection arose with prenatal tests using amniocentesis and ultrasound. These medical technologies were developed to detect genetic abnormalities such as spina bifida and Down syndrome. But they can also reveal the sex of the fetus—allowing for the abortion of a fetus of an undesired sex. Even among those who favor abortion rights, few advocate abortion simply because the parents do not want a girl. Nevertheless, in traditional societies with a powerful cultural preference for boys, this practice has become widespread.

Sex selection need not involve abortion, however. For couples undergoing *in vitro* fertilization (IVF), it is possible to choose the sex of the child before the fertilized egg is implanted in the womb. One method makes use of preimplantation genetic diagnosis (PGD), a procedure developed to screen for genetic diseases. Several eggs are fertilized in a petri dish and grown to the eight-cell stage (about three days). At that point the embryos are tested to determine their sex. Those of the desired sex are implanted; the others are typically discarded. Although few couples are likely to undergo the difficulty and expense of IVF simply to choose the sex of their child, embryo screening is a highly reliable means of sex selection. And as our genetic knowledge increases, it may be possible to use PGD to cull embryos carrying undesired genes, such as those associated with obesity, height, and skin color. The science-fiction movie *Gattaca* depicts a future

in which parents routinely screen embryos for sex, height, immunity to disease, and even IQ. There is something troubling about the *Gattaca* scenario, but it is not easy to identify what exactly is wrong with screening embryos to choose the sex of our children.

One line of objection draws on arguments familiar from the abortion debate. Those who believe that an embryo is a person reject embryo screening for the same reasons they reject abortion. If an eight-cell embryo growing in a petri dish is morally equivalent to a fully developed human being, then discarding it is no better than aborting a fetus, and both practices are equivalent to infanticide. Whatever its merits, however, this "pro-life" objection is not an argument against sex selection as such.

The latest technology poses the question of sex selection unclouded by the matter of an embryo's moral status. The Genetics & IVF Institute, a for-profit infertility clinic in Fairfax, Virginia, now offers a sperm-sorting technique that makes it possible to choose the sex of one's child before it is conceived. X-bearing sperm, which produce girls, carry more DNA than Y-bearing sperm, which produce boys; a device called a flow cytometer can separate them. The process, called MicroSort, has a high rate of success.

If sex selection by sperm sorting is objectionable, it must be for reasons that go beyond the debate about the moral status of the embryo. One such reason is that sex selection is an instrument of sex discrimination—typically against girls, as illustrated by the chilling sex ratios in India and China. Some speculate that societies with substantially more men than women will be less stable, more violent, and more prone to crime or war. These are legitimate worries—but the sperm-sorting company has a clever way of addressing them. It offers MicroSort only to couples who want to choose the sex of a child for purposes of "family balancing." Those with more sons than daughters may choose a girl, and vice versa. But customers may not use the technology to stock up on children of the same sex, or even to choose the sex of their firstborn child. (So far the majority of MicroSort clients have chosen girls.) Under restrictions of this kind, do any ethical issues remain that should give us pause?

The case of MicroSort helps us isolate the moral objections that would persist if muscle-enhancement, memory-enhancement, and height-enhancement technologies were safe and available to all.

It is commonly said that genetic enhancements undermine our humanity by threatening our capacity to act freely, to succeed by our own efforts, and to consider ourselves responsible—worthy of praise or blame—for the things we do and for the way we are. It is one thing to hit seventy home runs as the result of disciplined training and effort, and something else, something less, to hit them with the help of steroids or genetically enhanced muscles. Of course, the roles of effort and enhancement will be a matter of degree. But as the role of enhancement increases, our admiration for the achievement fades—or, rather, our admiration for the achievement shifts from the player to his pharmacist. This suggests that our moral response to enhancement is a response to the diminished agency of the person whose achievement is enhanced.

Though there is much to be said for this argument, I do not think the main problem with enhancement and genetic engineering is that they undermine effort and erode human agency. The deeper danger is that they represent a kind of hyperagency—a Promethean aspiration to remake nature, including human nature, to serve our purposes and satisfy our desires. The problem is not the drift to mechanism but the drive to mastery. And what the drive to mastery misses and may even destroy is an appreciation of the gifted character of human powers and achievements.

To acknowledge the giftedness of life is to recognize that our talents and powers are not wholly our own doing, despite the effort we expend to develop and to exercise them. It is also to recognize that not everything in the world is open to whatever use we may desire or devise. Appreciating the gifted quality of life constrains the Promethean project and conduces to a cer-

tain humility. It is in part a religious sensibility. But its resonance reaches beyond religion.

It is difficult to account for what we admire about human activity and achievement without drawing upon some version of this idea. Consider two types of athletic achievement. We appreciate players like Pete Rose, who are not blessed with great natural gifts but who manage, through striving, grit, and determination, to excel in their sport. But we also admire players like Joe DiMaggio, who display natural gifts with grace and effortlessness. Now, suppose we learned that both players took performance-enhancing drugs. Whose turn to drugs would we find more deeply disillusioning? Which aspect of the athletic ideal—effort or gift—would be more deeply offended?

Some might say effort: the problem with drugs is that they provide a shortcut, a way to win without striving. But striving is not the point of sports; excellence is. And excellence consists at least partly in the display of natural talents and gifts that are no doing of the athlete who possesses them. This is an uncomfortable fact for democratic societies. We want to believe that success, in sports and in life, is something we earn, not something we inherit. Natural gifts, and the admiration they inspire, embarrass the meritocratic faith; they cast doubt on the conviction that praise and rewards flow from effort alone. In the face of this embarrassment we inflate the moral significance of striving, and depreciate giftedness. This distortion can be seen, for example, in network-television coverage of the Olympics, which focuses less on the feats the athletes perform than on heartrending stories of the hardships they have overcome and the struggles they have waged to triumph over an injury or a difficult upbringing or political turmoil in their native land.

But effort isn't everything. No one believes that a mediocre basketball player who works and trains even harder than Michael Jordan deserves greater acclaim or a bigger contract. The real problem with genetically altered athletes is that they corrupt athletic competition as a human activity that honors the cultivation and display of natural talents. From this standpoint, enhancement can be seen as the ultimate expression of the ethic of effort and willfulness—a kind of high-tech striving. The ethic of willfulness and the biotechnological powers it now enlists are arrayed against the claims of giftedness.

The ethic of giftedness, under siege in sports, persists in the practice of parenting. But here, too, bioengineering and genetic enhancement threaten to dislodge it. To appreciate children as gifts is to accept them as they come, not as objects of our design or products of our will or instruments of our ambition. Parental love is not contingent on the talents and attributes a child happens to have. We choose our friends and spouses at least partly on the basis of qualities we find attractive. But we do not choose our children. Their qualities are unpredictable, and even the most conscientious parents cannot be held wholly responsible for the kind of children they have. That is why parenthood, more than other human relationships, teaches what the theologian William F. May calls an "openness to the unbidden."

May's resonant phrase helps us see that the deepest moral objection to enhancement lies less in the perfection it seeks than in the human disposition it expresses and promotes. The problem is not that parents usurp the autonomy of a child they design. The problem lies in the hubris of the designing parents, in their drive to master the mystery of birth. Even if this disposition did not make parents tyrants to their children, it would disfigure the relation between parent and child, and deprive the parent of the humility and enlarged human sympathies that an openness to the unbidden can cultivate.

To appreciate children as gifts or blessings is not, of course, to be passive in the face of illness or disease. Medical intervention to cure or prevent illness or restore the injured to health does not desecrate nature but honors it. Healing sickness or injury does not override a child's natural capacities but permits them to flourish.

Nor does the sense of life as a gift mean that parents must shrink from shaping and directing the development of their child. Just as athletes and artists have an obligation to cultivate their talents, so parents have an obligation to cultivate their children, to help them discover and develop their talents and gifts. As May points out, parents give their children two kinds of love: accepting love and transforming love. Accepting love affirms the being of the child, whereas transforming love seeks the well-being of the child. Each aspect corrects the excesses of the other, he writes: "Attachment becomes too quietistic if it slackens into mere acceptance of the child as he is." Parents have a duty to promote their children's excellence.

These days, however, overly ambitious parents are prone to get carried away with transforming love—promoting and demanding all manner of accomplishments from their children, seeking perfection. "Parents find it difficult to maintain an equilibrium between the two sides of love," May observes. "Accepting love, without transforming love, slides into indulgence and finally neglect. Transforming love, without accepting love, badgers and finally rejects." May finds in these competing impulses a parallel with modern science: it, too, engages us in beholding the given world, studying and savoring it, and also in molding the world, transforming and perfecting it.

Sorting out the lesson of eugenics is another way of wrestling with the ethics of enhancement. The Nazis gave eugenics a bad name. But what, precisely, was wrong with it? Was the old eugenics objectionable only insofar as it was coercive? Or is there something inherently wrong with the resolve to deliberately design our progeny's traits?

James Watson, the biologist who, with Francis Crick, discovered the structure of DNA, sees nothing wrong with genetic engineering and enhancement, provided they are freely chosen rather than state-imposed. And yet Watson's language contains more than a whiff of the old eugenic sensibility. "If you really are stupid, I would call that a disease," he recently told *The Times* of London. "The lower 10 percent who really have difficulty, even in elementary school, what's the cause of it? A lot of people would like to say, 'Well, poverty, things like that.' It probably isn't. So I'd like to get rid of that, to help the lower 10 percent." A few years ago Watson stirred controversy by saying that if a gene for homosexuality were discovered, a woman should be free to abort a fetus that carried it. When his remark provoked an uproar, he replied that he was not singling out gays but asserting a principle: women should be free to abort fetuses for any reason of genetic preference—for example, if the child would be dyslexic, or lacking musical talent, or too short to play basketball.

Watson's scenarios are clearly objectionable to those for whom all abortion is an unspeakable crime. But for those who do not subscribe to the pro-life position, these scenarios raise a hard question: If it is morally troubling to contemplate abortion to avoid a gay child or a dyslexic one, doesn't this suggest that something is wrong with acting on any eugenic preference, even when no state coercion is involved?

Consider the market in eggs and sperm. The advent of artificial insemination allows prospective parents to shop for gametes with the genetic traits they desire in their offspring. It is a less predictable way to design children than cloning or pre-implantation genetic screening, but it offers a good example of a procreative practice in which the old eugenics meets the new consumerism. A few years ago some Ivy League newspapers ran an ad seeking an egg from a woman who was at least five feet ten inches tall and athletic, had no major family medical problems, and had a combined SAT score of 1400 or above. The ad offered $50,000 for an egg from a donor with these traits. More recently a Web site was launched claiming to auction eggs from fashion models whose photos appeared on the site, at starting bids of $15,000 to $150,000.

On what grounds, if any, is the egg market morally objectionable? Since no one is forced to buy or sell, it cannot be wrong for reasons of coercion. Some might worry that hefty prices would exploit poor women by presenting them with an offer they couldn't refuse. But the designer eggs that fetch the highest prices are likely to be sought from the privileged, not the poor. If the market for premium eggs gives us moral qualms, this, too, shows that concerns about eugenics are not put to rest by freedom of choice.

A tale of two sperm banks helps explain why. The Repository for Germinal Choice, one of America's first sperm banks, was not a commercial enterprise. It was opened in 1980 by Robert Graham, a philanthropist dedicated to improving the world's "germ plasm" and counteracting the rise of "retrograde humans." His plan was to collect the sperm of Nobel Prize-winning scientists and make it available to women of high intelligence, in hopes of breeding supersmart babies. But Graham had trouble persuading Nobel laureates to donate their sperm for his bizarre scheme, and so settled for sperm from young scientists of high promise. His sperm bank closed in 1999.

In contrast, California Cryobank, one of the world's leading sperm banks, is a for-profit company with no overt eugenic mission. Cappy Rothman, M.D., a co-founder of the firm, has nothing but disdain for Graham's eugenics, although the standards Cryobank imposes on the sperm it recruits are exacting. Cryobank has offices in Cambridge, Massachusetts, between Harvard and MIT, and in Palo Alto, California, near Stanford. It advertises for donors in campus newspapers (compensation up to $900 a month), and accepts less than five percent of the men who apply. Cryobank's marketing materials play up the prestigious source of its sperm. Its catalogue provides detailed information about the physical characteristics of each donor, along with his ethnic origin and college major. For an extra fee prospective customers can buy the results of a test that assesses the donor's temperament and character type. Rothman reports that Cryobank's ideal sperm donor is six feet tall, with brown eyes, blond hair, and dimples, and has a college degree—not because the company wants to propagate those traits, but because those are the traits his customers want: "If our customers wanted high school dropouts, we would give them high school dropouts."

Not everyone objects to marketing sperm. But anyone who is troubled by the eugenic aspect of the Nobel Prize sperm bank should be equally troubled by Cryobank, consumer-driven though it be. What, after all, is the moral difference between designing children according to an explicit eugenic purpose and designing children according to the dictates of the market? Whether the aim is to improve humanity's "germ plasm" or to cater to consumer preferences, both practices are eugenic insofar as both make children into products of deliberate design.

The problem with eugenics and genetic engineering is that they represent the one-sided triumph of willfulness over giftedness, of dominion over reverence, of molding over beholding. Why, we may wonder, should we worry about this triumph? Why not shake off our unease about genetic enhancement as so much superstition? What would be lost if biotechnology dissolved our sense of giftedness?

From a religious standpoint the answer is clear: To believe that our talents and powers are wholly our own doing is to misunderstand our place in creation, to confuse our role with God's. Religion is not the only source of reasons to care about giftedness, however. The moral stakes can also be described in secular terms. If bioengineering made the myth of the "self-made man" come true, it would be difficult to view our talents as gifts for which we are indebted, rather than as achievements for which we are responsible. This would transform three key features of our moral landscape: humility, responsibility, and solidarity.

In a social world that prizes mastery and control, parenthood is a school for humility. That we care deeply about our children and yet cannot choose the kind we want teaches parents to be open to the unbidden. Such openness is a disposition worth affirming, not only within families but in the wider world as well. It invites us to abide the unexpected, to live with dissonance,

to rein in the impulse to control. A *Gattaca*-like world in which parents became accustomed to specifying the sex and genetic traits of their children would be a world inhospitable to the unbidden, a gated community writ large. The awareness that our talents and abilities are not wholly our own doing restrains our tendency toward hubris.

One of the blessings of seeing ourselves as creatures of nature, God, or fortune is that we are not wholly responsible for the way we are. The more we become masters of our genetic endowments, the greater the burden we bear for the talents we have and the way we perform. Today when a basketball player misses a rebound, his coach can blame him for being out of position. Tomorrow the coach may blame him for being too short. Even now the use of performance-enhancing drugs in professional sports is subtly transforming the expectations players have for one another; on some teams players who take the field free from amphetamines or other stimulants are criticized for "playing naked."

The more alive we are to the chanced nature of our lot, the more reason we have to share our fate with others. Consider insurance. Since people do not know whether or when various ills will befall them, they pool their risk by buying health insurance and life insurance. As life plays itself out, the healthy wind up subsidizing the unhealthy, and those who live to a ripe old age wind up subsidizing the families of those who die before their time. Even without a sense of mutual obligation, people pool their risks and resources and share one another's fate.

A lively sense of the contingency of our gifts—a consciousness that none of us is wholly responsible for his or her success—saves a meritocratic society from sliding into the smug assumption that the rich are rich because they are more deserving than the poor. Without this, the successful would become even more likely than they are now to view themselves as self-made and self-sufficient, and hence wholly responsible for their success. Those at the bottom of society would be viewed not as disadvantaged, and thus worthy of a measure of compensation, but as simply unfit, and thus worthy of eugenic repair. The meritocracy, less chastened by chance, would become harder, less forgiving. As perfect genetic knowledge would end the simulacrum of solidarity in insurance markets, so perfect genetic control would erode the actual solidarity that arises when men and women reflect on the contingency of their talents and fortunes.

Thirty-five years ago Robert L. Sinsheimer, a molecular biologist at the California Institute of Technology, glimpsed the shape of things to come. In an article titled "The Prospect of Designed Genetic Change" he argued that freedom of choice would vindicate the new genetics, and set it apart from the discredited eugenics of old.

To implement the older eugenics...would have required a massive social programme carried out over many generations. Such a programme could not have been initiated without the consent and co-operation of a major fraction of the population, and would have been continuously subject to social control. In contrast, the new eugenics could, at least in principle, be implemented on a quite individual basis, in one generation, and subject to no existing restrictions.

According to Sinsheimer, the new eugenics would be voluntary rather than coerced, and also more humane. Rather than segregating and eliminating the unfit, it would improve them. "The old eugenics would have required a continual selection for breeding of the fit, and a culling of the unfit," he wrote. "The new eugenics would permit in principle the conversion of all the unfit to the highest genetic level."

Sinsheimer's paean to genetic engineering caught the heady, Promethean self-image of the age. He wrote hopefully of rescuing "the losers in that chromosomal lottery that so firmly channels our human destinies," including not only those born with genetic defects but also "the 50,000,000 'normal' Americans with an IQ of less than 90." But he also saw that something bigger than improving on nature's "mindless, age-old throw of dice" was at stake. Implicit in technologies of genetic intervention was a more exalted place for human beings in the cosmos. "As we enlarge man's freedom, we diminish his constraints and that which he must accept as given," he wrote. Copernicus and Darwin had "demoted man from his bright glory at the focal point of the universe," but the new biology would restore his central role. In the mirror of our genetic knowledge we would see ourselves as more than a link in the chain of evolution: "We can be the agent of transition to a whole new pitch of evolution. This is a cosmic event."

There is something appealing, even intoxicating, about a vision of human freedom unfettered by the given. It may even be the case that the allure of that vision played a part in summoning the genomic age into being. It is often assumed that the powers of enhancement we now possess arose as an inadvertent by-product of biomedical progress—the genetic revolution came, so to speak, to cure disease, and stayed to tempt us with the prospect of enhancing our performance, designing our children, and perfecting our nature. That may have the story backwards. It is more plausible to view genetic engineering as the ultimate expression of our resolve to see ourselves astride the world, the masters of our nature. But that promise of mastery is flawed. It threatens to banish our appreciation of life as a gift, and to leave us with nothing to affirm or behold outside our own will.

Gene Therapies and the Pursuit of a Better Human

SARA GOERING

Cambridge Quarterly of Healthcare Ethics 9 (2000): 330–41.

Surely no one would dispute the claim that the aim of bettering humanity and/or our own children is morally acceptable. Indeed, most of us see as ideal a world in which every parent works toward improving the lot of his or her child, or the lot of all of our children. But while no one denies the importance of this quite general goal, we are still left with difficult issues about *how* we ought to proceed in addressing that goal. When we try to dodge diseases or disadvantages through genetic intervention, are we solving problems or just moving them to a different level?

How are we to decide what is to count as "bettering" children? Few of us would dispute the claim that eliminating Tay-Sachs disease or Lesch-Nyan syndrome or cystic fibrosis would count as an improvement for future generations. A future in which no one has to suffer from these debilitating diseases seems undeniably worth pursuing. On the other hand, disability rights advocates are quick to point out practical problems with holding this view without devaluing existing persons with those diseases. Even if we can conceptually distinguish between the value of individuals with disabilities and the relative value of bringing such individuals into existence given other options, in practice, public attitudes toward such individuals are likely to be prejudiced and will likely affect public financial support of the disabled.

Even if we could reach agreement about the value of genetically intervening for clear cases of debilitating disorders, there are some physiologically or genetically based conditions that offer disadvantages to children in our society that might not so clearly be candidates for intervention. What about cases in which the real cause of the disadvantage is located in unjustified societal prejudices or values? For instance, children who

are shorter than average (and grow into shorter than average adults) have a smaller statistical chance for success in classes and in athletics (and ultimately in the job market) because of the biased perception of them based on their inferior height. Physicians who offer growth hormone treatments treat the physiological symptoms of shortness as a way of solving the social problem for the child. But the community is then allowed to continue its arbitrary preference for taller people. In this case, society is at fault for creating the disadvantage—solving the real problem seems to require addressing societal values, *not* just engineering a way around the problem. This may seem obvious, since when height is the feature in question, there is no absolute advantage to be had, but only a relative advantage. There is no inherent value to being six feet tall, but it is advantageous if you are *taller* than others (within limits). But the same can be said of other features that do not rely on relative advantage, such as societal standards of beauty (having a symmetric face, hair in appropriate places and not in inappropriate places, etc.). Some interventions that appear to be beneficial for the recipient may not be real benefits after all if they leave the root of the disadvantages unaddressed.

Another difficult case is deafness. Most hearing people consider deafness to be a defect, a physiological problem that deserves medical attention if and when it is available. But at least a segment of the Deaf community values their physiology as different but equal to that of hearing people, and they may argue that the only reason that deafness confers any disadvantage in society (when it does), is because of unfair societal discrimination and the fact that society is set up for the benefit of the hearing. Indeed, a 1994 publication of the Denver Ear Institute notes that many deaf people consider deafness "a birthright to a distinctive and rewarding way of life." The Deaf community is rich and complex in terms of language, art, and social association. Deaf community advocates suggest that the Deaf are more appropriately considered a cultural and linguistic minority (on par, for instance, with Hispanic-Americans) than a disabled group. The availability of cochlear implants for deaf children has sparked the debate about the future of the Deaf community, and it will surely only be enflamed by the possibility of genetically engineering to avoid some forms of deafness. Segments of the dwarf community have made similar claims about the value of their genetic condition and problems with therapies that try to "rectify" it. Is the elimination of deafness or dwarfism a benefit, or is it a systematic destruction of special minority communities?

We might also ask ourselves about the case of homosexuality. Simon LeVay's announcement in 1991 of a statistical difference in the sizes of a particular hypothalamic nucleus between heterosexual males and homosexual males evoked a loud public debate about the relevance of genetic or biology-based explanations for homosexual lifestyles. If there is a genetic basis for homosexuality, then we must ask ourselves what to do about it. A homophobic parent might aspire to have this "defect" fixed, even though homosexuality itself does not bring about disadvantages; rather, homosexuals are often unfairly discriminated against by a society that arbitrarily devalues their lifestyle. Should we try to engineer a solution to this supposed "problem," or should we work to educate people that the only problem is within their unreasonable biases?

In general, then, it appears that we may not want to genetically treat (or eliminate) just any condition or trait that confers disadvantage to our children, especially when the disadvantages are not a direct result of the trait; rather, we need to find a reasonable decisionmaking process that will help to delineate what traits are acceptable candidates for genetic therapy or genetic engineering. The dominant paradigm in the literature for drawing this line has been a distinction between treatment and enhancement, based on standard medical practices. If we use the standard model of medical practice that relies on a principle of beneficence and is tied to a "normal" human capabilities model, then it seems justifiable (or perhaps even obligatory) for us to treat defects or diseases. But nothing follows about the permissibility of using genetic intervention for the purpose of mere enhancement. This distinction is intuitively appealing to doctors, genetic scientists, and the general public, including many medical ethicists, but it has been rejected more recently by ethicists on the basis of its vagueness.

According to the medical model, the basis for pursuing any genetic therapies is the relief of pain and suffering. W. French Anderson argues that genetic diseases that "produce significant suffering and premature death" ought to be the first candidates for genetic therapies, and then, if we succeed with those cases, we might be justified in extending genetic treatments to other diseases. He claims, however, that we should not undertake any genetic engineering for the purpose of enhancement. He offers two reasons why we should not engage in any enhancement engineering. First, he thinks that sort of engineering is "medically hazardous" because we are less sure about what "adding" a gene could do to the complex system compared to fixing an existing gene. Second, he believes that it is "morally precarious" because we don't have a clear way of determining what genes should be provided, who should receive them, and how to prevent discrimination against those who don't receive them. His proposal involves the claim that it is problematical for us to determine the details of enhancement engineering, but not problematical, and in fact defensible, for us to employ treatment of disease as a clear category for use of genetic engineering. This proposal is sound only if there is indeed no clear line between acceptable improvements and problematic ones, and if there is a clear line between treatment and enhancement. But is such a view defensible?

How are we to define "disease," if that is what we are allowed to treat? If we look more closely at the concepts of health and disease, we discover that the label "disease" is not metaphysically pure. Indeed, while we often assume that a disease is an objectively identifiable state, in fact, the identification of something as a disease is dependent at least in part on evaluative judgments of the physician or general society. Some commentators assume that the physiological conditions to be included under the label "disease" are ones that are identified either as abnormal or as dysfunctional relative to species norms. On this view, to be diseased is merely to exemplify a certain abnormal physiological state, whether or not it is disadvantageous or painful to the person. Anyone in any society could be objectively labeled as diseased simply by reference to his or her exemplification of the relevant physiological state. But this view does not stand up to difficult cases, as numerous commentators have pointed out. Disease is not simply a physiological state, but a physiological state that bears significantly on the functioning of the individual in his or her society. Colorblindness is not considered a significant disorder or disease in the United States, but in some places in Africa "in which the capacity to distinguish a great variety of shades of green is needed to function at a minimal level for survival" it is highly problematic. As Harlan Lane notes, alcohol use, tobacco addiction, large body weights, the need for eyeglasses, and hookworm infestation are all considered diseases in certain societies and not in others. The American medical system has recently medicalized many conditions that were not previously considered appropriate for "treatment," including "contraception, fertility, pregnancy, childbirth, child development, hyperactivity in children, reading difficulty, learning problems, drug addiction, criminality, child abuse, physical disability, exercise, hygiene, sleeplessness, diet, breast and nose size, wrinkles, baldness, obesity, and shortness." We view certain physical states as diseases because of our judgments about what is dysfunctional, and those judgments depend on our values and social norms, resources, and standard medical practices. These may differ across societies and across time periods, as well as within societies and time periods. Consider, for example, the fact that masturbation and homosexuality were both once identified as diseases. When we realize that the definition of disease is norm based, then we find that "the intuitively attractive reply that 'If we stick to curing disease and promoting health, all will be well' begins to lose its attraction." What counts as a disease depends on physiology but also on what the particular society values. Consequently, the line between treatment of disease and enhancement-directed engineering seems itself to rely on a rather fuzzy distinction.

There is also the further problem of defining when something is a disease in a society that agrees that a particular condition is not valuable. For instance, no one desires atherosclerosis and the heart attacks and strokes that often follow it. Evidence suggests that there is a gene that determines the body's ability to regulate blood cholesterol levels by production of low density lipoprotein (LDL) receptors on body cells. Inserting additional LDL receptor genes in otherwise normal individuals might reduce the probability for their developing atherosclerosis. But atherosclerosis is not so rigidly tied to genetic production of LDL receptors. Treatment could also take the form of reducing consumption of low density fat in the regular diet. Is genetic elimination of this "disposition" for heart disease rightly considered treatment or enhancement? Have we treated a condition that significantly contributes to much morbidity and mortality, or have we simply enhanced our systems so that we can be gluttonous, so that we can unrestrainedly eat according to our heart's desire rather than our body's needs? These difficult cases illustrate the difficulty of attempting to distinguish the treatment of disorder from creating enhancements. Given the problems with trying to force fit the genetic debate into these problematic categories, we ought to look for a new way to conceptualize the debate. What we care about is improving the lives of our children and future generations, but we are not certain what ought to clearly count as justifiable *genetic* improvement.

One possibility that I would like to propose involves using a famous sort of thought experiment in philosophy, proposed by John Rawls for devising a fair distributive justice scheme. From behind the veil of ignorance (which obscures each individual's detailed knowledge of his or her own position in society), Rawls has rational creatures attempt to figure out what basic rules of justice would be fair for all society. Because no one is certain if he or she will be at the lowest rung of the social ladder or at the highest one, Rawls believes that people in this "original position" would opt for rules of justice that require equal basic liberties and a "maximin" policy that requires any changes in distribution of goods to benefit the worst off in society as well as the ones who have reason to cause the change to occur.

What if we were to put ourselves behind the veil of ignorance in respect to our children's genetic makeup? That is, what if we tried to determine what traits we would desire for them, and what traits we would prefer for them not to have if we did not know the details of our society (that is, if we did not know the particular patterns of racial/sexual/gender discrimination that we find in our own society, or we did not know what society we would find ourselves in)? The veil of ignorance, then, is a way to conceal from us the particular biases that our society has for traits that are otherwise not genuinely physically desirable. When we put on this veil of ignorance, we assume that we do not know which society we will be living in—we do not know physical or social details about the majority class for instance. We then try to determine what physical traits would lead to clear advantages or disadvantages in *any* society. This test allows us to decide for our children and future generations what sorts of traits should *not* be genetically manipulated.

It seems that things like race and sexual preferences would be quickly eliminated as genetic engineering candidates, as well as cultural standards of beauty (including particular features as well as height) because they are only valued by particular societies. That is, if you live in a predominantly white society, having white skin would tend to confer advantages, but this would not be so in a predominantly black society. If there is no reason to prefer a particular trait from behind the veil of ignorance, then perhaps we should rule it out as a candidate for genetic engineering. Other things might be clear candidates for genetic intervention, because they would be disabilities (or bring disadvantages) for anyone in any society (e.g., conditions like Tay-Sachs or amino-deaminase deficiency).

Deafness would be more difficult—whether you need hearing depends on the social structure of society, and we can imagine a majority deaf society designed for the benefit of the deaf. Such societies are not completely imaginary. Although the deaf were not a majority, the history of Martha's Vineyard can be used as an illustration of what such a society might be like. But there is an asymmetry. If you are deaf in a world in which the norm is nondeaf, then you are likely to experience significant disadvantages, both in terms of social goods and physical safety, because most communication, transportation, and warning systems are designed for the hearing. However, if you are nondeaf in a world where deaf is the norm, then you are not so clearly disadvantaged. (This claim is not without contention. You might be more easily distracted, and there is the possibility of experiencing some kind of schizophrenic symptoms, since you might respond to stimuli not perceived by others. This sort of experience is not, however, borne out by the early childhood stories of hearing children raised in deaf families.) There is an asymmetric pattern of disability or disadvantage. The deaf individual might experience disadvantage in a hearing world, but the same might not be true (or at least not to the same extent) for the hearing person in a deaf world.

On the other hand, try height: the disability is symmetrical there. If you are tall in a short world, you hit your head often and cannot fit in cars or through doorways; if you are short in a tall world, you cannot reach the pedals or the countertops, etc. The feature of asymmetrical disadvantage might help to pick out factors that are worth changing genetically (or worth considering as candidates for genetic change). Perhaps changing the thing that "veiled" rational people agree would *always* be a detriment is permissible (or even required), as is changing what could not be a harm in *any* society (i.e., what involves asymmetrical conditions), but changing what finds its value only in the particular society should not be allowed.

While this suggestion is clearly susceptible to many of the criticisms of Rawls's work, it may at least help to figure out a way to start the difficult process of distinguishing between legitimate genetic intervention and discriminatory or arbitrary intervention. Furthermore, given limitations on our imaginations (whether we are behind the veil of ignorance or not), I would certainly propose that those who make policies on genetic therapies should represent a wide variety of physical abilities and conditions (so that we do not hastily presume, for instance, that deafness is a clear defect without first consulting with those who are deaf). Thus we must surely bring a fair representative sample to the table to consider these possible interventions. As Susan Wendell eloquently illustrates:

> The desire for perfection and control of the body, or for the elimination of differences that are feared, poorly understood, and widely considered to be marks of inferiority, easily masquerades as the compassionate desire to prevent or stop suffering. It is not only a matter of being deceived by others, but all too often a matter of deceiving ourselves. It is easy

to make the leaps from imagining that I would not want to live in certain circumstances to believing that no one would want to live in those circumstances, to deciding to prevent people from being born into those circumstances, to supporting proposals "mercifully" to kill people living in those circumstances—all without ever consulting anyone who knows life in those circumstances from experience.[1]

To ensure that such experience is taken into account, the ideal decisionmaking procedure would bring together a number of differently abled individuals who would first openly discuss the benefits and harms, delights and difficulties of living with various physical conditions (as a way to inform the rest of the group about conditions they may only understand superficially or peripherally). Then, each representative would perform the thought experiment suggested by the veil-of-ignorance strategy. While I do not claim that this strategy would produce *unanimous* agreement on appropriate candidates for genetic engineering, I do believe that it is likely to bring us closer to agreement on what traits we should *not* be genetically engineering. Furthermore, it should help us to uncover some of our societal biases regarding genetic and/or physical traits and to stretch our imaginations regarding how we might address these biases through nongenetic means. If we work to imagine societies where being short or deaf or homosexual is not a disadvantage (as it unfortunately is in our present society), then we may be able to apply that thinking to social structures in our present society.

Notes

1. Susan Wendell. *The Rejected Body: Feminist Philosophical Reflections on Disability.* (New York: Routledge, 1996), 156.

Jewish Reflections on Genetic Enhancement

JEFFREY H. BURACK

Journal of the Society of Christian Ethics 26, no. 1 (2006): 137–61.

As twenty-first-century Westerners in love with technology, many of us nonetheless are wary and fearful of genetic interventions that might make people taller, faster, stronger, or more aggressive or might make eyes bluer or hair blonder. As Jews, some of us may be especially hostile to such engineering because of its echoes of the recent past's murderous eugenics and because of the fear that it portends increasing veneration of models of humanness that look less and less like our image of ourselves. What about enhancements that are less superficial, however—those that aim at enhancing what we, as Jews, genuinely value in ourselves? What if genetic engineering could make us smarter, more thoughtful, better learners and scholars or more honest, hard working, and cooperative? What if we could be more compassionate and fair-minded; more beneficent and loving; more dutiful, humble, and devoted to seeking holiness? What, if anything, would be wrong with seeking to reshape ourselves in these ways?

Goals

How can offering Jewish reflections on social policy issues such as our stance toward genetic engineering be of use? This type of analysis typically serves one or more of four purposes:

- Advancing *halakhic* or intracommunity deliberation about which positions to take on matters of policy and personal behavior
- Contributing to public policymaking by offering a "Jewish position," to be considered alongside other religious and ethical perspectives
- Contributing to public understanding and discourse by reflecting on contemporary issues from the perspective of one wisdom tradition, or a version of it

- Helping Jews, whether they regard themselves as *halakhically* adherent or not, make choices for themselves regarding personal behavior and support for policy directions.

My purposes include neither of the first two: I make no claim to be generating either *halakhah* or a "Jewish position." Instead, I believe that refracting this contemporary issue through a Jewish lens may add clarity and substance to the wider secular discussion and that it will be of interest to individual Jews.

Example: Modafinil

To return to questions about human enhancement, I borrow a pharmacological example from Paul Root Wolpe's key paper on neuroenhancement.[1] Modafinil, a drug marketed since 2002 under the name Provigil®, is a psychostimulant that improves wakefulness and alertness. Unlike earlier stimulants, modafinil appears to have few side effects and low addiction potential and does not interfere with sleep. In fact, it is prescribed to reverse excessive sleepiness associated with conditions such as narcolepsy and sleep apnea. Modafinil's potential uses, however, go far beyond treating these disorders. Healthy users report increased alertness and attention to tasks. The U.S. military tested the drug in sleep-deprived helicopter pilots and found that it improved not only performance but also measures of well-being. Clearly there might be a wide market for nontherapeutic uses of such a drug—surely by persons who need to stay awake but also by those who simply could benefit from greater alertness.

Wolpe asks several questions regarding the appropriate uses of such a drug: "Should modafinil be prescribed solely as a medical drug, properly used only for those suffering from sleep pathology? . . . If so, third-party payers, including government programs, should cover it. Or, should it be classified as an over-the-counter drug, available to anyone who wants it? Or, should we create a class of drugs available only to those who can show legitimate social need, those whose fatigue might put others at risk, such as airline pilots, or truck drivers?" Wolpe goes on to ask whether we should restrict modafinil's use in other defined social settings, in which it might confer unfair advantages to some individuals, prevent acquisition of important learning skills in others, or lend itself to abuse. The yeshiva and the rabbinical seminary might be two such settings.

Why choose a pharmacological example to frame an essay about genetic enhancement? I have several reasons. First, to make the point that concerns about enhancement are not unique to genetic interventions. Second, because the sort of enhancement at issue, of mental clarity and acuity, is especially challenging from a Jewish point of view. Efforts to make our children taller or our athletes stronger are easy targets for critique; not so for serious efforts to improve qualities we value. Third, because such chemical enhancements already are with us, whereas for the moment their genetic analogues remain in the realm of science fiction. Our deliberations about available therapies will prepare the way for how we think about now-hypothetical genetic interventions.

These interventions may not remain hypothetical for long: Genetic intellectual enhancement has already occurred in mice. In 1999 scientists in Joe Tsien's Princeton lab inserted additional copies of the gene NR2B, which codes for a receptor for the neurotransmitter NMDA. The engineered mice remembered objects and spatial relations better and performed better on learning tasks than mice without the enhancement. In all the ways that we measure mouse intelligence, the NR2B-enriched mice were smarter.

Consider the laudable goal of learning more Torah. I am acutely aware of my modest—and deteriorating—powers of attention, concentration, and memory and the limits they place on my ability to learn. In the service of learning Torah, what could be wrong with taking modafinil or availing myself of the analogous gene therapy, such as getting myself an extra NR2B gene once it becomes available to humans? Like other religious and moral traditions, Judaism offers background beliefs and principles against which such questions are posed, including:

- An ontology of the meaning and purpose of human life
- Recommended aspirations and constraints on human desires
- Specific constraints on action in the pursuit of personal or collective goals, in the form of positive and negative commandments
- Mechanisms for deliberation about action—including rules about argument, appeals to authority, and the weights to be assigned to different consequences—and, in particular, about duty and responsibility.

Secular Critique

I highlight the chief concerns of the secular bioethics critique of genetic enhancement against these background Jewish beliefs. I draw a few examples from the Hastings Center's Enhancement Project, which produced a 1998 report on the subject. As an aside, I note that the cover of the report juxtaposes two drawings of a woman: presumably "before," with a big, perhaps Semitic nose, and "after," with bump and hook deleted, looking rather like Bette Davis. This illustration should remind us, lest we are tempted to feel morally superior, that as Jews we have been quick to avail ourselves of supposed enhancement technologies, and sometimes we have done so at least in part to appear or to be less "Jewish." Therefore it also is a reminder—superficial, perhaps, but clear—of the potential homogenizing power of these technologies to eliminate ethnic and other ancestral differences, whether voluntarily or coercively. The Hastings Center project identifies some of the implications of enhancement technology that should concern us. These implications include the following:

- Genetic technologies tamper inappropriately with what makes us essentially human and individual.
- Enhancement is an abuse of biomedical technology that properly is reserved for treatment, which aims to restore health and normal functioning.
- The very idea of enhancement valorizes specific conceptions of which human characteristics are normal and desirable, thereby devaluing persons who do not have them.
- The availability of such technologies within our present market-based economy would offend standards of distributive justice by exacerbating existing inequities in capacity and opportunity.
- Using technology to enhance ourselves may undermine the virtue of living and struggling with our imperfections.
- The availability of enhancement technologies promotes human aspirations that are ignoble and destructive and conflict with or undermine important social goals.
- Genetic interventions risk incalculable harm, foreseeable and not, and different in kind from the risks of other biomedical interventions.

Although all of these concerns find resonance in Jewish thought, I want to assert and try to explain some contrasts and suggest that Jewish concern focuses in somewhat different places. A Jewish view, for example, may be more permissive about social uses of technology but more restrictive about personal aspirations and behavior. I suggest that the concept at the core

of Jewish apprehensions about enhancement is *anavah*, or humility. We must be humble in our appreciation of human diversity and struggle, about our ability to know in detail what is genuinely expected of us, and about our ability to foresee the consequences and implications of our actions. Humility is threatened by the appeal of enhancement but in Judaism may be held in place by our sense of duty to God, self, and others.

Naturalism Versus Co-Creation

Despite avowedly secular roots, bioethics harbors an anxiety that tampering with our genetic essence is not our business. From the Christian and Greco-Roman traditions that preceded it, philosophical Anglo-American bioethics has inherited a strong naturalist bent that has been enhanced by its self-assigned role as critic of scientific biomedicine. Naturalism holds that we fundamentally are as given by God, nature, or evolution and that it is wrong to interfere with or try to change our quintessence. This attitude is reflected in the Edenic and Promethean myths, in which ultimate punishment is reserved for the crime of arrogating the creative spark or knowledge that should be reserved for the Divine. Oddly, although Judaism acknowledges a Creator and our own createdness, it does not seem to share this naturalist inclination. In Jewish tradition, what is fundamental to us, our creation in the Divine image, is something we cannot change no matter how we might try—so the essentialist concern is taken off the table. Regarding everything else, we are commanded to participate with God as co-creators, improving the world—which, after all, also is God's creation. We are reminded at every ritual occasion of our obligation to perform *tikkun olam*, healing and improvement of the given world. The first blessing to mark sacred time, on Shabbat or festivals, is a blessing on the light, which God has created but we re-create in smaller, human ways by kindling candles. The second is on wine—a self-conscious symbol of co-creation. God creates the vine and its fruit, but human intervention turns it into wine, symbol of celebration and conviviality. As an interesting side note, this particular co-creation is one we then use to alter our own consciousness. Far from being forbidden either the co-creation or its use for enhancement, we are commanded to do both. Moreover, the natural, God-given raw material alone simply will not do it.

Medicine, of course, is fundamentally *anti-naturalist*, in the sense that medicine's most basic function is not to allow disease processes to take their "natural" course. By no accident, then, have Jews and Western medicine shared a close historical relationship, as Elliott Dorff and others have pointed out. A basic attitude of Judaism is that God has given us the power to heal each other, just as God has given us anything else, and we are commanded directly to use that healing power. We do not worry so much about "playing God" with the natural world because by working to improve God's world, we are actually playing human beings, reverentially and according to the script given us. Nevertheless, we are acutely responsible for the consequences of those manipulations—all the more so because the objects of our actions never belong to us alone.

Substantive Moral Vision

The most basic difference between Judaism's moral framework and the dominant secular view is that although both are aspirational, Judaism tells us in some detail what we ought to aspire to. That is, it presumes and promotes a substantive vision of the purpose of human life and what gives life value. Although there probably are at least as many versions of this vision as there are Jews, I work from a general formulation that I hope is relatively uncontroversial, following the prophet Micah: "He has told you, O man, what is good, and what Adonai requires of you: only to do justice and to love goodness and to walk humbly with your God" (Micah 6:8). We are commanded to be just, kind, and

humble and to strive toward holiness through the imitation of God and through lives lived in consciousness of the Torah. We are called to act, to participate with the Divine and with our communities in *tikkun olam*. Fundamental to religious thought, and certainly to Jewish thought, is that we strive toward betterment of ourselves and the created world and that the characteristics of bettered selves and a better world can be agreed upon and described, at least in rough outline. A substantive moral framework, then, gives the concept of enhancement meaning independent of our personal desires. This point may seem obvious, but its impact on how we understand enhancement is enormous. The result is an explicit vision of what an enhanced human might be that is less ambiguous, and therefore less contestable, than what emerges from secular deliberation.

Enhancement implies a standard, norm, or goal against which the value of an object is judged. Sometimes the implied predicate seems obvious and univocal: A better tool is one that performs its specified task more easily or effectively. What does enhancing a person mean, however? What can it mean, without an agreed-upon set of standards for what makes a better person? Virtue or character ethics attempts to establish, or at least query, such standards. Contemporary biomedicine, however, typically invokes virtue ethics only in reference to physicians and other professionals, of whom we ask what dispositions might be desirable or appropriate. Such language generally is absent from discussion of the sort of choices individuals or communities should make about, for example, health care. Arguably, this is as it must be. Secular bioethics aims primarily at settling disputes and adjudicating competing claims among stakeholders in a deeply pluralistic society. Of necessity, then, it has difficulty establishing anything but procedural principles for collective deliberation and prudential principles for personal deliberation. The usual assumption is that individuals choose to maximize their ability to pursue their personal ends. Contrast, for example, the standard secular argument for why one should not smoke—foregoing short-term pleasure in the service of one's longer-term, but still personal, goals of a longer and healthier life—with the Jewish argument: that the body belongs to God, and the individual, as steward of the body, may not casually pollute it or cause it harm.

Obviously, even if every desired modification were permissible, not every desire should have its fulfillment socially guaranteed. With no point of view from which to answer the ontological question of what genuinely enhances us, however, secular bioethics has been preoccupied instead with the distinction between enhancement and treatment. Treatment is understood as the use of biomedical technology to remedy what we agree to consider a disease or injury, in contrast to mere enhancement, which is the use of that technology toward any other desired end. This heuristic is then put to work to decide what we should research, guarantee, pay for, and so on. Although we think we are deliberating about what enhancements are and are not, in fact we are worrying about which demands impose legitimate duty claims on the rest of us. In other words, the bioethical treatment–enhancement distinction tries to draw important normative implications from a conceptual and at least superficially value-neutral distinction—a project that Hume's is-ought problem would suggest may be impossible. From a Jewish perspective, however, to be enhanced means to be better suited to fulfill our human purpose. We have at least a general sense of what this is, and we have instruction manuals in the form of the Torah and its commentaries. From a secular perspective, we ask: Is this treatment or mere enhancement? From a Jewish perspective we ask instead: What is the goal of this intervention, and does it seek holiness? Does it serve us in our roles as caretakers and stewards of our bodies and our world?

Diversity and God's Image

I now turn to the "expressivist" critique of enhancement. This position, eloquently argued by Anita Silvers and others, holds that the very pursuit of biomedical enhancements, and even the willingness to regard nontherapeutic interventions as enhancements, expresses negative attitudes toward some existing persons. By valorizing specific human characteristics, seeking enhancement devalues and discriminates against disabled persons—or even those who simply have less of those characteristics. As human traits begin to appear optional, subject to being acquired or improved rather than merely allocated by the genetic lottery, there might be even greater stigma attached to not having them.

Judaism establishes a set of aspirations for human life and therefore seems inevitably to favor some forms of life over others. Does it therefore imply negative attitudes toward certain human characteristics and toward the persons who display them? Yes and no. A substantive ethical system certainly must attach positive moral valence to some characteristics and negative worth to others. In my view, however, the sort of threat Silvers and others see is minimized by three features of the Jewish view of human purpose and value: first, our universal creation *b'tzelem elohim*—that is, in the image of God; second, the nature of the actual qualities that are considered desirable, holy, and constitutive of that image; and third, the spirit of *anavah*, or humility, in which we must approach this analysis and our own self-improvement.

As Bernard Steinberg has put it, "In the cosmic context, differences of biological strength, social stature, economic power, and cultural achievement are reduced to secondary importance. These differences are marginal to the authentic center of human identity. Moreover, aware of the essential limitation of his finitude, the *hasid* knows, objectively speaking, that he is no more worthy than his neighbor. The standard of objectivity is not social convention but relation to God.[2] The source of human worth is the reflection of God's image, not any constellation of observable characteristics.

God's image is ineffable, but its manifestations are manifold. A lovely passage from Talmud

Sanhedrin tells us that when we mortals cast coins, usually with the face of a human ruler, we see precisely the same face on every coin. The Divine ruler, however, has cast countless images from a single original mold, and like snowflakes, every one of us is different. Furthermore, that original mold, of course, was itself fashioned in God's own image (*Sanhedrin* 4:5). Judaism's pantheon does not reflect human perfection, physical or otherwise: Jacob limps, Moses stutters, and families by and large are pretty dysfunctional. It may sound trite in our multicultural world, but as Rabbi Elliott Dorff has pointed out, Jews are commanded to celebrate difference and to respond to disability with gratitude rather than revulsion or disdain, praising God, *meshaneh ha-briyyot*, who creates us different.

Holding a shared conception of the Divine is not an invitation to discriminate when that very conception embraces the belief that all people share in it equally. In fact, such a belief should motivate social action to reduce discrimination. Consider, for example, obesity, or very short stature. Either can constitute a form of social disability, resulting in unpleasant and discriminatory treatment by other people and often a sense of diminished personal worth. Our obligation is not to change body shapes but to change social attitudes *about* body shapes because these very attitudes belie disrespect for some manifestations of the Divine image.

Self-Fulfillment

We fear that in trying to refashion themselves, people will choose bad things: characteristics that ultimately will make themselves and others less kind, compassionate, and humble and the social world less just and holy. There are genuine grounds for fearing such an inclination in contemporary American life. In his thoughtful book *Better Than Well*, Carl Elliott explores the American fascination with self-enhancement and self-creation. Elliott links this orientation to our founding hostility toward authority and tradition and subsequent emphasis on self-sufficiency. Elliott concludes, "We need to understand our-

selves as inheritors of a cultural tradition in which the significance of life has become deeply bound up with self-fulfillment. We need to understand . . . the paradoxical way in which a person can see an enhancement technology as a way to achieve a more authentic self, even as the technology dramatically alters his or her identity."[3] Furthermore, with self-fulfillment as the only end to which we all can universally agree, enhancement becomes more than just a desirable option. Elliott again: "Once self-fulfillment is hitched to the success of human life, it comes perilously close to an obligation—not an obligation to God, country, or family, but an obligation to the self. We are compelled to pursue fulfillment through enhancement technologies not in order to get ahead of others, but to make sure that we have lived our lives to the fullest."

There is a fascinating irony, however, in this worship of self-fulfillment. As opportunities for enhancement proliferate and as the changes we can potentially make become more profound, we are likely to become increasingly dissatisfied, both with the lot we are given in life and with our own efforts to improve it. In *The Paradox of Choice*, Barry Schwartz depicts the ways in which we are made miserable by the explosion of options in today's life—from which pair of jeans or television to buy to which career to pursue and whom to marry. As social affluence has progressively guaranteed that our basic needs are met, we attach greater and greater value to scarce goods and circumstances—regardless of their inherent or practical value. We can adopt one of two attitudes toward the multitude of choices we face. Schwartz cites Herbert Simon's distinction between "maximizers"—those who must make the very best choice of all those available—and "satisficers." Satisficers approach a choice with a list of the features they most want or need, go through the immediately available options until they find one that satisfies their requirements—and then stop there. Schwartz points out that the commitments and social ties that typically make us happiest are, in fact, those that constrain our choices—including marriage or other long-term love relationships, as well as child-rearing. He then demonstrates how people who are inclined to be maximizers are made increasingly unhappy by a growing range of choices. After all, they must review and compare every feature of each possible option to be sure the one they end up choosing is unsurpassed. Maximizers also take the results of their choices, particularly whether they ultimately find reason to regret them, as evidence of their personal worth. Finally, Schwartz points out, "the proliferation of options not only makes people who are maximizers miserable, but it may also make people who are satisficers into maximizers."[4]

Thus, substitution of self-fulfillment for an externally based conception of human worth, coupled with our increasingly affluent material culture, has led to an expanding and ultimately self-defeating sense that we not only can have and be all that we want but that we must do so. Failure to strive for maximal self-fulfillment has come to be regarded as a moral failing, a failure of imagination, will, effort, or talent. How much more this must be the case when we are considering opportunities not to buy blue jeans or televisions but to enhance ourselves or, worse, our children.

Giftedness

Against this background, we must read Michael Sandel's penetrating essay "The Case against Perfection." Sandel describes the allure of genetic enhancement as representing "a kind of hyper-agency—a Promethean aspiration to remake nature, including human nature, to serve our purposes and satisfy our desires.... And what the drive to mastery misses and may even destroy is an appreciation of the gifted character of human powers and achievements." Sandel wants to find "nonreligious" grounds for trying to preserve this sense of giftedness; he does so by pointing to the potential moral consequences of coming to view the shaping of ourselves as simply one more domain of consumer choice. "If bioengineering made the myth of the 'self-made man' come true, it would be difficult to view our talents as gifts for

which we are indebted, rather than as achievements for which we are responsible. This would transform three key features of our moral landscape: humility, responsibility, and solidarity." Sandel worries that, besides making us arrogant, the conviction that we can control our own and our children's destinies will unduly burden us with an excessive sense of our own responsibility for what we are, what we do, and what happens in the world around us. Ultimately, as a political philosopher Sandel is most concerned with the impact of such hubris on social solidarity. Our secular social contract hangs on the belief that our circumstances are not entirely under our control. Otherwise, why would persons who are prosperous, powerful, and beautiful owe anything at all to those who are less advantaged? Therefore, Sandel concludes, "A lively sense of the contingency of our gifts—a consciousness that none of us is wholly responsible for his or her success—saves a meritocratic society from sliding into the smug assumption that the rich are rich because they are more deserving than the poor."

I share Sandel's concern, but I raise two questions in response. First, the features Sandel enumerates—humility, a limited sense of personal responsibility, and social solidarity—are all important, attractive, and resonant with Jewish and other religious traditions. Why these three, however? Why are these moral attitudes particularly threatened by the rise of a maximizing attitude toward self-enhancement and the concomitant loss of a sense of giftedness? Second, if the reality is that we are rapidly gaining at least the technological means for this sort of control, what, if anything else, could preserve these moral features? Is the ground on which they stand really so shaky, or do they share some common foundation that might survive our growing ability to engineer ourselves?

Perhaps Sandel has simply put his finger on the three most important facets of moral thinking generally. Indeed, these concepts correspond to what Richard Shweder describes, on the basis of anthropological and cultural psychology studies, as the "big three" domains of moral reasoning across human civilizations: divinity, autonomy, and community. I make no claim that these concepts are exclusively or even especially Jewish; the fact that they are central to Jewish thought suggests, however, potential Jewish answers to the concerns I have raised. Again we can turn to the idea of humility. What may stop us from sliding clear off our moral landscape is the belief that there is no state of exaltation, perfection, or blessedness to which we can aspire and, upon reaching it, complete our work. In this sense, Judaism's strength may lie in the fact that its messianism is a process—an obligation of continuing effort and improvement—rather than a goal, a state to someday be reached. We should not fear improving ourselves; on the contrary, we are required to try to do so. Yet no matter how we may change,

there will be no less left to do. As Rabbi Tarfon was known to say, "You are not obliged to finish the task; neither are you free to neglect it" (*Pirkeh Avot* 2:21).

Notes

1. P. R. Wolpe, "Treatment, Enhancement, and the Ethics of Neurotherapeutics," *Brain and Cognition* 50 (2002): 387–95.
2. B. Steinberg, "Humility," in *Contemporary Jewish Religious Thought*, ed. A. A. Cohen and P. Mendes-Flohr (New York: Free Press, 1987).
3. C. Elliott, *Better Than Well: American Medicine Meets the American Dream* (New York: W. W. Norton, 2003).
4. B. Schwartz, *The Paradox of Choice: Why More Is Less* (New York: HarperCollins Publishers, 2004).

Transhumanist Values

NICK BOSTROM

From *Ethical Issues for the 21st Century*, edited by Frederick Adams. (Charlottesville, VA: Philosophical Documentation Center, 2003), 1–11.

1. What is Transhumanism?

Transhumanism is a loosely defined movement that has developed gradually over the past two decades. It promotes an interdisciplinary approach to understanding and evaluating the opportunities for enhancing the human condition and the human organism opened up by the advancement of technology. Attention is given to both present technologies, like genetic engineering and information technology, and anticipated future ones, such as molecular nanotechnology and artificial intelligence.

The enhancement options being discussed include radical extension of human health-span, eradication of disease, elimination of unnecessary suffering, and augmentation of human intellectual, physical, and emotional capacities. Other transhumanist themes include space colonization and the possibility of creating superintelligent machines, along with other potential developments that could profoundly alter the human condition. The ambit is not limited to gadgets and medicine, but encompasses also economic, social, institutional designs, cultural development, and psychological skills and techniques.

Transhumanists view human nature as a work-in-progress, a half-baked beginning that we can learn to remold in desirable ways. Current humanity need not be the endpoint of evolution. Transhumanists hope that by responsible use of science, technology, and other rational means we shall eventually manage to become posthuman, beings with vastly greater capacities than present human beings have.

Some transhumanists take active steps to increase the probability that they personally will survive long enough to become posthuman, for example by choosing a healthy lifestyle or by making provisions for having themselves cryonically suspended in case of de-animation. In contrast to many other ethical outlooks, which in practice often reflect a reactionary attitude to new technologies, the transhumanist view is guided by an evolving vision to take a more proactive approach to technology policy. This vision, in broad strokes, is to create the opportunity to live much longer and healthier lives, to enhance our memory and other intellectual faculties, to refine our emotional experiences and increase our subjective sense of well-being, and generally to achieve a greater degree of control over our own lives. This affirmation of human potential is offered as an alternative to customary injunctions against playing God, messing with nature, tampering with our human essence, or displaying punishable hubris.

Transhumanism does not entail technological optimism. While future technological capabilities carry immense potential for beneficial deployments, they also could be misused to cause enormous harm, ranging all the way to the extreme possibility of intelligent life becoming extinct. Other potential negative outcomes include widening social inequalities or a gradual erosion of the hard-to-quantify assets that we care deeply about but tend to neglect in our daily struggle for material gain, such as meaningful human relationships and ecological diversity. Such risks must be taken very seriously, as thoughtful transhumanists fully acknowledge.

Transhumanism has roots in secular humanist thinking, yet is more radical in that it promotes not only traditional means of improving human nature, such as education and cultural refinement, but also direct application of medicine and technology to overcome some of our basic biological limits.

2. Human Limitations

The range of thoughts, feelings, experiences, and activities accessible to human organisms presumably constitute only a tiny part of what is possible. There is no reason to think that the human mode of being is any more free of limitations imposed by our biological nature than are those of other animals. In much the same way as chimpanzees lack the cognitive wherewithal to understand what it is like to be human – the ambitions we humans have, our philosophies, the complexities of human society, or the subtleties of our relationships with one another – so we humans may lack the capacity to form a realistic intuitive understanding of what it would be like to be a radically enhanced human (a "posthuman") and of the thoughts, concerns, aspirations, and social relations that such humans may have.

Our own current mode of being, therefore, spans but a minute subspace of what is possible or permitted by the physical constraints of the universe. It is not farfetched to suppose that there are parts of this larger space that represent extremely valuable ways of living, relating, feeling, and thinking.

The limitations of the human mode of being are so pervasive and familiar that we often fail to notice them, and to question them requires manifesting an almost childlike naivete. Let's consider some of the more basic ones.

Lifespan

Because of the precarious conditions in which our Pleistocene ancestors lived, the human lifespan has evolved to be a paltry seven or eight decades. This is, from many perspectives, a rather short period of time. Even tortoises do better than that.

We don't have to use geological or cosmological comparisons to highlight the meagerness of our allotted time budgets. To get a sense that we might be missing out on something important by our tendency to die early, we only have to bring to mind some of the worthwhile things that we could have done or attempted to do if we had had more time. For gardeners, educators, scholars, artists, city planners, and those who simply relish observing and participating in the cultural or political variety shows of life, three score and ten is often insufficient for seeing even one major project through to completion, let alone for undertaking many such projects in sequence.

Human character development is also cut short by aging and death. Imagine what might have become of a Beethoven or a Goethe if they had still been with us today. Maybe they would have developed into rigid old grumps interested exclusively in conversing about the achievements of their youth. But maybe, if they had continued to enjoy health and youthful vitality, they would have continued to grow as men and artists, to reach levels of maturity that we can barely imagine. We certainly cannot rule that out based on what we know today. Therefore, there is at least a serious possibility of there being something very precious outside the human sphere. This constitutes a reason to pursue the means that will let us go there and find out.

Intellectual Capacity

We have all had moments when we wished we were a little smarter. The three-pound, cheese-like thinking machine that we lug around in our skulls can do some neat tricks, but it also has significant shortcomings. Some of these – such as forgetting to buy milk or failing to attain native fluency in languages you learn as an adult – are obvious and require no elaboration. These shortcomings are inconveniences but hardly fundamental barriers to human development.

Yet there is a more profound sense in the constraints of our intellectual apparatus limit our modes of mentation. I mentioned the chimpanzee analogy earlier: just as is the case for the great apes, our own cognitive makeup may foreclose whole strata of understanding and mental activity. The point here is not about any logical or metaphysical impossibility: we need not suppose that posthumans would not be Turing computable or that they would have concepts that could not be expressed by any finite sentences in our language, or anything of that sort.

The impossibility that I am referring to is more like the impossibility for us current humans to visualize an 200-dimensional hypersphere or to read, with perfect recollection and understanding, every book in the Library of Congress. These things are impossible for us because, simply put, we lack the brainpower. In the same way, we may lack the ability to intuitively understand what being a posthuman would be like or to grok the playing field of posthuman concerns.

Further, our human brains may cap our ability to discover philosophical and scientific truths. It is possible that failure of philosophical research to arrive at solid, generally accepted answers to many of the traditional big philosophical questions could be due to the fact that we are not smart enough to be successful in this kind of enquiry. Our cognitive limitations may be confining us in a Platonic cave, where the best we can do is theorize about "shadows", that is, representations that are sufficiently oversimplified and dumbed-down to fit inside a human brain.

Bodily Functionality

We enhance our natural immune systems by getting vaccinations, and we can imagine further enhancements to our bodies that would protect us from disease or help us shape our bodies according to our desires (e.g. by letting us control our bodies' metabolic rate). Such enhancements could improve the quality of our lives.

A more radical kind of upgrade might be possible if we suppose a computational view of the mind. It may then be possible to upload a human mind to a computer, by replicating *in silico* the detailed computational processes that would normally take place in a particular human brain. Being an upload would have many potential advantages, such as the ability to make back-up copies of oneself (favorably impacting on one's life-expectancy) and the ability to transmit oneself as information at the speed of light. Uploads might live either in virtual reality or directly in physical reality by controlling a robot proxy.

Sensory Modalities, Special Faculties, and Sensibilities

The current human sensory modalities are not the only possible ones, and they are certainly not as highly developed as they could be. Some animals have sonar, magnetic orientation, or sensors for electricity and vibration; many have a much keener sense of smell, sharper eyesight, etc. The range of possible sensory modalities is not limited to those we find in the animal kingdom. There is no fundamental block to adding say a capacity to see infrared radiation or to perceive radio signals and perhaps to add some kind of telepathic sense by augmenting our brains with suitably interfaced radio transmitters.

Humans also enjoy a variety of special faculties, such as appreciation of music and a sense of humor, and sensibilities such as the capacity for sexual arousal in response to erotic stimuli. Again, there is no reason to think that what we have exhausts the range of the possible, and we can certainly imagine higher levels of sensitivity and responsiveness.

Mood, Energy, and Self-Control

Despite our best efforts, we often fail to feel as happy as we would like. Our chronic levels of subjective well-being seem to be largely genetically determined. Life-events have little long-term impact; the crests and troughs of fortune push us up and bring us down, but there is little long-term effect on self-reported well-being. Lasting joy remains elusive except for those of us who are lucky enough to have been born with a temperament that plays in a major key.

In addition to being at the mercy of a genetically determined setpoint for our levels of well-being, we are limited in regard to energy, willpower, and ability to shape our own character in accordance with our ideals. Even such "simple" goals as losing weight or quitting smoking prove unattainable to many.

Some subset of these kinds of problems might be necessary rather than contingent upon our current nature. For example, we cannot both have the ability easily to break any habit and the ability to form stable, hard-to-break habits. (In this regard, the best one can hope for may be the ability to easily get rid of habits we didn't deliberately choose for ourselves in the first place, and perhaps a more versatile habit-formation system that would let us choose with more precision when to acquire a habit and how much effort it should cost to break it.)

3. The Core Transhumanist Value: Exploring the Posthuman Realm

The conjecture that there are greater values than we can currently fathom does not imply that values are not defined in terms of our current dispositions. Take, for example, a dispositional theory of value such as the one described by David Lewis. According to Lewis's theory, something is a value for you if and only if you would want to want it if you were perfectly acquainted with it and you were thinking and deliberating as clearly as possible about it. On this view, there may be values that we do not currently want, and that we do not even currently want to want, because we may not be perfectly acquainted with them or because we are not ideal deliberators. Some values pertaining to certain forms of posthuman existence may well be of this sort; they may be values for us now, and they may be so in virtue of our current dispositions, and yet we may not be able to fully appreciate them with our current limited deliberative capacities and our lack of the receptive faculties required for full acquaintance with them. This point is important because it shows that the transhumanist view that we ought to explore the realm of posthuman values does not entail that we should forego our current values. The posthuman values can be our current values, albeit ones that we have not yet clearly comprehended. Transhumanism does not require us to say that we should favor posthuman beings over human beings, but that the right way of favoring human beings is by enabling us to realize our ideals better and that some of our ideals may well be located outside the space of modes of being that are accessible to us with our current biological constitution.

Transhumanism promotes the quest to develop further so that we can explore hitherto inaccessible realms of value. Technological enhancement of human organisms is a means that we ought to pursue to this end. There are limits to how much can be achieved by low-tech means such as education, philosophical contemplation, moral self-scrutiny and other such methods proposed by classical philosophers with perfectionist leanings, including Plato, Aristotle, and Nietzsche, or by means of creating a fairer and better society, as envisioned by social reformists such as Marx or Martin Luther King. This is not to denigrate what we can do with the tools we have today. Yet ultimately, transhumanists hope to go further.

4. Basic Conditions for Realizing the Transhumanist Project

If this is the grand vision, what are the more particular objectives that it translates into when considered as a guide to policy?

What is needed for the realization of the transhumanist dream is that technological means necessary for venturing into the posthuman space are made available to those who wish to use them, and that society be organized in such a manner that such explorations can be undertaken without causing unacceptable damage to the social fabric and without imposing unacceptable existential risks.

Global Security

While disasters and setbacks are inevitable in the implementation of the transhumanist project (just as they are if the transhumanist project is not pursued), there is one kind of catastrophe that must be avoided at any cost:

> *Existential risk* – one where an adverse outcome would either annihilate Earth-originating intelligent life or permanently and drastically curtail its potential.

Several recent discussions have argued that the combined probability of the existential risks is very substantial. The relevance of the condition of existential safety to the transhumanist vision is obvious: if we go extinct or permanently destroy our potential to develop further, then the transhumanist core value will not be realized. Global security is the most fundamental and nonnegotiable requirement of the transhumanist project.

Technological Progress

That technological progress is generally desirable from a transhumanist point of view is also self-evident. Many of our biological shortcomings (aging, disease, feeble memories and intellects, a limited emotional repertoire and inadequate capacity for sustained well-being) are difficult to overcome, and to do so will require advanced tools. Developing these tools is a gargantuan challenge for the collective problem-solving capacities of our species. Since technological progress is closely linked to economic development, economic growth – or more precisely, productivity growth – can in some cases serve as a proxy for technological progress. (Productivity growth is, of course, only an imperfect measure of the relevant form of technological progress, which, in turn, is an imperfect measure of overall improvement, since it omits such factors as equity of distribution, ecological diversity, and quality of human relationships.)

Wide Access

It is not enough that the posthuman realm be explored by someone. The full realization of the core transhumanist value requires that, ideally, everybody should have the opportunity to become posthuman. It would be sub-optimal if the opportunity to become posthuman were restricted to a tiny elite.

There are many reasons for supporting wide access: to reduce inequality; because it would be a fairer arrangement; to express solidarity and respect for fellow humans; to help gain support for the transhumanist project; to increase the chances that you will get the opportunity to become posthuman; to increase the chances that those you care about can become posthuman; because it might increase the range of the posthuman realm that gets explored; and to alleviate human suffering on as wide a scale as possible.

The wide access requirement underlies the *moral urgency* of the transhumanist vision. Wide access does not argue for holding back. On the contrary, other things being equal, it is an argument for moving forward as quickly as possible. 150,000 human beings on our planet die every day, without having had any access to the anticipated enhancement technologies that will make it possible to become posthuman. The sooner this technology develops, the fewer people will have died without access.

5. Derivative Values

From these specific requirements flow a number of derivative transhumanist values that translate the transhumanist vision into practice.

To start with, transhumanists typically place emphasis on individual freedom and individual choice in the area of enhancement technologies. Humans differ widely in their conceptions of what their own perfection or improvement would consist in. Some want to develop in one direction, others in different directions, and some prefer to stay the way they are. It would be morally unacceptable for anybody to impose a single standard to which we would all have to conform. People should have the right to choose which enhancement technologies, if any, they want to use. In cases where individual choices impact substantially on other people, this general principle may need to be restricted, but the mere fact that somebody may be disgusted or morally affronted by somebody else's using technology to modify herself would not normally be a legitimate ground for coercive interference. Furthermore, the poor track record of centrally planned efforts to create better people (e.g. the eugenics movement and Soviet totalitarianism) shows that we need to be wary of collective decision-making in the field of human modification.

Another transhumanist priority is to put ourselves in a better position to make wise choices about where we are going. We will need all the wisdom we can get when negotiating the posthuman transition. Transhumanists place a high value on improvements in our individual and collective powers of understanding and in our ability to implement responsible decisions. Collectively, we might get smarter and more informed through such means as scientific research, public debate and open discussion of the future, information markets, and collaborative information filtering. On an individual level, we can benefit from education, critical thinking, open-mindedness, study techniques, information technology, and perhaps memory- or attention-enhancing drugs and other cognitive enhancement technologies. Our ability to implement responsible decisions can be improved by expanding the rule of law and democracy on the international plane. Additionally, artificial intelligence, especially if and when it reaches human-equivalence or greater, could give an enormous boost to the quest for knowledge and wisdom.

Given the limitations of our current wisdom, a certain epistemic tentativeness is appropriate, along with a readiness to continually reassess our assumptions as more information becomes available. We cannot take for granted that our old habits and beliefs will prove adequate in navigating our new circumstances.

Transhumanism advocates the well-being of all sentience, whether in artificial intellects, humans, and non-human animals (including extraterrestrial species, if there are any). Racism, sexism, speciesism, belligerent nationalism and religious intolerance are unacceptable. In addition to the usual grounds for deeming such practices objectionable, there is also a specifically transhumanist motivation for this. In order to prepare for a time when the human species may start branching out in various directions, we need to start now to strongly encourage the development of moral sentiments that are broad enough encompass within the sphere of moral concern sentiences that are constituted differently from ourselves.

Finally, transhumanism stresses the moral urgency of saving lives, or, more precisely, of preventing involuntary deaths among people whose lives are worth living. In the developed world, aging is currently the number one killer. Aging is also biggest cause of illness, disability and dementia. (Even if all heart disease and cancer could be cured, life expectancy would increase by merely six to seven years.) Anti-aging medicine is therefore a key transhumanist priority. The goal, of course, is to radically extend people's active health-spans,

not to add a few extra years on a ventilator at the end of life.

Since we are still far from being able to halt or reverse aging, cryonic suspension of the dead should be made available as an option for those who desire it. It is possible that future technologies will make it possible to reanimate people who have cryonically suspended. While cryonics might be a long shot, it definitely carries better odds than cremation or burial.

References

Lewis, D. "Dispositional Theories of value." *Proceedings of the Aristotelian Society Suppiement*, 63 (1989): 113–37.

Treatment, Enhancement, and the Ethics of Neurotherapeutics

PAUL ROOT WOLPE

Brain and Cognition 50 (2002): 387–95.

Introduction

The study of the brain has always promised more than just the cure of disease. Franz Joseph Gall's phrenology, which identified 27 faculties in the brain (such as valor, cunning, pride, ability to learn, ambition, and metaphysical perspicuity), was intended to detect the morally infirm and differentiate "higher" from "lower" races. Cesare Lombroso, the 19th Century "Father of Modern Criminology," argued that criminals were evolutionary throwbacks with "atavistic" brains and morphological features characteristic of lower races. Craniometry, the science of correlating brain size with intelligence, was used primarily to create intelligence hierarchies within and between races. Nobel Prize winning psychiatrist Antonio Egas Moniz

advanced lobotomy in the late 1930s and 1940s as a means of controlling aggressive or violent behavior. These efforts, and most that came after them, were suffused with moral assumptions and visions of desirable and undesirable human characteristics, but were believed by their proponents to represent the dispassionate pursuit of objective science.

Neuroscience today is also built on a series of fundamental assumptions about human nature and worth. It is not possible, and perhaps not desirable, to purge neuroscience of moral presuppositions, dealing as it does with fundamental aspects of identity, personality, free will, and other value-wrought concepts. As in the 19th and early 20th centuries, our scientific inquiry is guided by culturally determined standards of what traits we think are valuable to explore and what behaviors we think are desirable to control or eradicate. For example, imaging studies that look for morphological or functional differences in the orbitrofrontal cortex or the amygdala of "psychopaths" (usually defined as violent criminals with antisocial personality disorder) raise many of the same ethical and philosophical questions (if in much more sophisticated scientific packaging) as the science of earlier in the century. The attempt to localize criminality and explain it as the function of a specific pathologized section of the brain is itself an agenda of a particular cultural and historical moment, and one with significant moral implications.

Perhaps the most significant moral discussion in modern neuroscience has been directed at the use of pharmaceuticals to alter the fundamental cognitive and affective functions of the brain. The human desire to induce mental states through ingestion is, of course, as old as the discovery of fermentation (if not older, with the discovery of natural hallucinogens or stimulants), and so is moral debate about it. Nineteenth century America was particularly enamored of developing nutritional philosophies of health with a moral tinge, from the botanical medicine of Samuel Thompson to the non-stimulating diets developed by Will Kellogg (corn flakes were invented as a bland breakfast to avoid stirring up the passions in the morning) or Sylvester Graham (whose now-famous cracker was designed towards the same ends as corn flakes). For centuries, lay, folk, and professional movements in both Western and Eastern medicine have prescribed foods, herbs, and potions to induce proper physical and mental functioning. We still try to "eat right" to improve mood and general mental functioning, and use stimulants (caffeine), sedatives (alcohol), and mood enhancers (chocolate), and have built nutraceuticals (St. John's Wort, Kava, *Ginkgo biloba*) into a multi-billion dollar market. Yet, the debates about the proper use of these substances show no signs of abating.

The ability of the new range of pharmaceuticals to alter or target mood states, levels of cognition, or cognitive skills such as memory is one of the most promising and challenging developments of the 21st century. Drugs developed for some of our most intractable diseases now promise us the power not only to treat pathology, but to improve or augment otherwise average or typical functioning; not only to arrest the cognitive deterioration of Alzheimer's, for example, but to improve cognitive functioning in the healthy. Drugs developed for narcolepsy entice us with amphetamine-free wakefulness; drugs developed for depression promise to elevate our spirits in general and drugs developed for erectile dysfunction are sold freely on the web with only a nod to medical necessity. If history is any precedent, we will enthusiastically embrace these technologies, even as we agonize over whether or not we should do so.

Debate has already begun as to the implications of these technologies for defining the difference between treatment and enhancement. There are two fundamental questions that confront us. The first, more philosophical question of enhancement is about categorization: what do terms such as "average" or "normal" functioning, or even "disease" and "enhancement" mean when we can improve functioning across the entire range of human capability? Is the typical, occasional erectile dysfunction that most men experience a "disease" (or at least a condition worthy of medical attention) now that we have a treatment for it? If Prozac can lift everyone's mood, what then becomes "normal" or "typical" affect, and will grouchiness or sadness or inner struggle then be pathologized? And if we can all be happy and well-adjusted through Prozac, should insurance pay for everyone to reach that state of bliss? The second, related question addresses a broader social concern: should we encourage or discourage people to ingest pharmaceuticals to enhance behaviors, skills, and traits? What are the social (and economic, religious, psychological,...) implications of using drugs or other neurotechnologies to micromanage mood, improve memory, to maintain attentiveness or improve sexuality?

Neurotechnologies and the Enhancement Question

Human beings have always developed strategies and technologies to enhance their cognitive and affective functioning. We send our children to school, memorize poetry, develop training programs, meditate, enrich our word power, read novels, go to therapy, try to get a good night's sleep before exams, eat "brain food" such as fish, shut the door and turn off the music to study—all actions that, to one degree or another, are intended to create environments, inner states, or improved functioning that will encourage or support a desired level of neurological performance. We bang our heads, rub our temples, snap our fingers, and try to stop thinking directly about a topic to recall it to memory. In addition, we drink alcohol and caffeine, take Ritalin and Prozac, inhale nicotine, smoke marijuana, and use other pharmacological means to induce our brains to act in ways that we desire—to increase memory, stabilize mood, encourage creativity, or promote attentiveness.

The enhancement question, however, arises primarily in technologies that attempt to *directly* moderate the neurochemical, structural, or electrical components of the brain. The manipulation of brain function through learning, meditating, behavioral reinforcement, biofeedback, temple rubbing, or any other mechanism that either draws on the body's own resources, or manipulates the external environment to induce change do not raise the same ethical challenges. What characterizes the particular ethical currency of the enhancement debate today is the ability to bypass these types of activities and to change the brain directly.

Let us leaven our discussion with an example of a drug with the ability to enhance normal functioning: modafinil. Modafinil (2-(diphenylmethyl)-sulfinylacetamide) is a eugeroic (literally, "good arousal") drug that creates a wakeful, alert state

in those who take it. Early reports suggest that, unlike amphetamines, modafinil does not create a "buzz," does not cycle high and low, does not increase heart rate and blood pressure, and is non-addictive. Amphetamines create a dose-dependent impairment of the sleep cycle, so that one needs more and more amphetamines to stay awake, and is ultimately more fatigued. Modafinil not only does not disturb sleep, it only seems to cause wakefulness under conditions where vigilance is sought by the person who has taken it. Modafinil is generally prescribed for sleep disorders, such as narcolepsy and hypersomnia, and may be effective in the sleepiness that can accompany diseases such as Parkinson's.

Modafinil, marketed under the brand name Provigil, may eventually challenge Viagra in its appeal to off-label and black market usage. Also like Viagra, new sources have begun to tout the benefits of modafinil. A CBS News report trumpeted, "A Dream Come True? New Drug Tricks Brain To Be Awake" (CBS News 2002). The New York Times ran an article emphasizing the drug's potential in "a chronically sleep-deprived nation" (Goode 1998), and The New Yorker magazine ran a glowing piece asking whether "science can make regular sleep unnecessary" (Groopman 2001). Cephalon, the manufacturer, has done little to discourage the hype; in fact, the FDA recently cautioned Cephalon to be more careful in its claims about Provigil in its direct-to-consumer advertising (Los Angeles Times 2002).

Additionally, the potential of modafinil to be used for non-therapeutic purposes has been promoted in reports citing the armed services' interest in the drug for use in pilots. One study that came out of the United States Army Aeromedical Research Laboratory examined helicopter pilots who were exposed to two 40-h periods of continuous wakefulness separated by only one night of recovery sleep. When receiving modafinil, the pilots scored higher on tests of performance and physiological arousal than they did while on placebo, and also had improved self-ratings of vigor, energy, alertness, talkativeness, and confidence. It is not therefore surprising that the United States army, as well as a number of European armed forces, are already using monafidil; up until now, the standard issue wakefulness drug was Dexedrine, which cause all the side effects of amphetamines. The Department of Defense Advanced Research Projects Agency (DARPA), which is funding research into modafinil, justified the research by claiming:

> As combat systems become more and more sophisticated and reliable, the major limiting factor for operational dominance in a conflict is the warfighter. Eliminating the need for sleep while maintaining the high level of both cognitive and physical performance of the individual will create a fundamental change in warfighting and force employment, (quoted in Groopman 2001, 55).

The armed services are not employing the drug without at least some ethical reflection on the appropriate uses of pharmaceuticals as enhancement agents; as a United States Air Force report puts it: "The development of modafinil brings to light a crucial social question. What would be the impediment for its use, if a compound such as modafinil is more like caffeine than amphetamine in terms of safety, and yet, as effective as the amphetamines?" (Lyons & French 1991).

The "crucial social question" of Lyons and French already confronts us. The use of Viagra, for example, is common among men who would not qualify for a diagnosis of erectile dysfunction. Ritalin sales in certain school districts exceeds any reasonable estimate of children with ADHD that meets DSM-IV criteria. Kramer (1993) suggested that Prozac makes some patients "better than well," and prescriptions soared. Clearly, some of the top selling drugs in the world today are being used by patients who fit no traditional definition of pathology, yet still see in their own functioning a deficit that these drugs address.

Modafinil will likely follow the patterns of Viagra and Prozac, with areas of overprescribing, significant off-label usage, websites with cursory medical examination, and significant non-prescription sales. Still (or perhaps therefore?) policies need to be made, and so the enhancement question must be addressed. Should modafinil be prescribed solely as a medical drug, properly used only for those suffering from sleep pathology? If so third party payers, including government programs, should cover it. Or, should it be classified as an over-the-counter drug, available to anyone who wants it? Or, should we create a class of drugs available only to those who can show legitimate social need, those whose fatigue might put others at risk, such as airline pilots, or truck drivers? If so, we might see modafinil use as akin to reconstructive surgery, where payment is determined on perceived necessity. For those with severe injury or disfiguring birth defects, reconstructive surgery is medically justifiable and covered. For those electing to have surgery for cosmetic purposes, physicians are still free to offer it (or not), but no one is under a moral obligation to fund it. Finally, as a general social policy question, should we restrict modafinil's use in certain defined social settings, such as sports competitions (where those who use it will have an advantage), or in pediatric use (where students should be learning non-pharmaceutical attention skills), or in people in particularly high-stress jobs, such as airport traffic controllers (who might be tempted to abuse it)?

The Problems of Neurological Enhancement

The difficulty in deciding the questions of the correct use of neurological enhancers is, in part, a recognition that since we do not really understand the implications of enhancing neurological function, our strategies may backfire. The idea that attention is good, so increased attention is better, or that cognition is good, so increased cognition is better, may turn out to have unexpected consequences. Let us take as an example the effort to develop drugs targeted to improving memory in human beings. The improvement of memory sounds attractive in the abstract, and certainly is desirable for those suffering from Alzheimer's or other conditions that affect memory functions. But there are many unknowns in the use of such drugs in the cognitively intact.

The assumption is that memory drugs will simply increase the amount of memory we have available, leaving all other cognitive and affective processes unaffected. But in fact, memory is a selective, delicate process. There are experiences and data that our brains filters out. Our cognitive processes retain specific kinds of data, under specific circumstances, while other input is neglected. Who needs to remember the hours waiting in the Department of Motor Vehicles staring at the ceiling tiles, or to recall the transient amnesia following a personal trauma? Yet, we do not know whether memory enhancement drugs might impair our selectivity process. Might they improve our retention of all memories, even the traumatic or trivial memories that the brain tends to repress? Might we end up awash in memories that are troubling to us, unable to forget a painful past? And how might a memory drug affect associated mental processes—mood (which is closely connected to memory), or attentiveness (daydreaming is often fueled by a sudden recollection)? Perhaps evolution has stabilized at a particular level of memory capacity because more sacrifices a certain cognitive flexibility; a plastic brain may have advantages over one crammed with memory.

The concern is not only speculative. In 1999, scientists reported in *Nature* that they had genetically engineered mice with increased ability to perform learning tasks. The scientists inserted a gene in mouse zygotes that increased the production of the protein subunit NR2B, part of the NMDA receptor. The mice also displayed physiological changes in the hippocampus (associated with learning) when compared to nontransgenic mice. However, subsequent research seemed to indicate that the mice with enhanced NR2B seemed to have a greater sensitivity to pain. Though it may be that the mice do not feel the pain more acutely, just learn about pain more readily and thus seem to react to it more strongly, it is troubling that even the most preliminary research on memory enhancement has already raised the question of unexpected collateral effects. Perhaps there is a link we do not

understand between memory and pain, either at the structural or behavioral level. What other unexpected linkages might be discovered in attempts to change cognitive functions through induced physiological modification?

While most of the "cognitive enhancement" discussed in the literature focuses on memory or attentiveness, the range of cognitive abilities, of course, exceeds just these two traits. Learning, language, skilled motor behaviors, and "executive functions" (such as decision making, goal setting, planning, and judgment) are all part of general cognition, and a drug that managed to enhance a greater range of function (especially executive function) may be more desirable than one that narrowly enhanced memory alone. But if memory drugs alone have collateral affects, how much more so might a drug that influences a greater range of cognitive functioning?

It is not only the collateral effects of neurological enhancement that are troublesome, but also the nature of the change itself. For example, the progressive loss of cognitive function that characterizes Alzheimer's is usually described as constituting the "loss of personality" of the person with the disease. "Dad isn't Dad anymore" because his cognitive faculties as experienced by his loved ones are considered fundamental to who he is; loss of those functions are seen as loss of his essence. A general cognitive enhancement may have the same effect. Significantly improving our overall cognitive functioning may also alter aspects of our identity that are seen as fundamental to who we are. As Whitehouse et al. (1997, 16) write:

> Increased memory, new insights, and better reasoning could all lead to new values, new perspectives on one's relationships, and new sources of pleasure and irritation. That does not mean that the enhanced literally will lose their identities and become different people, any more than someone with Alzheimer's does. But in the figurative sense intended by caregivers of people with the disease, it may be that after some point the cognitively enhanced

will no longer be recognizable by those who knew them before their enhancement.

Research on patients with frontotemporal dementia, who demonstrate often dramatic changes in well-established patterns or religion, dress, style, and political philosophy, seems to indicate that some aspects of the self are functions of the frontal lobes. Lauren Slater, author of the memoir "Prozac Diary," writes that though Prozac relieved her of her symptoms, she no longer felt any desire to read the angst-ridden psychology and philosophy books that lined her bookshelf (Slater, 1998). Slater wonders what the loss of these books, that had once been sources of wisdom for her, meant for her sense of self: "who was I? Where was I? Everything seemed less relevant—my sacred menus, my gustatory habits, the narrative that had had so much meaning for me. Diminished." Even when she rediscovers her spiritual side later in the memoir, she now wonders if her calmer, more contemplative spirituality comes not from God, but from Prozac.

Neurological biotechnologies differ from others in that they ask us to explicitly consider the kind of "self" we want to have; or, to put it less dualistically, perhaps, the kind of self we want to be. For some, our astounding ability to manipulate our own biology is an integral part of who we are as human animals. For others, it is an affront to our humanity. This is an argument for which there are no right or wrong answers, emerging as it does from two philosophically different visions of human life. Yet therein lies the tension of the enhancement debate, and there is little doubt that the battlefield on which the debate will be waged next will be our ancient desire to control the workings of our own minds.

References

CBS News. "A Dream Come True? New Drug Tricks Brain to Be Awake; Military Is Interested." January 14, 2002. (http://www.ebsnews.com/now/story/0,1597,324299-412,00.shtml).

Goode, E. "New Hope for Losers in the Battle to Stay Awake." *New York Times,* November 3, 1998.

Groopman, J. "Eyes Wide open." *The New Yorker*, December 3, 1998, 52–57.

Los Angeles Times. EDA Reprimands 4 Drug Makers for Misleading Promotions." January 16, 2002. http://www.latimes.com/business/la-000004018janl 6.story?col=la-headlines-business.

Lyons, T. J., & French, J. "Modafinil: The Unique properties of a New Stimulant." *USAF School of Aerospace, Brooks TX, Science News Note*, 62 (1991), 432–35.

Slater, L. *Prozac diary*. New York: Random House, 1998.

Whitehouse, P. J., E. Juengst, M. Mehlman, and T. Murray. "Enhancing cognition in the intellectually intact." *Hastings Center Report*, Vol. 27, no. 3 (1997), 14–22.

Memory and Happiness

PRESIDENT'S COUNCIL ON BIOETHICS

From *Beyond Therapy: Biotechnology and the pursuit of Happiness*. http://www.bioethics.gov/reports/beyondtherapy/beyond_therapy_final_webcorrected.pdf (accessed March 30, 2008), 214-34.

At first glance, the pursuit of happiness—a forward-looking activity—might seem to have little to do with memory—the remembrance of things past. Yet a closer look reveals some deep connections. Could we be happy if we were unable to remember our own past, if we lived only day-to-day, one moment to the next? Could we be happy if we were unable to assimilate present experience into the remembered narrative of previous experience? Could we be happy in the absence of happy memories? Conversely, could we be happy in the presence of terrible memories, memories so traumatic and so life-altering that they cast a deep shadow over all that we do, today and tomorrow? As these questions imply, both our capacity to remember—our ability to recall and recollect—and the content of what we remember—the banked "traces" of specific past experiences—may well be crucial to our prospects for happiness.

A good memory is necessary even to do the little things that contribute to our happiness: preparing the foods we like, riding a bicycle, finding our way home or to the home of friends. Guiding us with little conscious effort, such memories are silently yet deeply part of who we are. Memory is also indispensable for our ability to learn new things: the name of a new acquaintance, the title of a new book, the contours of a new place. This forward-looking but memory-dependent readiness to capture and incorporate the not-yet-known and the not-yet-lived makes possible new pursuits, new associations, and new ways of getting along in the world—in a word, new ways of becoming happy.

Memory is important not only for retaining knowledge of what we can do. It is important also for allowing and enabling us to "know"—virtually without any deliberate effort on our part—*who we are*. Our memory, by its own activity, preserves for us the complex web of lived experiences that furnish our sense of self: the shared memories of living side-by-side with loved ones; the class long ago that changed our lives; the days we spent in sickness and celebration; our finest moments and most shameful acts. The memories and the "self" they shape are acquired over time. At each moment, our then-existing web of memories shapes the way we face and understand our everyday lives. But this web of memories is, paradoxically, not permanently fixed, unlike an image recorded on a photograph. As we give new meaning to old happenings and try to fit them within the larger narrative of our unfolding existence, it changes over the course of life. Our experiences at age sixteen will have a different meaning to us when remembered at age eighteen, and a very different meaning yet again when remembered at age fifty. As we grow older, memories become less vivid, but perhaps their significance becomes more clear; although they are less immediate, they are now part of the larger story of who we are. We can consciously re-examine the meaning of remembered events and, as a result, change *how* they are remembered. Yet the memories themselves set limits on how much can be re-written, and much of the "re-construction" or "re-membering" of our remembered lives results from *undirected* "editorial" work. Astonishingly, memory itself selectively retains and deletes, reconfigures and reintegrates, the experiences that comprise who we have been and, therefore, *are*. Our identity or sense of self emerges, grows, and changes. Yet, despite all the changes, thanks to the integrating powers of memory, our identity also, remarkably, persists *as ours*.

If the capacities of remembering are crucial for preserving the "my-ness" of any happiness that comes our way, the *content* of the memories are crucial for our happiness itself. We do not wish merely to remember having had satisfying experiences; we wish to remember them with satisfaction. We desire not only even-keeled memories, but also memories with feeling and with sense: we relish the memory of devoted parents, of first love, the birth of a child; we delight in recalling beautiful sights seen, good deeds done, worthy efforts rewarded. We especially want our memories to be not simply a sequence of disconnected experiences, but a narrative that seems to contain some unfolding purpose, some larger point from beginning to end, some aspiration discovered, pursued, and at least partially fulfilled.

Memory is central to human flourishing, in other words, precisely because we pursue happiness in time, as time-bound beings. We have a past and a future as well as a present, and being happy through time requires that these be connected in a meaningful way. If we are to flourish *as ourselves*, we must do so without abandoning or forgetting who we are or once were. Yet because our lives are time-bound, our happiness is always incomplete—always not-yet and on-the-way, always here but slipping away, but also always possible again and in the future. Our happiest experiences can be revivified. And, as we reminisce from greater distance and with more experience, even our painful experiences can often acquire for us a meaning not in evidence when they occurred.

The place of memory in the pursuit of happiness also suggests something essential about human identity, a theme raised in various places and in different ways throughout this report: namely, our identities are formed both by what we do and by what we undergo or suffer. We actively choose paths and do deeds fit to be remembered. But we also live through memorable experiences that we would never have chosen—experiences we often wish never happened at all. To some extent, these unchosen memories constrain us; though we may regret the shadows

they cast over our pursuit of happiness, we cannot simply escape them while remaining who we really are. And yet, through the act of remembering—the act of discerning and giving meaning to the past as it really was—we can shape, to some degree, the meaning of our memories, both good and bad.

The contribution of good memories to happiness, presented in this overly rosy account, makes clear how bad memories can undermine happiness, indeed, can cause misery. We can lose our memory through injury or illness; we can be plagued by terrifying, shameful, or guilty memories. Even for the fortunate and virtuous, life is not a bowl of cherries. To live, as we emphasized in the last chapter, is to age and decline, in memory as well as in muscle. To aspire is to risk disappointment. To love is to risk loss, and eventually to lose what one loves altogether in death. Bad memories, present inevitably to all of us, can not only mar present happiness; if sufficiently grave, they can overwhelm us and crush the prospect of seeking happiness any time in the future. Memory is not *always* a friend to happiness.

For this reason, people interested in happiness are interested, among other things, in better memories. Precisely because, in order to be happy, we need to be able to remember, we would like to find ways to keep our memory capacity intact, against the dangers of senility. Precisely because we desire happier memories, we might be tempted to "edit out," if we could, those memories that most disturb us or even to seek a new life history entirely. For understandable reasons, we might seek to restore the innocence or peace of mind that our actions or our sufferings have disrupted.

Until recently, the prospect of altering our remembrance of things past—and doing so with precision, getting the better memories we desire without compromising memory as a whole—was a mere fantasy. But in the near future that may not be so. Much memory research over the past decades has focused on finding the causes and then the remedies for forgetfulness, in the first instance to forestall or treat the senile dementias, but, in the second place, to prevent also the annoying lapses of memory in the elderly and middle-aged, who have trouble remembering, for example, where they left the house keys. Although the field is full of promise, there is little of practical value to report at the present time. Should such remedies for failing memories be found, their use would be welcomed by most people as a great boon. Assuming that there were no physical or mental side effects—a large assumption—there is little obvious reason to be concerned about the ethical or social implications.

Scientists have also sought ways to alter the *content* and *feeling tone* of specific memories, with the goal of helping people whose lives are crushed by remembered trauma. This research has yielded some novel pharmacological interventions, still rather limited in their effect but perhaps a harbinger of things to come, that change the way we remember the most emotionally affecting experiences of life, specifically by "numbing" the discomfort connected with the memory of our most painful experiences. The capacity to alter or numb our remembrance of things past cuts to the heart of what it means to remember in a human way, and it is this biotechnical possibility that we focus on here. Deciding when or whether to use such biotechnical power will require that we think long and hard about what it means to remember truthfully, to live in time, and to seek happiness without losing or abandoning our identity. The rest of this discussion of "memory and happiness" is an invitation to such reflection.

Biotechnology and Memory Alteration

It is a commonplace observation that, while some events fade quickly from the mind, emotionally intense experiences form memories that are peculiarly vivid and long-lasting. Not only do we recall such events long after they happened, but the recollection is often accompanied, in some measure, by a recurrence of the emotions aroused during the original experience.

A body of recent research on the formation of long-term memory has established two crucial facts about this phenomenon. First, immediately following a new experience there occurs a period of *memory consolidation*, during which some memories are encoded in the brain with more lasting impact than others. Second, strong emotional arousal is attended by the release of certain *stress hormones* (such as epinephrine, also known as adrenaline), and the presence or absence of these hormones in the brain during the period of memory consolidation greatly affects how strong and durable a memory is formed.

By the early 1990s, research on animals had shown that these stress hormones enhance the encoding of memories by activating the amygdala, a small almond-shaped region of the brain deep inside the temporal lobe. Experiments on rats showed that the memory of an experience can be strengthened if epinephrine (which produces high arousal) is injected into the amygdala immediately afterwards; conversely, such memory can be weakened by injecting into the amygdala drugs (called beta-blockers) that suppress the action of epinephrine.

Research with human subjects broadened these results and shed further light on the neuromodulatory processes that regulate the encoding of memories in the brain. Studies of patients with amnesia confirmed the crucial role of the amygdala in the consolidation of emotionally charged memories. People who have suffered damage to the amygdala typically have no difficulty remembering recent mundane events, but they do not exhibit the enhanced long-term memory normally produced by emotionally arousing experiences. Furthermore, a person with a damaged amygdala will typically recall emotional experiences *without* the normal repetition of the original emotion. In healthy subjects, fearful experiences are encoded with fearful memories, but subjects with amygdala damage often exhibit "abnormal fear response": they have difficulty learning to fear (and hence avoid) dangerous situations because they do not recall fearful events with the appropriate emotion. Evidently, the activation of the amygdala by stress hormones during highly emotional experiences leads to the encoding of memories that are not only more persistent but also more apt to return with the appropriate emotional accompaniment.

The results described above may help to explain what happens when, after living through particularly horrifying experiences, some people experience symptoms of PTSD. When a person experiences especially shocking or violent events (such as a plane crash or bloody combat), the release of stress hormones may be so intense that the memory-encoding system is over-activated. The result is a consolidation of memories both far stronger and more persistent than normal and also more apt, upon recollection, to call forth the intense emotional response of the original experience. In such cases, each time the person relives the traumatic memory, a new flood of stress hormones is released, and the experience may be so emotionally intense as to be encoded as a new experience. With time, the memories grow more recurrent and intrusive, and the response—fear, helplessness, horror—more incapacitating. As we shall see, drugs that might prevent or alleviate the symptoms of PTSD are among the chief medical benefits that scientists expect from recent research in the neurochemistry of memory formation.

In fact, the discovery of hormonal regulation of memory formation was quickly followed up by clinical studies on human subjects demonstrating that memory of emotional experiences can be altered pharmacologically. In one particularly interesting series of experiments, Larry Cahill and his colleagues showed that injections of beta-blockers can, by inhibiting the action of stress hormones, suppress the memory-enhancing effects of strong emotional arousal. The researchers showed their subjects a series of slides and told them one of two stories to explain the events depicted; one story was mundane and emotionally neutral, the other was tragic and emotionally gripping. Two weeks later, the participants were asked to recall the story, and those who had heard the emotionally arousing story were found—as expected—to recall what was depicted in the slides in far greater detail than those who had heard the mundane

version. The experiment was then repeated, except that half the participants were given an injection of the beta-blocker propranolol and half were injected with a saline placebo one hour before the slide show. What they found was that, after two weeks, those who had heard the more mundane version of the story had the same level of recollection regardless of whether they had received the beta-blocker or the placebo. But of the subjects who had heard the more arousing version of the story, only those receiving the placebo showed an enhanced level of recollection. Those who heard the arousing story after receiving the beta-blocker found it extremely sad and emotional at the time, but two weeks later they remembered it at the same emotional level as the group that had heard the neutral story.

Thus, taking propranolol appears to have little or no effect on how we remember everyday or emotionally neutral information. But when taken at the time of highly emotional experiences, propranolol appears to suppress the normal memory-enhancing effects of emotional arousal—while leaving the immediate emotional response unaffected. These results suggested the possibility of using beta-blockers to help survivors of traumatic events to reduce their intrusive—and in some cases crippling—memories of those events. In 2002 Roger K. Pitman and his colleagues published a pilot study reporting the use of propranolol administered to emergency room patients within six hours after a traumatic experience (mostly car accidents) and for an additional ten days thereafter. The patients—both those taking the drug and those taking placebos—were tested for their psychological and physiological response to a re-telling (with related images) of the traumatic event. One month after the event, those taking propranolol showed measurably lower incidence of PTSD symptoms than the control group. And three months later, while the PTSD symptoms of both groups had returned to comparable levels, the propranolol group showed measurably lower psycho-physiological response to "internal cues (that is, mental imagery) that symbolized or resembled the initial traumatic event."[1]

This study, while very preliminary, suggests that drugs may become available that will enable us not only to soften certain powerful memories but to detach them from the strong emotions evoked by the original experience. Propranolol and other currently available beta-blockers may not be able to do the whole job, and, until more evidence is acquired, we do well to regard them as weak precursors of subsequent drugs that might be more powerful and effective. Yet the prospect of such "memory numbing" drugs has already elicited considerable public interest in and concern about their potential uses in non-clinical settings: to prepare a soldier to kill (or kill again) on the battlefield; to dull the sting of one's own shameful acts; to allow a criminal to numb the memory of his or her victims. Some of these scenarios are perhaps far-fetched. But although the pharmacology of memory alteration is a science still in its infancy, the significance of this potential new power—to separate the subjective experience of memory from the truth of the experience that is remembered—should not be underestimated. It surely returns us to the large ethical and anthropological questions with which we began—about memory's role in shaping personal identity and the character of human life, and about the meaning of remembering things that we would rather forget and of forgetting things that we perhaps ought to remember.

Memory-Blunting: Ethical Analysis

If we had the power, by promptly taking a memory-altering drug, to dull the emotional impact of what could become very painful memories, when might we be tempted to use it? And for what reasons should we yield to or resist the temptation?

At first glance, such a drug would seem ideally suited for the prevention of PTSD, the complex of debilitating symptoms that sometimes afflict those who have experienced severe trauma. These symptoms—which include persistent re-experiencing of the traumatic event and avoidance of every person, place, or thing that might stimulate the horrid memory's return—can so burden mental life as to make normal everyday living extremely difficult, if not impossible. For those suffering these disturbing symptoms, a drug that could separate a painful memory from its powerful emotional component would appear very welcome indeed.

Yet the prospect of preventing (even) PTSD with beta-blockers or other memory-blunting agents seems to be, for several reasons, problematic. First of all, the drugs in question appear to be effective only when administered during or shortly after a traumatic event—and thus well before any symptoms of PTSD would be manifested. How then could we make, and make on the spot, the *prospective* judgment that a particular event is sufficiently terrible to warrant pre-emptive memory-blunting? Second, how shall we judge *which* participants in the event merit such treatment? After all, not everyone who suffers through painful experiences is destined to have pathological memory effects. Should the drugs in question be given to everyone or only to those with an observed susceptibility to PTSD, and, if the latter, how will we know who these are? Finally, in some cases merely witnessing a disturbing event (for example, a murder, rape, or terrorist attack) is sufficient to cause PTSD-like symptoms long afterwards. Should we then, as soon as disaster strikes, consider giving memory-altering drugs to all the witnesses, in addition to those directly involved?

These questions point to other troubling implications. Use of memory-blunters at the time of traumatic events could interfere with the normal psychic work and adaptive value of emotionally charged memory. A primary function of the brain's special way of encoding memories for emotional experiences would seem to be to make us remember important events longer and more vividly than trivial events. Thus, by blunting their emotional impact, beta-blockers or their successors would concomitantly weaken our recollection of the traumatic events we have just experienced. Yet often it is important, in the aftermath of such events, that at least someone remembers them clearly. For legal reasons, to say nothing of deeper social and personal ones, the wisdom of routinely interfering with the memories of trauma survivors and witnesses is highly questionable.

If the apparent powers of memory-blunting drugs are confirmed, some might be inclined to prescribe them liberally to all who are involved in a sufficiently terrible event. After all, even those not destined to come down with full-blown PTSD are likely to suffer painful recurrent memories of an airplane crash, an incident of terrorism, or a violent combat operation. In the aftermath of such shocking incidents, why not give everyone the chance to remember these events without the added burden of painful emotions? This line of reasoning might, in fact, tempt us to give beta-blockers liberally to soldiers on the eve of combat, to emergency workers en route to a disaster site, or even to individuals requesting prophylaxis against the shame or guilt they might incur from future misdeeds—in general, to anyone facing an experience that is likely to leave lasting intrusive memories.

Yet on further reflection it seems clear that not every intrusive memory is a suitable candidate for prospective pharmacological blunting. As Daniel Schacter has observed, "attempts to avoid traumatic memories often backfire":

> Intrusive memories need to be acknowledged, confronted, and worked through, in order to set them to rest for the long term. Unwelcome memories of trauma are symptoms of a disrupted psyche that requires attention before it can resume healthy functioning. Beta-blockers might make it easier for trauma survivors to face and incorporate traumatic recollections, and in that sense could facilitate long-term adaptation. Yet it is also possible that beta-blockers would work against the normal process of recovery: traumatic memories would not spring to mind with the kind of psychological force that demands attention

and perhaps intervention. Prescription of beta-blockers could bring about an effective trade-off between short-term reductions in the sting of traumatic memories and long-term increases in persistence of related symptoms of a trauma that has not been adequately confronted.[2]

The point can be generalized: in the immediate aftermath of a painful experience, we simply cannot know either the full meaning of the experience in question or the ultimate character and future prospects of the individual who experiences it. We cannot know how this experience will change this person at this time and over time. Will he be cursed forever by unbearable memories that, in retrospect, clearly should have been blunted medically? Or will he succeed, over time, in "redeeming" those painful memories by actively integrating them into the narrative of his life? By "rewriting" memories pharmacologically we might succeed in easing real suffering at the risk of falsifying our perception of the world and undermining our true identity.

Finally, the decision whether or not to use memory-blunting drugs must be made in the absence of clearly diagnosable disease. The drug must be taken right after a traumatic experience has occurred, and thus before the different ways that different individuals handle the same experience has become clear. In some cases, these interventions will turn out to have been preventive medicine, intervening to ward off the onset of PTSD before it arrives—though it is worth noting that we would lack even post hoc knowledge of whether any particular now-unaffected individual, in the absence of using the drug, would have become symptomatic. In other cases, the interventions would not be medicine at all: altering the memory of individuals who could have lived well, even with severely painful memories, without pharmacologically dulling the pain. Worse, in still other cases, the use of such drugs would inoculate individuals in advance against the psychic pain that *should* accompany their commission of cruel, brutal, or shameful deeds. But in all cases, from the defensible to the dubious, the use of such powers changes the character of human memory, by intervening directly in the way individuals "encode," and thus the way they understand, the happenings of their own lives and the realities of the world around them. Sorting out how and why this matters, and especially what it means for our idea of human happiness, is the focus of the more particular—albeit brief—ethical reflections that follow.

1. Remembering Fitly and Truly

Altering the formation of emotionally powerful memories risks severing what we remember from how we remember it and distorting the link between our perception of significant human events and the significance of the events themselves. It risks, in a word, falsifying our perception and understanding of the world. It risks making shameful acts seem less shameful, or terrible acts less terrible, than they really are.

Imagine the experience of a person who witnesses a shocking murder. Fearing that he will be haunted by images of this event, he immediately takes propranolol (or its more potent successor) to render his memory of the murder less painful and intrusive. Thanks to the drug, his memory of the murder gets encoded as a garden-variety, emotionally neutral experience. But in manipulating his memory in this way, he risks coming to think about the murder as more tolerable than it really is, as an event that should not sting those who witness it. For our opinions about the meaning of our experiences are shaped partly by the feelings evoked when we remember them. If, psychologically, the murder is transformed into an event our witness can recall without pain—or without *any* particular emotion—perhaps its moral significance will also fade from consciousness. If so, he would in a sense have ceased to be a genuine witness of the murder. When asked about it, he might say, "Yes, I was there. But it wasn't so terrible."

This points us to a deeper set of questions about bad memories: Would dulling our memory of terrible things make us too comfortable with the world, unmoved by suffering, wrongdoing, or cruelty? Does not the experience of hard truths—of the unchosen, the inexplicable, the tragic—remind us that we can never be fully at home in the world, especially if we are to take seriously the reality of human evil? Further, by blunting our experience and awareness of shameful, fearful, and hateful things, might we not also risk deadening our response to what is admirable, inspiring, and lovable? Can we become numb to life's sharpest sorrows without also becoming numb to its greatest joys?

These questions point to what might be the highest cost of making our memory of intolerable things more tolerable: Armed with new powers to ease the suffering of bad memories, we might come to see all psychic pain as unnecessary and in the process come to pursue a happiness that is less than human: an unmindful happiness, unchanged by time and events, unmoved by life's vicissitudes. More precisely, we might come to pursue such happiness by willingly abandoning or compromising our own truthful identities: instead of integrating, as best we can, the troubling events of our lives into a more coherent whole, we might just prefer to edit them out or make them less difficult to live with than they really are.

There seems to be little doubt that some bitter memories are so painful and intrusive as to ruin the possibility for normal experience of much of life and the world. In such cases the impulse to relieve a crushing burden and restore lost innocence is fully understandable: If there are some things that it is better never to have experienced at all—things we would avoid if we possibly could—why not erase them from the memory of those unfortunate enough to have suffered them? If there are some things it is better never to have known or seen, why not use our power over memory to restore a witness's shattered peace of mind? There is great force in this argument, perhaps especially in cases where children lose prematurely that innocence that is rightfully theirs.

And yet, there may be a great cost to acting compassionately for those who suffer bad memories, if we do so by compromising the truthfulness of how they remember. We risk having them live falsely in order simply to cope, to survive by whatever means possible. Among the larger falsehoods to which such practices could lead us, few are more problematic than the extreme beliefs regarding the possibility—and impossibility—of human control. Erring on the one side, we might come to imagine ourselves as having more control over our memories and identities than we really do, believing that we can be authors and editors of our memories while still remaining truly—and true to—ourselves. Erring on the other side, we might come to imagine that we are impotently in the grip of the past as we look to the future, believing that we can never learn to live with this particular memory or give it new meaning. And so we ease today's pain, but only by foreclosing, in a certain way, the possibility of being the kind of person who can live well with the whole truth—both chosen and unchosen—and the kind of person who can live well as himself.

2. The Obligation to Remember

Having truthful memories is not simply a personal matter. Strange to say, our own memory is not merely our own; it is part of the fabric of the society in which we live. Consider the case of a person who has suffered or witnessed atrocities that occasion unbearable memories: for example, those with firsthand experience of the Holocaust. The life of that individual might well be served by dulling such bitter memories, but such a humanitarian intervention, if widely practiced, would seem deeply troubling: Would the community as a whole—would the human race—be served by such a mass numbing of this terrible but indispensable memory? Do those who suffer evil have a duty to remember and bear witness, lest we all forget the very horrors that haunt them? (The examples of this dilemma need not be quite so stark: the memory of being embarrassed is a source of empathy for others who suffer embarrassment; the memory of losing a loved one is a source of empathy for those who experience a similar loss.) Surely, we cannot and should not force those who live through great trauma to endure its painful memory *for the benefit of the rest of us*. But as a community, there are certain events that we have an obligation to remember—an obligation that falls disproportionately, one might even say unfairly, on those who experience such events most directly. What kind of people would we be if we did not "want" to remember the Holocaust, if we sought to make the anguish it caused simply go away? And yet, what kind of people are we, especially those who face such horrors firsthand, that we can endure such awful memories?

3. Memory and Moral Responsibility

The question of how responsible we are or should be held for our memories, especially our memory failures, is a complicated one: Are remembering and forgetting voluntary or involuntary acts? To what extent should a man who forgets his child in a car, by mistake, be held "morally accountable" for his forgetting? Is remembering "something we do" or "something that happens to us"?

Hard as these questions are, this much seems clear: Without memory, both our own and that of others, the notion of moral responsibility would largely unravel. In particular, the power to numb or eliminate the psychic sting of certain memories risks eroding the responsibility we take for our own actions—since we would never have to face the harsh judgment of our own conscience (Lady Macbeth) or the memory of others. The risk applies both to self-serving uses of such a power (for example, drugs taken after a criminal act and before the next one) and to more ambiguous "social" uses (for example, drugs taken after killing in war and before killing again). Without truthful memory, we could not hold others or ourselves to account for what we do and who we are. Without truthful memory, there could be no justice or even the possibility of justice; without memory, there could be no forgiveness or the possibility of forgiveness—all would simply be *forgotten*.

Notes

1. Pitman, R. K., et al., "Pilot Study of Secondary Prevention of Posttraumatic Stress Disorder with Propranolol." *Biological Psychiatry,* 51 (2002): 189–92.
2. Schacter, D., *The Seven Sins of Memory: How the Mind Forgets and Remembers.* (New York: Houghton Mifflin, 2001), 183.

Genetic Dilemmas and the Child's Right to an Open Future

DENA S. DAVIS

Hastings Center Report 27, no.2 (1997): 7-15.

The profession of genetic counseling is strongly characterized by a respect for patient autonomy that is greater than in almost any other area of medicine. When moral challenges arise in the clinical practice of genetics, they tend to be understood as conflicts between the obligation to respect patient autonomy and other ethical norms, such as doing good and avoiding harm. Thus, a typical counseling dilemma exists when a person who has been tested and found to be carrying the gene for Tay-Sachs disease refuses to share that information with siblings and other relatives despite the clear benefits to them of having that knowledge, or when a family member declines to participate in a testing protocol necessary to help another member discover his or her genetic status.

This way of looking at moral issues in genetic counseling often leaves both the counselors and commentators frustrated, for two reasons. First, by elevating respect for patient autonomy above all other values, it may be difficult to give proper weight to other factors, such as human suffering. Second, by privileging patient autonomy and by defining the patient as the person or couple who has come for counseling, there seems no "space" in which to give proper attention to the moral claims of the future child who is the endpoint of many counseling interactions.

These difficulties have been highlighted of late by the surfacing of a new kind of genetic counseling request: parents with certain disabilities who seek help in trying to assure that they will have a child who shares their disability. The two reported instances are in families affected by achondroplasia (dwarfism) and by hereditary deafness. This essay will focus on deafness.

Such requests are understandably troubling to genetic counselors. Deeply committed to the principle of giving clients value-free information with which to make their own choices, most counselors nonetheless make certain assumptions about health and disability—for example, that it is preferable to be a hearing person rather than a deaf person. Thus, counselors typically talk of the "risk" of having a child with a particular genetic condition. Counselors may have learned (sometimes with great difficulty) to respect clients' decisions not to find out if their fetus has a certain condition or not to abort a fetus which carries a genetic disability. But to respect a parental value system that not only favors what most of us consider to be a disability, but actively expresses that preference by attempting to have a child with the condition, is "the ultimate test of nondirective counseling."

To describe the challenge primarily as one that pits beneficence (concern for the child's quality of life) against autonomy (concern for the parents' right to decide about these matters) makes for obvious difficulties. These are two very different values, and comparing and weighing them invites the proverbial analogy of "apples and oranges." After all, the perennial critique of a principle-based ethics is that it offers few suggestions for ranking principles when duties conflict. Further, beneficence and respect for autonomy are values that will always exist in some tension within genetic counseling. For all the reasons I list below, counselors are committed to the primacy of patient autonomy and therefore to nondirective counseling. But surely, most or all of them are drawn to the field because they want to help people avoid or at least mitigate suffering.

Faced with the ethical challenge of parents who wish to ensure children who have a disability, I suggest a different way to look at this problem. Thinking this problem through in the way I suggest will shed light on some related topics in genetics as well, such as sex selection. I propose that, rather than conceiving this as a conflict between autonomy and beneficence, we recast it as a conflict between parental autonomy and the child's future autonomy: what Joel Feinberg has called "the child's right to an open future."

New Challenges

The Code of Ethics of the National Society of Genetic Counselors states that its members strive to:

- Respect their clients' beliefs, cultural traditions, inclinations, circumstances, and feelings.
- Enable their clients to make informed independent decisions, free of coercion, by providing or illuminating the necessary facts and clarifying the alternatives and anticipated consequences.

Considering the uncertain and stochastic nature of genetic counseling, and especially in light of the difficulty physicians experience in sharing uncertainty with patients, it is remarkable that medical geneticists have hewed so strongly to an ethic of patient autonomy. This phenomenon can be explained by at least five factors: the desire to disassociate themselves as strongly as possible from the discredited eugenics movement; an equally strong desire to avoid the label of "abortionist," a realistic fear if counselors are perceived as advocates for abortion of genetically damaged fetuses; the fact that few treatments are available for genetic diseases; an awareness of the intensely private nature of reproductive decisions; and the fact that genetic decisions can have major consequences for entire families. As one counselor was quoted, "I am not going to be taking that baby home—they will."

The commitment to patient autonomy faces new challenges with the advances arising from the Human Genome Project. The example of hereditary deafness is reported by Walter E. Nance, who writes:

> It turns out that some deaf couples feel threatened by the prospect of having a hearing child and would actually prefer to have a deaf child. The knowledge that we will soon acquire [due to the Human Genome Project] will, of course, provide us with the technology that could be used to assist such couples in achieving their goals. This, in turn, could lead to the ultimate test of nondirective counseling. Does adherence to the concept of nondirective counseling actually require that we assist such a couple in terminating a pregnancy with a hearing child or is this nonsense[1]

Several issues must be unpacked here. First, I question Nance's depiction of deaf parents as feeling "threatened" by the prospect of a hearing child. From Nance's own depiction of the deaf people he encounters, it is at least as likely that deaf parents feel that a deaf child would fit into their family better, especially if the parents themselves are "deaf of deaf" or if they already have one or more deaf children. Or perhaps the parents feel that Deafness (I use the capital "D," as Deaf people do, to signify Deafness as a culture) is an asset—tough at times but worthwhile in the end—like belonging to a racial or religious minority.

Second, I want to avoid the issue of abortion by discussing the issue of "deliberately producing a deaf child" as distinct from the question of achieving that end by aborting a hearing fetus. The latter topic is important, but it falls outside the purview of this paper. I will focus on the scenario where a deaf child is produced without recourse to abortion. We can imagine a situation in the near future where eggs or sperm can be scrutinized for the relevant trait before fertilization, or the present situation in which preimplantation genetic diagnosis after in vitro fertilization allows specialists to examine the genetic makeup of the very early embryo before it is implanted.

Imagine a Deaf couple approaching a genetic counselor. The couple's goals are to learn more about the cause(s) of their own deafness, and, if possible, to maximize the chance that any pregnancy they embark upon will result in a Deaf child. Let us suppose that the couple falls into the 50 percent of clients whose Deafness has a genetic origin. The genetic counselor who adheres strictly to the tenets of client autonomy will respond by helping the couple to explore the ways in which they can achieve their goal: a Deaf baby. But as Nance's depiction of this scenario suggests, the counselor may well feel extremely uneasy about her role here. It is one thing to support a couple's decision to take their chances and "let Nature take its course," but to treat as a goal what is commonly considered to be a risk may be more pressure than the value-neutral ethos can bear. What is needed is a principled argument against such assistance. This refusal need not rise to a legal prohibition, but could become part of the ethical norms and standard of care for the counseling profession.

The path I see out of this dilemma relies on two steps. First, we remind ourselves why client autonomy is such a powerful norm in genetic counseling. Clients come to genetic counselors with questions that are simultaneously of the greatest magnitude and of the greatest intimacy. Clients not only have the right to bring their own values to bear on these questions, but in the end they must do so because they—and their children—will live with the consequences. As the President's Commission said in its 1983 report on Screening and Counseling for Genetic Conditions:

> The silence of the law on many areas of individual choice reflects the value this country places on pluralism. Nowhere is the need for freedom to pursue divergent conceptions of the good more deeply felt than in decisions concerning reproduction. It would be a cruel irony, therefore, if technological advances undertaken in the name of providing information to expand the range of individual choices resulted in unanticipated social pressures to pursue a particular course of action. Someone who feels compelled to undergo screening or to make particular reproductive choices at the urging of health care professionals or others or as a result of implicit social pressure is deprived of the choice-enhancing benefits of the new advances. The Commission recommends that those who counsel patients and those who educate the public about genetics should not only emphasize the importance of preserving choice but also do their utmost to safeguard the choices of those they serve.[2]

Now let us take this value of respect for autonomy and put it on both sides of the dilemma. Why is it morally problematic to seek to produce a child who is deaf? Being deaf does not cause one physical pain or shorten one's life span, two obvious conditions which it would be prima facie immoral to produce in another person. Deaf people might (or might not) be less happy on average than hearing people, but that is arguably a function of societal prejudice. The primary argument against deliberately seeking to produce deaf children is that it violates the child's own autonomy and narrows the scope of her choices when she grows up; in other words, it violates her right to an "open future."

The Child's Right to an Open Future

Joel Feinberg begins his discussion of children's rights by noticing that rights can ordinarily be divided into four kinds. First, there are rights that adults and children have in common (the right not to be killed, for example). Then, there are rights that are generally possessed only by children (or by "childlike" adults). These "dependency-rights," as Feinberg calls them, derive from the child's dependence on others for such basics as food, shelter, and protection. Third, there are rights that can only be exercised by adults (or at least by children approaching adulthood), for example, the free exercise of religion. Finally, there are rights that Feinberg calls "rights-in-trust," rights which are to be "saved for the child until he is an adult." These rights can be violated by adults now, in ways that cut off the possibility that the child, when it achieves adulthood, can exercise them. A striking example is the right to reproduce. A young child cannot physically exercise that right, and a teenager might lack the legal and moral grounds on which to assert such a right. But clearly the child, when he or she attains adulthood, will have that right, and therefore the child now has the right not to be sterilized, so that the child may exercise that right in the future. Rights in this category include a long list: virtually all the important rights we believe adults have, but which must be protected now to be exercised later. Grouped together, they constitute what Feinberg calls "the child's right to an open future."[3]

Feinberg illustrates this concept with two examples. The first is that of the Jehovah's Witness child who needs a blood transfusion to save his life but whose parents object on religious grounds. In this case, the parents' right to act upon their religious beliefs and to raise their family within the religion of their choice conflicts with the child's right to live to adulthood and to make his own life-or-death decisions. As the Supreme Court said in another (and less defensible) case involving Jehovah's Witnesses:

Parents may be free to become martyrs themselves. But it does not follow that they are free in identical circumstances to make martyrs of their children before they have reached the age of full and legal discretion when they can make that decision for themselves.[4]

The second example is more controversial. In 1972, in a famous Supreme Court case, a group of Old Order Amish argued that they should be exempt from Wisconsin's requirement that all children attend school until they are either sixteen years old or graduate from high school.[5] The Amish didn't have to send their children to public school, of course; they were free to create a private school of their own liking. But they framed the issue in the starkest manner: to send their children to any school, past eighth grade, would be antithetical to their religion and their way of life, and might even result in the death of their culture.

The case was framed as a freedom of religion claim on the one hand, and the state's right to insist on an educated citizenry on the other. And within that frame, the Amish won. First, they were able to persuade the Court that sending their children to school after eighth grade would potentially destroy their community.

Second, the Amish argued that the state's concerns—that children be prepared to participate in the political and economic life of the state—did not apply in this case. The Court listened favorably to expert witnesses who explained that the Amish system of home-based vocational training—learning from your parent—worked well for that community, that the community itself was prosperous, and that few Amish were likely to end up unemployed.

What only a few justices saw was that the children themselves were largely ignored in this argument. The Amish wanted to preserve their way of life. The state of Wisconsin wanted to make sure that its citizens could vote wisely and make a living. No justice squarely faced the question of whether the liberal democratic state owes all its citizens, especially children, a right to a basic education that can serve as a building block if the child decides later in life that she wishes to become an astronaut, a playwright, or perhaps to join the army. As we constantly hear from politicians and educators, without a high school diploma one's future is virtually closed. By denying them a high school education or its equivalent, parents are virtually ensuring that their children will remain housewives and agricultural laborers. Even if the children agree, is that a choice parents ought to be allowed to make for them?

From my perspective, the case was decided wrongly. If Wisconsin had good reasons for settling on high school graduation or age sixteen as the legal minimum to which children are entitled, then I think that the Amish children were entitled to that minimum as well, despite their parents' objections.

Is Creating a Deaf Child a Moral Harm?

Now, as we return to the example of the couple who wish to ensure that they bear only deaf children, we have to confront two distinctly different issues. The first is, in what sense is it ever possible to do harm by giving birth to a child who would otherwise not have been born at all? The second is whether being deaf rather than hearing is in fact a harm.

The first issue has been well rehearsed elsewhere. The problem is, how can it be said that one has harmed a child by bringing it into the world with a disability, when the only other choice was for the child not to have existed at all? In the case of a child whose life is arguably not worth living, one can say that life itself is a cruelty to the child. But when a child is born in less than ideal circumstances, or is partially disabled in ways that do not entail tremendous suffering, there seems no way to argue that the child herself has been harmed. This may appear to entail the conclusion, counter to our common moral sense, that therefore no harm has been done. "A wrong action must be bad for someone, but [a] choice to create [a] child with its handicap is bad for no one."[6]

All commentators agree that there is no purely logical way out of what Dan Brock calls the "wrongful handicap" conundrum. However, most commentators also agree that one can still support a moral critique of the parents' decision. Bonnie Steinbock and Ron McClamrock argue for a principle of "parental responsibility" by which being a good parent entails refraining from bringing a child into the world when one cannot give it "even a decent chance at a good life."[7]

I locate the moral harm differently, at least with respect to disabled persons wishing to reproduce themselves in the form of a disabled child. Deliberately creating a child who will be forced irreversibly into the parents' notion of "the good life" violates the Kantian principle of treating each person as an end in herself and never as a means only. All parenthood exists as a balance between fulfillment of parental hopes and values and the individual flowering of the actual child in his or her own direction. The decision to have a child is never made for the sake of the child—for no child then exists. We choose to have children for myriad reasons, but before the child is conceived those reasons can only be self-regarding. The child is a means to our ends: a certain kind of joy and pride, continuing the family name, fulfilling religious or societal expectations, and so on. But morally the child is first and foremost an end in herself. Good parenthood requires a balance between having a child for our own sakes and being open to the moral reality that the child will exist for her own sake, with her own talents and weaknesses, propensities and interests, and with her own life to make. Parental practices that close exits virtually forever are insufficiently attentive to the child as end in herself. By closing off the child's right to an open future, they define the child as an entity who exists to fulfill parental hopes and dreams, not her own.

Having evaded the snares of the wrongful handicap conundrum, we must tackle the second problem: is being deaf a harm? At first glance, this might appear as a silly question. Ethically, we would certainly include destroying someone's hearing under the rubric of "harm"; legally, one could undoubtedly receive compensation if one were rendered deaf through someone else's negligence. Many Deaf people, however, have recently been claiming that Deafness is better understood as a cultural identity than as a disability. Particularly in the wake of the Deaf President Now revolution at Gallaudet University in 1988, Deaf people have been asserting their claims not merely to equal access (through increased technology) but also to equal respect as a cultural minority. As one (hearing) reporter noted:

> So strong is the feeling of cultural solidarity that many deaf parents cheer on discovering that their baby is deaf. Pondering such a scene, a hearing person can experience a kind of vertigo. The surprise is not simply the unfamiliarity of the views; it is that, as in a surrealist painting, jarring notions are presented as if they were commonplace.[8]

From this perspective, the use of cochlear implants to enable deaf children to hear, or the abortion of deaf fetuses, is characterized as "genocide." Deaf pride advocates point out that as Deaf people they lack the ability to hear, but they also have many positive gains: a cohesive community, a rich cultural heritage built around the various residential schools, a growing body of drama, poetry, and other artistic traditions, and, of course, what makes all this possible, American Sign Language. Roslyn Rosen, the president of the National Association of the Deaf, is Deaf, the daughter of Deaf parents, and the mother of Deaf children. "I'm happy with who I am," she says, "and I don't want to be 'fixed.' Would an Italian-American rather be a WASP? In our society everyone agrees that whites have an easier time than blacks. But do you think a black person would undergo operations to become white?"

On the other side of the argument is evidence that deafness is a very serious disability. Deaf people have incomes thirty to forty percent below the national average. The state of education for the deaf is unacceptable by anyone's standards; the typical deaf student graduates from high school unable to read a newspaper.

However, one could also point to the lower incomes and inadequate state of education among some racial and ethnic minorities in our country, a situation we do not (or at least ought not) try to ameliorate by eradicating minorities. Deaf advocates often cite the work of Nora Ellen Groce, whose oral history of Martha's Vineyard, *Everyone Here Spoke Sign Language*, tells a fascinating story. For over two hundred years, ending in the middle of the twentieth century, the Vineyard experienced a degree of hereditary deafness exponentially higher than that of the mainland. Although the number of deaf people was low in noncomparative terms (one in 155), the result was a community in which deaf people participated fully in the political and social life of the island, had an economic prosperity on par with their neighbors, and communicated easily with the hearing population, for "everyone here spoke sign language." So endemic was sign language for the general population of the island that hearing islanders often exploited its unique properties even in the absence of deaf people. Old-timers told Groce stories of spouses communicating through sign language when they were outdoors and did not want to raise their voices against the wind. Or men might turn away and finish a "dirty" joke in sign when a woman walked into the general store. At church, deaf parishioners gave their testimony in sign.

As one Deaf activist said, in a comment that could have been directly related to the Vineyard experience, "When Gorbachev visited the U.S., he used an interpreter to talk to the President. Was Gorbachey disabled?" Further, one might argue that, since it is impossible to eradicate deafness completely even if that were a worthy goal, the cause of deaf equality is better served when parents who are proud to be Deaf deliberately have Deaf children who augment and strengthen the existing population. Many of the problems that deaf people experience are the result of being born, without advance warning, to hearing parents. When there is no reason to anticipate the birth of a deaf child, it is often months or years before the child is correctly diagnosed. Meanwhile, she is growing up in a world devoid of language, unable even to communicate with her parents. When the diagnosis is made, her parents first must deal with the emotional shock, and then sort through the plethora of conflicting advice on how best to raise and educate their child. Most probably, they have never met anyone who is deaf. If they choose the route recommended by most Deaf activists and raise their child with sign language, it will take the parents years to learn the language. Meanwhile, their child has missed out on the crucial development of language at the developmentally appropriate time, a lack that is associated with poor reading skills and other problems later.

Further, even the most accepting of hearing parents often feel locked in conflict with the Deaf community over who knows what is best for their child. If Deafness truly is a culture rather than a disability, then raising a deaf child is somewhat like white parents trying to raise a black child in contemporary America (with a background chorus of black activists telling them that they can't possibly make a good job of it!). Residential schools, for example, which can be part of the family culture for a Deaf couple, can be seen by hearing parents as Dickensian nightmares or, worse, as a "cultlike" experience in which their children will be lost to them forever.

By contrast, deaf children born to Deaf parents learn language (sign) at the same age as hearing children. They are welcomed into their families and inculcated into Deaf culture in the same way as any other children. Perhaps for these reasons, by all accounts the Deaf of Deaf are the acknowledged leaders of the Deaf Pride movement, and the academic crème de la crème. In evaluating the choice parents make who deliberately ensure that they have Deaf children, we must remember that the statistics and descriptions of deaf life in America are largely reflective of the experience of deaf children born to hearing parents, who make up the vast majority of deaf people today.

But if Deafness is a culture rather than a disability, it is an exceedingly narrow one. One factor that does not seem clear is the extent to which children raised with American Sign Language as their first language ever will be completely comfortable with the written word. (Sign language itself has no written analogue and has a completely different grammatical structure from English.) At present, the conflicted and politicized state of education for the deaf, along with the many hours spent (some would say "wasted") on attempting to teach deaf children oral skills, makes it impossible to know what is to blame for the dismal reading and writing skills of the average deaf person. Some deaf children who are raised with sign language from birth do become skilled readers. But there is reason to question whether a deaf child may have very limited access to the wealth of literature, drama, and poetry that liberals would like to consider every child's birthright.

Although Deaf activists rightly show how many occupations are open to them with only minor technological adjustments, the range of occupations will always be inherently limited. It is not likely that the world will become as Martha's Vineyard, where everyone knew sign. A prelingually deafened person not only cannot hear, but in most instances cannot speak well enough to be understood. This narrow choice of vocation is not only a harm in its own sake but also is likely to continue to lead to lower standards of living. (Certainly one reason why the Vineyard deaf were as prosperous as their neighbors was that farming and fishing were just about the only occupations available.)

Either Way, A Moral Harm

If deafness is considered a disability, one that substantially narrows a child's career, marriage, and cultural options in the future, then deliberately creating a deaf child counts as a moral harm. If Deafness is considered a culture, as Deaf activists would have us agree, then deliberately creating a Deaf child who will have only very limited options to move outside of that culture, also counts as a moral harm. A decision, made before a child is even born, that confines her forever to a narrow group of people and a limited choice of careers, so violates the child's right to an open future that no genetic counseling team should acquiesce in it. The very value of autonomy that grounds the ethics of genetic counseling should preclude assisting parents in a project that so dramatically narrows the autonomy of the child to be.

Coda

Although I rest my case at this point, I want to sketch out some further ramifications of my argument. Are there other, less obvious, ways in which genetic knowledge and manipulation can interfere with the child's right to an open future?

The notion of the child's right to an open future can help in confronting the question of whether to test children for adult-onset genetic diseases, for example Huntington disease. It is well known that the vast majority of adults at risk for Huntington disease choose not to be tested. However, it is not uncommon for parents to request that their children be tested; their goals may be to set their minds at rest, to plan for the future, and so on. On one account, parental authority to make medical decisions suggests that clinicans should accede to these requests (after proper counseling about possible risks). A better account, in my opinion, protects the child's right to an open future by preserving into adulthood his own choice to decide whether his life is better lived with that knowledge or without.

Finally, a provocative argument can be made that sex selection can be deleterious to the child's right to an open future. I am ignoring here all the more obvious arguments against sex selection, even when accomplished without abortion. Rather, I suspect that parents who choose the sex of their offspring are more likely to have gender-specific expectations for those children, expectations that subtly limit the child's own individual flowering. The more we are able to control our children's characteristics (and the more time, energy, and money we invest in the outcome), the more invested we will become in our hopes and dreams for them. It is easy to sympathize with some of the reasons why parents might want to ensure a girl or boy. People who already have one or two children of one sex can hardly be faulted for wanting to "balance" their families by having one of each. And yet, this ought to be discouraged. If I spent a great deal of time and energy to get a boy in the hope of having a football player in the family, I think I would be less likely to accept it with good grace if the boy hated

sports and spent all his spare time at the piano. If I insisted on having a girl because I believed that as a grandparent I would be more likely to have close contact with the children of a daughter than of a son, I think I would be find it much harder to raise a girl who saw motherhood as a choice rather than as a foregone conclusion. Parents whose preferences are compelling enough for them to take active steps to control the outcome, must, logically, be committed to certain strong gender-role expectations. If they want a girl that badly, whether they are hoping for a Miss America or the next Catherine McKinnon, they are likely to make it difficult for the actual child to resist their expectations and to follow her own bent.

Notes

1. Walter E. Nance, "Parables," in *Prescribing Our Future: Ethical Challenges in Genetic Counseling*, ed. Dianne M. Bartels, Bonnie S. LeRoy, and Arthur L. Caplan (New York: Aldine De Gruyter, 1993), 92.

2. President's Commission for the Study of Ethical Problems in Biomedical and Behavioral Research, *Screening and Counseling for Genetic Conditions: A Report on the Ethical, Social, and Legal Implications of Genetic Screening, Counseling, and Education Programs* (Washington, DC: Government Printing Office, 1983), 56.

3. Joel Feinberg, "The Child's Right to an Open Future," in *Whose Child? Children's Rights, Parental Authority, and State Power*, ed. William Aiken and Hugh LaFollette (Totowa, NJ: Littlefield, Adams 1980), 124–53.

4. *Prince v. Massachusetts,* 321 U.S. 158 (1944), at 170.

5. *Wisconsin v. Yoder,* 406 U.S. 205 (1972).

6. Dan Brock, "The Non-Identity Problem and Genetic Harms," *Bioethics* 9, no. 3/4 (1995): 269–75, at 271.

7. Bonnie Steinbock and Ron McClamrock, "When is Birth Unfair to the Child?" *Hastings Center Report* 24, no. 6 (1994): 15–21, at p. 17.

8. Edward Dolnick, "Deafness as Culture," *The Atlantic Monthly* 272 no. 3 (1993): 37–53.

Extending Preimplantation Genetic Diagnosis

Medical and Non-Medical Uses

JOHN A. ROBERTSON

Journal of Medical Ethics 29 (2003): 213–16.

Debate about new reproductive technologies often cites preimplantation genetic diagnosis (PGD)—the technique by which early human embryos are genetically screened for selection for transfer to the uterus—as a practice that needs close ethical, legal, and social scrutiny. The use of PGD is growing, as are the indications for it. This article describes medical and nonmedical extensions of PGD, and discusses the ethical, legal, and policy issues which they raise.

PGD and Its Prevalence

PGD has been available since 1990 for testing of aneuploidy in low prognosis in vitro fertilisation (IVF) patients, and for single gene and X linked diseases in at risk couples. One cell (blastomere) is removed from a cleaving embryo and tested for the genetic or chromosomal condition of concern. Some programmes analyse polar bodies extruded from oocytes during meiosis, rather than blastomeres. Cells are then either karyotyped to identify chromosomal abnormalities, or analysed for single gene mutations and linked markers.

Physicians have performed more than 3000 clinical cycles of PGD since 1990, with more than 700 children born as a result. The overall pregnancy rate of 24% is comparable to assisted reproductive practices which do not involve embryo or polar body biopsy.

More than two thirds of PGD has occurred to screen out embryos with chromosomal abnormalities in older IVF patients and in patients with a history of miscarriage.

Several new indications for PGD single gene mutational analysis have recently been reported. New uses include PGD to detect mutations for susceptibility to cancer and for late onset disorders such as Alzheimer's disease. In addition, parents with children needing hematopoietic stem cell transplants have used PGD to ensure that their next child is free of disease and a good tissue match for an existing child. Some persons are also requesting PGD for gender selection for both first and later born children, and others have speculated that selection of embryos for a variety of non-medical traits is likely in the future.

PGD is ethically controversial because it involves the screening and likely destruction of embryos, and the selection of offspring on the basis of expected traits. While persons holding right to life views will probably object to PGD for any reason, those who view the early embryo as too rudimentary in development to have rights or interests see no principled objection to all PGD. They may disagree, however, over whether particular reasons for PGD show sufficient respect for embryos and potential offspring to justify intentional creation and selection of embryos. Donation of unwanted embryos to infertile couples reduces this problem somewhat, but there are too few such couples to accept all unwanted embryos, and in any event, the issue of selecting offspring traits remains.

Although ethical commentary frequently mentions PGD as a harbinger of a reproductive future of widespread genetic selection and alteration of prospective offspring, its actual impact is likely to be quite limited. Even with increasing use the penetrance of PGD into reproductive practice is likely to remain a very small percentage of the 150 000 plus cycles of IVF performed annually throughout the world. Screening for susceptibility and late onset diseases is limited by the few diseases for which single gene predispositions are known. Relatively few parents will face the need to conceive another child to provide an existing child with matched stem cells. Nor are non-medical uses of PGD, other than for gender, likely to be practically feasible for at least a decade or more. Despite the limited reach of PGD, the ethical, legal, and policy issues that new uses raise, deserve attention.

New Medical Uses

New uses of PGD may be grouped into medical and non-medical categories. New medical uses include not only screening for rare Mendelian diseases, but also for susceptibility conditions, late onset diseases, and HLA matching for existing children.

Embryo screening for susceptibility and late onset conditions are logical extensions of screening for serious Mendelian diseases. For example, using PGD to screen out embryos carrying the p53 or BRCA1&2 mutations prevent the birth of children who would face a greatly increased lifetime risk of cancer, and hence require close monitoring, prophylactic surgery, or other preventive measures. PGD for highly penetrant adult disorders such as Alzheimer's or Huntington's disease prevents the birth of a child who will be healthy for many years, but who in her late 30s or early 40s will experience the onset of progressive neurological disease leading to an early death.

Although these indications do not involve diseases that manifest themselves in infancy or childhood, the conditions in question lead to substantial health problems for offspring in their thirties or forties. Avoiding the birth of children with those conditions thus reflects the desire of parents to have offspring with good prospects for an average life span. If PGD is accepted to exclude offspring with early onset genetic diseases, it should be accepted for later onset conditions as well.

PGD for adult onset disorders does mean that a healthy child might then be born to a person with those conditions who is likely to die or become incompetent while the child is dependent on her. But that risk has been tolerated in other cases of assisted reproduction, such as intrauterine insemination with sperm of a man who is HIV positive, IVF for women with cystic fibrosis, and use of gametes stored prior to cancer therapy. As long as competent caregivers will be available for the child, the likely death or disability of a parent does not justify condemning or stopping this use, anymore than that reproduction by men going off to war should be discouraged.

A third new medical indication—HLA matching to an existing child—enables a couple to have their next child serve as a matched hematopoietic stem cell donor for an existing sick child. It may also ensure that the new child does not also suffer from that same disease. The availability of PGD, however, should not hinge on that fact, as the Human Fertilisation and Embryology Authority, in the UK, now requires. A couple that would coitally conceive a child to be a tissue donor should be free to use PGD to make sure that that child will be a suitable match, regardless of whether that child is also at risk for genetic disease. Parents who choose PGD for this purpose are likely to value the new child for its own sake, and not only for the stem cells that it will make available. They do not use the new child as a "mere means" simply because they have selected HLA matched embryos for transfer.

Non-Medical Uses of PGD

More ethically troubling has been the prospect of using PGD to screen embryos for genes that do not relate to the health of resulting children or others in the family. Many popular accounts of PGD assume that it will eventually be used to select for such non-medical traits as intelligence, height, sexual orientation, beauty, hair and eye colour, memory, and other factors. Because the genetic basis of those traits is unknown, and in any case is likely to involve many different genes, they may not be subject to easy mutational analysis, as Mendelian disease or susceptibility conditions are. Aside from gender, which is identifiable through karyotyping, it is unrealistic to think that non-medical screening for other traits, with the possible exception of perfect pitch, will occur anytime soon.

Still, it is useful to consider the methodology that ethical assessment of non-medical uses of PGD, if available, should follow. The relevant questions would be whether the proposed use serves valid reproductive or rearing interests; whether those interests are sufficient to justify creating and destroying embryos; whether selecting for a trait will harm resulting children; whether it will stigmatise existing persons, and whether it will create other social harms.

To analyse how these factors interact, I discuss PGD for sex selection and for children with perfect pitch. Similar issues would arise with PGD for sexual orientation, for hair and eye color, and for intelligence, size, and memory.

PGD for Gender Selection

The use of medical technology to select the sex of offspring is highly controversial because of the bias against females which it usually reflects or expresses, and the resulting social disruptions which it might cause. PGD for gender selection faces the additional problem of appearing to be a relatively weak reason for creating and selecting embryos for discard or transfer.

The greatest social effects of gender selection arise when the gender of the first child is chosen. Selection for first children will overwhelmingly favour males, particularly if one child per family population policies apply. If carried out on a large scale, it could lead to great disparities in the sex ratio of the population, as has occurred in China and India through the use of ultrasound screening and abortion. PGD, however, is too expensive and inaccessible to be used on a wide scale for sex selection purposes. Allowing it to be used for the first child is only marginally likely to contribute to societal sex ratio imbalances. But its use is likely to reflect cultural notions of male privilege and may reinforce entrenched sexism toward women.

The use of PGD to choose a gender opposite to that of an existing child or children is much

less susceptible to a charge of sexism. Here a couple seeks variety or "balance" in the gender of offspring because of the different rearing experiences that come with rearing children of different genders. Psychologists now recognise many biologically based differences between male and female children, including different patterns of aggression, learning, and spatial recognition, as well as hormonal differences. It may not be sexist in itself to wish to have a child or children of each gender, particularly if one has two or more children of the same gender.

Some feminists, however, would argue that any attention to the gender of offspring is inherently sexist, particularly when social attitudes and expectations play such an important role in constructing sex role expectations and behaviours. Other feminists find the choice of a child with a gender different from existing children to be morally defensible as long as "the intention and consequences of the practice are not sexist", which is plausibly the case when gender variety in children is sought. Desiring the different rearing experiences with boys and girls does not mean that the parents, who have already had children of one gender, are sexists or likely to value unfairly one or the other gender.

Based on this analysis the case is weak for allowing PGD for the first child, but may be acceptable for gender variety in a family. With regard to the first child, facilitating preferences for male firstborns carries a high risk of promoting sexist social mores. It may also strike many persons as too trivial a concern to meet shared notions of the special respect due preimplantation embryos. A proponent of gender selection, however, might argue that cultural preferences for firstborn males should be tolerated, unless a clearer case of harm has been shown. If PGD is not permitted, pregnancy and abortion might occur instead.

The case for PGD for gender variety is stronger because the risk of sexism is lessened. A couple would be selecting the gender of a second or subsequent children for variety in rearing experiences, and not out of a belief that one gender is privileged over another. Gender selection in that case would occur without running the risks of fostering sexism and hurting women.

The question still arises whether the desire for gender variety in children, even if not sexist, is a strong enough reason to justify creating and discarding embryos. The answer depends on how strong an interest that is. No one has yet marshalled the evidence showing that the need or desire for gender variety in children is substantial and important, or whether many parents would refrain from having another child if PGD for gender variety were not possible. More evidence of the strength and prevalence of this need would help in reaching a conclusion. If that case is made, then PGD for gender variety might be acceptable as well.

PGD for Perfect Pitch

Perfect or "absolute" pitch is the ability to identify and recall musical notes from memory. Although not all great or successful musicians have perfect pitch, a large number of them do. Experts disagree over whether perfect pitch is solely inborn or may also be developed by early training, though most agree that a person either has it or does not. It also runs in families, apparently in an autosomal dominant pattern. The gene or genes coding for this capacity have not, however, been mapped, much less sequenced. Because genes for perfect pitch may also relate to the genetic basis for language or other cognitive abilities, research to find that gene may be forthcoming.

Once the gene for perfect pitch or its linked markers are identified, it would be feasible to screen embryos for those alleles, and transfer only those embryos that test positive. The prevalence of those genes is quite low (perhaps three in 100) in the population, but high in certain families. Thus only persons from those families who have a strong interest in the musical ability of their children would be potential candidates for PGD for perfect pitch. Many of them are likely to take their chances with coital conception and exposure of the child to music at an early age. Some

couples, however, may be willing to undergo IVF and PGD to ensure musical ability in their child. Should their request be accepted or denied?

As noted, the answer to this question depends on the importance of the reproductive choice being asserted, the burdens of the selection procedure, its impact on offspring, and its implications for deselected groups and society generally. The strongest case for the parents is if they persuasively asserted that they would not reproduce unless they could select that trait, and they have a plausible explanation for that position. Although the preference might appear odd to some, it might also be quite understandable in highly musical families, particularly ones in which some members already have perfect pitch. Parents clearly have the right to instill or develop a child's musical ability after birth. They might reasonably argue that they should have that right before birth as well.

If so, then creating and discarding embryos for this purpose should also be acceptable. If embryos are too rudimentary in development to have inherent rights or interests, then no moral duty is violated by creating and destroying them. Some persons might think that doing so for trivial or unimportant reasons debases the inherent dignity of all human life, but having a child with perfect pitch will not seem trivial to parents seeking this technique. Ultimately, the judgment of triviality or importance of the choice within a broad spectrum rests with the couple. If they have a strong enough preference to seek PGD for this purpose and that preference rationally relates to understandable reproductive goals, then they have demonstrated its great importance to them. Only in cases unsupported by a reasonable explanation of the need—for example, perhaps creating embryos to pick eye or hair colour, should a person's individual assessment of the importance of creating embryos be condemned or rejected.

A third relevant factor is whether musical trait selection is consistent with respect for the resulting child. Parents who are willing to undergo the costs and burdens of IVF and PGD to have a child with perfect pitch may be so overly invested in the child having a musical career that they will prevent it from developing its own personality and identity. Parents, however, are free to instill and develop musical ability once the child is born, just as they are entitled to instill particular religious views. It is difficult to say that they cross an impermissible moral line of risk to the welfare of their prospective child in screening embryos for this purpose. Parents are still obligated to provide their child with the basic education and care necessary for any life plan. Wanting a child to have perfect pitch is not inconsistent with parents also wanting their child to be well rounded and equipped for life in other contexts.

A fourth factor, impact on deselected groups, is much less likely to be an issue in the case of perfect pitch because there is no stigma or negative association tied to persons without that trait. Persons without perfect pitch suffer no stigma or opprobrium by the couple's choice or public acceptance of it, as is arguably the case with embryo selection on grounds of gender, sexual orientation, intelligence, strength, size, or other traits. Nor is PGD for perfect pitch likely to perpetuate unfair class advantages, as selection for intelligence, strength, size, or beauty might.

A final factor is the larger societal impact of permitting embryo screening for a non-medical condition such as perfect pitch. A valid concern is that such a practice might then legitimise embryo screening for other traits as well, thus moving us toward a future in which children are primarily valued according to the attractiveness of their expected characteristics. But that threat is too hypothetical to justify limiting what are otherwise valid exercises of parental choice. It is highly unlikely that many traits would be controlled by genes that could be easily tested in embryos. Gender is determined by the chromosome, and the gene for perfect pitch, if ever found, would be a rare exception to the multifactorial complexity of such traits. Screening embryos for perfect pitch, if otherwise acceptable, should not be stopped simply because of speculation about what might be possible several decades from now.

PGD for Other Non-Medical Traits

The discussion of PGD for perfect pitch illustrates the issues that would arise if single gene analysis became possible for other traits, such as sexual orientation, hair or eye colour, or height, intelligence, size, strength, and memory. In each case the ethical assessment depends on an evaluation of the importance of the choice to the parents and whether that choice plausibly falls within societal understandings of parental needs and choice in reproducing and raising children. If so, it should usually be a sufficient reason to create and screen embryos. The effect on resulting offspring would also be of key moral importance. Whether selection carries a public or social message about the worth of existing groups should also be addressed.

Applying this methodology might show that some instances of non-medical selection are justified, as we have seen with embryo selection for gender variety and perhaps for having a child with perfect pitch. The acceptability of PGD to select other non-medical traits will depend on a careful analysis of the relevant ethical factors, and social acceptance of much greater parental rights to control the genes of offspring than now exists.

Conclusion

Although new indications are emerging for PGD, it is likely to remain a small part of reproductive practice for some time to come. Most new indications serve legitimate medical purposes, such as screening for single gene mutations for late onset disorders or susceptibility to cancer. There is also ethical support for using PGD to assure that a child is an HLA match with an existing child.

More controversial is the use of PGD to select gender or other non-medical traits. As with medical uses, the acceptability of non-medical screening will depend upon the interests served and the effects of using PGD for those purposes. Speculations about potential future non-medical uses should not restrict new uses of PGD which are otherwise ethically acceptable.

CASES

DNAdirect.com: Direct-to-Consumer Marketing of Genetic Tests

"Your genes. Your health. Your choices." At the DNAdirect website you can choose from a rich menu of genetic testing options. You can get tested for Alpha-1 Antitrypsin Deficiency, blood-clotting disorders, breast and ovarian cancer, and diabetes risk. These tests look for certain changes in chromosomes, genes, or proteins that are associated with particular inherited diseases, and claim to determine your vulnerability to certain diseases, based on your genetic profile. You can also test your response to certain drugs. And you can get information about ethnicity, ancestry, and paternity. At DNAdirect, each test costs between about two hundred and three thousand dollars. Just take a swab from the inside of your mouth and send it in, along with your credit card number. A treasure trove of information is just a mouse-click away.

DNAdirect is just one of a slew of online companies that offer direct-to-consumer genetic testing. Traditionally these tests have only been available through health care providers, but as testing gets cheaper and as the number of genetic tests expands, these services are increasingly available to the public, often without the involvement of medical professionals.

Proponents believe these tests offer individuals an opportunity to take their health into their own hands in a way never before possible. Armed with information about potential risk factors and predispositions, people can lower their risks through lifestyle choices and can be alert for signs and symptoms of diseases for which they are at risk. Another advantage of these tests is that individuals can gather personal genetic information without involving their health insurance companies or their doctors—the information stays out of their medical records and cannot be used against them.

Still, direct-to-consumer genetic testing has many critics. Perhaps the primary concern is the quality of the testing. Many of the genetic tests offered directly to consumers are inaccurate, and there is currently no oversight of these genetic testing companies. There is no way to know which companies are legitimate, and whether the information you receive is reliable. Furthermore, consumers may have trouble distinguishing between tests that are widely accepted by medical professionals and those whose validity has not been established. Consumers may not know which tests are clinically useful and which are not (and which are, in essence, a waste of money).

The privacy that these personalized services seems to offer is appealing; the public really does fear that their genetic information may be used against them. But there is some debate about whether or not fears about genetic discrimination are well-founded. Experts argue that actual instances of discrimination based on genetic information are extremely rare. The concern over genetic privacy is overblown, they say, and does not outweigh the potential problems of these personalized tests. Indeed, the very privacy that people gain has a dark side: without the involvement of doctors or trained genetic counselors, people may not be able to interpret and act wisely upon the genetic information in their hands.

DNAdirect promises that its "board-certified medical genetics experts" will provide web-enabled tools, information, and phone counseling to its customers. Still, many of the companies offering genetic testing do not also offer counseling, or offer counseling by people who are not properly qualified. Interpreting genetic information can be extremely complex. People may make potentially serious decisions—such as whether to have children—based on the genetic information they receive, so the possibility of misinterpretation is serious. Genetic testing may also give the mistaken impression that the risk of getting a disease is directly related to one's genetic makeup. But the etiology of disease is complex, and genetic factors play only a partial role. Diabetes, for example, may have an important genetic component, but environmental factors such as lifestyle also play a large role.

Discussion Questions

1. What kind of access should consumers have to genetic tests?
2. Many doctors believe that patients should not be allowed to purchase genetic tests without also receiving counseling with the test results. Is this overly paternalistic?
3. Do individuals have a right to their own genetic information?

Sources

Gene Tests [informational website funded by the National Institutes of Health]. http://www.genetests.org/ (accessed May 7, 2008).

Gollust, Sarah E., Sara Chandros Hull, Benjamin S. Wilfond. "Limitations of Direct-to-Consumer Advertising for Genetic Testing." *JAMA* 288 (2002): 1762–67.

Williams, Shawna and Gail Javitt. "Direct-to-Consumer Genetic Testing: Empowering or Endangering the Public?" Genetics and Public Policy Center. 2007. http://www.dnapolicy.org/images/issuebriefpdfs/2006_DTC_Issue_Brief.pdf (accessed May 7, 2008).

Wolfberg, Adam J. "Genes on the Web—Direct-to-Consumer Marketing of Genetic Testing." *New England Journal of Medicine* 355, no. 6 (2006): 543–45.

Playing God in the West, but Not in the East

A common moral objection to biotechnology and genetic engineering is that we are "playing God"—we are tinkering with the Stuff of Life, with God's Creation. John Tierney reported in the *New York Times* that many scientists from the United States and Europe are fleeing to Asia, where biotechnology and genetic engineering, including stem cell research, do not meet the same moral and legal resistance. The sorts of playing-God criticisms so frequent in the West do not seem to have much purchase in the East. There is little resistance to genetic engineering, and embryos do not have such a contested moral status. Indeed, China, India, and Singapore have laws supporting embryo cloning for medical research. When Hwang Woo Suk of South Korea reported that he had successfully cloned a human embryo, he justified his research as consistent with the Buddhist doctrine of reincarnation. Although Hwang was accused of scientific fraud, his research agenda was nevertheless given moral support by the head of South Korea's largest Buddhist order, who said that Hwang and other Korean scientists should not be guided by Western ethics.

Tierney suggests that the openness to genetic research in Asia rests, in large part, on a different view of divinity and the afterlife. The concern about "playing God" really does not exist in Asian cultures. Biologist Lee Silver has mapped biotechnology policies around the world, and found that those countries in which Asian religions (e.g., Buddhism and Hinduism) prevail have a permissive and positive approach to embryo and genetic research. "Most people in Hindu and Buddhist countries have a root tradition in which there is no single creator God. Instead there may be many gods, and there is no master plan for the universe."

Discussion Questions

1. Do these cultural differences suggest that bioethics is relative to culture? Why or why not?
2. How do you understand the term, "playing God"? What, if anything, is wrong with playing God?
3. What secular concepts correspond to the concerns implied by the playing-God metaphor?
4. Are there concepts in Asian religions analogous to the concerns implied by the playing-God metaphor?

Sources

Silver, Lee M. *Challenging Nature: The Clash of Science and Spirituality at the New Frontiers of Life*. New York: Ecco Press, HarperCollins, 2006.

Tierney, John. "Are Scientists Playing God? It Depends on Your Religion." *New York Times*, November 20, 2007.

Myriad Genetics and the BRCA-2 Gene

Every year, almost 200,000 women will be diagnosed with breast cancer. A small percentage of these cases are hereditary. In the 1990s, scientists found that the hereditary form of the disease is often caused by a mutation in one of two genes, which have been named the BRCA-1 and BRCA-2 genes (for "breast cancer 1 and 2"). Genetic mutations on either of these genes greatly increase a woman's chance of developing breast cancer—she will have a greater than eighty percent chance of getting the disease within her lifetime. A diagnostic test that can identify a mutation on either of these two genes is invaluable to doctors and patients. Armed with knowledge from these tests, women and their doctors can choose the most effective treatment strategy. (Men with BRCA mutations can get breast cancer, too, and a BRCA mutation can be passed on to the children, so men can also benefit from diagnostic tests on the BRCA genes.)

Myriad Genetics, a U.S. biopharmaceutical company, in collaboration with the University of Utah, was the first to sequence the BRCA-1 gene, and in 1994 applied for and obtained patent protection for the isolated DNA coding of the BRCA-1 polypeptide. Myriad and its collaborators went on to sequence and then patent BRCA-2. The patents cover not only the sequence of each gene, but any use of the sequence, or knowledge about it, to develop diagnostic tests or therapies. Myriad enforced its patent, asking all researchers and laboratories involved in research or clinical trials on BRCA-1 and -2 to immediately stop their work. Myriad developed and marketed its own diagnostic test—BRCAnalysis© , which it sells to patients for about nine hundred dollars. Myriad also developed the BRCA Risk Calculator, which is available online. Under pressure and criticism,

Myriad subsequently allowed National Institutes of Health researchers access to the diagnostic BRCA tests for half the commercial price.

Myriad's BRCA patents have been challenged, both on legal and moral grounds. The legal arguments center on technicalities (related, for example, to the novelty of the invention). The moral opposition runs deeper. One of the main concerns is that Myriad's patents may limit research and innovation on diagnostic tests for breast cancer, thus potentially denying many benefits to women with BRCA mutations. A broader moral claim is that it is wrong for any one person or group to own pieces of the human genome. In Myriad's defense, biomedical and pharmaceutical research is driven by private industry, and the potential for profit—primarily through patenting new discoveries—is what keeps the wheels turning.

Discussion Question

1. Should individuals or corporations be able to patent a genetic sequence?

Sources

Betti, Christopher J. "Diagnostic Genetic Technologies Left Stranded on First Base: A Need to Unwind the Protection Afforded Gene Patents." *Journal of the DuPage County Bar Association*. 2005. http://www.dcba.org/brief/aprissue/2005/art30405.htm (accessed May 9, 2008).

Myriad Genetics. http://www.myriad.com/; and http://www.myriadtests.com/provider/brca-risk-calculator.htm (accessed May 9, 2008).

World Intellectual Property Organization. "Bioethics and Patent Law: The Case of Myriad." 2006. http://www.wipo.int/wipo_magazine/en/2006/04/article_0003.html (accessed May 9, 2008).

Mo Money[1]

In 1976, John Moore, an Alaskan pipeline worker, sought treatment for hairy-cell leukemia at the University of California. His doctors

---

[1] The original version of this case was prepared at the Goizueta Business School, Emory University, by Jennifer Dellapina under the supervision of George D. Randels, Jr. The case has been adapted for use here.

removed his spleen, which had grown from a half pound to over fourteen pounds, and he recovered.

Moore did not know that his doctor had been harvesting white blood cells from his spleen for use in developing an "immortal" cell line. Moore's cells were so valuable because, once cultured, they behaved unusually: the "Mo line," as the doctors called it, was able to produce blood proteins capable of fighting immunosuppressive diseases. Moore also did not know that the university had been granted a patent on this new "invention." He became suspicious when his doctors continued to encourage him to provide cell samples, and in 1983 pressured him to sign over all rights to his cells. (He refused.) The Mo line was sold to a biotechnology company for 1.7 million dollars and could eventually generate more than 3 billion dollars.

Moore sued his doctor and the University of California for stealing his property. This was the first time an individual had legally staked a claim of ownership over tissues and cells. Moore said that he had been "essence-raped." He had no objection to genetic research but felt that he should benefit from any profits derived from the Mo line, since his unique cells were required to develop it.

The California Supreme Court ruled against John Moore, saying that his spleen ceased to be his property once it left his body. John Locke, in *Two Treatises of Government*, writes that "labour . . . puts the difference of value on every thing," inferring that when we mix our labor with an object, it becomes our property. The Court adapted this theory when it determined that it was the manipulation of the cells, rather than some magical curative power in the cells themselves, that made the cell line valuable. Thus, John Moore was not entitled to financial rewards from the continued sale of the cell line. Moore did receive a small settlement; a lower court was to determine if the doctors had obtained Moore's consent before patenting the cell line.

In the dissenting opinion, Justice George wrote,

Unlike the gizzards of domestic poultry, the spleens of human beings do not come within the definition of "goods." Property is acquired by 1. Occupancy; 2. Accession; 3. Transfer; 4. Will; or 5. Succession. A spleen is not "personal property" which the patient, to avoid sale by the hospital as unclaimed property, must claim within "a period of 180 days following the departure of the owner from the hospital."

In Moore's case, none of these five acts took place; neither his spleen, nor his cells nor any other body part, falls under the definition of property.

By definition, individual rights end with death. But John Moore is still alive, and his case set a precedent in genetic patenting cases. In 1991, the U.S. Department of Commerce applied for a cell line patent that was derived from a Panamanian woman. While studying the Guaymi Indians in a Panamanian rain forest, U.S. researchers discovered that a member of the tribe carried a retrovirus that could be altered and used to treat leukemia and AIDS. The woman was unaware that her cells were about to be patented. When another research group discovered the process, they alerted the Guaymi General Congress, who then protested at a meeting of the United Nations. The United States withdrew the patent application.

Physicians and geneticists are thankful for the cell lines they have been able to secure; a tissue sample taken from a cancerous cervix in 1951 produced cells that have successfully been grown in test tubes and currently live in hundreds of labs around the world. These cells have helped scientists extensively in the study of human illnesses.

Discussion Questions

1. Do you agree with the California Supreme Court's decision that Moore's spleen, and the cell line derived from it, were not his property?

2. Can a person be said to own pieces of his or her body? If so, which pieces?

3. Should cell lines be patentable?

Sources

Skloot, Rebecca. "Taking the Least of You." *New York Times Magazine*, April 16, 2006. http://www.nytimes.com/2006/04/16/magazine/16tissue.html?pagewanted=2

Consumer Eugenics

Dr. Jeffrey Steinberg operates the Fertility Institutes of Los Angeles and Las Vegas, where couples around the world can come to choose the sex of their offspring. They come to Steinberg's clinics because sex-selection is illegal in many countries, but not in the United States. The Fertility Institutes have contracted with a travel service "that can assist with all travel, lodging, transportation and other arrangements at very attractive negotiated rates."

Steinberg's clinics utilize preimplantation genetic diagnosis (PGD) to screen embryos for gender, and then implant either male or female embryos, depending upon the patient's preference. They guarantee that the sex-selection process will be accurate. Previously, the Fertility Institutes had used a pre–*in vitro* fertilization (IVF) sperm sorting technique that is less reliable, but did not involve the creation and destruction of unwanted embryos.

Although it is well known that families in China and India prefer sons—even to the point of aborting female fetuses—Steinberg says that his clients as a whole balance out each other. While the Chinese like boys, the Canadians like girls.

Discussion Questions

1. Do you think that this is an ethical use of PGD?
2. Would the Fertility Institutes' previous method of sperm sorting before IVF be ethically preferable to using PGD?

Sources

Johnson, Carla K. "Wealthy Go to U.S. to Choose Baby's Sex." *Washington Post*, June 14, 2006. http://www.washingtonpost.com/wp-dyn/content/article/2006/06/14/AR2006061401477_pf.html (accessed June 18, 2006).

The Fertility Institutes, "Helping Couples Become Family." http://www.fertility-docs.com (accessed June 1, 2008).

Williams Syndrome and PGD

Williams syndrome is a rare neurodevelopmental disorder caused during meiosis by the loss of a strand of about twenty-five genes on the double helix, including an important gene called LIMK1. This genetic accident leads to a miswiring of the brain. Children born with Williams syndrome have cognitive deficits ranging from mild to quite severe, and will typically have an IQ around sixty. Like children born with Down syndrome, Williams children have characteristic facial features, which are often described as "elfin": a small upturned nose, long upper lip, wide mouth, and small chin. They often have small and widely spaced teeth. Most individuals with Williams syndrome have heart and blood vessel problems, sometimes mild but sometimes severe enough to require surgery.

Adults with Williams syndrome usually require some help with daily living. As David Dobbs puts it, "many with Williams have so vague a concept of space . . . that even as adults they will fail at six-piece jigsaw puzzles, easily get lost, draw like a preschoolers and struggle to replicate a simple T or X shape built with a half-dozen building blocks." Yet as Dobbs also notes, it is not these cognitive limitations that really define people with Williams syndrome. Instead, it is their personality. They are extremely friendly and gregarious, and can and will talk to anyone. Their language skills are very nearly normal. They have no fear of strangers, and no social inhibitions. Parents often describe their Williams syndrome child with terms like joyous and delightful. The downside of their gregariousness is that they lack a nuanced understanding of social interactions, and fail to "read" facial expression and subtle conversational markers. They also often fail to develop deep and sustained friendships.

Over the past decade, scientists working in the field of molecular cytogenetics have developed new ways to identify chromosomal abnormalities, greatly expanding the possibilities for prenatal genetic diagnosis. These new techniques include fluorescence *in situ* hybridization (FISH) and comparative genomic hybridization (CGH), and have made it possible to identify submicroscopic aberrations, including microdeletion syndromes such as Williams syndrome.

According to the Kleberg Cytogenetics Laboratory at the Baylor College of Medicine, which offers "FISH-based assay for identifying the deletion on 7Q11.23 associated with Williams syndrome," over ninety percent of individuals with Williams syndrome "have a deletion of the elastic gene on the long arm of chromosome 7 detectable with this FISH assay."

At the present time, there is no cure for Williams syndrome.

Discussion Questions

1. Would it be ethical for a couple to perform prenatal genetic testing for Williams syndrome? Would preimplantation genetic screening of embryos during IVF be ethical?
2. Do the particulars of a genetic disorder matter when discussing the morality of prenatal testing? For example, is Williams syndrome different from Down syndrome or autism spectrum disorder? And are these disorders different from something like Huntington's or Tay-Sachs or sickle-cell trait? Why?

Sources

Dobbs, David. "The Gregarious Brain." *The New York Times Magazine*, July 8, 2007.

Kleberg Cynogenetics Laboratory. "Williams Syndrome, FISH Analysis." http://www.bcm. edu/geneticlabs/tests/cyto/williams.html (accessed May 9, 2008).

Shaffer, Lisa G., and Bassem A. Bejjani. "A Cytogeneticist's Perspective on Genomic Microassays." *Human Reproduction Update*, 10, no. 3 (2004): 221–26.

Williams Syndrome Association. http://www. williams-syndrome.org/ (accessed May 9, 2008).

Better Brains Through "Chemistry"

In a commentary published in the journal *Nature*, two Cambridge University researchers reported that a number of their colleagues admitted to using prescription drugs to enhance their ability to work. Two of the most popular drugs among academics are Adderall, a stimulant prescribed for attention-deficit/hyperactivity disorder, and Provigil, a drug that promotes wakefulness and is prescribed for narcolepsy. In the flood of letters that followed this revelation, many academics reported that they, too, had used these drugs to improve their performance at work. They were able to work longer hours, focus for longer periods on their research or writing, and be far more productive overall than without the help of the medications. The off-label use of these drugs by college and even high school students is also widespread.

Discussion Questions

1. What are the moral similarities and differences between cosmetic surgery for breast enhancement and "brain enhancement" with Adderall or Provigil? Between the use of anabolic steroids by athletes and the use of brain stimulants by academics?
2. Is it cheating for a student or professor to make use of brain enhancement?
3. Would it be ethical for a physician to prescribe Provigil to a college professor who wanted a leg up on his colleagues?
4. Would you take a cognitive enhancer?

Source

Sahakian, Barbara, and Sharon Morein-Zamir. "Professor's Little Helper." *Nature* 450, no. 20 (2007): 1157–59.

Therapeutic Forgetting

The drug propranolol is a beta blocker long used in the treatment of hypertension. Recent research has suggested new possibilities for its use. Propranalol has been shown to influence emotional processing in the brain, particularly the processing of emotional memories. Not only can the drug inhibit the brain's "replay" of bad memories, it appears to block the storing of emotional memories in the first place. Research with American soldiers in Iraq suggests that propanalol may prevent post traumatic stress disorder, if the drug is taken right after a traumatic event. The drug works by blocking the flow of adrenaline, which acts to solidify memories.

Discussion Questions

1. The President's Council on Bioethics (in "Memory and Happiness") warns against the use of memory-blunting drugs like propranalol. What are their primary concerns? Are their concerns justified?
2. Does the President's Council use a slippery slope argument? (An effective one?)
3. Would you take a pill for therapeutic forgetting?
4. Assuming propranolol were approved for use in therapeutic forgetting, should it be prescribed only to the victims of trauma? Or should anyone have access? Who should decide which memories are bad enough to wipe away?

Sources

Davis, Jeanie Lerche. "Forget something? We wish we could." *WebMD*. Apr. 9, 2004. http://www.webmd.com/anxiety-panic/features/forget-something-we-wish-we-could (accessed June 22, 2008).

Kolber, Adam J. "Therapeutic Forgetting: The Legal and Ethical Implications of Memory Dampening." *Vanderbilt Law Review* 59 (2006): 1561. Available at SSRN: http://ssrn.com/abstract=887061.

Soul Catcher 2025

Researchers at British Telecommunications (BT) are at work on a microchip that would be implanted in the skull just behind the eye, and that would record a person's thoughts and feelings. If all goes well, the "Soul Catcher" should be ready for use by 2025.

According to futurologists at BT, the human brain processes about ten terabytes of data—adding up the lifetime flow of impulses from the optical nerve, and nerves in the ears, nose, tongue, and skin—over an average eighty-year lifespan (equivalent to the storage capacity of 7,142,857,142,860,000 floppy discs). Within thirty years, computer memory and miniaturization technology will probably have advanced to the point where ten terabytes can be stored on a single chip. A person's whole life experience could be captured and stored on a tiny sliver of silicon.

Dr. Chris Winter of BT's Artificial Life team has said of the Soul Catcher technology, "This is the end of death." The Soul Catcher would be able to record and then play back on a computer all of a person's life experiences. Combining this experiential record with a record of a person's genes, "we could recreate a person physically, emotionally, and spiritually." He continued, "The implanted chip would be like an aircraft's black box, and would enhance communications beyond current concepts. For example, police would be able to use it to relive an attack, rape or murder, from the victim's point of view, to help catch the criminal" (Human Rights Watch 2008).

Peter Cochrane, Head of Advanced Applications and Technology for BT, had this to say about the future of cybernetics (human-machine interface technology):

When we have the choice to implant several terabytes of additional memory into our skull . . . we have to think carefully about this and what it means. But I suspect it may be less of a threat than those people taking anabolic steroids to enhance their muscles. . . . It is very strange that people find it acceptable to promote and employ silicone implants and undergo cosmetic surgery while they worry about silicon implants which potentially can save our lives and amplify our thought processes.

Cochrane sees the Soul Catcher as a logical extension of other human-machine interface technologies that have medical applications, particularly in repairing communication. For example, we use "external" body monitoring and repair technologies such as hearing aids. A variety of "internal" technologies have also been developed. Cochlear implants can restore some hearing to the profoundly deaf. A microtransmitter implanted into the brain has allowed a paraplegic to communicate directly with a computer through thinking, and retinal implants, in which a tiny electronic chip implanted in the eye would deliver electrical impulses to the retina, are currently under development for treating people with macular degeneration.

Discussion Questions

1. Does the Soul Catcher technology strike you as ethically problematic?
2. Is the Soul Catcher qualitatively different from other cybernetic technologies such as cochlear or retinal implants?
3. One can imagine various ethically troubling applications of the Soul Catcher technology (e.g., the CIA recording and examining people's private thoughts as envisioned in the Tom Cruise movie *Minority Report*; an evil scientist downloading his lifetime experiences and transplanting his "soul" into a newborn). Does the possibility for misapplication create a strong "slippery slope" argument against the development of such technology?
4. Respond to Cochrane's suggestion that implants that are designed to "amplify our thought processes" are morally superior to implants or enhancements designed to improve our looks.

Sources

Human Rights Watch, Project Freedom. "British Telecom and the Mark of the Beast." 2008.

http://www.mindcontrolforums.com/pro-freedom.co.uk/the_beast.html (accessed May 8, 2008).

Cochrane, Peter. "The Future of Cybernetics." Interview on (ABC News.com). http://www.cochrane.org.uk/opinion/archive/interviews/cybernetics.php (accessed May 8, 2008).

Be More Than You Can Be

From a presentation by Michael Goldblatt, Director of the Defense Sciences Office (DSO) of the Defense Advanced Research Project Agency (DARPA).

Imagine soldiers having no physical limitations. . . .

What if, instead of acting on thoughts, we had thoughts that could act? Indeed, imagine if soldiers could communicate by thought alone . . . or communications so secure there is zero probability of intercept. Imagine the threat of biological attack being inconsequential. And contemplate, for a moment, a world in which learning is as easy as eating, and the replacement of damaged body parts as convenient as a fast food drive-through.

As impossible as these visions sound or as difficult you might think the task would be, these visions are the everyday work of the Defense Sciences Office. . . .

Enhanced human performance . . . is born from the realization that with the emphasis on technology in the battle space the human is rapidly becoming "the weakest link." Soldiers having no physical, physiological, or cognitive limitations will be key to survival and operational dominance in the future.

The exoskeleton initiative will provide mechanical augmentation extending individual performance. Metabolically dominant warfighters of the future will be able to keep their cognitive abilities intact, while not sleeping for weeks. They will be able to endure constant, extreme exertion and take it in stride. Success in metabolic engineering will be visible, because I will be the first volunteer to be transformed. The Biovision's tools are the enabling technologies necessary to make the revolution real.

Discussion Questions

1. Do you find the enhancement of soldiers to be ethically acceptable?
2. Would you evaluate these enhancements differently if they would be utilized by civilians rather than soldiers?
3. Goldblatt is quite enthusiastic about these enhancement projects. What are some possible dangers that might accompany them?
4. How do you think Sandel, Burack, and Bostrom would evaluate the DSO's projects?

Source

Michael Goldblatt. "Defense Sciences Office (DSO), Office Overview." http://www.darpa.mil/ darpatech2002/presentations/dso_pdf/speeches/ GOLDBLAT.pdf (accessed June 1, 2008).

CHAPTER 8

The Environmental Turn in Bioethics

INTRODUCTION

The word "bioethics" suggests an ethics concerned with *bios*, or life. This, indeed, is what American biochemist Van Rensselaer Potter had in mind when he coined the term. He conceived of ethics as a dialogue between medical science and values, the ultimate purpose of which is to protect and nurture life on earth. Bioethics, in Potter's formulation, is a "bridge." It is a bridge not only between a scientific orientation and a values orientation, but it is also a bridge to the future. Our survival depends on being able to bring values and science together, allowing values to shape the scientific enterprise in ways both sustainable and humane.

For most of its life as an academic field, bioethics has veered away from this broad Potterian vision. It has instead remained focused on the narrower enterprise of medicine, without explicitly placing this enterprise within its larger context of planetary health. It is a truism, of course, that there can be no enduring health without a healthy home planet. But this necessary natural substrate of human health has been largely invisible and taken for granted, both by health professionals and by bioethicists.

Times have been changing, though, and bioethics is finally taking what might be called "the environmental turn." Environmental decline, or "change" if you prefer the more neutral description, is now impinging on everything we do, personally and professionally. Although environmental problems were certainly real and pressing at the birth of bioethics, they have lately begun to shape consciousness and conversation in more central ways. For example, thirty years ago few people worried about global warming, and many were downright skeptical. Now in the view of most scientists, climate change is a reality, not a prediction. Its effects on human health are real and documented, and it shapes many of our individual and collective decisions. It is also beginning, in small ways, to shape the conversation about health, medicine, and medical ethics.

Scholars and activists are trying to return bioethics to its environmental roots, and by doing so maintain its relevance in the twenty-first century by bringing the field into connection again with the big question of human survival. Ethicists and health professionals are exploring what an environmentally sustainable health care system might look like, how doctors might take environmental values seriously within their practice, how climate change might shape the conversation about health care priorities, what concepts from ecosystem science are applicable to the conversation about human health, and whether the moral vocabulary developed within the field of environmental ethics might have something to offer bioethics.

The environmental turn in bioethics is still in its infancy. You will notice that a number of the essays in this chapter are of the agenda-setting variety, and work with large themes like sustainable health as opposed to highly focused ethical problems (as in, for example, the end-of-life area, where a well-developed literature explores questions about artificial nutrition and hydration). There is an effort under way to define the scope of the issues, to lay out broad themes, and to challenge big ideas, like what "health" means and what the core values and concerns of bioethics should be. This is an exciting area of bioethics to work in, and one likely to blossom over the next few years. The discussion will certainly become more focused over time, as we struggle to deal with the particulars of climate change and carbon footprints, green design of hospitals, and balancing individual and environmental harms and benefits of particular therapies and technologies.

Redefining Bioethics, Redefining Health

Van Rensselaer Potter conceptualized bioethics as a field devoted to the value dimensions of human flourishing within the context of planetary health. The first section of three readings focuses on the meaning and scope of bioethics as a field of moral inquiry, and each asks in a different way that bioethics expand out toward a broader, Potterian vision. At the same time, each of the readings challenges us to rethink what, exactly, is meant by health, and what values health embodies.

Writer and farmer **Wendell Berry**, one of the country's most eloquent and prolific environmentalists, explores the meaning of health. Health, of course, is a primary moral focus of the field of bioethics. Although there has been considerable debate within bioethics about how to define health, the dialogue has worked under the assumption that health is an individual possession. Berry notes that the root meaning of health is wholeness, and he asks us to see health not as an isolated and personal possession, but rather as something that connects us with others, including nonhuman others. As the title of his essay argues, health is membership in community. He says, "I believe that community—in the fullest sense: a place and all its creatures—is the smallest unit of health and that to speak of the health of an isolated individual is a contradiction in terms." Berry also sets the stage for a bigger bioethics conversation by noting that health is intimately connected with many other aspects of our lives: it is connected to patterns of consumption, to lifestyle, to the vitality of our ecosystems, to our relationships with others, and to what people on the other side of the world are doing.

Ted Schettler, science director of the Science and Environmental Health Network, brings us more explicitly into conversation about medicine. He asks, "How would a more ecological vision of health, and of medicine, look?" Like Berry and Potter, Schettler notes that human health cannot be viewed in isolation from the ecosystems upon which humans depend. There is abundant evidence (if common sense were not compelling enough) that stable, healthy ecosystems are foundational to human health, and that degradation of these ecosystems negatively impacts human well-being. Ecological health, he says, "embraces the deeply fundamental complex relationships that collectively influence human and environmental health." Schettler foreshadows some themes from the third section of our chapter readings ("Sustainable Health Care") when he argues that the health care sector has a moral responsibility to address ecological realities, for example, by addressing its own multiple contributions to environmental degradation.

The final reading in the first section, by **Jessica Pierce and Andrew Jameton**, explores new ways of thinking about bioethics, particularly in light of ideas borrowed from environmental philosophy. Pierce and Jameton's *The Ethics of Environmentally Responsible Health Care* (2006) offered the first and most comprehensive philosophical defense of sustainability in health. This excerpt from their book explores how the core moral principles and norms of bioethics must shift to accommodate environmental values. They explore how the principles of respect for autonomy, beneficence, nonmaleficence, and justice might evolve in light of an overarching commitment to sustainability, and they offer some new principles to enrich the moral vocabulary of bioethics.

Health and the Environment

Science is, by nature, value-laden. There are no "facts," if facts are taken to be objective entities, devoid of human perspective. Scientists cannot ignore the value dimension of their work, or do so only at the peril of humanity. This, indeed, was Potter's central message: scientists must recognize and proactively address the moral dimensions of their work. The converse is also true: moral reflection must connect with reality, empirical data, real experiences, and the facts of the situation under discussion. Just as science without values may be blind, so values without science can be vague, loose, even dangerous. One of the strengths of bioethics as a field of applied and practical philosophy has been the willingness of philosophers to learn about particular diseases and medical treatments, the intricacies of genetic germ line therapy, or the realities of a life as an Alzheimer's patient. Bioethicists and health professionals who want to engage environmental questions must seek with equal resolve to understand the realities of the environmental issues facing the world today. This is a task of Herculean proportions, given the scope of the problems at hand and the breadth of scientific expertise involved. But armed with some knowledge, moral reflection is likely to be more mature and more useful.

There is a huge and growing empirical literature on how human health and environmental health are linked. This section offers a very brief introduction to some of these connections. You will notice that the three short articles are empirical rather than philosophical: they establish some of the background knowledge that informs the conversation about environmental responsibilities in health care. A wealth of information on health and the environment is available on the Internet, and we have noted in the chapter bibliography some of the best informational sites. What we want you to take from these readings is this: human health depends in a multitude of fundamental ways on healthy, functioning ecosystems; the world's ecosystems are under severe strain, and degradation of these natural systems is already negatively impacting health in many ways; these threats to health are likely to become more serious in the future. These facts establish the moral imperative that shapes environmental bioethics.

The environmental issues that pose the most serious threats to health include climate change, depletion of the ozone layer, water scarcity, deforestation, degradation of marine ecosystems, and the dynamics of human population growth and migration. The essay by epidemiologist **Anthony McMichael** and his colleagues gives an overview of the challenge to human health from global environmental changes, focusing in particular on climate change. This is emerging as one of the most important challenges to health, and ultimately (as we see in the next section of readings) to health care. Although the authors focus mainly on describing the problem, they do suggest a few ways in which health professionals might respond.

In a most general sense, we rely on healthy ecosystems to provide us with the essentials of life: oxygen, water, food, shelter. These "ecosystem services" are the various processes by which the environment provides us with sustenance and protection. To borrow a metaphor from medicine, these are nature's "life support" services. These include the pollination of crops by bees and other pollinating insects, the dispersal of seeds by birds, moderation of temperatures, cleaning and detoxifying of water, and protection from the sun's ultraviolet rays. In their short article "Embedded in Nature," **Eric Chivian**, founder and director of the Center for Health and the Global Environment at Harvard, and **Aaron Bernstein** focus on the services provided by biodiversity and offer evidence that human activities are driving many species to extinction. In particular, they note how the loss of biodiversity deprives us of potentially useful tools in medicine and medical research. Some of the most promising new drugs are developed based on what we learn from unusual species.

Sustainable Health Care

Our readings so far have explored an "ecological" vision of health and of bioethics, as well as some of the many interconnections, both positive and negative, between health and the environment. This next section moves more clearly into philosophical analysis and asks, What are the moral challenges posed to medicine by environmental realities? Should environmental responsibility be one of the moral principles that guide medicine, and, if so, how comfortably will environmentally shaped values such as sustainability sit alongside traditional medical ethics values such as respect for autonomy? What would a more sustainable health care system look like, and how might the integration of environmental values transform the doctor-patient relationship?

Consider the real and symbolic landscape of a large academic medical center, located in a large urban area in Anywhere, U.S.A. Sitting by the window on the fifth floor of the newly built and well-appointed forty-two million dollar cancer treatment center, I look out upon the blackened smokestack of the medical center's incinerator. I make sure the window is shut tight, because I do not like the thought of miniscule carcinogenic particulates floating down from the smokestack toward my inhaling lungs. There is, of course, a deep irony here in this health care landscape, one that forms a central motif in the work of **Andrew Jameton and Jessica Pierce** on environmental ethics in health care. Health care, although ostensibly committed to protecting and promoting human health, is itself a dangerously unhealthy business. Health care practices are environmentally unsustainable and polluting.

In "Sustainable Health Care and Emerging Ethical Responsibilities," they argue that health care institutions as a whole, and medical professionals as individuals, have a moral obligation to consider the environmental effects of their activities and soften environmental impacts wherever possible. This moral obligation is based, first of all, in the fundamental commitment of medicine to human well-being. Ethical arguments for sustainability in health care also arise from our obligation not to harm others, from our responsibilities for the welfare of future generations and of nature, and from a commitment to social justice. This reading outlines the basis and contours of the argument for sustainability in health care.

Jameton and Pierce argue, on the practical side, for a careful life-cycle analysis of the raw materials of health care; this is part of a larger project of determining health care's ecological footprint and then figuring out how to make it smaller. Health care has both downstream and upstream environmental costs. Downstream costs include waste and pollution (e.g., from burning of fossil fuels, incineration of plastics), while upstream costs include the extraction of raw materials and the various ecological costs of manufacture and shipping. On the philosophical side, Jameton and Pierce ask their readers to consider some of the moral tensions raised by sustainability. One of the biggest of these is limits. Ecological constraints set limits, whether we respect them or not, on the scale and accessibility of health care. One possible response to limits is restricting access to high-cost, high-tech care, especially when marginally useful. Health care would focus instead on high-impact, low-cost health services such as preventive care and immunizations.

"Medicine After Oil," by **Daniel Bednarz**, also speaks to the question of sustainable health, and narrows the moral focus to the particular issue of medicine's profound reliance on oil—an essentially unsustainable, politically volatile, and environmentally damaging material. Bednarz considers the prospect of "peak oil" for medicine. Peak oil refers to the theory that at some point in time global oil production will reach its peak—its maximum level of production—after which it will enter a period of terminal decline in production and upward spiral in cost. Oil production, on this theoretical model, follows a bell curve, and once we reach the high point it is all downhill. Unfortunately, oil production will peak and then decline, but demand will continue to grow. A shortfall in oil production would be catastrophic for the world economy. On a smaller scale, Bednarz argues that health care is utterly dependent upon oil, and so a crash in production would signal the collapse of health care. Rather than sitting back and waiting for the inevitable crash, we can and should use the prospect of peak oil as a catalyst for creating a more sustainable and cost-effective health care system.

Although it seems important to engage environmental concerns within health care, the marriage of environmental values with the traditional values of medical ethics will not necessarily be a happy one. Some worry that the infiltration of environmental values into medical ethics will erode in dangerous ways the core values that respect and protect patients. **Paul Carrick**, for example, explores the tension between the value of environmental preservation and the value of individual life saving. He notes that environmental values may be at odds with end-of-life care that focuses solely on the needs of the patient at hand. Bedside values conflict with larger goals. Carrick uses the philosophy of *deep ecology* as a foil against which to test the strength of our commitment to the sick and dying. The ethical ideal in deep ecology is to become a mature and "expansive" self who identifies not only with all of humanity, but with all of nature. The burdens of end-of-life care may press upon the conscience of this deep-ecological patient, who may decide that prolonging his or her own life through treatments is selfish and harmful to other living beings. For Carrick, this burden of conscience is unethical, particularly when it falls on the most vulnerable. Bedside values, in his view, trump environmental ones.

We come, finally, full circle to some of the questions posed in chapter 2. How, if at all, should doctors and other health professionals respond to the environmental crisis? Do physicians have a primary obligation to their patients? Or to the ecosystems that ultimately sustain health? The **American Medical Association's** "Declaration of Professional Responsibility" is about the commitment of physicians to the "health of humanity." It is interesting that ecosystem health is not explicitly mentioned in the declaration, nor does the declaration explicitly connect the health of humanity to the health of ecosystems. The declaration speaks, instead, of bioterrorism, the AIDS pandemic, and the potential misuse of genetic science. The AMA describes the Declaration as "a public reaffirmation of physicians' dedication to the ideals and obligations of the profession. These ideals and obligations transcend physician roles and specialties, professional associations, geographic boundaries, and political differences, uniting all physicians in a community of service to humankind" (CEJA Report 5-I-01). As you read the Declaration, notice what moral responsibilities it affirms.

The final reading is a short policy statement, also from the **American Medical Association**, on "Stewardship of the Environment." What is interesting here, first of all, is the language of stewardship, which has been all but absent from the other readings in this chapter, although the ideal of stewardship has been a central theme in the literature of environmental ethics. Second, this statement raises questions about the usefulness of ethics policy. The recommendations of this policy are so broad that they lack teeth. Physicians are encouraged, for example, to include discussion of "these issues" when appropriate with patients. But nothing more is said about what exactly they might discuss or what an appropriate opportunity might look like. Would it be appropriate, for example, to engage in a discussion of resource scarcity and waste with an eighty-five-year-old man considering cardiac bypass graft surgery for an old and failing heart? Or when counseling a couple with six children who want *in vitro* fertilization so they can add a seventh?

As you read the essays and case studies in this chapter, take care to notice other ways in which these broad environmental issues connect with issues covered in earlier chapters. How might environmental constraints color the conversation about reproduction: Is the right to family planning, contraception, and abortion

Websites of Interest

Consortium for Conservation Medicine. http://www.conservationmedicine.org/

Center for Health and the Global Environment at Harvard Medical School. http://chge.med.harvard.edu/

The Green Health Center. http://www.unmc.edu/green/

Science and Environmental Health Network. http://www.sehn.org/

International Society of Doctors for the Environment. http://201.216.215.170/isde.org/

Health and Environment Alliance. http://www.env-health.org/a/2220

The Climate and Health Council. http://www.climateandhealth.org/

Hospitals for a Healthy Environment. http://www.h2e-online.org/

Canadian Association of Physicians for the Environment. http://www.cape.ca/

Health Care Without Harm. http://www.noharm.org/us

a central environmental value? Or would a principle of respect for all life suggest a stronger opposition to abortion? How do we balance the need to limit resource use with care for individual patients, particularly when such care verges toward the futile or merely symbolic? How do we balance the needs of patients with an obligation to care for the environment? Should health care be radically downsized? How can research help and hinder our efforts to make health care more sustainable?

REFERENCES AND FURTHER READING

Auerbach, Paul S. "Physicians and the Environment." *JAMA* 299, no. 8 (2008): 956–58.

Ausubel, Kenny, and J.P. Harpignies, eds. *Ecological Medicine: Healing the Earth, Healing Ourselves*. San Francisco: Sierra Club Books, 2004.

Benatar, Solomon R., A.S. Daar, and Peter A. Singer. "Global Health Ethics: The Rationale for Mutual Caring." *International Affairs* 79 (2003):107–38.

Bernstein, Aaron, and David S. Ludwig. "The Importance of Biodiversity to Medicine." *JAMA* 300, no. 19 (2008): 2297–99.

Bush, Roger W. "Reducing Waste in US Health Care Systems." *JAMA* 297, no. 8 (2007): 871–74.

Cox, Stanley. "Big Medicine's Malignant Growth." *Alternet* February 22, 2006. http://www.alternet.org/module/printversion/32413 (accessed February 8, 2008).

Epstein, Paul R., and Greg Guest. "International Architecture for Sustainable Development and Global Health." In *Globalization, Health, and the Environment: An Integrated Perspective*. Ed. Greg Guest. Lanham, MD: Altamira Press, 2005. 239–258.

Germain, Adrienne. "Population and Reproductive Health: Where Do We Go Next?" *American Journal of Public Health*, 90, no. 12 (2000): 1845–47.

Gill, Mike, Fiona Godlee, Richard Horton, and Robin Stott. "Doctors and Climate Change." *British Medical Journal* 335 (2007):1104–5.

Gostin, Lawrence O. "Why Rich Countries Should Care About the World's Least Healthy People." *JAMA* 298, no. 1 (2007): 89–92.

Haines, Anthony, R.S. Kovats, D. Campbell-Lendrum, and C. Corvalan. "Climate Change and Human Health: Impacts, Vulnerability, and Mitigation." *Lancet* 367 (2006): 2101–9.

Herschel, Elliott. *Ethics for a Finite World*. Golden, CO: Fulcrum Publishing, 2005.

Holtz, Timothy, and S. Patrick Kachur. "The Reglobalization of Malaria" In *Sickness and Wealth: The Corporate Assault on Global Health*. Ed. Meredith Fort, Mary Anne Mercer, and Oscar Gish. Boston: South End Press, 2004. 131–143.

Kaebnick, G.E. "On the Sanctity of Nature." *Hastings Center Report* 30, no. 5 (2000): 16–23.

Lubchenco, Jane. "Entering the Century of the Environment." *Science* 279 (1998): 491–97.

McMichael, Anthony J., A. Nyong, and C. Corvalan. "Global Environmental Change and Health: Impacts, Inequalities, and the Health Sector." *British Medical Journal*, 336 (January 26, 2008): 191–94.

Patz, Jonathan A., Holly K. Gibbs, Jonathan A. Foley, Jamesine V. Rogers, and Kirk R. Smith. "Climate Change and Global Health: Quantifying a Growing Ethical Crisis." *EcoHealth* 4, no. 4 (2007): 397–405.

Pierce, Jessica, and Andrew Jameton. *The Ethics of Environmentally Responsible Health Care*. New York: Oxford University Press, 2004.

Potter, Van R. *Global Bioethics: Building on the Leopold Legacy*. East Lansing: Michigan State University Press, 1988.

_____. 1971. *Bioethics: A Bridge to the Future*. Englewood Cliffs, NJ: Prentice-Hall, 1971.

Ryan, Maura. "Beyond a Western Bioethics?" *Theological Studies* 65 (2004): 158–77.

Whitehouse, Peter J. "The Rebirth of Bioethics: Extending the Original Formulations of Van Rensselaer Potter." *American Journal of Bioethics* 3, no. 4 (2003): W26–W31.

DISCUSSION QUESTIONS FOR THE READINGS

Health Is Membership

1. What does Berry mean when he says, "Health is membership"? Do you agree?

2. In what sense is Berry's vision of health ecological? What other definitions of health have you come across in this book, and how do they differ from Berry's?

Toward an Ecological View of Health: An Imperative for the Twenty-First Century

1. Why, according to Shettler, must medicine and public health work together? What specific changes to medicine does he recommend?

2. What does a "new bioethic" for the twenty-first century need to accomplish?

3. How would you compare Shettler's view of medicine's moral agenda with the professional ethic developed in chapter 2 (by, for example, Wynia et al. and Miller, Brody, and Chung)?

New Ways of Thinking About Bioethics

1. Give some examples of how traditional moral principles in bioethics are expanded and modified by ecological values. For example, how do Pierce and Jameton understand "harm"? How is the principle of respect for autonomy modified?

2. Which of the two environmental philosophies discussed in this essay seems most promising in relation to the ethics of health care? What might it have to offer?

3. Compare the argument of Pierce and Jameton with that of Shettler. Where is there agreement? Divergence?

4. How do Pierce and Jameton define a viable bioethics?

Global Environmental Change and Health: Impacts, Inequalities, and the Health Sector

1. What major global environmental problems are impacting health? Which of these do the authors consider most critical to address and why?

2. What do the authors mean by "adaptive" strategies? What adaptive strategies should be taken to lessen health risks from environmental change?

3. What are some of the interconnections between environmental degradation, poverty, and social inequalities?

Embedded in Nature: Human Health and Biodiversity

1. What is biodiversity? Why is it important to human health?
2. Give three specific examples from the reading of how biodiversity is related to health care. Can you think of other examples? You might look on the following websites: http://es.epa.gov/ncer/biodiversity/ and http://www.ecology.org/biod/.

Sustainable Health Care and Emerging Ethical Responsibilities

1. How are health and environment linked? How are health care and environment linked?
2. What are three ethical tensions raised by a commitment to sustainable health care? Can you think of other ethical tensions?
3. Do you agree that the Hippocratic principle requires sustainable practices in health care?

Medicine After Oil

1. What is "peak oil"? (You may have to look on the Internet for the answer.)
2. In what ways is the health care system dependent on oil? How might peak oil impact the delivery of health care?
3. What solutions does Bednarz offer to the peak oil crisis?

Deep Ecology and End-of-Life Care

1. Why does Carrick think that expanding moral attention to the global environment will downgrade our respect for individual patients? Do you agree with his argument?
2. Do Carrick's concerns about deep ecology apply to all ecological perspectives? Do they apply to any of the readings you have done so far in this chapter? (Do Berry, Shettler, or Pierce and Jameton downgrade respect for human individuals?)

Declaration of Professional Responsibility: Medicine's Social Contract with Humanity

1. Which of these principles represent the "centuries-old ethic" of medicine, and which represent new responsibilities for the twenty-first century?
2. Which of the nine commitments is most controversial?
3. The declaration states that for physicians, "Humanity is our patient." Is this too broad an interpretation of the scope of physician responsibility? Or too narrow? (What about "the planet is our patient"?)

Stewardship of the Environment

1. Which of the seventeen points would you consider to be of primary importance for physicians?
2. Does this statement suggest any shifts in the physician-patient relationship?

READINGS

Health Is Membership

WENDELL BERRY

From *Another Turn of the Crank: Essays by Wendell Berry* (Washington, DC: Counterpoint, 1995), 86–100.

From our constant and increasing concerns about health, you can tell how seriously diseased we are. Health, as we may remember from at least some of the days of our youth, is at once wholeness and a kind of unconsciousness. Disease (dis-ease), on the contrary, makes us conscious not only of the state of our health but of the division of our bodies and our world into parts.

The word "health," in fact, comes from the same Indo-European root as "heal," "whole," and "holy." To be healthy is literally to be whole; to heal is to make whole. I don't think mortal healers should be credited with the power to make holy. But I have no doubt that such healers are properly obliged to acknowledge and respect the holiness embodied in all creatures, or that our healing involves the preservation in us of the spirit and the breath of God.

If we were lucky enough as children to be surrounded by grown-ups who loved us, then our sense of wholeness is not just the sense of completeness in ourselves but also is the sense of belonging to others and to our place; it is an unconscious awareness of community, of having in common. It may be that this double sense of singular integrity and of communal belonging is our personal standard of health for as long as we live. Anyhow, we seem to know instinctively that health is not divided.

Of course, growing up and growing older as fallen creatures in a fallen world can only instruct us painfully in division and disintegration. This is the stuff of consciousness and experience. But if our culture works in us as it should, then we do not age merely into disintegration and division, but that very experience begins our education, leading us into knowledge of wholeness and of holiness. I am describing here the story of Job, of Lazarus, of the lame man at the pool of Bethesda, of Milton's Samson, of King Lear. If our culture works in us as it should, our experience is balanced by education; we are led out of our lonely suffering and are made whole.

In the present age of the world, disintegration and division, isolation and suffering seem to have overwhelmed us. The balance between experience and education has been overthrown; we are lost in experience, and so-called education is leading us nowhere. We have diseases aplenty. As if that were not enough, we are suffering an almost universal hypochondria. Half the energy of the medical industry, one suspects, may now be devoted to "examinations" or "tests"—to see if, though apparently well, we may not be latently or insidiously diseased.

If you are going to deal with the issue of health in the modern world, you are going to have to deal with much absurdity. It is not clear, for example, why death should increasingly be looked upon as a curable disease, an abnormality, by a society that increasingly looks upon life as insupportably painful and/or meaningless. Even more startling is the realization that the modern medical industry faithfully imitates disease in the way that it isolates us and parcels us out. If, for example, intense and persistent pain causes you to pay attention only to your stomach, then you must leave home, community, and family and go to a sometimes distant clinic or hospital, where you will be cared for by a specialist who will pay attention only to your stomach.

Or consider the announcement by the Associated Press on February 9, 1994, that "the incidence of cancer is up among all ages, and researchers speculated that environmental exposure to cancer-causing substances other than cigarettes may be partly to blame." This bit of news is offered as a surprise, never mind that the environment (so called) has been known to be polluted and toxic for many years. The blame obviously falls on that idiotic term "the environment," which refers to a world that surrounds us but is presumably different from us and distant from us. Our laboratories have proved long ago that cigarette smoke gets inside us, but if "the environment" surrounds us, how does *it* wind up inside us? So much for division as a working principle of health.

This, plainly, is a view of health that is severely reductive. It is, to begin with, almost fanatically individualistic. The body is seen as a defective or potentially defective machine, singular, solitary, and displaced, without love, solace, or pleasure. Its health excludes unhealthy cigarettes but does not exclude unhealthy food, water, and air. One may presumably be healthy in a disintegrated family or community or in a destroyed or poisoned ecosystem.

So far, I have been implying my beliefs at every turn. Now I had better state them openly.

I take literally the statement in the Gospel of John that God loves the world. I believe that the world was created and approved by love, that it subsists, coheres, and endures by love, and that, insofar as it is redeemable, it can be redeemed only by love. I believe that divine love, incarnate and indwelling in the world, summons the world always toward wholeness, which ultimately is reconciliation and atonement with God.

I believe that health is wholeness. For many years I have returned again and again to the work of the English agriculturist Sir Albert Howard, who said, in *The Soil and Health*, that "the whole problem of health in soil, plant, animal, and man [is] one great subject."

I am moreover a Luddite, in what I take to be the true and appropriate sense. I am not "against technology" so much as I am for community. When the choice is between the health of a community and technological innovation, I choose the health of the community. I would unhesitatingly destroy a machine before I would allow the machine to destroy my community.

I believe that the community—in the fullest sense: a place and all its creatures—is the smallest unit of health and that to speak of the health of an isolated individual is a contradiction in terms.

We are now pretty clearly involved in a crisis of health, one of the wonders of which is its immense profitability both to those who cause it and to those who propose to cure it. That the illness may prove incurable, except by catastrophe, is suggested by our economic dependence on it. Think, for example, of how readily our solutions become problems and our cures pollutants. To cure one disease, we need another. The causes, of course, are numerous and complicated, but all of them, I think, can be traced back to the old idea that our bodies are not very important except when they give us pleasure (usually, now, to somebody's profit) or when they hurt (now, almost invariably, to somebody's profit).

This dualism inevitably reduces physical reality, and it does so by removing its mystery from it, by dividing it absolutely from what dualistic thinkers have understood as spiritual or mental reality.

A reduction that is merely theoretical might be harmless enough, I suppose, but theories find ways of getting into action. The theory of the relative unimportance of physical reality has put itself into action by means of a metaphor by which the body (along with the world itself) is understood as a machine. According to this metaphor—which is now in constant general use—the human heart, for example, is no longer understood as the center of our emotional life or even as an organ that pumps; it is understood as "a pump," having somewhat the same function as a fuel pump in an automobile.

If the body is a machine for living and working, then it must follow that the mind is a machine for thinking. The "progress" here is the reduction of mind to brain and then of brain to computer. This reduction implies and requires the reduction of knowledge to "information." It requires, in fact, the reduction of everything to numbers and mathematical operations.

This metaphor of the machine bears heavily upon the question of what we mean by health and by healing. The problem is that like any metaphor, it is accurate only in some respects. A girl is only in some respects like a red rose; a heart is only in some respects like a pump. This means that a metaphor must be controlled by a sort of humorous intelligence, always mindful of the exact limits within which the comparison is meaningful. When a metaphor begins to control intelligence, as this one of the machine has done for a long time, then we must look for costly distortions and absurdities.

Of course, the body in most ways is not at all like a machine. Like all living creatures and unlike a machine, the body is not formally self-contained; its boundaries and outlines are not so exactly fixed. The body alone is not, properly speaking, a body. Divided from its sources of air, food, drink, clothing, shelter, and companionship, a body is, properly speaking, a cadaver, whereas a machine by itself, shut down or out of fuel, is still a machine. Merely as an organism (leaving aside issues of mind and spirit) the body lives and moves and has its being, minute by minute, by an interinvolvement with other bodies and other creatures, living and unliving, that is too complex to diagram or describe. It is, moreover, under the influence of thought and feeling. It does not live by "fuel" alone.

A mind, probably, is even less like a computer than a body is like a machine. As far as I am able to understand it, a mind is not even much like a brain. Insofar as it is usable for thought, for the association of thought with feeling, for the association of thoughts and feelings with words, for the connections between words and things, words and acts, thought and memory, a mind seems to be in constant need of reminding. A mind unreminded would be no mind at all. This phenomenon of reminding shows the extensiveness of mind—how intricately it is involved with sensation, emotion, memory, tradition, communal life, known landscapes, and so on. How you could locate a mind within its full extent, among all its subjects and necessities, I don't know, but obviously it cannot be located within a brain or a computer.

Where the art and science of healing are concerned, the machine metaphor works to enforce a division that falsifies the process of healing because it falsifies the nature of the creature needing to be healed. If the body is a machine, then its diseases can be healed by a sort of mechanical tinkering, without reference to anything outside the body itself. This applies, with obvious differences, to the mind; people are assumed to be individually sane or insane. And so we return to the utter anomaly of a creature that is healthy within itself.

The modern hospital, where most of us receive our strictest lessons in the nature of industrial medicine, undoubtedly does well at surgery and other procedures that permit the body and its parts to be treated as separate things. But when you try to think of it as a place of healing—of reconnecting and making whole—then the hospital reveals the disarray of the medical industry's thinking about health.

In healing, the body is restored to itself. It begins to live again by its own powers and instincts, to the extent that it can do so. To the extent that it can do so, it goes free of drugs and mechanical helps. Its appetites return. It relishes food and rest. The patient is restored to family and friends, home and community and work.

This process has a certain naturalness and inevitability, like that by which a child grows up, but industrial medicine seems to grasp it only tentatively and awkwardly. For example, any ordinary person would assume that a place of healing would put a premium upon rest, but hospitals are notoriously difficult to sleep in. They are noisy all night, and the routine interventions go on relentlessly. The body is treated as a machine that does not need to rest.

You would think also that a place dedicated to healing and health would make much of food. But here is where the disconnections of the industrial system and the displacement of industrial humanity are most radical. Sir Albert Howard saw accurately that the issue of human health is inseparable from the health of the soil, and he saw too that we humans must responsibly occupy our place in the cycle of birth, growth, maturity, death, and decay, which is the health of the world. Aside from our own mortal involvement, food is our fundamental connection to that cycle. But probably most of the complaints you hear about hospitals have to do with the food, which, according to the testimony I have heard, tends to range from unappetizing to sickening. Food is treated as another unpleasant substance to inject. And this is a shame. For in addition to the obvious nutritional link between food and health, food can be a pleasure. People who are sick are often troubled or depressed, and mealtimes offer three opportunities a day when patients could easily be offered something to look forward to. Nothing is more pleasing or heartening than a plate of nourishing, tasty, beautiful food artfully and lovingly prepared. Anything less is unhealthy, as well as a desecration.

Why should rest and food and ecological health not be the basic principles of our art and science of healing? Is it because the basic principles already are technology and drugs? Are we confronting some fundamental incompatibility between mechanical efficiency and organic health? I don't know. I only know that sleeping in a hospital is like sleeping in a factory and that the medical industry makes only the most tenuous connection between health and food and no connection between health and the soil. Industrial medicine is as little interested in ecological health as is industrial agriculture.

A further problem, and an equally serious one, is that illness, in addition to being a bodily disaster, is now also an economic disaster. This is so whether or not the patient is insured. It is a disaster for us all, all the time, because we all know that personally or collectively, we cannot continue to pay for cures that continue to get more expensive. The economic disturbance that now inundates the problem of illness may turn out to be the profoundest illness of all. How can we get well if we are worried sick about money?

I wish it were not the fate of this essay to be filled with questions, but questions now seem the inescapable end of any line of thought about health and healing. Here are several more:

1. Can our present medical industry produce an adequate definition of health? My own guess is that it cannot do so. Like industrial agriculture, industrial medicine has depended increasingly on specialist methodology, mechanical technology, and chemicals; thus, its point of reference has become more and more its own technical prowess and less and less the health of creatures and habitats. I don't expect this problem to be solved in the universities, which have never addressed, much less solved, the problem of health in agriculture. And I don't expect it to be solved by the government.

2. How can cheapness be included in the criteria of medical experimentation and performance? And why has it not been included before now? I believe that the problem here is again that of the medical industry's fixation on specialization, technology, and chemistry. As a result, the modern "health care system" has become a way of marketing industrial products, exactly like modern agriculture, impoverishing those who pay and enriching those who are paid. It is, in other words, an industry such as industries have always been.

3. Why is it that medical strictures and recommendations so often work in favor of food processors and against food producers? Why, for example, do we so strongly favor the pasteurization of milk to health and

cleanliness in milk production? (Gene Logsdon correctly says that the motive here "is monopoly, not consumer health.")

4. Why do we so strongly prefer a fat-free or a germ-free diet to a chemical-free diet? Why does the medical industry strenuously oppose the use of tobacco, yet complacently accept the massive use of antibiotics and other drugs in meat animals and of poisons on food crops? How much longer can it cling to the superstition of bodily health in a polluted world?

5. How can adequate medical and health care, including disease prevention, be included in the structure and economy of a community? How, for example, can a community and its doctors be included in the same culture, the same knowledge, and the same fate, so that they will live as fellow citizens, sharers in a common wealth, members of one another?...

Toward an Ecological View of Health

An Imperative for the Twenty-First Century

TED SCHETTLER

Nature's goods and services are the ultimate foundations of life and health, even though in modern societies this fundamental dependency may be indirect, displaced in space and time, and therefore poorly recognized.

—Lee Jong-wook, Director-General 2003–2006, World Health Organization, *Ecosystems and Human Well-Being: Health Synthesis* (a report of the Millennium Ecosystem Assessment, United Nations Environment Program)

People's views of what health is differ. One dominant view, common in the medical profession, considers health to be the absence of disease. The World Health Organization maintains that health is a state of complete physical, mental, and social well-being and not merely the absence of disease or infirmity. Public health emphasizes the well-being of communities and the qualities of relationships among individuals as essential indicators of health. An ecologist might add features of entire ecological systems in which individuals and communities of many species live in dynamic interaction as being critical to health.

Farmer, ecologist, and author Wendell Berry thinks of health as membership. Berry says that health is wholeness and believes that the community is the smallest unit to which the concept of health applies. To speak of the health of an isolated individual is a contradiction, he says. Aldo Leopold, ecologist and author of *Sand County Almanac*, insisted that the integrity of the entire biotic community is critical. Health, he said, is maintenance of the capacity for self-renewal.

Ethical decision making tends to follow underlying definitions and assumptions. Now we know that past assumptions have led us into hazardous terrain. Considerable evidence tells us that we live in a world that is essentially new and different. Assumptions, worldviews, and ethical frameworks based on a past that no longer exists may not serve us well. Indeed, the long-term quality of human life and ultimately of survival is likely to depend on widespread adoption of a more integrated view of human health as embedded in an ecological framework. This expanded view of health will need to find expression throughout cultural and social institutions, including the medical and public health professions and the courts.

An Essentially New World

In 2005, the United Nations released the Millennium Ecosystem Assessment, which is the largest evaluation of the health of the earth's ecosystems ever attempted.

Among the findings:

- In the past fifty years, humans have changed ecosystems more rapidly and extensively than in any comparable period of time in human history.
- Approximately sixty percent of the ecosystem services examined, from regulation of air quality to purification of water, are being degraded or used unsustainably.
- Between one third and one half of the land surface of the earth has been transformed by human activity.
- The changes have contributed to substantial net gains in human well-being and economic development for many people.
- These gains, however, have been achieved at growing costs in the form of the degradation of many ecosystem services, increased risks of nonlinear changes, exacerbation of poverty for many groups of people, and growing disparities and inequities.
- In the past fifty years, the world's human population has increased from 2.4 billion to 6.4 billion people. Much of this growth has occurred in increasingly large cities where mega-slums proliferate. Mega-slums are incubators of new and reemergent diseases that can quickly travel across the world via air travel. Greed, inequity, poor planning, and disrespect for human rights create the slums and tend to intensify degradation of ecosystems and their services.

Changes in ecosystems increase the likelihood of nonlinear, accelerating, abrupt, and potentially irreversible changes with important consequences for human well-being. Growing pressures from over-harvesting, climate change, invasive species, and nutrient loading push ecosystems toward thresholds that they would not otherwise encounter.

- Economic globalization forges ahead without concomitant investment in a global public health infrastructure. This is a formula for catastrophe.
- Large numbers of plant and animal species have been driven to extinction, and most marine fisheries are severely depleted. More than half the world's coral reefs are threatened by human activities. Loss of species and genetic diversity decreases the resilience of ecosystems (the level of disturbance that an ecosystem can undergo without crossing a threshold to a different structure or functioning).
- Positive carbon balance (net increase of carbon released into the atmosphere and oceans) has resulted in global climate change, greenhouse gas effects, and increased acidification of oceans, threatening the marine food web.
- Anthropogenic nitrogen fixation from fertilizer production and use and fossil-fuel combustion exceeds all natural terrestrial processes combined. Nitrous oxides are greenhouse gas and ozone precursors. Nitrates contaminate ground and surface water and, along with phosphorous, cause eutrophication of marine and fresh-water systems, algal blooms, attendant health risks, and fish depletion. (Eutrophication refers to an increase in the concentration of plant nutrients such as phosphorus and nitrogen in an aquatic ecosystem, which often results in excessive plant growth and decay and consequent oxygen depletion.)
- Over the past fifty years, there has been an accelerated release of artificial chemicals into the environment, many of which are long-lived and transformed into by-products whose behaviors, synergies, and impacts are not well known. Humans

are at risk from inorganic and organic pollutants present in food and water.

Ironically, much of this damage is the direct or indirect result of human attempts to utilize ecosystem services that provide food, water, timber, fiber, and fuel. Indeed, since the beginning of life on earth, all organisms have modified their environments and, in turn, have been changed themselves. But humans have embarked on an unprecedented experiment of energy and resource dissipation rather than exchange and renewal. As a result, the ecological systems that have supported life as we know it are unraveling.

Implications for Ethics

Medical Ethics

Medical ethics largely addresses the rights of individuals and the obligation of practitioners to provide competent care with compassion. The Principles of Medical Ethics of the American Medical Association state that although the physician is to contribute to the improvement of the community and the betterment of public health, the individual patient is of paramount concern.

Public Health Ethics

A number of ethical concepts are relevant to public health, including communitarianism, civil liberties, human rights, social justice, and others. From the communitarian perspective, public health ethics are based on recognizing that individual liberty and, indeed, human existence rely heavily upon the interdependent communities to which we all belong. Exclusive pursuit of private interest erodes the network of social environments on which we depend. Individual autonomy requires maintenance of the institutions of civil society where citizens in solidarity learn respect for others as well as self-respect.

Public health ethics often encounters the tension that sometimes arises between individual and public interests. Conflicting views about how best to deploy limited social resources in the interest of public health are common. Relationships among rights, duties, and responsibilities demand attention.

Bioethics

Bioethics is often confused with medical ethics, but the two are really quite different. With an emphasis on individuals, medical ethics predominately addresses autonomy, beneficence, nonmaleficence, and distributive justice. Bioethics has a more expansive perspective in which humans are situated within larger complex ecological systems that also deserve moral consideration.

Oncologist Van Rensselaer Potter from the University of Wisconsin introduced the term *bioethics* in 1970. He saw the concept as biology, combined with diverse humanistic knowledge, forging a science that sets a system of medical and environmental priorities for acceptable survival. Potter asserted that any ethic for the human species has to be based on the possibility of severely degraded quality of life—even human extinction—and that each of us has the capacity to figure out how we ought to live, to avoid the fate of most other species.

Potter was strongly influenced by ecologist Aldo Leopold and geneticist C. H. Waddington. For Leopold, land was a collective organism—not merely soil, but "a fountain of energy flowing through a circuit of soils, plants, and animals." People, he said, are "plain members of the biotic community." Leopold argued that a thing was right when it tends to preserve the integrity, stability, and beauty of the biotic community. It was wrong when it did otherwise. He thought that ethics and beauty should play an important role in deciding how to live on the earth. With a nod to Darwin he said, the breeding of ethics is as yet beyond our powers. All science can do is to safeguard the environment in which ethical mutations might take place.

Geneticist C. H. Waddington thought that "what is demanded of each generation is a theory of ethics which is neither mere rationalization of existing prejudices, nor a philosophical discourse so abstract as to be irrelevant to the practical problems with which mankind is faced at that time emphasis." For Waddington, a kind of biological wisdom would enable us to judge between different ethical rules. Leopold, Potter, and Waddington were keenly aware that modern humans had existed on earth for mere moments in the deep time of billions of years of other life forms. Biological wisdom, they knew, would be necessary to prolong our stay with meaningful quality.

In 1978, philosopher Hans Jonas concluded that modern technology has introduced actions, objects, and consequences of such novel scale that the framework of former ethics can no longer contain them. Jonas argued that the power of our technologies and actions to reach far into time and space is sufficient to establish a moral responsibility to future generations. This is not, he pointed out, an assertion about the rights of future generations but rather a claim about our responsibilities to them.

The Millennium Ecosystem Assessment shows that much human behavior reflects little recognition of responsibilities to future generations or even to people alive today, particularly when they live in some remote place or are otherwise marginalized. We draw down the earth's natural capital, squander resources into scarcity, and contaminate ecosystems with synthetic chemicals and other industrial waste. We seem unable to recognize natural planetary limits, failing to restore life-support systems. Indeed, this pattern of behavior typifies many of our social and most of our economic institutions. The health care sector, for example, not only treats people whose illnesses are in part or wholly attributable to environmental conditions but also contributes in many ways to environmental degradation that fosters ill health.

Medicine and Public Health

At the beginning of the twentieth century, the quality of medical education and practice was poorly regulated. The *Flexner Report*, commissioned by the Carnegie Foundation in 1910, concluded that medical practice was not sufficiently informed by science and that medical education should be designed so that physicians would be well grounded in science and the

pathophysiology of disease. Along with other social, cultural, economic, and political forces, adoption of these recommendations helped to shape the trajectory of twentieth-century medicine. The scientific understanding of the origins of disease dramatically advanced, and physicians increasingly organized, acquiring substantial power and authority. Medicine became solidified as a largely male profession. This professionalism and gender bias helped to accelerate the divergence of the paths of medicine and public health already under way. Broadly speaking, medicine focused primarily on the pathophysiology and treatment of diseases, while public health emphasized prevention and the conditions in which disease developed.

Once translated into medical interventions, advances in biomedical understanding led to improved outcomes of many diseases. At the same time, improvements in sanitation, working conditions, housing, nutrition, care for poor people, and infectious-disease prevention dramatically improved the public's health. Differing approaches to human disease were justified in part by competing worldviews and ethical frameworks, which were, in turn, reflected in political decisions. For most of the twentieth century, medicine would dominate public health in the competition for resources and authority.

Technological achievements that emerged out of what is now a vast medical-industrial complex have come at a steep price. In the United States, as a percentage of gross domestic product, medical expenditures grew from five percent in 1970 to sixteen percent in 2005. The Centers for Medicare and Medicaid Services expects this to increase to twenty percent by 2017. This relentless growth was predictable. Disease has become a commodity subject to market forces, and disease care is a major driver of economic growth. Products and services are manufactured, bought, and sold. At the same time, public health expenditures designed to prevent disease have been funded much more modestly. According to the Centers for Disease Control, beginning in the 1980s expenditures for core public health functions actually declined, and in 1993 represented only about 1.6 percent of total health care expenditures.

The United States spends far more per capita than any other country in the world on health care. Capital equipment, buildings, operations, material throughput, transportation, water and electricity demands, and pharmaceuticals contribute significantly to these growing expenses. A large and growing environmental footprint of this medical-industrial complex has direct and indirect impacts on human health throughout the world.

According to the U.S. Department of Energy, medical facilities spend 5.3 billion dollars annually on energy, and rank second only to the food-service industry in intensity of energy usage. The health care sector generates thousands of tons of waste each day—including toxic materials and chemicals—and still relies heavily on incineration to "treat" portions of the waste stream, including pathological and chemotherapy waste. Waste incineration releases hazardous pollutants into the air or concentrates them in ash from which they find their way into the ambient environment after disposal. Pharmaceutical products or by-products are discarded or excreted into sewerage systems, contaminating surface waters and drinking water throughout the United States.

Health care food-procurement supports an industrial agricultural system heavily reliant on fossil fuels in production and transport. These practices cause air and water pollution, climate change, biodiversity loss, topsoil erosion, and eutrophication of surface waters, and adversely impact the social and economic fabric of rural communities. Moreover, this dominant agricultural system produces a diet that is calorie rich, lacks the appropriate mix of micro- and macro-nutrients, and promotes obesity, diabetes, cancer, neurodegeneration, and other adverse health outcomes treated in those same health care facilities.

Overtreatment and Suboptimal Health

Despite ever increasing expenditures, by almost any measure the health status of Americans is inferior to that of people in most other countries in the developed world. The United States ranks fifteenth in life expectancy and nearly last, compared with other developed countries, in infant mortality. A recent study concluded that, based on self-reported illnesses and biological markers of disease, late-middle-aged U. S. residents are much less healthy than their counterparts in Great Britain for diabetes, hypertension, heart disease, myocardial infarction, stroke, lung disease, and cancer. These differences exist at all points of socioeconomic status, despite the United States spending more than twice as much per capita on medical care as the United Kingdom.

Asthma, neurodevelopmental disorders, some kinds of cancer, some birth defects, mental illness, obesity, diabetes, premature births, and newly emerging and some recurrent infectious diseases are all increasing in the United States and throughout much of the world. These trends result from direct and indirect impacts of multiple interacting factors acting within a changing ecosocial environment—factors such as dietary inadequacies or excesses; exposure to toxic chemicals and pollutants in air, water, or food; inadequate exercise; exposure to recurring or emerging infectious agents; and social and economic inequities and deprivation.

Despite their predominantly systemic origins, diseases are generally viewed by the health care sector as problems in individuals to be treated with drugs, procedures, and personal behavioral changes. Moreover, to the extent that they address disease prevention at all, most health care professionals focus their efforts on well-established, proximate causes of disease—like blood pressure screening—rather than more distal or structural causes—like inadequate food access or poverty. Even so, much of the technical response to illness is of unproven benefit and often outright dangerous. Wennberg et al. estimate that as much as thirty percent of medical care paid for by Medicare as well as private insurers is useless and unnecessary, and some is dangerous. In 1999, the Institute of Medicine estimated that medical errors are responsible for nearly 100,000 deaths in the United States each year. More health care clearly does not mean better health.

Beyond the Medicine-Public Health Divide: Toward an Ecological View of Health

When viewed as separate domains, many relationships among individual, public, and ecological health are either unapparent or ignored. Artificial boundaries drawn for professional, social, political, or economic reasons tend to obscure their intimate interrelationships. Viewed as nested spheres, however, vivid patterns begin to emerge. Individual health cannot be realized independent of public and ecological health. Similarly, public and ecological health depend to a large degree on the health of individuals.

These relationships suggest ways forward. Instead of ignoring and often facilitating the degradation of ecological systems on which human health depends, both medical and public health practitioners have unrealized opportunities to transform their practices and embrace responsible, restorative membership in a larger planetary community. Since current and future generations of humans are fundamentally dependent on environmental quality and ecosystem services for their well-being, the health care and public health sectors have both opportunities and responsibilities to address these realities by modifying practices and modeling behavior. What we might call "ecological health practice" will favor interventions that can solve multiple problems without creating new ones and take into account intimate relationships in an integrated ecosocial model. This is what Wendell Berry calls "solving for pattern."

Implications for Health Care and Public Health

Most immediately, health care providers and public health institutions can modify their practices in order to reduce impacts on public and environmental health. Attention to material flows, purchasing practices, waste disposal, energy and water consumption, and building design have begun to constrain the growth of the environmental footprint of the medical-industrial complex. Many medical institutions are beginning to address the links between industrial agricultural practices, farm policy, human disease, and

adverse ecosocial impacts by preferentially purchasing sustainably grown food and otherwise supporting local growers.

However, efforts toward environmentally responsible health care will not be sufficient if they do not explicitly confront the inexorable growth of the entire enterprise. Current measures will result in only marginal gains. Serious, prolonged attention to the scope, scale, and appropriateness of health care services, seen through an expanded lens of bioethics that embraces the fundamental interconnections among individual, public, and environmental health, is required. Brownlee and others show that we need not sacrifice our current health and, based on experience in other countries, can actually expect to achieve improved health status. Cutting back on unnecessary and often harmful services is an obvious first step. Beyond that, however, by focusing on policies and interventions proven to prevent many diseases and promote well-being, we can eliminate the need for many resource-consuming, environmentally degrading health care practices.

A focus on disease prevention will inevitably challenge many social, economic, and political traditions—particularly in the United States. Many upstream causes of disease are built into the fabric of contemporary society and will require structural changes if they are to be reduced. With few exceptions, however, the health care sector has few incentives to drive the social change necessary for disease prevention, having become well funded and firmly established in circumstances as they are. The public health sector struggles at the margin, is underfunded, and may run the risk of being co-opted by political ideology into a medical model that emphasizes personal responsibility, privatization, and the dominance of market forces. Yet without change that reflects the new realities of today's world, medical and public health ethics will erode the very basis of their existence. They cannot remain viable if they continue to ignore the profound interconnectedness of individuals, families, and communities with the larger natural world.

It is increasingly clear that the world of the twenty-first century requires a new bioethic that builds on and recontextualizes twentieth century medical and public health ethics. Ethics may embody what we believe and value, but surely must also be informed by what we know to be true. If people are to survive on earth with lives of quality, all institutional sectors, including health care and public health, will need to take a hard look at objective data and, led by biological wisdom, give moral consideration to entire ecosocial systems as well as their human participants. A new bioethic will emphasize interdependence and interconnectedness, duties and responsibilities as well as rights, and will celebrate humans as members of complex communities. The alternative is to plan for a past that no longer exists, while ignoring a future that will not be denied.

References

Banks, J., M. Marmot, Z. Oldfield, and J. Smith. "Disease and Disadvantage in the United States and in England." *Journal of the American Medical Association* 295, no. 17 (2006): 2037–45.

Berry, W. "Health Is Membership." In *Another Turn of the Crank*, 86–109. Washington, DC: Counterpoint.

Brownlee S. *Overtreated: Why Too Much Medicine Is Making Us Sicker and Poorer*. New York: Bloomsbury USA, 2007.

Flexner, A., 1910. Medical Education in the United States and Canada. Carnegie Foundation for Higher Education. Available at: http://www.carnegiefoundation.org/publications/pub.asp?key=43&subkey=977

HEALTH CARE BUILDINGS How do they use energy and how much does it cost? at http://www.eia.doe.gov/emeu/consumptionbriefs/cbecs/pbawebsite/health/health_howuseenergy.htm

Jameton, A. "Environmental Health Ethics." In *Environmental Health: From Global to Local*, edited by H. Frumkin. San Francisco: Jossey-Bass. 143–169

Jonas, H. *The Imperative of Responsibility: In Search of an Ethics for the Technological Age*. Chicago: University of Chicago Press, 1984.

Leopold, A. *A Sand County Almanac*. New York: Oxford University Press, 1949.

Marmot, M. "Social Determinants of Health Inequalities." *Lancet* 365, no. 9464. (2005): 1099–1104.

MMWR weekly. June 09, 1995 / 44(22);421, 427–429; Estimated Expenditures for Core Public Health Functions – Selected States, October 1992-September 1993 Available at: www.cdc.gov/mmwr/preview/mmwrhtml/00037197.htm

Pierce, J., and A. Jameton. *The Ethics of Environmentally Responsible Health Care*. New York: Oxford University Press, 2003.

Potter, V. R. *Global Bioethics*. East Lansing: Michigan State University Press, 1988.

"Recent trends in infant mortality in the United States" at http://www.cdc.gov/nchs/data/databriefs/db09.htm and CIA. The World Factbook at http://www.cia.gov/library/publications/the-world-factbook/rankorder/2102rank.html

United Nations Environment Program (UNEP). "Millennium Ecosystem Assessment." 2005. http://millenniumassessment.org/en/products.aspx (accessed July 16, 2006).

Waddington, C. H. (1960). *The ethical animal*. London: George Allen & Unwin.

Wennberg JE, Fisher ES, Skinner JS. "Geography and the debate over Medicare reform." *Health Affairs* (Millwood). Suppl Web Exclusives: W96-114.

New Ways of Thinking About Bioethics

JESSICA PIERCE AND ANDREW JAMETON

From *The Ethics of Environmentally Responsible Health Care* (New York: Oxford University Press, 2004), 111–125.

Since the field of bioethics emerged some four decades ago, much has changed in the world of health care and in the larger world that health care serves. The most important of these changes—the increasingly stressed state of the global ecosystem and the attendant decline in both ecosystem and human health—have immense relevance to health care. In its 40-year life, bioethics has proven itself a resilient and responsive field, able to stay abreast of the moral dimensions of technological and organizational changes within medicine. Mirroring the insularity of medicine, however, bioethics so far has not integrated environmental concerns into its dominant theoretical approaches. Nevertheless, we are hopeful that it will continue to transform its ways of thinking, and that it will become a vocal public advocate for the movement toward sustainable health by drawing forth the profound connections between health and the natural world.

Ethics seeks to answer the question "How ought we to live?" An abundance of empirical information links health and environment. For the many people who strive to live a good life, a moral framework is needed to establish the relevance of this information, particularly for those thinking about the good life in the context of health care. Because the thinking that has thus far shaped bioethics has limitations that hold back this move toward sustainability, while environmental ethics has explored how to widen the circle of moral perception to include nature, a dialogue between the two is necessary and should prove fruitful.

What Might Environmental Philosophy Offer to Bioethics?

In 1967, historian Lynn White, Jr., published an article in *Science* entitled "The Historic Roots of Our Ecologic Crisis." White argued that one

reason the environmental crisis has developed is that Christianity fostered a belief that nature exists solely as a resource for humans. Societies exploit nature partly because their religious and philosophical traditions regard the natural world as little more than a vast collection of raw materials. Since the 1960s, a rich and perceptive body of literature has developed around this question of how the dominant worldview, the conglomeration of beliefs and attitudes about nature that has developed within Western thought, shapes our troubled relationship to nature.

Like many other contemporary scholars, William Leiss argues that destructive attitudes toward nature were crystallized during the Enlightenment by the development of modern science, which gave birth to the dream that humans would achieve complete mastery over nature. Philosophy rationalized and legitimized the drive to master nature: the sharp division of the world into spiritual (the human mind, the noumenal world) and material (nature, the phenomenal world) encouraged humans to view nature as usable machinery, without any spiritual animation. The growth of capitalism, particularly the agenda of increasing human material well-being by exploiting natural resources, was closely tied to this philosophical trend.

According to Leiss, mastery over nature "has been a more or less tacit presupposition of modern ideologies within their systems of explicit rationalization for concepts such as individual freedom, social justice, economic development through market forces, imperialism, and élite or class privilege." Humanity's entitlement to dominate nature, "a subterranean theme that runs throughout the collective consciousness of the modern era," is a grounding presupposition of the moral philosophy that has shaped bioethics. Although scholars in bioethics have challenged a number of tacit assumptions in modern philosophy's theoretical edifice, the exploitative attitude toward nature has seldom been one of them.

As the field of environmental ethics developed during the 1970s and 1980s, and as environmental problems became more pronounced, environmental philosophers began to challenge these assumptions about the human relationship to nature and to see that the concepts and methods of philosophy were themselves limiting factors in adequately addressing environmental problems. Philosophers began to explore more radical approaches: *biocentrism* argues that all living things deserve moral consideration; *ecocentrism* moves attention to the value of whole ecosystems. A more comprehensive overview of environmental philosophy as it relates to bioethics would also include *deep ecology, social ecology*, and *ecofeminism*.

Biocentrism

Paul Taylor characterizes biocentrism as "biocentric egalitarianism": in principle, all living beings have equal inherent worth and an equal right to pursue their own form of flourishing. A life-centered ethic, in contrast to an anthropocentric one, entails "prima facie moral obligations that are owed to wild plants and animals themselves as members of Earth's biotic community." Other things being equal, humans are morally bound to protect wild plants and animals or promote their good for their own sake. Our duties to protect biodiversity, to seek to maintain balance in ecosystems, and to slow global warming are rooted in obligations to individual entities.

The ground of the obligation to protect and promote the good of living entities stems, in Taylor's theory, from two interconnected concepts that together are the basis of respect for nature. First, every organism has a good of its own, which humans—the only moral agents—can either thwart or promote by our actions. This good Taylor defines as the full development of an entity's "biological powers," or its capacity to cope with its environment and live out its full life cycle. Compare this rich notion of an entity's good to the standard debate about animal research, which connects the good of a living thing almost entirely to its sentience or its capacity to feel pain.

The second of Taylor's key concepts is inherent worth. A living entity is worthy of being preserved for its own sake and therefore deserves moral consideration. Taylor draws a parallel between an attitude in human ethics of respect for persons and in environmental ethics of respect for nature. "When we adopt an attitude of respect for persons as the proper (fitting, appropriate) attitude to take toward all persons as persons, we consider the fulfillment of the basic interests of each individual to have intrinsic value." The attitude of respect for nature is an ultimate or fundamental commitment—there is no higher norm to which it refers. As Taylor says, "It sets the total framework for our responsibilities toward the natural world."

Ecocentrism

Ecocentrism, or *holism*, is the view that the biosphere as an interconnected whole has moral standing. Beginning from the science of ecology, it sees the world as an integrated web of parts and relationships. One cannot sensibly value just "life" or the lives of individual creatures as in biocentrism, because the whole organic process involves death and decay. There must be some other locus of value. Homeostasis, equilibrium, and integrity are normative principles from which we can derive our obligations to nature. In Aldo Leopold's now famous phrase, "A thing is right when it tends to preserve the integrity, stability, and beauty of the biotic community. It is wrong when it tends otherwise."

The roots of Leopold's "land ethic," which he articulated in the final chapter of *A Sand County Almanac*, lie in evolutionary theory and ecology. Influenced by David Hume and Adam Smith, Charles Darwin argued that ethics rests upon human "sentiments." The bonds of familial and parental affections are shared by all mammals, and this expanded circle of social sentiments proved to be an effective adaptive strategy for the human species. "All ethics so far evolved," says Leopold, "rest upon a single premise: that the individual is a member of a community of interdependent parts." As we come to understand (through ecology) our connection to the biotic community, it is natural that our moral sentiments should extend to it. "The land ethic simply enlarges the boundaries of the community to include soils, waters, plants, and animals, or collectively: the land...."

Leopold grounds his land ethic in what he calls "ecological conscience." We can be ethical, he says, only in relation to "something we can see, feel, understand, love, or otherwise have faith in." Leopold uses the story of Odysseus to argue this point: When Odysseus returned from Troy, he hanged a dozen female slaves whom he suspected of betraying him. For Odysseus, this was an ethical course of action, since slaves were property, not people. Similarly, many today fail to extend moral obligation to the land because they see it as mere property. Just as our moral sensibilities have expanded to include all humans, we need to extend the moral community to include the land upon which and within which we live. So the first task in talking about responsibilities to nature is to establish nature as something we can see, feel, understand, and love.

Ecocentrism does not displace responsibilities to individual entities, including people, but incorporates them—though holistic concerns may take priority. Leopold and other ecocentrists have used a metaphor of tree rings, or expanding concentric circles, and argued for the accretion of new, larger rings, with duties to human community, especially to family, forming the core.

Naturalistic Ethics

The wealth of ecologically related principles promises great potential for extending the agenda of bioethics. The ecological perspective on ethics allows the ethics of health care to cohere with a more relevant ethic guiding human conduct generally during this century of globalization and environmental crisis, and helps avoid a con-

centration on the conduct of health professionals and patients isolated from the larger changes in our global condition. Grounding human morality in an ecological framework radically alters our relationships to each other and to the larger biotic community. It leads us to identify different, often new, moral problems and facilitates the movement toward a culture that respects nature's limits, that consumes modestly and shares nature's now-fragile bounty broadly, deeply, and convivially. It is within this kind of worldview that the notion of sustainable health will most comfortably find a home. But this wealth of new ideas challenges the essential drive in philosophical theory for parsimony of concepts and principles.

The first major enterprise in medical ethics, and perhaps the project that most helped it coalesce into a coherent discipline, resulted from an act of Congress establishing the National Commission for the Protection of Human Subjects of Biomedical and Behavioral Research. Its best-known publication, *The Belmont Report*, published in 1979, set forth three principles to guide the ethical conduct of research: respect for persons, beneficence, and justice. As Albert Jonsen remembers it, these three principles "came to mind almost unbidden" (Baker et al. 1999, 266). Because the principles were fluid and offered a framework for exploring moral problems rather than a rigid moral calculus, they served well the discussion of dilemmas created by rapid technological change in medicine. Medical ethics had discovered itself.

Although these concepts are vague, retaining this common vocabulary serves a practical purpose as bioethics takes on the more inclusive moral challenges of our deteriorating habitat. Problem-solving application of accepted principles and methods to new situations and conditions can begin immediately. Without much reflection on theory or principles, bioethicists, clinicians, and patients can more intuitively integrate a fresh consciousness of their global situation that might lead them to make different decisions simply because their understanding of the facts is so different. For example, patients might be more willing to limit care; clinicians might gently discourage expensive care that simply prolongs dying; ethicists might write more about problems relating to materials and services. The principles and grounding of ethics will not have changed dramatically, only our perception of the reality around us.

The central principles that have thus far guided bioethics remain relevant, though specification of the principles will need to reflect awareness of environmental responsibility. Beauchamp and Childress argue that "specification holds out the possibility of a continually expanding normative viewpoint that is faithful to initial beliefs (which are not renounced) and that tightens rather than weakens coherence among the full range of accepted norms." Norms are not, as they note, meant to be static, but can evolve and find shape as we face new moral dilemmas, or as our perceptions of old moral dilemmas change. The norms widely accepted in medical ethics discussion and practice can evolve in response to the environmental challenge.

Just as a core set of values evolved to respond to the needs of the developing field of bioethics, another set has evolved in environmental ethics: sustainability, a fair distribution of environmental benefits and burdens, modesty of consumption, responsibility to nature and to future generations. In our view, this set of principles, the principles of sustainability, should become central guiding principles of discussion in health-care ethics. So, we propose here to discuss how the conventional framework might effectively be modified by and integrated with ecological concepts.

Beneficence and Nonmaleficence

Health Care Without Harm, which campaigns to reduce toxic hospital wastes, uses as its slogan "First, do no harm." Although HCWH's practical agenda is conservative—for example, better separation of health-care wastes, phaseout of health care products containing polyvinyl chloride (PVC)—their use of the principle of nonmaleficence is actually quite radical, and

takes the principle far beyond its traditional functions in medical ethics. "Do no harm," suggests that health professionals' responsibilities to avoid harm extend beyond the bedside and beyond the health-care setting. Health professionals must avoid harming the community and the natural environment.

Likewise, the principle of beneficence, which has been used in bioethics to inform doing good for the patient, takes on a much different meaning when used in an environmental context. If a clinician must take into account not only his or her patient's good, but also the good of the factory worker who assembled the thermometer that the nurse is reading, and the good of those who might be exposed to the waste products of the thermometer once it is discarded, the range of application of the principle has broadened dramatically.

Bioethics has certainly explored issues where beneficence and nonmaleficence extend beyond the bedside. The sticky problem of quarantine for individuals with infectious illness such as tuberculosis raises the issue of preventing harm to the community. Childhood vaccinations usually pose small risks to a child in exchange for protecting the community's health as well as the child's. Some bioethicists have raised the question of whether physicians have obligations to the community at large, with actions such as working to prevent human rights abuses or providing free or low-cost care for the poor.

Bioethics has not yet seriously grappled with the background volume of harm, both practical and philosophical, brought to attention by the environmental discussion. Although there is discussion in the biomedical literature about how best to define harm, there is a broad level of implicit agreement that, in the context of medicine, *harms* can only be done to humans. The same assumption underlies the principle of doing good. These presuppositions lay out a moral system in which nonhuman forms of life, as well as inanimate nature, lack moral value. They may be relevant to a discussion about morality, but only in their utility or disutility to humans. Animal research is the only bioethics context we are aware of in which nonmaleficence has been extended beyond our own species.

Strong responsibilities to the environment *can* be established within a strictly "human-centered" view. Global warming, for example, poses potential risks of grave harm to humans, regardless of whether we care about the survival of nature *per se* (although of course we are dependent on it as well). But there are compelling reasons for considering a more robust understanding of harms and benefits.

The public, together with most of us in bioethics, usually celebrates the technological benefits and promise of medicine as though they were separable from the destructiveness of the society that supports health care and helped compensate for it. But Western civilization, especially in the United States, is probably the most destructive civilization in the history of humankind. This destructiveness cannot be appreciated fully if we focus largely on the short-term interests of individuals and their immediate communities, as we normally do when we consider beneficence and nonmaleficence in bioethics. According to environmental ethics, additional considerations must be taken into account: the good of future human generations, of people around the world, of nonhuman species, and of earth's ecosystems, which are collective entities that cannot be reduced to the individuals that compose them.

Moreover, the harm that we are doing is mostly a collective harm. If we examine each individual decision one by one, we usually highlight the benefits to be achieved in the care of a single patient, and we discount or disregard the harm done during the life cycle of the materials we use to achieve this good. In so doing, we are acting like sensible utilitarians and choosing an action where the good clearly seems to outweigh the costs. But in doing so, we are also adopting, as ethicists, a consumerist perspective that gives moral weight only to one link of the whole chain of consequences of an action. Since health care, and society at large, collectively causes harm of a similar kind millions of times over (such as carbon emissions and toxic waste), each tiny bit of harm adds up to the great cumulative disaster of climate change and the global ecological crisis.

When we realize that the technology of health care—which can be neither developed nor applied without intensive use of oil, mining, and chemistry, with all their side effects—is environmentally destructive, we must recognize that our normal way of assessing beneficence disregards the precariousness of the earth's situation and its relationship to the technology of medicine. Worse, we are unable to do so in part because of our anthropocentrism.

When the full cost to the life of the earth is put into the balance, everyday decisions unquestioned by ethicists and regarded as rational and even praiseworthy may be seen as questionable and possibly maleficent. If nonmaleficence is viewed from an environmental perspective in the form of the precautionary principle, many health care activities probably do at least as much harm to the world as good.

Autonomy, Coercion, and Participation

Autonomy has not always held the primacy of place in philosophy that it now commands in bioethics. In early moral philosophy, personal autonomy was not central but functioned, in Albert Jonsen's words, as a "prop for arguments about moral accountability and responsibility" since there had to be some sense of free will in order to make humans responsible for their own actions. Even Kant, who is often hailed as the father of autonomy, bound it to a concept of universal law determining human decisions. Yet autonomy has gradually taken hold as the moral trump card in much contemporary work in bioethics. The principle of autonomy, in its modern form, articulates the core commitment of liberal theory to personal freedom and to the idea that individuals have the right to make choices for themselves, based on their own values and goals. Now environmental questions challenge both the standard meaning of autonomy and its primacy of place in bioethics.

There are several respects in which environmental concerns press for a more nuanced principle of autonomy. The tension that was implicit in the notion of autonomy as understood by Kant and others needs to be rediscovered. Autonomous individuals exist as members of a moral community who share common ends. This community needs to expand to place humans within their biotic community. With a shift in thinking, personal choice can be understood in the context of belonging to and feeling responsible to the biological as well as the human community.

Some may suspect that this reframing of autonomy is an attempt to sugar-coat certain forms of coercion. Perhaps, within health care, there is some truth to this. A sustainable health-care system will undoubtedly limit the choices of both patients and physicians. But patients and physicians alike are already coerced by prevailing interventionist standards and by the ready availability of heroic "life saving" treatments and drugs. And people already need to be coaxed and prodded into healthier lifestyles, conserving health-care products, and forgoing expensive and marginally useful treatments. It may turn out that there is no increase in the level of coercion, if its direction shifts from forcing expansion to supporting stewardship and modest health-care consumption.

For the concept of autonomy to be richly nuanced so that it can guide respect for human dignity while avoiding its crude application as a catch all for personal choice, it must be placed in proper relationship to the concept of connection. *Connection*, or interdependency, is a common motif in the environmental literature. The images of circularity, balance, and webs recur frequently, both as description and as normative ideals. Ecology is based on the study of connections between elements in a living system, including humans. The world is a "whole Earth community." Principles of ecological design prioritize "working with nature" and "harmony with nature": connection is built into design, with closed loops of production, waste transformed into energy, and humans integrated into biotic communities.

Although in conventional bioethics obligations derive from the sincere convictions of the autonomous individual, the ecological concept of obligation is more intimately grounded in connection than is autonomy. Connectedness is about "binding" and is closely related to the idea of community; communities are a stronger ground of obligation than the beliefs of individuals. Inclusion in a community is the main source of moral obligation. Not only does the idea of interconnection place us in community, but it also expands the concept of community. From an ecological perspective, we are global citizens and members of a biotic community.

If one's "self" is defined by and through relationships, this connectedness can also be seen as being at odds with conceptions of the self as autonomous. Both feminist and environmental writings have explored such interconnected conceptions of the self. Environmental philosophers amplify this alternative view by suggesting that the "self" is more appropriately defined through relationship not only with other people, but also with nature. Warwick Fox's *Toward a Transpersonal Ecology* is the most sustained treatment of the "ecological self." One of the more interesting implications of a "transpersonal self" (a "wide, expansive, or field-like conception of the self") is that: "Care flows naturally if the 'self' is widened and deepened so that protection of free Nature is felt and conceived as protection of ourselves...."

It is tempting to romanticize the idea of humans in community with nature, but nature plays a significant role in unpleasant human experiences of disease, suffering, and death. Humans are hosts to a vast number of parasites living in our intestines, on our skin, in our hair. Many of these interrelationships are symbiotic and quite necessary to our health, while others we rightly label as diseases. Yet even disease, as biologist René Dubos is famous for saying, is part of the overall harmony of nature. It is important that while treating the disease element as an intruder, we think ecologically: the most obvious tie that binds us with the rest of life is the inevitability of death, disease, and decay. It has already been well argued in bioethics that we need not equate death with failure and that palliation of suffering should sometimes outweigh efforts to save lives. An ecological perspective adds to this argument the ability to make death more meaningful in a large biological context.

Nevertheless, the expression of self-control—of controlling desires for material goods, of making choices in light of the needs of the whole community—is a clear and strong expression of self-determination. So how should the individual be included in an ecological perspective on health-care decision-making? A shift in thinking needs to occur so that the articulation of personal choice is understood inside the context of duties to each other and to nature. Autonomy is not necessarily threatened by this contextualization: individual choice can be an expression of belonging in and feeling responsible to the human and biological community.

For autonomy to be maximized in a sustainable context, individuals need to be able to participate, and feel that they are participating, in the decisions that set social priorities to protect humans and nature. The language of individual participation is similar to the language of individual autonomy. Both concepts offer the patient a voice in health-care decisions. But the language of participation is more communitarian; it lacks the implications of individual separateness found in the language of autonomy. Where clinician and consumer disagree, for example, the language of autonomy leads to a power struggle over whose opinion should dominate. Indeed, "Who should decide?" has been one of the major questions in health care ethics. In contrast, the language of participation is a language of inclusion. The question of who should decide, then, can be answered flexibly, depending on what needs to be decided.

Justice, Equality, and Balance

Basic political and material equality is a prominent feature of the modern concept of justice. Yet, for several reasons, an ecological point of view does not so obviously entail equality. Even though all people face a common global environmental dilemma, people in different regions and conditions experience this circumstance very differently. Nor is saying that we are all interconnected to say that we are all equal. If strict material equality were insisted upon, and the ability of the environment to support human life fell to a low level, then survival and equality would become mutually inconsistent. Even in good times, the ideal of equality fits poorly with basic concepts of ecological community. Since animals and plants are part of our community, we need to consider the fundamental differences among species as basic to rules on how to treat them. Given the distinctness of the ecological roles of species and their radically differing capacities for pleasure and pain, it is probably best not to use equality as the central concept for understanding justice in the whole ecological community.

In the world of nature, however, the concept of justice has a close affinity to the Platonic ideal of justice as harmony. A healthy ecosystem is one that *justifies*—that is, balances or harmonizes—the complex relationships among its components. Since all creatures in an ecosystem are interdependent, attributing excessively high standing to a conscious élite of large organisms is problematic unless the élite, like Plato's guardians, are living modestly and thinking of the welfare of the whole.

These classical conceptions of justice also connect human health to justice. A healthy person's body is also a "just" one, with its harmony and temperance realized as homeostasis. In this sense ecological medicine contains a commitment to justice, and bioethics can reframe the problem of justice as an effort to balance the fundamental elements of ecological balance: preservation of ecosystems, maintenance of community and population health, and care for the individual. A healthy and sustainable balance of resources allocated among these three spheres would be a just one as well.

Philosophers writing about justice in health care have often focused on distinctions that acquiesce in dissimilar treatment of individuals. Once that step has been taken, there is little in doctrines of equality to make it clear that extreme differences in allocation of resources are problematic. But if we accept the principle that everyone in the world has an equal claim to the earth's commons and resources, then we can justly claim that everyone has an equal entitlement to the use of Earth's atmosphere, so the agenda of equalizing industrial output of carbon becomes one of central moral significance. The concept of justice as balance then comes into play. Rather than leaving ourselves without a way of attacking extreme disparities that stem from the principle of autonomy, we can hold that for the sake of harmony and balance, only small differences in access to resources should be tolerated.

Are sustainability and justice necessarily related? If one omits concern for the welfare and interests of future generations, then one can imagine an unsustainable world that meets the criteria of justice for a short time. This world may be efficient, meet people's needs, and allocate resources and power equally, but only until Earth's ecosystem collapses. If one believes that justice includes the needs and interests of future generations, however, then a just world must also be sustainable. To state the relationship the other way around, if the world is unsustainable then it is also unfair, at least to future generations and to nature's great ecosystem.

There are additional connections and disconnections between sustainability and justice. The most obvious is efficiency in the use of global resources. Since the largest sustainable gains in efficiency can be achieved by leveling down consumption by those who are well off, and the pressure for reducing overall consumption is great, greater material equality is the surest route to sustainability. This strategy is consistent with a Rawlsian perspective on justice. Rawls argued that it was morally acceptable to allocate more resources to some people if it in fact helped the condition of the worst off. He made this argument with the assumption that economic growth would result; but in the contracting economy, growth is economically impossible, and thus Rawls must be run in reverse: we must first take from the better off in order to increase resources available to the worst off.

The potential conflict between meeting basic human needs and preserving nature presents a difficult practical challenge for environmentalism. Holmes Rolston III raises poignant questions about meeting the needs of the poor when doing so may involve wiping out habitat for tigers. But if the needs of the poor are to be met for any extended period of time, it is necessary to preserve the ecological stability of the regions where they live. A right to environmental protection should be regarded as one element of basic human rights, since a sound ecology is also a condition of human health. As with the Rawlsian argument, this means that economic change during the environmental crisis must involve a combination of leveling down of wealth and income for the best off with a leveling up of the worst off.

Justice and Modesty

Bioethics has dwelt primarily on the medical problems of individuals in clinical settings—more specifically, on the moral questions that arise in academic medical centers. The clinical setting has controlled the discourse. As we note above, this narrowly focused gaze limits opportunities to discuss crucial questions about the environment and about justice, questions that are inherent in contemporary medical procedures and technologies. Ethical conversation about justice in the access of patients to therapies has tended to focus on the benefits and monetary costs to individuals and their families; more distant environmental expenditures in the life cycle of medical products recede to the background.

The parameters of bioethical discussion of high-cost therapies were set about 40 years ago in the Seattle debate over access to dialysis. Machines were too scarce and their use too expensive for distribution to all who needed them. The question of justice centered on *deservingness*. Bioethicists criticized allocation criteria explicitly based on merit, behavior, or social class, and on the whole supported criteria such as medical need or prospects for recovery. But these more neutral principles still resulted in a vast disparity in the levels of health care available to different economic classes. The exclusion of some people from services, and the inclusion of others, remains a premise underlying the discussion of justice in medical care.

Working for the most part in medical centers with highly paid health professionals, and addressing the clinical problems of patients able to afford them, bioethicists have tended to accept wide differences in care and have been willing to perform philosophical work that justifies those differences. A more global perspective opens the prospect of grappling with what Paul Farmer labels "the leading ethical question of our times"—the immense disparities in public health around the world.

But environmental philosophies are ready at hand to save the moral life of bioethics. Such philosophies generally view overconsumption as not only destructive of our habitat but a moral failing in itself, and they prescribe *modesty* as a tonic for the spiritual emptiness engendered by the endless pursuit of material goods. The permaculture ethic, for example, calls for "active conservation, ethics and frugal use of resources, and 'right livelihood.'" Deep ecology promotes a philosophy of "simple in means, rich in ends." The writings of Thoreau are an early articulation of voluntary simplicity. A surprisingly widespread desire to live modestly is evidenced by the popularity of Duane Elgin's book *Voluntary Simplicity*, first published in 1981. It advocates three interconnected tenets: frugal consumption, ecological awareness, and personal growth. Like permaculture and deep ecology, voluntary simplicity responds to the need to protect nature and at the same time heals the malaise of a materialistic lifestyle. By consuming less and worrying less about what we want to buy, we have more time and energy to spend with our children, family, and friends and to enjoy games, music, and other wholesome activities. It is only a small step to conclude that a simple life requires a modest system of medical care.

The notion of *modesty* is about having "enough." But what is enough? The question suggests why the element of personal growth is considered a central tenet of simple living. Maturity is marked by the ability to distinguish between needs and desires, and between personal and community needs.

Conclusion

A viable bioethics informed by environmental philosophy will

- be able to include an account of the value of the natural world,
- have some mechanism for balancing human health needs with the needs of nature,
- appreciate that the proper context of bioethics is global in scope,
- commit us to a strong principle of justice that demands a leveling in the distribution of resources and risks, and that aims toward modesty and adequacy for all, and
- have ecological sustainability as a core evaluative principle.

Those who are attuned to the state of our planetary health and to the living conditions of people around the world may feel an overwhelming sense of helplessness and hopelessness. The problems humanity faces seem so complex and so serious that it is hard know how—or even whether—to take action. Our inevitable complicity in the death of nature and the suffering of distant others may cause so much moral discomfort that simple avoidance seems the only psychologically bearable response.

But it is not necessary to adopt a stance of despair. Millions of people around the world are working toward reconciling human needs with the limits of the earth. All of us have a moral responsibility to become aware of how our actions affect others globally, human and nonhuman alike, and how our daily lives are likely to shape the future. We have a responsibility to educate ourselves and others, and to do some careful thinking about what we need and do not need, who we care about and how we mean to care for them. If we feel a commitment to promoting and maintaining human health, we must take the state of the natural environment immediately and carefully into account. We must embrace sustainable health for humans and for the ecosystems we depend on for survival.

Global Environmental Change and Health

Impacts, Inequalities, and the Health Sector

A. J. MCMICHAEL, A. NYONG, AND C. CORVALAN

British Medical Journal 336 (Jan 26, 2008): 191–194.

Human actions are changing many of the world's natural environmental systems, including the climate system. These systems are intrinsic to life processes and fundamental to human health, and their disruption and depletion make it more difficult to tackle health inequalities. Indeed, we will not achieve the UN millennium development health goals if environmental destruction continues. Health professionals have a vital contributory role in preventing and reducing the health effects of global environmental change.

Problems of Focus

In 2000 the United Nations set out eight development goals to improve the lives of the world's disadvantaged populations. The goals seek reductions in poverty, illiteracy, sex inequality, malnutrition, child deaths, maternal mortality, and major infections as well creation of environmental stability and a global partnership for development. One problem of this itemisation of goals is that it separates environmental considerations from health considerations. Poverty cannot be eliminated while environmental degradation exacerbates malnutrition, disease, and injury. Food supplies need continuing soil fertility, climatic stability, freshwater supplies, and ecological support (such as pollination). Infectious diseases cannot be stabilised in circumstances of climatic instability, refugee flows, and impoverishment.

The seventh millennium development goal also takes a limited view of environmental sustainability, focusing primarily on traditional localised physical, chemical, and microbial hazards. Those hazards, which are associated with industrialisation, urbanisation, and agriculture in lower income countries, remain important as they impinge most on poor and vulnerable communities. Exposure to indoor air pollution, for example, varies substantially between rich and poor in urban and rural populations. And the World Health Organization estimates that a quarter of the global burden of disease, including over one third of childhood burden, is due to modifiable factors in air, water, soil, and food. This estimated environment related burden is much greater in low income than high income countries overall (25% versus 17% of deaths—and widening further to a two-fold difference in percentages between the highest and lowest risk countries). Heavy metals and chemical residues contaminate local foods, urban air pollution causes premature deaths, and waterborne enteric pathogens kill two million children annually.

These relatively localised environmental health hazards, though, are mostly remediable.

Meanwhile, a larger scale, less remediable, and potentially irreversible category of environmental health hazard is emerging. Human pressures on the natural environment, reflecting global population growth and intensified economic activities, are now so great that many of the world's biophysical and ecological systems are being impaired. Examples of these global environmental changes include climate change, freshwater shortages, loss of biodiversity (with consequent changes to functioning of ecosystems), and exhaustion of fisheries. These changes are unprecedented in scale, and the resultant risks to population health need urgent response by health professionals and the health sector at large.

Who Will Be Affected

The health effects of global environmental change will vary between countries. Loss of healthy life years in low income African countries, for example, is predicted to be 500 times that in Europe. The fourth assessment report of the Intergovernmental Panel on Climate Change concluded that adverse health effects are much more likely in low income countries and vulnerable subpopulations. These disparities may well increase in coming decades, not only because of regional differences in the intensity of environmental changes (such as water shortages and soil erosion), but also because of exacerbations of differentials in economic conditions, levels of social and human capital, political power, and local environmental dependency.

These differential health risks also reflect the wider issue of access to global and local "public goods." Most of the world's arable land has now been privatised; stocks of wild species (fish, animals, and wild plants) are declining as population pressures and commercial activities intensify; and freshwater is increasingly becoming subject to market pricing. Social policies should therefore pay particular attention to the health inequalities that flow from unequal access to environmental fundamentals.

Availability of safe drinking water illustrates the point about access to what, historically, was common property: 1.1 billion people lack safe drinking water, and 2.6 billion lack basic sanitation. Beyond diarrhoeal disease, water related health risks also arise from chemical contamination—such as arsenic as a cause of skin pigmentation, hyperkeratosis, cardiovascular disease, neuropathy, and cancer.

Role of Social Conditions

The relation of environmental impoverishment to health risks and inequalities is complex. Environmental degradation impairs health, while health deficits (for example, malnutrition or depletion of the workforce from AIDS) can amplify environmental mismanagement. This causes inequalities in both health endangering exposures and health outcomes.

India provides a good example of the complexity of these relations. The country's average life expectancy is relatively low but is expected to improve with industrialisation and modernisation. Industrialisation is contributing to the rapid increase of coal burning in India, and the resultant addition to global emissions and climate change amplifies health risks worldwide. These health risks will affect the world's most vulnerable populations.

The risks to population health from environmental change have far reaching implications for prevention strategies (fig. 8.1). Global changes result in loss of natural resources. Resolution of these risks therefore requires a different approach from that used for the more familiar challenges presented by time limited and reversible local environmental contamination.

Climate Change and Health

Human induced global climate change is now an acknowledged reality. We have taken a long time to recognise the resultant health risks, current and future, and their unequal effects around the world, but the topic is now attracting much attention. Risks to health will arise by direct and indirect pathways and will reflect changes in both average climate conditions and in climatic variability. The main risks are:

- Effects of heat waves and other extreme events (cyclones, floods, storms, wildfires)
- Changes in patterns of infectious disease
- Effects on food yields
- Effects on freshwater supplies
- Impaired functioning of ecosystems (for example, wetlands as water filters)
- Displacement of vulnerable populations (for example, low lying island and coastal populations)
- Loss of livelihoods.

Extreme weather events, infection, and malnutrition will have the greatest health effects in poor and vulnerable populations (box 8.1). In sub-Saharan Africa over 110 million people currently live in regions prone to malaria epidemics. Climate change could add 20–70 million to this figure by the 2080s (assuming no population increase, and including forecast malaria reductions in West Africa from drying). Any such increase would exacerbate poverty and make it harder to achieve and sustain health improvements.

Some links between climate change and human health are complex. For example, the predicted drying in sub-Saharan Africa could increase the incidence of HIV infection, as impoverished

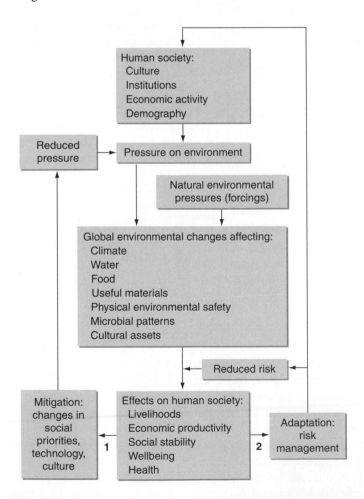

Figure 8.1

■ Relations between human induced global environmental changes affect health and social policy responses. True primary prevention (path 1) reduces or eliminates the human pressures on environment. A more defensive type of prevention is attained through adaptive interventions to lessen risk (path 2), particularly in vulnerable communities.

Box 8.1 Africa and Climate Change

Africa is very vulnerable to climate change because of other environmental and social stresses. The economy depends critically on agriculture, which accounts for two thirds of the workforce and up to half of household incomes and food.

- Climate models predict regional increases in mean temperatures of several degrees centigrade by 2100, a decline in summer rainfall in southern and northern Africa and some increase in west and east Africa. Drying, plus the demands of population growth and economic development, will exacerbate regional water scarcity
- Falls in crop yields due to 1-2°C warming by 2050 would add an estimated 12 million additional Africans to the 200 million currently undernourished

- Extreme events such as flooding change will affect food availability by damaging roads, storage, and markets—floods in 2000 in Mozambique damaged about 10% of farmland and 90% of irrigation, displaced two million people, and affected up to 1.5 million livelihoods (mostly in poor rural areas)
- Livestock viral diseases such as east coast fever, foot and mouth disease, blue tongue virus, Rift valley fever are climate sensitive. Regional increases in temperature and rainfall could affect tsetse fly habitat and hence trypanosomiasis in livestock
- Climate change and agricultural downturn in Africa may force populations to move, generating conflicts over territory. Pastoralists forced to search for grazing land because of wells drying up may partly explain the Darfur crisis in Sudan

---

rural farming families move to cities where conditions foster sex work and unsafe sex.

The recent report of the Global Environmental Change and Human Health project gives a good summary of the major categories of current and predicted health effects of global environmental changes other than climate change.

Roles for Doctors and Other Health Professionals

The spectrum of potential strategies to reduce health risks is wide, commensurate with the diversity of threats to health posed by climate change and other global environmental changes. Local policies and actions, both to mitigate environmental change at source and to adapt to existing and unavoidable risks to health, will often need support from health attuned policies at provincial, national, and international levels. For example, community programmes to mosquito-proof houses will need to be reinforced by improvements in the national surveillance of infectious diseases and in outbreak warning systems.

Doctors and other health professionals have particular knowledge, opportunity, and, often, political leverage that can help ensure—through advocacy or direct participation—that preventive actions are taken. Actions include promoting public understanding, monitoring and reporting the health effects of environmental change, and proposing and advocating local adaptive responses (box 8.2).

Various websites list and discuss actions for doctors to take, both individually and collectively (box 8.3). For example, the US Centers for Disease Control and Prevention lists 11 functions for the public health system and practitioners for responding to climate change. And Doctors for the Environment Australia has run a successful, continuing, national campaign of patient education by distributing posters and pamphlets for use in doctors' waiting rooms.

Box 8.2 How Health Professionals Can Promote Adaptive Strategies

- Public education, especially through healthcare settings such as doctors' waiting rooms and hospital clinics
- Preventive programmes—eg, vaccines, mosquito control, food hygiene and inspection, nutritional supplementation
- Health care (especially mental health and primary care) for communities affected by environmental adversity

- Surveillance of disease (especially infectious disease) and key risk factors
- Forecasting future health risks from projected climate change
- Forecasting future health risks and gains from mitigation and adaptation strategies
- Health sector workforce training and in-career development

Strategies That Extend Beyond Health Sector:

- Early warning systems for impending extreme weather (eg, heatwaves, storms)
- Neighbourhood support schemes to protect the most vulnerable people

- Climate-proofed housing design, urban planning, water catchment, and farming practices
- Disaster preparedness, including capacity of the health system

Box 8.3 Environmental websites helpful for doctors and other health professionals

Centers for Disease Control and Prevention (US) (www.cdc.gov/nceh/climatechange)

Doctors for the Environment Australia (www.dea.org.au)

Global environmental change and human health project (www.essp.org/en/joint-projects/health.html)

Intergovernmental Panel on Climate Change (www.ipcc.ch)

International Society of Doctors for the Environment (www.isde.org)

Medact UK (www.medact.org/env_climate_change.php)

Adaptive Strategies to Lessen Health Risks

Many local actions can be taken to reduce the vulnerability of communities and populations. These will vary considerably between different regions of the world, and in relation to prevailing socioeconomic conditions and available resources. During Australia's recent prolonged drought (2001–7), some rural health doctors reported that fostering and supporting communal activities (community choirs, social gatherings, financial advisory networks, etc.) increased local resilience against depression associated with loss of livelihood.

Climate change and other large scale environmental changes are unlikely to cause entirely new diseases (although they may contribute to the emergence of new strains of viruses and other microbes that can infect humans). Rather, they will alter the incidence, range, and seasonality of many existing health disorders. Hence, existing healthcare and public health systems should provide an appropriate starting point for adaptive strategies to lessen health effects.

Preventive Action

Although adaptive strategies will minimise the effects of climate change, the greater public health preventive challenge lies in stopping the process of climate change. This requires bold and far sighted policy decisions at national and international levels, entailing much greater emissions cuts than were being proposed a decade ago.

Scientists have concluded that we need to prevent atmospheric carbon dioxide concentrations exceeding 450–500 ppm to avoid the serious, perhaps irreversible, damage to many natural systems and ecological processes that a global average temperature increase of 2–3°C would cause. This requires early radical action as today's concentrations are approaching 390 ppm (compared with 280 ppm before industrialisation). Health professionals, acting through citizens' or professional organisations, have both the opportunity and responsibility to contribute to resolving this momentous issue. Improving awareness of the problem is the first step. Since 1993, doctors from 14 countries (including six low income countries) have had a central role in the Intergovernmental Panel on Climate Change's assessment of the health effects of climate change. We should also add this topic, including its relevance to health professional activity, to the medical curriculum.

The health sector, meanwhile, must minimise greenhouse gas emissions from its own infrastructure, especially hospitals. Health researchers should act to minimise greenhouse gas emissions from their own studies.

Conclusion

The Stern report, in 2006, highlighted the potentially great damage to the world's economic system from unconstrained climate change. The greater risk, however, is to the vitality and health of all species, including humans, if current trends continue to weaken the earth's life support systems. The health professions have a crucial role in promoting public understanding of this fundamental association and health protecting responses to it.

Embedded in Nature

Human Health and Biodiversity

ERIC CHIVIAN AND AARON S. BERNSTEIN

Environmental Health Perspectives 112, no. 1 (2004): A120.

A loss of global biodiversity, namely a reduction in the variety of life on Earth, is rarely given much attention by physicians or environmental scientists. Like most people, they do not spend much time thinking about their relationship to other life forms, and they generally act, unknowingly, as if human beings were separate from the rest of nature—as if we could change the composition of the atmosphere and degrade the land and the oceans without these alterations having much effect on us. It is this disconnect that is at the core of the global environmental crisis—that policy makers and the public by and large do not understand that their health and lives are ultimately dependent on other species and on the integrity of the planet's ecosystems, and, as a result, they do not appreciate the urgent need to protect the natural world.

Approximately 1.7 million species have been identified on Earth and given Linnaean names, but there may be 10 times that number in all, and perhaps many times more if we include microbial diversity. Species interact with each other and with their physical and chemical environments to make up ecosystems such as forests and wetlands. Stratospheric ozone depletion, pollution, the introduction of alien species, the overharvesting of species, and increasingly global climate change all threaten biodiversity and thus ecosystem function. However, the degradation, reduction, and fragmentation of habitats on land, in fresh water, and in the oceans are the greatest threats. All of these factors are the result of human activity and are driven by unsustainable consumption, especially in the industrialized world, and rising human populations. Together they have disrupted grassland, river, lake, coral reef, and other ecosystems at alarming levels, and have raised the rate of species extinctions to 100 and, by some estimates, even to 1,000 times natural background rates.

The loss of species deprives us of invaluable tools for biomedical research that provide insights into how human cells and organ systems function in health and illness, and precludes our developing important new medicines for currently untreatable human diseases. Cone snails, a large genus of some 500 species that live mostly in tropical coral reefs and mangroves, are a case in point. These remarkable creatures capture their prey by lancing them with a harpoon coated with a cocktail of toxic peptides, which bind to an enormous variety of ion channels and receptors on cellular membranes throughout the animal kingdom. Each species may make as many as 100 distinct toxins, so there may be as many as 50,000 different ones in all. One hundred or so of these toxins have been studied to date and have demonstrated such selectivity for specific receptors that some have been used, for example, to help characterize subtypes of nicotinic acetylcholine receptors in mammalian heart muscle, leading to a better understanding of the mechanisms that control heart rate and contractility.

Others are being developed as medicines, including a painkiller possibly 1,000 times more potent than morphine but that does not cause tolerance or addition. This painkiller may soon come on the market in Europe for the treatment of severe, chronic pain, a condition that often defies treatment with opiates such as morphine because of tolerance. Other cone snail toxins are being investigated for treating intractable epilepsy, for preventing nerve cell death when there is inadequate circulation and for the early diagnosis and treatment of small cell carcinomas of the lung, one of the most aggressive human cancers. Cone snails may contain the largest and most clinically important pharmacopoeia of any genus in nature, and yet, as coral reefs and mangroves are in danger of being destroyed, so are they.

The importance of biodiversity to human health is particularly well illustrated by some human infectious diseases. Lyme disease, the most common vectorborne disease in the United States, is a prime example. When high levels of vertebrate-species diversity exist in a Lyme disease area, the risk of getting Lyme disease is lessened. One reason is that some of the vertebrates that are bitten by infected ticks, the vectors which transmit the Lyme bacteria, are "dead end" hosts—poorly able or incapable of passing on the bacteria and continuing the disease cycle. This effectively "dilutes" the disease agent and makes it less likely for an infected tick to transmit the disease to a human. Another reason this diversity is beneficial is that some vertebrate species compete with the main Lyme reservoir host or carrier (the white-footed mouse in the eastern United States), whereas others are predators—in both cases keeping mice populations low and reducing disease risk. This buffering effect conferred by biodiversity may also apply to other human infectious diseases such as West Nile encephalitis, cutaneous and visceral leishmaniasis, African trypanosomiasis, and Chagas disease.

Finally, and most importantly, ecosystems provide the life support systems for all life, including human life, on Earth. Not only do they give us food and fuel, but ecosystems, among other things, purify air and fresh water, bind and detoxify poisonous substances, break down wastes and recycle nutrients on land and in the oceans, pollinate crops and natural vegetation, make soils fertile, and store carbon, mitigating human-caused climate change. We tend to take these services for granted and generally do not recognize that we cannot live without them. Nor do we understand many ecosystem services well enough to recreate them, not knowing what species are necessary for the services to work and in what proportions, or whether for some services there are essential or "keystone" species without which ecosystems would cease to function. Human activity may now be altering some ecosystems in destructive ways that we are unaware of and that could lead to a collapse of their functioning.

The importance of recognizing how biodiversity affects human health and how it is increasingly threatened by human activity will only increase in coming years. Physicians and environmental scientists will need to understand these interconnections because they will be called upon to explain them to policy makers and the public. Such knowledge will also be critically important in clinical medicine, particularly in relation to the emergence and spread of some human infectious diseases.

Sustainable Health Care and Emerging Ethical Responsibilities

ANDREW JAMETON AND JESSICA PIERCE

From *Life Support: The Environment and Human Health*, edited by Michael McCally, (Cambridge, MA: MIT Press, 2002), 285–93.

The declining condition of the natural environment is beginning to affect the health of populations in many parts of the world. As a result, health care professionals and organizations need to consider the long-term environmental costs of providing health care and to reduce the material and energy consumption of the health care industry. This may seem a surprising conclusion, given that average human health has, for the most part, improved in recent decades despite environmental decline. As indicated in the World Health Organization's fiftieth anniversary report the average life expectancy at birth worldwide has increased rapidly (from 46 years in 1958 to an unprecedented 66 years in 1998), the rate of death among children under five has decreased, more people than ever before have access to at least minimal health care services as well as safe water and sanitation. New vaccinations and medications await wide distribution.

Yet these achievements are fragile. In the long term, human health requires a healthy global ecosystem. About 25 percent of health problems are already environmental in origin. There is no realistic way or current technology available to replace declining natural ecosystem services (e.g., climate stabilization, water purification, waste decomposition, pest control, seed dispersal, soil renewal, pollination, biodiversity, and protection against solar radiation) that are essential to health. Although public health experts increasingly recognize the significant role the environment plays in public health, it is less well recognized that personal health care services also depend significantly on and have consequences for the environment.

Linking Health Care and the Environment

Health care figures both as a solution to environmental decline and as a problem. Increasing health problems generated by environmental decline will require medical treatment. At the same time, health care services also damage the environment. In the United States, such services generate over 3 million tons of solid waste per year. As with other service industries such as hotels and restaurants, hospitals consume energy in heating, cooling, manufacturing, and transportation. They occupy large, complex buildings surrounded by concrete and asphalt surfaces; they use high-volume food services, laundry, high-speed transportation, and paper, packaging, and disposable supplies. Health services also pose unique problems, including the use of pharmaceutical and biological products with complex manufacturing processes, environmentally significant precursors, and potentially toxic bodily by-products of medications, as well as complex and hazardous solid, air, and water emissions, including toxic, infectious, and radioactive wastes.

Environmental costs are most evident at the downstream end of health care: the by-products that leave the system as waste. The problems of medical waste, particularly infectious materials (e.g., human tissues and blood) and biohazardous agents (e.g., heavy metals and radioactive isotopes), are fairly well understood and regulated. Still, several groups are exploring additional sources of environmental harm. Health Care Without Harm, a coalition of activists and health care organizations, has advocated the elimination of mercury from health care products. They encourage the separation of polyvinyl chloride (PVC) plastics from the collection of infectious wastes because, during the common practice of incinerating infectious wastes, carcinogenic dioxins are released when PVC products are included. Most recently, and more controversially, the coalition has begun warning patients and health care professionals against the use of vinyl intravenous bags containing phthalate plasticizers, which may leach toxins into patients' bodies.

The Sustainable Hospitals Project of the Lowell Center for Sustainable Production, in Lowell, Massachusetts, is also working on pollution prevention in health care facilities. It is focusing attention on alternatives to products that contain potentially harmful materials such as latex, PVC, and mercury, particularly through influencing purchasing practices within hospitals. The Green Health Center project at the University of Nebraska Medical Center is exploring the ethical principles relevant to providing environmentally sound, high-quality health care.

Not as well understood, yet perhaps more important than pollution downstream from health care services, are the environmental effects upstream from health care delivery. Health care services rely on an enormous array of natural resources, including common and rare metals, naturally occurring pharmaceutical precursors, rubber, petroleum, biomass, and water. Intravenous pumps, x-ray films, latex gloves—each of these common hospital items requires complex manufacturing processes with attendant environmental effects, many of which are felt on the other side of the world. The environmental costs of natural-resource consumption in health care have not been carefully studied, so the degree to which health care activities contribute to environmental deterioration is difficult to assess. However, because health care services represent a significant sector of intensive North American economies, health care shares responsibility for the environmental problems created by the acquisition, processing, and transportation of natural resources required to make the supplies and energy used by consumers.

Sustainable Health Care

If the earth's ecosystem is to continue to support human health, each community needs to maintain public health and provide health care in ways that will sustain the earth's ecosystem. By many accounts, the environmental crisis results from a combination of population growth, consumption patterns, and technology choices. That world population growth must be slowed, and probably reversed, to avoid overwhelming the earth's natural systems has been recognized by many. Less well recognized, but equally important, is that the billion members of the world's consumer class threaten future human welfare with their material, and energy-intensive, lifestyles. One way to represent the scale of consumption is to use the ecological "footprint": an estimate of the amount of space it takes to generate the energy, food, pasture, consumer goods, and so on that it takes to maintain each of us. The Ecological Footprints of Nations Study calculates that "humanity as a whole uses over one-third more resources and ecoservices than what nature can regenerate." The United States has a footprint of 9.6 hectares per capita, whereas Canada's average per capita footprint is 7.2 hectares, still well over the 1.7 hectares globally available per capita.

Large-scale health care systems, such as those in Canada and the United States, depend on wealthy economies to sustain them. But wealthy economies are unsustainable and must scale down their overall consumption of materials and energy. If wealthy industrialized societies as a whole are unsustainable, then so are the health care systems housed by these societies. And if the material scale of these economies is to be reduced, so must the scale of health care. The degree of reduction needed is extremely uncertain, but "Factor X" debates in Europe have set goals for overall reduction of national throughput by factors of one-half, one-fourth, one-tenth, and even smaller fractions of current material and energy consumption. These levels of reduction are likely to prove very challenging. Indeed, it is extremely unlikely that any imaginable new technology could achieve these reductions in resource consumption without a substantial reduction in the supply of consumer products as well. Although no empirical data show that the scale of consumption of natural resources required by industrialized health care systems is ecologically unsustainable, current levels of consumption may challenge our ability to provide health care for future generations. We should thus examine how we can reduce the scale of health care to more modest, sustainable levels.

The environmental impact of health care and the puzzle of sustainability raise ethical questions regarding health care's environmental stewardship. Concern for the health of the earth's ecosystems suggests that health care institutions and practitioners should reassess their practices in order to soften or eliminate harmful effects. At the same time, they have to balance their environmental responsibilities with their obligations to serve the immediate needs of patients. Addressing the issue of balance requires combining considerations from both medical ethics and environmental ethics.

The field of medical ethics has focused largely on principles of human autonomy and issues surrounding benefit to individual patients. It has made significant contributions to our understanding of bedside care, decision making with patients, and the use of new health care technologies. Although some bioethicists have discussed issues with environmental implications—such as new technologies, genetic engineering, overpopulation, and treatment of animals—few ethicists have linked bedside concerns to the larger context of global environmental well-being. Meanwhile, the field of environmental ethics has grown extensively, but with little attention to medicine and health care. It is time for environmental ethics and medical ethics to reopen a dialogue and seek an ethically appropriate balance between immediate individual health needs and sustainability.

The ethical argument for considering sustainability in health care arises from basic ethical commitments common to environmental and medical ethics. First, today's generations have responsibilities for the welfare of future generations. Along with society at large, health care should accept a responsibility to meet current needs in ways modest and clean enough to be sustainable for centuries. Second, humans have a responsibility toward the natural world for the sake of both nature and ourselves. Indeed, action to reduce the impact of humans on nature is urgent; the World Wide Fund for Nature estimates an overall decline of 30 percent in the state of nature since 1970. Third, because about 80 percent of the world's wealth benefits only 20 percent of its people, the vast majority have very little. Poverty is one of the main factors contributing to poor health, and it reduces the ability of populations to cope with environmental decline. Justice and sustainability require that health care services be more equitably allocated on a global scale.

But why should the world's wealthy consumer classes, who spend roughly 90 percent of all of the dollars spent on health care in the world, be sensitive to ethical principles suggesting that they should reduce their consumption of health care materials and services? Two shifts in standard moral concepts with which people are commonly educated might help here. First, many environmental philosophers work from a concept of personal identity that appreciates individuals as strongly connected with all humans, creatures, and the natural world in a cyclical flow of materials and energy. The concept of "ecosystem health" draws on the close relationship of human health to the condition of nature and makes it conceptually immediate to think of human health as dependent on ecosystem health. This more holistic self-concept can help individuals to accept an extended sense of responsibility through an appreciation of connectedness with others and the natural world.

Second, part of our sense of personal identity and integrity depends on our ability to assume responsibilities for others, and so a moral conversation conscious of the need for people to meet their responsibilities could help to fulfill more completely the humanness of individuals. This Kantian approach ultimately rests the freedom of the individual on his or her ability to fulfill his or her sense of duty. In health care ethics, it would thus become acceptable to expand the ethics conversation over "What does this patient want?" to include "How can we help this patient fulfill his or her sense of responsibility?" Principles of environmental responsibility and awareness of environmental effects need to be built into health care education and decisions at every level.

Key Ethical Tensions

To establish an ethical balance between environmental concerns and a commitment to patient care, three major dilemmas must be addressed: the individual versus the whole, sustainability versus social justice, and sustainability versus health.

The Individual Versus the Whole

The Hippocratic principle of "do no harm" has strongly influenced the ethics of health care. This principle also requires that health care maintain sustainable practices and avoid harm to both humans and the natural world. Although medicine is already rife with dilemmas in which avoiding harm to patients results in harm or burdens to others, broadening our ethical responsibilities to include nature and future generations will undoubtedly intensify such conflicts. Perhaps the most difficult will be the inevitable conflicts between the individual and the whole. In medical ethics, the tendency has been to emphasize the responsibility of the health care provider to the individual patient—the relationship of trust; the need for the physician to keep the patient's benefit foremost. Global environmental concerns press physicians and other health care professionals to ask first "How will this commitment to care for patients place long-term burdens on the sustainability of health care?"

Sustainability Versus Social Justice

Environmental sustainability and social justice are mutually reinforcing goals, and both are vital elements of population health. Yet the easy alliance of these two extraordinarily idealistic goals arouses a deeper sense of unease. The scale of these questions is so broad, and the empirical data available on their interrelationships so minimal, that one can only speculate. Can industrialized countries in the Northern Hemisphere support their high levels of health care consumption without exploiting or ignoring widespread poverty, environmental degradation, ill health, and suffering in poorer regions of the world? The scope of the world's present distributive injustice—and the sheer number of people struggling to live with almost nothing—coupled with the profound constraints of our already-stressed ecosystems call into question our ability to achieve both sustainability and justice. We may have to ask which should have primacy.

Sustainability Versus Health

The need for limits suggests potential problems for maintaining good health conditions in the long term. As the 1993 World Bank Development Report showed, health improvement in the twentieth century was closely linked to economic development. Improved health and life expectancy were afforded by industrial and technological growth that stabilized food supplies, processed sewage, cleaned and transported water, developed vaccines, improved education, established health records and surveillance, and devised effective medical technologies.

However, seeking gains in human health and welfare through aggressive economic development without regard for environmental effects may guarantee the ecological disaster already at our doorstep. Indeed, the increasing intensity of the agricultural, industrial, and energy sectors of the economy can be connected with increasing public health problems. And if the world's most developed economies reduce their overall consumption of natural resources and materials to achieve sustainability, and if their health service industries thereby accomplish parallel reductions, will these health services become less effective? There is some evidence from less developed nations that good public health can be maintained on minimal resources when these resources are appropriately directed at basic public health infrastructures such as clean air and water, sanitation, education, and stable food supplies. Will hospitals and clinics in the most highly technological and developed economies be able to learn to treat patients effectively while using fewer natural resources? If a significant scaling down of the health care sector is necessary, this may mean that some acutely ill individuals needing costly therapies will not receive treatment. Will the already troubling ethical issues of rationing high-tech care necessarily be extended to an even wider range of health care services?

Prescriptions

Health care professionals can offer leadership both in devising environmentally sound health care practices and in articulating the principles of sustainable health. Jane Lubchenco has urged scientists to undertake a new social contract to redirect the research enterprise from immediate social benefits toward a sustainable biosphere. Similarly, health care professionals need to include environmental care among their primary ethical obligations. This obligation can first be expressed by increasing consciousness of environmental issues in the education of health care professionals and patients, but it must eventually lead to appreciable reductions in the material scale of the world's most advanced health care services. Health care professionals will thus have to become actively involved in the ethical debates concerning balancing environmentally responsible health care with clinical services.

If the bright vision of the World Health Organization's fiftieth year is to be sustained, bioethics and health policy must begin to speak with one voice both to the needs of individuals and to the limitations of nature. Because earth's biological systems are necessary for human well-being, our medical pursuit of health must not diminish the abundance and vitality of the natural world.

Medicine After Oil

It Could Be Distributed a Lot More Democratically

DANIEL BEDNARZ

Orion (July/August 2007): 72–73.

The scale and subtlety of our country's dependency on oil and natural gas cannot be overstated. Nowhere is this truer than in our medical system.

Petrochemicals are used to manufacture analgesics, antihistamines, antibiotics, antibacterials, rectal suppositories, cough syrups, lubricants, creams, ointments, salves, and many gels. Processed plastics made with oil are used in heart valves and other esoteric medical equipment. Petrochemicals are used in radiological dyes and films, intravenous tubing, syringes, and oxygen masks. In all but rare instances, fossil fuels heat and cool buildings and supply electricity. Ambulances and helicopter "life flights" depend on petroleum, as do personnel who travel to and from medical workplaces in motor vehicles. Supplies and equipment are shipped—often from overseas—in petroleum-powered carriers. In addition there are the subtle consequences of fossil fuel reliance. A recently retired doctor informs me, "In orthopedics we used to set fractures mostly by feel and knowing the mechanics of how the fractures were created. I doubt that many of the present orthopedists could do a good job if you took away their [energy-powered] fluoroscope or X-ray."

Despite this enormous vulnerability, public discussions of health care routinely ignore the prospect of peak oil. The proposed reforms, which seek to cover more people while holding down escalating costs, amount to little more than fiscal maneuvers. They take no notice of ecological resource constraints that will set limits on our ability to give people access to medical care.

The coming scarcity of fossil fuels, on top of inflationary costs in medicine (the prices of oil and natural gas are approximately four times

what they were in 1999 and rising) and the expenses of treating Baby Boomers (a cohort twice the size of its predecessor), could overwhelm a medical system already in crisis. We can avoid collapse, however, by reducing medicine's present consumption of energy and creating a health-care system that reflects our actual relationship to resources. Ironically, peak oil can be a catalyst for creating a health-care system that is cost-effective, ecologically sustainable, and congruent with a democratic social ethos.

At present we have a tiered health-care system. At the top is a Ferrari model of care that reflects our affluence, fascination with technology, and extravagance. Ferrari care has made possible the treatment of rare life-threatening diseases and expensive procedures like organ transplants, but it has also been used for esoteric and often redundant testing and vanity procedures such as botox injections. At the bottom is a jalopy model serving over 50 million un- and underinsured Americans who very often receive no treatment, defer treatment until their condition cannot be ignored, or face economic ruin when they seek adequate care. If the two tiers persist after peak oil, they will eventually be preserved by force—armed guards at gated medical facilities— for the few able to pay, while the rest of Americans are relegated to the jalopy and faced with overt rationing, triage, and curtailment of medical care. Such an outcome would be an overt contravention of democratic values—most Americans tell pollsters they believe that health care is a human right, not a privilege awarded those with higher income.

What then should we do? The best democratic option is to replace both the Ferrari and the jalopy with a Honda. The post-peak Honda health-care model will of necessity operate with fewer overall resources and less energy than today's health-care system, and at lower cost. But it need not result in poorer quality of care. Although the United States spends more on health than any other nation—per capital health-care costs in this country are three times those in Great Britain and more than twice those in Canada—we do not have the best health outcomes. A study in the *Journal of the American Medical Association* in 2006, for example, reported that "white, middle-aged Americans—even those who are rich—are far less healthy than their peers in England."

The commonsensical Honda model will emphasize public health—the prevention of disease and the promotion of health within the population as a whole—over treatment medicine, which focuses on restoring health to chronically or acutely ill individuals. Typically accomplished through the diffusion of information, low-cost therapies, and the promotion of healthful nutrition and lifestyle, preventive medicine allows people to avoid or postpone disease, and to stay clear of the costliest and most energy-intensive sectors of the medical system—doctors' offices, pharmacies, and the hospital. In the Honda model, treatment medicine would continue, but its role would be brought into better balance with the vastly more cost-effective and energy-efficient mode of preventive health care.

The public health system arose in the early decades of the last century as a response to fears of infectious diseases in our country's crowded cities. Its outlook is inherently egalitarian—if the entire community is not protected, then no one's health is assured. Public health is no longer the force it was when it sent "ladies in white uniforms" into communities to preach the Gospel of Germs, explaining the relationship between hygiene and disease prevention. Today, public health is overburdened and underfunded, receiving about 5 percent of health-care dollars, with the balance going to treatment medicine and to biomedical research.

Despite funding inadequacies, public health is in place and functioning. Public health workers, for example, educate about and test for HIV/AIDS and other sexually transmitted diseases; they interdict infectious diseases like avian flu; they create emergency plans to deal with a variety of disaster scenarios; they monitor waste management and air and water quality. No new system needs to be invented or institutionalized to meet the health-care challenges of the coming energy transition, or, for that matter, those of climate change.

Already, some public health officials are beginning to address peak oil's effect on health care. On the national level, the Center for Environmental Health at the Centers for Disease Control is investigating impacts of petroleum scarcity on pharmaceuticals. In Congress, a Peak Oil Caucus led by Roscoe Bartlett (R-MD) and Tom Udall (D-NM), is looking into the health risks posed by economic decline and mass unemployment, which peak oil is likely to trigger. At the local level, Indianapolis's Marion County Health Department is the first in the country to begin planning for maintaining public health services under differing scenarios of energy scarcity.

Late though the hour is, we can still avert the worst health consequences of an energy downturn, but doing so will require transforming our entire health-care system. The elitist impulse to perpetuate Ferrari care for the explicit benefit of the few at the expense of the many will persist after peak oil, and substantial citizen action will be needed to put into effect the affordable, egalitarian Honda model. Medicine itself could play a central role in this effort, by educating those who are unaware of the sweeping changes peak oil will initiate. Reprising its inaugural campaign against germs, public health could become a platform for disseminating a Gospel of Energy Conservation. For the most part, the medical community is as naïve about peak oil as the rest of the citizenry. As one public health official told me after hearing about medicine's reliance on oil, "Oh my, I never thought of it that way. This is serious."

Deep Ecology and End-of-Life Care

PAUL CARRICK

Cambridge Quarterly of Healthcare Ethics 8 (1999): 107–17, 250–56.

Whoever wishes to pursue properly the science of medicine, must proceed thus. First he ought to consider what effects each season of the year can produce . . . The next point is the hot winds and the cold, especially those that are universal . . . He must consider the properties of the waters . . . The soil, too, whether bare and dry or wooded and watered . . . Through these considerations . . . [the physician] will have full knowledge of each particular case, will succeed best in securing health, and will achieve the greatest triumphs in the practice of his art.

—*Hippocrates, 5th Century B.C.*
Airs Waters Places

Introduction

Physicians and nurses caring for terminally ill patients are expected to center their moral concerns almost exclusively on the needs and welfare of the dying patient and the patient's family. But what about the relationship of traditional medical ethics to the emerging new theories of environmental ethics, like deep ecology? As we glide into the twenty-first century, can anyone seriously doubt that the mounting global concerns of environmental ethics will eventually influence the ethics of medicine too?

For example, suppose physicians were to integrate the core values of an ecocentric environmental ethic like deep ecology into contemporary North American norms of healthcare for the dying. How would this shift affect the attitudes and treatment decisions of caregivers toward the terminally ill? Specifically, would the medical community's adoption of the deep ecology ethic help or hurt the interests of the dying and their families?

In particular, suppose the dying patient were a partisan of the deep ecology philosophy of the Norwegian philosopher Arne Naess.[1] Would this dying patient then feel some added pressure to opt for voluntary active euthanasia? In fact, does deep ecology implicitly encourage the notion that the terminally ill should quit life early in order to conserve medical and other valuable resources in a world as over-populated by humans as ours? And would the adoption of a global environmental ethic such as deep ecology diminish or reinforce the autonomy of the dying patient?

In pursuing these issues, I am going to focus on conflicts between the scope of traditional anthropocentric medical ethics and global ecocentric environmental ethics. My thesis is that in its noble effort to upgrade the value of non-human animal and plant life and to redirect our moral attention to caring for the broader biotic community, deep ecology in effect downgrades the value of human individuals living now. This is particularly so for those who are aged, chronically sick, and terminally ill. To be sure, I will raise questions about what I call the tendency toward "environmental paternalism." I will argue that we should be cautious of importing global environmental ethical theories into our healthcare ethics precisely because these environmental theories, often with the best intentions, may undermine respect for individual human life.

My plan of inquiry is threefold. First, I will introduce the case study of Mildred Vanderwall, a terminally ill patient. This case will illustrate some possible moral stresses and conflicts experienced by patients newly diagnosed with Alzheimer's disease and flirting with suicide. Second, I will explicate and critically discuss some of the leading concepts and principles associated with Naess's deep ecology program. I will suggest how this program, should it become influential in society, might affect the attitudes and medical choices of caregivers and terminally ill patients. Last, I will extrapolate from this case to explore some of the larger implications of the deep ecology ethic for healthcare ethics generally. Admittedly, it is bold to imagine that physicians or patients will become deep ecologists or environmental partisans any time soon. Even so, by exploring the cross currents of environmental ethics and healthcare ethics, this essay reveals some of the particulars of their uneasy marriage.

The Case of Mildred Vanderwall

Mildred Vanderwall, age 61, was recently diagnosed with Alzheimer's disease. She is in the early stages and may live for 8 to 10 years before Alzheimer's takes her life.

An accomplished symphony musician and a divorced mother of three adult children, Mildred's failing memory led her to resign her violinist position two months ago with the Cleveland Symphony Orchestra. She took early retirement, declining a European tour that was to have begun later in the year.

Just last month, Mildred was informed by her personal physician, Dr. Stanley Rosenbaum, of the inevitable course of Alzheimer's. She intends to live independently as long as she can. As her powers slip, she intends to move into a nursing care facility. She is frightened by the hopelessness of her diagnosis, a diagnosis currently shared by four million Americans nationwide. Yet she has vowed not to be a burden to her adult children. The thought of suicide has entered her head.

Mildred learns that there is no single test for Alzheimer's. She learns that it is diagnosed by ruling out all other likely diseases. She also learns that there is no cure, and that only one drug, Tacrine, is FDA-approved specifically for Alzheimer's. She discovers that Tacrine slows somewhat the onslaught of the debilitating symptoms. Mildred tries to comprehend that she will in time become a total stranger to herself—she will experience a total loss of her core identity, her sense of being human in the world.

This unalterable fact depresses her. The option of suicide never completely fades even though she is being treated with the antidepressant Zoloft™. She is also currently in individual counseling biweekly with a geriatric psychotherapist.

Fundamentally, Mildred Vanderwall believes in God; she is a practicing Lutheran. Though she has flirted with thoughts of suicide, four months have now passed since Mildred received her Alzheimer's diagnosis. Following a personal visit by her pastor, Reverend Turner, she now feels opposed to both voluntary active euthanasia and physician-assisted suicide. She feels this would be for her a cowardly and sinful way out. (Her rejection of physician-assisted suicide also conforms to current Lutheran church doctrine.)

End-of-Life Decisions

In exploring some of the links between traditional medical ethics and environmental ethics, and with an eye toward anticipating some of the ethical implications of physician-assisted suicide for the terminally ill (an option recently reviewed and denied by the U.S. Supreme Court), I begin with three observations.

First, Mildred's opposition to voluntary active euthanasia for the terminally ill is defensible on moral if not also on religious grounds. I will offer a brief sketch of this defense shortly and at least show that it cannot be easily dismissed.

Second, stock environmental ethics concerns about the global impact of human overpopulation, or worries about depleting limited medical or other resources resulting from longterm care of Alzheimer's patients like Mildred, challenge but do not defeat moral resistance to voluntary active euthanasia.

Third, one of the primary benefits to discussions of medical ethics derived from environmental ethics is that the latter's broader, global concerns invite us to weigh more carefully several significant metaphysical questions that are seldom introduced by medical ethics investigations alone. These grand questions include:

1) Where does humanity fit into the general scheme of things?

2) What, if any, moral obligations to end their lives do the infirm or dying elderly owe to future, unborn generations?

3) What moral consideration do humans owe to nonhuman life, like hemlock trees, antelope, or chimpanzees with whom we share this planet?

A Metaphysical Mind-Shift

Arne Naess and his leading American disciples, Bill Devall and George Sessions, have sketched or hinted at tentative answers to these three questions. In an effort to explicate the core ideas of the deep ecology mindset, let us turn to their theses.

For example, in answer to (1), Where does humanity fit into the general scheme of things?, their *doctrine of biocentric equality* asserts that humanity is not privileged: people are only a part of nature.[2] Humanity has no greater or lesser inherent value as a life form than any other living thing.[3]

In answer to (2), What, if any, moral obligations to end their lives do the infirm or dying elderly owe to future, unborn generations?, the deep ecology view suggests that the infirm elderly and dying may owe to future generations of humans (and other nonhuman life forms too) the moral duty not to linger when the quality of their lives is profoundly reduced by the ravages of disease. Why? Because to prolong human life when that life is not capable any longer of reaching its species-defined potential—due to disease or decrepitude—contradicts the deep ecology ideal of the mature "ecological self," a self that all must strive to attain. As Devall and Sessions clarify, in deep ecology "the sense of self requires a further maturity and growth, an identification which goes beyond humanity to include the nonhuman world" and our impact as humans on that world.[4]

That is, one must think beyond one's own selfish needs in the present to the needs of nonhumans and other life forms and what is best for the posterity of the earth in the long run. This consti-

tutes a radical new vantage point from which to experience oneself in relation to other beings and to nature. If adopted by healthcare professionals, this perspective also implies that those nurturing the dying need to rethink whether their support and resources might be better spent nurturing the larger, equally valuable biotic community. No doubt to some this sort of question smacks of inhumane, environmental hubris. But to others it marks a long overdue correction in the resetting of global healthcare priorities. For example, is it not much more fiscally and environmentally prudent to encourage physician-assisted suicide for the dying rather than to encourage the dying to hang on in their usual misery or reduced quality of life?

For reasons to be explored below, I personally remain skeptical of the therapeutic implications of deep ecology for the humane practice of medicine.

Finally, in answer to (3), What moral considerations do humans owe to non-human life?, it follows from Naess's deep ecology framework that the moral duties that humans owe to nonhumans may at times be equivalent in moral force to those duties that humans customarily owe only to each other. To elaborate:

> *Biocentric equality* is intimately related to all-inclusive *self-realization* in the sense that if we harm the rest of Nature then we are harming ourselves. There are no boundaries and everything is interrelated. But insofar as we perceive things as individual organisms or entities, the insight draws us to respect all human and non-human individuals in their own right as parts of the whole without feeling the need to set up hierarchies of species with humans on top.[5]

To further summarize, Naess's deep ecology "eco-sophy" (as he dubs it) declares that human communities will live in cooperation with nature provided that at least two conditions are met: (1) each person's self-identification with nature is regularly practiced as a set of personal habits; and (2) the biocentric equality of all living things is accepted as a moral starting point.

Again, self-realization means that each individual's spiritual growth must transcend the isolated, competitive human ego, maturing to experience the oneness and harmony of the entire biotic community. Relatedly, biocentric egalitarianism means that all living things, including humans, plants, animals, and even rivers, mountains, and ecosystems, are of equal moral worth, of equal intrinsic value. The revolutionary ethical credo is that humans are not above or outside of nature. Nor should humans continue to view themselves in such a pre-Darwinian, ignorant way.

Moreover, no account of the deep ecology philosophy would be complete without mention of Naess's formula for right living:

"Rich life, simple means."

In a 1995 essay Naess states that this aphorism "suggests for medical bioethics a strengthening of preventive medicine, and a reduced reliance on technologically advanced treatments—especially if they require large investments of resources and energy." He concludes, "Medical bioethics can learn from ecological bioethics the need for a moral vision that can reorder its priorities."[6]

Respect for Human Life

Let us return to the case of Mildred Vanderwall. We recall her eventual opposition to voluntary active euthanasia, especially following her discussion with her pastor. At least two sturdy arguments can be marshaled in support of Mildred's rejection of voluntary active euthanasia. The first is the secular respect for human life argument. The second is the theological sanctity of human life argument. Although Mildred adheres to the theological version especially, each has deep roots in our Western ethical heritage.

The secular version of the respect for human life argument says that human life has moral worth in and of itself. Why? Precisely because human life is the highest known form of life. Furthermore, human life is asserted to have a basic dignity, intelligence, and autonomy setting it apart from all other creatures. Therefore, to willfully destroy human life—except possibly in self-defense or to prevent an even greater evil—is wrong. But voluntary active euthanasia willfully destroys a human life. Therefore, it is wrong. On this particular argument, the act of killing a person is not wrong because it produces a social disutility like, say, removing a gainfully employed citizen from the tax rolls. Rather, it is wrong because human life is inherently valuable, irrespective of what people can or cannot contribute to their society.

What about the theological sanctity of human life argument, which also condemns voluntary active euthanasia? A standard version of this argument arises from the notion that human life is a gift from God. For example, Aquinas writes, "it belongs to God alone to pronounce sentence of death or life.. . ."[7] We are, in effect, trustees of this unique life. According to this argument, then, human life is a divine-like, special gift. Therefore, to willfully end one's own life via active euthanasia offends God. Indeed, such human ingratitude is morally repugnant and sinful. It falls far short of God's moral law as expressed in the Old and New Testaments.

Of course, some philosophers would dismiss this and similar theological arguments. For one thing, they demand a compelling proof for the existence of a purposive, caring God of the sort this argument requires. However, it deserves repeating that this is a theological argument, not a philosophical one. Hence, as Tom Beauchamp has pointed out, *if* theology provides reasons that are valid *independently* of philosophy, as a variety of religious traditions have insisted (for example, revealed truths, miracles, prophecies, etc.), then philosophical objections to such arguments are far from fatal.[8] For this reason, Mildred Vanderwall's religious objections to voluntary active euthanasia cannot be discounted. She has a fair point if one grants that there may indeed exist theological, revealed truths in our universe.

Yet how different these two arguments look—the secular respect for human life argument and the theological sanctity of human life argument—when weighed against the implied force of Naess's deep ecology program. As I will show, deep ecology tends to undermine these arguments.

Take, for example, two related claims. The first claim is that long-term care of doomed Alzheimer's patients is morally questionable because it squanders valuable and limited medical and other resources. These resources could be more usefully pressed into the service of the biotic community elsewhere. For example, according to one study, Mildred and her family will incur individual expenses exceeding $213,000 during the usual 4 years between diagnosis and death from Alzheimer's.

The second claim is that long-term care of doomed Alzheimer's patients is morally questionable because in the wake of global human overpopulation, the dying aged are too great a burden on the entire ecosystem—fellow humans, other living things, the whole planet.

So on this account not only is there nothing wrong morally with voluntary active euthanasia for those who are terminally ill, should a patient like Mildred elect it. What's more, there may be a prima facie duty to quit life in such terminally ill circumstances based on global environmental considerations such as air, land, and water pollution; deforestation; ozone depletion; global warming; loss of biodiversity. That is, most of this environmental destruction and biological impoverishment identifies the swelling human population as a major cause of these ecological ills.

To be sure, the balancing and regulation of human populations, human goods and services, and their global impact ultimately involve questions of individual human worth and distributive justice. For example, should we redistribute our healthcare resources away from those who are hopelessly ill and toward those who are healthy, those who are recovering, and the young?

Deep Ecology and Healthcare Ethics

To briefly explore the force of this last query, consider that deep ecologists (as opposed to shallow, strictly human-centered ecologists, in Naess's language) assert that our dominant Western world view is responsible for much of the world's current environmental degradation. Therefore, we need an alternative world view to the flawed Judeo-Christian or capitalist-dominated perspective held by most medical practitioners in the richer, first world nations. Part of the alternative world view of deep ecology is borrowed from Eastern philosophies like Hinduism, Buddhism, and Taoism.[9] These are oriental religious traditions that tend to see humans as fully integrated into nature rather than dominating nature (as in the typically Western schema). Another part of deep ecology's alternative world view is taken from the pages of evolutionary biology and scientific ecology: namely, the notion that all life forms function as an interdependent holistic web, no part of which is completely isolated from any other.

In this section, I shall show how deep ecology's alternative world view, coupled with a pair of its central platform principles, pushes terminally ill patients in the direction of physician-assisted suicide.

Naess and Sessions have articulated a platform of eight "eco-philosophical" principles as both a summary and a decidedly pacifistic call to arms. These eight principles are designed to provide a core platform around which the eclectic deep ecology movement can be deployed worldwide by local and regional activists, who sometimes call themselves "eco-warriors."[10] With an eye to the moral endorsement or condemnation of voluntary active euthanasia for Alzheimer's or other terminal patients, only two of these eight principles will be investigated here:

4. The flourishing of human life and cultures is compatible with a *substantial decrease* of the human population. The flourishing of non-human life requires such a decrease. [population reduction principle]

7. The ideological change [needed] is mainly that of appreciating life quality . . . rather than [humans] adhering to a high standard of living.. . . [life quality principle][11]

These two crucial social policy norms associated with the deep ecology program together have often-overlooked implications for the humane practice of medicine.

How do Naess and Sessions defend the population reduction principle? Their starting point is that high human population growth rates in many developing countries will ultimately diminish the quality of life for millions of people across the globe.

Like many areas of debate in environmental law and public policy, these two principles are easily adapted to consequentialist (or results-based) reasoning. For example, the *population reduction principle* tacitly alludes to the fact that in less than 60 years our human population is projected to almost double, going from 6.3 billion today to perhaps over 10 billion by the year 2050.

What's more, the related *life quality principle* almost certainly invites a consequentialist argument favoring a prima facie duty for the terminally ill to seek a form of voluntary active euthanasia. Again, this life quality principle asserts that the quality of human life must be our chief moral concern, not the mere quantity. In addition, this principle is compatible with a cost-benefit perspective according to which prolonging a nonproductive human life unjustly drains limited medical and other resources[12] This last claim may be asserted even though, ironically, the whole notion of what a life worth living is defies any precise definition by strictly quantitative methods of assessment.

We are now ready to uncover the more opaque implications of the deep ecology framework. I suggest that, overall, unanswered momentous questions and conflicting moral duties abound.

Deep Ecology and Patient Care

Broadly construed, how would the deep ecology philosophy of Arne Naess, George Sessions, and William Devall reshape Western medicine? Specifically, how would this philosophy challenge the time-tested quartet of bioethical principles: autonomy, beneficence, justice, and nonmaleficence?[13] Would patients and their caregivers be better or worse off were the deep ecology paradigm shift to go through?

Autonomy

Take the concept of patient *autonomy*. This notion requires that the competent patient be understood as a self-determining agent of his or her own aims, goals, or destiny. In my view, under the influence of deep ecology this concept would now be regularly overridden by what I have dubbed *ecological paternalism*. By ecological paternalism, I mean that the proposed actions of an individual or group may be overridden by an informed judgment of the long-term negative consequences likely to result from these proposed actions on the local, regional, or global environment.

Incidentally, who would be licensed to make this patient care judgment? Perhaps a specially trained and duly appointed, environmentally sensitive hospital committee of some sort. Or alternatively, a deep ecology healthcare expert—that is, someone highly educated in the nuances of holistic environmental philosophy and medicine. Or someone who would competently and compassionately monitor a hospital's global environmental interests within the patient care matrix of curing and caring? In any case, such critically important questions about the chain of command and scope of medical decision-making are studiously ignored by the proponents of deep ecology. This is most peculiar, for the individual patient and his or her medical team would certainly be required to yield to the directives of a higher moral authority associated with the utopian thinking of these deep ecology visionaries.

To illustrate, take the case of George, a lung cancer patient who wishes to amuse himself in the last 6 months of his life by taking his favorite chain saw and cutting down a dozen old-growth hemlock trees situated on 10 acres of land he owns in Pine Grove, Pennsylvania. Neither George nor anyone else would be using these cut trees. Nor does George intend them to be used. His aim is simply to engage in some exercise and sheer fun by cutting down these hemlocks that he owns. Because no "vital needs" of George would be served (to employ Naess's and Sessions's vague phrase), and because the trees are of equal worth due to the principle of biocentric equality, George's joyful chainsawing must be overruled and condemned as morally wrong.[14] Typical of the deep ecology gestalt, the environment and specifically the old-growth hemlocks are in this scenario a more important consideration than the individual's psychological and physical wants. This, even though the satisfaction of these wants may be completely legal and—on a traditional anthropocentric ethical yardstick— morally unobjectionable.

Beneficence

Beneficence, the notion that the physician must try to practice good deeds primarily for the sake of his patient's health and welfare, will need to be modified by deep ecology, too. How so? Because its moral scope of concern will now be expanded to include not just the patient but the entire surrounding biosphere within which the patient lives, works, and plays. So beneficence is, in effect, redefined to mean *biospherical beneficence*.

But what does this mean? Consider Jake, another terminally ill, competent patient. Jake has colorectal cancer. He refuses to quit smoking because at age 80 he still really likes "his smokes," as he affectionately calls them. Legally blind and growing weaker in the last two months of his life, smoking is one of life's few remaining pleasures. But the deep ecologist attending physician would overrule Jake's autonomous desire to continue smoking in the last weeks of his life. He would also overrule the hospice nurses who wink at Jake's smoking. This despite the fact that their own sense of beneficence toward this particular patient's psychological needs is for them the morally decisive factor here. The nurses are required to confiscate Jake's cigarettes, which displeases him greatly and conflicts his caregivers.

It will no longer wash to say, beneficently and with an eye also to preserving Jake's sense of autonomy, "let the old gentleman smoke." Why confiscate the cigarettes? Because secondhand smoke is polluting too many living things—not to mention the unhealthy physical effects on Jake's

lungs and heart. Also, the carbon monoxide and other harsh pollutants in secondhand smoke are in the aggregate threatening to deplete the ozone layer. They contribute, also, to acid rain.

So the old anthropocentric healthcare ethic is adjusted to ask, What is good for the patient's immediate environment, his household, his surrounding community, and the entire biosphere?

These global considerations would easily override Jake's option to smoke, and that of all similarly situated patients.

Justice

Then there is the thorny concept of *justice*. By *justice*, in this context, I mean primarily the duty to render each person what is his or her due. In healthcare settings, the concept of justice presents a variety of rich applications and extensions. For example, allocating transplantable organs or other scarce medical resources in some fair manner of distribution, or ensuring that every citizen has adequate access to medical care. So how does the deep ecology program redirect our concern about justice, especially distributive justice? In my opinion, it does so in at least two ways.

First, deep ecology increases our sensitivity about what constitutes a just response to the needs of nonhuman animals or plants. As we saw in the case of George, we should not encourage a terminally ill patient to amuse himself by cutting down old-growth trees even on his own property. This is so not simply because such conduct is wasteful of trees. That would be a mere instrumental reason; it still ignores the alleged inherent worth of the trees as valuable beings in and of themselves. What's more, following from deep ecology's twin principles of *self-realization* and *biocentric equality*, this conduct is blameworthy because it is unjust both to the trees and to the patient's own sense of his discerning "ecological self," to use Naess's mysterious metaphysical language.

Second, deep ecology increases the sensitivity of the first world peoples living in the Northern, developed nations to the often unhealthy living conditions of the people in the Southern, developing nations. For example, consider that 99% of all infectious diseases occur in the developing nations.[15] Also, in these same countries, 80% of all diseases are caused by consuming water contaminated with pathogens or pollution.[16] The point is that since deep ecology's eight platform principles also declare (in principle 1) that "the well-being and flourishing of human and nonhuman life on earth have value in themselves," and that "these values are *independent of* the usefulness of the nonhuman world to human purposes," our concept of justice must widen dramatically.[17] It must now include not only what is due to each citizen living in his or her own society. It must also include what is due to all humans living anywhere on the planet. So what is due to starving Ethiopians or malnourished Haitian children becomes as pressing a question morally as what is due to the endangered elephant or bald eagle.

Nonmaleficence

Lastly, there is the keystone value of healthcare ethics, *nonmaleficence*. "[H]elp or at least do no harm," the Hippocratic physician implored over 2,000 years ago.[18] This is still sound advice in the age of high technology medicine. Moreover, this specific imperative of nonmaleficence (or noninjury) is no less crucial for palliative care of the terminally ill than it is for acute care patients awaiting, say, a kidney transplant. What, then, is the likely reframing of this notion of nonmaleficence if we imagine a paradigm shift in contemporary medicine toward an ecocentrically oriented deep ecology?

Quite simply, it is this: we must broaden our moral commitment of nonmaleficence, parallel to our broadened moral commitment of beneficence, in order to include the entire planet within the scope of our moral concern. It is imperative that we avoid injuring members of the human community in the practice of medicine, to be sure. Yet the deep ecology gestalt further asserts that all members of the biotic community, including nonhuman animals, plants, and even natural elements, deserve some moral consideration from every caregiver too. Unfortunately, such a sweeping scope of moral concern for the prima facie duty of nonmaleficence is highly impracticable.

To take but one example, deep ecology would in one stroke condemn almost all animal experimentation now crucially facilitating much of biomedicine's search for cures to a variety of insidious human diseases. To deep ecologists, this animal research is morally questionable: it causes physical and psychological injury to innocent creatures. Most are killed. In fact, virtually all such research animals are sacrificed in the caged wheels of biomedical progress (an estimated 17 to 22 million animals annually in the United States alone).[19]

Deep Ecology and Euthanasia

I conjectured that Naess's deep ecology program would endorse active voluntary euthanasia for any terminally ill patient who is competent, hurting, and agreeable to a somewhat earlier than usual exit from the ravages of his or her disease. I argued further that this endorsement follows from Naess's population reduction principle and life quality principle. It also follows from Naess's belief that the human population must be significantly reduced in order to bring into healthier balance all life forms with which *Homo sapiens* share this planet.

What, then, about involuntary euthanasia? Could Naess consistently endorse this draconian measure? He could not, for at least two reasons. First, Naess is on record as opposing the practices of Nazi medicine and Nazi culture. He states, "As deep ecologists, we take a natural delight in diversity as long as it does not include crude, intrusive forms like Nazi culture, that are destructive to others."[20] Second, he opposes despotic measures of any sort, especially those crushing to life. He writes, "For deep ecology, there is a core democracy in the biosphere . . . We have the goal not only of stabilizing human population but also of reducing it to a sustainable minimum without revolution or dictatorship."[21]

It comes as little surprise, therefore, that following from these persistent concerns about human overpopulation, the deep ecologists are forced by their principles to endorse the practice of passive voluntary euthanasia for the terminally ill as morally acceptable. Why? Because by declining to use the often high tech, costly rescue procedures involved in prolonging or sustaining the lives of those who are critically ill, aged, or dying, the ecologically mature medical community prudently signals to all persons the importance of conforming to the deep ecology credo, "rich life, simple means." In so doing, it is hoped that each person will live into old age for as long as nature, and the ecologically sensitive application of biomedicine, warrant. Ideally, each person will flourish at any stage along life's continuum. This will be accomplished by obtaining, when required, lower tech medical intervention; the discipline of a balanced diet (preferably vegetarian); the norms of preventive medicine; and the personal habits of regular exercise and sound hygiene—until that critical point in the life span of each individual is reached when to further coax life along one would have to resort to possibly futile, often painful, and usually expensive medical therapies.

Conclusion

I conclude with this caveat: theories of environmental ethics cannot and should not be ignored by biomedicine. Doubtless there is much to learn from these global calculations. But practically speaking, the jury remains out on the worth of the deep ecology program, and on an array of other ecocentric theories, for the humane practice of medicine. For when an environmental theory pressures the terminally ill to quit life in favor of the global claims of ecological paternalism, then the dignity, autonomy, and inherent value of that dying patient's life are diminished. As the earlier case of Mildred Vanderwall showed, a person's higher sense of duty to the individual worth of each human being, or to God, cannot be dismissed.

Moreover, as we saw, mere appeals to ecologically paternalistic concerns—such as the alleged negative impact of human overpopulation, or the alleged misallocation of scarce medical resources—that lead to judgments affecting how we care for those who are aged, frail, and dying, *do not* automatically trump either the secular or theological variants of the respect for human life principle. This principle has animated much of the caring tradition in the Western healing arts since the time of Hippocrates. Indeed, to yield that precious ground to any of the environmental philosophers today would amount to increasingly experiencing the patient as a mere means to some fanciful ecological Utopia. Again, if the dying patient is construed as a mere means, that patient is dispensable.

Precisely because the deep ecology program threatens to ignore patient autonomy in favor of environmental paternalism, and precisely because it tacitly cheapens the value of individual human life, deep ecology sows the seeds of a potentially misanthropic program of medical care. Therefore, it ought to be resisted.

Notes

1. Naess, A. "The Shallow and the Deep, Long-Range Ecology Movements: A Summary." *Inquiry* 16 (1973): 95–100. Naess, A. *Ecology, Community, and Lifestyles.* Edited and translated by D. Rothenberg. Cambridge: Cambridge University Press, 1989. Devall, B. and G. Sessions. *Deep Ecology: Living as if Nature Mattered.* Salt Lake City, UT: Peregrine Smith Books, 1985. Sessions, G. "Deep Ecology as World View." In *World Views and Ecology* Edited by M.E. Tucker and J.A. Grim, 207–27. Lewisburg, PA: Bucknell University Press, 1993.
2. See note 1, Devall, *Sessions* 1985:65–73.
3. See note 1, Devall, Sessions 1985:71. The authors state, "The *refusal* to acknowledge that some life forms have greater or lesser intrinsic value than others . . . runs counter to the formulations of some ecological philosophers and New Age writers." (Emphasis added).
4. See note 1, Devall, Sessions 1985:67.
5. See note 1, Devall, Sessions 1985:68.

6. Naess A. "Deep ecology." In *Encyclopedia of Bioethics*, rev. ed., edited by W.T. Reich, 687–88. New York: Macmillan, 1995, at p. 688.

7. Aquinas, T. *Summa Theologica* II-II, Q. 64, Art.5. For a critique of Aquinas' argument, see Beauchamp, T. "Suicide." In *Matters of Life and Death: New Introductory Essays in Moral Philosophy*, 3rd ed., edited by T. Regan, 69–120. New York: McGraw Hill, 1993. See also in that same volume: Singer, P. "Animals and the Value of Life." Ch. 8, 280–321; Callicott, JB. "The Search for an Environmental Ethic." Ch. 9, 322–82.

8. See note 7, Beachamp 1993:86.

9. Seed, J.J. Macy, P. Fleming, and A. Naess. *Thinking Like a Mountain: Towards a Council of All Beings*. Philadelphia: New Society Publishers, 1988, 19–30. Reprinted in *Environmental Ethics and Policy Book: Philosophy, Ecology, Economics*, edited by D. VanDeVeer and C. Pierce, 222–6. Belmont, CA: Wadsworth Publishing, 1994.

10. See note 9, VanDeVeer, Pierce 1994:238–46. Environmental activists associated with the worldwide "ecology movement" hold diverse environmental philosophies. For a concise overview, see note 7, Callicott 1993. See also Desjardin, J. *Environmental Ethics*. Belmont, CA: Wadsworth Publishing, 1993, 211–63. Desjardin's discussion of distinctions between deep ecology, social ecology, and ecofeminism are particularly instructive at pp. 236–39. See also note 1, Devall, Sessions 1985:17–39.

11. See note 1, Devall, Sessions 1985:70; Naess 1989:Ch. 1.

12. Naess does not explicitly endorse a cost-benefit analysis approach. His philosophy is eclectic and pluralistic, having more in common with the ethics of Gandhi and Kant than with the utilitarians Bentham and Mill. However, no philosopher can regulate how his philosophy will be interpreted, adapted, or even misused by others. In weighing the social as well as the strictly logical implications of deep ecology for healthcare ethics at the end-of-life, it is fair to speculate on even unintended outcomes.

13. Beauchamp, T. and J. F. Childress. *Principles of Biomedical Ethics*. 4th ed. New York: Oxford University Press, 1994, 120–394.

14. Devall, B., and G. Sessions. *Deep Ecology: Living as If Nature Mattered.* Salt Lake City, UT: Peregrine Smith Books, 1985, 71. See also Naess, A. *Ecology, Community, and Lifestyle.* Edited and translated by D. Rothenberg. Cambridge: Cambridge University Press, 1989. Naess and Sessions admit: "The term 'vital need' is left deliberately vague to allow for considerable latitude in judgment" (p. 71). In my view, their failure to operationalize or at least provide necessary conditions for this concept, is the Achilles' heel of their account. Distinguishing in detail between "needs," "wants," and "relative needs," is also largely ignored.

15. Brown, I. R., D. Flavin, and H. Kane. *Vital Signs 1966: The Trends That Are Shaping Our Future.* New York: W. W. Norton, 1996, 130–1.

16. See note 15, Brown, Flavin, Kane 1996, 130–1.

17. See note 14, Devall, Sessions 1985:70 emphasis.

18. Carrick, P. *Medical Ethics in Antiquity: Philosophical Perspective on Abortion and Euthanasia.* Boston: Kluwer Academic Publishers, 1985, 156–8.

19. Office of Technology Assessment. *Alternatives to Animal Use in Research, Testing, and Education.* Washington, DC: U.S. Government Printing Office, 1986.

20. See note 14, Devall, Sessions 1985:75–6.

21. See note 14, Devall, Sessions 1985:75–6.

Declaration of Professional Responsibility

Medicine's Social Contract with Humanity

AMERICAN MEDICAL ASSOCIATION

http://www.arria-assn.org/ama/upload/mm/369/declaration.pdf

Preamble

Never in the history of human civilization has the well being of each individual been so inextricably linked to that of every other. Plagues and pandemics respect no national borders in a world of global commerce and travel. Wars and acts of terrorism enlist innocents as combatants and mark civilians as targets. Advances in medical science and genetics, while promising great good, may also be harnessed as agents of evil. The unprecedented scope and immediacy of these universal challenges demand concerted action and response by all.

As physicians, we are bound in our response by a common heritage of caring for the sick and the suffering. Through the centuries, individual physicians have fulfilled this obligation by applying their skills and knowledge competently, selflessly and at times heroically. Today, our profession must reaffirm its historical commitment to combat natural and man-made assaults on the health and well being of humankind. Only by acting together across geographic and ideological divides can we overcome such powerful threats. Humanity is our patient.

Declaration

We, the members of the world community of physicians, solemnly commit ourselves to:

 I. Respect human life and the dignity of every individual.

 II. Refrain from supporting or committing crimes against humanity and condemn all such acts.

 III. Treat the sick and injured with competence and compassion and without prejudice.

 IV. Apply our knowledge and skills when needed, though doing so may put us at risk.

 V. Protect the privacy and confidentiality of those for whom we care and breach that confidence only when keeping it would seriously threaten their health and safety or that of others.

 VI. Work freely with colleagues to discover, develop, and promote advances in medicine and public health that ameliorate suffering and contribute to human well-being.

 VII. Educate the public and polity about present and future threats to the health of humanity.

 VIII. Advocate for social, economic, educational, and political changes that ameliorate suffering and contribute to human well-being.

 IX. Teach and mentor those who follow us for they are the future of our caring profession.

We make these promises solemnly, freely, and upon our personal and professional honor.

(Adopted by the House of Delegates of the American Medical Association in San Francisco, California on December 4, 2001.)

Stewardship of the Environment

AMERICAN MEDICAL ASSOCIATION

Policy H-135.973

The AMA: (1) encourages physicians to be spokespersons for environmental stewardship, including the discussion of these issues when appropriate with patients; (2) encourages the medical community to cooperate in reducing or recycling waste; (3) encourages physicians and the rest of the medical community to dispose of its medical waste in a safe and properly prescribed manner; (4) supports enhancing the role of physicians and other scientists in environmental education; (5) endorses legislation such as the National Environmental Education Act to increase public understanding of environmental degradation and its prevention; (6) encourages research efforts at ascertaining the physiological and psychological effects of abrupt as well as chronic environmental changes; (7) encourages international exchange of information relating to environmental degradation and the adverse human health effects resulting from environmental degradation; (8) encourages and helps support physicians who participate actively in international planning and development conventions associated with improving the environment; (9) encourages educational programs for worldwide family planning and control of population growth; (10) encourages research

and development programs for safer, more effective, and less expensive means of preventing unwanted pregnancy; (11) encourages programs to prevent or reduce the human and environmental health impact from global climate change and environmental degradation. (12) encourages economic development programs for all nations that will be sustainable and yet nondestructive to the environment; (13) encourages physicians and environmental scientists in the United States to continue to incorporate concerns for human health into current environmental research and public policy initiatives; (14) encourages physician educators in medical schools, residency programs, and continuing medical education sessions to devote more attention to environmental health issues; (15) will strengthen its liaison with appropriate environmental health agencies, including the National Institute of Environmental Health Sciences (NIEHS); (16) encourages expanded funding for environmental research by the federal government; and (17) encourages family planning through national and international support. (CSA Rep. G, I-89; Amended: CLRPD Rep. D, I-92; Amended: CSA Rep. 8, A-03; Reaffirmed in lieu of Res. 417, A-04)

CASES

Malaria and DDT

For many people, the three letters "DDT" are an iconic symbol of toxic chemicals run amuck in the natural environment, and a vivid reminder that lack of foresight in the use of chemicals can have tragic consequences. Yet DDT's dirty

history stands in odd contrast to its rebirth, in the twenty-first century, as a symbol of hope for millions of people suffering and dying from a largely preventable disease.

DDT (dichlorodiphenyl-trichloroethane) was first synthesized in 1874, but only came into widespread use during World War II, where it was employed by the military to control the spread of insect-borne diseases like malaria and typhus among the troops. When the war ended, DDT became available on the civilian market, and it quickly became a popular agricultural pesticide. In the early days of DDT, thousands upon thousands of tons were sprayed on crops throughout the United States and Europe.

The golden days of DDT came to an end in 1962, with the publication of Rachael Carson's *Silent Spring*. Carson documented the ecological devastation wrought by the widespread use of DDT and other synthetic chemicals, and posed links between pesticides and sharp declines in populations of birds and other wildlife. She also suggested links between DDT and human cancer.

DDT belongs to a group of chemicals called persistent organic pollutants (POPs), so-called because they persist, or "bioaccumulate," in the environment. POPs are stored in the body fat of animals, and their presence is magnified through the food chain, so that predatory species at the top of the food chain, including humans, often have very high concentrations of the chemicals in their blood and body fat. After *Silent Spring*, DDT became synonymous with environmental destruction. DDT was banned in the United States and many European countries in the 1970s.

Despite its bad reputation among environmentalists, DDT is considered by many public health experts to be one of the most important weapons against the global spread of malaria. Malaria causes more suffering and loss of life than almost any other disease. There are estimated to be at least three hundred million acute cases of malaria each year, and the disease kills more than a million people every year, most of them young children. Although spraying with DDT will not, by itself, end malaria, its appropriate use is considered vital to combating the disease and reducing the number of malaria deaths. Data on indoor spraying suggest that when used in small quantities, DDT is cheap, effective, and remarkably safe.

In 2006, the World Health Organization (WHO) endorsed widespread use of DDT across Africa. Although DDT has been in use in a number of African countries, WHO recommended that spraying be expanded into more geographic regions, and that it be combined with the use of insecticide-treated bed nets. Dr. Arata Kochi, the head of WHO's global malaria program, believes that DDT is the most effective insecticide against the *Anopheles* mosquitoes, whose bite carries the protozoan parasites that cause malaria. According to WHO, DDT poses negligible health risks when sprayed in small amounts on the inner walls of people's homes (Dugger 2006).

The nonprofit group Beyond Pesticides has publicly opposed WHO's policy, calling it shortsighted and dangerous. According to Beyond Pesticides, "Given the well-documented adverse health effects associated with DDT's toxic properties, and its persistence, the international community has a social responsibility to reject the use of this chemical and practice sound and safe pest management practices at the community level that prevent insect-borne diseases like malaria." Research on POPs suggests that even miniscule amounts can have widespread reverberations within biological systems.

Proponents of DDT-based malaria control argue that the amount of DDT sprayed within homes is very small, and is probably quite safe for the human inhabitants. Whether or not this is true, DDT arguably represents some level of threat to wildlife. The larger reverberations within ecosystems are not thoroughly understood, but research since the 1960s has confirmed Carson's claims that DDT is toxic to many species of birds. Metabolites of DDT interfere with calcium absorption, and eggshells become so thin that they break before chicks have a chance to develop. DDT has been linked, as just one example, to the dramatic decline of bald eagles and peregrine falcons.

The Precautionary Principle

The so-called precautionary principle is often referred to in discussions of environmental ethics and public health policy. One commonly cited formulation of the principle reads: "Where there are threats of serious or irreversible environmental damage, lack of full scientific certainty shall not be used as a reason for postponing cost-effective measures to prevent environmental degradation" (United Nations). The precautionary principle suggests that even inaction is a form of action. Furthermore, uncertainty cannot form a valid justification for inaction, since failure to act is a form of action (failure to respond to climate change, for example, is to endorse the status quo as an appropriate course of action).

Discussion Questions

1. How, if at all, should we weigh the survival of birds against human needs?
2. What guidance might the precautionary principle offer in response to this case?
3. Does it matter, morally speaking, that the harms caused by malaria are tangible and immediate, while harms to the environment may be more nebulous and long-term?
4. What other factual information would you want to collect in considering the wisdom of WHO's malaria control program?

Sources

Dugger, Celia W. "W.H.O. Supports Wider Use of DDT to Combat Malaria." *New York Times*, September 16, 2006.

Beyond Pesticides. "Groups say DDT use for malaria control threatens public health." 2006. http://www.beyondpesticides.org/news/daily_news_archive/2006/09_15_06.htm (accessed February 1, 2008).

Physicians and the Environmental Imperative

Dr. Paul S. Auerbach argued in the February 28, 2008, issue of *JAMA* that physicians must confront today's most pressing global issue: the state of the environment. After outlining the links between various environmental issues and threats to human health, he argues that physicians, in their professional role, must respond to the environmental imperative—they have a moral responsibility to increase their awareness of and involvement with environmental issues.

> By virtue of their knowledge and experience, physicians are rightfully concerned about individual and population health. However, medicine's focus on pathogens and disease processes may be misguided compared with the potential loss of life that may result from such environmental eventualities as the melting of the polar ice caps. The time has come to consider broadening what the medical profession must learn, expanding awareness by educating physicians about the best environmental science. Given the hypothetical and known links of global climate change to human health, and the increasing concern that this change is accelerating, medicine must be involved in any proposed mediation. ... Every physician should strive to be a physician for the environment.

Discussion Questions

1. Do you agree with Auerbach that physicians have a moral responsibility to become aware of and involved with environmental issues?
2. Auerbach's "environmental imperative" is based on the principle that physicians must be concerned with widespread loss of life resulting from environmental decline. In a sense,

physician responsibility is extended out to the whole planet. Can you think of some scenarios in which addressing the "environmental patient" would conflict with a physician's duty to benefit his or her particular patients?

3. Which should take moral priority in a physician's clinical decision making—the individual patient or the stability of ecosystems? Why?

Source

Auerbach, Paul S. "Physicians and the Environment." *JAMA* 299, no. 8 (2008): 956–58.

Population Connection

The current world population sits at just over 6.6 billion. In the past fifty years, human numbers have increased at breakneck speed—increasing more in the past fifty than in the previous four million years combined. There is some evidence that the population explosion that has brought us, over the past three centuries, to our current numbers is beginning to abate. Still, despite declining birth rates, the United Nations predicts that global numbers will reach about nine billion by 2050, before growth begins to really level off.

Explosive population growth is considered by many scientists and policymakers to be one of the main drivers of environmental degradation, alongside patterns of consumption and technology use. Global warming, loss of forests, water scarcity, species extinction, toxic pollution—all of these are exacerbated by growing human populations.

Discussion Questions

1. How should environmental constraints influence how doctors counsel patients about their reproductive decisions?

2. With less than five percent of the world's population, the United States consumes roughly twenty-five percent of the world's resources, and ranks highest in the world for carbon emissions. Some argue that people in highly consumptive societies like the United State have a stronger obligation to limit their reproduction, since one child consumes so much and has such a large ecological footprint, relative to children in other parts of the world. How would you assess this argument?

3. Consider the views of the Pontifical Council for the Family, a group that assists the pope in his jurisdiction over the Catholic Church.

The council urges Christians and all people of good will to educate themselves on the many ways the population-control movement uses the media to project economic and demographic statistics that are both simplistic and inexact.... The "anti-baby" mentality, so characteristic of population control programs, refuses to acknowledge God as the sole creator of life, and thus contributes to the culture of death.... In the words of Pope Paul VI, "You must strive to multiply bread so that it suffices for the tables of mankind, and not favor an artificial control of birth.... in order to diminish the number of guests at the banquet of life" (Nienstedt 2008).

What is your reaction? How would you relate this to the statements in the previous case?

4. Is there a morally neutral or purely scientific stance on the issue of population? If yes, what is it?

Source

Nienstedt, John C. "Facing Down the New Paradigm: The Family Planning Agenda of the United Nations' 'Millennial Goals'." *Crisis Magazine*. http://crisismagazine.com (accessed February 1, 2008). "The Population Institute." www.populationinstitute.org (accessed February 25, 2008).

Sustainable Trials

The carbon footprint of health care includes not only the activities of health care institutions like hospitals and clinics, but also the footprint of the machinery that functions behind and in support of these institutions. One substantial engine in this health care machinery is clinical research.

The Sustainable Trials Study Group, convened by the London School of Hygiene and Tropical Medicine, set out to assess the carbon costs of clinical research, with an eye toward eventually reducing greenhouse gas emissions. They began with a case study on one particular clinical trial, the U.K. Medical Council's so-called CRASH trial. This trial investigated the effect of corticosteroids on death and disability in adults with head injury.

The carbon audit of the trial took into account some of the following facts: The drug used in the trial was manufactured in the United States by Pfizer, and the placebo was made in France. Both drug and placebo were shipped to and packaged in Wales. The packaged drugs and placebos were then sent to London for distribution to hospitals in forty-nine different countries. The audit also took into consideration the coordination of the study by researchers, travel by researchers to participating countries, and the recruitment of patients. The Trials Study Group concluded that the CRASH trial generated about 630 tons of carbon dioxide equivalents, about the carbon cost of 525 roundtrip flights between London and New York.

Anthony J. McMichael and Hilary J. Bambrick note, in a commentary on the Sustainable Trials Study Group: "The notion of utility poses a challenge for research ethics. Each well-designed clinical trial has the potential to reduce morbidity or mortality, or both. Should that anticipated health benefit be assessed against the long-term health (and other) risks from climate change?"

Discussion Questions

1. What do McMichael and Bambrick mean by "utility"? What does utility have to do with the carbon footprint of research?
2. How would you answer McMichael and Bambrick's question?

Sources

McMichael, Anthony J., and Hilary J. Bambrick. "Greenhouse-gas costs of clinical trials." *The Lancet* 369 (May 12, 2007): 1584–85.
Sustainable Trials Study Group. "Towards Sustainable Clinical Trials." *British Medical Journal* 334 (2007):671–73.

Asthma Inhalers and Ozone

In 2006, the U.S. Food and Drug Administration announced that albuterol inhalers containing chlorofluorocarbon (CFC) propellants would be banned beginning in 2009, in accordance with a global agreement called the Montreal Protocol. The Montreal Protocol suggested a gradual phaseout of the CFC-containing consumer products, because CFCs deplete the stratospheric ozone layer. In the 1980s, scientists discovered a large hole in the ozone layer over Antarctica. They hypothesized that depletion of the ozone layer would pose a direct threat to human health and survival, since stratospheric ozone protects the earth from the sun's ultraviolet radiation. Decreased ozone protection would lead to increased exposure to UVA and UVB radiation. Albuterol inhalers containing CFC will be replaced with devices that use the ozone-safe propellant hydrofluoroalkane (HFA).

Unlike the old inhalers, for which inexpensive generics have long been available, the new ozone-friendly inhalers are covered by patents. This means the new inhalers will cost thirty to sixty dollars more than the older CFC-containing generic versions. The new inhalers use different drugs than many of the old devices. Commonly used over-the-counter inhalers such as Primatene Mist contain the drug epinephrine, whereas the new HFA inhalers contain albuterol. Epinephrine inhalers may no longer be available.

Many doctors are in favor of the transition to a new generation of inhalers—not for environmental reasons, but for medical ones. They see the transition as an opportunity to encourage the use of inhalers containing albuterol, which can help prevent asthma attacks rather than just address symptoms. The older, over-the-counter CFC inhalers such as Primatene Mist were designed for "rescue" breathing—they address symptoms, but not the underlying disease. Since Primatene Mist and other similar inhalers are available without a prescription, some doctors are concerned that asthmatics are self-diagnosing and self-treating, rather than seeking medical treatment for their asthma.

Some patient advocates argue that Primatene Mist and similar products provide an important stopgap treatment for people caught without their inhalers, who cannot see their doctors immediately. These over-the-counter inhalers may also be the only medicine available to those who cannot afford or do not want to see a doctor. Asthma is disproportionately common among low-income people, who tend to breathe dirtier air and be exposed to agents such as dust mites and cockroaches, which are associated with asthma attacks. These populations are often uninsured; thus, the high cost of inhalers will be most painfully felt by the very populations who need them most. According to federal officials, the new policy could translate into an additional cost of ninety-five dollars a year for the 1.25 million uninsured patients with asthma.

Consumer reactions have been mixed. A woman quoted in the *New York Times*—an upper-middle-class mother with two asthmatic children—said that the small increase in cost was worth protecting the environment. "For me," she said, "that's a small price to pay for a clean environment." But another patient interviewed for the same story thought the move away from CFC-containing devices was "straining at gnats": the burden on patients was too great, relative to the small amount of CFCs in each inhaler (Pollack 2006b). Yet another worried that the move would disproportionately burden the poor.

Discussion Questions

1. How should environmental harms, even small ones, weigh against benefits to individual patients? Is it fair to weigh the accumulated risks of many inhalers against cost and convenience for an individual patient?

2. What social justice issues does this case raise?

3. How should financial cost be weighed against environmental protection? Is ninety-five dollars per patient per year too much?

4. A "commons" problem is one in which there is a conflict between individual interests and the common good. Is this an example of a commons problem?

Sources

American Lung Association. "CFC-Free Inhalers: Time to Make the Switch." http://www.lungusa.org/site/pp.asp?c = dvLUK9OoE&b = 2222599 (accessed February 13, 2008).

Pollack, Andrew. "Expected Ban on Primatene Mist Raises Some Concerns." *New York Times*, May 12, 2006a.

——. "The Higher Cost of Breathing." *New York Times*, May 12, 2006b.

Tarkan, Laurie. "Rough Transition to a New Asthma Inhaler." *New York Times*, May 13, 2008.

U.S. Environmental Protection Agency. "Ozone Layer Depletion." http://www.epa.gov/ozone/strathome.html (accessed February 23, 2008).

Mussels on Prozac

Trace amounts of many pharmaceutical compounds have been found in rivers and streams throughout the United States. It also is likely that aquatic species are absorbing at least some of these chemicals. The effects of these chemicals on aquatic species are only now being studied, and very little is known at this point. But many scientists are already deeply concerned.

For example, research presented recently to the American Chemical Society showed that fluoxetine, more commonly known as the antidepressant Prozac, caused female mussels to prematurely release their larvae. This is unlikely to make the female mussels happy: larvae released too early are not viable, and will quickly perish. Of the three hundred or so known species of freshwater mussels, about seventy percent are already extinct, endangered, or in steep decline.

Scientists worry that pharmaceutical contamination may further hasten their demise. Mussels play a vital role in the healthy functioning of streams and rivers. They filter water, and are an important food source for fish, muskrats, and other animals. Trouble for the mussels will signal trouble for other species as well.

Mussels are, to rivers and streams, rather like the canary in a coal mine. Mussels eat by straining microorganisms out of hundreds upon hundreds of gallons of water, so any contaminants in the water are likely to pass through their bodies. If the mussels are in trouble, it is usually a sign of deeper problems that may not yet be visible. Therefore, the research on Prozac in mussels is troubling to those who worry about the health of our waterways. Indeed, traces of Prozac have also been found in other aquatic species like frogs and fish.

And it is not just Prozac. Low levels of a wide variety of pharmaceutical compounds, from aspirin to antibiotics to estrogen, have been found in surface waters, both in the United States and around the world. Many of these pharmaceuticals affect the endocrine systems of aquatic species: they disrupt hormones, and thus can affect development and behavior. Studies have found, for example, that estrogen (found in birth control pills) causes changes in gender expression (the "masculinization" of female fish and "feminization" of male fish). The widespread phenomenon of deformed frogs is attributed to endocrine-disrupting chemicals in the environment. Some scientists worry that chronic exposure by water-dwelling creatures to very low levels of the chemicals could accumulate slowly and go unnoticed until damage is irreversible.

There is no evidence that the traces of chemicals in the water are harmful to humans, but neither is there evidence to the contrary. Concern about the problem is relatively new, and no careful studies have yet been conducted. Although scientists do not know how serious the problem is, so far, these substances—what the Environmental Protection Agency calls "emerging contaminants"—have been found almost everywhere scientists have looked. Scientists do not yet know what exposure to these substances, especially in combination, might mean.

Pharmaceuticals wind up in waterways either through direct disposal (dumping unused or expired pills down the drain or into the trash can) or through residuals found in human excrement, both of which make their way through the wastewater system and back into streams and rivers.

The problems for aquatic creatures are likely to become more acute. Prescription drug use is on the rise. According to market analysis of the prescription drug industry, the percentage of prescriptions purchased in the United State grew by seventy percent in the decade from 1993–2003. The average number of prescriptions for each person increased from 7.8 to 11.8, according to the Kaiser Family Foundation (p. 1). At this point in time, very few pharmacies will accept unused prescriptions (though the number of take-back centers is beginning to grow). Many people will begin taking a drug, only to stop because of unpleasant side effects or simply out of laziness or forgetfulness. People who are prescribed an antibiotic will often, contrary to instructions, stop taking the pills when they start feeling better. Sometimes a patient may try five or six different drugs for a particular condition before finding the best fit. Doctors rarely give patients instructions about what to do with unused pills. All in all, this translates into a huge number of pills sitting in people's medicine cabinets, or winding up in their trashcans or toilets.

Discussion Questions

1. Some psychiatrists are concerned about what they see as the epidemic use of mood-enhancing or -stabilizing drugs like Prozac for what might be called "the human condition" (occasional stress, unhappiness, existential discomfort, or personal dissatisfaction) as opposed to the appropriate use of such drugs for clinical depression. How might consideration

of "need" enter into the discussion of pharmaceuticals and the environment?

2. Should the ultimate fate of a pharmaceutical product be part of the consideration, by patient and doctor, about whether and what drugs to take?

Sources

American Medical Association House of Delegates. Resolution 411 (A-06): "Safe Disposal of Unused Pharmaceuticals." http://www.ama-assn.org/ama1/pub/upload/mm/471/41/a06.doc (accessed September 15, 2006).

Dean, Cornelia. "Drugs Are in the Water. Does it Matter?" *New York Times*, April 3, 2007.

Daughton, Christian G., and Thomas A. Ternes. "Pharmaceuticals and Personal Care Products in the Environment: Agents of Subtle Change." *Environmental Health Perspectives Supplements* 107, no. 56 (1999): 907–38.

"Ingredient in Prozac Increases Risk of Extinction for Freshwater Mussels." *Science Daily*, 2006. http://www.sciencedaily.com/releases/2006/09/060914153812.htm (accessed September 15, 2006).

Jensen, Ric. "Scientists Explore If Pharmaceuticals Alter Quality of Rivers, Streams." Texas Water Resources Institute. 2004. http://twri.tamu.edu/newsarticles.php?view=2004–05–05 (accessed September 15, 2006).

Kaiser Family Foundation. "Prescription Drug Trends." 2007. http://www.kff.org/rxdrugs/upload/3057_06.pdf (accessed May 20, 2008).

United States Environmental Protection Agency, National Exposure Research Laboratory Environmental Sciences. "PPCPs as Environmental Pollutants: Pharmaceuticals and Personal Care Products in the Environment: Overarching Issues and Overview." By Christian G. Daughton. 2006. http://www.epa.gov/esd/chemistry/phrama/book-summary.htm (accessed September 15, 2006).

United States Geological Survey. "Emerging Contaminants in the Environment." 2007. http://toxics.usgs.gov/regional/emc/ (accessed May 6, 2009).

"What Every American Can Do to Prevent Misuse of Prescription Drugs." 2007. http://www.whitehousedrugpolicy.gov/pda/022007.html (accessed February 14, 2008).